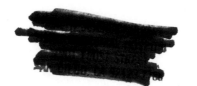

PLASTIC SURGERY

Indications, Operations, and Outcomes

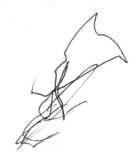

Bruce M. Achauer, MD, FACS
Professor of Surgery,
Division of Plastic Surgery,
University of California Irvine,
California College of Medicine,
Orange, California

Elof Eriksson, MD, PhD, FACS
Joseph E. Murray Professor of Plastic and Reconstructive Surgery,
Harvard Medical School;
Chief, Division of Plastic Surgery,
Brigham and Women's Hospital;
Chief, Division of Plastic Surgery,
Children's Hospital,
Boston, Massachusetts

Bahman Guyuron, MD, FACS
Clinical Professor of Plastic Surgery,
Case Western Reserve University,
Cleveland, Ohio;
Medical Director,
Zeeba Medical Campus,
Lyndhurst, Ohio

John J. Coleman III, MD, FACS
Professor of Surgery;
Chief of Plastic Surgery;
Staff Physician,
Indiana University Medical Center;
Director, Pediatric Burn Unit;
Staff Physician,
Riley Children's Hospital;
Staff Physician,
Wishard Memorial Hospital,
Indianapolis, Indiana

Robert C. Russell, MD, FRACS, FACS
Clinical Professor of Surgery,
Division of Plastic Surgery,
Southern Illinois University School of Medicine,
Springfield, Illinois

Craig A. Vander Kolk, MD, FACS
Associate Professor of Plastic Surgery;
Director, Cleft and Craniofacial Center,
Johns Hopkins University School of Medicine,
Baltimore, Maryland

PLASTIC SURGERY

Indications, Operations, and Outcomes

Volume Four
Hand Surgery

EDITOR
Robert C. Russell, MD, FRACS, FACS
Clinical Professor of Surgery,
Division of Plastic Surgery,
Southern Illinois University School of Medicine,
Springfield, Illinois

OUTCOMES EDITOR
Edwin G. Wilkins, MD, MS
Associate Professor of Plastic Surgery,
University of Michigan Health Systems,
Ann Arbor, Michigan

MANAGING EDITOR
Victoria M. VanderKam, RN, BS, CPSN
Clinical Nurse, Division of Plastic Surgery,
University of California Irvine Medical Center,
Orange, California

ILLUSTRATIONS BY
Min Li, MD
Indiana University School of Medicine,
Department of Surgery, Section of Plastic Surgery,
Indianapolis, Indiana

with 6279 *illustrations, including* 963 *in color, and* 18 *color plates*

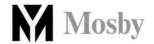 Mosby

A Harcourt Health Sciences Company

St. Louis   London   Philadelphia   Sydney   Toronto

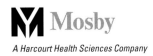

A Harcourt Health Sciences Company

Acquisitions Editor: Richard Zorab
Developmental Editor: Dolores Meloni
Project Manager: Carol Sullivan Weis
Senior Production Editor: Karen Rehwinkel
Designers: Dave Zielinski/Mark Oberkrom

Mosby, Inc.
A Harcourt Health Sciences Company
11830 Westline Industrial Drive
St. Louis, Missouri 63146

Printed in the United States of America

Volume 4 ISBN 0-8151-0999-7
Set ISBN 0-8151-0984-9

00 01 02 03 04 GW/MVY 9 8 7 6 5 4 3 2 1

Contributors

BRUCE M. ACHAUER, MD, FACS
Professor of Surgery,
Division of Plastic Surgery,
University of California Irvine,
California College of Medicine,
Orange, California

GREGORY J. ADAMSON, MD
Clinical Instructor of Orthopedics,
University of Illinois College of Medicine at Peoria;
Staff, St. Francis Medical Center,
Peoria, Illinois

GHADA Y. AFIFI, MD
Clinical Assistant Professor,
Division of Plastic Surgery,
Department of Surgery,
Loma Linda University Medical Center and Children's
    Hospital;
Attending Surgeon, Plastic Surgery,
Jerry L. Pettis Memorial Veterans Affairs Medical Center,
Loma Linda, California;
Private Practice,
Newport Beach, California

RICHARD D. ANDERSON, MD
Plastic Surgery Staff,
Scottsdale Healthcare Hospitals;
Private Practice,
Scottsdale, Arizona

JAMES P. ANTHONY, MD
Associate Professor of Surgery,
Division of Plastic Surgery,
University of California–San Francisco,
San Francisco, California

HÉCTOR ARÁMBULA, MD
Professor of Plastic Surgery,
Postgraduate Division of Medicine,
Universidad Nacional Autonoma de Mexico;
Chairman, Plastic Surgery Service,
Hospital de Traumatologia Magdalena de las Salinas,
Instituto Mexicano del Seguro Social, IMSS,
Mexico City, Mexico

LOUIS C. ARGENTA, MD
Julius A. Howell Professor and Chairman,
Department of Plastic Surgery,
Wake Forest University School of Medicine;
Professor and Chairman,
Department of Plastic and Reconstructive Surgery,
North Carolina Baptist Hospital,
Winston-Salem, North Carolina

DUFFIELD ASHMEAD IV, MD
Assistant Clinical Professor of Plastic Surgery and
    Orthopedics,
University of Connecticut School of Medicine,
Farmington, Connecticut;
Director, Division of Hand Surgery,
Connecticut Children's Medical Center,
Hartford, Connecticut

CHRISTOPHER J. ASSAD, BS, MD, FRCSC
Plastic and Reconstructive Surgeon;
Associate Staff,
Halton Health Care Services Corporation,
Milton District Hospital,
Milton, Ontario, Canada

THOMAS J. BAKER, MD
Professor of Plastic Surgery–Voluntary,
University of Miami School of Medicine;
Senior Attending Physician,
Mercy Hospital,
Miami, Florida

TRACY M. BAKER, MD
Instructor in Plastic Surgery,
University of Miami School of Medicine,
Miami, Florida

JUAN P. BARRET, MD
Professor, Rijksuniversiteit Groningen;
Plastic and Reconstructive Surgeon,
University Hospital Groningen,
Groningen, The Netherlands

MUNISH K. BATRA, MD
Assistant Clinical Instructor–Voluntary,
Division of Plastic Surgery,
University of California–San Diego Medical Center,
San Diego, California;
Private Practice,
Del Mar, California

BRUCE S. BAUER, MD, FACS
Associate Professor of Surgery,
Northwestern University Medical School;
Head, Division of Plastic Surgery,
The Children's Memorial Hospital,
Chicago, Illinois

STEPHEN P. BEALS, MD, FACS, FAAP,
Assistant Professor of Plastic Surgery,
Mayo Medical School;
Adjunct Professor,
Department of Speech and Hearing Science,
Arizona State University;
Craniofacial Consultant,
Barrow Neurological Institute
Phoenix, Arizona

MICHAEL S. BEDNAR, MD
Associate Professor,
Department of Orthopedic Surgery and Rehabilitation,
Stritch School of Medicine,
Loyola University–Chicago,
Maywood, Illinois

RAMIN A. BEHMAND, MD
Chief Resident,
Division of Plastic and Reconstructive Surgery,
University of Michigan Hospitals,
Ann Arbor, Michigan

RUSSELL W. BESSETTE, DDS, MD
Clinical Professor of Plastic Surgery,
State University of New York–Buffalo,
School of Medicine;
Executive Director of Research,
Sisters Hospital,
Buffalo, New York

MARINA D. BIZZARRI-SCHMID, MD
Instructor in Anesthesia,
Harvard Medical School;
Anesthesiologist,
Brigham and Women's Hospital,
Boston, Massachusetts

GREG BORSCHEL, MD
Plastic Surgery Resident,
University of Michigan Hospitals,
Ann Arbor, Michigan

MARK T. BOSCHERT, MS, MD
Attending Physician,
St. Joseph Health Center;
Private Practice,
St. Charles, Missouri,
Attending Physician,
Barnes-St. Peters Hospital,
St. Peters, Missouri

JOHN BOSTWICK, MD, FACS
Professor and Chairman of Plastic Surgery,
Emory University School of Medicine;
Chief of Plastic Surgery,
Emory University Hospital,
Atlanta, Georgia

J. BRIAN BOYD, MB, ChB, MD, FRCSC, FACS
Professor of Surgery,
The Ohio State University College of Medicine,
Columbus, Ohio;
Chairman of Plastic Surgery,
Cleveland Clinic–Florida,
Fort Lauderdale, Florida

WILLIAM R. BOYDSTON, MD, PhD
Pediatric Neurosurgeon,
Children's Healthcare of Atlanta,
Scottish Rite Children's Hospital,
Atlanta, Georgia

KARL H. BREUING, MD
Instructor in Surgery,
Harvard Medical School;
Attending Physician, Plastic Surgery,
Brigham and Women's Hospital;
Attending Physician, Plastic Surgery,
Children's Hospital;
Attending Physician, Plastic Surgery,
Faulkner Hospital;
Attending Physician, Plastic Surgery,
Dana Farber Cancer Institute,
Boston, Massachusetts

FORST E. BROWN, MD
Emeritus Professor of Plastic Surgery,
Dartmouth Medical School,
Hanover, New Hampshire;
Consultant,
Veterans Administration Hospital,
White River Junction, Vermont

RICHARD E. BROWN, MD, FACS
Clinical Associate Professor;
Hand Fellowship Director,
Division of Plastic Surgery,
Southern Illinois University School of Medicine,
Springfield, Illinois

MARIE-CLAIRE BUCKLEY, MD
Plastic Surgery Fellow,
University of Minnesota Medical School,
Division of Plastic and Reconstructive Surgery,
Minneapolis, Minnesota

GREGORY M. BUNCKE, MD, FACS
Clinical Assistant Professor of Surgery,
University of California–San Francisco,
San Francisco, California;
Clinical Assistant Professor of Surgery,
Stanford University,
Stanford, California;
Co-Director, Division of Microsurgery,
California Pacific Medical Center,
San Francisco, California

HARRY J. BUNCKE, MD
Clinical Professor of Surgery,
University of California–San Francisco,
San Francisco, California;
Associate Clinical Professor of Surgery,
Stanford Medical School,
Stanford, California;
Director, Microsurgical Transplantation–Replantation
  Service,
California Pacific Medical Center–Davies,
San Francisco, California

RUDOLF BUNTIC, MD
Clinical Instructor,
Division of Plastic Surgery,
Stanford University,
Stanford, California;
Attending Microsurgeon,
California Pacific Medical Center,
San Francisco, California

ELISA A. BURGESS, MD
Resident in Plastic Surgery,
Oregon Health Sciences University,
Portland, Oregon

FERNANDO D. BURSTEIN, MD
Clinical Associate Professor,
Plastic and Reconstructive Surgery,
Emory University School of Medicine;
Chief, Plastic and Reconstructive Surgery;
Co-Director, Center for Craniofacial Disorders,
Scottish Rite Children's Medical Center,
Atlanta, Georgia

GRANT W. CARLSON, MD
Professor of Surgery,
Emory University School of Medicine;
Chief of Surgical Services,
Crawford Long Hospital;
Chief of Surgical Oncology,
Emory Clinic,
Atlanta, Georgia

JAMES CARRAWAY, MD, AB
Professor of Plastic Surgery;
Chairman, Division of Plastic Surgery,
Eastern Virginia Medical School,
Norfolk, Virginia

STANLEY A. CASTOR, MD
Plastic Surgery Staff Physician,
The Watson Clinic,
Lakeland, Florida

BERNARD CHANG, MD
Director, Plastic and Reconstructive Surgery,
Mercy Medical Center,
Baltimore, Maryland

YU-RAY CHEN, MD
Professor, Department of Plastic Surgery,
Chang Gung University Medical School
Tao-Yuan, Taiwan;
Superintendent and Attending Surgeon,
Department of Plastic Surgery,
Chang Gung Memorial Hospital,
Taipei, Taiwan

ANDREAS CHIMONIDES, BS, MD
Staff Physician,
Butler Memorial Hospital,
Butler, Pennsylvania;
Staff Physician,
St. Francis Medical Center;
Staff Physician,
University of Pennsylvania Medical Center–St. Margaret's
    Hospital,
Pittsburgh, Pennsylvania

MARK A. CODNER, MD
Clinical Assistant Professor,
Emory University School of Medicine;
Private Practice,
Atlanta, Georgia

I. KELMAN COHEN, MD
Professor of Surgery;
Director, Wound Healing Center,
Medical College of Virginia,
Virginia Commonwealth University,
Richmond, Virginia

MYLES J. COHEN, MD
Clinical Assistant Professor of Surgery,
University of Southern California School of Medicine;
Attending Physician,
Cedars Sinai Medical Center,
Los Angeles, California

STEVEN R. COHEN, MD
Associate Clinical Professor,
Division of Plastic and Reconstructive Surgery,
University of California Medical Center–San Diego;
Chief, Craniofacial Surgery,
Children's Hospital of San Diego,
San Diego, California

VICTOR COHEN, MD
Resident Physician,
McGill University Health Center,
McGill University School of Medicine,
Montreal, Quebec, Canada

JOHN J. COLEMAN III, MD, FACS
Professor of Surgery;
Chief of Plastic Surgery;
Staff Physician,
Indiana University Medical Center;
Director, Pediatric Burn Unit;
Staff Physician,
Riley Children's Hospital;
Staff Physician,
Wishard Memorial Hospital,
Indianapolis, Indiana

LAWRENCE B. COLEN, MD
Associate Professor of Plastic and Reconstructive Surgery,
Eastern Virginia Medical School,
Norfolk, Virginia

E. DALE COLLINS, MD, MS
Assistant Professor of Surgery,
Dartmouth Medical School,
Hanover, New Hampshire;
Medical Director, Comprehensive Breast Program,
Dartmouth-Hitchcock Medical Center,
Lebanon, New Hampshire

MATTHEW J. CONCANNON, MD, FACS
Assistant Professor;
Director of Hand and Microsurgery,
University of Missouri,
Columbia, Missouri

BRUCE F. CONNELL, MD
Clinical Professor of Surgery,
University of California Irvine,
California College of Medicine,
Orange, California

AISLING CONRAN, MD
Assistant Professor, Clinical Anesthesia,
University of Chicago,
Chicago, Illinois

PAUL C. COTTERILL, BS, MD, ABHRS,
Honorary Lecturer,
Sunnybrook Hospital,
Department of Dermatology,
University of Toronto,
Toronto, Ontario, Canada

KIMBALL MAURICE CROFTS, MD
Staff Physician,
Utah Valley Regional Medical Center,
Provo, Utah;
Staff Physician,
Timpanogos Regional Hospital,
Orem, Utah;
Staff Physician,
Mt. View Hospital,
Payson, Utah;
Staff Physician,
Sevier Valley Hospital,
Richfield, Utah

LISA R. DAVID, MD
Assistant Professor,
Department of Plastic and Reconstructive Surgery,
Wake Forest University School of Medicine;
Attending Physician,
North Carolina Baptist Hospital,
Winston-Salem, North Carolina

WILLIAM M. DAVIDSON, AB, DMD, PhD
Professor and Chairman,
Department of Orthodontics,
University of Maryland Dental School;
Associate Staff, Dentistry,
Johns Hopkins Hospital,
Baltimore, Maryland

MARK A. DEITCH, MD
Assistant Professor of Surgery,
Division of Orthopedic Surgery,
University of Maryland School of Medicine,
Baltimore, Maryland

MARK D. DeLACURE, MD, FACS
Chief, Division of Head and Neck Surgery and Oncology;
Associate Professor of Otolaryngology–Head and Neck
    Surgery,
Department of Otolaryngology;
Associate Professor of Reconstructive Plastic Surgery,
Institute of Reconstructive Plastic Surgery,
Department of Surgery,
New York University School of Medicine,
New York, New York

VALERIE BURKE DeLEON, MA,
Department of Cell Biology and Anatomy,
Johns Hopkins University School of Medicine,
Baltimore, Maryland

JOHN Di SAIA, MD
Assistant Clinical Professor,
Division of Plastic Surgery,
University of California Irvine,
California College of Medicine,
Orange, California

RICHARD V. DOWDEN, MD
Clinical Assistant Professor,
Case Western Reserve University,
Cleveland, Ohio

CRAIG R. DUFRESNE, MD, FACS
Clinical Professor of Plastic Surgery,
Georgetown University,
Washington, DC;
Plastic Surgery Section Chief;
Co-Director, Center for Facial Rehabilitation,
Fairfax Hospital,
Inova Hospital System,
Fairfax, Virginia

FELMONT F. EAVES III, MD, FACS
Assistant Clinical Professor,
University of North Carolina,
Chapel Hill, North Carolina;
Attending Physician,
Charlotte Plastic Surgery Center;
Attending Physician,
Carolinas Medical Center;
Attending Physician,
Presbyterian Hospital;
Attending Physician,
Mercy Hospital,
Charlotte, North Carolina

PHILIP EDELMAN, MD
Associate Professor of Medicine;
Director, Toxicology and Clinical Services,
Division of Occupational and Environmental Medicine,
George Washington University School of Medicine,
Washington, DC

ERIC T. EMERSON, MD
Private Practice,
Gastonia, North Carolina

TODD B. ENGEN, MD
Clinical Faculty,
University of Utah School of Medicine,
Salt Lake City, Utah;
Clinical Director,
Excel Cosmetic Surgery Center,
Orem, Utah

BARRY L. EPPLEY, MD, DMD
Assistant Professor of Plastic Surgery,
Indiana University School of Medicine,
Indianapolis, Indiana

ELOF ERIKSSON, MD, PhD, FACS
Joseph E. Murray Professor of Plastic and Reconstructive
    Surgery,
Harvard Medical School;
Chief, Division of Plastic Surgery,
Brigham and Women's Hospital;
Chief, Division of Plastic Surgery,
Children's Hospital,
Boston, Massachusetts

GREGORY R.D. EVANS, MD, FACS
Professor of Surgery;
Chair, Division of Plastic Surgery,
University of California Irvine,
California College of Medicine
Orange, California

JEFFREY A. FEARON, MD, FACS, FAAP
Director, The Craniofacial Center,
North Texas Hospital for Children at Medical City Dallas,
Dallas, Texas

LYNNE M. FEEHAN, MS, PT
Senior Hand Therapist,
Hand Program,
Workers' Compensation Board of British Columbia,
Richmond, British Columbia, Canada

RANDALL S. FEINGOLD, MD, FACS
Assistant Clinical Professor, Plastic and Reconstructive
    Surgery,
Albert Einstein College of Medicine,
Bronx, New York;
Attending Surgeon,
Long Island Jewish Medical Center,
New Hyde Park, New York;
Chief, Division of Plastic Surgery,
North Shore University Hospital at Forest Hills,
Forest Hills, New York

ROBERT D. FOSTER, MD
Assistant Professor in Residence,
Division of Plastic and Reconstructive Surgery,
University of California–San Francisco,
San Francisco, California

FRANK J. FRASSICA, MD
Professor of Orthopedic Surgery and Oncology,
Johns Hopkins University School of Medicine,
Baltimore, Maryland

ALAN E. FREELAND, MD
Professor, Department of Orthopedic Surgery;
Director, Hand Surgery Service,
The University of Mississippi Medical Center,
Jackson, Mississippi

MENNEN T. GALLAS, MD
Junior Faculty Associate,
University of Texas M.D. Anderson Cancer Center,
Houston, Texas

BING SIANG GAN, MD, PhD, FRCSC
Assistant Professor,
Departments of Surgery and Pharmacology-Toxicology,
University of Western Ontario;
Staff Surgeon,
Hand and Upper Limb Centre;
Staff Surgeon,
St. Joseph's Health Centre,
London, Ontario, Canada

WARREN L. GARNER, MD
Associate Professor of Surgery,
University of Southern California;
Associate Professor of Plastic Surgery;
Director, LAC & USC Burn Center,
Los Angeles, California

DAVID G. GENECOV, MD
Attending Surgeon,
International Craniofacial Institute,
Dallas, Texas

GEORGE K. GITTES, MD
Associate Professor,
Department of Surgery,
University of Missouri–Kansas City;
Holder and Ashcraft Chair of Pediatric Surgical Research,
Children's Mercy Hospital,
Kansas City, Missouri

JEFFREY A. GOLDSTEIN, MD
Associate Professor of Surgery,
Case Western Reserve University;
Medical Director, Craniofacial Center;
Chief of Plastic and Reconstructive Surgery,
Rainbow Babies and Children's Hospital,
Cleveland, Ohio

HECTOR GONZALEZ-MIRAMONTES, MD
Private Practice,
Guadalajara, Mexico

LAWRENCE J. GOTTLIEB, MD
Professor of Clinical Surgery,
University of Chicago,
Pritzker School of Medicine,
Chicago, Illinois

MARK S. GRANICK, MD
Professor of Surgery;
Chief of Plastic Surgery,
MCP-Hahnemann University,
Philadelphia, Pennsylvania

FREDERICK M. GRAZER, MD, FACS
Associate Clinical Professor,
Division of Plastic Surgery,
University of California Irvine,
California College of Medicine;
Staff Physician,
University of California Irvine Medical Center,
Orange, California;
Clinical Professor of Surgery,
The Pennsylvania State University Milton S. Hershey
    Medical Center College of Medicine,
Hershey, Pennsylvania;
Staff Physician,
Hoag Memorial Hospital Presbyterian,
Newport Beach, California

JON M. GRAZER, MD, MPH
Staff Physician,
Hoag Memorial Hospital Presbyterian,
Newport Beach, California;
Staff Physician,
Western Medical Center,
Santa Ana, California

JUDITH M. GURLEY, MD
Assistant Professor of Surgery,
Division of Plastic and Reconstructive Surgery,
Washington University School of Medicine;
Attending Physician,
St. Louis Children's Hospital;
Attending Physician,
Shriner's Hospital for Children,
St. Louis, Missouri

BAHMAN GUYURON, MD, FACS
Clinical Professor of Plastic Surgery,
Case Western Reserve University,
Cleveland, Ohio;
Medical Director,
Zeeba Medical Campus,
Lyndhurst, Ohio

HONGSHIK HAN, MD
Plastic Surgery Resident,
Division of Plastic Surgery,
Northwestern University Medical School,
Chicago, Illinois

ROBERT A. HARDESTY, MD
Professor,
Loma Linda University School of Medicine;
Medical Staff President;
Chief of Plastic Surgery,
Loma Linda University Medical Center,
Loma Linda, California

MAUREEN HARDY, PT, MS, CHT
Clinical Assistant Professor,
University of Mississippi Medical Center;
Director, Hand Management Center,
St. Dominic Hospital,
Jackson, Mississippi

ALAN SCOTT HARMATZ, BS, MD
Assistant Professor of Surgery,
University of Vermont College of Medicine,
Burlington, Vermont;
Attending Physician,
Maine Medical Center,
Portland, Maine

STEPHEN U. HARRIS, MD
Staff Physician,
Nassau County Medical Center,
East Meadow, New York;
Staff Physician,
North Shore Hospital,
Manhasset, New York;
Staff Physician,
Winthrop University Hospital,
Mineola, New York;
Plastic Surgeon,
Long Island Plastic Surgical Group,
Garden City, New York

ROBERT J. HAVLIK, MD
Associate Professor of Surgery,
Indiana University School of Medicine,
Indianapolis, Indiana

DETLEV HEBEBRAND, MD, PhD
Attending Physician,
Hand and Burn Center,
Bergmannsheil Clinic,
Ruhr University,
Bochum, Germany

MARC H. HEDRICK, MD
Assistant Professor of Surgery and Pediatrics,
Division of Plastic and Reconstructive Surgery,
University of California–Los Angeles School of Medicine,
Los Angeles, California

DOMINIC F. HEFFEL, MD
Resident, General Surgery,
University of California–Los Angeles Center for Health
    Sciences,
Los Angeles, California

CHRIS S. HELMSTEDTER, MD
Director of Orthopedic Oncology–Southern California,
Kaiser Permanente,
Baldwin Park, California;
Assistant Clinical Professor, Orthopedics and Surgery,
University of Southern California School of Medicine,
Los Angeles, California

VINCENT R. HENTZ, MD
Professor of Functional Restoration (Hand Surgery),
Stanford University School of Medicine,
Stanford, California

JEFFREY HOLLINGER, DDS, PhD
Professor, Biology and Biomedical Health Engineering;
Director, Center for Bone Tissue Engineering,
Carnegie Mellon University,
Pittsburgh, Pennsylvania

HEINZ-HERBERT HOMANN, MD
Attending Physician,
Hand and Burn Center,
Bergmannsheil Clinic,
Ruhr University,
Bochum, Germany

CHARLES E. HORTON, MD, FACS, FRCSC
Professor of Plastic Surgery,
Eastern Virginia Medical School,
Norfolk, Virginia;
Clinical Professor of Surgery,
Medical College of Virginia,
Richmond, Virginia

CHARLES E. HORTON, Jr., MD
Assistant Professor of Urology,
Eastern Virginia Medical School;
Chief, Department of Urology,
Children's Hospital of the King's Daughters,
Norfolk, Virginia

ERIC H. HUBLI, MD, FACS, FAAP
Craniomaxillofacial Surgeon,
International Craniofacial Institute,
Dallas, Texas

ROGER J. HUDGINS, MD
Assistant Professor,
Morehouse University School of Medicine;
Chief of Pediatric Neurosurgery,
Children's Healthcare of Atlanta,
Scottish Rite Children's Hospital,
Atlanta, Georgia

LAWRENCE N. HURST, MD, FRCSC
Professor and Chairman,
Division of Plastic Surgery,
The University of Western Ontario;
Chief, Division of Plastic Surgery
London Health Sciences Centre, University Campus,
London, Ontario, Canada

ETHYLIN WANG JABS, MD
Dr. Frank V. Sutland Professor of Pediatric Genetics;
Professor of Pediatrics, Medicine, and Plastic Surgery,
John Hopkins University School of Medicine,
Baltimore, Maryland

MOULTON K. JOHNSON, MD
Associate Professor of Orthopedic Surgery,
University of California–Los Angeles,
Los Angeles, California

GLYN JONES, MD, FRCS, FCS
Associate Professor of Plastic Surgery;
Chief of Plastic Surgery,
Crawford Long Hospital,
Emory Clinic,
Atlanta, Georgia

NEIL F. JONES, MD
Professor, Division of Plastic and Reconstructive Surgery,
Department of Orthopedic Surgery,
University of California–Los Angeles;
Chief of Hand Surgery,
University of California–Los Angeles Medical Center,
Los Angeles, California

JESSE B. JUPITER, MD
Professor of Orthopedic Surgery,
Harvard Medical School;
Head, Orthopedic Hand Service,
Massachusetts General Hospital,
Boston, Massachusetts

M.J. JURKIEWICZ, MD, DDS
Professor of Surgery, Emeritus,
Emory University School of Medicine,
Atlanta, Georgia

MADELYN D. KAHANA, MD
Associate Professor of Anesthesiology and Pediatrics,
The University of Chicago Hospital,
Chicago, Illinois

CHIA CHI KAO, MD
Fellow, Department of Reconstructive and Plastic Surgery,
University of Southern California,
Los Angeles, California

AJAYA KASHYAP, MD
Assistant Professor,
University of Massachusetts Medical Center,
Worcester, Massachusetts;
Attending Plastic Surgeon,
Metrowest Medical Center,
Framingham, Massachusetts

JULIA A. KATARINCIC, MD
Consultant, Department of Orthopedic Surgery,
Mayo Clinic,
Rochester, Minnesota

DANIEL J. KELLEY, MD
Assistant Professor;
Director, Head and Neck Oncology/Skull Base Surgery,
Department of Otolaryngology and Bronchoesophagology,
Temple University School of Medicine,
Philadelphia, Pennsylvania

KEVIN J. KELLY, DDS, MD
Associate Professor,
Department of Plastic Surgery,
Vanderbilt University School of Medicine;
Director, Craniofacial Surgery,
Department of Plastic Surgery,
Vanderbilt Medical Center,
Nashville, Tennessee

PRASAD G. KILARU, MD
Clinical Assistant Professor of Surgery,
University of Southern California–Los Angeles,
Los Angeles, California;
Staff Physician,
City of Hope National Medical Center,
Duarte, California

GABRIEL M. KIND, MD
Assistant Clinical Professor,
Department of Surgery,
Division of Plastic and Reconstructive Surgery,
University of California–San Francisco;
Assistant Director of Research;
Assistant Fellowship Director,
The Buncke Clinic,
San Francisco, California

BRIAN M. KINNEY, MD, FACS, MSME
Clinical Assistant Professor of Plastic Surgery,
University of Southern California–Los Angeles;
Former Chief,
Century City Hospital,
Los Angeles, California

ELIZABETH M. KIRALY, MD
Fellow, Hand and Microvascular Surgery,
University of Nevada School of Medicine,
Department of Surgery,
Division of Plastic Surgery,
Las Vegas, Nevada

JOHN O. KUCAN, MD
Professor of Surgery,
Institute of Plastic Surgery,
Southern Illinois University School of Medicine,
Springfield, Illinois

M. ABRAHAM KURIAKOSE, MD, DDS, FACS
Assistant Professor of Otolaryngology,
Division of Head and Neck Surgery,
Department of Otolaryngology,
New York University School of Medicine;
Attending Surgeon,
New York University Medical Center,
New York, New York

AMY L. LADD, MD
Associate Professor,
Division of Hand and Upper Extremity,
Department of Functional Restoration,
Stanford University;
Chief, Hand and Upper Extremity Clinic,
Lucile Salter Packard Children's Hospital,
Stanford, California

PATRICK W. LAPPERT, MD
Assistant Professor of Surgery,
Uniformed Services University of the Health Sciences,
Bethesda, Maryland;
Chief, Department of Plastic Surgery,
Naval Medical Center,
Portsmouth, Virginia

DON LaROSSA, MD
Professor of Plastic Surgery,
The University of Pennsylvania School of Medicine;
Staff Physician,
Hospital of The University of Pennsylvania;
Senior Surgeon,
Children's Hospital of Philadelphia,
Philadelphia, Pennsylvania

DAVID L. LARSON, MD
Professor and Chair of Plastic and Reconstructive Surgery,
Medical College of Wisconsin,
Milwaukee, Wisconsin

DONALD R. LAUB, Jr., MS, MD
Assistant Professor,
Departments of Surgery and Orthopedics,
University of Vermont;
Attending Plastic and Hand Surgeon,
Fletcher Allen Health Care,
Burlington, Vermont

MICHAEL LAW, MD
Fellow, Microsurgery,
University of Southern California–Los Angeles,
Division of Plastic Surgery,
Los Angeles, California

W. THOMAS LAWRENCE, MPH, MD
Professor and Chief,
Section of Plastic Surgery,
University of Kansas Medical Center,
Kansas City, Kansas

W.P. ANDREW LEE, MD, FACS
Assistant Professor of Surgery,
Harvard Medical School;
Chief of Hand Service,
Department of Surgery,
Massachusetts General Hospital,
Boston, Massachusetts

SALVATORE LETTIERI, MD
Senior Associate Consultant,
Mayo Clinic,
Division of Plastic and Reconstructive Surgery,
Rochester, Minnesota

JAN S. LEWIN, PhD
Assistant Professor and Director,
Speech Pathology and Audiology Section,
University of Texas M.D. Anderson Cancer Center,
Houston, Texas

TERRY R. LIGHT, MD
Dr. William M. Scholl Professor;
Chairman, Department of Orthopedic Surgery and
    Rehabilitation,
Stritch School of Medicine,
Loyola University–Chicago,
Maywood, Illinois

SEAN LILLE, MD
Research Professor,
Department of Chemistry and Biochemistry,
Arizona State University,
Tempe, Arizona;
Research Scientist,
Mayo Clinic–Scottsdale,
Scottsdale, Arizona;
Private Practice,
Phoenix, Arizona

TED LOCKWOOD, MD
Associate Clinical Professor,
University of Kansas Medical School;
Assistant Clinical Professor,
University of Missouri–Kansas City Medical School,
Kansas City, Missouri

MICHAEL T. LONGAKER, MD, FACS
John Marquis Converse Professor of Plastic Surgery Research;
Director of Surgical Research,
New York University School of Medicine;
Attending Plastic Surgeon,
New York University Medical Center,
New York, New York

H. PETER LORENZ, MD
Assistant Professor of Plastic Surgery,
University of California–Los Angeles School of Medicine,
Los Angeles, California

GEORGE L. LUCAS, MD
Professor and Chairman,
Orthopedic Surgery;
Program Director,
University of Kansas–Wichita;
Orthopedic Surgeon,
Via Christi Hospital;
Orthopedic Surgeon,
Wesley Medical Center,
Wichita, Kansas

PETER J. LUND, BS, MD
Orthopedic/Hand Surgery,
Methodist Volunteer General Hospital,
Martin, Tennessee

STEVEN D. MACHT, MD, DDS
Clinical Professor of Plastic Surgery,
George Washington University,
Washington, DC

JOHN S. MANCOLL, MD
Private Practice,
Fort Wayne, Indiana

GREGORY A. MANTOOTH, MD
Chief Resident,
Division of Plastic and Reconstructive Surgery,
Indiana University,
Indianapolis, Indiana

BENJAMIN M. MASER, MD
Community Physician,
Department of Functional Restoration,
Stanford University,
Stanford, California

BRUCE A. MAST, MD
Assistant Professor,
Department of Surgery,
Division of Plastic and Reconstructive Surgery,
University of Florida;
Chief, Section of Plastic Surgery,
Malcolm Randall Gainesville Veterans Administration
    Medical Center,
Gainesville, Florida

ALAN MATARASSO, MD
Clinical Associate Professor of Plastic Surgery,
Albert Einstein College of Medicine;
Surgeon,
Manhattan Eye, Ear, Throat Hospital,
New York, New York

G. PATRICK MAXWELL, MD
Assistant Professor of Plastic Surgery,
Vanderbilt University;
Director, Institute for Aesthetic Surgery,
Baptist Hospital,
Nashville, Tennessee

MICHAEL H. MAYER, MD
Physician and Surgeon,
Plastic and Reconstructive Surgery,
Portland, Oregon

TRACY E. McCALL, MD
Chief Plastic Surgery Resident,
State University of New York,
Health Science Center at Brooklyn,
Brooklyn, New York

ROBERT L. McCAULEY, MD
Chief, Plastic and Reconstructive Surgery,
Shriners Burns Hospital Galveston;
Professor of Surgery and Pediatrics,
University of Texas Medical Branch,
Galveston, Texas

LAWRENCE R. MENENDEZ, MD
Associate Professor, Clinical Orthopedics;
Associate Professor, Department of Surgery,
Division of Tumor and Endocrine,
University of Southern California;
Chief of Orthopedics,
Kenneth Norris Jr. Cancer Hospital,
Los Angeles, California

FREDERICK J. MENICK, MD
Private Practice,
Tucson, Arizona

WYNDELL H. MERRITT, MD, FACS
Clinical Assistant Professor of Surgery,
Medical College of Virginia,
Richmond, Virginia

BRYAN J. MICHELOW, MBBCh, FRCS
Clinical Assistant Professor,
Case Western Reserve University,
Cleveland, Ohio

SCOTT R. MILLER, MD
Clinical Instructor of Plastic Surgery,
University of California–San Diego,
San Diego, California;
Attending Surgeon,
Scripps Memorial Hospital,
La Jolla, California

TIMOTHY A. MILLER, MD
Professor,
University of California–Los Angeles;
Chief, Plastic Surgery,
Wadsworth Veterans Administration Medical Center,
Los Angeles, California

FERNANDO MOLINA, MD
Professor, Plastic, Aesthetic, and Reconstructive Surgery;
Head, Division of Plastic and Reconstructive Surgery,
Hospital General Dr. Manual Gea Gonzalez,
Mexico City, Mexico

ROBERT E. MONTROY, MD
Associate Clinical Professor,
Division of Plastic Surgery,
University of California Irvine,
California College of Medicine,
Orange, California;
Chief, Plastic Surgery Section;
Assistant Chief, Spinal Cord Injury/Disease Health Care
    Group,
Department of Veterans Affairs Medical Center,
Long Beach, California

THOMAS S. MOORE, MD
Clinical Professor of Plastic Surgery,
Indiana University School of Medicine;
Chairman, Department of Plastic Surgery,
St. Vincent Hospital,
Indianapolis, Indiana

FARAMARZ MOVAGHARNIA, DO
Plastic Surgeon;
Staff Physician,
Emory Northlake Regional Medical Center,
Atlanta, Georgia

ARIAN MOWLAVI, MD
Plastic Surgery Resident,
Southern Illinois University School of Medicine,
Springfield, Illinois

JOSEPH E. MURRAY, MD
Emeritus Professor of Surgery,
Harvard Medical School,
Boston, Massachusetts

THOMAS A. MUSTOE, MD
Professor and Chief, Division of Plastic Surgery,
Northwestern University Medical School,
Chicago, Illinois

ARSHAD R. MUZAFFAR, MD
Chief Resident,
Department of Plastic Surgery,
University of Texas Southwestern Medical Center,
Parkland Memorial Hospital,
Dallas, Texas

NASH H. NAAM, MD, FACS
Clinical Professor,
Department of Plastic and Reconstructive Surgery,
Southern Illinois University School of Medicine,
Springfield, Illinois;
Director, Southern Illinois Hand Center,
Effingham, Illinois

SATORU NAGATA, MD, PhD
Visiting Professor,
Division of Plastic Surgery,
University of California Irvine,
California College of Medicine,
Orange, California;
Department Director,
Reconstructive Plastic Surgery,
Chiba Tokushukai Hospital,
Narashinodai, Funabashi, Chiba, Japan

DANIEL J. NAGLE, MD
Associate Clinical Professor of Orthopedic Surgery,
Northwestern University Medical School;
Attending Hand and Microsurgeon,
Northwestern Memorial Hospital,
Chicago, Illinois

FOAD NAHAI, MD, FACS
Private Practice,
Atlanta, Georgia

DAVID T. NETSCHER, MD, FACS
Associate Professor,
Division of Plastic Surgery,
Baylor College of Medicine;
Chief, Plastic Surgery,
Veterans Affairs Medical Center,
Houston, Texas

MICHAEL W. NEUMEISTER, MD
Assistant Professor;
Plastic Surgery Program Director;
Chief, Microsurgery and Research,
Southern Illinois University School of Medicine;
Director, Hyperbaric Oxygen Unit,
Co-Director, Regional Burn Unit,
Memorial Medical Center,
Springfield, Illinois

RONALD E. PALMER, MD
Clinical Assistant Professor,
University of Illinois College of Medicine at Peoria,
Peoria, Illinois

FRANK A. PAPAY, MS, MD, FACS, FAAP
Assistant Clinical Professor,
The Ohio State University College of Medicine,
Columbus, Ohio;
Staff Surgeon;
Head, Section of Craniofacial and Pediatric Plastic Surgery,
The Cleveland Clinic Foundation,
Department of Plastic and Reconstructive Surgery,
Cleveland, Ohio

ROBERT W. PARSONS, MD
Professor Emeritus in Plastic Surgery and Pediatrics,
University of Chicago,
Pritzker School of Medicine,
Chicago, Illinois

WILLIAM C. PEDERSON, MD, FACS
Clinical Associate Professor,
Department of Surgery and Orthopedic Surgery,
University of Texas Health Science Center–San Antonio,
San Antonio, Texas

LINDA G. PHILLIPS, MD
Professor of Plastic Surgery;
Chief, Division of Plastic Surgery,
University of Texas Medical Branch,
Galveston, Texas

GEORGE J. PICHA, MD, PhD, FACS
Clinical Assistant Professor,
Division of Plastic Surgery,
Case Western Reserve University,
Cleveland, Ohio;
Private Practice,
Lyndhurst, Ohio

JEFFREY C. POSNICK, DMD, MD, FRCSC, FACS
Clinical Professor, Plastic Surgery, Pediatrics, Oral and
    Maxillofacial Surgery, and Otolaryngology/Head and Neck
    Surgery,
Georgetown University,
Washington, DC;
Director, Posnick Center for Facial Plastic Surgery,
Chevy Chase, Maryland

JASON N. POZNER, MD
Private Practice,
Boca Raton, Florida

STEFAN PREUSS, MD
Fellow, Plastic and Reconstructive Surgery,
Harvard Medical School;
Staff Physician,
Brigham and Women's Hospital;
Staff Physician,
Children's Hospital,
Boston, Massachusetts

JULIAN J. PRIBAZ, MD
Associate Professor of Surgery;
Program Director,
Harvard Plastic Surgery Residency Training Program,
Harvard Medical School;
Associate Surgeon,
Brigham and Women's Hospital;
Associate Surgeon,
Children's Hospital,
Boston, Massachusetts

C. LIN PUCKETT, MD, FACS
Professor and Head, Division of Plastic Surgery,
University of Missouri,
Columbia, Missouri

OSCAR M. RAMIREZ, MD
Clinical Assistant Professor,
Johns Hopkins University School of Medicine;
Clinical Assistant Professor,
University of Maryland,
Baltimore, Maryland;
Director,
Esthétique International,
Plastic Surgical Center,
Timonium, Maryland

GERALD V. RAYMOND, MD
Assistant Professor,
John Hopkins University School of Medicine;
Neurologist,
Kennedy Krieger Institute,
Baltimore, Maryland

RILEY REES, MD
Professor of Plastic and Reconstructive Surgery,
University of Michigan Medical Center;
Chief, Plastic Surgeon Section,
Veterans Administration Medical Center,
Ann Arbor, Michigan,
Associate,
Chelsea Community Hospital,
Chelsea, Michigan

DANIEL REICHNER, MD
Plastic Surgery Resident,
University of California Irvine,
California College of Medicine,
Orange, California

JOAN RICHTSMEIER, MA, PhD
Professor, Department of Cell Biology and Anatomy,
Department of Plastic Surgery,
Johns Hopkins University School of Medicine,
Baltimore, Maryland

DAVID RING, MD
Fellow, Orthopedic Hand Service,
Massachusetts General Hospital,
Boston, Massachusetts

THOMAS L. ROBERTS III, MD
Associate Clinical Professor of Surgery,
Medical University of South Carolina at Spartanburg,
Spartanburg, South Carolina

ROD J. ROHRICH, MD, FACS
Professor and Chairman,
Department of Plastic Surgery,
University of Texas Medical Center at Dallas,
Dallas, Texas

LORNE E. ROTSTEIN, MD, FRCSC, FACS
Associate Professor,
Department of Surgery,
University of Toronto;
Staff Surgeon,
Princess Margaret Hospital,
The Toronto General Hospital University Health Network,
Toronto, Ontario, Canada

J. PETER RUBIN, MD
Fellow in Plastic Surgery,
Harvard Medical School,
Boston, Massachusetts

ROBERT C. RUSSELL, MD, FRACS, FACS
Clinical Professor of Surgery,
Division of Plastic Surgery,
Southern Illinois University School of Medicine,
Springfield, Illinois

A. MICHAEL SADOVE, MD
Professor of Surgery (Plastics),
Indiana University School of Medicine;
Chief, Plastic Surgery,
James Whitcomb Riley Hospital for Children,
Indianapolis, Indiana

KENNETH E. SALYER, MD
Adjunct Professor, Department of Orthodontics,
Baylor College of Dentistry,
Baylor University,
Dallas, Texas;
Clinical Professor, Department of Surgery,
Division of Plastic and Reconstructive Surgery,
University of Texas Health Science Center at San Antonio,
San Antonio, Texas;
Founding Director,
International Craniofacial Institute,
Cleft Lip and Palate Treatment Center,
Dallas, Texas

NICOLAS SASTRE, MD
Professor of Plastic Surgery,
Postgraduate Division of Medical Faculty,
Universidad Nacional Autonoma de Mexico;
Chairman, Plastic Surgery Department,
Hospital General de Mexico,
Mexico City, Mexico

STEPHEN A. SCHENDEL, MD, DDS
Professor and Head, Division of Plastic and Reconstructive
    Surgery;
Chairman, Department of Functional Restoration,
Stanford University,
Stanford, California

STEPHEN B. SCHNALL, MD
Associate Professor of Clinical Orthopedics,
University of Southern California School of Medicine,
Los Angeles, California

ALAN E. SEYFER, MD
Chief, Plastic Surgery,
Professor of Surgery, Anatomy, and Cell Developmental
    Biology,
Oregon Health Sciences University;
Chief, Plastic Surgery,
Doernbecher Childrens Hospital;
Staff Surgeon,
Shriners' Hospital for Crippled Children;
Portland Veterans Administration Medical Center,
Portland, Oregon

JATIN P. SHAH, MD, FACS, FRCS, FDSRCS
Professor of Surgery,
Weill Medical College,
Cornell University;
E.W. Strong Chair in Head and Neck Oncology;
Chief, Head and Neck Service,
Memorial Sloan-Kettering Cancer Center,
New York, New York

ARTHUR SHEKTMAN, MD
Attending Surgeon,
Newton-Wellesley Hospital,
Newton, Massachusetts;
Attending Surgeon,
St. Elizabeth's Medical Center,
Boston, Massachusetts

RANDY SHERMAN, MD
Professor and Chief,
Division of Plastic and Reconstructive Surgery,
University of Southern California–Los Angeles;
Chief, Plastic Surgery,
University of Southern California University Hospital;
Chief, Plastic Surgery,
Los Angeles County Hospital,
Los Angeles, California

PETER P. SIKO, MD
Research Manager,
The Buncke Clinic,
San Francisco, California

CARL E. SILVER, MD
Professor of Surgery,
Albert Einstein College of Medicine;
Chief, Head and Neck Surgery,
Montefiore Medical Center,
Bronx, New York

JEFFREY D. SMITH, MD
Clinical Fellow in Surgery,
Harvard Medical School;
Chief Resident, Plastic Surgery,
Brigham and Women's Hospital;
Chief Resident, Plastic Surgery,
Children's Hospital,
Boston, Massachusetts

NICOLE ZOOK SOMMER, MD
Plastic Surgery Resident,
Southern Illinois University School of Medicine,
Springfield, Illinois

RAJIV SOOD, MD
Associate Professor of Plastic Surgery,
Indiana University Medical Center;
Chief, Plastic Surgery Section,
Wishard Memorial Hospital,
Indianapolis, Indiana

CAROL L. SORENSEN, PsyD
Adjunct Professor of Psychology,
Concordia University,
Irvine, California

PANAYOTIS N. SOUCACOS, MD, FACS
Professor and Chairman,
Department of Orthopedics,
University of Ioannina School of Medicine,
Ioannina, Greece

MYRON SPECTOR, BS, MS, PhD
Professor of Orthopedic Surgery (Biomaterials),
Harvard Medical School;
Director of Orthopedic Research,
Department of Orthopedic Surgery,
Brigham and Women's Hospital,
Boston, Massachusetts

MELVIN SPIRA, MD, DDS
Professor of Surgery,
Division of Plastic Surgery,
Baylor College of Medicine,
Houston, Texas

HANS U. STEINAU, MD
Professor, Department of Plastic Surgery,
Director, Clinic for Plastic Surgery,
Hand and Burn Center,
Bergmannsheil Clinic,
Ruhr University,
Bochum, Germany

PETER J. STERN, MD
Professor and Chairman,
Department of Orthopedic Surgery,
University of Cincinnati College of Medicine,
Cincinnati, Ohio

BERISH STRAUCH, MD
Professor and Chairman,
Department of Plastic Surgery,
Albert Einstein College of Medicine,
Montefiore Medical Center,
Bronx, New York

JAMES M. STUZIN, MD
Clinical Assistant Professor of Plastic Surgery–Voluntary,
University of Miami School of Medicine;
Senior Attending Physician,
Mercy Hospital,
Miami, Florida

MARK R. SULTAN, MD
Associate Clinical Professor of Surgery,
Columbia University;
Chief, Division of Plastic Surgery,
Beth Israel Medical Center,
New York, New York

WILLIAM M. SWARTZ, MD, FACS
Clinical Associate Professor,
Department of Surgery,
University of Pittsburgh,
Pittsburgh, Pennsylvania

JULIA K. TERZIS, MD, PhD, FRCSC
Professor, Department of Surgery,
Division of Plastic and Reconstructive Surgery;
Director, Microsurgery Program,
Eastern Virginia Medical School,
Microsurgical Research Center,
Norfolk, Virginia

VIVIAN TING, MD
Resident in General Surgery,
University of Rochester Medical Center,
Strong Memorial Hospital,
Rochester, New York

BRYANT A. TOTH, MD, FACS
Assistant Clinical Professor of Surgery,
Department of Surgery,
University of California–San Francisco;
Attending Surgeon,
California Pacific Medical Center,
San Francisco, California;
Chief, Division of Plastic Surgery,
Children's Hospital of Northern California,
Oakland, California

LAWRENCE C. TSEN, MD
Assistant Professor of Anesthesia,
Harvard Medical School;
Attending Anesthesiologist,
Department of Anesthesiology,
Perioperative and Pain Medicine,
Brigham and Women's Hospital,
Boston, Massachusetts

MARTIN G. UNGER, MD, FRCSC, ABCS, ABHRS
Clinical Teacher and Lecturer,
University of Toronto;
Chief of Plastic Surgery,
One Medical Place Hospital,
Toronto, Ontario, Canada

ALLEN L. VAN BEEK, BS, MD
Clinical Associate Professor,
University of Minnesota,
Department of Surgery,
Minneapolis, Minnesota

VICTORIA M. VANDERKAM, RN, BS, CPSN
Clinical Nurse, Division of Plastic Surgery,
University of California Irvine Medical Center,
Orange, California

CRAIG A. VANDER KOLK, MD, FACS
Associate Professor of Plastic Surgery,
Director, Cleft and Craniofacial Center,
Johns Hopkins University School of Medicine,
Baltimore, Maryland

NICHOLAS VEDDER, MD
Associate Professor,
University of Washington,
Seattle, Washington

MARIOS D. VEKRIS, MD
Orthopedic Attending Surgeon,
Ioannina University Hospital,
Ioannina Medical School,
Ioannina, Greece

PETER M. VOGT, MD, PhD
Associate Professor;
Attending Physician,
Hand and Burn Center,
Bergmannsheil Clinic,
Ruhr University,
Bochum, Germany

JEFFREY D. WAGNER, MD
Associate Professor of Surgery,
Department of Surgery,
Division of Plastic and Reconstructive Surgery,
Indiana University School of Medicine,
Indianapolis, Indiana

ROBERT L. WALTON, MD, FACS
Professor of Surgery,
University of Chicago School of Medicine;
Chief, Section of Plastic Surgery,
University of Chicago Hospitals,
Chicago, Illinois

BERNADETTE WANG, MD
Fellow, Hand and Microsurgery,
Curtis National Hand Center,
Union Memorial Hospital,
Baltimore, Maryland

H. KIRK WATSON, MD
Director, Connecticut Combined Hand Surgery Fellowship;
Assistant Clinical Professor of Orthopedics, Rehabilitation,
    and Plastic Surgery,
Yale University School of Medicine,
New Haven, Connecticut;
Clinical Professor, Department of Orthopedics,
University of Connecticut School of Medicine,
Farmington, Connecticut;
Senior Staff,
Hartford Hospital;
Connecticut Children's Medical Center,
Hartford, Connecticut

M. SHARON WEBB, MD, PhD, JD
Attorney-at-Law,
Boston, Massachusetts

DENTON D. WEISS, LCDR, MC, USNR
Department of Plastic Surgery,
Naval Medical Center Portsmouth,
Portsmouth, Virginia

KATHLEEN J. WELCH, MD, MPH
Instructor in Anesthesia,
Harvard Medical School;
Director of Plastic Surgical Anesthesia,
Brigham and Women's Hospital,
Boston, Massachusetts

DEBORAH J. WHITE, MD
Staff Physician,
Scottsdale Healthcare,
Scottsdale, Arizona

GORDON H. WILKES, BS, MD, FRCSC
Clinical Professor of Surgery,
University of Alberta;
Chief of Surgery,
Misericordia Hospital,
Edmonton, Alberta, Canada

J. KERWIN WILLIAMS, MD
Clinical Associate Professor,
Division of Plastic Surgery,
Emory University School of Medicine;
Attending Physician,
Pediatric and Craniofacial Associates,
Atlanta Plastic Surgery,
Atlanta, Georgia

TODD WILLIAMS, MD
Chief Plastic Surgery Fellow,
Southern Illinois University School of Medicine,
Institute for Plastic and Reconstructive Surgery,
Springfield, Illinois

PETER D. WITT, MD, FACS
Associate Professor of Plastic Surgery;
Director, Pediatric Plastic Surgery,
Sutherland Institute,
University of Kansas School of Medicine,
Kansas City, Kansas

JOHN F. WOLFAARDT, BDS, MDent, PhD
Professor,
Faculty of Medicine and Dentistry,
University of Alberta;
Director, Craniofacial Osseointegration and Maxillofacial
    Prosthetic Rehabilitation Unit,
Misericordia Hospital,
Edmonton, Alberta, Canada

WILLIAM A. ZAMBONI, MD
Professor and Chief,
Division of Plastic Surgery,
University of Nevada School of Medicine,
Las Vegas, Nevada

JAMES E. ZINS, MD
Chairman, Department of Plastic Surgery,
The Cleveland Clinic Foundation,
Cleveland, Ohio

ELVIN G. ZOOK, MD
Professor of Plastic Surgery,
Southern Illinois University School of Medicine;
Chairman, Department of Plastic Surgery,
Memorial Medical Center,
Springfield, Illinois

RONALD M. ZUKER, MD, FRCSC, FACS, FAAP
Professor of Surgery,
University of Toronto;
Head, Division of Plastic Surgery,
The Hospital for Sick Children,
Toronto, Ontario, Canada

*To my parents, Harry Ellsworth and Helen Marjorie Russell,
who provided me the opportunity to pursue a career in medicine,
thank you*

"Life breaks all men, but some become strong in the broken places."
Ernest Hemingway

General Preface

This large project is dedicated to our colleagues who have contributed individual chapters to this textbook. Those who write chapters for books know that they are the unsung heroes of the medical publishing business. The chapter authors are recognized experts in their fields who have given their time in an effort to communicate their knowledge to the rest of the world. This unselfish work involves a long time commitment and a multistaged process. We would not have plastic surgery textbooks if it were not for the many people who give so freely of their time and expertise. We thank each of our chapter authors; this project is by you and for you, and we hope that you are proud of the finished product.

Plastic Surgery: Indications, Operations, and Outcomes was envisioned as a comprehensive overview of the entire discipline of plastic surgery. The concept was to create a practical book that would be useful for plastic surgeons in practice and for those in training. Each clinical chapter follows a standard format as closely as possible; the chapters first describe the indications for surgery, then discuss the operation of choice, including procedural details, and finally present outcomes information when available.

A project such as this has a history of its own. Bruce Achauer started the process in 1992 by talking to publishers and potential coeditors. He has provided leadership throughout the project. Working together, Achauer, Elof Eriksson, and Bahman Guyuron determined the title, focus, outline, and editors. In the fall of 1995, Achauer, Eriksson, and Guyuron signed a contract with Mosby, agreeing that they would edit the textbook. Jack Coleman, Bob Russell, and Craig Vander Kolk agreed to serve as volume editors.

Early on it was decided that the authors would focus on outcomes as much as possible, although we knew full well that there was little information on outcomes in plastic surgery. The goal was to increase awareness of this need and guide readers to begin thinking toward measuring outcomes. Ed Wilkins accepted the challenge of serving as outcomes editor.

The actual writing of the text began in 1996. The entire process of writing and editing took several years and involved a long-term commitment. The publishing business, like many others, has undergone tremendous change, including consolidation and the creation of larger firms from several companies. There was also an inevitable change of personnel during the process. Although Mosby started the project, Harcourt Health Sciences completed it. Throughout the years, our editorial staff has been extremely helpful.

Many individuals have been involved with this project. We extend our gratitude to the following people: John DeCarville and Bob Hurley, who captured our vision from the start and fully embraced it; Richard Zorab, Senior Editor, and Dolores Meloni, Senior Developmental Editor, of Harcourt Health Sciences, who saw the project through to its fruition; our tireless production staff of Carol Weis, Project Manager, and Florence Achenbach, Rick Dudley, Karen Rehwinkel, Christine Schwepker, and David Stein, Production Editors; and finally, Victoria VanderKam, who was willing to do anything necessary to see this project through.

It has been a fabulous experience, and we are grateful for the opportunity to participate. We thank everybody (authors, illustrators, and editors) for their commitment, hard work, and friendship and for creating this excellent textbook for plastic surgery.

BRUCE M. ACHAUER
ELOF ERIKSSON
BAHMAN GUYURON
JOHN J. COLEMAN
ROBERT C. RUSSELL
CRAIG A. VANDER KOLK

Preface to the Fourth Volume

Hand surgery has been practiced for years by many different kinds of surgeons with a variety of interests. The specialty came of age during the last 30 years as more surgeons limited their practice to hand surgery. The majority of general, plastic, and orthopedic residency programs still include hand surgery as part of the required training and test residents' knowledge of the specialty in board examinations. The decision by the American Boards of Surgery, Plastic Surgery, and Orthopedic Surgery to jointly offer a Certificate of Added Qualification (CAQ) in Hand Surgery awarded to diplomats who have completed an additional year of training and passed the required examination has legitimized the practice of hand surgery as a recognized subspecialty.

The increased interest in hand surgery has greatly advanced our understanding of the pathophysiologic changes and disease processes that affect the hand, leading to new treatment methods and technological advancements. The operating microscope is now used to repair nerves and small blood vessels, making digital and limb replantation and revascularization and free tissue transfers everyday procedures. The endoscope now provides a minimally invasive technique for examination and, in some cases, repair of wrist injuries. New and improved prosthetics and internal fixation devices have changed the way we treat fractures and reconstruct joints. The majority of extremity sarcomas are now treated by compartmental resection and reconstruction rather than amputation. These options were not available 30 years ago.

The geometric expansion of our medical knowledge has recently been tempered by a desire to verify and substantiate our medical and surgical protocols with outcome data, which seek to document the validity of our treatments. This volume of *Plastic Surgery: Indications, Operations, and Outcomes* is an attempt to summarize the principles and practice of hand surgery at the beginning of the twenty-first century and present existing outcome data. It should therefore be useful for students, residents, fellows, and practicing hand surgeons alike.

Any medical textbook that recommends and describes treatment modalities is attempting to hit a moving target. Current recommendations are always unstable and evolve as new knowledge or technological advances improve our understanding and provide us with better ways to treat patients. In short, the questions never change, only the answers.

This text has many outstanding contributors and chapters and literally takes the reader from anatomy through reflex sympathetic dystrophy. The color plates depicting fresh cadaver dissections in Chapter 94 are a wonderful addition to the standard anatomic drawings also included in the text. Each chapter presents the most up-to-date information available on the given subject and presents available outcome information regarding the recommended treatment options. Not surprisingly, creating the first comprehensive medical text including an outcomes section highlighted the dearth of true outcome instruments or data presently available, and we hope this revelation will stimulate the reader as much as it has the authors and editor to further develop this information. As physicians, we all believe that what we do is in the best interest of our patients, but we need to prove it to insurance companies, HMOs, lawyers, and the patients.

I have personally read all 42 chapters in this section several times and wish to apologize now for any mistakes, ambiguities, or misunderstandings that will inevitably surface after publication. I had the last editorial review and accept all responsibility for any escaped errors or omissions.

I wish to personally thank all of the contributing authors, their typists, and my own office staff for their efforts to complete this volume. Finally, I wish to thank the editors and staff at Mosby for their dedication to producing a quality textbook.

I hope you will learn as much about hand surgery reading this textbook as I did editing it.

ROBERT C. RUSSELL

Outcomes Preface

At the dawn of a new millennium, we are witnessing the most dramatic overhaul of the American health care system in more than a century. Health care reform is well underway, driven by economic and political forces within both the public and private sectors. The watchwords of this not-so-quiet revolution, terms such as *efficiency, cost-effectiveness,* and *value,* reflect the new demand by payers that health care interventions deliver measurable benefit at reasonable costs. Contrary to long-standing traditions in the United States, exactly what constitutes a "reasonable" cost is determined not by those who provide health care but rather by those who foot the bill. The growing emphasis on cost-effectiveness, or "value" for every dollar spent, is forcing providers to fundamentally rethink traditional patterns of care. In this brave new world, medical decisions are made only after the perceived benefits have been weighed against the risks *and* costs of treatment.

Recent reforms also reflect changes in the traditional standards by which we have assessed the effectiveness of care. Treatment options are no longer being judged simply in terms of morbidity and mortality. Instead, interventions are evaluated by studying their impacts on long-term functioning, well-being, and quality of life. This new emphasis on measurement of outcomes from the "patient's viewpoint" is of particular interest to plastic surgeons. Unlike cardiac or transplant surgeries, aesthetic and reconstructive procedures usually do not produce life-saving results. Instead, plastic surgeons endeavor to bestow more subtle benefits on their clientele, improving their body image, psychosocial well-being, and physical functioning. Lest plastic surgeons downplay the significance of their work, it is important to note that health services researchers and payers now evaluate the value of health care interventions in terms of quality-adjusted life years (QALYs) contributed. Interventions that substantially improve quality of life may be viewed as comparable (or superior) to treatment options that increase longevity.

Clearly, assessment of patient-centered outcomes is of critical importance not only to plastic surgeons but to all health care providers. Outcomes data are playing increasingly important roles in determining which treatment modalities are supported by payers and managed care providers. Research assessing the results and costs of care also may determine where and by whom that care is delivered. Outcomes studies also provide key information to patients and providers to assist in medical decision-making. In managing health care delivery systems, outcomes data (such as patient satisfaction) identify potential targets for quality improvement efforts and provide meaningful yardsticks with which to assess progress.

Given the growing importance of assessing and reporting patient-centered results of care, the chapter authors of this textbook have included "Outcomes" sections where appropriate. Available data on a diverse array of outcomes parameters are referenced. However, as the reader will note, considerable gaps still exist in our knowledge of surgical outcomes, particularly in the areas of quality of life and cost analyses. While we attempt to summarize existing outcomes data in each chapter, we also have endeavored to highlight some areas in which more research is needed. For many aesthetic and reconstructive problems and procedures, the quantity of unanswered research questions dwarfs our current body of knowledge. It is the hope of the volume authors and editors that some of the issues raised in these chapters will stimulate new outcomes studies to answer these questions.

EDWIN G. WILKINS

Contents

VOLUME TWO CRANIOMAXILLOFACIAL, CLEFT, AND PEDIATRIC SURGERY
Craig A. Vander Kolk, Editor

VOLUME THREE HEAD AND NECK SURGERY
John J. Coleman III, Editor

VOLUME FOUR   HAND SURGERY
Robert C. Russell, Editor

PART I

GENERAL PRINCIPLES

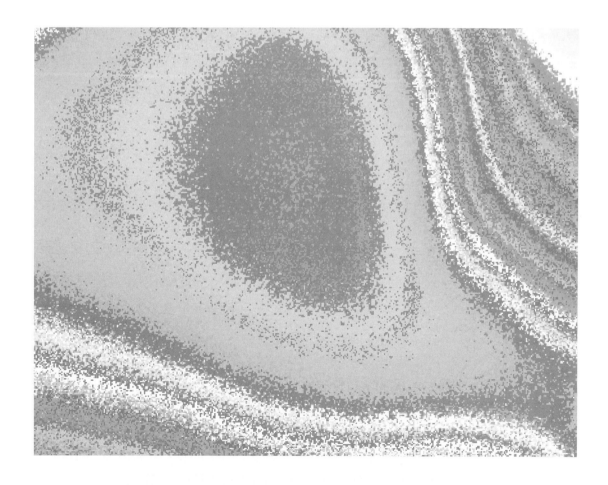

CHAPTER 94

Function, Anatomy, and Biomechanics

Nash H. Naam
Myles J. Cohen
Moulton K. Johnson

INTRODUCTION

The human hand is a complex organ comprised of a number of different tissues, with a high degree of functional specialization that permits the hand to fulfill its main roles of prehension and cognition. The combined actions of the shoulder, elbow, forearm, and wrist provide the hand with a wide range of spatial positioning. A thorough knowledge of hand anatomy and biomechanics is essential for the hand surgeon.

SKIN AND SUBCUTANEOUS TISSUE

The striking difference between the skin on the dorsum of the hand and that of the palm is an example of the high specialization of hand structures necessary to fulfill their specific functions. The dorsal skin is thin, mobile, and elastic, with loose areolar tissue between it and an investing layer of fascia. This design permits increased joint mobility. The palmar skin, by contrast, is thick and relatively immobile, providing stability for grip and pinch functions.[45] The palmar skin is fixed to the underlying palmar fascia, digital tendon sheaths, and skeleton by a series of osseous cutaneous ligaments.

The palmar skin has multiple transverse flexion creases that correspond to the sites of skin folding when the hand is closed. The skin adheres to the underlying fascia at these creases, with minimal intervening fatty tissue. The thenar crease marks the junction of the relatively fixed skin in the center of the palm and the more mobile skin covering the thenar eminence. It corresponds to the radial edge of the palmar aponeurosis. The palmar creases do not exactly correspond to the underlying joints (Figure 94-1).

The palmar skin shows multiple cutaneous striations of papillary ridges, which are more well developed in areas used for grasp. They assume a concentric orientation in the pulp, producing fingerprints unique to each individual. Apart from

their legal importance, these ridges serve to improve the contact between the skin and an object during grasping to prevent slipping and they also play a role in the tactile functions of the digits by virtue of the distribution of Meissner's corpuscles, which are found only in glabrous skin.[17,45]

THE RETINACULAR SYSTEM

The retinacular system of the hand has several important functions. The attachment of the retaining ligaments to the skin of the hand enhances its stability and helps form the skin creases. It also provides fascial compartments for hand structures, such as tendons, vessels, and nerves.

PALMAR FASCIA

The palmar fascia can be divided into three components: midpalmar, thenar, and hypothenar (Figure 94-2 and Plate 1).

The Midpalmar Fascia
The midpalmar fascia is triangular in shape. Its proximal end is attached to the palmaris longus or to the palmar surface of the transverse carpal ligament (TCL) in the absence of the palmaris longus. It extends distally to the base of the fingers and is composed of longitudinal, transverse, and vertical fibers. The longitudinal fibers may be classified as *superficial* or *deep*.[25,48]

The Longitudinal Fibers
The superficial longitudinal fibers constitute the pretendinous bands immediately palmar to the flexor tendons and their sheaths. They become wider as they extend toward the fingers. They diverge as they approach the metacarpophalangeal (MCP) joints. The central-most fibers parallel the flexor tendons of the long and ring fingers. The band to the index finger angles radially around the radial side of the index

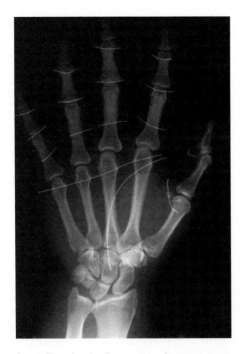

Figure 94-1. The distal palmar crease lies just proximal to the ulnar MCP joints, with the proximal palmar crease being situated more proximally and more developed in its radial end. The middle digital crease lies at the level of the PIP joint, the distal digital crease is located just distal to the DIP joint, and the proximal digital crease lies along the level of the mid-shaft of the proximal phalanx.

MCP joint, whereas the fibers to the small finger angle around the ulnar side of the small finger. The pretendinous bands are attached to the dermis of the palmar skin. The majority of the superficial fibers end at the palmar skin creases, and a few distal fibers mix with the transverse subcutaneous band of the natatory ligament. The skin pits that are seen in Dupuytren's contracture are related to fibrosis of the midpalmar fascia at the level of the distal palmar creases or the natatory ligaments at the level of the proximal digital creases.[37,52,53] The deep longitudinal fibers pass distally beneath the natatory ligament to insert into the lateral digital sheet.

The Vertical Fibers

A deep vertical paratendinous system divides the midpalmar space into several compartments through which the digital flexor tendons, lumbrical muscles, digital nerves, and vessels pass. The superficial vertical fibers pierce the palmar fat pad to anchor the skin to the palmar aponeurosis. The septa of Legueu and Juvara[30,52] originate from the palmar fascia at the level of the proximal edge of the flexor tendon sheath and pass dorsally between the lateral surfaces of the A1 pulleys and the digital neurovascular bundles. They attach to the deep transverse metacarpal ligament at the point of insertion into the volar plate of the MCP joint.

The Transverse Fibers

The transverse fibers are thin, strong, shiny fibers that run transversely deep to the pretendinous bands in the distal palm

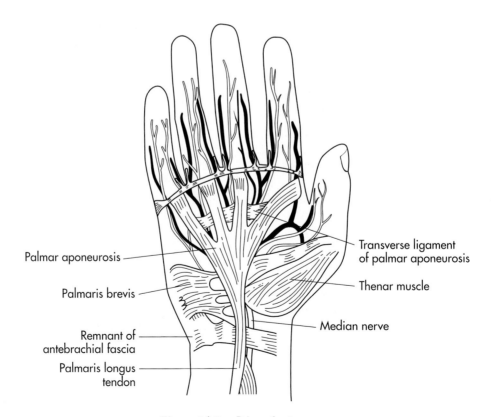

Palmar aponeurosis

Palmaris brevis

Remnant of antebrachial fascia

Palmaris longus tendon

Transverse ligament of palmar aponeurosis

Thenar muscle

Median nerve

Figure 94-2. Palmar fascia.

just proximal to the A1 pulley. The vertical fibers pass between the transverse fibers, forming the A0 pulley. Zancolli notes that there is no connection between the transverse and the pretendinous fibers.[52,53] The former are not involved in Dupuytren's contracture.

The Natatory Ligaments

The natatory ligaments are composed of transverse fibers that run transversely distal to the superficial transverse ligament at the palmar surface of the interdigital commissure. The proximal border extends from the ulnar border of the small finger to the radial border of the index finger. It then occasionally extends to the proximal digital crease of the thumb. It fuses distally with the digital fascia at the base of each finger and continues with the fascia covering the digital neurovascular bundles. Contracture of the natatory ligament in Dupuytren's contracture results in limitation of abduction of the digits. In the thumb it may result in limitation of abduction and extension.[25,37,46,53]

RETAINING LIGAMENTS OF THE DIGITS

The main function of the retaining ligaments is to stabilize the skin and the extensor mechanism of the digits and support the neurovascular bundles (Figure 94-3).

GRAYSON'S LIGAMENT

The fibers of Grayson's ligament pass transversely from the volar aspect of the flexor tendon sheath to the skin. The ligament lies on the same plane in the digits as the natatory ligament in the hand. This ligament forms the palmar wall of the compartment through which the neurovascular bundles pass. It prevents the bundles from bowstringing during finger flexion.[25,46,52,53] It also stabilizes the palmar skin in grasp.

CLELAND'S LIGAMENT (DORSAL DIGITAL SEPTUM)

Cleland's ligaments are subcutaneous ligaments that originate from the digital skeleton and pass laterally to attach to the digital skin.[25,27] The major bundles as described by Cleland are present around the proximal interphalangeal (PIP) joint. Their fibers originate from the distal third of the proximal phalanx and the base of the middle phalanx, diverging away from the joint to be attached to the skin of the proximal and middle phalanges. The minor bundles are shorter, strong fibers that originate from the lateral aspect of the distal interphalangeal (DIP) joint and insert into the overlying skin laterally and

dorsally. All of the fibers of these ligaments pass dorsally to the neurovascular bundles.[25,27]

TRANSVERSE RETINACULAR LIGAMENT OF LANDSMEER

The short, wide, obliquely-directed fibers of the transverse retinacular ligament of Landsmeer extend along the lateral side of the PIP joint superficial to the collateral ligament. The ligaments originate from the volar plate and the flexor tendon sheath in the area of the A1 pulley. They extend dorsally, where they attach to the lateral margin of each lateral band. The transverse retinacular ligament pulls the lateral bands volarly during digital flexion. During extension, they limit the dorsomedial displacement of the lateral bands. These ligaments therefore play an important role in preventing a swan-neck deformity (Figure 94-4).[25,27,46]

OBLIQUE RETINACULAR LIGAMENT OF LANDSMEER

The oblique retinacular ligaments (ORLs) are attached proximally to the distal metaphysis of the proximal phalanx at the distal bony attachment of the A2 pulley. The ligaments run distally under the transverse retinacular ligament to join the

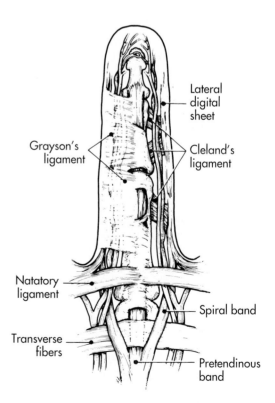

Figure 94-3. Schematic illustration of digital fascia showing Grayson's and Cleland's ligaments. (From McFarlane RM: Dupuytren's contracture. In Green DP [editor]: *Operative hand surgery,* ed 3, New York, 1993, Churchill Livingstone.)

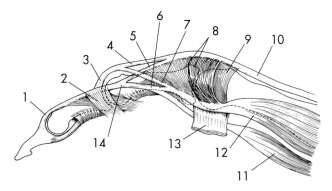

Figure 94-4. Diagrammatic representation of the extensor system. *1*, Terminal extensor tendon; *2*, transverse and oblique retinacular ligaments; *3*, central slip of the extensor tendon; *4*, middle band of the common extensor tendon; *5*, lateral band of the common extensor tendon; *6*, lateral band of interossei; *7*, middle band of the interossei; *8*, dorsum of the interossei; *9*, sagittal band; *10*, common extensor tendon; *11*, lumbrical muscle; *12*, interosseous muscle; *13*, transverse intermetacarpal ligament; *14*, lateral extensor tendon. (From Valentin P: Physiology of extension of the fingers. In Tubiana R [editor]: *The hand*, vol 1, Philadelphia, 1981, WB Saunders.)

lateral conjoined band to form the terminal conjoined extensor tendon, which inserts into the base of the distal phalanx (see Figure 94-4 and Plate 2). Each ORL lies volar to the axis of PIP-joint motion and through its attachment to the conjoined tendon passes dorsal to the DIP joint.[24,27,45]

The flexor digitorum profundus (FDP) initiates flexion at the DIP joint during flexion, producing tightness of the ORLs, which, because of their position volar to the axis of PIP-joint motion, increases the flexion moment at the PIP joint, contributing to the synchronized flexion of the PIP and the DIP joints. The ORL, in conjunction with the volar plate, the flexor digitorum superficialis (FDS) and the flexor tendon sheath, helps prevent hyperextension of the PIP joint during extension.[46,53]

MUSCLES AND TENDONS OF THE FOREARM, WRIST, AND HAND

EXTRINSIC MUSCLES

Extensors

SUPERFICIAL LAYER. In the forearm the superficial layer consists of four muscles: the extensor digitorum communis (EDC), the extensor digiti minimi (EDM), the extensor carpi ulnaris (ECU), and the anconeus (Figure 94-5 and Plate 3). The muscles of the superficial layer share a common extensor origin at the lateral epicondyle.

The Extensor Digitorum Communis. The EDC is the most radial of the superficial group of tendons as it passes distally toward the wrist.[24,40,49,52,53] It divides into four slips at the

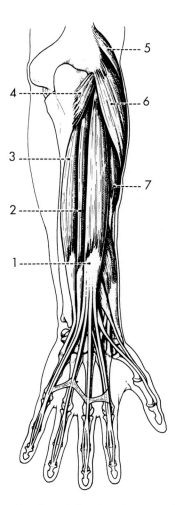

Figure 94-5. Muscles of the dorsal aspect of the forearm. *1*, Extensor digitorum communis; *2*, extensor digiti minimi; *3*, extensor carpi ulnaris; *4*, anconeus; *5*, brachioradialis; *6*, extensor carpi radialis longus; *7*, extensor carpi radialis brevis. (From Valentin P: Extrinsic muscles of the hand and wrist: an introduction. In Tubiana R [editor]: *The hand*, vol 1, Philadelphia, 1981, WB Saunders.)

distal third of the forearm. The tendons enter the fourth dorsal compartment under the extensor retinaculum. The tendons are interconnected on the dorsal aspect of the hand by the variable junctura tendinum. The most consistent of these connect the ring finger tendon to the tendons of the long and little fingers. Usually a thin junctura joins the middle and index common extensor passing over the extensor indicis proprius (EIP). The tendons insert in the dorsal hood extensor mechanism. The tendon to the little finger is variable and may be represented by only a thin tendon slip. Occasionally the tendon may give a slip to the dorsal capsule of the MCP joint at the base of the finger, forming an insertion at the dorsal aspect of the base of the proximal phalanx.

The muscle receives its nerve supply from the posterior interosseous nerve. It extends the MCP joint primarily through the function of the sagittal bands and in conjunction with the intrinsics also extends the interphalangeal (IP) joints.

The Extensor Digiti Minimi. The EDM arises from the common extensor origin and the intermuscular septum.[24,40,49,52,53] It passes distally between the EDC and the ECU. It passes to the little finger through the fifth dorsal compartment. The tendon is larger than the EDC tendon of the little finger and frequently is composed of two or more slips. It passes ulnar to the EDC, uniting with it just proximal to the MCP joint. It assists in extending the little finger in conjunction with the EDC. Innervation is through the posterior interosseous nerve.

Extensor Carpi Ulnaris. The ECU arises from the common extensor origin and from the dorsal aspect of the ulna.[24,40,49,52,53] It is a long muscle with rather short fibers.[7] The tendon enters the hand through the sixth dorsal compartment. It has a constant relationship with the head of the ulna, passing through a groove just dorsal to the ulnar styloid. The tendon inserts into the ulnar aspect of the base of the fifth metacarpal. The muscle is supplied by the posterior interosseous nerve. It is a powerful wrist extensor and ulnar deviator in both pronation and supination. The tendon is an important stabilizer of the head of the ulna and the distal radioulnar joint.[16,47]

THE DEEP LAYER. The deep layer consists of four muscles: the abductor pollicis longus (APL), the extensor pollicis brevis (EPB), the extensor pollicis longus (EPL), and the EIP.

Abductor Pollicis Longus. The APL originates from the dorsal aspect of the radius, the dorsoradial aspect of the ulna, and the interosseous membrane. It runs obliquely around the dorsoradial aspect of the radius, coursing over the radial wrist extensors to insert on the lateral aspect of the first metacarpal. It gives off a slip at its insertion to the trapezium and another slip to the APB. The tendon runs in the first dorsal compartment accompanied by the EPB, in which it may have two, three, or more tendon slips.[23,27,48] The muscle is supplied by the posterior interosseous nerve. This muscle has several functions. It abducts the thumb through a tendon slip to the APB and extends the thumb with a tendon insertion onto the base of the first metacarpal. It functions as an extensor rather than a palmar abductor of the first metacarpal. It also radially deviates the wrist and stabilizes the trapeziometacarpal joint.[7,53]

Extensor Pollicis Brevis. The EPB originates from the dorsal aspect of the radius distal to the origin of the APL and from the interosseous membrane.[8,26] It courses obliquely toward the radial side of the wrist parallel, just distal, and then dorsal to the APL. Both muscles pass superficial to the extensor carpi radialis longus (ECRL), extensor carpi radialis brevis (ECRB), and brachioradialis in the distal forearm. The tendon of the EPB passes through the first dorsal compartment and then runs dorsal to the first metacarpal and inserts on the dorsal surface of the base of the proximal phalanx of the thumb. The tendon inserts into the extensor hood of the thumb at the MCP joint in the majority of cases. The tendon has a bony attachment to the base of the first metacarpal in 20% of cases,[8] and occasionally it inserts into the base of the distal phalanx. Fre-

quently the tendon is separated from that of the APL by a fibrous septum in the first dorsal compartment. It is therefore critical to release and observe all tendon slips during surgical release of the first dorsal compartment in DeQuervain's tenosynovitis. Failure to identify the separate compartment of the EPB may result in persistent symptoms after release. The muscle may also be absent in some cases.[8,23] It is innervated by the posterior interosseous nerve.

Extensor Pollicis Longus. The EPL arises from the dorsal aspect of the middle third of the ulna and the interosseous membrane. Part of the fleshy muscle belly lies underneath the extensor retinaculum in the third dorsal compartment. As the tendon emerges from the third dorsal compartment, it curves radially around Lister's tubercle, obliquely crossing the ECRL and ECRB tendons as it passes toward the dorsal aspect of the MCP joint of the thumb. It forms the ulnar dorsal border of the anatomic snuff box (Plate 4). The tendon receives the aponeurotic insertion of the abductor pollicis brevis (APB) and the adductor pollicis (AP) before inserting into the base of the distal phalanx on the dorsal aspect of the thumb (Plate 5).

The muscle is supplied from the posterior interosseous nerve. The EPL has complex functions based on the joint involved. It is an extensor of the IP and MCP joints. It is an adductor and extensor of the trapeziometacarpal joint. It acts as a supinator of the thumb metacarpal and it also aids in extension and radial deviation of the wrist. The tendon thus has a unique function, which is to pull the whole thumb toward the plane of the hand (retroposition).[7]

Extensor Indicis Proprius. The EIP muscle arises from the dorsal surface of the distal third of the ulna distal to the origin of the EPL and the dorsal aspect of the interosseous membrane.[7,24,40,49] Its tendon passes through the fourth dorsal compartment deep to the EDC. It passes to the ulnar side of the EDC tendon to the index finger at the level of the second metacarpal and unites with it at the level of the extensor hood at the MCP joint.[40] The tendon may be absent, and occasionally there may be a separate slip to the long or the ring fingers. It is supplied by the posterior interosseous nerve. It facilitates independent index finger extension when the other fingers are flexed. It is a relatively weak muscle but is very useful as a donor tendon for transfers.[7]

THE LATERAL COMPARTMENT. The lateral compartment consists of the supinator, the brachioradialis, the ECRL, and the ECRB.[49] The latter three muscle bellies form the mobile wad of Henry, an important landmark in the proximal forearm.

Brachioradialis. The brachioradialis originates from the proximal two thirds of the lateral supracondylar ridge of the humerus and the intermuscular septum proximal to the origin of the ECRL.[7,40,49,53] The muscle lies on the radial aspect of the forearm, crossing the ECRL, pronator teres (PT), and the radial surface of the radius. The tendon inserts into the styloid process of the radius and through a thin aponeurotic fascia into the antebrachial fascia. This aponeurotic insertion has to be divided if the tendon muscle unit is to be used as a tendon transfer.

The brachioradialis is the most proximal muscle supplied by the radial nerve in the forearm. It flexes the elbow joint, supinates the fully pronated forearm, and can be a weak pronator of the fully supinated forearm.[7]

Extensor Carpi Radialis Longus. The ECRL arises from the distal third of the lateral supracondylar ridge of the humerus and the lateral epicondyle. It passes distally at the radial side of the ECRB and passes with it through the second dorsal compartment to the radial side of Lister's tubercle. The tendon inserts into the dorsoradial aspect of the base of the second metacarpal. Sometimes the tendon gives a slip to be inserted with the ECRB. This may result in difficulty harvesting the ECRL during a tendon transfer.[7] The muscle is supplied by the radial nerve. It acts as a wrist extensor and radial deviator. Many everyday activities, such as hammering nails or fishing, require alternating movements of radial wrist extension and ulnar wrist flexion. The ECRL and the flexor carpi ulnaris (FCU) are the two main muscles that act as reciprocal antagonists that alternately contract in such activities.[7]

Extensor Carpi Radialis Brevis. The ECRB originates from the lateral epicondyle. The muscle belly passes between the ECRL and the EDC. Its tendon passes through the second dorsal compartment on the ulnar side of the ECRL to insert on the dorsal aspect of the base of the third metacarpal. This insertion is closer to the long axis of the hand, making the ECRB a more effective wrist extensor. It is the only wrist extensor that does not produce radial or ulnar deviation.[7,40,49,53] It is innervated by the radial nerve.

The extensor retinaculum is the thickened distal-most portion of the dorsal antebrachial fascia. It is formed by oblique and transverse fibers coursing transversely across the dorsal aspect of the wrist, passing over all of the extensor tendons.[25,52,53] It is about 2 to 3 cm long and 4 to 6 cm wide. On the radial side, the extensor retinaculum joins the antebrachial fascia, covering the flexor carpi radialis (FCR) and the base of the thenar muscles. On the ulnar side it extends over the ECU tendon and the distal ulna to join with the antebrachial fascia and the TCL over the pisiform to attach to the pisiform and triquetrum. Multiple fibrous septa extend from the extensor retinaculum to attach to the distal radius and ulna, forming six osteofibrous compartments for the passage of extensor tendons. The extensor retinaculum has two layers, superficial and deep, which are more identifiable at the ulnar end. The deep layer forms the floor of the tendinous tunnels on the dorsal aspect of the wrist.[25,53] The extensor retinaculum is located proximal to the TCL. Its distal margin corresponds to the proximal fibers of the TCL at the level of the proximal pole of the pisiform. Thus the proximal pole of the pisiform serves as a landmark to the proximal edge of the TCL and the distal edge of the extensor retinaculum. The extensor retinaculum acts as a powerful pulley, preventing bowstringing of extensor tendons during wrist extension. It also stabilizes the ECU tendon during pronation and supination by maintaining the close relationship of the ECU tendon with the head of the

ulna.[16] The part of the extensor retinaculum in the sixth dorsal compartment also serves as an important stabilizer of the distal radioulnar joint (DRUJ).[16]

Each of the extensor tendons is surrounded by a synovial sheath as they pass beneath the extensor retinaculum beginning at their musculotendinous junction and extending variably to the midcarpus and bases of the metacarpals.

Flexors

THE SUPERFICIAL LAYER. The muscles of the superficial layer are the PT, the FCR, the palmaris longus (PL), and the FCU (Figure 94-6). They originate from the medial epicondyle of the humerus by the common flexor pronator origin.

Pronator Teres. The PT is the most radial of the superficial muscles.[24,40,48,53] It passes distally and radially to insert through a flat tendon on the radial aspect of the mid-radius. It pronates the forearm, wrist, and hand with the elbow extended. The PT is valuable as a tendon transfer for wrist extension in patients with radial nerve palsy. A strip of the

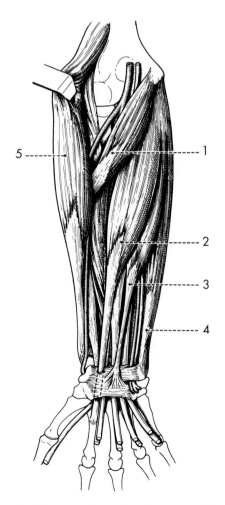

Figure 94-6. Flexor muscles in the volar aspect of the forearm, the superficial layer. *1,* Pronator teres; *2,* flexor carpi radialis; *3,* palmaris longus; *4,* flexor carpi ulnaris; *5,* brachioradialis. (From Valentin P: Extrinsic muscles of the hand and wrist: an introduction. In Tubiana R [editor]: *The hand,* vol I, Philadelphia, 1981, WB Saunders.)

periosteum from the distal radius is usually harvested in continuity with the end of the tendon to increase its length.

Flexor Carpi Radialis. The FCR originates from the medial epicondyle of the humerus and the common flexor pronator origin just lateral to the PT.[24,40,48,53] It becomes tendinous at the mid-forearm level and crosses the wrist within its own osteofibrous tunnel under the crest of the trapezium to insert into the volar aspect of the base of the index finger metacarpal (see Figure 94-6). Sometimes it is inserted into the flexor retinaculum, especially when the PL is absent. The muscle is supplied by the median nerve. Its main function is flexion of the wrist. It is a weak elbow flexor and also helps in radial deviation of the wrist.

Palmaris Longus. The PL originates from the flexor pronator origin. The muscle belly is small, and a long, thin tendon runs superficial to the TCL to attach to the apex of the palmar aponeurosis. It is absent in 10% to 15% of patients. The palmaris longus is an ancillary flexor of the wrist and is a dispensable tendon that can be used as a tendon transfer or graft. Care should be exercised in harvesting this tendon to protect the median nerve just deep to it or the palmar cutaneous branch of the median nerve just radially.

Flexor Carpi Ulnaris. The FCU has two heads, a humeral and an ulnar head. The humeral head arises from the medial epicondyle and is the most medial of the four superficial muscles. The ulnar head arises from the medial border of the olecranon and the upper part of the dorsal border of the ulna. The two heads are united by a tendinous arch, called *Osborne's ligament,* under which passes the ulnar nerve.[24,49] The muscle itself is a long, fleshy muscle with short, parallel, obliquely running fibers that insert into the strong central tendon nearly to its insertion on the pisiform (see Figure 94-6). The tendon insertion extends into the palmar aspect of the base of the fifth metacarpal and sometimes the fourth metacarpal and the hook of the hamate. Some fibers may extend to the medial side of the TCL, forming a roof for the ulnar artery and nerve.[23] The FCU is supplied by the ulnar nerve. It is a powerful flexor and ulnar deviator of the wrist. It provides a stabilizing effect on the wrist, and in its role as a flexor it is important for hand-tool use. The FCU may be used as a tendon transfer in radial nerve palsy cases to restore finger extension. However, the muscle does not have the excursion necessary to restore full finger extension.

THE INTERMEDIATE LAYER. The intermediate layer consists mainly of the flexor digitorum superficialis (FDS).

Flexor Digitorum Superficialis. The FDS originates from three separate heads: (1) the humeral head, which arises from the medial epicondyle at the common flexor pronator origin; (2) an ulnar head from the medial border of the coronoid process of the ulna; and (3) a radial head from the oblique muscular line of the radius, which runs from the bicipital tuberosity to the anterior border of the radius. Some fibers frequently originate from the medial collateral ligament of the

elbow joint.[48,53] An aponeurotic arch that connects the radial to the ulnar head passes over the median nerve and the ulnar artery.[48] The muscle splits into four tendons: two superficial, which run to the long and ring fingers, and two deep, which run to the index and small fingers. The unit to the long finger is the most independent. The ring finger unit is somewhat independent, but the index-and small-finger tendons do not have the same degree of independence. The tendons pass through the carpal tunnel underneath the TCL. The long-finger tendon lies to the radial side of the ring finger, whereas the index-and small-finger tendons lie deep to the other two. The flexor superficialis tendon to the small finger is most ulnar, it is quite variable, and sometimes it is absent. The muscle is supplied by the median nerve.[24,40,49,53]

THE DEEP LAYER. The deep layer consists of two muscles, the flexor digitorum profundus (FDP) on the ulnar side and the flexor pollicis longus (FDL) on the radial side (Figure 94-7).

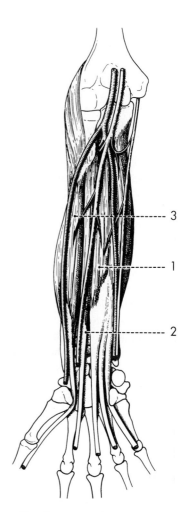

Figure 94-7. The flexor muscles at the volar aspect of the forearm, the deep layer. *1,* Flexor digitorum profundus; *2,* the tendon to the index finger; *3,* flexor pollicis longus. (From Valentin P: Extrinsic muscles of the hand and wrist: an introduction. In Tubiana R [editor]: *The hand,* vol 1, Philadelphia, 1981, WB Saunders.)

Flexor Digitorum Profundus. The FDP is a large, flat muscle that originates from (1) the volar and ulnar aspects of the proximal two thirds of the ulna, (2) the dorsal aspect of the ulna and the septum that separates the profundus from the FCU, (3) the ulnar half of the interosseous membrane alongside the origin of the FPL, and (4) occasionally from the radius, slightly distal to the bicipital tuberosity.[25,40,48] The index finger component is the most independent. The degree of independence decreases from radial to ulnar. The profundus tendons lie on the floor of the carpal tunnel beneath the superficialis tendons. The lumbrical muscles originate from the radial side of the profundus tendons in the palm, though they may in part arise more proximally within the carpal tunnel.

The radial half of the profundus muscle is supplied by the median nerve, whereas the ulnar half is supplied by the ulnar nerve.

Flexor Pollicis Longus. The FPL originates mainly from the middle third of the volar aspect of the radius. An anatomic variant may occur when an accessory muscle belly originates from the medial border of the coronoid process or the medial epicondyle of the humerus, called the *accessory muscle of Gantzer*.[24,52] The tendon passes through the carpal tunnel on its radial side adjacent and just deep to the plane of the median nerve and it bends around the trapezium, running between the two heads of the flexor pollicis brevis (FPB) and then between the two sesamoids when present, to insert into the distal phalanx of the thumb. An intertendinous band may connect the FPL to the profundus tendon of the index finger.[14,23] When present, this may prevent independent flexion of the thumb or index finger with extension of the other. This sometimes causes pain in the distal forearm and it is the cause of Linburg's syndrome.

Flexor Tendons in the Digits

The FDS and FDP tendons pass through the carpal tunnel and the palm with the superficialis tendons volar to the profundus position (Plate 6). The tendons then enter the flexor tendon sheath at the level of the distal end of the metacarpals just proximal to the MCP joints. The superficialis tendon splits into radial and ulnar halves at the level of the base of the proximal phalanx, and the profundus tendon passes through the superficialis tendon. Each half of the superficialis tendon flattens and rotates 180 degrees around the sides of the profundus tendon to become dorsal where the two slips decussate, forming the chiasma tendinum of Camper, before they insert into the lateral crest of the volar surface of the middle phalanx.

The profundus tendon passes through the superficialis tendon and continues distally across the DIP joint. The tendon inserts into the volar aspect of the proximal half of the distal phalanx. Occasionally a second band inserts into the volar plate of the DIP joint.[15]

Function of the Superficialis and Profundus Tendons

The superficialis and profundus tendons are pure flexors of the finger joints.[7] The superficialis tendon has a longer moment arm at the MCP joint because it lies superficial to the profundus tendon. The superficialis slips lie on each side of and beneath the profundus tendon at the PIP joint, thus having a smaller moment arm than the profundus at this joint. The superficialis slips, however, are able to bowstring slightly, increasing their moment arm.[7]

At the wrist the TCL acts as a pulley for the flexor tendons in the carpal tunnel. It maintains all the flexor tendons in the central position of the wrist, preventing palmar and ulnar displacement, especially during wrist flexion and ulnar deviation.

A retinacular structure proximal to the flexor tendon sheath at the level of the distal third of the metacarpals is comprised of the superficial transverse metacarpal ligament and the ligaments of Juvara and Legeue.[36,53] Manske refers to it as the "palmar aponeurosis pulley."[36] Hunter[19] notes that this preannulus system may prevent bowstringing or lateral shifts of flexor tendons after trigger-finger release of the A1 pulley.

FLEXOR TENDON SHEATHS OF THE FINGERS AND THE THUMB

The flexor tendon sheath is composed of retinacular and membranous portions. The retinacular portion of the flexor tendon sheath—the pulley system of the fingers and the thumb—are essential for optimum flexor tendon function. They enhance the ability of the flexor tendons to produce full digital flexion.

The retinacular portion of the flexor tendon sheath together with the volar surface of the phalanges form a fibroosseous canal with a synovial lining. It begins at the head of the metacarpal and extends to the base of the distal phalanx. The system of annular and cruciate pulleys along the digits holds the flexor tendons in the sheath close to the digital skeleton, minimizing the moment arm at each joint.[29,32]

The synovial sheath consists of visceral and parietal layers, which fuse at each end of the flexor tendon sheath and are contiguous at the vinculae. The visceral layer forms the epitenon of the flexor tendons. The parietal layer forms the membranous portion of the sheath and lines the inner surface of each pulley. The synovial sheath provides a closed cavity containing synovial fluid, which helps the tendon glide and provides tendon nutrition.[29,33,35]

Annular Pulleys

The annular pulleys are thickened fibrous bands that prevent bowstringing of the flexor tendons during finger flexion (Plates 7 and 8). There are five annular pulleys (Figure 94-8; see Plate 8).

The A1 pulley is approximately 10 mm long and is located at the level of the MCP joint and the base of the proximal phalanx. It is primarily attached to the volar plate, with the distal part attached to the base of the proximal phalanx.[21,53] The A2 pulley is the strongest and the longest annular pulley, measuring approximately 17 mm.[49] It is attached to bony

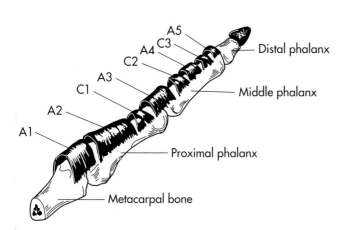

Figure 94-8. The annular and cruciate pulley system of the flexor tendon sheath.

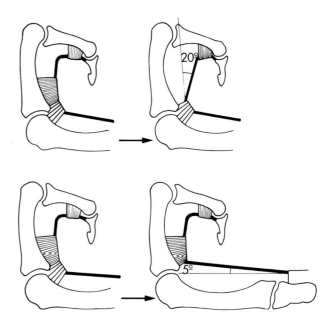

Figure 94-9. The effect of A1 and A2 pulleys on the flexor tendons during finger flexion. (From Simmons BP, delaKaffiniere JY: Physiology of finger flexion. In Tubiana R [editor]: *The hand*, vol 1, Philadelphia, 1981, WB Saunders.)

longitudinal ridges at the lateral margins of the proximal half of the proximal phalanx.[53] The A3 pulley is a short, relatively thin band that is approximately 3 mm long. It supports the tendons across the PIP joint, where it is attached to the lateral edges of the volar plate. The A4 pulley attaches to bony ridges at the mid-portion of the middle phalanx and averages 8 mm in length. The A5 pulley is a very thin, short pulley attached to the edges of the volar plate of the DIP joint and is frequently absent.

The A2 and A4 pulleys are the most important for optimum flexor tendon function. After lacerations, every attempt should be made to preserve or reconstruct these two pulleys.[10,11,19,29]

Cruciate Pulleys

The cruciate pulleys are thin, flexible pulleys with crisscrossing fibers. There are three pulleys: C1, C2, and C3 (see Figure 94-8). C1 and C3 are the more frequently found cruciate pulleys (see Plates 7 and 8).

The C1 pulley is located between the A2 and A3 pulleys. The C2 pulley is located proximal to the A4 pulley, and the C3 pulley lies between the A4 and A5 pulleys. The cruciate pulleys, because of their flexibility, have the ability to retain the flexor tendons without restricting the full flexion of the joints.[10,11,19-21,53]

FLEXOR TENDON SHEATH OF THE THUMB

The pulley system in the thumb is somewhat different. There are two annular pulleys, A1 and A2, and one oblique pulley (Plate 9).[10,11,49] The A1 pulley is located at the level of the MCP joint and is attached laterally to the volar plate and to the base of the proximal phalanx. The oblique pulley is at the level of the shaft of the proximal phalanx. It is approximately

11 mm in length and extends obliquely in a distal and radial direction. The distal A2 pulley is 10 mm long and is attached at the lateral edges of the volar plate of the IP joint.

Functions of the Flexor Tendon Pulley System

The pulley system is essential for achieving full digital flexion. The mechanisms by which the pulleys assist the flexor tendons include the following:

1. The pulleys maintain the flexor tendons close to the skeletal system, preventing them from "bowstringing" during joint flexion without interfering with joint movements. The strong A2 and A4 pulleys maintain the flexor tendons close to the bony structures at the level of the phalangeal shafts. However, at the level of the digital joints, the pulley system allows slight bowstringing of the flexor tendons with digital flexion.[20,32,42,53]

2. The pulley system helps to distribute the flexor tendon excursion across the digital joints. The relative amount of bowstringing of the flexor tendons across the joints determines the moment arm of each tendon at that joint. The relative amount of individual tendon excursion required for a given arc of motion will be proportional to the moment arm. The loss of a pulley mechanism, for instance, will result in an increased moment arm because of bowstringing, resulting in a net increase in the amount of tendon excursion required to flex the joint (Figure 94-9).[7,42]

Mechanism of Finger Flexion

Simple finger flexion is a complex movement that requires the interaction of several tendons and structures[7,21,42,52,53] At the initiation of flexion, the FDP tendon is the primary digital flexor. The first joint to flex is the PIP joint. The MCP joint is resisted in the initial stages of flexion by the extrinsic extensor mechanism and by the intrinsics. The tension increases in the intrinsics with progressive flexion of the PIP joint, resulting in flexion of the MCP joint.[42,53] Flexion of the DIP joint is limited by the ORL. As the PIP joint flexes, the tension in the ORL decreases, allowing the DIP joint to be flexed by the action of the FDP (Figure 94-10).[42,53]

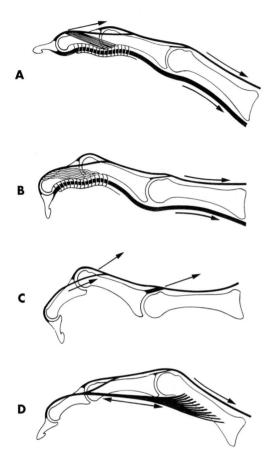

Figure 94-10. **A,** The oblique retinacular ligament is taut in extension of the PIP joint, preventing flexion of the DIP joint. **B,** Release of the retinacular ligament allows flexion of the DIP joint. **C,** Clawing of the finger as a result of absence of the volar force. **D,** Hyperextension of the MCP joint is prevented by the viscoelastic resistance of the intrinsics. (From Simmons BP, delaKaffiniere JY: Physiology of finger flexion. In Tubiana R [editor]: *The hand,* vol 1, Philadelphia, 1981, WB Saunders.)

Figure 94-11. The vincular system of blood supply to the flexor tendons in the flexor tendon sheath.

Blood Supply to the Flexor Tendons

The flexor tendons are vascularized from three sources: the point of bony insertion, the vincular system, and the vessels in the palm (Plate 10). The tendons are surrounded in the palm by a paratenon. The tendons are supplied in this loose connective tissue by numerous segmental blood vessels from the superficial palmar arch.[19,21,23,53] The tendons receive a segmental blood supply in the digital flexor sheath through the vincular system (Figure 94-11).[19,24] These vincula act as mesenteric bands carrying a relatively extensive network of vessels to both tendons. The vincula brevia are located close to the insertion point of each tendon. The superficialis tendon has a large vinculum near the PIP joint just proximal to its insertion. The vinculum longum of the profundus tendon actually pierces the superficialis tendon close to the level of the PIP joint (see Figure 94-11). The intratendinous blood vessels course primarily in the dorsal portion of each tendon and are at greater risk with placement of dorsal sutures when repairing lacerations. Focal areas of decreased vascularity have been identified in the superficialis tendon proximal to Camper's chiasm and in the profundus tendon between the vinculum longum and the vinculum breve,[19] potentially jeopardizing healing of lacerations in these areas.

FLEXOR TENDON NUTRITION. The flexor tendons in the distal forearm and palm receive their nutritional supply through vascular perfusion from longitudinally oriented blood vessels from the surrounding paratenon. The flexor tendons have a dual source of nutrition inside the tendon sheath by vascular perfusion through the vincular system and diffusion of nutrients from the synovial fluid. Most studies suggest that diffusion is more important than perfusion within the digital sheath.[19,33,35]

INTRINSIC MUSCLES OF THE FINGERS

INTEROSSEI

Most anatomists describe three palmar interossei and four dorsal interossei (Figure 94-12).

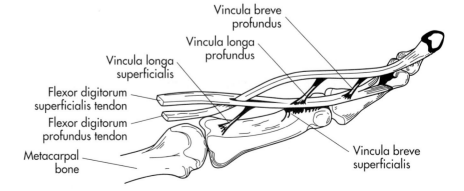

Vincula breve profundus

Vincula longa profundus

Vincula longa superficialis

Flexor digitorum superficialis tendon

Flexor digitorum profundus tendon

Metacarpal bone

Vincula breve superficialis

Palmar Interossei

Each palmar interosseous muscle originates as a single muscle belly from the anterior aspect of its respective metacarpal on the surface facing the axis of the third metacarpal (Plate 11). The first palmar interosseous is therefore located between the second and third metacarpals. It inserts on the ulnar side of the index finger. The second is located between the third and fourth metacarpals and inserts on the radial side of the ring finger, and the third palmar interosseous is located between the fourth and fifth metacarpal and inserts on the radial side of the small finger. The emerging tendon crosses just palmar to the axis of the MCP joint dorsal to the deep transverse metacarpal ligament. The main insertion of the palmar interossei is into the extensor hood.[40,50,53]

Dorsal Interossei

There are four dorsal interossei located in the four intermetacarpal spaces (see Plate 3). Each originates from the two metacarpals that bound the space and inserts into the side of the corresponding digit near the axis of digital rotation. The first and second dorsal interossei insert on the radial sides of the index and long fingers, whereas the third and fourth dorsal interossei insert on the ulnar sides of the long and ring fingers, respectively.

The muscles and insertions of the dorsal interossei are variable. There may be two muscle bellies, one superficial and one deep as viewed from the dorsum of the hand. The superficial muscle belly, when present, courses distally and its tendon passes beneath the sagittal band to insert on the bony tubercle at the base of the proximal phalanx. The deep head passes distally superficial to the sagittal band, forming a tendinous aponeurosis, which inserts into the extensor hood of the respective digit (Figure 94-13).[40,50,53] The deep tendon that inserts into the base of the proximal phalanx runs between the capsule of the MCP joint and the sagittal band.[53] The main insertion of the first dorsal interosseous muscle is to the radial base of the proximal phalanx of the index finger. The third dorsal interosseous inserts primarily into the aponeurosis. All the interossei are supplied by the deep branch of the ulnar nerve.

FUNCTION OF THE INTEROSSEI. The multiple complex functions of interosseus muscles were studied by electromyography.[50,53] Their functions include flexion of the MCP joint, extension of the IP joints, digital adduction and abduction, digital rotation for prehension, and, to a minor degree, centralization of the extensor tendons over the metacarpal head. The interossei act solely as adductors and abductors when the digits are fully extended. The dorsal interossei act as IP-joint extensors only in MCP-joint flexion. The palmar interossei adduct and the dorsal interossei abduct the fingers. Side-to-side movement in the index finger can also be produced by alternate contraction of the EDC and the EIP. The side-to-side movements of the ulnar-three digits, however, are entirely produced by the interossei.[52,53] Rotational movements of the fingers are extremely important during fine precision digital prehension. This fine rotation movement allows the fingers to place the pulp in an optimum position for the best contact with the object. The interosseous muscles also stabilize the proximal phalanx of each digit during pinch and grip prehension by preventing MCP-joint hyperextension and centralize the extensor tendons over the metacarpal heads by their attachment to the transverse fibers of the extensor hood.

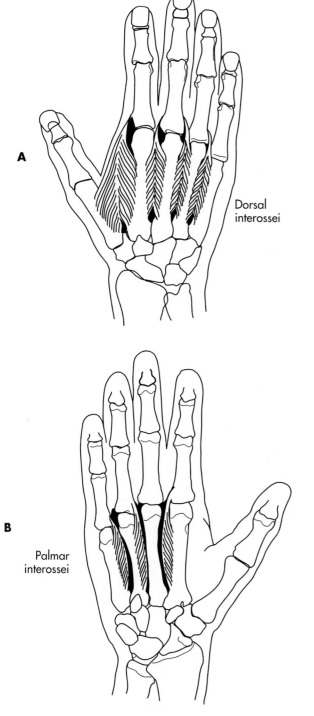

A

Dorsal interossei

B

Palmar interossei

Figure 94-12. A, The dorsal interossei function as the finger abductor. **B,** The palmar interossei function as adductor of the fingers.

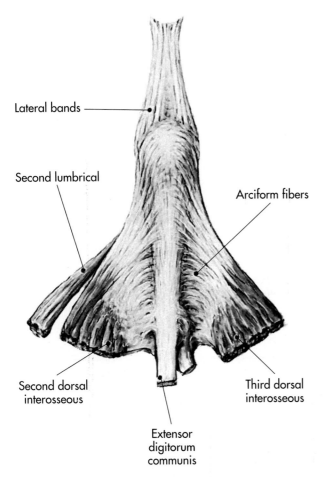

Lateral bands

Second lumbrical

Arciform fibers

Second dorsal interosseous

Third dorsal interosseous

Extensor digitorum communis

Figure 94-13. The extensor system of the long finger after being removed from the phalanges and the MCP joint showing the attachment of the dorsal interosseous muscles. (From Posner MA, Kaplan EB: Osseous and ligamentous structures. In Spinner M [editor]: *Kaplan's functional and surgical anatomy of the hand,* ed 3, Philadelphia, 1984, JB Lippincott.)

THE LUMBRICALS

There are four lumbrical muscles (Plate 12; see also Plate 2). They are the only skeletal muscles in the body that do not have any direct bony attachment. They function as a connector between the FDP and the extensor mechanisms.[50,53]

The lumbricals originate from the FDP tendons in the palm. The first and second lumbricals are attached to the radial side of the profundus tendon of the index and middle fingers, respectively, whereas the third and fourth are attached to the two adjacent profundus tendons of the middle and ring and the ring and little fingers. When the fingers are flexed, the origin of the lumbricals may retract into the carpal tunnel and may reach as far proximally as the distal end of the radius.

The muscle fibers take their origin on the profundus tendons and course toward the radial side of the digits, crossing to the radial side of each MCP joint. A narrow, flattened tendon emerges from the muscle at this level to join the radial edge of the extensor aponeurosis (see Figure 94-13). The two

radial lumbricals join the two dorsal interossei, whereas the two ulnar lumbricals join the two palmar interossei.[50,52,53]

The radial-two lumbricals are supplied by the median nerve through branches from the digital nerves of the first and second web spaces (Plate 13). The two ulnar lumbricals are supplied on their deep surfaces by fibers from the deep motor branch of the ulnar nerve.

Function of the Lumbricals

The main function of the lumbricals is to facilitate extension of the IP joints. The lumbricals can extend the IP joints in any position of the MCP joint.[50] Clawing of the index and long fingers does not occur in patients with ulnar nerve palsy because the radial-two lumbricals innervated by the median nerve remain functional. The lumbrical muscles have a high concentration of proprioceptive receptors, which indicates their important role in balancing the forces between the flexor and extensor mechanisms of the fingers.[50]

Explanation of the Claw Hand Deformity

The finger is a four-link, three-joint system. Elimination of intrinsic muscles removes the key balancing forces that control the distal links. The intrinsics pass volar to the MCP flexion axis and dorsal to the IP joints. They act to balance the extrinsic extensor force at the MCP joint, preventing hyperextension. As the MCP joint extends, the intrinsics are placed under greater tension, enhancing their ability to extend the IP joints through their insertions into the extensor hood.

Paralysis of the intrinsic interossei and lumbrical muscles results in a significant reduction in MCP-joint flexion force. In active extension, the MCP joint is subject to an unbalanced extensor force through the extrinsic extensor muscles. The MCP joint is pulled into hyperextension. The extrinsic extensor is tethered by the sagittal bands, thus its excursion is applied primarily to the MCP joint. The reduced excursion available for the PIP and DIP joints results in decreased extensor moment at these more distal joints. As the MCP joint hyperextends, it places the flexor tendons under greater tension, which is now applied to the PIP and DIP joints. The claw deformity is the result of this force imbalance. A claw hand deformity does not occur when both the intrinsic and extrinsic flexor muscles are paralyzed.

INTRINSIC MUSCLES OF THE THUMB

Abductor Pollicis Brevis

The abductor pollicis brevis is the most superficial muscle of the thenar eminence (see Plate 7). It originates from the TCL and the PL, and may receive an additional slip from the APL. The tendon is adherent to the radial side of the MCP joint capsule of the thumb. A few fibers join the tendon of the FPB and insert into the radial sesamoid. The rest of the fibers join the extensor expansion of the thumb.[26] Some fibers also insert into the radial side of the base of the proximal phalanx dorsal and distal to the insertion of the FPB.[1]

Flexor Pollicis Brevis

The FPB originates by two heads (Plate 14). The superficial head originates from the anterior and distal edge of the TCL, the anterior surface of the FCR tendon sheath, and the crest of the trapezium. The deep head originates from the anterior surface of the trapezoid and the capitate proximal to the insertion of the oblique head of the adductor pollicis.[26] The two heads unite, forming an arch for the passage of the FPL. The tendon inserts into the lateral sesamoid and the lateral tubercle of the base of the proximal phalanx.[26,40]

The Opponens Pollicis

The opponens pollicis originates from the transverse carpal ligament deep to the fibers of the APB, the ridge of the trapezium, and the capsule of the trapeziometacarpal joint. The muscle inserts directly into the radial border of the first metacarpal.

Adductor Pollicis

The AP originates from two heads (Plate 15). The oblique head originates from the dorsal wall of the carpal tunnel, including the ligaments covering the capitate and the trapezoid and the tunnel of the FCR. The transverse head originates from the volar aspect of the third metacarpal from the neck to the base. The two heads converge and the fibers rotate to create a small tendinous arch, either in the oblique or transverse head or between the two heads, for passage of the deep branch of the ulnar nerve and the deep palmar arch. The rotation of the fibers allows the transverse head to insert mainly into the medial sesamoid of the MCP joint, and the fibers of the oblique head insert into the extensor expansion. Another extension is inserted into the ulnar tubercle of the base of the proximal phalanx.[1,26,40]

The APB and opponens pollicis are supplied by the median nerve. The FPB is mainly supplied by the median nerve, but the deep fibers have a dual innervation from both the median and ulnar nerves. The AP is supplied by the deep branch of the ulnar nerve. Numerous variations in the innervation of the thenar muscles have been noted, such as the Riché-Cannieu and Martin-Gruber anastomosis. This probably explains the variable residual activity of the thenar muscles after median nerve injuries in some patients.[2,23,26]

Biomechanics of Thumb Motion

The thumb is uniquely equipped to perform its major function, which is opposition. The special arrangement of the bony structures and associated muscles allows the thumb to perform that function.[53] Opposition itself is a complex movement, with the ultimate goal of bringing the pulp of the thumb across the palm to meet the pulp of the other digits. Three distinct components, including projection, adduction, and pronation, are present when analyzing the complex movement of thumb opposition. Projection of the trapezio-metacarpal joint is essentially a combination of flexion and abduction. Adduction of the thumb column and pronation bring the pulp of the thumb close to the pulp of the other digits. Pronation occurs mainly by rotation of the thumb metacarpal at the trapeziometacarpal joint. The overall rotation is enhanced by flexion of the MCP and IP joints.[52,53]

Release of the thumb after opposition, which Zancolli calls *retroposition,* is also a complex movement requiring abduction, supination, and extension. The EPL is the main muscle responsible for retroposition.[52,53] The intrinsic muscles of the thumb are generally the motor muscles of opposition, whereas the extrinsics are the motor muscles of retroposition.[52,53]

Function of the Thenar Muscles

The thenar muscles work in harmony to achieve the complex movements of the thumb. The movement of opposition is initiated by the combined action of the APB and opponens pollicis muscles. The combined action of these muscles moves the thumb into the position of abduction, flexion, and pronation. The FPB is essentially a flexor of the trapeziometa-carpal joint, producing a lesser amount of projection and no rotation. But it also flexes, radially deviates, and pronates the MCP joint. Its action therefore completes the movement of opposition.[26,52,53]

The AP pulls the thumb toward the second metacarpal. It produces this movement by acting on the trapeziometacarpal joint. It also acts at the level of the MCP joint where it flexes, ulnarly deviates, and supinates that joint. It also has some effect on extension of the IP joint and plays an important role in the pulp-to-side or key pinch.

EXTENSOR APPARATUS OF THE FINGERS

The common extensor tendon divides at the level of the proximal half of the proximal phalanx into three slips, one central and two lateral (see Plates 2 and 12). The central slip attaches to the dorsal aspect of the base of the middle phalanx.

The intrinsic tendons of the interossei on the ulnar side and the interossei and the lumbricals on the radial side form the aponeuroses, or wing tendons (see Figure 94-13). The lumbrical tendon is usually located on the most lateral part of the radial wing tendons. The lateral slip of the common extensor origin joins the tendons of the intrinsics, forming the lateral bands on the dorsolateral aspect of the PIP joint (Figure 94-14).

The lateral bands on the two sides of the extensor hood decussate and join together at the level of the distal part of the middle phalanx and with the ORL form the terminal or conjoined tendon, which inserts on the dorsal aspect of the base of the distal phalanx (see Figure 94-4).[49,50]

SAGITTAL BAND

The sagittal band functions as a passive stabilizer for the extensor tendon over the MCP joint (see Figure 94-14 and

Plate 2). The distal part of the sagittal band is covered by the transverse fibers of the interosseous hood. The sagittal band passes on each side of the MCP joint, reaching volarly to attach to the volar plate of the MCP joint.[53] The sagittal band helps to stabilize the common extensor tendon during flexion and hyperextension. It also limits the proximal excursion of the common extensor tendon and is the primary extensor of the MCP joint. As the extrinsic extensor contracts, its force is transmitted to the sagittal bands, which lift the base of the proximal phalanx, extending the MCP joint and allowing transmission of extrinsic excursion distally to the PIP and DIP joints.

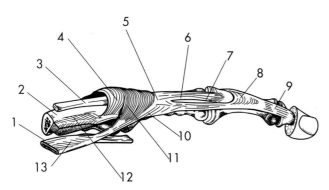

Figure 94-14. The extensor apparatus of the finger. *1,* Flexor digitorum profundus tendon; *2,* metacarpal bone; *3,* tendon of extensor digitorum; *4,* interosseous hood; *5,* lateral slip; *6,* central slip; *7,* insertion of middle extensor tendon; *8,* triangular ligament; *9,* insertion of terminal extensor tendon; *10,* lateral band; *11,* insertion of lumbrical muscle to dorsal hood; *12,* interosseous muscle; *13,* lumbrical muscle.

TRIANGULAR LIGAMENT

The triangular ligament is formed by the transverse fibers that connect the lateral bands at the level of the proximal part of the middle phalanx (see Figure 94-14 and Plate 12). The triangular ligament may limit volar and lateral shifting of the lateral bands during flexion. The ligament is attenuated in a boutonniere deformity, contributing to volar subluxation of the lateral bands.[53]

TRAPEZIOMETACARPAL JOINT

The trapeziometacarpal joint is often described as a biconcave saddle joint (Figure 94-15). The proximal articular surface is mainly concave in the radioulnar direction and convex in the dorsopalmar direction. The base of the first metacarpal is asymmetrical, but the central part is saddle-shaped and surrounded by radial and ulnar slopes. It is concave in a dorsopalmar direction and convex radioulnarly. The base of the first metacarpal has volar and dorsal beaks. The volar beak is longer and has no ligament attachment.[41,52,53] The stability of the trapeziometacarpal joint is dependent on the surrounding muscles and ligaments.

LIGAMENTS

Anterior Oblique Ligament
The anterior oblique ligament (AOL) is the most important stabilizing capsular ligament. It runs obliquely from the palmar tubercle of the trapezium to the palmar tubercle of the first

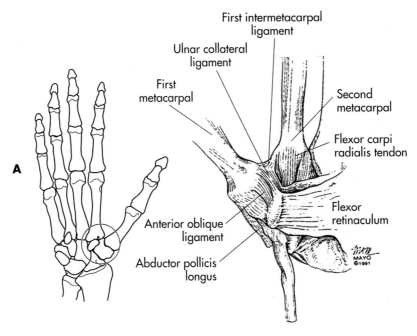

Figure 94-15. A, Palmar view of the trapeziometacarpal joint. *Continued*

metacarpal base. This ligament is responsible for retaining the intraarticular fracture fragment of the base of the first metacarpal in a Bennett's fracture. It becomes attenuated in advanced trapeziometacarpal arthritis, which allows radial subluxation of the base of the first metacarpal.[22,41,52]

Posterior Oblique Ligament

The posterior oblique ligament (POL) is a strong dorsal ligament represented by a long band that runs in a fan-shaped fashion from the dorsoulnar tubercle of the trapezium to the palmar tubercle of the metacarpal base. This ligament is taut in opposition and full abduction.[22,53]

Dorsoradial Ligament

The dorsoradial ligament is an intracapsular ligament that extends from the dorsoradial tubercle of the trapezium to the dorsoradial aspect of the base of the first metacarpal. The ligament becomes taut in thumb adduction and is lax in abduction. Although frequently normal in many cases of early osteoarthritis, it is attenuated in advanced degenerative arthritis.[22,52]

First Intermetacarpal Ligament

The first intermetacarpal ligament is a very strong extracapsular ligament that is attached to the bases of the first and second metacarpals. The distal end of the ECRL tendon runs between the intermetacarpal ligament and the POL. It is elongated in trapeziometacarpal arthritis, allowing radial subluxation of the base of the first metacarpal.[52,53]

Ulnar Collateral Ligament

The ulnar collateral ligament is an extracapsular ligament that runs obliquely from the TCL to the palmar ulnar tubercle of the base of the first metacarpal. It becomes tight in extension, abduction, and pronation.[22]

MOVEMENTS OF THE TRAPEZIOMETACARPAL JOINT

There are essentially two types of movements at the trapeziometacarpal joint; simple movements such as abduction, adduction, extension, and flexion and complex movements such as opposition and retroposition. Zancolli[52,53] notes that simple movements occur at the saddle joint, but the complex movements also involve the articulation between the convex spheroidal surface of the trapezium with the radial slope of the base of the first metacarpal.[53] The flexion-extension axis passes through the trapezium in a radioulnar direction, whereas the abduction-adduction axis passes through the metacarpal base in a dorsopalmar direction.

Opposition represents an ulnarly and palmarly directed circumduction movement with axial rotation and pronation of the first metacarpal, whereas retroposition represents a radially and dorsally directed circumduction movement with supination of the first metacarpal. Opposition and retroposition require axial rotation of the thumb. The thumb rotates as a cone, with the apex at the crossing of the flexion-extension and abduction-adduction axes at the base of the metacarpal.[41,52,53]

THE METACARPOPHALANGEAL JOINT OF THE THUMB

The main function of the MCP joint is to position and simultaneously provide stability for the thumb in the power grip.[1] The MCP joint of the thumb therefore is somewhat

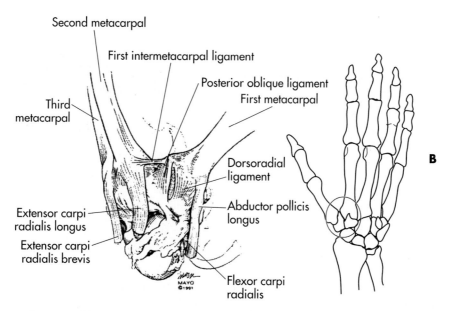

Second metacarpal
First intermetacarpal ligament
Posterior oblique ligament
First metacarpal
Third metacarpal
Dorsoradial ligament
Extensor carpi radialis longus
Extensor carpi radialis brevis
Abductor pollicis longus
Flexor carpi radialis

B

MAYO ©1991

Figure 94-15, cont'd. B, Dorsal view of the trapeziometacarpal joint. (From Imaeda T, An K-N, Cooney WP, et al: J Hand Surg [AM] 18:226-231, 1993.)

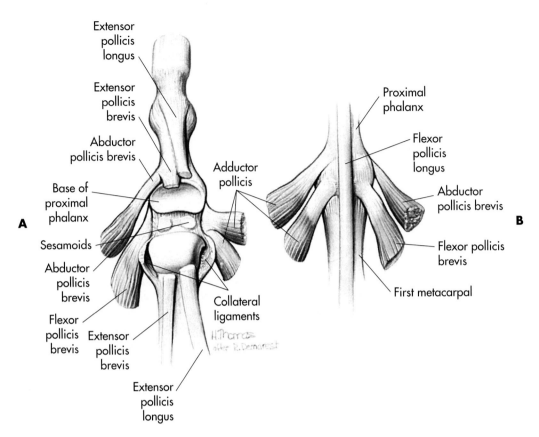

Figure 94-16. **A,** The inside of the MCP joint of the right thumb, viewed from the dorsal aspect after removal of the dorsal capsule. Note the presence of the sesamoids in the volar plate. **B,** The MCP joint of the right thumb, viewed from the volar aspect. (From Kaplan EB, Riordan DC: The thumb. In Spinner M [editor]: *Kaplan's functional and surgical anatomy of the hand,* ed 3, Philadelphia, 1984, JB Lippincott.)

different from the MCP joints of the fingers. The range of flexion of the thumb MCP joint is less than that of the finger MCP joints. Two sesamoid bones are usually present in the volar plate. The radial sesamoid is normally larger than the ulnar sesamoid. The two sesamoid bones are connected by transverse fibers. A tunnel adherent to those fibers is present for the passage of the FPL tendon (Figure 94-16). The articular surface of the head of the first metacarpal is trapezoidal in shape, with the volar aspect being wider than the dorsal aspect. The articular surface extends more volarly to provide articulation to the two sesamoid bones and the volar plate.[1,40,52,53]

LIGAMENTS AND MUSCLES

The collateral ligaments are similar to the collateral ligaments of the other MCP joints. The ulnar collateral ligament is thicker than the radial ligament. Its main part stretches from the tubercle of the ulnar aspect of the metacarpal head to the volar ulnar aspect of the base of the proximal phalanx next to the insertion of the adductor tendon. The accessory collateral ligament (ACL) extends volarly and inserts into the ulnar aspect of the volar plate and the ulnar sesamoid. The radial collateral ligament (RCL) is attached to the radial side of the base of the proximal phalanx just behind the insertion of the

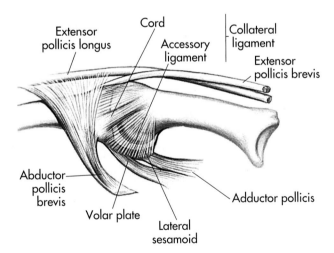

Figure 94-17. The MCP joint of the right thumb, viewed from the radial side. (From Kaplan EB, Riordan DC: The thumb. In Spinner M [editor]: *Kaplan's functional and surgical anatomy of the hand,* ed 3, Philadelphia, 1984, JB Lippincott.)

FPB. The accessory ligament is attached to the radial border of the volar plate and to the radial sesamoid. The collateral ligaments are taut in flexion and relaxed in extension, whereas the accessory collateral ligaments are stretched in extension and relaxed with flexion (Figure 94-17).[1,26] The volar plate is an

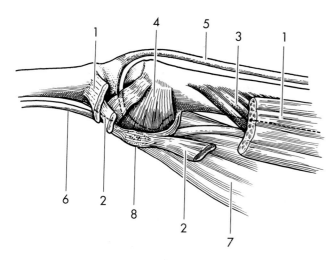

Figure 94-18. The radial aspect of the MCP joint of the thumb. *1,* Abductor pollicis brevis; *2,* the two heads of the flexor pollicis brevis; *3,* opponens pollicis; *4,* the two parts of the radial collateral ligament; *5,* extensor pollicis brevis; *6,* flexor pollicis longus; *7,* adductor pollicis; *8,* the volar plate and the radial sesamoid. (From Aubriot JH: The metacarpophalangeal joint of the thumb. In Tubiana R [editor]: *The hand,* vol 1, Philadelphia, 1981, WB Saunders.)

important fibrous structure that prevents hyperextension. The edges provide attachment for the first annular pulley, the thenar muscles, and the collateral ligaments. The volar plate extends from the volar aspect of the neck of the first metacarpal to the volar base of the proximal phalanx.[1,26,40]

Several muscles attach to the sides of the MCP joint (see Figure 94-16). The adductor aponeurosis on the ulnar side passes over the edge of the volar plate and the ulnar sesamoid to the ulnar border of the EPL tendon. That aponeurosis is responsible for the Stener's lesion associated with rupture of the ulnar collateral ligament, which comes to lie superficial to the aponeurosis. In this event the ligament is typically avulsed distally. The proximal margin of the aponeurosis displaces distally and radially, trapping the distal end of the ligament superficial to its insertion. The adductor pollicis muscle has two other insertions, one to the volar part of the aponeurosis and through it to the volar plate and the ulnar sesamoid and another insertion on the ulnar aspect of the base of the proximal phalanx.

The insertions of the thenar muscles are on the radial side of the thumb. The deep head of the FPB inserts into the radial border of the volar plate and to the radial sesamoid, whereas the superficial head inserts on the radial aspect of the base of the proximal phalanx. The APB aponeurosis inserts into the extensor hood radially. It also inserts into the radial side of the base of the proximal phalanx dorsal and distal to the insertion of the flexor pollicis brevis (Figure 94-18).[1,25]

INTERPHALANGEAL JOINT OF THE THUMB

The IP joint of the thumb plays an important role in the overall activity of bringing the pulp of the thumb toward the

other digits in opposition. As the IP joint of the thumb goes from extension to flexion it rotates into pronation about 5 to 10 degrees. This is primarily the result of the dissimilar shape of the two phalangeal condyles of the proximal phalanx. The ulnar condyle protrudes more dorsally and ulnarly than the radial condyle. This results in rotation of the distal phalanx on its longitudinal axis as it moves from extension to flexion. The overall pronation of the thumb therefore occurs at the three main joints: the trapeziometacarpal, the MCP and the IP.[1,26]

DIGITAL JOINTS

METACARPOPHALANGEAL JOINT

The MCP joint is a multiaxial condyloid joint, which allows a relatively wide range of motion. The metacarpal head is asymmetrically shaped, being wider on the volar aspect with its longest diameter in an anteroposterior direction. The articular cartilage covers about three fourths of its spherical anteroposterior surface. It articulates with the base of the proximal phalanx, which is oblong in shape with its longest axis perpendicular to the long axis of the metacarpal head. This arrangement facilitates flexion-extension and abduction and adduction of the joint. The base of the proximal phalanx matches the metacarpal head in radial-to-ulnar configuration. However, in the anteroposterior configuration it covers only about one third of the condylar surface of the head of the metacarpal. The two collateral ligaments and the volar plate form a strong fascial three-sided support for the MCP joint (Figure 94-19).[12,40] The capsule is relatively lax and it allows significant motion at the joint with some degree of distraction.

Volar Plate

The volar plate reinforces the volar part of the capsule. Its proximal membranous portion is attached to the volar aspect of the neck of the metacarpal. The distal part is cartilaginous and is attached to the volar side of the base of the proximal phalanx. The thick cartilaginous part is an important factor in preventing hyperextension of the MCP joint. The sides of the volar plate are the sites of attachment of the ACLs, the transverse intermetacarpal ligaments, the first annular pulley, and the septa of Legeue and Javara.[12,40,52,53]

Collateral Ligaments

The collateral ligaments on the radial and ulnar sides of each joint are very thick ligaments with an average length of about 12 to 14 mm (see Figure 94-19). Each ligament is composed of two parts: the main MCP part (collateral ligament proper), which is located dorsal and distal, and the accessory metacarpoglenoid part, which is located palmar and proximal. The fibers of the ligament originate from a tuberosity on the dorsolateral aspect of the metacarpal head. The fibers then run obliquely, distally, and volarly. The fibers of the proper collateral ligament insert into the lateral tubercle of the base of the proximal phalanx near its volar surface. These fibers pass

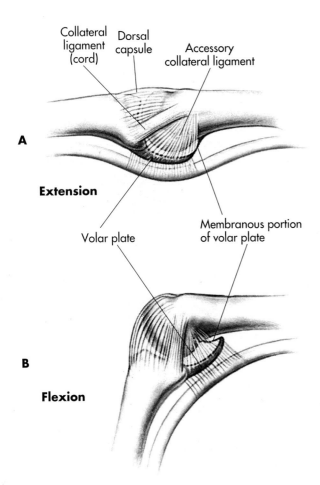

Figure 94-19. MCP joint demonstrating the collateral ligaments and the volar plate in extension **(A)** and flexion **(B)**. (From Posner MA, Kaplan EB: Osseous and ligamentous structures. In Spinner M [editor]: *Kaplan's functional and surgical anatomy of the hand,* ed 3, Philadelphia, 1984, JB Lippincott.)

dorsal to the flexion-extension axis of the joint. The metacarpal head is broader on the palmar side and the ligaments have a tendency to diverge more and become tight as flexion increases.[12] The collateral ligaments are therefore taut when the joint is flexed and become lax during extension. This allows more lateral movement of the MCP joint in extension and stabilization in flexion. Prolonged immobilization of the MCP joints in extension can result in fibrosis and shortening of the relaxed collateral ligaments, leading to loss of MCP-joint flexion.

The metacarpoglenoid fibers, or accessory ligaments, are triangular structures that originate from the same tuberosity with the MCP fibers. The fibers fan out from that attachment toward the lateral border of the volar plate. The ACL lies volar to the flexion-extension axis of the MCP joint. Its fibers are therefore taut in extension and lax in flexion. The terminal fibers of the ACL pierce the transverse metacarpal ligament and fuse with the flexor tendon sheath. Their main function is to maintain the stability of the flexor tendons during flexion.[12]

Movements of the Metacarpophalangeal Joint

Three different types of movement occur at the MCP joint. The flexion-extension movement is the main movement of the

joint and it has a typical range of 80 to 100 degrees. The joint also allows radial and ulnar deviation that occurs in a frontal plane and can be performed voluntarily. The third movement is axial rotation, which is more marked in border digits. Axial rotation is a passive movement that occurs as a result of the asymmetry of the collateral ligaments. The RCL runs more obliquely and is attached very close to the joint, whereas the ulnar collateral ligament is directed more vertically and is attached more proximally on the metacarpal head.[12]

PROXIMAL INTERPHALANGEAL JOINT

The geometric structure of the bones of the PIP joint and the attached soft tissue allow the movements to be limited to one plane (flexion-extension) while preventing rotation or lateral movements.

The articular surface of the head of the proximal phalanx is trapezoidal in shape, with the palmar aspect almost twice the width of the dorsal aspect. The condyles of the head of the proximal phalanx are symmetrical and therefore the axis of motion is essentially a single transverse axis through the tuberosities on the lateral aspects of the head of the proximal phalanx at the attachment of the collateral ligament. A shallow anteroposterior groove exists between the two condyles. There is slight variation in the groove in each digit that allows convergence of the fingers toward the scaphoid tubercle when they are flexed into a fist position. The distal articular surface is the base of the middle phalanx, which is wider in a radial ulnar direction than the dorsal volar direction. It has two fossae that correspond to the condyles of the proximal phalanx and are separated by a smooth anteroposterior ridge that corresponds to the anteroposterior groove of the head of the proximal phalanx. The base of the middle phalanx is significantly shorter in anteroposterior diameter than the head of the proximal phalanx. That allows only about one half of the articular surface of the proximal phalanx to be covered by the base of the middle phalanx. The rest of the articular surface of the head of the proximal phalanx is in contact with the volar plate. The volar plate of the PIP joint contributes to enlarging the total surface area available to articulate with the larger size of the proximal articular surface.[7,51]

The dorsal capsule is very thin and lax on the dorsal surface of the joint. This is reinforced by the extensor mechanism on the dorsal aspect of the joint.

Volar Plate

The volar plate has a strong distal attachment to the volar base of the middle phalanx (Figure 94-20). The main attachment is on the two lateral parts of this volar border that provide attachment for the ACLs, whereas the central part of the insertion is more loosely attached to the periosteum. This allows retraction of the volar plate from the base of the middle phalanx when the joint is flexed. The proximal attachment of the volar plate is, however, more complex. The proximal part, which is thin and membranous, is attached to the volar aspect of the proximal phalanx and through the checkrein ligaments to each side of the volar aspect of the proximal phalanx.[51] The

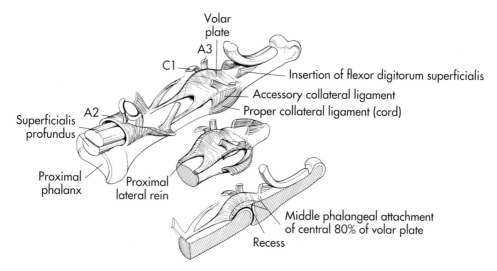

Figure 94-20. The volar aspect of the PIP joint, showing the relationship of the volar plate to the flexor tendons and the flexor sheath. (From Posner MA, Kaplan EB: Osseous and ligamentous structures. In Spinner M [editor]: *Kaplan's functional and surgical anatomy of the hand,* ed 3, Philadelphia, 1984, JB Lippincott.)

checkrein ligaments extend from the lateral proximal volar plate to two ridges on the volar lateral surfaces of the proximal phalanx named by Watson[51] the *assembly lines.* Several other structures are attached to these ridges, including the flexor tendon sheath, Cleland's ligament, the oblique retinacular ligament, and the transverse retinacular ligament.

The palmar surface of the volar plate is lined with the synovial cells of the parietal portion of the membranous sheath. The volar plate is connected on the volar side with the flexor tendon sheath. The thickness of the volar plate in that area is 1.5 mm, which increases the moment arm of the superficialis tendon by 25%.[7] All of the volar structures, including the volar plate, the flexor tendons, and the flexor tendon sheath, are important in preventing hyperextension of the PIP joint.

Collateral Ligaments
The radial and ulnar collateral ligaments are strong, 2- to 3-mm thick bands that are attached proximally to the lateral tubercle on each side of the head of the proximal phalanx along the flexion-extension axis of the joint. Each ligament extends distally and volarly to attach to the lateral beveled surface of the base of the middle phalanx. The more volar fibers run in a more oblique course to attach to the sides of the volar plate. These fibers represent the ACLs. The tension of the collateral ligaments is essentially the same whether the joint is flexed or extended. This constant tension prevents lateral movement in the PIP joints, whether they are in a position of flexion or extension. The collateral ligaments and the volar plate form a three-sided fascial structure to suspend the head of the proximal phalanx.[12]

DISTAL INTERPHALANGEAL JOINT

The bony structure of the DIP joint and the soft tissue attachments are very similar to those of the PIP joint. The FDP

is the only flexor. The capsule on the dorsal aspect is so closely attached to the extensor tendon that it is virtually impossible to separate them.

The condyles of the head of the middle phalanx are asymmetrical in width, length, and projection, resulting in a deviation of the long axis of the distal phalanx from that of the middle phalanx. This is true except in the long finger, in which the long axis of both phalanges is the same. The adjacent fingers therefore have a tendency to deviate toward the central digit, with the distal phalanx of the index finger inclined ulnarward and those of the ring and little fingers inclined radially. There are no lateral or rotational movements.[7,12,40]

FUNCTION, ANATOMY, AND BIOMECHANICS OF THE WRIST

The wrist is a complex, multiarticulated linkage system between the forearm and the hand. The multiarticulated pattern allows a wide range of motion that serves to increase the function of the hand.[44] The articulation of the distal radius to the proximal carpal row forms the radiocarpal joint. The distal articular surface of the radius is triangular in shape, with the apex being the styloid process and the base being the ulnar (sigmoid) notch that articulates with the head of the ulna at the DRUJ. The concave distal articular surface is divided by an anteroposterior ridge into a radical triangular fossa for the articulation with the scaphoid (scaphoid fossa) and a quadrangular-shaped ulnar fossa for articulation with the lunate (lunate fossa).[40,44] The triangular fibrocartilage, which articulates with the triquetrum, completes the proximal articular surface of the radiocarpal joint and is attached to the distal margin of the ulnar notch (sigmoid notch).

The distal articular surface of the radius is tilted in two planes. In the sagittal plane there is a palmar tilt that averages 11 degrees, whereas in the frontal plane there is a volar inclination that averages 26 degrees.[6,44] The sigmoid notch is a concave facet that has three margins: palmar, dorsal, and distal. The palmar and dorsal margins provide attachment to the distal radioulnar ligaments, whereas the palmar and dorsal edges of the distal margin provide attachment to the palmar and dorsal radioulnar ligaments of the triangular fibrocartilage.[4,6,39,44]

The carpal bones are grouped into two transverse rows: the proximal carpal row consisting of scaphoid, lunate, triquetrum, and pisiform and the distal carpal row of trapezium, trapezoid, capitate, and hamate. The pisiform is not actually a part of the wrist joint, and most anatomists consider it a sesamoid bone in the FCU tendon. Each carpal bone has several articular surfaces for articulation with neighboring bones.[40,44]

The radiocarpal joint is formed by the distal radius and the triangular fibrocartilage, forming a biconcave proximal articular surface articulating with the distal smooth biconvex surface that is formed by the scaphoid, lunate, and triquetrum, and the connecting interosseous ligaments.[40,44]

The mid-carpal joint is the articulation between the proximal and distal carpal rows. The convex distal articular surface of the scaphoid radially articulates with the trapezium and the trapezoid. This is a typical gliding joint. The ulnar distal surface of the scaphoid, the lunate, and the triquetrum articulate with the capitate and the hamate, forming a diarthroidal-type joint. Sometimes the lunate has a separate facet distally to articulate with the hamate. The mid-carpal joint therefore comprises two different types of articulations, which adds to the complexity of that joint.[4,44,52,53]

The pisotriquetral joint is a separate entity being isolated from the radiocarpal and the mid-carpal joints. Occasionally, communications with the radiocarpal joint exist.

ANATOMY OF WRIST LIGAMENTS

The capsules of the radiocarpal and the midcarpal joints are reinforced by dorsal, volar, and interosseous ligaments. The volar ligaments are thicker and stronger. All of the ligaments are intracapsular and the interosseous ligaments are intraarticular (Figures 94-21 and 94-22).[4,43,44,52,53]

Volar Radiocarpal Ligaments
RADIOSCAPHOCAPITATE LIGAMENT. The radioscaphocapitate ligament arises from the volar and the radial aspects of the radial styloid process and runs distally and volarly to attach in a groove in the waist of the scaphoid (see Figure 94-21). It then continues distally to attach to the center of the volar aspect of the capitate. The fibers intermingle with the ulnocapitate ligament.[4,5,43,44]

RADIOLUNATE LIGAMENT. The radiolunate ligament is sometimes called the *volar radiotriquetral ligament* and originates from a rough triangular facet in the volar aspect of the

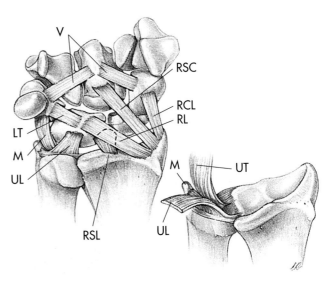

Figure 94-21. The palmar extrinsic wrist ligaments. *LT,* Lunotriquetral ligament; *M,* ulnocarpalmeniscus; *RCL,* radial collateral ligament; *RL,* radiolunate ligament; *RSC,* radioscaphocapitate ligament; *RSL,* radioscapholunate ligament; *UL,* ulnolunate ligament; *V,* V ligament. (From Taleisnik J: *The wrist,* New York, 1985, Churchill Livingstone.)

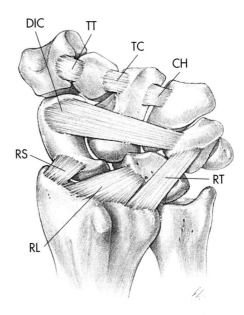

Figure 94-22. Dorsal wrist ligaments. *CH,* Capitohamate; *DIC,* dorsal intercarpal; *PT,* trapeziotrapezoid; *RS, RL, RT,* radioscaphoid, radiolunate, and radiotriquetral fascicles of the dorsal radiocarpal ligament; *TC,* trapeziocapitate. (From Taleisnik J: *The wrist,* New York, 1985, Churchill Livingstone.)

distal radius. It extends volar to the proximal pole of the scaphoid and the scapholunate joint to end in the volar aspect of the lunate.[5,43,44] Burger[4,5] calls this ligament the *long radiolunate ligament.*

THE RADIOSCAPHOLUNATE LIGAMENT (LIGAMENT OF TESTUT). The radioscapholunate ligament originates from a small tubercle on the volar margin of the distal radius. It then extends distally to attach to the proximal pole of the

scaphoid and to the scapholunate interosseous ligament. Some fibers extend to the lunate. This ligament is relatively weak, with minimal stabilizing effect (see Figure 94-21).[4,5,43,44]

SHORT RADIOLUNATE LIGAMENT. The short radiolunate ligament is ulnar to the radioscapholunate ligament. This ligament originates from the lunate fossa and attaches distally to the proximal volar margin of the lunate.[4,5]

Ulnocarpal Ligaments

ULNOTRIQUETRAL LIGAMENT. The ulnotriquetral (UT) ligament extends from the palmar aspect of the palmar distal radioulnar ligament to the palmar surface of the triquetrum.

ULNOLUNATE LIGAMENT. The ulnolunate (UL) ligament originates with the UT ligament from the palmar distal radioulnar ligament, which is a part of the triangular fibrocartilage. Its fibers course obliquely to attach to the palmar surface of the lunate.[4,5,16]

Dorsal Ligaments

DORSAL RADIOCARPAL LIGAMENT. The dorsal radiocarpal ligament originates from the dorsal margin of the distal radius and extends distally and ulnarly to attach to the dorsal aspect of the triquetrum (see Figure 94-22). Some fibers attach to the dorsal aspect of the lunate and occasionally to the capitate.[52,53] The ligament is reinforced by fibers from the extensor retinaculum (see Figure 94-22).[37,43]

Intercarpal Ligaments

The intercarpal ligaments connect the bones in the same carpal row (interosseous ligaments) or the two carpal rows (mid-carpal ligaments).

INTEROSSEOUS LIGAMENTS. The two main interosseous ligaments of the proximal carpal row are the scapholunate and the lunotriquetral interosseous ligaments. These ligaments are attached to the dorsal, proximal, and palmar margins of the corresponding articular surfaces.[3,4,43] They separate the radiocarpal from the mid-carpal joints. They are reinforced by fibers from the capsular ligaments. Histologic evaluation of the interosseous ligaments identifies the structure of the dorsal and volar parts to be composed of collagen fascicles, whereas the proximal parts are entirely fibrocartilaginous and are avascular without innervation.[3,43]

The bones in the distal carpal row are interconnected by a system of short, thick transversely-oriented interosseous ligaments that allow minimal intercarpal translational motion.[4,43] This is especially true for the capitohamate joint. The palmar ligaments are usually thick and the dorsal ligaments are thin.

MIDCARPAL LIGAMENTS

Palmar Mid-Carpal Ligament. The palmar mid-carpal ligament (*Poirier's ligament,* or *V ligament*) originates from the neck of the capitate and fans out proximally into two distinct fascicles to attach to the scaphoid and the triquetrum (see Figure 94-21).[4,43,44,53] This ligament has an important

stabilizing effect on the capitate. The radial portion also plays a role in supporting the distal pole of the scaphoid.[44]

Dorsal Intercarpal Ligament. As described by Taleisnik,[43] the dorsal intercarpal ligament extends from the dorsal aspect of the triquetrum to the scaphoid. Some fibers may extend to the trapezium and the trapezoid.[43]

BIOMECHANICS OF THE WRIST

The movements of the wrist are very complex because they include both the radiocarpal and mid-carpal joints and some movements between the individual carpal bones. Several attempts have been made to group individual carpal bones into separate units to understand carpal kinematics. One concept uses the anatomic configuration of the carpal bones into proximal and distal carpal rows. This concept depends on the somewhat similar movements of the bones of each row of carpal bones.[19,40] Another concept favored by Taleisnik[44] arranges the carpal bones into vertical columns: the lateral mobile column, which is composed of the scaphoid; the central flexion-extension column, which is essentially composed of the lunate, trapezium, trapezoid, capitate, and hamate; and the medial rotation column, which is composed of the triquetrum. A third concept, introduced by Lichtman,[31] describes the carpal bones as an oval ring with two mobile links at the scaphotrapezial and triquetrohamate joint that allows reciprocal motion between the proximal and distal carpal rows in radial and ulnar deviation.

Wrist Kinematics

The main movements of the wrist are palmar flexion-dorsiflexion and radioulnar deviation. Combinations of these movements produce circumduction. The axis of palmar flexion-dorsiflexion is a transverse axis that passes through the head of the capitate. A separate axis for radial and ulnar deviation also passes through the head of the capitate. A functional axis of wrist motion combines some ulnar deviation with palmar flexion and radial deviation with dorsiflexion.[4,44,53]

The proximal carpal row undergoes certain changes as a unit during radial and ulnar deviation. The individual bones of the proximal carpal row, however, display a tendency toward individual motion.[18,44] The scaphoid assumes a palmar-flexed position in radial deviation and through the strong scapholunate interosseous ligament pulls the lunate into a palmar-flexed position as well (Figure 94-23, *A*). Generally speaking, the lunate has more tendency to dorsiflex as a result of its shorter dorsal aspect.[44] The lunate, in addition to the effect of the scaphoid, is also influenced by the capitate. The capitate has a tendency to dorsiflex during radial deviation and that results in pushing the lunate into a palmar-flexed position (Figure 94-23, *B*).[44,53] The triquetrum moves distally on the hamate during ulnar deviation, assuming a low position (Figure 94-23, *C*). The triquetrum itself becomes dorsiflexed, pulling the lunate into a dorsiflexed position. The opposite occurs in radial deviation. As the triquetrum advances proximally on the hamate, it assumes a palmar-flexed position, and through the intact lunotrique-tral ligament it pulls the lunate into a palmar-flexed position (Figure 94-23, *D*). The lunate is therefore influenced by the tendency of the scaphoid and the triquetrum to palmar flex with radial deviation.[18,44,53] The distal carpal row moves as a unit with the hand through the strong carpometacarpal (CMC) attachment.[44]

The degree of involvement of the radiocarpal and the mid-carpal joints in the palmar flexion-dorsiflexion arc of

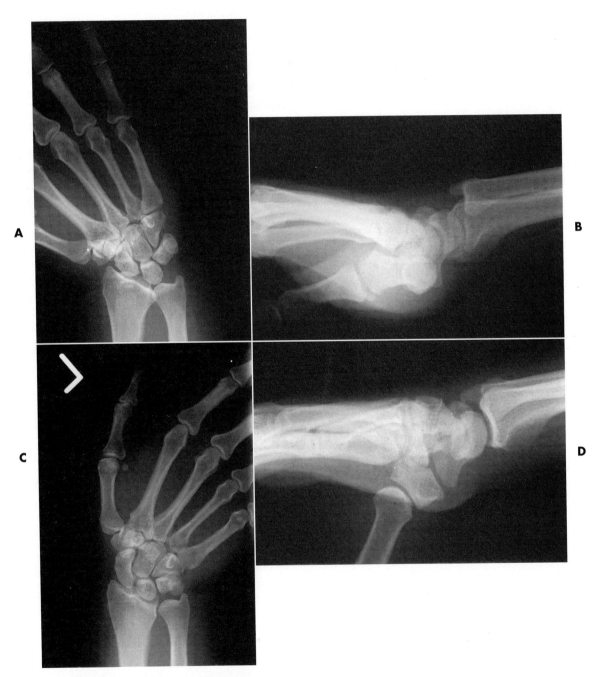

Figure 94-23. **A,** PA view of the wrist in radial deviation. The proximal carpal row is palmar flexed. The triquetrum is in high position, being more proximal in relation to the hamate. The lunate is triangular in shape, and the scaphoid is palmar-flexed with a foreshortened appearance. **B,** Lateral radiograph of the wrist in radial deviation. The lunate and the scaphoid are palmar-flexed. **C,** PA view the wrist in ulnar deviation. The proximal carpal row is dorsiflexed. The scaphoid is in a more vertical position, the lunate is trapezoidal in shape, and the triquetrum is in the low position. **D,** Lateral radiograph of the wrist in ulnar deviation. The lunate is dorsiflexed and the capitate is palmar-flexed.

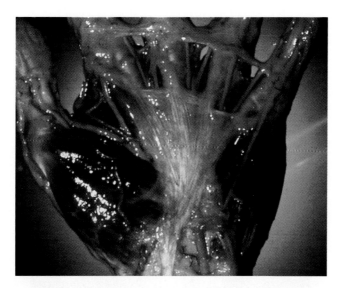

Plate 1. Palmar aponeurosis showing the pretendinous bands and their bifurcating fibers. (From Johnson MK, Cohen MJ: *Hand atlas*, Springfield, Ill, 1975, Charles C. Thomas. Courtesy of Myles J. Cohen and Moulton K. Johnson.)

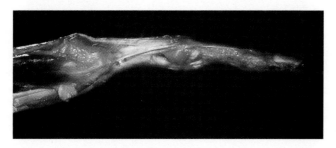

Plate 2. Lateral view of the MCP, PIP, and the DIP joints. Note the sagittal band and the ORL and the attachment of the interossei and lumbricals to the extensor hood. (From Johnson MK, Cohen MJ: *Hand atlas*, Springfield, Ill, 1975, Charles C. Thomas. Courtesy of Myles J. Cohen and Moulton K. Johnson.)

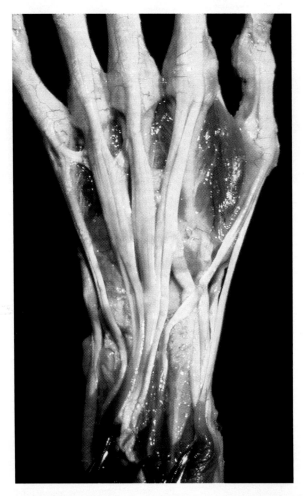

Plate 3. The extensor tendons and dorsal interossei on the dorsal aspect of the wrist and the hand after removal of the extensor retinaculum. Note the arrangements of the extensor tendons according to their compartment. (From Johnson MK, Cohen MJ: *Hand atlas*, Springfield, Ill, 1975, Charles C. Thomas. Courtesy of Myles J. Cohen and Moulton K. Johnson.)

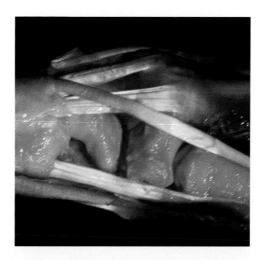

Plate 4. The anatomic snuffbox being bound by the EPL dorsally and the APL and EPB volarly. Note the scaphoid and the scaphotrapezial joint in the anatomic snuffbox. (From Johnson MK, Cohen MJ: *Hand atlas*, Springfield, III, 1975, Charles C. Thomas. Courtesy of Myles J. Cohen and Moulton K. Johnson.)

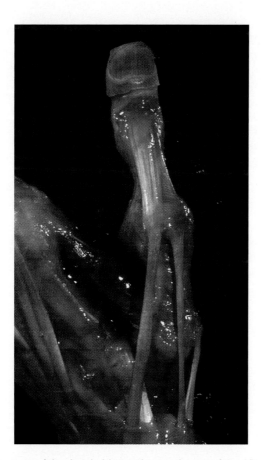

Plate 5. The dorsal aspect of the thumb. Notice the attachment of the APL, the EPB, and the EPL tendons. (From Johnson MK, Cohen MJ: *Hand atlas*, Springfield, III, 1975, Charles C. Thomas. Courtesy of Myles J. Cohen and Moulton K. Johnson.)

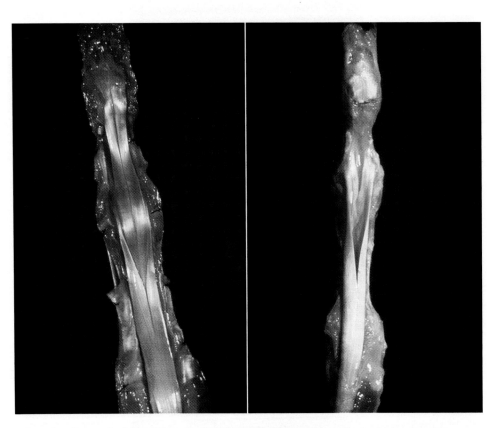

Plate 6. Camper's chiasm. Note the splitting of the FDS tendon slips and how the slips rotate around the FDP tendon before inserting into the volar aspect of the base of the middle phalanx. (From Johnson MK, Cohen MJ: *Hand atlas*, Springfield, Ill, 1975, Charles C. Thomas. Courtesy of Myles J. Cohen and Moulton K. Johnson.)

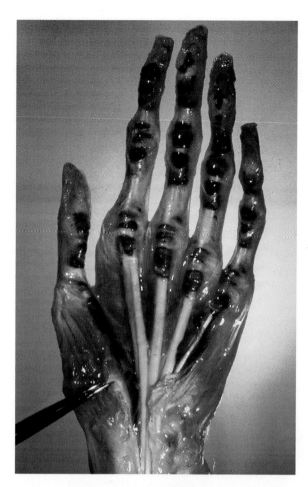

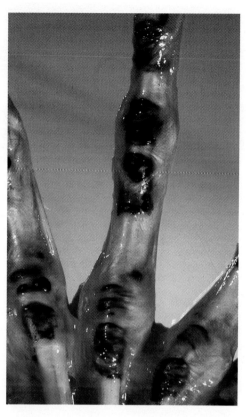

Plate 7. The flexor tendon sheath and the membranous and retinacular portions of the fingers and the thumb. (From Johnson MK, Cohen MJ: *Hand atlas*, Springfield, Ill, 1975, Charles C. Thomas. Courtesy of Myles J. Cohen and Moulton K. Johnson.)

Plate 8. The flexor tendon sheath and the annular pulley system. (From Johnson MK, Cohen MJ: *Hand atlas*, Springfield, Ill, 1975, Charles C. Thomas. Courtesy of Myles J. Cohen and Moulton K. Johnson.)

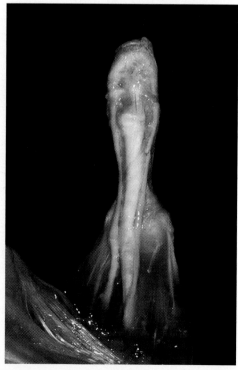

Plate 9. The volar aspect of the thumb. Note the FPL tendon in the flexor tendon sheath between the two sesamoid bones. (From Johnson MK, Cohen MJ: *Hand atlas*, Springfield, Ill, 1975, Charles C. Thomas. Courtesy of Myles J. Cohen and Moulton K. Johnson.)

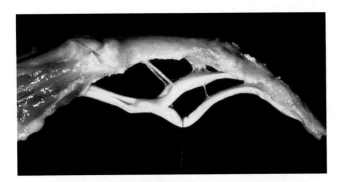

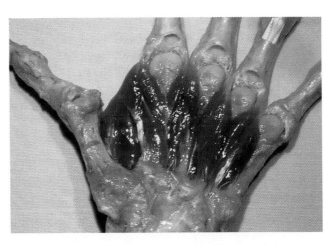

Plate 10. The FDS and FDP tendons and the vincula system. (From Johnson MK, Cohen MJ: *Hand atlas*, Springfield, Ill, 1975, Charles C. Thomas. Courtesy of Myles J. Cohen and Moulton K. Johnson.)

Plate 11. The palmar interossei after removal of the adductor pollicis. (From Johnson MK, Cohen MJ: *Hand atlas*, Springfield, Ill, 1975, Charles C. Thomas. Courtesy of Myles J. Cohen and Moulton K. Johnson.)

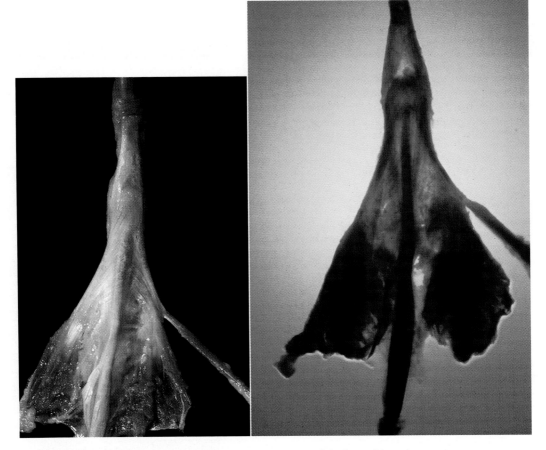

Plate 12. The extensor mechanism of the dorsal aspect of the finger. Note the common extensor tendon over the dorsal aspect of the MCP joint and the sagittal bands with the attachment of the lumbricals and the interossei. (From Johnson MK, Cohen MJ: *Hand atlas*, Springfield, Ill, 1975, Charles C. Thomas. Courtesy of Myles J. Cohen and Moulton K. Johnson.)

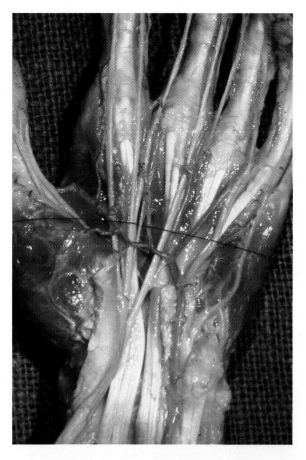

Plate 13. The ulnar artery and the superficial palmar arch with its branches. Note the median nerve and its branches. The bifurcation of the common digital arteries is located more distal than the bifurcation of the common digital nerves. (From Johnson MK, Cohen MJ: *Hand atlas*, Springfield, Ill, 1975, Charles C. Thomas. Courtesy of Myles J. Cohen and Moulton K. Johnson.)

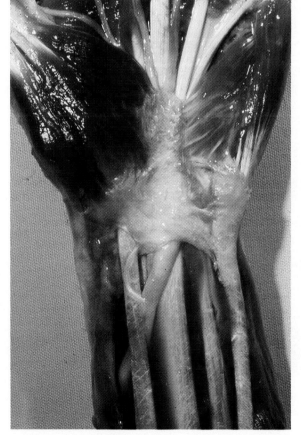

Plate 14. The flexor retinaculum and the thenar and hypothenar muscles. (From Johnson MK, Cohen MJ: *Hand atlas*, Springfield, Ill, 1975, Charles C. Thomas. Courtesy of Myles J. Cohen and Moulton K. Johnson.)

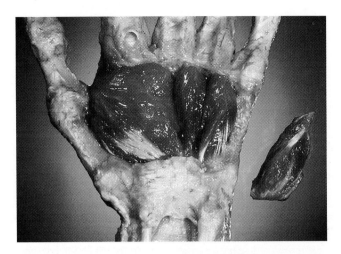

Plate 15. The palmar interossei and the adductor pollicis. (From Johnson MK, Cohen MJ: *Hand atlas*, Springfield, Ill, 1975, Charles C. Thomas. Courtesy of Myles J. Cohen and Moulton K. Johnson.)

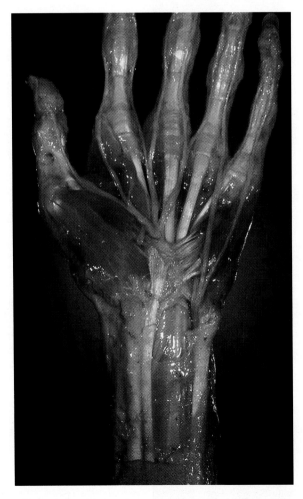

Plate 16. The median and the ulnar nerves and their branches. (From Johnson MK, Cohen MJ: *Hand atlas*, Springfield, Ill, 1975, Charles C. Thomas. Courtesy of Myles J. Cohen and Moulton K. Johnson.)

motion is still controversial.[18] However, it is fair to say that both the radiocarpal and the mid-carpal joints contribute significantly to the range of palmar flexion-dorsiflexion motion of the wrist.

Disruption of the strong scapholunate interosseous ligament causes scapholunate dissociation and removes the influence of the scaphoid on the lunate. The scaphoid then assumes a palmar-flexed position and the lunate and triquetrum become relatively dorsiflexed. If the lunotriquetral ligament is torn, the lunate rotates into palmar flexion with the scaphoid during radial deviation, and the triquetrum assumes a relatively dorsiflexed position. It appears that during radial deviation the scaphoid is the primary rotational element, pulling the whole proximal row into palmar flexion. The triquetrum is the main rotational element during ulnar deviation, pulling the proximal carpal row into dorsiflexion.[52,53]

DISTAL RADIOULNAR JOINT

The DRUJ is a diarthroidal trochoid articulation between the head of the ulna and the sigmoid notch of the distal radius.[6,13,16,40] The two articular surfaces are seldom completely parallel because the average inclination of the ulnar seat is 20 degrees, whereas that of the sigmoid notch is only 7 degrees.[6,13,16,47] The articular surface of the ulnar head is covered by articular cartilage over an average of 111 degrees, whereas the sigmoid notch has only articular coverage of 71 degrees. The radius of the distal ulnar articular surface is one third less than that of the sigmoid notch.[6,13,16,47] The contact between the articular surfaces is maximal at neutral forearm rotation in which 60% of the articular surface of the sigmoid notch is in contact with the ulnar head. That contact becomes only 10% in extremes of rotation.[6,13,16,47]

STABILIZING SOFT TISSUE STRUCTURES OF THE DISTAL RADIOULNAR JOINT

The DRUJ acquires its stability through the support of the surrounding soft tissue structures. The most important stabilizing structures are the triangular fibrocartilage, the ulnocarpal ligaments, the ECU tendon and its sheath, the pronator quadratus, and the radioulnar interosseous membrane.[6,13,16,39,47]

Triangular Fibrocartilage
The triangular fibrocartilage (TFC) is part of the triangular fibrocartilage complex (TFCC) and is considered the most important stabilizer of the DRUJ. It also serves as a load-transferring structure by transmitting approximately 18% of the load across the wrist joint.[6,13,16,39] The TFC consists of two components: the articular disc and the distal radioulnar ligaments.

The articular disc is a biconcave fibrocartilaginous structure that separates the ulnar dome from the ulnar carpus. It varies in thickness according to the degree of ulnar variance, being thicker in ulnar-minus wrists.

The two distal radioulnar ligaments originate respectively from the palmar and dorsal edges of the distal radius, blending with the peripheral fibers of the articular disc. They extend ulnarly to attach mainly to the fovea, but some fibers travel distally to attach to the styloid process of the ulna.[13,16] The distal radioulnar ligaments play an important role in the stability of the DRUJ. Their role in stabilization is controversial, and most investigators have concluded that the palmar ligament is taut during pronation, preventing dorsal translation of the ulna, and the dorsal ligament is tightened in supination, restricting the tendency of the distal ulna to translate palmarly.[13] Other researchers, however, found that the palmar ligament is tighter in supination and the dorsal ligament tightens in pronation.[6,16]

Ulnocarpal Ligaments
Two groups of longitudinally oriented fibers emerge from the palmar edge of the TFC (Figure 94-24). One group extends directly to attach to the palmar surface of the triquetrum, forming the ulnotriquetral (UT) ligament; the other group courses obliquely to attach to the palmar surface of the lunate, forming the ulnolunate (UL) ligament. These ligaments provide stability to the DRUJ and maintain axial alignment between the ulna and the ulnar carpus.[4,5,16]

The ECU tendon and sheath also provide dynamic stability to the DRUJ. They resist the tendency of the ulna to translate dorsally during pronation and palmarly during supination. The pronator quadratus, by virtue of its transverse position between the radius and the ulna, acts as a mechanical factor, preventing any lateral displacement and increasing the coaptation between the radius and the ulna.[6,16] The radioulnar interosseous membrane also plays an important role in the stability of the DRUJ. It is an important stabilizer, preventing separation between the radius and the ulna, and is a load-transfer structure, preventing distal and proximal migration.[13,16,47]

Biomechanics of the Distal Radioulnar Joint
The main function of the DRUJ, in conjunction with the proximal radioulnar joint (PRUJ), is to provide forearm rotation. The movements of pronation and supination are not simple rotations of the radius about the ulna. There is an element of dorsopalmar translation associated with the rotation. Therefore, in pronation the radius rotates and translates palmarly, and in supination the radius rotates and translates dorsally.[13,16,39] The relative length of the radius and ulna changes with forearm rotation. With supination, the ulna appears relatively shorter than in pronation, a fact that must be considered in assessing ulnar variance.

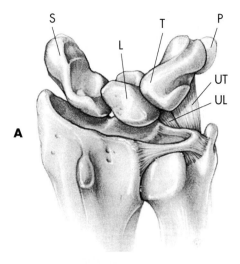

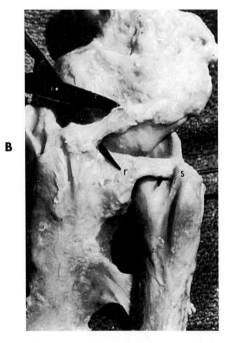

Figure 94-24. **A,** The triangular fibrocartilage and the V-shaped ulnocarpal ligament. **B,** The triangular fibrocartilage and the ulnocarpal ligaments as shown in anatomic section. The scissors are placed under the distal radiotriquetral ligament. *L,* Lunate; *P,* pisiform; *S,* scaphoid; *T,* triquetrum; *UL,* ulnocarpal ligament; *UT,* ulnotriquetral ligament; *r,* radius; *s,* ulnar styloid. (From Bowers WH: The distal radioulnar joint. In Green DP [editor]: *Operative hand surgery,* ed 3, New York, 1993, Churchill Livingstone.)

NERVE SUPPLY OF THE HAND

MEDIAN NERVE AT THE WRIST AND IN THE HAND

The median nerve at the wrist lies deep to the PL between that tendon and the FCR (Plates 13, 14, and 16). The palmar cutaneous branch originates from the radial side of the nerve about 5 to 7 cm proximal to the wrist and runs along the FCR.

It passes superficial to the TCL to supply the proximal part of the palm. The median nerve enters the carpal tunnel superficial to the digital flexor tendons, which are deep to it (Figure 94-25).[28,35,40] The median nerve divides into its terminal branches close to the distal end of the carpal tunnel. The pattern and the exact site of division vary.[28,33] The digital branches supply the radial and the ulnar sides of the thumb, index, and long fingers and the radial side of the ring finger.

The motor branch of the median nerve usually originates from the radial side, with the other division at the distal end of the carpal tunnel. It is not uncommon, however, for the motor branch to originate more proximally within the carpal tunnel or from the volar or the ulnar side of the nerve, crossing superficial to the main trunk before reaching the thenar muscles. That position makes the thenar motor branch vulnerable to injury during carpal tunnel release.[28] The motor branch loops around the distal edge of the transverse carpal ligament before piercing the fibrous septum that separates the mid-palmar space from the thenar space. Sometimes the motor branch has a separate fibrous tunnel as it enters into the thenar muscles.[28,34] It gives a branch to the superficial head of the FPB and then supplies the entire APB and the opponens pollicis.

The common digital branches from the median nerve in the palm run deep to the superficial palmar arch but become superficial to the digital vessels as they approach the base of the digits.[2,40] The digital branch to the radial side of the index finger supplies the first lumbrical, and the common digital nerve to the index and long web space supplies a branch to the second lumbrical.[2,40] The branch that supplies sensation to the radial side of the thumb often crosses superficial to the volar aspect of the MCP joint, where it may be vulnerable to injury during trigger-thumb release.[2,34]

ULNAR NERVE

The ulnar nerve accompanies the ulnar artery in the distal forearm (see Plates 13 and 16). The ulnar nerve gives off a dorsal cutaneous branch about 5 to 7 cm proximal to the styloid process of the ulna that pierces the fascia and winds around the ulnar aspect of the forearm to supply the dorsal aspect of the ulnar side of the hand. It also supplies the dorsal aspect of the small finger and the ulnar side of the ring finger to the level of the PIP joint. Occasionally it supplies the entire dorsal surface of the small finger.[2,40]

The ulnar nerve divides into deep and superficial branches in the proximal part of the palm at the level of Guyon's canal. The superficial branch supplies the palmaris brevis and then divides into two branches, one to the ulnar side of the little finger and the other to the adjoining surface of the ring and little fingers. Sometimes this branch may occasionally have communicating fibers with the most ulnar digital branches of the median nerve.[2,40] These anomalous

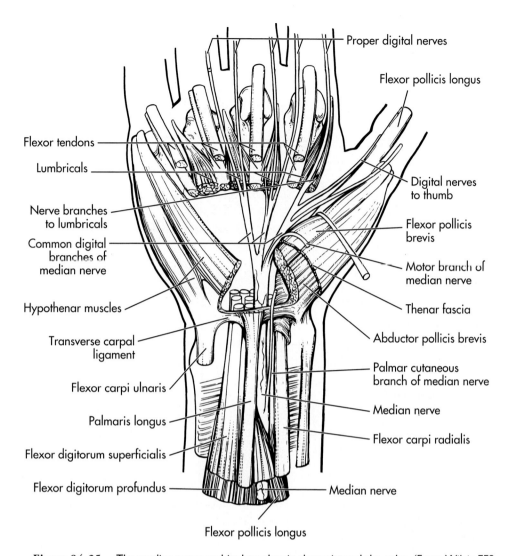

Figure 94-25. The median nerve and its branches in the wrist and the palm. (From Wilgis EFS, Kaplan EB: The blood and the nerve supply of the hand. In Spinner M [editor]: *Kaplan's functional and surgical anatomy of the hand,* ed 3, Philadelphia, 1983, JB Lippincott.)

branches can be injured, especially during endoscopic carpal tunnel release.

The deep branch and the ulnar artery pass underneath a fibrotic arch made by the origin of the flexor digiti minimi (FDM). It then accompanies the deep palmar arch, passing between the abductor digiti minimi (ADM) and the FDM, where it gives branches to the hypothenar muscles.[2,53] It runs radially deep to the palmar interosseous fascia and the mid-palmar space and ends by passing between the two heads of the AP. It innervates the interosseous muscles and the two ulnar lumbricals. The interossei branches enter the muscles on the palmar surface, and the lumbrical branches enter on the dorsal side (Figure 94-26).[53]

Guyon's Canal
Guyon's canal begins at the level of the proximal edge of the TCL. The floor of the canal is triangular in shape and formed by the TCL and the pisohamate ligament. The pisiform and

the distal fibers of the FCU tendon form the ulnar wall of the canal. The radial wall is formed by the hook of the hamate. The roof of the canal is formed by the volar carpal ligament, which is reinforced with the fibers from the insertion of the FCU on the pisiform.[9,53] The ulnar artery is radial to the ulnar nerve in the canal of Guyon (see Figure 94-26).

Superficial Radial Nerve
The superficial branch of the radial nerve passes between the tendons of the brachioradialis and the ECRL near the mid-forearm and pierces the deep fascia to become subcutaneous. It runs toward the anatomic snuff box superficial to the APL and the EPB. The nerve divides, giving distal sensory branches to the dorsal surface of the proximal phalanges to the level of the PIP joint of the index and long fingers, the radial half of the ring finger, and the dorsal aspect of the thumb to the level of the IP joint. It also supplies the dorsal aspect of the radial part of the hand.[2,40,53]

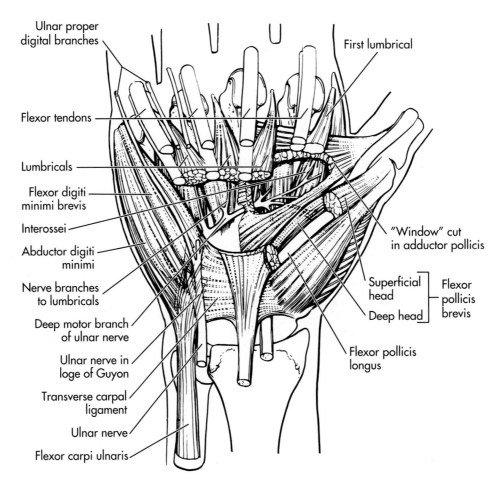

Figure 94-26. The course and the branches of the deep branch of the ulnar nerve. Note the branches to the interossei and the ulnar-two lumbrical muscles. (From Wilgis EFS, Kaplan EB: The blood and the nerve supply in the hand. In Spinner M [editor]: *Kaplan's functional and surgical anatomy of the hand*, ed 3, Philadelphia, 1984, JB Lippincott.)

BLOOD SUPPLY OF THE HAND

The hand is supplied by a system of anastomotic arches that frequently show anatomic variations. The main arterial supply is through the radial and ulnar arteries, with contributions from other blood vessels, including the anterior interosseous artery, its dorsal branch, and sometimes the median artery.[27,40,52,53]

RADIAL ARTERY

The radial artery at the wrist is located anteromedial to the APL and the EPB tendons. The artery then passes deep to those tendons and the EPL to cross the anatomic snuffbox. The artery enters the palm between the two heads of the first dorsal interosseous muscle and is then covered by the AP. Just before going underneath the AP, it gives off the princeps pollicis artery, which divides into the two digital arteries of the thumb. The radial artery then runs medially between the interosseous muscles and the AP to become the main

component of the deep palmar arch. The radial artery also gives off a dorsal carpal branch, which anastomoses with the dorsal carpal branch of the ulnar artery to form the dorsal carpal arch.[40,53]

ULNAR ARTERY

The ulnar artery lies radial to the tendon of the FCU at the level of the wrist (see Plate 13). It passes with the ulnar nerve superficial to the TCL into the canal of Guyon. The artery gives off its deep branch at that level, which accompanies the deep branch of the ulnar nerve under the origin of the FDM. It then passes between the transverse and oblique parts of the AP to lie dorsal to the AP, where it gives off the deep branch that joins the radial artery, forming the deep palmar arch. The ulnar artery then forms the superficial palmar arch. The artery also gives off the dorsal ulnar carpal artery, which passes beneath the tendon of the FCU and the ECU to join the dorsal radial carpal branch, forming the dorsal carpal arch.[23,40,53]

DORSAL CARPAL ARCH

The dorsal carpal arch is formed by the anastomosis of the radial and ulnar dorsal carpal arteries. It also receives branches from the dorsal branch of the anterior interosseous artery. It gives off dorsal metacarpal branches to the second, third, and fourth intermetacarpal spaces. They may be joined by perforating arteries running dorsally from the deep palmar arch through the intermetacarpal spaces.

The first dorsal metacarpal artery supplying the dorsal aspects of the thumb and index finger usually arises from the radial artery before it passes between the two heads of the first dorsal interosseous muscle.[40,53]

SUPERFICIAL PALMAR ARCH

The superficial palmar arch lies just distal to the transverse carpal ligament, where it is vulnerable to injury during a carpal tunnel release. It is formed by the anastomosis of the ulnar artery and the superficial branch of the radial artery. It gives off the common digital arteries that usually run superficial to the nerve branches. The common digital arteries divide at the base of the fingers distal to the division of the nerves to give off the digital arteries, which lie dorsal to the digital nerves in the digits. Many variations have been noted in the superficial palmar arch.[23,48] The median artery occasionally contributes significantly to the formation of the superficial palmar arch.

DEEP PALMAR ARCH

The deep palmar arch is formed at the level of the metacarpal bases by the anastomosis of the radial artery and the deep branch of the ulnar artery. It gives off metacarpal branches to the second, third, and fourth intermetacarpal spaces. It also gives off dorsal perforating branches to join the dorsal metacarpal arteries. The deep palmar arch is also subject to considerable anatomic variations.[23,48,53]

REFERENCES

1. Aubriot JH: The metacarpophalangeal joint of the thumb. In Tubiana R (editor): *The hand,* vol 1, Philadelphia, 1981, WB Saunders.
2. Backhouse KM: Nerve supply in the arm and hand. In Tubiana R (editor): *The hand,* vol 1, Philadelphia, 1981, WB Saunders.
3. Berger RA: The gross and histologic anatomy of the scapholunate interosseous ligament, *J Hand Surg [Am]* 21:170-178, 1996.
4. Berger RA: The ligaments of the wrist: a current overview of anatomy with considerations of their potential functions, *Hand Clin* 13(1):63-82, 1997.
5. Berger RA, Landsmeer JMF: The palmar radiocarpal ligaments: a study of adult and fetal human wrist joints, *J Hand Surg [Am]* 15:847-854, 1990.
6. Bowers WH: The distal radioulnar joint. In Green DP, Hotchkiss RN, Pederson WC (editors): *Operative hand surgery,* ed 4, New York, 1999, Churchill Livingstone.
7. Brand PW, Hollister A: *Clinical mechanics of the hand,* ed 2, St. Louis, 1993, Mosby, pp 254-352.
8. Brunelli GA, Brunelli GR: Anatomy of the extensor pollicis brevis muscle, *J Hand Surg [Br]* 17:267-269, 1992.
9. Denman EE: The anatomy of the space of Guyon, *Hand* 10:69-76, 1978.
10. Doyle JR: Anatomy of the finger flexor tendon sheath and pulley system, *J Hand Surg [Am]* 13:473-484, 1988.
11. Doyle JR: Anatomy of the flexor tendon sheath and pulley system: a current review, *J Hand Surg [Am]* 14:349-351, 1989.
12. Dubousset JF: The digital joints. In Tubiana R (editor): *The hand,* vol 1, Philadelphia, 1981, WB Saunders.
13. Ekenstam FW af, Hagert CG: Anatomical studies on the geometry and stability of the distal radioulnar joint, *Scand J Plast Reconstr Surg* 19:17, 1985.
14. Fahrer M: Interdependent and independent actions of the fingers. In Tubiana R (editor): *The hand,* vol 1, Philadelphia, 1981, WB Saunders.
15. Gad P: The anatomy of the volar parts of the capsules of the finger joints, *J Bone Joint Surg* 49B:362, 1967.
16. Garcia-Elias M: Soft tissue anatomy and relationships about the distal ulna, *Hand Clin* 14(2):165-176, 1998.
17. Glicenstein J, Dardour JC: The pulp: anatomy and physiology. In Tubiana R (editor): *The hand,* vol 1, Philadelphia, 1981, WB Saunders.
18. Green DP: Carpal dislocations and instabilities. In Green DP (editor): *Operative hand surgery,* ed 3, New York, 1993, Churchill Livingstone.
19. Hunter JM: Anatomy of flexor tendons: pulley, vencular, synovia and vascular structures. In Spinner M (editor): *Kaplan's functional and surgical anatomy of the hand,* ed 3, Philadelphia, 1984, JB Lippincott.
20. Hunter JM, Cook JF Jr: The pulley system: rationale for reconstruction. In Strickland JW, Steichen JB (editors): *Difficult problems in hand surgery,* St. Louis, 1982, Mosby.
21. Idler RS: Anatomy and biomechanics of digital flexor tendons, *Hand Clin* 1(1):3-11, 1985.
22. Imaeda T, Ann K-N, Cooney WP, Linscheid R: Anatomy of trapeziometacarpal ligaments, *J Hand Surg [Am]* 18:226-231, 1993.
23. Kaplan EB: Anatomical variations of the forearm and the hand. In Tubiana R (editor): *The hand,* vol 1, Philadelphia, 1981, WB Saunders.
24. Kaplan EB, Hunter JM: The muscles and the tendon systems of the fingers. In Spinner M (editor): *Kaplan's functional and surgical anatomy of the hand,* ed 3, Philadelphia, 1984, JB Lippincott.
25. Kaplan EB, Milford LW: The retinacular system of the hand. In Spinner M (editor): *Kaplan's functional and surgical anatomy of the hand,* ed 3, Philadelphia, 1984, JB Lippincott.
26. Kaplan EB, Riordan DC: The thumb. In Spinner M (editor): *Kaplan's functional and surgical anatomy of the hand,* ed 3, Philadelphia, 1984, JB Lippincott.

27. Landsmeer JMF: *Atlas of anatomy of the hand,* Edinburgh, 1976, Churchill Livingstone.

28. Lanz V: Anatomic variations of the median nerve in the carpal tunnel, *J Hand Surg [Am]* 2:44-53, 1977.

29. Leddy JP: Flexor tendons: acute injuries. In Green DP (editor): *Operative hand surgery,* ed 3, New York, 1993, Churchill Livingstone.

30. Legueu MMF, Juvara E: Des aponeurosis de la paume de la main, *Bull Soc Anat Paris* May:393, 1892.

31. Lichtman DM, Schneider JR, Swafford AR, Mack GR: Ulnar midcarpal instability: clinical and laboratory analysis, *J Hand Surg [Am]* 6:515-523, 1981.

32. Lin G-T, Amadio PC, Ann K-N, Cooney WP: Functional anatomy of the human digital flexor pulley system, *J Hand Surg [Am]*14:949-956, 1989.

33. Lundborg G: Experimental flexor tendon healing without adhesion formation: a new concept of tendon nutrition and intrinsic healing mechanisms, *Hand* 8:235-238, 1976.

34. MacKinnon SE, Dellon AL: *Surgery of the peripheral nerve,* New York, 1988, Thieme Medical Publishers, p 152.

35. Manske PR, Lesker PA: Nutrient pathways of flexor tendons in primates, *J Hand Surg [Am]* 7:436-444, 1982.

36. Manske PR, Lesker PA: Palmar aponeurosis pulley, *J Hand Surg [Am]* 8:259-263, 1983.

37. McFarlane RM: Dupuytren's contracture. In Green DP (editor): *Operative hand surgery,* ed 3, New York, 1993, Churchill Livingstone.

38. Mizuceki T, Ikuta Y: The dorsal carpal ligaments: their anatomy and function, *J Hand Surg [Br]* 14:91-98, 1989.

39. Palmer AK, Werner FW: The triangular fibrocartilage complex of the wrist: anatomy and function, *J Hand Surg* 6:153-161, 1981.

40. Pick TP, Howden R (editors): *Gray's anatomy: descriptive and surgical,* New York, 1978, Crown Publishers.

41. Pieron AP: The first carpometacarpal joint. In Tubiana R (editor): *The hand,* vol 1, Philadelphia, 1981, WB Saunders.

42. Simmons BP, delaKaffiniere JY: Physiology of flexion of the fingers. In Tubiana R (editor): *The hand,* vol 1, Philadelphia, 1981, WB Saunders.

43. Taleisnik J: The ligaments of the wrist, *J Hand Surg [Am]* 1:110, 1976.

44. Taleisnik J: *The wrist,* New York, 1985, Churchill Livingstone.

45. Thomine JM: The skin of the hand. In Tubiana R (editor): *The hand,* vol 1, Philadelphia, 1981, WB Saunders.

46. Thomine JM: The development and anatomy of the digital fascia. In Hueston JT, Tubiana R (editors): *Dupuytren's disease,* ed 2, Edinburgh, 1985, Churchill Livingstone.

47. Tolat AR, Stanley JK, Trail IA: A cadaveric study of the anatomy and stability of the distal radioulnar joint in the coronal and transverse planes, *J Hand Surg [Br]* 21:587, 1996.

48. Tountas C, Bergman R: Anatomic variations of the upper extremities, New York, 1993, Churchill Livingstone.

49. Valentin P: Extrinsic muscles of the hand and wrist: an introduction. In Tubiana R (editor): *The hand,* vol I, Philadelphia, 1981, WB Saunders.

50. Valentin P: The interossei and the lumbricals. In Tubiana R (editor): *The hand,* vol I, Philadelphia, 1981, WB Saunders.

51. Watson HK, Light TR, Johnson TR: Check rein resection for flexion contracture of the middle joint, *J Hand Surg [Am]* 4:67-71, 1979.

52. Zancolli EA: *Structural and dynamic basis of hand surgery,* ed 2, Philadelphia, 1979, JB Lippincott.

53. Zancolli EA, Cozzi EP: *Atlas of surgical anatomy of the hand,* New York, 1992, Churchill Livingstone.

CHAPTER

Embryology

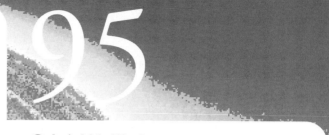

Gabriel M. Kind

INTRODUCTION

Detailed studies of the embryologic development of human limbs were done as early as the 1870s, but the quest for complete understanding of the complex biochemical processes that result in limb formation continues to this day. Much of this information may seem unessential for the practicing surgeon. A familiarity with this topic, however, is quite useful for those clinicians dealing with pediatrics in general and congenital hand problems in particular. The ubiquity of antenatal ultrasound[15,47] has resulted in an increasing number of diagnoses now being made well before birth, which has extended the role of the consultant even further.

The remarkable development of the human hand occurs during a relatively brief period of embryonic life. There is extensive cell migration and multiplication from the third to the sixth postovulatory week as limb formation takes place. The next 2 weeks is the period of limb bud differentiation. Embryogenesis is complete by the eighth week of development. All final structures are present and are undergoing differential growth from that point until birth. Most congenital deformities of the upper limb, therefore, occur as the result of an insult to the embryo in the third to the eighth week of intrauterine development. The exceptions to this are those deformities that are the result of external or mechanical forces, such as compression of the uterus, ischemic events, or amniotic bands. With this time frame in mind, the International Federation of Societies for Surgery of the Hand has modified a classification of congenital hand deformities first proposed by Swanson.[60] A more detailed discussion of congenital hand deformities can be found in Chapter 99.

UPPER LIMB FORMATION: AN OVERVIEW

The human upper extremity develops from small buds consisting of mesenchymal cells covered by a shell of ectoderm. These are first detectable adjacent to the eighth to tenth somites in the third postovulatory week. The thickened ectoderm overlying the bud is known as the *apical ectodermal ridge* (AER). It has been shown in chick embryos that the ridge forms in response to a signal from the flank mesoderm.[16] Initial limb bud formation is not formed by cellular proliferation but by a decrease in the proliferation of the surrounding tissue.[55] The limb buds appear as small protrusions at each end of the Wolffian ridge, a bilateral longitudinal crest of tissue (Figure 95-1). The limb buds grow rapidly after their appearance, as mesenchymal cells at the base of the bud differentiate into the various tissues that become a limb (Figure 95-2).

The AER appears to play a significant role in bud outgrowth, and this has been the subject of numerous investigations. There is a "progress zone" of undifferentiated mesoderm cells maintained at the end of the AER (Figure 95-3). There is interdependence between the AER and this underlying mesoderm such that without the AER, mesenchymal differentiation and limb formation does not occur, whereas AER formation depends on signals from the underlying mesenchyme. When the AER is cut away from a developing chick limb bud, the bud stops growing and a truncated limb will result.[59,64] Transplanted presumptive limb mesenchyme from the Wolffian ridge to the flank results in AER formation, and an additional limb develops.[28]

Skeletal structures develop sequentially in a proximal to distal axis. A severely truncated limb will result when the AER is removed early in development (Figure 95-4, *A*), whereas removal later will result in lack of distal structures only. The AER appears to control limb-growth sequencing, but it does not control what type of structure is formed because this is determined by the mesenchyme. This has been shown in experiments in which mesoderm and ectoderm were exchanged between hindlimbs and forelimbs and in another in which the AER was exchanged between limb buds of different developmental stages. The mesoderm and not the ectoderm in each case determines the type of tissue formed.[51,73]

An additional signaling region has been demonstrated in the thickened ectoderm at the posterior limb bud margin. This "zone of polarizing activity" (ZPA) appears to determine the anteroposterior morphology of the limb (Figure 95-5). The mechanism by which this signaling takes place is as yet unresolved. Cells in the ZPA are histologically indistinguishable from surrounding cells. Their location has been determined by transplanting small blocks of tissue to other

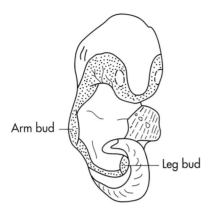

Figure 95-1. Drawing of an embryo 4.2 mm long, approximately day 32. The stippled area represents the ectodermal ring. The caudal portion of the ring constitutes the Wolffian ridge, which is a crest of mesoderm that separates the upper and lower limb buds. The upper limb bud will form opposite the eighth to tenth somites.

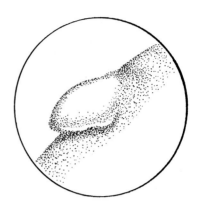

Figure 95-2. The early upper limb bud, approximately day 32.

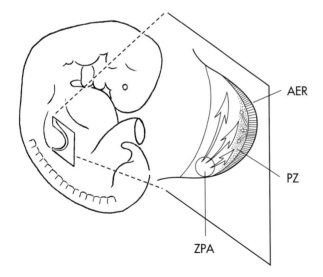

Figure 95-3. The early limb bud consists of an outer layer of ectoderm called the *apical ectodermal ridge* (AER), which is thought to have a dynamic relationship with two signaling regions: the progress zone (PZ) and the zone of polarizing activity (ZPA). Signals from the ridge *(small arrows)* maintain the progress zone, which causes the limb bud to grow distally. Additional ridge signals maintain the ZPA, which releases a signal *(large arrows)* that maintains the progress zone. The ZPA also produces morphogens that control anteroposterior relationships.

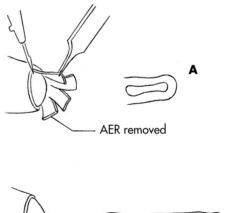
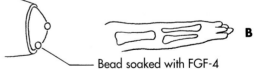

Figure 95-4. **A,** After experimental removal of the AER from an early upper limb bud, a truncated limb with just a humerus develops. **B,** Simultaneous application of beads soaked in FGF-4 to the posterior and apical bud margins will result in the formation of a limb with a humerus, radius, ulna, and digits. However, although FGF-4 is able to mimic the signals from the AER, it fails to perform the mechanical function of the ridge, and the handplate formed in this limb becomes cylindrical, resulting in digits that are bunched together.

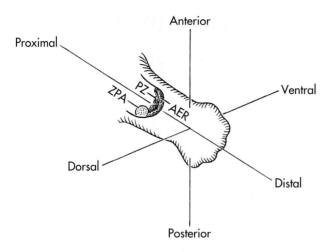

Figure 95-5. The zone of polarizing activity determines anteroposterior morphogenesis, presumably by a diffusible morphogen. The progress zone appears to affect proximodistal positioning.

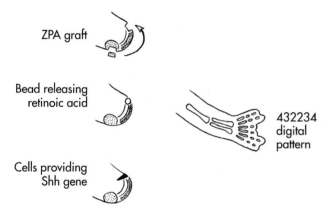

Figure 95-6. Experimental grafting to the anterior limb bud of either a polarizing region, a bead releasing retinoic acid, or cells expressing the Sonic hedgehog (Shh) gene will result in a duplicate production of digits in a mirror-image pattern (432234).

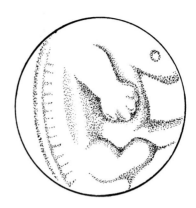

Figure 95-7. The limbs of an embryo at approximately postovulatory day 42. The digital rays are clearly evident in the handplate, which is more advanced than the foot.

locations. A digit or digits will form if the ZPA is transplanted,[25,26] depending on the amount of tissue grafted and the length of time it is in contact with the limb bud (Figure 95-6, *A*). A digit 2 will form when approximately 30 ZPA cells are grafted, whereas approximately 70 cells produce a digit 3 and greater than 100 are required to produce a digit 4.[64] Similarly, a graft of ZPA cells left in place for 15 hours will induce the formation of an extra digit 2; but if left for 17 to 24 hours, a digit 3 will form.[57] The digit closest to the polarizing region is always more posterior in character than those farther away.[66] This explains the resulting mirror-image–type limbs produced by ZPA transplantation to the anterior limb bud (Figure 95-6, *B*).

The signals responsible for these effects appear to be carried by either a long-range morphogen or by short-range cell-to-cell interactions. There are experimental data that support each theory. In either case, induced structures are derived from host tissue and therefore the ZPA can be thought of as a true signaling region. Interestingly, these signals appear to be similar across vertebrate species because cells from the posterior margin of many different vertebrates, including humans, will induce wing formation when transplanted to the anterior wing bud margin in the chick.[20,33,68]

Hand and Phalangeal Formation

The hand plate becomes recognizable at the end of the limb bud at approximately 33 days postovulation in the 7- to 9-mm embryo.[45] The spinal nerves are present at this time at the root of the upper limb bud, and mesenchymal condensations are forming to create the skeleton of the upper limb. The brachial plexus has formed by 37 days, and the radial and median nerves reach the elbow. A mesenchymal humerus, radius, and ulna are identifiable.

Phalangeal formation becomes evident by approximately day 41 (Figure 95-7). The AER has become a flattened layer at the distal end of the hand paddle at this stage. Portions of this rim degenerate, which results in cell death and web-space formation. The tissue beneath the intact portions of the AER continues to condense, resulting in the formation of the digits (Figure 95-8). The radial, ulnar, and median nerves have reached the hand plate by this time.

Apoptosis, or *programmed cell death* (PCD), appears to play a significant role in embryologic development. This process appears to be genetically determined and controlled by cellular interactions rather than any external force.[30,72] Regions of cell death have been identified at the anterior and posterior margins of the chick limb bud, as well as between the radius and ulna.[52]

Phalangeal formation is an example of PCD (Figure 95-9). It has been shown in rodents that there is a zone of cell death that occurs around the first digit. This PCD results in a zone of

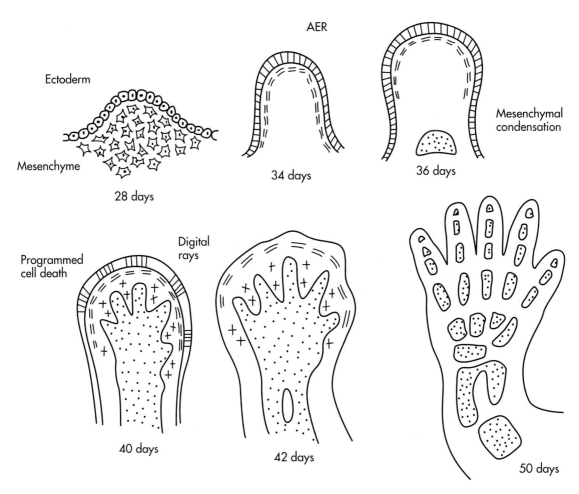

Figure 95-8. Schematic of the normal development of the human upper limb, in numbers of days postovulation.

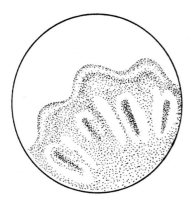

Figure 95-9. The hand of a 42-day embryo, showing formation of the interdigital space. This is an example of apoptosis, or programmed cell death.

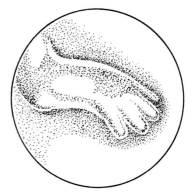

Figure 95-10. This drawing of the hand of an 11-week embryo shows the complete development of the phalanges and the interdigital spaces.

necrosis, which reduces the size of the first digit by decreasing the mesodermal component. An increase in the size of this zone of necrosis will result in a reduction in the size of the adjoining second and third digits, whereas a reduction in this zone will result in an enlargement of the first digit.[53]

An interdigital mesenchyme PCD begins proximally and serves to clear the web spaces of soft tissue. The PCD appears to be particularly intense along the radial and ulnar borders of the hand, and may serve to prevent formation of supernumerary digits.[30,35] Aberrant patterns of PCD are thought to result in polydactyly or syndactyly deformities.[37,54]

The interdigital spaces are cleared, and five digits are clearly discernible by the end of the eighth week (Figure 95-10) and fingernails can be seen by week 17 (Figure 95-11).

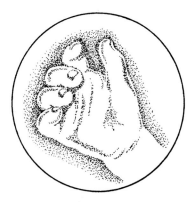

Figure 95-11. This drawing of a 17-week embryo shows the presence of well-developed fingernails.

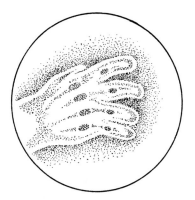

Figure 95-12. The hand of a 12-week fetus demonstrates ossification of the central portions of the tubular bones. Also note the lack of ossification of the carpus.

Skeletal Development

Bone formation occurs first as a condensation of mesoderm that chondrifies in the fifth postovulatory week. The central areas of the proximal tubular bones chondrify first, followed by ossification approximately a week later (Figure 95-12). Distal progression of chondrification and then ossification occurs. The humerus begins to ossify in the sixth week. During this time the phalanges are undergoing chondrification. The distal phalanges typically ossify before the proximal phalanges (Figure 95-13). Ossification and remodeling continue throughout the remainder of fetal life and into the postnatal period.[3,23,58,69]

The carpus is the one exception to the proximal to distal rule of chondrification and ossification. The carpal bones do not chondrify until the seventh week. The scaphoid, lunate, and pisiform bones usually begin as two distinct condensations that fuse much later, whereas the trapezium, trapezoid, and capitate develop in their original form. All of the other carpal bones reach their final configuration through a complex sequence of migration and fusion.[7] The carpus has a low rate of differential growth and usually does not begin to ossify until after birth. Carpal ossification, for this reason, is a useful postnatal marker for skeletal development and can be used clinically to estimate the age of the child.[46]

The upper and lower limbs are developmentally parallel to each other at 6 weeks. This relationship, however, has changed by 8 weeks as the preaxial limb border moves from a cranial to a more medial position (Figure 95-14). The mechanism of this change is poorly understood, but it is believed to involve growth of all of the limb components, especially the skeletal and articular structures of the shoulder girdle.[45]

Joint development occurs as early as the sixth week, when joint capsular structures are found before joint separation. Synovial mesenchyme with embryonal blood vessels form between the periosteum and the joint capsule. Chondrocytes condense during the seventh week, forming two dense plates separated by synovium. These plates are the precursors of articular cartilage.[24] Joint motion must occur for joints to develop beyond this point. Chick embryos paralyzed at this stage develop flat articular surfaces and joint spaces obliterated

by fibrous tissue.[18] Cavitation is present by the end of the eighth week in the human shoulder, elbow, and radioscaphoid joints; cavitation in the hand joints occurs somewhat later.

Peripheral Nerve Development

Bardeen and Lewis[2] demonstrated in 1901 that all of the nerves to the upper limb pass through a cervicobrachial plexus that is present at the base of the limb bud by the fourth postovulatory week. The major peripheral nerves, as previously mentioned, are identifiable in the developing limb at the elbow by 37 days and at the wrist by 41 days.[13] Chick embryo experiments have confirmed the observation that the peripheral nerves are not present in the primitive limb bud but develop after the limbs have formed. Mixed motor and sensory nerve trunks in chick embryos enter the limb as a "pioneer growth cone,"[32] which becomes surrounded by mesenchyme. This mesenchyme forms a perineural sheath, through which the nerve axons sprout branches to individual muscles.

The process by which individual muscles become innervated has been the subject of many experiments. The removal of somitic mesoderm results in limbs that lack muscles and nerve branches to the absent muscles, whereas the remaining nerves are otherwise normal.[4] This suggests that the presence of muscle is not the stimulus for nerve development. Removal of the neural tube results in the absence of motor nerve formation, but sensory nerves develop normally. Destruction of the neural crest results in normal motor nerves but absent sensory nerves.[32] Thus the presence of motor nerves is not necessary for sensory nerve formation to occur, and vice versa.

Peripheral Vascular Development

There is rapid development of the major arteries of the upper limb from the third to the eighth postovulatory week. Metabolic gradients result in increasing vascularity of myogenic areas and avascularity of chondrogenic areas.[63] The limb has developed an axial artery by the fifth week. This rudimentary brachial artery gives off an interosseous and a median artery on the volar surface of the limb.[38] During the sixth week an ulnar artery forms and progresses to the hand to form the deep palmar arch. The radial artery is formed on the

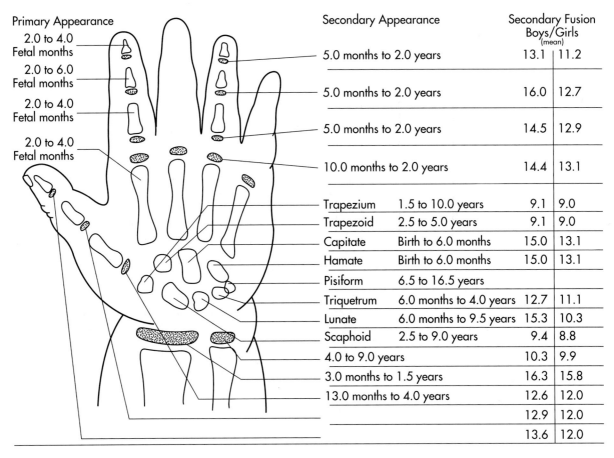

Primary Appearance		Secondary Appearance		Secondary Fusion Boys/Girls (mean)	
2.0 to 4.0 Fetal months		5.0 months to 2.0 years		13.1	11.2
2.0 to 6.0 Fetal months		5.0 months to 2.0 years		16.0	12.7
2.0 to 4.0 Fetal months		5.0 months to 2.0 years		14.5	12.9
2.0 to 4.0 Fetal months		10.0 months to 2.0 years		14.4	13.1
	Trapezium	1.5 to 10.0 years		9.1	9.0
	Trapezoid	2.5 to 5.0 years		9.1	9.0
	Capitate	Birth to 6.0 months		15.0	13.1
	Hamate	Birth to 6.0 months		15.0	13.1
	Pisiform	6.5 to 16.5 years			
	Triquetrum	6.0 months to 4.0 years		12.7	11.1
	Lunate	6.0 months to 9.5 years		15.3	10.3
	Scaphoid	2.5 to 9.0 years		9.4	8.8
		4.0 to 9.0 years		10.3	9.9
		3.0 months to 1.5 years		16.3	15.8
		13.0 months to 4.0 years		12.6	12.0
				12.9	12.0
				13.6	12.0

Figure 95-13. The time of appearance of primary and secondary ossification centers in the hand, and the average time of fusion of secondary centers.[3] There is a significant amount of variation, and times of appearance and fusion can also be altered in the presence of congenital anomalies.[58]

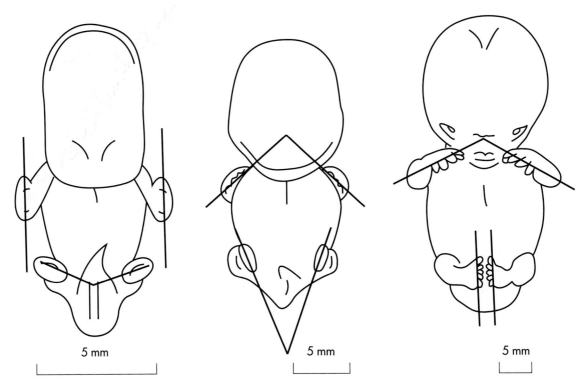

Figure 95-14. Ventral views of embryos at decreasing magnifications show the change in the orientation of the limbs to the trunk during the last 2 weeks of embryogenesis. Embryos are shown at approximately 41, 48, and 56 days, respectively.

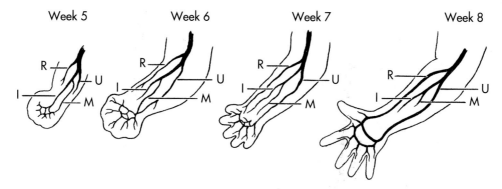

Figure 95-15. The development of the major vessels within the upper limb from the fifth through the eighth week after ovulation. The median *(M)* and interosseous *(I)* arteries provide the early blood supply. The ulnar artery *(U)* then forms from the median artery to become the dominant vessel to the hand. The radial artery is the last to develop, and following its formation the median and interosseous arteries undergo a relative decrease in size. The interosseous artery persists in the adult on the interosseous membrane and terminates at the wrist, whereas the median artery persists as a nutrient vessel found on the ventral surface of the median nerve. This artery persists as the major conduit to the hand in a small number of people.

preaxial side of the limb around the end of the seventh week (Figure 95-15). The ulnar and radial arteries enlarge as the median and interosseous arteries undergo a relative decrease in size. The median artery persists as the main supply for the median nerve, and the interosseous artery persists as a variable-sized vessel on the volar side of the interosseous membrane, terminating at the carpus. All of these vessels display a significant amount of variability.[12]

Muscle Development

Upper limb muscles form from "blastema," or masses of mesenchymal tissue. These blastema consist of myoblasts that originate from limb bud mesenchyme or that migrate from the somite. Muscle blastema form on the dorsal and ventral side of the limb to give origin to the extensor and flexor muscle groups, respectively. Every upper extremity muscle is identifiable by the eighth postovulatory week.

Experimental studies suggest that muscle blastema differentiation is under the influence of local forces, rather than the somite of origin or any neural input.[5] Differentiation occurs in a proximal to distal direction, as is the case with skeletal development. Once the blastemas have divided and the muscles attach to their skeletal origin, their tendons develop separately.[56] A tendon will degenerate if it fails to join its muscle belly, whereas a muscle can survive without a tendon if the muscle is innervated.[22,27,29] A tendon that fails to insert on its corresponding bone will attach to the nearest bone, tendon, or fascia.

The understanding of forearm and hand muscle differentiation has been significantly advanced by the work of Cihak.[6-9] The blastema of the volar superficial muscles of the forearm begins to differentiate before that of the deeper muscles. Differentiation begins in the fifth week and is complete by the eighth week. The flexor digitorum superficialis (FDS) develops from the superficial palmar blastema and migrates proximally to its origin. During this migration the median nerve comes to lie on the deep surface of the muscle bellies of the FDS.

The intrinsic muscles of the hand develop from five embryonic muscle layers: the interossei dorsalis accessorii, the intermetacarpals, the flexor breves profundi, the contrahentes, and the lumbricals. These develop from a common intrinsic blastema during the sixth and seventh week. The interossei muscles form from various contributions of the three most dorsal of these layers: the interossei dorsalis accessorii, the intermetacarpals, and the flexor breves profundi.[9] The contrahentes is a more palmar structure that becomes the adductor pollicis (Figure 95-16). The lumbricals form as a sheet at the level of the carpus and give rise to the tendons of the flexor digitorum profundus during the sixth week. The lumbricals have inserted onto the dorsal aponeuroses of the fingers by the end of the sixth week.

The flexor breves profundi gives rise to both the thenar and hypothenar muscles. The superficial layer becomes the abductor pollicis brevis, the radial portion becomes the opponens pollicis, and the deep portion becomes both heads of the flexor pollicis brevis. These muscles are all innervated by the median nerve, except for the deep head of the flexor pollicis brevis, which is innervated by a branch of the ulnar nerve that passes through the adductor pollicis.

The most ulnar flexor breves profundi become the hypothenar muscles. The abductor digiti minimi forms late in the sixth week, and the opponens digiti minimi and the flexor digiti minimi form in the middle of the seventh week.

Genetic Encoding and Molecular Responses

There is experimental evidence that several regulatory molecules are expressed by genes of the apical ectodermal ridge. The fibroblast growth factors (FGF), which appear to have a significant role in the signaling between the AER and the underlying mesenchyme, are by far the most thoroughly understood of these molecules.

The molecule FGF-4 is found in the AER of early mouse limb buds. Application of FGF-4, both in vitro and in vivo, has been shown to maintain proliferation of cells in a bud that

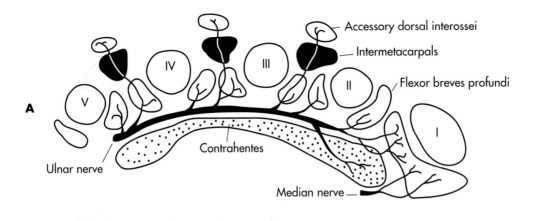

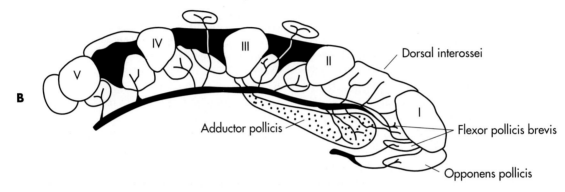

Figure 95-16. Cross-section through an embryonic **(A)** and an adult **(B)** palm showing the intrinsic muscle layers and their innervation. Note the formation of the interossei from various combinations of the accessory dorsal interossei, the intermetacarpals, and the flexor breves profundi, and the regression of the contrahentes into the adductor pollicis.

would otherwise have stopped growing after experimental ridge removal[42-44] (see Figure 95-4, *B*). Furthermore, there is evidence that FGF-4 maintains polarizing activity.[70] Application of FGF-4 to the apical and posterior limb bud margin maintains polarizing activity if the ridge is removed. This polarizing activity preserves the progress zone, allowing continued proximal to distal growth. A limb that grows as the result of FGF-4 mimicking the signal from the ridge, however, is not normal. The handplate becomes cylindrical, and the resulting digits are bunched together (see Figure 95-4, *B*). These data suggest that FGF-4 acts to link growth and pattern formation during limb development.

The FGF-2 molecule, like FGF-4, is able to maintain polarizing activity in culture.[1] When FGF-2 is applied in vivo to the anterior limb bud margin via a retrovirus, it causes additional limb elements to be formed.[49] This appears to be mediated through proliferation of precursor cells and not by alteration of anterior limb bud cells. Beads soaked in FGF-1, FGF-2, or FGF-4 and placed in the presumptive flanks of chick embryos induce the formation of ectopic limb buds, which can develop into complete limbs.[11]

The FGF-8 molecule is a more recently identified fibroblast growth factor that is expressed in the ectoderm of the prospective limb bud territory in both the mouse and chick embryo.[13,34] Mesodermal FGF-8 appears to induce limb forma-

tion by causing FGF-8 gene expression in the ectoderm. Secretion of FGF-8 by the ectoderm appears to initiate limb bud formation. Purified FGF-8 will substitute for the AER in maintaining mouse limb bud outgrowth. Thus FGF-8 appears to be a key regulator of limb induction, initiation, and development.

Signals from the AER apparently control the expression of several regulatory proteins. Msx-1 and Msx-2 are widely expressed in vertebrate embryos. Msx-1 is strongly expressed in the mesenchyme and weakly expressed in the AER, whereas Msx-2 is found weakly in the mesenchyme and more strongly in the AER. Studies have shown that changes in the expression of these genes can occur rapidly.[10,14,50] This supports the idea of a continuous interplay between the AER and the mesenchyme during the growth of the limb bud.

Signals from the AER are apparently necessary for the proper expression of the HOX genes. The Hox are 38 genes present in higher vertebrates that encode proteins responsible for the establishment of cell identity along the anteroposterior body axis.[35] There is a correlation between the relative position of these genes along the chromosome and the axial level of the limb bud in which they are expressed. More 3' genes are expressed in the forelimb and the 5' genes are expressed in the hind limb bud. The HOX genes are expressed in a complex pattern that appears to result from the response of limb mesoderm to the Sonic hedgehog (see below). The specific responses are dependent on the temporal context of the mesoderm receiving the signal, and not simply the signal alone.[40]

The HOX genes appear to function in determining the timing and extent of local growth rates. When HOXD13 was disrupted in the mouse, distal limb growth was retarded.[17] Recent evidence demonstrates that synpolydactyly is caused by expansions of the polyalanine segment in the amino-terminal region of HOXD13.[39]

Retinoic acid is an endogenously produced hydrophobic molecule present in the developing limb bud that acts by binding and activating nuclear receptors. There is a higher concentration in the posterior region near the zone of polarizing activity, and undifferentiated limb buds have demonstrably higher concentrations than more differentiated limb buds.[61,62] Retinoic acid applied to the chick limb bud will produce duplicate wing patterns similar to those seen after grafts from the polarizing zone (see Figure 95-6).[65,67] Both ZPA grafting and retinoic acid application display dose-dependence. The dose of applied retinoic acid required to produce a full set of digits is similar to the concentration of endogenous retinoic acid.[55] These data support the idea that retinoic acid plays a role in limb development, but the nature of this role is not completely understood.

The Sonic hedgehog (Shh) is a vertebrate homologue of the Drosophila segment polarity gene hedgehog.[48] There is evidence to suggest that Shh is the endogenous polarizing signal. Shh RNA co-localizes with ZPA activity, and Shh is also expressed in the posterior mesenchyme of limb buds and zebrafish pectoral fin buds.[19,31] Retinoic acid application to the anterior wing limb bud activates Shh expression in the underlying mesenchyme.[21] Anterior wing bud grafting with cells transfected with the Shh coding region produces wing duplications similar to those produced by ZPA grafting or retinoic acid treatment (see Figure 95-6).

These findings suggest that the Shh patterns the anteroposterior limb axis.[48] Tickle proposed that Shh may be the signal that maintains the progress zone of the AER while simultaneously acting as a positional signal along the anteroposterior axis[64] (see Figure 95-3).

SUMMARY

Formation of the human upper limb in the embryo is essentially complete by the eighth week of postovulatory life. Advances in experimental embryology and related fields have provided a greater understanding of the complex processes involved in fetal limb development. Future work will hopefully continue to expand this knowledge and ultimately permit the clinical application of experimental embryology to diagnose and treat congenital extremity malformations.

REFERENCES

1. Anderson R, Landry M, Muneoka K: Maintenance of ZPA signaling in cultured mouse limb bud cells, *Development* 117:1421-1433, 1993.
2. Bardeen CR, Lewis WH: Development of the limbs, body-wall and back in man, *Am J Anat* 1:1, 1901.
3. Caffey J: *Pediatric x-ray diagnosis: a textbook for students and practitioners of pediatrics, surgery and radiology,* ed 7, Chicago, 1978, Year Book Medical Publishers.
4. Chevallier A, Kieny M, Mauger A: Limb-somite relationship: effect of removal of somitic mesoderm on the wing musculature, *J Embryol Exp Morph* 43:263, 1978.
5. Chevallier A, Kieny M, Mauger A: Limb-somite relationship: origin of the limb musculature, *J Embryol Exp Morph* 41:245, 1977.
6. Cihak R: Connections of the abductor pollicis longus and brevis in the ontogenesis of the human hand, *Folia Morphol* 20:102, 1972.
7. Cihak R: Ontogenesis of the skeleton and intrinsic muscles of the human hand and foot, *Ergeb Anat Entwicklungsgesch* 46:1, 1972.
8. Cihak R: Reduction of insertion of M. interosseous dorsalis accessorius in human ontogenesis, *Folia Morphol* 21:228, 1973.
9. Cihak R: Differentiation and rejoining of muscular layers in the embryonic hand. In Bergsma D, Wicklind L (editors): *Morphogenesis and malformation of the limb,* vol 13, New York, 1977, Alan R. Liss.
10. Coelho CND, Krabbenhoft KM, Upholt WB, et al: Altered expression of the chicken homeobox-containing genes Ghox-7 and Ghox-8 in the limbbuds of limbless mutant embryos, *Development* 113:1487-1493, 1991.
11. Cohn MJ, Izpisua-Belmonte JC, Abud H, et al: Fibroblast growth factors induce additional limb development from the flank of chick embryos, *Cell* 80(5):739-746, 1995.
12. Coleman SS, Anson BJ: Arterial patterns in the hand, *Surg Gynecol Obstet* 113:409, 1961.
13. Crossley PH, Minowada G, MacArthur CA, et al: Roles for FGF-8 in the induction, initiation, and maintenance of chick limb development, *Cell* 84(1):127-136, 1996.
14. Davidson DR, Crawley A, Hill RE, et al: Position-dependent expression of two related homeobox genes in developing vertebrate limbs, *Nature* 352:429-431, 1991.
15. Deschamps F, Teot L, Benningfield C, et al: Ultrasonography of the normal and abnormal antenatal development of the upper limb, *Ann Hand Upper Limb Surg* 11:389-400, 1992.
16. Dhouailly D, Kieny M: The capacity of the flank somatic mesoderm of early bird embryos to participate in limb development, *Dev Biol* 28:162-175, 1972.
17. Dolle P, Dierich A, LeMeur M, et al: Disruption of the Hoxd-13 gene induces localized heterochrony leading to mice with neotenic limbs, *Cell* 75:431-441, 1993.
18. Drachman DB, Sokoloff L: The role of movement in embryonic joint development, *Dev Biol* 12:401, 1966.

19. Echelard Y, Epstein DJ, St-Jacques B, et al: Sonic hedgehog, a member of a family of putative signaling molecules, is implicated in the regulation of CNS polarity, *Cell* 75:14417-14430, 1993.

20. Fallon JF, Crosby GM: Polarizing zone activity in limb buds of amniotes. In Balls M, Ede DA, Hincliffe JR (editors): *Vertebrate Limb and Somite Morphogenesis,* Cambridge, 1977, Cambridge University Press.

21. Francis PH, Richardson MK, Brickell PM, et al: Bone morphogenetic proteins and a signalling pathway that controls patterning in the developing chick limb, *Development* 120:209-218, 1994.

22. Graham JH, Stephens TD, Siebert GR, et al: Determinants in the morphogenesis of muscle tendon insertions, *J Pediatr* 101:8255, 1982.

23. Gray DJ, Gardner E, O'Rahilly R: The prenatal development of the skeleton and joints of the human hand, *Am J Anat* 101:169-223, 1957.

24. Haines RW: The development of joints, *J Anat* 81:33, 1947.

25. Hinchliffe JR, Sansom A: The distribution of the polarizing zone (ZPA) in the legbud of the chick embryo, *J Embryol Exp Morph* 86:169-175, 1985.

26. Honig L, Summerbell D: Maps of strength of positional signalling activity in the developing chick wing, *J Embryol Exp Morph* 87:163-174, 1985.

27. Jacob HJ, Christ B: On the formation of muscular pattern in the chick limb. In Merker HJ, Nau H (editors): *Teratology of the limbs,* Berlin, 1980, Walter de Gruyter and Co.

28. Kieny M: Variation de la capacite inductrice du mesoderme et de la competence dee l'ectoderme au cours de l'induction primaire du bourgeon de membre chez l'embryon de poulet, *Arch Anat Microsc Morphol Exp* 57:401-418, 1968.

29. Kieny M, Chevallier A: Anatomy of tendon development in the embryonic chick wing, *J Embryol Exp Morph* 49:153, 1979.

30. Kimura S, Shiota K: Sequential changes of programmed cell death in developing fetal mouse limbs and its possible roles in limb morphogenesis, *J Morphol* 229(3):337-346, 1996.

31. Krauss S, Concordet J-P, Ingham PW: A functionally conserved homolog of the Drosophila segment polarity gene *hh* is expressed in tissues with polarizing activity in zebrafish embryos, *Cell* 75:1431-1444, 1993.

32. Lewis J, Al-Ghaith L, Swanson G, et al: The control of axon outgrowth in the developing chick wing. In Fallon J, Caplan A (editors): *Limb development and regeneration,* part A, New York, 1983, Alan Liss Inc.

33. MacCabe JA, Parker BW: Polarizing activity in the developing limb of the Syrian hamster, *J Exp Zool* 195:311-317, 1976.

34. Mahmood R, Bresnick J, Hornbruch A, et al: A role for FGF-8 in the initiation and maintenance of vertebrate limb bud outgrowth, *Curr Biol* 5(7):797-806, 1995.

35. McGinnis W, Krumlauf R: Homeobox genes and axial patterning, *Cell* 68:283-302, 1992.

36. Menkes B, Deleanu M: Leg differentiation and experimental syndactyly in chick embryo, *Revue Roumaine d'Embryologie et de Cytologie, Serie d'embryologie,* 1:69-74, 1964.

37. Milaire J: Aspects of limb morphogenesis in mammals. In DeHaan RL, Ursprung H (editors): *Organogenesis,* New York, 1965, Holt, Rinehart, Winston.

38. Mrazkova O: Ontogenesis of arterial trunks in the human forearm, *Folia Morph* 21:193, 1973.

39. Muragaki Y, Mundlos S, Upton J, et al: Altered growth and branching patterns in synpolydactyly caused by mutations in HOXD13, *Science* 272:548-551, 1996.

40. Nelson CE, Morgan BA, Laufer E, et al: Analysis of Hox gene expression in the chick limb bud, *Development* 122(5):1449-1466, 1996.

41. Nilsson L, Hamberger L: *A child is born,* New York, 1990, Delacorte Press.

42. Niswander L, Martin GR: Fgf-4 expression during gastrulation, myogenesis, limb and tooth development in the mouse, *Development* 114:755-768, 1992.

43. Niswander L, Martin GR: FGF-4 and BMP-2 have opposite effects on limb growth, *Nature* 361:68-71, 1993.

44. Niswander L, Tickle C, Vogel A, et al: FGF-4 replaces the apical ectodermal ridge and directs outgrowth and patterning of the limb, *Cell* 75:579-587, 1993.

45. O'Rahilly R, Gardner E: The timing and sequence of events in the development of the limbs in the human embryo, *Anat Embryol* 148:1-23, 1975.

46. O'Rahilly R, Gardner E, Gray DJ: The skeletal development of the hand, *Clin Orthop* 13:42-50, 1959.

47. Ploeckinger-Ulm B, Ulm MR, Lee A, et al: Antenatal depiction of fetal digits with three-dimensional ultrasonography, *Am J Obstet Gynecol* 175: 571-574, 1996.

48. Riddle RD, Johnson RL, Laufer E, et al: Sonic hedgehog mediates the polarizing activity of the ZPA, *Cell* 75:1401-1416, 1993.

49. Riley BB, Savage MP, Simandl BK, et al: Retroviral expression of FGF-2 (bFGF) affects patterning in chick limb bud, *Development* 118:95-104, 1993.

50. Robert B, Lyons G, Simandl BK, et al: The apical ectodermal ridge regulates Hox-7 and Hox-8 gene expression in developing chick limb buds, *Genes Dev* 5:2363, 1991.

51. Rubin L, Saunders JW Jr: Ectodermal-mesodermal interactions in the growth of limb buds in the chick embryo: constancy and temporal limits of the ectodermal induction, *Dev Biol* 28:94-112, 1972.

52. Saunders JW, Gasseling MT, Saunders LC: Cellular death in morphogenesis of the avian wing, *Dev Biol* 5:147-148, 1962.

53. Scott WJ: Physiological cell death in normal and abnormal rodent limb development. In Persud TV (editor): *Advances in the study of birth defects,* vol 3, Baltimore, 1979, University Park Press.

54. Scott WJ, Ritter EJ, Wilson JG: Delayed appearance of ectodermal cell death as a mechanism of polydactyly induction, *J Embryol Exp Morphol* 42:93, 1977.

55. Searls RL, Janners MY: The initiation of limb bud outgrowth in the embryonic chick, *Dev Biol* 24:198-213, 1971.

56. Shellswell WG, Wolpert L: The pattern of muscle and tendon development in the chick wing. In Balls M, Ede DA, Hincliffe JR (editors): *Vertebrate limb and somite morphogenesis,* Cambridge, 1977, Cambridge University Press.

57. Smith JC: The time required for positional signalling in the chick wing bud, *J Exp Embryol Morph* 52:105-113, 1980.

58. Stuart HC, Pyle SI, Cornol J, et al: Onsets, completions and spans of ossification in the 29 bone growth centers of the hand and wrist, *Pediatrics* 29:237, 1962.

59. Summerbell D: A quantitative analysis of the effect of excision of the AER from the chick limb bud, *J Embryol Exp Morph* 32:651-660, 1974.

60. Swanson AB, Swanson GG, Tada K: A classification for congenital limb malformation, *J Hand Surg* 8:693-702, 1983.

61. Thaller C, Eichele G: Identification and spatial distribution of retinoids in the developing chick limb bud, *Nature* 327:625-628, 1987.

62. Thaller C, Eichele G: Isolation of 3,4-didehydroretinoic acid: a novel morphogenetic signal in the chick wing bud, *Nature* 345:815-819, 1990.

63. Tickle C: Experimental embryology as applied to the upper limb: review article, *J Hand Surg* 12B:294, 1987.

64. Tickle C, Eichele G: Vertebrate limb development, *Annu Rev Cell Biol* 10:121-152, 1994.

65. Tickle C, Lee J, Eichele G: A quantitative analysis of the effect of all-trans-retinoic acid on the pattern of chick wing development, *Dev Biol* 109:82-95, 1985.

66. Tickle C, Summerbell D, Wolpert L: Positional signalling and specification of digits in chick limb morphogenesis, *Nature* 254:199-202, 1975.

67. Tickle C, Alberts B, Wolpert L, et al: Local application of retinoic acid to the limb bud mimics the action of the polarizing region, *Nature* 296:564-666, 1982.

68. Tickle C, Shellswell G, Crawley A, et al: Positional signalling by mouse limb polarizing region in the chick limb bud, *Nature* 259:396-397, 1976.

69. Upton J: Congenital anomalies of the hand and forearm. In McCarthy J (editor): *Plastic surgery,* vol 8, Philadelphia, 1990, WB Saunders.

70. Vogel A, Tickle C: FGF-4 maintains polarizing activity of posterior limb bud cells in vivo and in vitro, *Development* 119:199-206, 1993.

71. Wolpert L: Positional information, pattern formation, and morphogenesis. In Connelly TG (editor): *Morphogenesis and pattern formation,* New York, 1981, Raven Press.

72. Yasuda M: Normal and abnormal morphogenesis of the hand, *Orthop Surg Traumatol* 34:915-921, 1991.

73. Zwilling E: Ectoderm-mesoderm relationship in the development of the chick embryo limb bud, *J Exp Zool* 128:423-441, 1955.

Examination of the Hand

Michael W. Neumeister

INTRODUCTION

Phylogenetically, the hand has evolved to prosper as an organ of immense importance for mankind, most notably for its intricate functions in daily activities and its expressive role in nonverbal communication. The hand has been promoted as a symbol for peace, friendship, authority, welcoming, and power. Each specific action of the hand relies on the finely tuned biomechanical interplay of the intrinsic and extrinsic musculotendinous forces. The skeleton and its stabilizing ligaments provide a framework for the hands or fingers to grasp, pinch, squeeze, oppose, grip, and manipulate. The skin houses an enormous consortium of sensory receptor sites that allow sensory communication between the environment and the cerebral cortex. The hand thus acts as our tactile eyes, a function that is appreciated by all people, but none more so than the surgeon who uses this tool to examine patients and to perform surgery.[62] The blind use their hands to read; persons who are aphasic use their hands to communicate with others. The thumb offers prehensile grip and further differentiates man from his lower evolutionary rivals. The American Medical Association's *Guidelines to the Evaluation of Permanent Impairment* considers the loss of a thumb to be equivalent to a 40% to 50% reduction in total hand function and a 36% reduction of upper extremity function.[2] The hand contributes 90% to the function of the upper extremity. Considering the hand's role in the labor force, entertainment, art, literature, and passion, it behooves us, as hand surgeons, to fully define the normal and pathologic boundaries in each patient that we examine as he or she presents with various ailments. The complicated architecture and biomechanics of the hand demand a thorough understanding of anatomy, physiology, and pathophysiology.

Examination of the hand should commence with the patient seated directly across from the examiner. Both hands are placed on the examining table and examined identically and sequentially (Figure 96-1). This allows for a comparative analysis and objectivity in the interpretation of the examination. Celsus' classical description of the cardinal signs of inflammation—calor, dolor, tumor, rubor—are as pertinent today as they were in the first century AD, and the examiner should be observant of these signs, as well as masses, swelling, and tenderness. The fingernails, skin, muscles, tendons, bones, and joints are all integral parts of the functional hand and as such should be assessed individually and as a composite structure.

SKIN

The hand has two major types of skin. The dorsal surface of the hand has pliable, relatively thin, nonglabrous skin. Its texture is consistent with that of the forearm and arm, although in relative terms there is a limited amount of subcutaneous fat on the dorsum of the hand. The dorsal skin creases denote the position of the underlying joints (Figure 96-2).[12,49] Immediately below the dermis is a layer of subcutaneous fat that houses small branches of dorsal cutaneous nerves and vessels that arise from a deeper plane. The larger vessels and nerves lie between the loose areolar plane and the overlying subcutaneous fat. The larger veins are usually visible on the dorsum of the hand and fingers. The extensor tendons are situated volar to the dorsal veins and nerves and dorsal to the metacarpal and phalangeal bones of the hand. In contrast to the palmar skin, there are no vertical septa connecting the underlying tissues to the dorsal skin. This becomes significant in inflammatory, infectious, or edematous states that often manifest with marked swelling of the back of the hand and/or fingers instead of the palmar side. This mandates the need for a thorough examination of both sides of the hand, despite observing swelling of only the dorsum. This pliable skin compensates for the increased convexity of the distal transverse arch of the hand when making a fist or during prehension.[12] There is a relative redundancy of skin over the phalangeal joints to allow appropriate unopposed flexion at each joint. The dorsal skin has a variable number of skin appendages, hair follicles, and sebaceous glands. Their density tapers to rather sparse concentrations on the distal aspects of the fingers. There are numerous sweat glands on all areas of the dorsal skin.

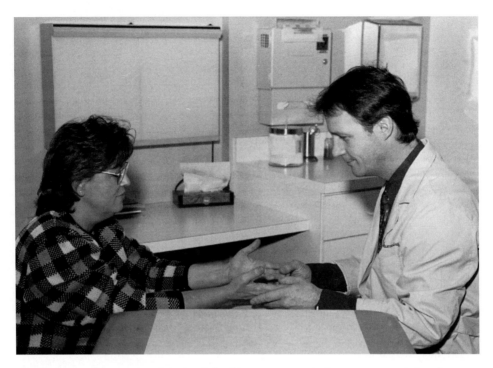

Figure 96-1. Examination of the hand should commence with the patient seated directly across from the examiner. Both hands are examined identically and sequentially for comparative analysis. Bracelets and wrist watches should be removed.

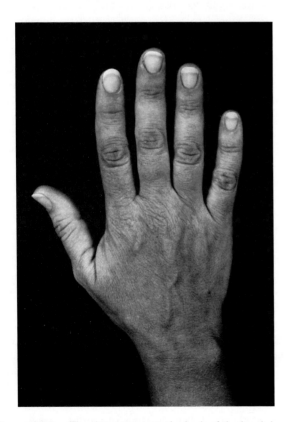

Figure 96-2. The skin creases on the back of the hand denote the location of the underlying joints. A greater redundancy of skin is noted at the MCP joints and the proximal IP joints to compensate for their arch of rotation.

The glabrous skin on the palm and volar fingers is a unique tactile surface of the body that communicates a multitude of information about our environment to the cerebrum.[38,55,82] This thickened, imprinted skin is laden with layers of cornified epithelium and covers the palm and volar lateral aspect of the digits. The mid-axial line in the fingers demarcates the volar glabrous skin from nonglabrous dorsal skin, although there is a tendency for the glabrous skin to creep dorsally distal to the distal interphalangeal (DIP) joint. Sympathetically innervated eccrine sweat glands are abundant in the glabrous skin in contrast to a complete lack of hair follicles or sebaceous glands.[55]

The prominent creases on the palm of the hand are ramifications of the underlying fascia and joints (Figure 96-3).[12,69] The flexion creases on the volar surface of the fingers extend to the mid-lateral aspect of the digit. One crease is usually present just proximal to the DIP joint. There are invariably two creases at the proximal interphalangeal (PIP) joint and one or two creases at the distal palmar digital junction, which translates to the middle of the proximal phalanx in the skeletal plane.[49] A line connecting the lateral ends of each joint's flexion crease denotes the mid-axial line (Figure 96-4). Subcutaneous fat is almost completely void at the site of the digital creases. Minor injury at these sites may allow bacteria to penetrate the underlying flexor sheaths or cause damage to the neurovascular bundles in these areas.[49] A relative abundance of fat is present between the creases.

Each web space has a dorsal-to-palmar obliquity. The distal palmar crease extends from the web space of the index and long

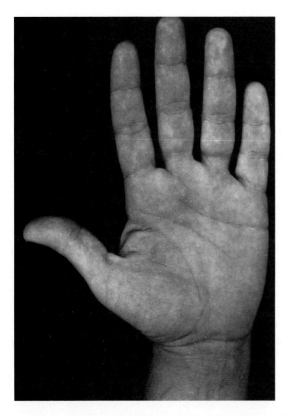

Figure 96-3. The imprinted glabrous skin on the palmar surface of the hand is distinct from the pliable skin on the dorsum of the hand. The prominent creases of the palm are ramifications of the underlying fascia and joints.

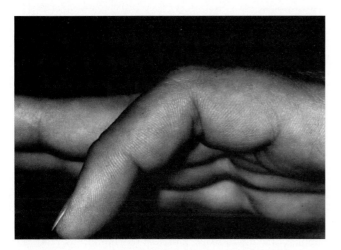

Figure 96-4. The mid-axial line is formed by connecting the lateral terminal creases of each joint's flexion endpoint. This line forms the border of the glabrous and nonglabrous skin of the fingers.

fingers to the ulnar side of the palm at the level of the metacarpal necks. The proximal palmar crease is usually 1 to 2 cm proximal to the distal crease, but starts at the radial border of the palm and extends ulnarly for a variable distance.[49] These transverse palmar creases compensate for flexion of the metacarpophalangeal (MCP) joints.[41,51] The A1 pulley and the leading edge of the decussation of the flexor digitorum sublimis tendon are present at this level. The fingertips touch the

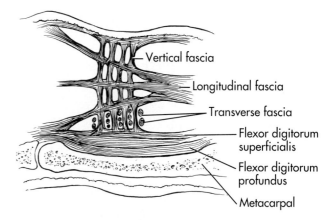

Figure 96-5. There are four layers of fascia in the palm: the deep fascia over the intrinsics, the superficial transverse fascia, the vertical fascia, and the longitudinal fascia. The dense condensations of fascia decrease the pliability of the palmar skin.

palm at the level of the transverse creases during fist formation. The crease at the base of the thenar eminence merges distally with the proximal palmar crease. This is accentuated during opposition of the thumb. This crease also corresponds to the course of the radial digital nerve to the index finger. The second longitudinal crease of the palm compensates for the increased palmar concavity created by thumb opposition or fist formation. This crease courses from the base of the long finger to the radial edge of the hypothenar eminence.

There are four layers of fascia in the palm (Figure 96-5).* The deep fascia overlies the intrinsic muscles at the metacarpal level. The superficial transverse fascia (of Skoog)[70] extends from the ulnar side of the little finger to the radial side of the index finger and is located just proximal to the MCP joints. The vertical septa of Legueu and Juvara appear to arise from this transverse fascia and in essence compartmentalize the palm's fat in the subcutaneous plane.[47] Two other systems of vertical fibers contribute to anchoring the palm skin to the underlying fascia and tendon sheaths and bones: the vertical fibers of the deep layer of the longitudinal fascia (McGouther's fibers) and the fibers between the transverse fascia and the tendon sheaths.[57] There is a higher concentration of the vertical septa around the palmar creases in the mid-palm. The skin of the palm is therefore quite immobile, with little plasticity.[34,57,73] The concentration of vertical fibers is minimal over the hypothenar eminence and even less over the thenar eminence, resulting in relative laxity of the skin in these areas. The functional significance of the vertical septa is brought to light during grasping and gripping maneuvers, in which a stable palmar surface is required. The palmar skin, without stable creases, would bunch and potentially hinder the ability to grasp objects.

The longitudinal fascia of the palm has a variety of components (Figure 96-6).[34,69] The longitudinal condensations into the digits lie palmar to the transverse fibers and form the pretendinous bands that eventually bifurcate at the MCP level to contribute to the spiral bands of Gosset.[28,34] Digital

*References 6, 28, 31, 34, 47, 54, 56, 73.

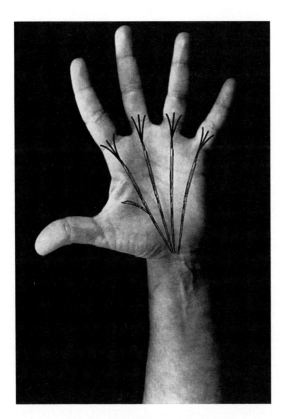

Figure 96-6. The longitudinal fascia of the palm has a variety of components. Tributaries of the fascia progress to the digits, the palmar dermis, the flexor sheath, and underlying fascia.

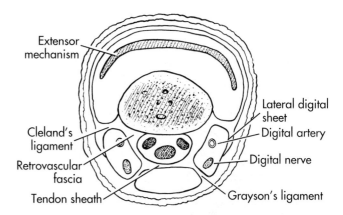

Figure 96-7. The fascia of the digits is composed of Cleland's ligaments, Grayson's ligaments, the retrovascular fascia, and the lateral sheet.

A critical analysis of the integument should precede any other aspect of the clinical examination of the hand. The skin's color, contour, pliability, texture, and turgor must be observed. The fingerprints, creases, and fat pads are noted and palpated. Irregularities, masses, tenderness, and the presence of sweating are recorded. Sensation, range of motion, and motor function are subsequently tested.

NERVES

The ulnar nerve enters the wrist radial to the flexor carpi ulnaris (FCU) but dorsal and ulnar to the ulnar artery. The nerve travels through Guyon's canal, which is bound by the flexor retinaculum or carpal ligament on its floor, the pisiform and pisofascial ligament ulnarly, the hook of the hamate radially, and a thin fascial condensation superiorly.[32,45,56,60] The motor branch of the hypothenar muscles is given off within the canal. The ulnar nerve terminates as a superficial, deep branch at the end of Guyon's canal (Figure 96-8). The superficial branch supplies motor innervation to the palmaris brevis muscle and sensation to the ulnar palm, little finger, and the ulnar side of the ring finger. The deep motor branch supplies the interosseous muscles, the lumbricals, and the adductor and deep head of the flexor pollicis brevis (FPB). The dorsal cutaneous branch of the ulnar nerve arises from the ulnar nerve on average approximately 6 cm proximal to the head of the ulna and passes between the ulna and FCU to supply sensation to the dorsum of the hand and the ulnar two digits.[11] A branch of this nerve crosses transversely across the wrist to supply sensation to the dorsal skin of the wrist. The ulnar nerve in the forearm travels between the flexor digitorum superficialis (FDS) and flexor digitorum profundus (FDP) muscles and innervates the FDP to the little and ring fingers.

The median nerve also courses between the FDS and FDP muscles in the forearm, although more radially than the ulnar

extensions of the fascia pass deep to the natatory ligament and the neurovascular bundles. The longitudinal fascia is continuous with the thenar and hypothenar fascia.[69] Other fibers of the longitudinal fascia have superficial insertions into the dermis distal to the MCP joint and midway between the distal and proximal palmar creases.[57] The deepest layer of the longitudinal fascia passes on either side of the flexor sheath.[69]

The spiral band is a fibrous condensation formed from the pretendinous band, natatory ligament, and vertical septa.[28] Distal to the natatory ligaments, the spiral bands progress to the digits as the lateral digital sheet. The natatory ligament runs transversely as a continuous 1-cm wide strip at the level of the web space from the ulnar side of the little finger to its termination in the first web space and proximal thumb crease as the distal commissural ligament of Grapow.[29] The natatory ligament gives off distal fibers to the spiral band to help form the lateral digital sheet. The digital fascia of the fingers has been described as retaining ligaments of the skin or the extensors (Figure 96-7).[58,69] Cleland's ligaments are fascial condensations that arise from the area of the assembly line on the phalanx and pass dorsal to the neurovascular bundles in an oblique fashion to terminate in the dermis of the skin.[15] Grayson's ligament is a thinner fascia that arises from the flexor sheath and courses volar to the neurovascular bundles enroute to the overlying dermis.[30] The neurovascular bundle is further encased by the fascia of the lateral digital sheet and the retrovascular fascia on its lateral and dorsal medial sides, respectively.[30,34,70,75] These fibers likely have insertions to the bone and skin along their course.

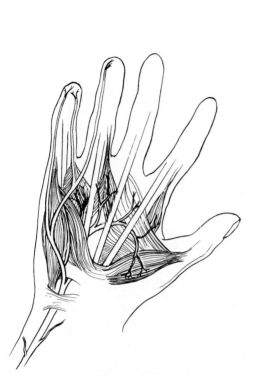

Figure 96-8. The ulnar nerve travels through Guyon's canal and terminates as a superficial and deep branch. The hypothenar muscles, interossei, ulnar two lumbricals, and the deep head of the FPB muscle are supplied by the ulnar nerve. Sensation of the ulnar side of the palm and dorsum and the ulnar one and a half digits is also provided by the ulnar nerve.

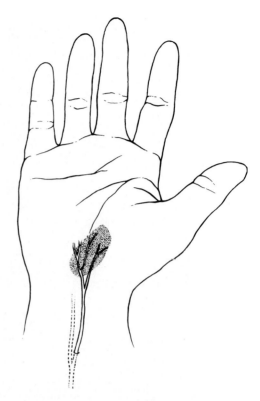

Figure 96-9. The palmar cutaneous branch of the median nerve provides sensibility in an ellipse at the base of the thenar eminence.

nerve. Before entering the carpal tunnel, the median nerve emerges from between the FDS tendons and the flexor carpi radialis (FCR) deep to the palmaris longus (PL). The palmar cutaneous branch of the median nerve diverges from the radial side of the median nerve approximately 6 to 10 cm proximal to the flexor retinaculum.[61] This sensory branch travels superficial to the retinaculum within a separate tunnel to supply an ellipse of skin over the base of the thenar eminence (Figure 96-9). The nerve is not affected in carpal tunnel syndrome but can be injured by a palmar incision between the PL and FCR. The median nerve innervates the pronator teres (PT), FCR, PL, and FDS muscles. The anterior interosseous nerve arises from the dorsal ulnar aspect of the median nerve at the distal end of the cubital fossa. This nerve travels along the interosseous membrane to its termination in the pronator quadratus muscle. Along its course, the anterior interosseous nerve innervates the FDP to the index and long fingers, the flexor pollicis longus (FPL), and the pronator quadratus muscle. The functional significance of interruption of the anterior interosseous nerve becomes manifest in a decreased pinch strength of the index finger and thumb. The examination and assessment of the function of the anterior interosseous nerve is performed by isolating the FDP of the index finger and the FPL of the thumb while the patient actively flexes the distal phalanx of each digit. The examiner asks the patient to pinch the tips of the index finger and thumb together. This posture, sometimes referred to as the "O" sign, is unable to be achieved if there is complete

disruption of the anterior interosseous nerve (Figure 96-10). Alternatively, weakness of this nerve can be elicited by forcing the examiner's finger through the "O" sign as the patient resists. The examiner's finger easily passes through the flexed index finger and thumb distal phalanx if anterior interosseous nerve function is impaired.

The median nerve trifurcates at the distal end of the carpal tunnel and sends common digital nerves to the thumb, index, and long fingers, and the radial aspect of the ring finger (Figure 96-11). The most ulnar common digital nerve bifurcates at the level of the MCP joint to course up the radial side of the ring finger and the ulnar side of the long finger, respectively, as their digital nerves. The central common nerve also bifurcates at the level of the MCP joint between the index and long fingers, progressing as digital nerves to the radial side of the long finger and ulnar side of the index finger. The most radial common nerve bifurcates almost immediately on exiting the carpal tunnel and sends digital nerves to the thumb and the radial side of the index finger. The digital nerve of the finger travels in a plane bound by Cleland's ligament, Grayson's ligament, the lateral digital sheet, and a retrovascular fascial condensation. Dorsal branches course from the digital nerve at the level of the PIP and DIP joints to supply the dorsal skin over the middle and distal phalanx of the index, long, ring, and small fingers (Figure 96-12).

The radial nerve divides into the deep motor branch, the posterior interosseous nerve, and the superficial radial branch at the level of the proximal forearm. The superficial radial nerve travels immediately under the brachioradialis until it reaches the junction of the proximal two thirds and distal one third of the forearm, where it pierces the antibrachial fascia and

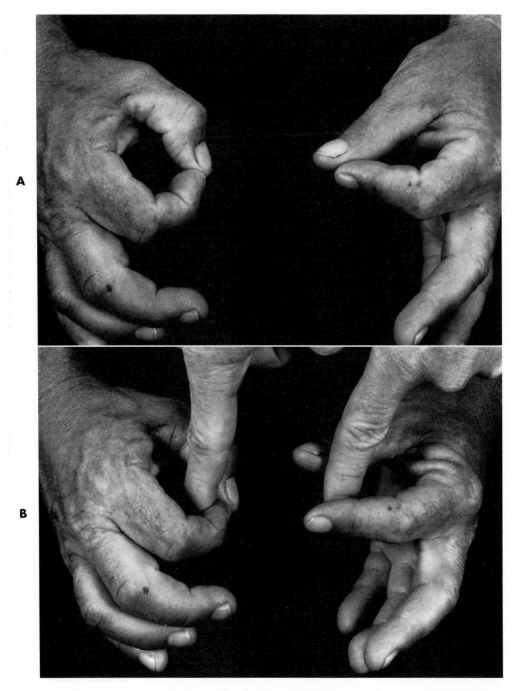

Figure 96-10. **A,** Functional loss of the anterior interosseous nerve results in an inability to flex the distal phalanx of the index finger and the thumb. The patient is unable to maintain the "O" sign. **B,** The examiner's finger is easily pulled through the "O" sign.

emerges in a subcutaneous plane between the brachioradialis and the extensor carpi radialis longus (ECRL) tendons.[61] Multiple branches of the superficial radial nerve provide sensation to the dorsum of the radial side of the hand; the ring, long, and index fingers; and the thumb (Figure 96-13).

The three major nerves of the hand are the conduits between the cerebrum and the skin's specialized receptors (Figure 96-14). There are three types of sensory receptors in the skin of the hand: thermoreceptors that mediate changes in skin temperature; mechanoreceptors that mediate changes in pressure, touch, and movement; and nociceptors that mediate information related to pain).[38,53,55] A large subpapillary neural network is concentrated in the glabrous skin of the palm and fingers to relay information about the environment to the cerebrum, which interprets the perception of "sensation." The sensory receptors are either encapsulated or are present as free nerve endings. The free nerve endings are myelinated and nonmyelinated and course from the subpapillary plexus to the epidermis.[38] These nerve endings lie between epidermal cells up to the layer of the stratum granulosum.[55]

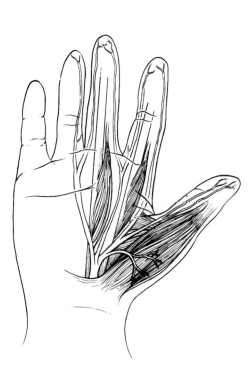

Figure 96-11. The median nerve trifurcates at the distal end of the carpal tunnel to innervate the radial two lumbricals and the thenar musculature and provide sensation to the thumb, index finger, long finger, and the radial half of the ring finger.

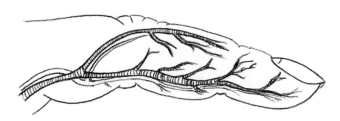

Figure 96-12. Dorsal branches of the digital nerves pass from the common volar digital nerve beginning at the level of the PIP joint to supply the dorsal skin distally.

The hair follicles are supplied by a basketlike arrangement of free nerve endings. Free nerve endings are usually nociceptors and thermoreceptors.

The perception of mechanical stimuli to the skin of the hand is mediated by rapidly adapting and slowly adapting mechanoreceptors (Figure 96-15). The rapidly adapting receptors are serviced by myelinated A fibers.[55] They include the Pacinian and Meissner corpuscles, which both mediate moving touch and vibration.[38] These receptors respond to the onset of a mechanical stimulus. The Pacinian corpuscles are situated in the connective tissue, usually along nerve trunks.[52,55] A single myelinated fiber serves each Pacinian corpuscle. There may be as many as 120 Pacinian corpuscles on the palmar surface of each finger.[89] Pacinian corpuscles are not present in the hairy skin on the back of the hand. Meissner corpuscles are encapsu-

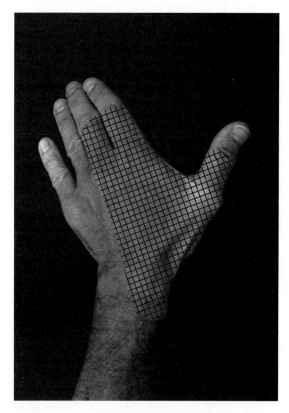

Figure 96-13. The superficial radial nerve supplies sensation of the dorsum of the radial hand, ring finger, long finger, index finger, and thumb.

lated mechanoreceptors situated in the dermal papillary ridges of the skin. The number of Meissner corpuscles varies in the hand, ranging from 20 on the fingertip to 5 per square millimeter on the palm.[90]

The Merkel cell neurite complexes are slowly adapting mechanoreceptors that mediate constant touch and pressure through myelinated fibers. The Merkel cell disks lie in the epidermis at the layer of the stratum germinativum.[38]

The corpuscles of Ruffini and Krause are poorly understood mechanoreceptors found in the deep dermis or subcutaneous tissue.[55] The thinly encapsulated Ruffini corpuscles are slowly adapting mechanoreceptors that respond to deformational changes in the surrounding collagen. The Krause corpuscles also have a poorly defined capsule and are considered rapidly adapting receptors of mechanical deformation.[55]

Sensibility and stereognosis pertain to the ability to feel and the perception of understanding or recognizing the contours of objects by the sense of touch.[86] Sensation, on the other hand, is a cerebral understanding or perception of the information sent to the brain from the sensory end organs.[86] Sensibility may be affected by intrinsic and extrinsic factors (Table 96-1).

The clinical tests of sensation are predominantly designed to clarify thresholds and function of sensibility. Tubiana et al[80] have grouped sensibility testing into three main categories: threshold tests, functional tests, and objective tests. The threshold tests include temperature, pressure, touch, vibration, and sharp stimulus. The functional tests include two-point discrim-

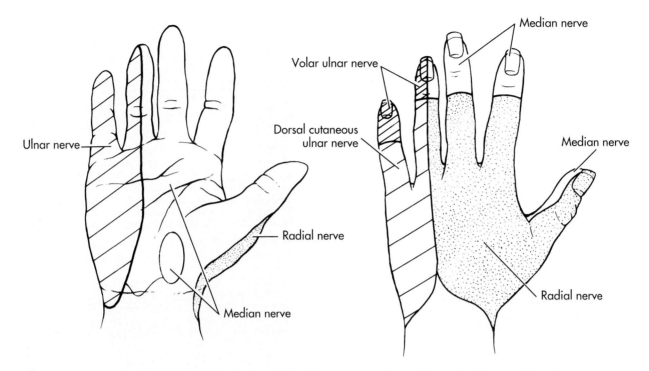

Figure 96-14. The ulnar, median, and radial nerves provide sensibility to the fingers and hand in a characteristic distribution.

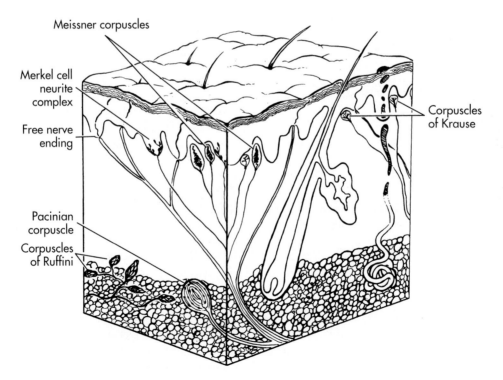

Figure 96-15. The perception of mechanical stimuli of the skin is mediated by various mechanoreceptors. Pacinian corpuscles, Meissner corpuscles, Merkel cell neurite complex, corpuscles of Ruffini and Krause, and free nerve endings all play an intricate role in the perception of sensation.

Table 96-1.
Classification of Sensory Recovery

GRADE	RECOVERY OF SENSIBILITY
S0	No recovery of sensibility in the autonomous zone of the nerve
S1	Recovery of deep cutaneous pain sensibility with the autonomous zone of the nerve
S1+	Recovery of superficial pain sensibility
S2	Recovery of superficial pain and some touch sensibility
S2+	As in S2, but with overresponse
S3	Recovery of pain and touch sensibility with disappearance of overresponse*
S3+	As in S3, but localization of the stimulus is good and there is imperfect recovery of two-point discrimination*
S4	Complete recovery*

From Dellon AL: *Evaluation of sensibility and re-education of sensation in the hand,* Baltimore, 1991, Williams and Wilkins.
*These classifications were modified to include classic two-point discrimination ranges as follows: S3 has two-point discrimination greater than 15 mm; S3+ includes 7- to 15-mm range; S4 includes 2- to 6-mm range.

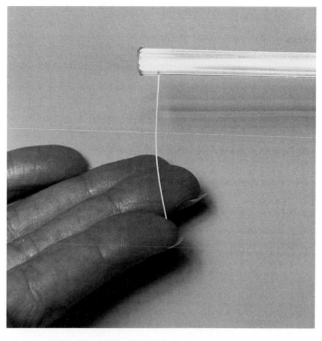

Figure 96-16. The Semmes-Weinstein monofilament test for sensibility is performed with the hand secured on a flat or immobile surface and the palm and digit tested sequentially to create sensibility mappings. Normal sensibility in the fingers localizes pressures in probes between 2.44 and 2.83.

ination and stereognosis. The objective tests include object manipulation. A fourth group to be included in sensibility tests includes sudomotor function (sympathetic).

Examination of hand sensibility must follow a systematic and consistent approach. Gross sensation is extremely subjective and does not allow documentation of progress or regeneration or functional impairment of the nerve. A discussion of more appropriate means of testing sensation follows. The importance of a detailed and well-documented evaluation of the sensibility of the hand cannot be overstated. Evaluation of the median, ulnar, and radial nerves is observed by sensory testing and mapping of their characteristic areas of innervation.

LIGHT TOUCH AND PRESSURE

The Semmes-Weinstein monofilament testing is the most accurate means of evaluating light touch and deep pressure.[9,10,71,86,87] The complete kit contains 20 nylon monofilaments mounted in Lucite rods. Mini kits with five monofilaments are also available. The filaments have a constant length but increasing diameters and are marked with numbers ranging from 1.56 to 6.65. These numbers represent logorhythmic quotients of the force in milligrams required for the filament to bend or buckle when pressing against the skin of the finger.[86] The monofilaments are applied perpendicular to the skin with the patient's view obstructed. The patient responds when the monofilament induces a sensation. Two out of three responses must coincide to be considered accurate for that site. Normal sensibility in the fingers localizes pressure in probes between 2.44 and 2.83.[71,86] The hand is secured on a flat, immobile surface to prevent retraction or inadvertent movement and to provide a constant counterforce during testing (Figure 96-16). The palm and each digit are tested identically and sequentially to create sensibility mappings. Both hands should be tested to provide control and comparison values.

Two-point discrimination tests are a reliable and easy method of evaluating the quality of sensibility in the fingers and hand.[8,22,23,52,53] MacKinnon and Dellon[53] have popularized two-point testing with the easy-to-use calibrated Disk-Criminator (Figure 96-17). Two-point discrimination tests are performed in two different ways. Static and dynamic two-point discrimination tests evaluate innervation density of slowly adapting group-A beta nerve fibers and rapidly adapting group-A beta nerve fibers, respectively.[23] The hand is supported and secured to prevent inadvertent movement. The patient's view is obstructed, and the Disk-Criminator is placed on the finger with the prongs in line with the longitudinal axis of the digital nerves (Figure 96-18). This helps prevent crossover assessment of the opposite digital nerve. The prong should be touched lightly on the area in question and should proceed in a distal to proximal direction. Random sequences of one or two prongs are performed to guarantee accurate testing.

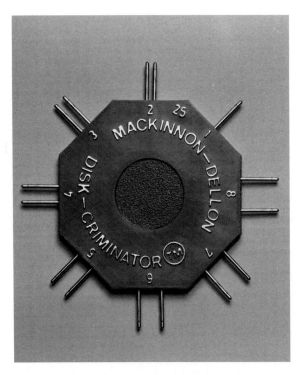

Figure 96-17. The MacKinnon-Dellon calibrated Disk-Criminator used for two-point discrimination tests.

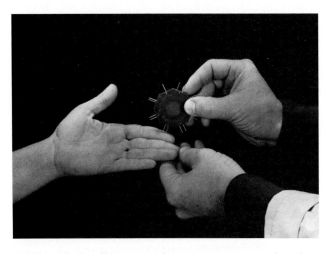

Figure 96-18. Two-point discrimination is tested with a Disk-Criminator with the prongs in line with the longitudinal access of the digital nerves. Each side of the digits should be tested identically and sequentially. The patient's view should be obstructed during the test to prevent untoward bias.

Seven out of ten identical responses at one setting are considered appropriate to designate a two-point discrimination value.[86] The normal static two-point discrimination is 2 to 5 mm on the volar fingertips, 7 to 10 mm at the base of the palm, 7 to 12 mm on the dorsum of the digits, and 10 to 25 mm on the forearm.[8,9,14,23,86] There is a high level of reliability of static two-point discrimination tests, although concerns do arise because the test requires patient compliance and cooperation and examiner consistency. Varying the pressure on the

Disk-Criminator's prongs when placed on the skin may not accurately delineate one-prong versus two-prong measurements, but rather the difference between light versus heavy pressure. The patient's responses may be somewhat inaccurate or confusing without appropriate care and attention to technique when performing this test.

Dynamic two-point discrimination testing is performed from proximal to distal, with normal values being 2 mm at the distal volar fingertip. Alternating one or two prongs while recording the response achieved most frequently (usually 7 out of 10) denotes the patient's discrimination.[86] Dynamic two-point discrimination returns before static two-point discrimination after sensory nerve injury.

Sensibility testing is used to evaluate afferent and efferent sensory pathways.[9,53] Predictable sensory recovery patterns of the nerves after surgery have been reported.[53,68] Dellon noted the return of pain perception first followed by vibration at 30 H$_z$, moving light touch, static light touch, and finally vibration at 256 H$_z$.[23,53] Two-point discrimination is the last modality to return.[9,23] The Tinel's sign denotes axonal regeneration.[56,76,78] It is often elicited in areas of chronic nerve compression or regenerating nerves after trauma. The Tinel's sign may not be perceived immediately after nerve repair, but may take 4 to 6 weeks to develop.[86] The continuous distal advancement of this sign is an indication of appropriate nerve regeneration. The sign is detected with a gentle tap of the examiner's finger over the sensory nerve. The patient perceives tingling or "pins and needles" distal to the provoked site in the cutaneous distribution of the nerve in question. A vibrometer (biophysometer) is a hand-held, variable amplitude, fixed frequency vibrator that may give more quantitative results in vibration testing and assessment of a Tinel's sign.[21,36] The entire course of the nerve in the hand should be evaluated in this manner to elicit potential sites of compression. The most common sites in the hand are over the carpal ligament for median nerve compression (carpal tunnel syndrome) and over Guyon's canal (ulnar nerve compression).[27,53] The superficial radial nerve may be compressed at its exit between the tendons of the brachioradialis and the ECRL. A Tinel's sign may be elicited at this site on the distal forearm. Other provocative maneuvers to evaluate nerve irritability or compression are the Phalen's test and direct compression over the site in question (Figure 96-19).[66] The examiner passively flexes the patients wrist for approximately 60 seconds or until the patient remarks on dysesthesia in the fingers or thumb. Direct compression of the median nerve just proximal to the carpal ligament will also reproduce the dysesthesia of carpal tunnel syndrome. Similar provocative tests are performed just proximal to Guyon's canal for ulnar nerve compression and over the distal radial forearm for compression of the superficial radial nerve (Wartenberg's syndrome).[84]

A system for documenting the recovery of a nerve after trauma, repair, or grafting has been formatted for sensory and motor recovery, respectively.[20] Tables 96-1 and 96-2 illustrate the classification of sensory and motor recovery. MacKinnon and Dellon modified the sensory classification to include the evaluation of two-point discrimination such that

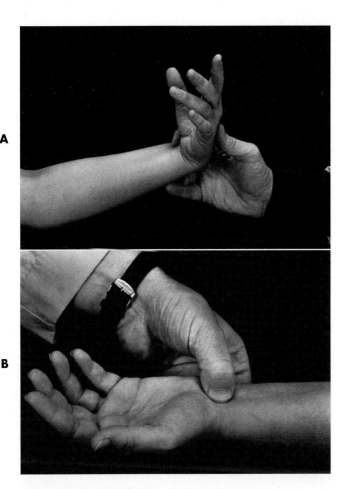

A

B

Figure 96-19. **A,** Phalen's test is performed with the wrist in extreme flexion. The reproduction of the compressive symptoms should be noted within the first 60 seconds. **B,** Compression over the site in question should reproduce the symptoms.

GRADE	MOTOR RECOVERY
M0	No contraction
M1	Return of perceptible contraction in the proximal muscle
M2	Return of perceptible contraction in both proximal and distal muscles
M3	Return of function in both proximal and distal muscles to such a degree that all important muscles are sufficiently powerful to act against gravity
M4	All muscles act against strong resistance and some independent movements are possible
M5	Full recovery in all muscles

Table 96-2.
Classification of Motor Recovery

From Dellon AL: *Evaluation of sensibility and re-education of sensation in the hand,* Baltimore, 1991, Williams and Wilkins.

patients with S3 have a two-point discrimination greater than 15 mm, S3+ a two-point discrimination between 7 mm and 15 mm, and S4 a two-point discrimination between 2 mm and 6 mm and denotes normal sensibility.[20]

SYMPATHETIC FUNCTION TESTING

The hand's sympathetic nervous system modulates sweat response, vasoconstriction, vasodilatation, and pilomotor activity. The sympathetic tests (sudomotor) do not assess functional sensibility but rather provide objective methods to test for sympathetic nerve function in noncompliant or poorly motivated patients.[59,86] There are four broad categories that need to be addressed when evaluating sympathetic function in the hand, namely trophic changes, sweat response, vasomotor activity, and pilomotor function. Trophic changes to the integument are observed after complete denervation and are identified through inspection and palpation of the skin and fingernails. The distal finger pulp may atrophy, creating a tapering of the fingers.[14] The poor vascular tone may be responsible for this so called "pencil pointing" affect.[9,86] The capillary ridges of the

epidermis atrophy and render the skin smooth and silky feeling, often leaving glabrous skin almost devoid of fingerprints after denervation. Hair follicles lose tone and, subsequently, their hair.[86] The erectile pilomotor function is lost. Chronic sympathetic denervation leads to dryness, scaling, and, occasionally, fissuring of the skin. The fingernails become brittle, a symptom that may be related to a decrease in water content within the nail plate. The growth of the nail is attenuated. Atrophy of the distal fingertip can lead to hook-nail deformity.[86] Occasionally, trauma to the hand has secondary manifestations on the nail growth. A transverse ridge of the nail can often be observed after injury to the hand or finger or after a systemic illness, and is likely a manifestation of a temporary change in the normal physiology of the germinal matrix. A temporal relationship between the injury and the nail ridge can be calculated because the ridge grows out as the nail grows at a rate of approximately 1 mm per week.

Lost vasomotor regulation is reflected in the skin color and temperature. The skin takes on a bluish or mottled appearance that may alternate with a pink, warm hand because of the loss of the heat regulatory capacity. Several sudomotor tests are usually performed in the clinic or hand-therapy unit.

The Ninhydrin printing test was first described by Moberg[59] and is considered the test most accurate to objectively assess sympathetic function.[4,9,65,86] The hand is cleaned thoroughly with soap and water and isopropyl alcohol. After air drying, the hand is placed palm up under a lamp for approximately 20 minutes. An imprint of the palm is then obtained by placing the hand on porous paper (i.e., bond paper).[86] The paper is sprayed with Ninhydrin and allowed to dry overnight. A purple pattern should appear on the paper if normal sweating response is intact. The individual's unaffected hand is used as a control.

The wrinkle test was first described by O'Rain.[63] The hands are completely submerged in a bowl of lukewarm water for approximately 20 to 30 minutes. The skin is subsequently examined for any degree of wrinkling or pruning. There is a strong correlation with wrinkling and sweating, although the exact mechanism by which the wrinkling occurs is still ill defined. The O'Riain wrinkle test has varying reliability depending on the nature of the sudomotor injury.[67] The examiner or therapist is also not able to quantify the degree of wrinkling.

The denervated hand is rendered susceptible to trauma and ulcerations because of the inability to perceive pain. The testing of pain is usually performed with a pin prick. Enough pressure is required to slightly indent the skin but not enough to cause bleeding.[80] The unaffected hand is used as a control. The patient acknowledges the testing by appropriate "sharp" or "dull" responses, and the affected areas are mapped.

Vibration perception testing utilizes tuning forks with varying cycles per second H_z to stimulate selected nerve and end organs. Pacinian corpuscles are stimulated by 256 H_z tuning forks and Meissner corpuscles respond to 30 H_z tuning forks.[14,86] Either end of the tuning fork can be used in the testing, but the examiner should always use the same end to provide consistency. The pronged end of the tuning fork may be more appropriate for the pulp of the fingertips or palm because of the extent of the overlying tissue. The fingers are tested in a distal to proximal direction until the patient senses the vibration.[21]

Temperature perception can be easily tested in the hand-therapy unit with the aid of temperature-specific probes. The hot and cold probes are usually 115° F and 40° F, respectively.[86] The fingers are tested from distal to proximal. The appropriate response and the lapsed time between application of the stimulus and the perception of hot and cold is recorded.

THE MOBERG PICK-UP TEST

Stereognosis is the ability to recognize or identify objects based solely on the sense of touch. Moberg[59] described a pick-up test that required the patient to identify 10 small objects without the aid of vision. The objects are placed in a container and the patient is timed as he or she moves the objects from one container to another. The patient is subsequently blindfolded and the test repeated. The patient is asked to identify the objects as he or she places them into the second container. The Moberg pick-up test is applicable for patients with combined median and ulnar nerve palsies.[59] The test has less significance in patients with isolated ulnar nerve palsy because most can identify objects using the intact sensation of the median nerve–innervated radial three digits. The ulnar two digits are taped down when testing the median nerve alone.

BONES AND JOINTS

The metacarpal bones form the skeletal framework of the hand, articulating proximally with the carpus and distally with the phalanges. Two transverse arches of the hand are the direct result of the interrelationships of the metacarpals and the carpus.[18,50,80] The proximal carpometacarpal (CMC) arch has a dorsal convexity that is greater on the radial side than the ulnar side.[12] The first metacarpal is angled approximately 45 degrees from the second metacarpal (angle of separation) in the sagittal plane. The thumb rests anatomically with the pulp facing the radial side of the long finger's distal phalanx. The trapezial metacarpal joint is unique in that it is a biconcavoconvex joint.* This configuration allows for complex, multiplaned movements, such as circumduction of the thumb.[37] The angle of circumduction denotes the extreme range of motion of the thumb (Figure 96-20).[35,80] This angle, which is usually 135

---

*References 5, 7, 19, 25, 40, 44, 61.

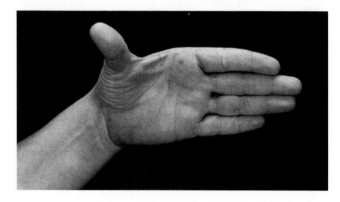

Figure 96-20. The angle of circumduction is measured at the patient's maximum angle of intersection between the plane of the second and third metacarpals and the plane of the first and second metacarpals. This angle is usually around 130 degrees.

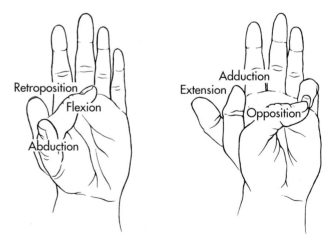

Figure 96-21. The thumb is able to perform a variety of different motions, including flexion, extension, adduction, abduction, retroposition, and opposition. It is through these movements that prehension is possible.

degrees, is measured by placing the back of the hand on the table, having the patient maximally circumduct the thumb, and measuring the intersection angle between the plane of the second and third metacarpals and the plane of the first and second metacarpals.[3] Traditionally the motion of the thumb encompasses flexion, extension, adduction, abduction, retroposition, and opposition (Figure 96-21).

THE FIRST CARPOMETACARPAL JOINT

The capsule of the first CMC joint is redundant and loose. The ligamentous support allows the thumb's wide circumduction through a broad range of motions. The range of motion of the first metacarpal is limited by the adductor muscle and fascia and the first dorsal interosseous muscle and fascia.

The stabilizing ligaments of the first CMC joint include the intracapsular and extracapsular ligaments. The strongest and perhaps most important ligament is the extracapsular anterior oblique CMC ligament, which inserts from the palmar ulnar tubercle (Beak) of the first metacarpal and wraps obliquely around the base of the metacarpal to insert on the anterior crest of the trapezium.[64] The integrity of this strong ligament is lost through attrition in basilar joint arthritis and leads to subluxation of the first metacarpal.[13,79]

Subluxation of the metacarpal on the trapezium is often accompanied by hyperextension of the MCP joint of the thumb and adduction of the metacarpal. The intercarpal ligaments with attachments to the base of the first and second metacarpals also act as a checkrein for the motion of this first metacarpal bone.

The first metacarpal internally rotates (counter clockwise in the ulnar direction) on adduction and externally rotates (clockwise) on abduction. These conjoint movements facilitate pulp-to-pulp pinch of the thumb with the other digits.[17] Kuczynski[43] notes the resting position of the thumb is 60 degrees from a line through the heads of the stable central second and third metacarpals.

The examiner must put the thumb through a full range of motion to fully assess the metacarpal range of motion. The base of the first metacarpal is easily palpated when the thumb is in the adducted position. The "step off" of the metacarpal off the trapezium when the thumb is adducted vanishes as the thumb is brought into abduction, flexion, or opposition. Inflammation of the metacarpotrapezial joint can be elicited through a number of provocative maneuvers, including palpation, the grind test, and the crank test. The grind test is perhaps the most clinically reliable. The examiner grasps the distal metacarpal between his or her thumb and index finger and an axial load is applied to the metacarpotrapezial joint while rotating the metacarpal at its base. Crepitus and/or tenderness is elicited if significant arthritis is present. The crank test applies an axial load to the metacarpotrapezial joint during flexion and extension of the metacarpal.

The second metacarpal is much more restricted in its motion than the first metacarpal. There is virtually no movement at the second CMC joint because of the ligamentous attach-ments to the third metacarpal, the trapezoid, and the capitate bones. The ECRL tendon may be palpated at the base of the second metacarpal. The extensor pollicis longus (EPL) tendon courses obliquely just proximal to the base of the second metacarpal as it wraps around Lister's tubercle and heads toward the thumb MCP joint. The third metacarpal moves a few degrees in flexion and extension but it is also restricted by the strong intercarpal and CMC ligaments.[60] The base of the third metacarpal is not as prominent as the second metacarpal. A slight depression at the base denotes the articulation with the capitate bone. The extensor carpi radialis brevis (ECRB) inserts into the base of the third metacarpal. The fourth and fifth metacarpals have a greater mobility at their base, enjoying 10 degrees and 20 degrees of anteroposterior movement, respectively.[60] Each has articulation with the hamate bone. The oblique articulation of the fifth metacarpal with the hamate allows the opponens digiti minimi (ODM) muscle to radially rotate the metacarpal while flexing it forward. The extensor carpi ulnaris (ECU) inserts onto the dorsal ulnar aspect of the base of the fifth metacarpal. Fractures of its base (reverse Bennett's fracture) are often responsible for the displacement of the fifth metacarpal in a dorsoulnar direction.

The distal metacarpal arch also supports a dorsal convexity.[12,80] The arch is at the level of the MCP joints. Opposition of the thumb to the little finger will increase the convexity of the arch, whereas hyperextension of all MCP joints will render the arch almost flat. The changes in the arch configuration are secondary to the increased range of motion of the distal metacarpals. The metacarpals may be palpated along the entire dorsal surface while the finger is observed for signs of irregularities, masses, or tenderness. The stability of the bases is examined by cupping the patient's hand and bimanually loading each CMC joint. The metacarpal heads should be readily visible on full flexion of the fingers. The third metacarpal head is usually the most prominent (Figure 96-22). The third metacarpal is the longest bone in the hand, followed by the second, fourth, fifth, and first metacarpals, respectively. Volar displacement of the metacarpal head after neck fractures results in loss of knuckle prominence, which is often seen with boxer's fractures.

The MCP joints are examined for deformity, inflammation, dislocation, stability, and range of motion. The stability of the MCP joints of the fingers is dependent on the collateral and accessory ligaments, the deep metacarpal ligament, volar plate, sagittal band, and extrinsic forces of the flexor and extensor tendons and the abductor and adductors of the fingers.[70,77] The normal distal transverse arch should be observed in the resting position (see Figure 96-22). The extensor tendon should be identified over the central portion of the metacarpal head. The fingers are parallel in extension and point toward the scaphoid tubercle in flexion (Figure 96-23).

Stability of each joint is tested in extension and in flexion. The examiner stabilizes the metacarpal bone while deviating the proximal phalanx in the opposite direction (Figure 96-24). There will be a greater deviation in extension than in flexion. The MCP joint of the thumb is similar to that of the fingers except that there is less motion in the ulnar/radial direction

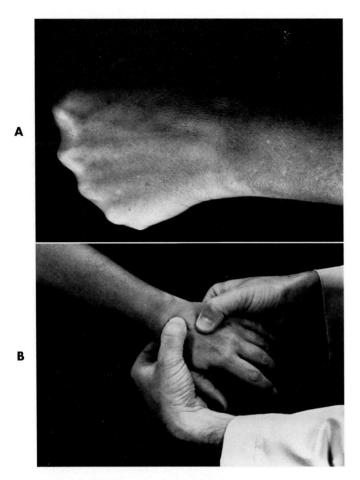

Figure 96-22. **A,** The third metacarpal is the longest bone in the hand, followed by the second, fourth, fifth, and first metacarpals, respectively. **B,** The CMC joints are evaluated individually by a bimanual examination. The third metacarpal head is usually the most prominent of the knuckles when making a fist.

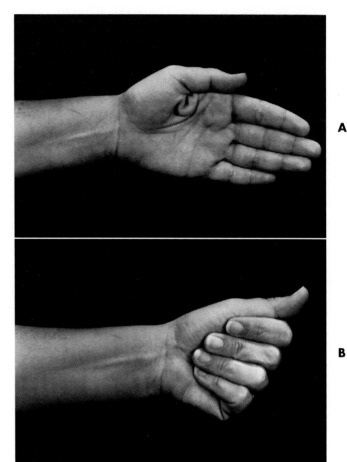

Figure 96-23. **A,** The fingers are parallel in extension. **B,** The fingernails diverge in a line pointing to the scaphoid tubercle during flexion of the fingers.

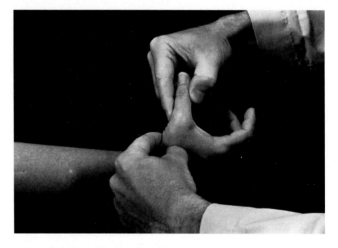

Figure 96-24. The stability of the joint is tested in flexion and extension against resisted opposition by the examiner. A distinct endpoint should be noted on passive motion of the joint.

and in extension/flexion because of the constraints of the radial and ulnar collateral ligaments. The ulnar collateral ligament is extremely important to the MCP joint of the thumb because it is constantly stressed by the forces of pinch. The stability of the ulnar collateral ligament should be tested with the thumb in flexion and in extension. The examiner will note a definite endpoint on deviating the thumb to the radial side. Loss of the integrity of the ulnar collateral ligament (gamekeeper's or skier's thumb) will lead to a greater deviation and lack of an appropriate endpoint. The normal endpoint on radial deviation is in the range of 30 to 45 degrees.[24]

The tubercle on the dorsal/radial side of the index metacarpal head is easily palpable. This bony prominence marks the insertion of the radial collateral ligament.[61] The collateral ligaments tighten during flexion of the MCP joint and are relaxed in extension. This allows greater lateral mobility of the proximal phalanx in extension. There is virtually no lateral motion of the proximal phalanx during MCP flexion. This phenomenon relates to the cam effect of the metacarpal head because of its greater volar width.

The collateral ligaments of the PIP joints are taut in extension because of their oblique orientation.[12] Therefore there is more stability for the interphalangeal (IP) joints in

extension. The thick volar plate and checkrein ligaments offer stability on the palmar side of the joints. The central slip courses over the capsule on the extensor side of the PIP joint to inset into the base of the middle phalanx.[61] The collateral, accessory collateral, and transverse retinacular ligaments provide lateral stability to the PIP joints.

The stability of the DIP joint is similar to that of the PIP joint. The terminal extensor tendon courses over the capsule of the DIP joint to terminate on the dorsal base of the distal phalanx. The FDP tendon lies palmar to the volar plate and inserts on the volar aspect of the base of the distal phalanx. The DIP joint moves solely in a flexion and extension plane. The average active range of motion for the distal phalanx is approximately 80 degrees.[80] There is usually an additional passive extension at this joint of 20 to 30 degrees.

MUSCLES

THE INTRINSICS

There are 18 intrinsic muscles in the hand, including seven interosseous, four lumbricals, four thenar muscles (adductor pollicis [AP], abductor pollicis brevis [APB], flexor pollicis brevis [FPB], opponens pollicis [OP]), and three hypothenar muscles (adductor digiti quinti, abductor digiti quinti, and opponens digiti quinti). These muscles were phylogenetically the first motors for the fingers.[72] The interosseous muscles are divided into two groups: four dorsal and three volar muscles. The dorsal interosseous muscles are abductors and weak flexors of the proximal phalanges of the index, long, and ring fingers. The first, second, and fourth dorsal interosseous muscles have superficial and deep muscle bellies with corresponding medial and lateral tendons.[72] The medial tendon travels under the sagittal band and inserts into the lateral tubercle of the base of the proximal phalanx. This musculotendinous unit is responsible for abduction of the digits on the metacarpal and is also a weak flexor of the proximal phalanx. The lateral tendon courses superficial to the sagittal band to continue as the lateral band of the finger's extensor apparatus. This lateral tendon acts in conjunction with the extensor apparatus to flex the proximal phalanx at the MCP joint while extending the middle and distal phalanges at the PIP and DIP joints, respectively. The first dorsal interosseous muscle has its origin on the radial side of the second metacarpal and inserts as two heads into the base of the index finger's proximal phalanx and into the radial lateral band of the finger.[61] The first dorsal interosseous muscle is innervated by the last motor branch of the ulnar nerve. The function and strength of the first dorsal interosseous muscle is tested by having the patient place the ulnar side of both hands on the examination table such that the radial side of index finger is facing up (Figure 96-25). The patient is asked to raise the index finger toward the ceiling. Resistance by the examiner is applied to the finger to observe the strength.

The second dorsal interosseous muscle arises from the adjacent shafts of the second and third metacarpals. This muscle is also supplied by the ulnar nerve. The second dorsal interosseous muscle is tested by having the patient place his or her hand palm down on the examination table. The patient spreads all the fingers against resistance (Figure 96-26).

The third dorsal interosseous muscle has its origin on the adjacent third and fourth metacarpals and inserts on the ulnar side of the long finger. The fourth dorsal interosseous muscle

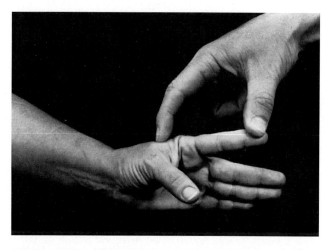

Figure 96-25. The first dorsal interosseous muscle is tested by having the patient move the finger in a radial direction against resistance from the examiner. The examiner can palpate the mass of the first dorsal interosseous muscle during this procedure.

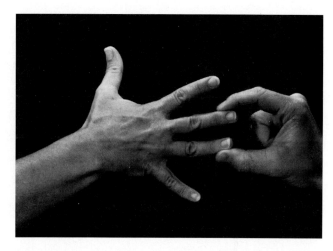

Figure 96-26. The second dorsal interosseous muscle is tested by having the patient place his or her hand palm down while spreading the fingers against resistance.

originates from the adjacent fourth and fifth metacarpals and inserts to the ulnar side of the ring finger. These latter two dorsal interosseous muscles are supplied by the ulnar nerve. Their function is tested by having the patient spread and close the fingers against resistance.

The volar interosseous muscles are all innervated by the ulnar nerve and function to adduct and weakly flex the index, ring, and little fingers toward the long finger. The first volar interosseous muscle has its origin from the volar lateral shaft to the second and third metacarpals.[61] This interosseous muscle inserts into the ulnar lateral band of the index finger. The second and third interosseous muscles arise from the adjacent shafts of the third/fourth and fourth/fifth metacarpals to insert on the radial lateral bands of the ring and little fingers, respectively.[61] The volar interosseous muscles are examined by placing a paper between the digits and having the patient hold the fingers tightly together as the examiner tries to withdraw the paper while noting the degree of resistance. The test is performed sequentially between each of the fingers and is compared to the contralateral hand.

The lumbrical muscle (*Lumbricus* means "wormlike") is perhaps the most interesting of the intrinsic hand muscles. Described as the "work horse" of the extensor apparatus, the lumbrical was observed by Smith[73] to be the only muscle in the body that "is able to relax the tendon of its own antagonist." The four lumbricals are palmar to the volar interosseous muscles and arise in zone III from the radial side of the FDP tendons to the index, long, ring, and little fingers.[61] The lumbricals of the index and long fingers are innervated by the median nerve, and the ring-and little-finger lumbricals are innervated by the ulnar nerve. Each lumbrical inserts at an angle of approximately 40 degrees into the radial lateral band of each finger.[73] Contraction of the lumbrical muscle pulls the radial lateral band proximally and simultaneously draws the FDP tendon distally. Relaxation of the FDP tendon decreases its antagonistic force, and therefore resistance on the lateral bands and extensor apparatus is decreased. The lateral bands can then extend the IP joints and flex the MCP joints. The

lumbricals also aid in MCP joint flexion. Continued contraction of the FDS and FDP tendons also contributes to MCP flexion. The long flexors contribute to MCP flexion only after the IP joints are flexed.

The mass action of the lumbrical and interossei intrinsics draws the MCP joint into flexion and the PIP and DIP joints into extension.[33,73] The position is known as the "intrinsic plus." The intriguing and complex harmony between the interossei, lumbricals, and long extrinsic tendons relies on their balanced interplay to provide unbridled function of each finger. The foreshortening of the lumbricals through voluntary or involuntary contraction will draw the fingers into a resting intrinsic-plus position. Stiffness of the digits may be related to joint degeneration; capsular, ligamentous, or skin contracture; long tendon adhesions; or intrinsic tightness. The test for intrinsic tightness or contracture is performed as follows: the examiner brings the proximal phalanx passively into extension. The IP joints will passively extend with intrinsic tightness (Figure 96-27). Resistance to active or passive flexion of the PIP and DIP joints is exhibited secondary to the taut lateral bands.

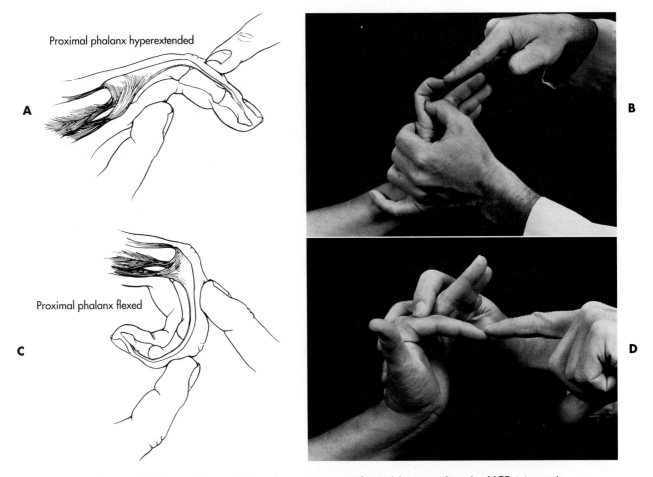

Figure 96-27. **A,** The intrinsic tightness test is performed by extending the MCP joint and attempting to passively flex the PIP joint. Tight intrinsic muscles offer resistance to active and passive flexion of the PIP joints. **B,** This patient has normal intrinsic muscles, allowing active and passive IP joint flexion while the MCP joint is held in hyperextension. **C,** Passive flexion of the MCP joint removes tension from the intrinsics and allows passive motion of the IP joints. **D,** This patient has extrinsic tendon adhesions that prevent active and passive IP joint flexion when the MCP joint is held in flexion.

bands. This is in contrast to extrinsic tightness (extensor adhesions) that allows passive range of IP motion with the MCP joint extended. Passive flexion of the MCP joint takes tension off the intrinsics despite their tightness, allowing passive and active motion of the IP joints. Extrinsic tendon adhesions, however, will prevent flexion of the IP joint when the MCP joint is flexed. Examination of the hand should also note two other finger deformities (the boutonniere and swan-neck deformities) that are related to imbalance of the intrinsic and extrinsic forces.

The Boutonniere Deformity

The boutonniere deformity is characterized by PIP-joint flexion and hyperextension at the MCP and DIP joints. The boutonniere deformity usually results from division or attenuation of the central slip with separation from the transverse retinacular ligament. The lateral bands migrate volar to the PIP-joint axis of rotation and, in essence, act as flexors. The flexor digitorum sublimis tendon has less resistance and flexes the PIP joint. The lateral bands and the oblique retinacular ligaments contract with time, preventing normal extension at the PIP joint. The distal phalanx is drawn into hyperextension through the action of the contracted lateral bands and oblique retinacular ligament. Later the head of the proximal phalanx is trapped dorsal to the retaining lateral bands, preventing reduction of the deformity. The MCP joint develops a compensatory hyperextension through the action of the sling effect of the sagittal band as the extensor tendon transfers forces through it (Figure 96-28). The initial evaluation of the boutonniere deformity should include assessment of the active and passive range of motion of the DIP and PIP joints while observing the reducibility of the deformity. The distal phalanx is examined for oblique retinacular tightness by passively extending the PIP joint while attempting to passively flex the distal phalanx. If the oblique retinacular ligament and lateral bands are severely contracted, the distal

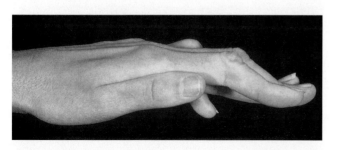

Figure 96-28. The boutonniere deformity is characterized by flexion of the PIP joint and hyperextension at the DIP joint. The lateral bands migrate volar to the pivotal axis of the PIP joint, becoming a flexor force at this joint. Foreshortening of the lateral bands draws the distal phalanx further into extension through the terminal tendon.

phalanx will be unable to flex. The examiner then flexes the PIP joint. This relaxes the lateral bands and oblique retinacular ligament, allowing the distal phalanx to now passively and actively flex.

The Swan-Neck Deformity

The swan-neck deformity is characterized by PIP joint hyperextension and DIP joint flexion. With time, the functional loss is related to loss of range of motion at the PIP joint. A swan-neck deformity may be secondary to disruption of the terminal extensor tendon from the distal phalanx or to pathology around the PIP joint, including volar-plate laxity, increased forces through the intrinsics, or loss of the FDS insertion. Lacerations or disruptions of the terminal tendon result in a relative proximal foreshortening of the extensor mechanism, which allows the lateral bands to migrate dorsally. The unopposed action of the FDP tendon draws the distal phalanx into flexion. The PIP-joint volar plate stretches, creating a swan-neck deformity.

Alternatively, instability around the PIP joint may be the primary source of a swan-neck deformity. The volar-plate laxity promotes hyperextension at the PIP joint. The transverse retinacular ligament stretches as the triangular ligament shortens, allowing the lateral bands and oblique retinacular ligament to displace dorsally. The lateral bands tighten with time and become unable to traverse the condyles of the proximal phalanx during flexion. The normal harmony of finger flexion in which the distal phalanx flexes after the middle phalanx is lost.[46] The distal phalanx flexes first until the FDP overpowers the dorsal PIP structures. The terminal tendon attenuates and the unopposed action of the FDP results in a flexion deformity at the DIP joint. The examiner should observe the active and passive range of motion of the DIP and PIP joints. Fixed deformities at the joints are noted as the fingers are ranged passively. Intrinsic muscle tightness, volar subluxation of the proximal phalanx, and evidence of trauma to the finger may lead to a swan-neck deformity. Careful examination of these structures is warranted to determine the cause. Palpation of the middle phalanx may identify a fracture healed in hyperextension, which can manifest as a swan-neck deformity.

Paralysis of the intrinsic muscles, as happens in low ulnar or median nerve palsy, alters the delicate balance of the motor units of each finger.[74] The extrinsic extensors, acting unopposed at the MCP joint, draw the proximal phalanx into extension. The volar plate stretches and the extensors pull the proximal phalanx into hyperextension. Landsmeer[46] observed the progressive horizontal displacement of the sagittal band with further hyperextension of the proximal phalanx. The excursion of the central slip is blocked, permitting the unopposed action of the FDS and FDP tendons to draw the middle and distal phalanges into flexion. This is known as "intrinsic minus position" or "claw hand." Wrist flexion increases the deformity through a tenodesis effect. The intrinsic paralysis not only affects the resting position of the fingers but also their function. Grasp is severely compromised. The normal synchronous motion of MCP flexion, followed respectively by DIP- and PIP-joint flexion, is lost. The flexion of the MCP joint in intrinsic paralysis occurs after flexion of the other joints caused by continued contraction of the FDS and FDP tendons.

The adductor pollicis (AP) muscle is a thin, fan-shaped muscle in the interosseous adductor compartment of the first web space. The terminal branch of the radial artery commonly passes through the two heads of the adductor origin. The oblique head has it origin at the base of the second and third metacarpal bones and the capitate bone. The palmar surface of the third metacarpal serves as the origin for the transverse head of the adductor.[61] The two heads converge to insert as a tendon, which may contain a sesamoid bone on the ulnar side of the base of the proximal phalanx. The adductor muscle is innervated by the deep branch of the ulnar nerve. The muscle acts to adduct the thumb and assists in its opposition.

THE EXTRINSICS

The flexor digitorum sublimis is innervated by the median nerve in the forearm and is primarily responsible for flexion of the PIP joint. The flexor digitorum sublimis tendon inserts via two slips onto the volar aspect of the proximal two thirds of the middle phalanx. The ulnar nerve innervates the little and ring fingers' FDP, and the anterior interosseous nerve supplies the long and index fingers. The FDP tendon inserts onto the base of the distal phalanx. The primary function of the profundus tendon is to flex the distal phalanx. Continued contraction of the FDP tendon contributes to the flexion of the PIP and MCP joints.

The flexor digitorum sublimis and FDP tendons flex the phalanx by a direct pulling action. The more proximal joints, however, are flexed through a sling effect established by the pulley system of the fingers. The long flexors travel in a fibroosseous canal that is strengthened by eight pulleys along the finger. There are five annular pulleys (A1 through A5) and three cruciate pulleys (C1 through C3).[61] The pulleys prevent

bow stringing of the long flexor tendons during flexion. The A2 and A4 pulleys over the proximal and middle phalanges, respectively, are most important in preserving the tendon's moment arm and the patient's subsequent grip strength.

The resting tone of the long tendons in the hand fosters a characteristic cascade of finger flexion that should be inspected before manipulating the hand during the examination. The composite finger flexion increases from the index finger to the little finger (Figure 96-29). Any deviation from the cascade usually signifies disruption of the long flexors. The exceptions to this rule may include adhesions, joint contractures, or proximal nerve injuries that alter the natural harmony of the resting biomechanics of the hand (Figure 96-30).

The integrity of the flexor digitorum sublimis and profundus tendons should be examined independently and in tandem. The patient places his or her hand palm up on the examination table with the fingers extended and the examiner holds the other three fingers in extension. The FDP is tested with the MCP and PIP joints stabilized while the patient attempts to flex the distal phalanx (Figure 96-31). The flexor

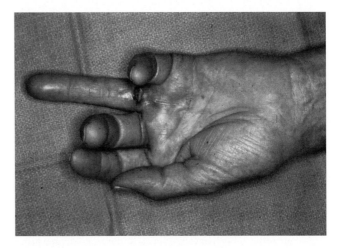

Figure 96-30. Loss of continuity of the flexor tendons results in a loss of the normal cascade of finger flexion.

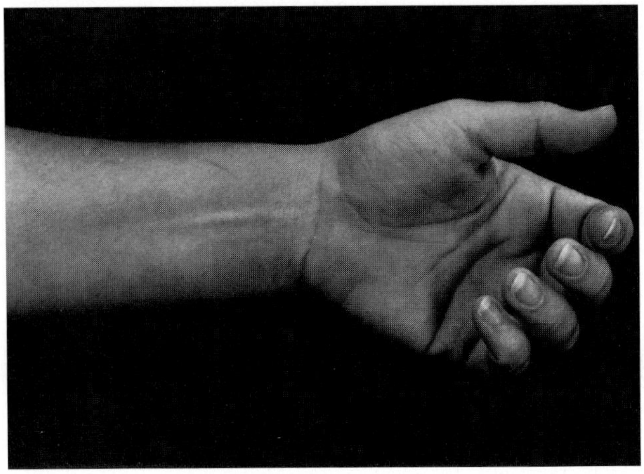

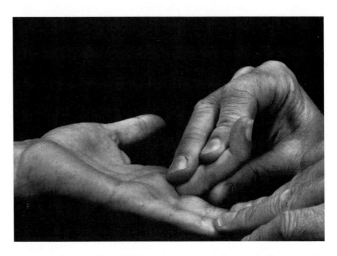

Figure 96-29. The resting cascade of finger flexion illustrates the increasing composite finger flexion from the index to the little fingers.

Figure 96-31. The FDP tendon is tested individually with the MCP and PIP joints in extension while the patient attempts to flex the distal phalanx.

digitorum sublimis is then examined. The PIP and MCP joints are released and the patient again flexes the finger while the distal phalanges of the remaining digits are held in full extension (Figure 96-32). The PIP joint, and to a minor degree the MCP joint, should flex during this second procedure. The distal phalanx does not flex because of the quadrigia affect of the FDP tendons.[49,83] Approximately 20% of patients may not have a flexor digitorum sublimis tendon to the little finger and therefore will have limited or no PIP flexion when testing this muscle.[61]

Extension of the fingers recruits both the extrinsic and intrinsic muscles. The long extensors of the fingers include the extensor digitorum communis (EDC), extensor indicis proprius (EIP), and extensor digiti quinti (EDQ). The EDC and the EIP are innervated by the posterior interosseous nerve. Each finger receives an EDC tendon. The EIP merges with the EDC of the index finger as they insert into the extensor expansion under the sagittal band. The index finger is the most independent digit, which is partially attributable to the dual extensors and the paucity of juncture tendinea that interconnect the ulnar three digital extensors.[42]

Extensor tendons that are easily identifiable as they diverge on the back of the hand are centralized over the MCP joints and remain so in extension and flexion. Loss of the integrity of the sagittal bands through attrition or trauma results in subluxation usually into the ulnar gutters of the extensor tendons. The MCP joints are put through active and passive range-of-motion exercises. Subluxing extensor tendons may be centralized in full MCP extension but translocate ulnarly in full flexion. Eventually, active extension is lost. The patients are able, however, to maintain extension of the fingers when they are passively put in this position. The ulnar three digits are more commonly affected with extensor tendon subluxations. Patients presenting with an inability to extend the ulnar two or three digits should be thoroughly evaluated to rule out other causes of this deformity, including ruptured extensor tendons, posterior interosseous nerve palsy, volar dislocation of the proximal phalanx, intrinsic tightness, and flexor contractures of the skin, tendon, volar plate, and collateral ligaments.

The long extensor tendons pass under the sagittal band and merge with the extensor expansion over the dorsum of the proximal phalanx to terminate on the dorsal surface of the base

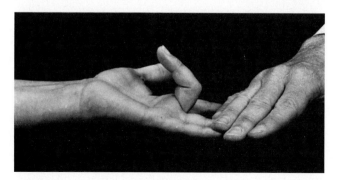

Figure 96-32. The FDS tendon is examined by mobilizing the other fingers in extension, including the distal phalanges, while the patient attempts to flex the involved finger.

of the middle phalanx (see Figure 96-28).[79] A few fibers diverge before this termination to join with the lateral bands. The proximal phalanx is brought into extension by the sling affect of the sagittal bands. Contracting the long extensors causes the tendon to lift the sagittal band that, because of its attachment to the volar plate, extends the proximal phalanx. Full extension of the fingers renders the MCP joints in a neutral or slightly hyperextended position. Flexion of the IP joints during this maneuver allows the MCP joint to hyperextend even more. This occurs because the tension is taken off the intrinsics and the long extensors can draw back the proximal phalanx further.[73]

The intrinsic muscles also use the sling principle to some extent to flex the MCP joint. The proximal phalanx is pulled into flexion through direct insertion of the interosseous muscles but also through the pull of the lateral bands that coalesce with the extensor expansion.

THE THENAR MUSCLES

The intrinsic muscles of the thumb are chiefly responsible for thumb opposition. The APB, FPB, and opponens brevis, which make up the thenar eminence, are all supplied by the recurrent motor branch in the median nerve.[61] The FPB has a superficial and deep head. The deep head is commonly supplied by a branch of the ulnar nerve. The FPB chiefly acts to flex the thumb at the CMC and MCP joints. The superficial head of the FPB is also a weak abductor, whereas the deep head is a weak adductor. The opponens pollicis muscle lies deep to the APB and radial to the FPB. The insertion along the full length of the radial side of the first metacarpal allows this muscle to pull the first metacarpal through an ulnar, clockwise rotation, bringing the thumb into the center of the palm. This movement of opposition is very important in grasping objects and allowing pulp-to-pulp communication of the thumb and the other digits. The APB muscle is the most superficial muscle of the thenar eminence. A radial sesamoid bone lies within the conjoint tendon of the APB and FPB muscles.

THE EXTRINSICS OF THE THUMB

There are four extrinsic muscles that influence the movement of the thumb: three in the dorsal compartments and one in the flexor surface. The FPL is innervated by the anterior interosseous nerve. The tendon, which is the most radial structure in the carpal tunnel, inserts on the palmar surface of the base of the distal phalanx of the thumb. The FPL is the only muscle to flex the phalangeal joint of the thumb. Continued contractions assist in flexion of the MCP and CMC joints.

The three dorsal extrinsic muscles that affect the thumb lie deep to the extensor muscles of the fingers in the forearm. The abductor pollicis longus (APL), extensor pollicis brevis (EPB), and EPL muscles have been termed "outcropping" muscles because they emerge from under the muscles of the fourth dorsal compartment (EDC and EIP) to veer radially over the

ECRL and ECRB.[61] The APL muscle, innervated by the posterior interosseous nerve, acts to abduct and extend the first metacarpal at the CMC joint. The APL lies within the first dorsal compartment along with the EPB tendon, which is often separated from the APL by a fibrous septum. The EPL, like the EPB, is innervated by the posterior interosseous nerve and acts to extend the thumb at the MCP and CMC joints. The EPL also extends to the IP joint. Its tendon passes within the third dorsal compartment, wraps around Lister's tubercle of the radius to course ulnarly to the EPB to the distal phalanx. The direction of pull of the EPL allows it to act as an adductor of the thumb, as well as an extender. The EPL over the carpus forms the ulnar boundary of the anatomic snuffbox, and the EPB and APL form the radial boundary. Pulsations of the superficial terminal branch of the radial artery can be palpated within the anatomic snuffbox.

The complex movement of the thumb should be examined in isolation and in composite movement. During examination of the thumb, attention must be paid to the thenar eminence, the first web space, and the resting position of the thumb. Atrophy, contractures, and abnormal resting positions are signs of musculoskeletal or neural compromise. The resting position of the thumb should be in the circumduction plane. Interruption of any of the three major nerves that supply the muscles of the thumb will affect the thumb's resting position. A median nerve palsy renders the thumb devoid of its intrinsic abduction and opposition. The APL muscle will take over some of the abduction properties of the first metacarpal, although this action is weakened. The thumb therefore takes on a position of adduction. The thenar eminence appears atrophied. Interruption of the ulnar nerve renders the thumb devoid of its intrinsic adductors (first dorsal interosseous muscle, adductor pollicis, and the deep head of the FPB).[85] Loss of the thumb intrinsic muscles creates an imbalance in the function of the extrinsic muscles, with loss of flexor stability. The patient compensates for this lack of adduction by utilizing the FPL and

index FDP. There is a characteristic flexion of the DIP and IP joints of these digits when attempting pinch (Froment's sign) (Figure 96-33).[26] The loss of thumb MCP stability results in hyperextension of this joint (Jeannes' sign).[39]

Posterior interosseous nerve palsy results in an inability of the thumb to extend. The unopposed activity of the FPL draws the MCP and IP joints into flexion. The adductors pull the thumb toward the index finger, leading to an adduction contracture.

The CMC, MCP, and IP joints are passively and actively put through range-of-motion exercises. The patient is asked to perform pulp-to-pulp pinch with each finger while the examiner observes the ease and extent of opposition (Figure 96-34). Each thumb function is tested in isolation. The APB is tested as the patient pushes against resistance while the thumb is in the abducted position (Figure 96-35). The opponens pollicis muscle is similarly tested with the thumb more circumducted (Figure 96-36). The adductors are evaluated as the patient pinches a paper between the thumb and index finger. Significant resistance should be observed when pulling the paper (Figure 96-37). The FPB function is assessed with the thumb MCP joint in flexion and resistance applied volarly

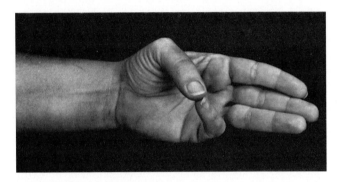

Figure 96-34. Opposition of the thumb is observed with pulp-to-pulp pinch of the thumb to each fingertip.

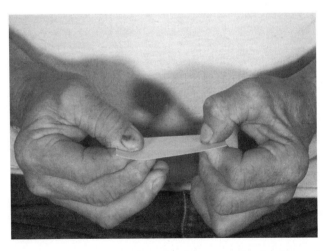

Figure 96-33. Froment's sign. Compensation for loss of strength in adduction is performed by overactivity of the FPL and index FDP.

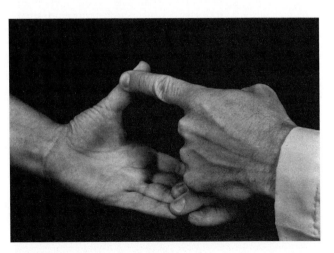

Figure 96-35. The APB muscle originates from the flexor retinaculum, scaphoid, and trapezium and inserts on the lateral side of the base of the proximal phalanx of the thumb. This muscle abducts the thumb and assists in opposition. In testing the APB, the patient pushes against resistance while the thumb is in an abducted position.

(Figure 96-38). The MCP joint of the thumb is stabilized in neutral, and the patient is asked to bend the IP joint against resistance to test FPL function (Figure 96-39).

The extensors are examined with the patient's hand palm down on the examining table. The thumb is actively extended. The EPL, EPB, and APL can be palpated as they define the anatomic snuffbox (Figure 96-40).[48] Each muscle tendon unit is then tested in isolation by applying resistance to the site immediately distal to the insertion of this tendon (Figure 96-41).

Occasionally there is an anomalous communication between the FPL and the FDP to the index finger. This may be a true communication with an aberrant tendon connecting

the FPL in the distal forearm to the index FDP (Lindburg).[49] A pseudocommunication may also occur. Occasionally, synovial hypertrophy between the FPL and index FDP tendons may simulate a true tendinous communication. In either case, these aberrant communications are observed as the patient flexes the distal phalanx of the thumb, producing an inadvertent flexion of the distal phalanx of the index finger. This may be a source of discomfort at the base of the thenar eminence or within the radial wrist. This communication is tested with the ulnar three digits stabilized as the patient opposes his or her thumb to the MCP joint of the little finger, producing flexion of the DIP joint of the index finger (Figure 96-42).

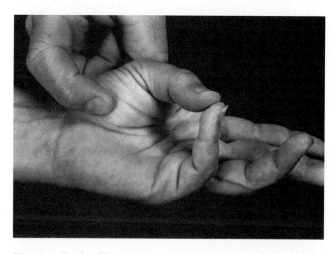

Figure 96-36. The opponens pollicis muscle originates from the flexor retinaculum and trapezium and inserts on the lateral half of the volar surface of the first metacarpal. The opponens pollicis muscle rotates the first metacarpal ulnarly into opposition. The muscle is tested against resistance with the thumb in a circumducted position.

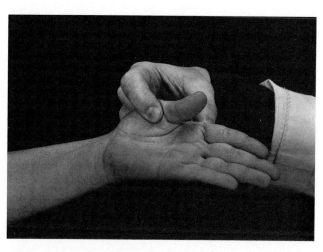

Figure 96-38. The FPB muscle originates from the flexor retinaculum, scaphoid bone, and trapezium and inserts onto the base of the proximal phalanx of the thumb, thereby acting to abduct the thumb and assist in opposition. The muscle is tested with the thumb MCP joint in flexion and resistance is applied volarly.

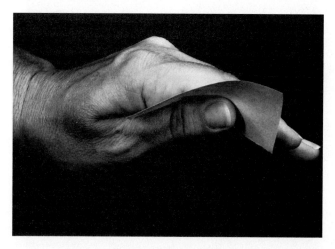

Figure 96-37. The thumb's adductors (first dorsal interosseous muscle, adductor pollicis, and the deep head of the FPB) are evaluated as the patient pinches paper between the thumb and index finger.

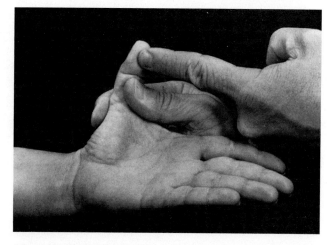

Figure 96-39. The FPL tendon is responsible for flexing the distal phalanx of the thumb. The MCP joint is stabilized as the patient flexes the IP joint.

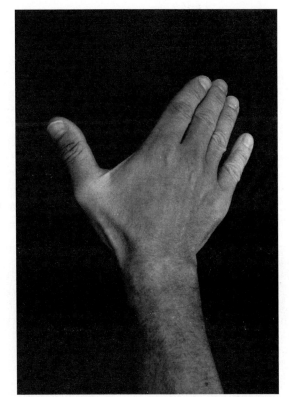

Figure 96-40. The anatomic snuffbox is defined by the APL and EPB radially and the EPL ulnarly.

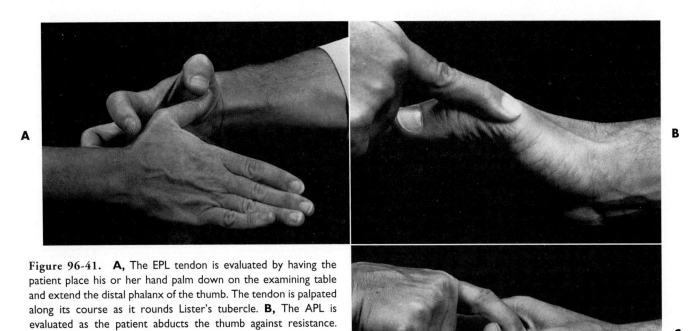

A

B

C

Figure 96-41. **A,** The EPL tendon is evaluated by having the patient place his or her hand palm down on the examining table and extend the distal phalanx of the thumb. The tendon is palpated along its course as it rounds Lister's tubercle. **B,** The APL is evaluated as the patient abducts the thumb against resistance. **C,** The EPB is examined by applying resistance to the dorsal aspect of the proximal phalanx while the patient attempts to extend the proximal phalanx.

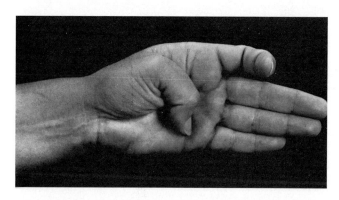

Figure 96-42. The anomalous communication between the FPL and the index FDP is tested as the examiner stabilizes the ulnar three digits. The patient opposes his thumb to the MCP joint of the little finger. Flexion of the distal phalanx of the index finger will be apparent if the anomalous communication exists.

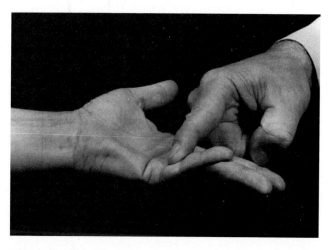

Figure 96-44. The flexor digiti quinti muscle originates from the hook of hamate and flexor retinaculum inserting on the base of the proximal phalanx of the little finger. This muscle flexes the little finger at the MCP joint and is tested by flexing the MCP joint.

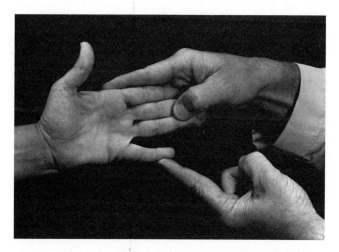

Figure 96-43. The abductor digiti quinti muscle originates from the pisiform bone and the pisohamate ligament inserting onto the base of the proximal phalanx and extensor expansion. The muscle acts to flex the MCP joint and abduct the little finger. Examination of the muscle is performed with the finger abducted against resistance.

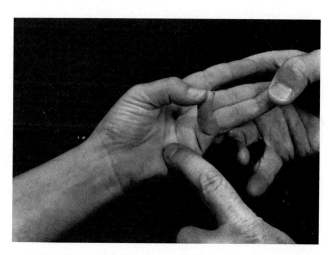

Figure 96-45. The opponens digiti minimi muscle originates from the hook of hamate and flexor retinaculum and inserts along the volar surface of the fifth metacarpal. The muscle radially rotates the fifth metacarpal. The opponens digiti minimi muscle is tested by performing a pulp-to-pulp pinch with the little finger to the thumb.

THE HYPOTHENAR MUSCLES

The hypothenar muscles form the ulnar palmar eminence in the hand, which is comprised of the abductor digiti minimi, flexor digiti minimi brevis, and the opponens digiti minimi.[61] Each muscle is innervated by the ulnar nerve. The abductor digiti minimi is responsible for abduction of the little finger and, to a minor degree, flexion at the MCP joint. The flexor digiti minimi brevis lies radial to the abductor digiti minimi. The flexor digiti minimi flexes the MCP joint. The opponens digiti minimi lies deep to the other two hypothenar muscles and flexes the fifth metacarpal while rotating it in a radial direction. The hypothenar muscles act

together to increase the convexity of the distal palm on gripping. The abductor digiti minimi is tested by placing the back of the patient's hand on the examining table while the little finger is abducted against resistance (Figure 96-43). The flexor digiti quinti is examined by flexing the MCP joint while the finger is adducted. The IP joints must be kept in extension (Figure 96-44). The opponens digiti minimi muscle is tested by performing a pulp-to-pulp pinch with the little finger to the thumb (Figure 96-45).

The palmaris brevis muscle is often a mere rudimentary muscle situated under the skin and subcutaneous tissue over the ulnar aspect of the carpal ligament and hypothenar eminence. The palmaris brevis originates from the flexor retinaculum and the palmar aponeurosis at the expansion of the palmaris brevis tendon. This muscle inserts into the dermis of the ulnar palm. The function is limited but the palmaris brevis may aid in deepening the convexity of the proximal palm during grip.[61] Adequate isolation of the muscle is difficult and the functional examination of the palmaris brevis is meaningless.

THE VASCULAR SYSTEM

The ulnar artery originates in the cubital fossa as the larger terminal branch of the brachial artery. The ulnar nerve is medial to the ulnar artery, which travels between the flexor digitorum sublimis and FDP muscles. The FCU muscles protect the neurovascular bundle medially until it enters Guyon's canal. The ulnar artery bifurcates into a deep and superficial branch at the distal end of Guyon's canal. The palmar branch travels through the hypothenar muscles to form the deep palmar arterial arch, which is the communicating vascular segment between the ulnar and radial arteries. The deep palmar arch lies palmar to the volar interosseous muscles at the level of the proximal metaphysis of the metacarpals.[88]

The radial artery arises in the cubital fossa as a smaller branch of the brachial artery. The artery travels between the brachioradialis and the supinator/flexor muscle mass, becoming more superficial in the distal forearm, lying just radial to the FCR tendon. A small, superficial branch continues to travel over the flexor retinaculum through the thenar muscles. This artery eventually merges with the superficial palmar vascular arch. The larger, deeper branch of the radial artery veers radiodorsally at the wrist, coursing under the APL, EPB, and the EPL tendons in the base of the anatomic snuffbox between the first and second metacarpals to eventually pierce through the two heads of the first dorsal interosseous muscle and the adductor muscle and merge with the deep palmar vascular arch. Perforating branches of the deep palmar arch travel between the metacarpals to the dorsum of the hand and are the communicating vascular supply that joins the ulnar and radial arteries at a level approximately 1.5 to 2 cm distal to the deep palmar arch. The superficial palmar arch lies superficial to the flexor digitorum sublimis and FDP tendons. Four common digital vessels arise from the superficial arch, which in turn bifurcates at the level of the MCP joints to supply corresponding radial and ulnar sides of adjacent digits.[16] The thumb receives its blood supply from branches of the radial artery as it passes through the first web space and occasionally from branches of the superficial arch.[3]

The hands and fingers are assessed for color, turgor, capillary refill, and trophic changes. Complete disruption of vascular inflow renders the skin white, cold, and devoid of capillary refill. Turgor is diminished. A blue, mottled finger

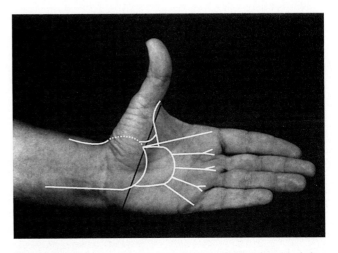

Figure 96-46. The location of the superficial palmar arch lies in a line between the base of the extended thumb to the point approximately 1 cm distal to the hook of hamate. The deep palmar arch is approximately 1.5 cm to 2 cm proximal to the superficial arch.

or hand with brisk capillary refill may indicate compromise of venous outflow or hyperactivity of the sympathetic nervous system. Chronic vascular insufficiency leads to loss of hair on the dorsum of the hand, shiny skin, atrophy of the fat pads, and nail-plate changes.

Examination of the radial and ulnar arteries includes palpation of pulses at the wrist. The digital vessels are usually palpable as well on the volar aspect of each side of the finger or thumb. The superficial palmar arch lies in a line between the base of the extended thumb to a point 1 cm distal to the hook of Hamate (Figure 96-46). The deep palmar arch is approximately 1.5 to 2 cm proximal to the superficial arch. The contribution of the radial and ulnar arteries to the vascularity of the hand is assessed by the Allen's test.[1] The integrity of the palmar vascular arch can also be evaluated with this test. The Allen's test is performed as the patient makes a tight fist. The radial and ulnar arteries are occluded by the examiner (Figure 96-47). The patient opens and closes the fist approximately four times to help exsanguinate the hand. The examiner keeps the radial artery occluded and releases the ulnar artery. This procedure is repeated by occluding the ulnar artery and releasing the radial artery. The return of blood flow into the hand and fingers is observed as a pink hyperemia. Normally, this should return within 3 to 5 seconds. Any delay in refilling is recorded, and any area with a lack of reperfusion may indicate a loss of continuity of the palmar vascular arches.

Ischemic changes, such as ulcerations, mottling, pain, and tenderness, may be the result of arterial occlusion, ectatic vessels, or endarteritis obliterans secondary to systemic autoimmune disorders such as Raynaud's disease or scleroderma. Ulnar hammer syndrome represents an occlusion of the ulnar artery within the palm (usually Guyon's canal). Pain and tenderness in the ulnar palm is the most common presentation. Ischemia of digits may also manifest, particularly if the ulnar

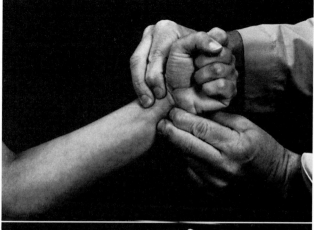

A

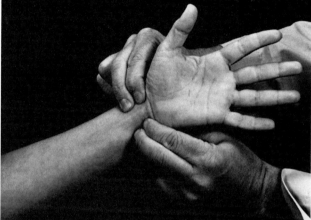

B

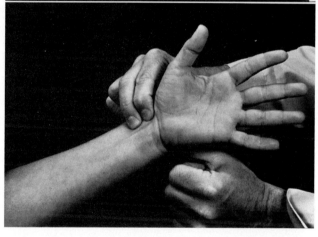

C

Figure 96-47. A, An Allen's test is performed by occluding both the radial and ulnar arteries with the hand in a clinched position. **B,** The patient is asked to open and shut the fist three or four times. The compression on the radial artery is released and the return of blood flow to the hand is observed. **C,** The procedure is performed again, this time releasing the ulnar artery compression first.

artery is the predominant artery supplying the fingers and there is a lack of continuity between the radial artery and the ulnar artery. Occlusion within the vascular arches of the palm may present similarly. Ancillary tests used to examine the hand's vascularity include Doppler studies, oximeters, angiograms, and cold immersion tests.

REFERENCES

1. Allen EV: Thromboangiitis obliterans: methods of diagnosis of chronic occlusive arterial lesions distal to the wrist, with illustrative cases, *Am J Med Sci* 178:237-244, 1929.

2. American Medical Association: Extremities, spine and pelvis. In *Guides to the evaluation of permanent impairment,* ed 14, Chicago, 1995, the Association.

3. Ames EL, Bissonette M, Acland R, et al: Arterial anatomy of the thumb, *J Hand Surg [Br]* 18:427-436, 1993.

4. Aschan W, Moberg E: The Ninhydrin fingerprint test used to map out partial lesions to hand nerves, *Acta Chir Scand* 123:365-370, 1962.

5. Ateshian GA, Rosenwasser MP, Mow VC: Curvature characteristics and congruence of the thumb carpometacarpal joint: differences between female and male joints, *J Biomech* 25(6): 591-607, 1992.

6. Bade H, Schubert M, Koebke J: Functional morphology of the deep transverse metacarpal ligament, *Anat Anz* 176(5):443-450, 1994.

7. Barmakion JT: Anatomy of the joints of the thumb, *Hand Clin* 8(4)683-691, 1992.

8. Bell-Krotoski JA: Advances in sensibility evaluation, *Hand Clin* 7:3, 1991.

9. Bell-Krotoski JA: Sensibility testing: current concepts in rehabilitation of the hand. In Hunter JM, Mackin EJ, Callahan AD (editors): *Rehabilitation of the hand: surgery and therapy,* ed 4, St. Louis, 1996, Mosby, pp 109-128.

10. Bell-Krotoski JA, Weinstein S, Weinstein C: Testing sensibility including touch-pressure, two-point discrimination, point localization and vibration, *J Hand Ther* 6(2):114-123, 1993.

11. Botte MJ, Cohen MS, Lavernia CJ, et al: The dorsal branch of the ulnar nerve: an anatomic study, *J Hand Surg [Am]* 15:603-607, 1990.

12. Boyes JH: The normal hand. In Boyes JH (editor): *Bunnell's surgery of the hand,* ed 5, Philadelphia, 1970, JB Lippincott.

13. Burton RI, Pellegrini VD: Surgical management of basal joint arthritis of the thumb. Part II. Ligament reconstruction with tendon interposition arthroplasty, *J Hand Surg [Am]* 11:324-332, 1986.

14. Callahan AD: Sensibility assessment: prerequisites and techniques for nerve lesions in continuity and nerve lacerations. In Hunter JM, Mackin EJ, Callahan AD (editors): *Rehabilitation of the hand: surgery and therapy,* ed 4, St. Louis, 1996, Mosby.

15. Cleland J: On the cutaneous ligaments of the phalanges, *J Anat Physio* 12:526, 1878.

16. Coleman SS, Anson BT: Arterial patterns in the hand based upon a study of 650 specimens, *Surg Gynecol Obstet* 113: 408,1961.

17. Cooney WP, An KN, Daube JR, Askew L: Electromyographic analysis of the thumb: a study of isometric forces in the pinch and grasp, *J Hand Surg [Am]* 10:202, 1985.

18. Cooney WP, Chao EYS: Biomechanical analysis of static forces in the hand during hand function, *J Bone Joint Surg* 59A:27, 1997.

19. Dahhan P, Fischer L, Alliey Y: The trapezoimetacarpal articulation, *Anat Clin* 2:43, 1980.

20. Dellon AL: *Evaluation of sensibility and re-education of sensation in the hand,* Baltimore, 1981, Williams & Wilkins.

21. Dellon AL: The vibrometer, *Plast Reconstr Surg* 71:427-431, 1983.

22. Dellon AL, MacKinnon SE, Brosby P: Reliability of two-point discrimination measurements, *J Hand Surg [Am]* 12:693-696, 1987.

23. Dellon ES, Mourey R, Dellon AL: Human pressure perception values for constant and moving one-and two-point discrimination, *Plast Reconstr Surg* 90:112, 1992.

24. Dray GI, Eaton RG: Dislocations and ligament injuries in the digits. In Green SP (editor): *Operative hand surgery,* ed 2, New York, Churchill Livingstone,1988.

25. Eaton RG, Littler JW: A study of the basal joint of the thumb, *J Bone Joint Surg* 51A:661, 1969.

26. Froment J: Paralysie des muscles de la main et troubles de la prehension, *J Med Lyon,* 1920.

27. Gelberman RH, Szabo RM, Williamson RV, Dimick MP: Sensibility testing in peripheral nerve compression syndromes, *J Bone Joint Surg* 65A:632, 1983.

28. Gosset J: Dupuytren's disease and the anatomy of palmodigital aponeurosis. In Hueston J, Tubiana R (editors): *Dupuytren's disease,* ed 2, Edinburgh, 1985, Churchill Livingstone.

29. Grapow M: Die anatomic und physiologische betentung der palmar aponourose, *Archiv far anatomic and physiologie leipzig, anatomiscle abtheilung* 2-3:143-158, 1887.

30. Grayson J: The cutaneous ligaments of the digits, *J Anat* 75:164, 1941.

31. Gupta R, Allen F, Tan V, et al: The effect of shear stress on fibroblasts derived from Dupuytren's tissue and normal palmar fascia, *J Hand Surg [Am]* 23(5):945-950, 1998.

32. Guyon F: Note sur une disposition anatomique progare a la face onterieure de la region di poignet et non encore decrite par le decteur, *Bull Soc Anat Paris* 6:184-186, 1861.

33. Holguin PH, Rico AA, Gomez LP, Munuera LM: The coordinate movement of the interphalangeal joints: a cinematic study, *Clin Orthop* 362:117-124, 1999.

34. Holland AJ, McGouther DA: Dupuytren's disease and the relationship between the transverse and longitudinal fibers of the palmar fascia: a dissection study, *Clin Anat* 10:97-103, 1997.

35. Hollister A, Buford WL, Myers LM, et al: The axes of rotation of the thumb carpometacarpal joint, *J Orthop Res* 10(3):454-460, 1992.

36. Horch K, Hardy M, Jimenez S, et al: An automated tester for evaluation of cutaneous sensibility, *J Hand Surg [Am]* 17:829-837, 1992.

37. Imaeda T, An KN, Cooney WP: Functional anatomy and biomechanics of the thumb, *Hand Clin* 8(1)9-16, 1992.

38. Jakubovic HR, Ackerman AB: Structure and function of skin: development, morphology, and physiology. In Moschella SL, Hurley HJ (editors): *Dematology,* ed 3, Philadelphia, 1992, WB Saunders.

39. Jeanne: La deformation du pouce dans la paralyse du cubital, *Bulliten et Memoires de la societe churgical de Paris* 703-719, 1915.

40. Kapandji AI: Clinical evaluation of the thumb's opposition, *J Hand Ther* 5:102-106, 1992.

41. Kaplan EB: Anatomy and kinesiology of the hand. In Flynn JE (editor): *Hand surgery,* ed 2, Philadelphia, 1975, Williams & Wilkins.

42. Ketchum LD, Thompson D, Peacock G, et al: Forces generated by intrinsic muscles of the index finger, *J Hand Surg* 2:571, 1978.

43. Kuczynski K: CMC joint of the human thumb, *J Anat* 118:119, 1974.

44. Kuczynski K: The thumb and the saddle, *Hand* 7:120, 1975.

45. Landsmeer JMF: *Atlas of anatomy of the hand,* Edinburgh, 1976, Churchill Livingstone.

46. Landsmeer JMF: The coordination of finger joint motion, *J Bone Joint Surg* 45A:1654-1662, 1963.

47. Legueu F, Juvara E: Des aponevrosis de la paume de la main, *Bull Soc Anat Paris* 6:383-400, 1892.

48. Lindburg RM, Comstock BE: Anomalous tendon slips from the flexor pollicis longus to the flexor digitorum profundus, *J Hand Surg* 4(1),79-83, 1979.

49. Lister G: *The hand: diagnosis and indications,* ed 3, Edinburgh, 1993, Churchill Livingstone.

50. Littler JW: The physiology and dynamic function of the hand, *Surg Clin North Am* 4:259, 1960.

51. Lu TW, O'Connor JJ: Bone position estimation from skin marker coordinates using global optimisation with joint constraints, *J Biomech* 32(2):129-134, 1999.

52. Mackinnon SE, Dellon AL: Two-point discrimination tester, *J Hand Surg [Am]* 10:906, 1985.

53. Mackinnon SE, Dellon AL: Diagnosis of nerve injury. In *Surgery of the peripheral nerve,* New York, 1988, Thieme Medical Publishers.

54. Manske P, Lester P: Palmar aponeurosis pulley, *J Hand Surg* 8:259-265, 1983.

55. Martin JH: Somatic sensory system I: receptor physiology and submodality coding. In Kandel ER, Schwarz JH (editors): *Principles of neural science,* North-Holland, 1982, Elsevier.

56. McFarlane RM, Mayer JR, Hugill JV: Further observations on the anatomy of the ulnar nerve at the wrist, *Hand* 8:115, 1976.

57. McGouther D: The microanatomy of Dupuytren's contracture, *The Hand* 14:215-236, 1982.

58. Milford LW: *Retaining ligaments of the digits of the hand,* Philadelphia, 1968, WB Saunders.

59. Moberg E: Objective methods for determining the functional value of sensibility in the hand, *J Bone Joint Surg* 40A:454-476, 1958.

60. Moldaver J: Tinel's sign: its characteristics and significance, *J Bone Joint Surg* 60A:412-413, 1978.

61. Moore KL: *Clinically oriented anatomy,* ed 2, Baltimore, 1985, Williams & Wilkins.

62. Nelson DL: The importance of the physical examination, *Hand Clin* 13(1):13-15, 1997.

63. O'Rain S: New and simple test of nerve function in the hand, *Br Med J* 22:612, 1973.

64. Pellegrini VD: Osteoarthritis of the trapeziometacarpal joint: the pathophysiology of articular cartilage degeneration. Part I. Anatomy and physiology of the aging joint, *J Hand Surg [Am]* 16:967-974, 1991.

65. Perry JF, Hamilton GF, Lachenbruch PA, et al: Protective sensation in the hand and its correlation to the Ninhydrin sweat test following nerve laceration, *Am J Phys Med* 53:133, 1974.

66. Phalen GS: Spontaneous compression of the median nerve at the wrist, *JAMA* 145:1128, 1951.

67. Phelps P, Walker E: Comparison of the finger wrinkling test results to established sensory tests in peripheral nerve injury, *Am J Occup Ther* 31:9, 1977.

68. Rosen B: Recovery of sensory and motor function after nerve repair: a rationale for evaluation, *J Hand Ther* 9(4):315-327, 1996.

69. Ryan GM: Palmar fascial complex anatomy and pathology in Dupuytren's disease, *Hand Clin* (2)15:1, 73-86, 1999.

70. Ryan GM, Murray D, Chung K, et al: The extensor retinacular system at the metacarpophalangeal joint: anatomical and histological study, *J Hand Surg [BR]* 22:585-590, 1997.

71. Schulz LA, Bohannon RW, Morgan WJ: Normal digit tip values for the Weinstein enhanced sensory test, *J Hand Ther* 11(3):200-205, 1998.

72. Skoog T: The transverse elements of the palmar aponeurosis in Dupuytren's contracture, *Scand J Plast Reconstr Surg* 1:51, 1967.

73. Smith RJ: Intrinsic contracture. In Green DP (editor): *Green's operative hand surgery,* ed 2, New York, 1988, Churchill Livingstone.

74. Srinivasan H: Patterns of movement of the totally intrinsic-minus fingers, *J Bone Joint Surg* 58A(6):777-791, 1976.

75. Stacke HG: *The palmar fascia,* Edinburgh, 1973, Churchill Livingstone.

76. Sunderland S, Bradley KC: Rate of advance of Hohmann-Tinel sign in regenerating nerves, *Arch Neurol Physchiat* 62:650, 1952.

77. Takagoshi H, et al: Fibrous structure and connection surrounding the metacarpophalangeal joint, *Acta Med Okayama* 52(1): 19-26, 1998.

78. Tinel J: The "tingling" sign in peripheral nerve lesions, *Presse Med* 47:388, 1915.

79. Tomaino MH, Pellegrini VD, Burton RI: Arthroplasty of the basal joint of the hand, *J Bone Joint Surg* 77A(3):346-355, 1995.

80. Tubiana R, Thomine JM, Mackin E: *The examination of the hand and wrist,* St. Louis, 1996, Mosby.

81. Valentin P: The interossei and lumbrical. In Tubiana R (editor): *The hand,* vol 2, Philadelphia, 1985, WB Saunders.

82. Vallbo AB, Joansson RS: The tactile sensory innervation of the glabrous skin of the human hand. In Gordon G (editor): *Active touch,* Oxford, 1978, Pergamon Press.

83. Verdan C: Syndrome of the quadrigia, *Surg Clin North Am* 40:425, 1960.

84. Wartenberg R: Cheiralgia paresthetica (isolierte neuritis des ramus superficialis nerve radialis), *Z Ges Neurol Psychiatr* 141:145-155, 1932.

85. Wartenberg R: A sign of ulnar palsy, *JAMA* 112:16-88, 1938.

86. Waylett-Randall J: Sensibility evaluation and rehabilitation, *Orthop Clin North Am* 19:1,43-56, 1988.

87. Weinstein S: Fifty years of somatosensory research: from Semmes-Weinstein monofilaments to the Weinstein Enhanced Sensory Test, *J Hand Ther* 6:11-22, 1993.

88. Weinzweig N, Starker I, Sharzer L, Fleegler E: Revisitation of the vascular anatomy of the lumbrical and interosseous muscles, *Plast Reconstr Surg* 99(3)785-790, 1997.

89. Winklemann RK: Nerve endings in normal and pathologic skin, Springfield, Ill, 1960, Charles C. Thomas.

90. Zrubecky G: *Die hand, das tastorgan des menschen,* Stuttgart, 1960, Ferdinand Enke.

CHAPTER 97

Anesthesia for Hand Surgery

Aisling Conran
Madelyn D. Kahana

INTRODUCTION

Anesthetic options for hand surgery include intravenous (IV) sedation combined with a local field block, regional neural blockade, or general anesthesia. The risks, benefits, and contraindications for these choices are presented, as is a review of the neuroanatomy and the sensory distribution of the brachial plexus. Toxic doses of local anesthetics and signs and symptoms of an accidental intravascular injection are discussed. Supplemental peripheral nerve blocks, necessary when a regional anesthetic is incomplete, are also described.

REGIONAL VERSUS GENERAL ANESTHESIA

The choice of anesthesia is based on the patient's comorbid medical conditions, his or her informed consent for the general or regional anesthetic, and the site and length of the planned surgery. A history of coronary artery disease, congestive heart failure, significant chronic obstructive pulmonary disease (COPD), or renal or hepatic dysfunction will influence the choice of regional versus general anesthesia.[13,14,16] Children and adults who lack the emotional maturity to cooperate with placement of a regional block require a general anesthetic.

Monitored anesthesia care with supplemental local anesthesia is appropriate for consenting patients whose surgical pain can be controlled with a digital or field block (Figure 97-1). This is a good option in the emergent patient with a full stomach, for whom little or no sedation is given. Moderate levels of sedation that are appropriate for a patient who has fasted will increase the risk of aspiration in a patient who has not fasted.

REGIONAL ANESTHESIA OF THE ARM AND HAND

Regional anesthesia of the arm and hand consists of either intravenous regional anesthesia (a Bier block) or brachial plexus blockade, which may be performed at various levels

(Table 97-1). Each technique has specific advantages and disadvantages. The site of surgery, the ability of the patient to comfortably position the affected arm, and the possible complications of the individual block determine the optimal procedure in a given patient. The use of a tourniquet also needs to be considered when making this decision.

An understanding of the anatomy of the brachial plexus is necessary to effectively perform regional blocks on patients (Figure 97-2). The plexus is divided into roots, trunks, divisions, cords, and peripheral nerves based on anatomic landmarks. The roots include C5 to C8, T1, and variably C4 and/or T2. The trunks—superior, middle, and inferior—are arranged in a vertical fashion between the anterior and middle scalene muscles. Each trunk divides at the lateral edge of the first rib to form anterior and posterior divisions. These divisions pass posterior to the midportion of the clavicle. The cords are found within the axilla. The cords are formed by combinations of the above divisions and are named for their relationship to the axillary artery. The anterior divisions of the superior and middle trunks form the lateral cord. The posterior divisions of all three trunks become the posterior cord. The anterior division of the inferior trunk forms the medial cord. As the cords pass the lateral border of the pectoralis minor muscle they divide into the peripheral nerves. The lateral cord gives rise to the musculocutaneous nerve and a portion of the median nerve. The medial cord produces a contribution to the median nerve and gives rise to the ulnar, medial antebrachial, and medial brachial cutaneous nerves. The posterior cord becomes the radial and axillary nerves (Figure 97-3).

An axillary block is frequently performed for hand and forearm surgery. An easily identified landmark—the axillary artery—and a reliable orientation of the nerves around the artery aid in performing this procedure accurately. Safety is also an advantage of this technique. The patient, however, must be able to abduct the arm for the block to be performed. Hyperabduction may decrease the sensation of the axillary arterial pulse secondary to occlusion by the humeral head. The axillary block may be performed with a transarterial approach, a nerve stimulator, paresthesias, or a multiple-injection technique.[9,10] The radial nerve is posterior to the axillary artery, the ulnar nerve is inferior, and the median nerve is superior (Figure 97-4).

Typically, 40 ml of local anesthetic is used for the block. The musculocutaneous nerve is sometimes missed with this approach to the brachial plexus because this nerve leaves the sheath before it enters the axilla. The musculocutaneous nerve may be blocked by injecting 5 ml of local anesthetic into the body of the coracobrachialis muscle. Tourniquet pain may be covered by blocking the intercostobrachial nerve (T2 innervation) via an extended skin wheal overlying the

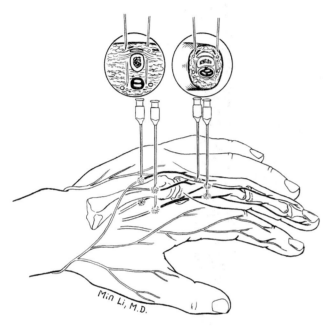

Figure 97-1. Digital nerve block; techniques at base of finger and between metacarpals.

axillary artery. As with any nerve block, hematoma and infection are risks, but they are rare complications. The ease of compressing the axillary artery contributes to the low level of this complication.[2,3,15]

The supraclavicular block can be performed without abduction of the arm and provides excellent anesthesia for elbow, forearm, and hand surgery. The brachial plexus is made up of vertically arranged trunks at this level so that none of the peripheral nerves has left the sheath. Paresthesias may be elicited or a nerve stimulator technique is utilized. Pneumothorax occurs in 0.5% to 0.6% of patients, and symptoms may not occur until hours after block placement. Patients with significant respiratory disease may not tolerate this complication, and therefore this block should not be performed in these patients.

The neurovascular bundle is identified at the midpoint of the clavicle, where it is sandwiched between the clavicle and the first rib. The patient should be supine, with the head turned away. The arm on which surgery is to be performed should be adducted, with the hand extended to the ipsilateral knee. Several landmarks are important for use of the brachial plexus block: identification of the midpoint of the clavicle, the posterior border of the sternocleidomastoid (SCM) (identified by having the patient raise his or her head), and the interscalene groove (identified by palpating the posterior border of the SCM and then rolling the palpating fingers over the anterior scalene muscle into the groove), and palpation of the subclavian artery (Figure 97-5). Typically 30 ml of local anesthetic is needed to complete this block.[15]

The infraclavicular approach offers the advantages of a supraclavicular block: providing blockade of the musculocutaneous and axillary nerves with a much lower incidence of pneumothorax. The arm may be in any position, which is an advantage in a patient with a painful fracture or arthritis. No

Table 97-1.
Neural Blockade of the Upper Extremity

BLOCK/SITE OF SURGERY	ADVANTAGES	NERVE MOST LIKELY MISSED	COMPLICATIONS & PROBLEMS
Axillary block/hand, forearm	Ease, safety, reliability	Musculocutaneous	Intravascular injection
Supraclavicular/hand, forearm, elbow	Arm in any position		0.5% pneumothorax, 46%-60% phrenic nerve block
Infraclavicular/hand, forearm, elbow	Blocks musculocutaneous and axillary nerves reliably		Increased risk of intravascular injection
Bier block/hand, forearm	Ease of administration, rapid recovery, rapid onset, muscle relaxation, controllable		Accidental or early deflation of tourniquet may lead to intravascular injection, tourniquet pain, postoperative pain; necessary to exsanguinate painful extremity

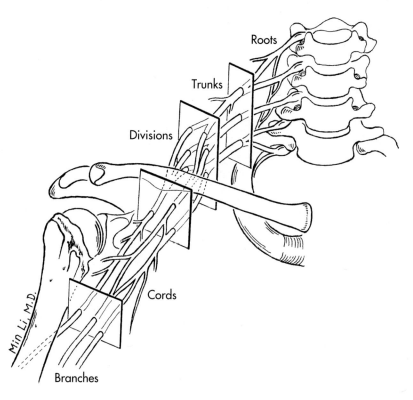

Figure 97-2. Roots, trunks, divisions, cords, and branches of the brachial plexus.

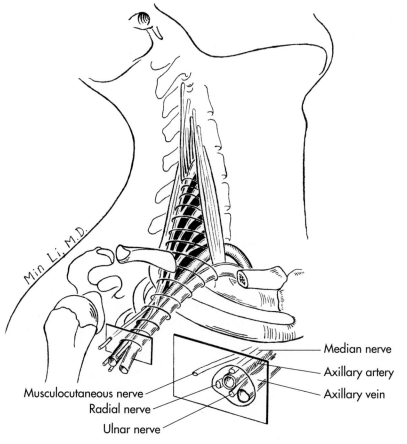

Figure 97-3. Brachial plexus sheath with cross-sectional anatomy at the level of the axillary nerve block.

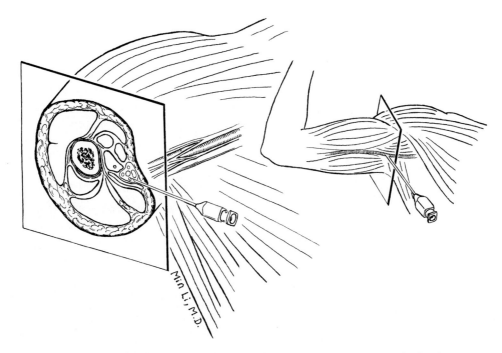

Figure 97-4. Axillary nerve block; needle insertion and anatomy at this level.

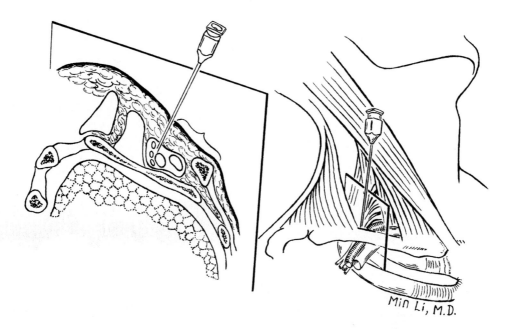

Figure 97-5. Anatomy and technique of the supraclavicular block.

palpable landmarks necessitates the use of a nerve stimulator in the performance of this block, which is done 2 cm inferior to the midpoint of the clavicle and directing the needle laterally (Figure 97-6). Again, 30 ml of local anesthetic is required to perform a successful block.[3,15]

The Bier block, named for German surgeon August Bier, has many advantages, including ease of administration, reproducibility, muscle relaxation, and rapid onset and recovery. This block has a duration of approximately 90 minutes. The block is performed through an IV catheter placed distally in the operative arm. Another IV catheter is required in a separate extremity for fluids, sedation, antibiotics, and other medications. The arm is exsanguinated and the tourniquet inflated. The local anesthetic, 4 to 6 mg/kg of 0.5% lidocaine without epinephrine, is administered slowly. The onset of anesthesia is about 5 minutes.[15] The normal single dose of lidocaine is 200 mg (60 ml).

Problems with the Bier block include the risk of intravascular spread of local anesthetic with early (<25 minutes) or accidental release of the tourniquet. The use of large volumes

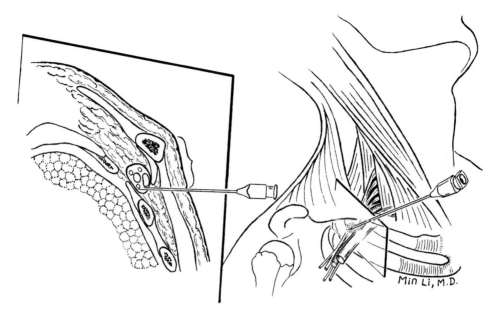

Figure 97-6. Landmarks and technique of the infraclavicular block.

of local anesthetics increases the possibility of a toxic dose. The use of bupivacaine is *not recommended* for IV regional anesthesia because of cardiovascular toxicity. Tourniquet pain can be a problem, usually after 1 hour, but can be mitigated by the use of a double tourniquet. When tourniquet pain occurs, the distal cuff is inflated over anesthetized skin and only then is the proximal tourniquet deflated. This technique ensures maintenance of the block while providing another 30 to 40 minutes free of tourniquet pain. The rapid recovery from the Bier block, advantageous to the ambulatory surgical patient, can be problematic if another source of pain control is not instituted early in the postoperative period. The necessity of exsanguinating a painful extremity is a distinct disadvantage of this block.[3,15]

The interscalene block provides excellent anesthesia for shoulder surgery because it also blocks the cervical plexus. This block, however, frequently misses the ulnar nerve and therefore it is largely inadequate for hand surgery.[3,15]

Blocks should be tested before the performance of surgery. The sensory innervation of the hand is made up of three nerves: radial, ulnar, and median. The radial nerve innervates the radial dorsum of the hand and the dorsum of the thumb, index, and middle fingers, as well as the radial half of the ring finger up to the distal interphalangeal (DIP) joints. The median nerve provides sensation to the nail beds and palmar surface of these fingers. The ulnar nerve provides sensation to the ulnar half on both the palmar and dorsal surfaces of the ring finger and the entire sensation of the little finger (Figure 97-7). Blockade of the specific nerves can be demonstrated by testing the skin in the areas described above, or the motor innervation of these peripheral nerves may be examined. A block of the musculocutaneous nerve is demonstrated by having the patient flex his biceps. The patient's inability to perform this task indicates that the musculocutaneous nerve is

blocked. If the patient is unable to extend at the elbow, the radial nerve, which provides innervation to the triceps, is blocked. The radial nerve also provides the innervation for supination and extension of the wrist and fingers (Figure 97-8, *A-B*). Having the patient oppose his or her thumb and little finger demonstrates the innervation by the ulnar nerve, as does flexion of the wrist and adduction of all fingers (Figure 97-8, *B-C*). If the patient is able to touch his or her thumb to the index finger, the median innervation is intact.[3]

If, after testing the block, it becomes apparent that one peripheral nerve was missed, supplemental peripheral nerve blocks may be performed (Table 97-2). The radial, median, and ulnar nerves may be supplemented at both the wrist or elbow. The risk of intraneural injection is increased with peripheral blockade, in which 3 to 5 ml of local anesthetic is injected in the immediate vicinity of the peripheral nerve. The radial nerve at the elbow is found at the anterior aspect of the lateral epicondyle, lateral to the biceps tendon. A field block is performed at the wrist of the multiple peripheral branches of the radial nerve at the base of the extensor pollicis longus tendon (2 ml) and then with 1 ml across the "anatomic snuffbox" (Figure 97-9). The median nerve may be blocked at the elbow where it is medial to the brachial artery, with the artery medial to the biceps tendon. The median nerve may be blocked at the wrist between the flexor carpi radialis and palmaris longus tendons, approximately 2 cm from the palm. The ulnar nerve is located posterior to the medial epicondyle (Figure 97-10, *A*). Injection of local anesthetic at this site, however, can produce neuritis, and therefore it is recommended that the injection of 3 to 5 ml of local anesthetic be made at a point 3 to 5 cm proximal to the elbow. The ulnar nerve may also be blocked on the radial side of the flexor carpi ulnaris tendon (Figure 97-10, *B*). Because anesthesia is

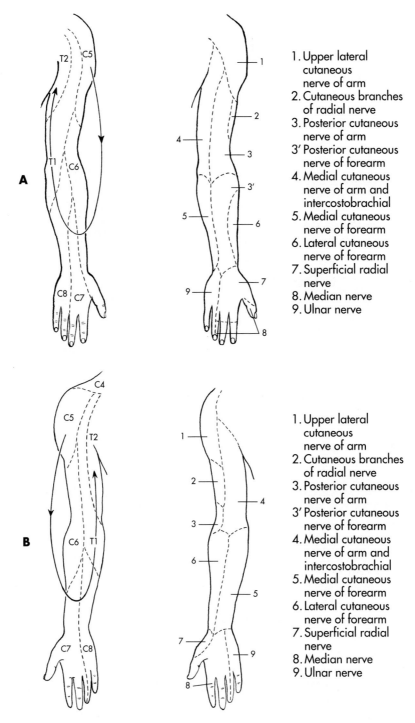

1. Upper lateral
   cutaneous
   nerve of arm
2. Cutaneous branches
   of radial nerve
3. Posterior cutaneous
   nerve of arm
3' Posterior cutaneous
   nerve of forearm
4. Medial cutaneous
   nerve of arm and
   intercostobrachial
5. Medial cutaneous
   nerve of forearm
6. Lateral cutaneous
   nerve of forearm
7. Superficial radial
   nerve
8. Median nerve
9. Ulnar nerve

1. Upper lateral
   cutaneous
   nerve of arm
2. Cutaneous branches
   of radial nerve
3. Posterior cutaneous
   nerve of arm
3' Posterior cutaneous
   nerve of forearm
4. Medial cutaneous
   nerve of arm and
   intercostobrachial
5. Medial cutaneous
   nerve of forearm
6. Lateral cutaneous
   nerve of forearm
7. Superficial radial
   nerve
8. Median nerve
9. Ulnar nerve

Figure 97-7. A and **B,** Cutaneous nerve supply of the upper extremity.

provided *only* to the hand when peripheral nerve blocks are performed at the wrist or elbow, and because the wrist block is simpler and more effective, the wrist location is preferred.[3,15]

LOCAL ANESTHETIC PHARMACOLOGY

The injection site, dose, addition of a vasoconstricting agent, and the pharmacologic properties of the drug determine systemic absorption of the local anesthetic.

A comparison of blood concentrations of local anesthetics after various sites of administration reveals the highest peak levels after intercostal blocks, followed in decreasing order by caudal, epidural, and brachial plexus blocks, and subcutaneous injections.[12] The maximum blood level of local anesthetic drugs is also related to the total dose of drug administered for any particular block, and for most drugs this relationship is linear. Epinephrine (5 μg/ml) decreases the rate of absorption of the local anesthetic because it causes vasoconstriction. This is particularly true with brachial plexus blockade.[13,14]

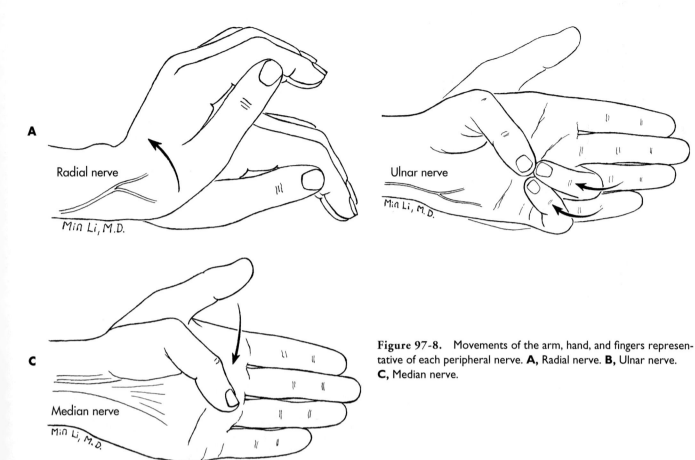

Figure 97-8. Movements of the arm, hand, and fingers representative of each peripheral nerve. **A,** Radial nerve. **B,** Ulnar nerve. **C,** Median nerve.

Table 97-2.
Peripheral Nerve Blocks

NERVE	ELBOW	WRIST	SENSATION
Radial	Anterior aspect of the lateral epicondyle, lateral to the biceps tendon	Base of the extensor pollicis longus tendon and across the "anatomic snuffbox"	Lateral aspect of the dorsum of the hand (thumb side), proximal portion of the thumb, index, middle, and lateral half of the ring fingers
Median	Medial to brachial artery, which is medial to biceps tendon	Between carpi radialis and palmaris longus tendon	Palmar aspects of thumb, index, middle, and radial half of the ring finger
Ulnar	Posterior to the medial epicondyle, 3-5 cm proximal	Radial side of the carpi ulnaris tendon	Ulnar side of the hand, little, and ring fingers

There are two classes of local anesthetics: esters and amides. Esters undergo hydrolysis in the plasma by pseudocholinesterase, whereas amides undergo hepatic degradation. Patient age also influences the metabolism of these drugs. The half-life of lidocaine is 80 minutes in volunteers ages 22 to 26, but 138 minutes in persons ages 61 to 71.[13] Newborn infants have immature hepatic enzyme systems and prolonged elimination of lidocaine and bupivacaine. Patients with poor liver function or decreased hepatic blood flow, including patients with congestive heart failure, will have a significantly prolonged half-life of amide local anesthetics.[13]

Systemic reactions to local anesthetics primarily involve the central nervous (CNS) and cardiovascular (CVS) systems. The CNS is generally more sensitive to local anesthetic toxicity and,

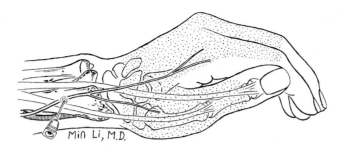

Figure 97-9. Landmarks and needle insertion for the radial nerve block at the wrist.

as such, reactions will be clinically apparent there first. The more potent the local anesthetic, the more likely it will induce CNS toxicity. Hypercarbia, hypoxia, and acidosis will decrease the seizure threshold in the brain and enhance the likelihood of CNS toxicity. Using the lowest dose (minimum concentration and volume) for the desired block also aids in reducing this risk.[5] The patient who develops CNS toxicity may experience dizziness, light-headedness, tinnitus, circumoral numbness, metallic taste in the mouth, loss of consciousness, muscular twitching, and convulsions. These signs of CNS excitation are then followed by signs of CNS depression, respiratory

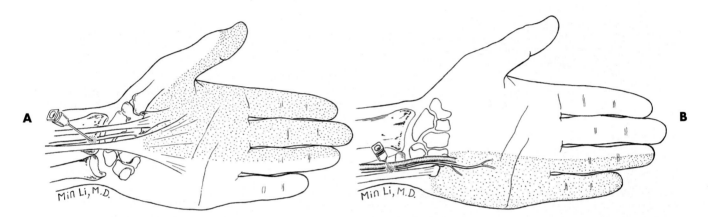

Figure 97-10. Landmarks and needle insertion for median **(A)** and ulnar **(B)** nerve blocks at the wrist.

Table 97-3.
Local Anesthetics: Toxic Doses

TYPE OF LOCAL ANESTHETIC	DRUG	MAXIMAL SINGLE DOSE (ADULTS)	MAXIMAL DOSE/KG (~60 KG)	ONSET	DURATION (MINUTES)	CC:CNS DOSE RATIO
Esters	Tetracaine	100 mg	2.5 mg/kg	Slow	60-180	
Amides	Lidocaine (with epinephrine)	300 mg 500 mg	5 mg/kg 7 mg/kg	Rapid	60-120	7.1 ± 1.1
	Mepivacaine (with epinephrine)	400 mg 500 mg	7 mg/kg 8.3 mg/kg	Slow	90-180	
	Bupivacaine	175 mg	3 mg/kg	Slow	240-480	3.7 ± 0.5
	Ropivacaine	250 mg	4 mg/kg	Slow	300-480	

Data from Stoelting RK: Local anesthetics. In *Pharmacology and physiology in anesthetic practice*, ed 2, Philadelphia, 1991, JB Lippincott, p 150; ropivacaine information from package insert; per kg and mepivacaine dosing from Bonica JJ: Regional analgesia/anesthesia. In *The management of pain*, Philadelphia, 1990, Lea & Febiger, p 1890; epinephrine dosing from Covino BG: Clinical pharmacology of local anesthetic agents. In Cousins MJ, Bridenbaugh PO (editors): *Neural blockade*, ed 2, St. Louis, 1988, JB Lippincott, p 112.

depression, and respiratory arrest.[11] Even low plasma concentrations of local anesthetics are associated with restlessness, vertigo, tinnitus, numbness of the tongue, and circumoral numbness. With moderate local anesthetic plasma concentrations, there is slurred speech and skeletal muscle twitching. High plasma concentrations result in convulsions, coma, and cardiorespiratory arrest.[5,6]

Constant communication with the patient will aid in recognition of this developing complication. If toxicity is suspected, one *must* stop injecting the local anesthetic and begin to assess and support the airway, breathing, and circulation. Benzodiazepines or sodium thiopental (50 to 100 mg intravenously) will treat seizure activity.[1,6,8,12,13]

Local anesthetics also decrease the rate of firing of the Purkinje fibers and ventricular muscle because of a decrease in the availability of fast sodium channels. The rate of recovery from this decrease is slower with bupivacaine than with lidocaine. Local anesthetics prolong conduction time in the heart and produce a long PR interval and a widened QRS complex. Extremely high concentrations of local anesthetics will depress the sinus node, leading to sinus bradycardia and ultimately sinus arrest. In addition to their effects on the fast sodium channels, local anesthetics also exert a direct myocardial depressant action that is dose dependent. Bupivacaine can produce ventricular fibrillation and other arrhythmias secondary to inhibition of fast sodium channels and slow calcium channels.[4,6] The cardiovascular collapse to CNS toxic dose ratio (CC:CNS) has been calculated for both lidocaine and bupivacain (Table 97-3). The dose of lidocaine required to produce cardiovascular collapse in sheep is seven times that needed to produce CNS toxicity. The CC:CNS dose ratio for bupivacaine is about half of that of lidocaine. That is, the dose of bupivacaine required for cardiovascular collapse in sheep is only about 3.5 times the dose needed to produce signs of CNS toxicity, a much narrower window of safety than is seen with lidocaine.[6] The same is thought to be true in humans.

Ropivacaine, a long-acting local anesthetic like bupivacaine, was developed to be more cardioprotective than bupivacaine. The reversal of the fast sodium channel blockade is shorter with ropivacaine than with bupivacaine. In addition, intravenous ropivacaine is cleared more quickly than intravenous bupivacaine. Both factors suggest decreased toxicity with ropivacaine as compared with bupivacaine, but current data are limited.

The toxicity of local anesthetics is additive, not synergistic. This is an important concept to remember because local anesthetics are often combined to take advantage of other pharmacokinetic properties. For example, with its rapid onset chloroprocaine is sometimes combined with bupivacaine, which has a prolonged duration of action.

In addition to their toxic effects, it is important to remember that ester local anesthetics may produce allergic reactions because they are derivatives of para-aminobenzoic acid (PABA), a known allergen, or contain a preservative, methylparaben, whose chemical structure is similar to PABA. Both PABA and methylparaben are thought to be offending agents. Allergy to amide local anesthetics is rare. Adverse reactions to local anesthetics are often the result of high plasma concentrations or the rapid absorption of epinephrine in the local anesthetic rather than a true allergic reaction. If a patient does have an allergy to a local anesthetic, he will have cross-sensitivity to other drugs in the same class. For example, an allergy to procaine, an ester, will place the patient at risk for an allergic reaction to tetracaine, also an ester, but not necessarily to bupivacaine, an amide local anesthetic.[12]

SUMMARY

Brachial plexus blockade is beneficial in the ambulatory surgical patient because the patient's postoperative pain is also well controlled. A successful regional block will provide hours of postoperative analgesia. In addition, patients with a regional block are able to resume enteral intake more quickly than those who are given a general anesthetic, facilitating their tolerance of oral pain medications and their discharge home.

An IV technique and regional brachial plexus blocks are effective in providing anesthesia of the hand for surgery. Appropriate blocks include the Bier block; axillary, supraclavicular, and infraclavicular blocks; and peripheral nerve blocks. Each block has individual advantages and disadvantages and is not without potential complications. Toxicity with local anesthetics may occur with these blocks secondary to the large drug doses (volumes and/or concentrations) used. Particular attention needs to be paid when these blocks are placed in small adults (<50 kg) or children.

REFERENCES

1. Auroy YA, Narchi P, Messiah A, et al: Serious complications related to regional anesthesia, *Anesthesiology* 87(3):479-486, 1997.
2. Bonica JJ: *The management of pain,* Philadelphia, 1990, Lea & Febiger, p 1890.
3. Bridenbaugh LD: The upper extremity somatic blockade. In Cousins MJ, Bridenbaugh PO (editors): *Neural blockade in clinical anesthia and management of pain,* ed 2, Philadelphia, 1988, JB Lippincott.
4. Bruelle P, Lefrant J, de la Coussaye JE, et al: Comparative electrophysiologic and hemodynamic effects of several amide local anesthetic drugs in anesthetized dogs, *Anesth Analg* 82:648-656, 1996.
5. Cohn SJ: Mepivacaine. In Roizen MF, Fleisher LA (editors): *Essence of anesthesia practice,* Philadelphia, 1997, WB Saunders.
6. Covino BG: Clinical pharmacology of local anesthetic agents. In Cousins MJ, Bridenbaugh PO (editors): *Neural blockade in clinical anesthesia and management of pain,* ed 2, Philadelphia, 1988, JB Lippincott.
7. Eisenach JC: Regional anesthesia: vintage bordeaux, *Anesthesiology* 87(3)467-469, 1997.

8. Feldman HS: Toxicity of local anesthetic agents. In Rice SA, Fish KJ (editors): *Anesthetic toxicity,* New York, 1994, Raven Press.

9. Pearce HD, Lindsay D, Leslie K: Axillary plexus block in two hundred consecutive patients, *Anaesth Intens Care* 24:453-458, 1996.

10. Pere P, Pitkanen M, Tuominen M, et al: Clinical and radiological comparisons of perivascular and transarterial techniques of axillary brachial plexus block, *Br J Anaesth* 70:276-279, 1993.

11. Reisner LS: Bupivacaine. In Roizen MF, Fleisher LA (editors): *Essence of anesthesia practice,* Philadelphia, 1997, WB Saunders.

12. Stoelting RK: *Pharmacology and physiology in anesthetic practice,* ed 2, Philadelphia, 1991, JB Lippincott, pp 148-169.

13. Strichartz GR, Berde CB: Local anesthetic toxicity. In Miller RD (editor): *Anesthesia,* ed 4, New York, 1994, Churchill Livingstone.

14. Tucker GT, Moore DC, Bridenbaugh PO, et al: Systemic absorption of mepivacaine in commonly used regional block procedures, *Anesthesiology* 37:277-287, 1972.

15. Wedel DJ: Nerve blocks. In Miller RD (editor): *Anesthesia,* ed 4, New York, 1994, Churchill Livingstone.

16. Weeks PM: Hand injuries, *Curr Probl Surg* 30(8):749-750, 1993.

CHAPTER

Therapeutic Management of Hand Trauma

Lynne M. Feehan
Maureen Hardy

INTRODUCTION

The intent in this chapter is to take the reader inside the clinic and head of a hand therapist. Despite differences in style and technique, we all face similar challenges in rehabilitating patients with hand injuries. The therapist's perspective on the processes of rehabilitation and disablement is discussed and applied to hand therapy. The value of an outcome-oriented, patient-centered perspective has been advanced because we believe it is helpful to avoid "seeing" an elephant, as the four blind men did who described only the part they felt. We suggest all clinicians look at results from the patient's perspective and evaluate the impact of clinical interventions on the total person—in other words, "looking at" and managing the whole elephant.

The scope of therapeutic evaluation covers everything from the evaluation of tissue-specific dysfunction to the overall functional abilities of the affected individual. Suggested therapeutic intervention strategies are based on the principles of wound healing and early functional reactivation. Splinting, modalities, and exercise and functional reactivation programs are reviewed because these are the three most commonly used therapeutic "tools." Therapeutic management strategies for four common problems—primary tendon repairs, closed proximal interphalangeal (PIP)–joint trauma, nerve compression, and hand fractures—are also presented.

Finally, a generic overview of the process of outcome measurement as it applies to hand rehabilitation is presented. Outcome research in hand therapy is lacking, and we advance the argument that all clinicians need to be more aware of the importance of using outcome measurements as a way of evaluating the efficacy of hand-therapy interventions.

HAND THERAPY

Hovering over an operating room during a surgical procedure on the hand provides a universal perspective (Figure 98-1). On one side of the toweled curtain is the sterile field, with the involved arm exposed. This arm, with its complex anatomy and function, is really quite similar to all other arms. Even the occasional anatomic variations are well known. On the other side of the curtain is someone unique—there is not another human being who has the same physiologic, psychologic, and social mix. This anesthetized patient lying on the operating room table will awaken to manifest his or her own unique personality. Hand therapy is the arena for "managing" concerns or issues emanating from both sides of the curtain, with *management* in this case meaning to lead, guide, and maneuver the therapeutic process in a predefined direction.

HAND THERAPIST: TEACHER, COACH, PARENT

It is difficult to describe a hand therapist in generic terms. However, some common attributes that define a "good" hand therapist include the following:

- Clinical experts in the therapeutic management of patients with hand and upper-extremity problems
- Active learners and critical consumers, absorbing new information and evaluating it on its scientific and clinical merit
- Open minded and adaptable to new ways of seeing and doing things
- Skilled communicators, freely and effectively sharing their perspective and insights with all involved in patient management
- A combination of *teacher* and *coach,* someone who is continually striving to teach oneself and others while coaxing and cheering patients on to achieve their maximal potential

Therapeutic or clinical excellence has one additional quality: approaching patient management much like good *parents* would approach their children. An excellent clinician looks to the future, planning (and worrying) about the growth and independence of the person he or she has come to know,

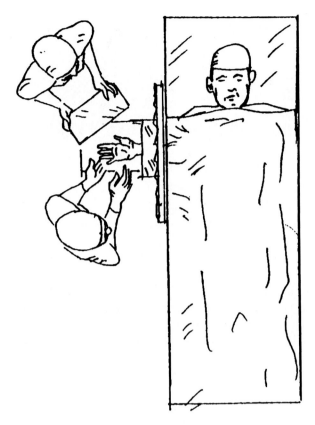

Figure 98-1. Hand therapy: the arena for managing concerns or issues emanating from both sides of the curtain.

and anticipating and guiding with the intent of prevention first and foremost in his or her thoughts.

THE REHABILITATION PROCESS: ASSISTING INDIVIDUALS IN THEIR FUNCTIONAL RECOVERY

How does hand therapy differ from hand surgery? The surgeon and therapist are both trying to help the same hand-injured person, but they view patient management from different perspectives. Therapists manage patients from a rehabilitation perspective in which rehabilitation is a process of recovery from some aspect of physical, psychologic, or social dysfunction. Therapists, as rehabilitation professionals, are persons assisting individuals in their functional recovery.

Hand therapy is the subspecialty within physical rehabilitation that assists individuals in their recovery from hand or upper-extremity physical dysfunction. Hand therapists primarily manage the physical aspect of a person's dysfunction, but they also need to have an appreciation of psychosocial functioning. Not only will the patient's psychosocial status influence therapeutic management, but therapeutic interventions will also affect psychosocial well-being.

THE HAND THERAPIST'S PERSPECTIVE: DETERMINING THE FUNCTIONAL IMPACT OF THE HAND INJURY

Determining the "physical-functional" implications of a traumatic hand injury requires a multidimensional view of the problem (Figure 98-2). Hand therapists look beyond the injury-healing process and also evaluate different levels of functional impairment experienced by the hand-injured patient.

THE INJURY-HEALING PROCESS

A traumatic hand injury is followed by a wound-healing response (Figure 98-2, *A*). The complicated biologic process that occurs during wound healing is constantly changing over time. Managing a person's hand injury based on the biologic status of the healing tissues at the time of intervention is called the *wound-healing principle* (see principles of treatment).[36]

LEVELS OF FUNCTIONAL IMPACT

An individual's ability to function within each one of the domains of physical, psychologic, and social functioning can also be subdivided into three separate but interrelated levels of functional abilities[87]:
1. Functional abilities *inside* the person at the cell/tissue/organ/system level
2. Functional abilities *of* the person at the specific task/activity level
3. Functional abilities *outside* the person at the performance of normal life roles level

The terminology adopted by the World Health Organization[100] states that dysfunction inside the person is an *impairment*, dysfunction of the person is a *disability*, and dysfunction outside the person is a *handicap*. The traumatic hand-injury healing process affects all three levels of a person's functional abilities.

Impairment
Impairment, the initial physical-functional effect of the injury healing process, occurs inside the person, influencing the normal functional abilities of the affected cells, tissues, organs, or body systems. A traumatic hand injury may influence such normal functions as tendon glide, muscle strength, joint stability, or hand sensibility (Figure 98-2, *B*). Hand therapists use their knowledge of normal tissue anatomy, physiology, and function to help recover tissue and hand function in individuals who have sustained a traumatic hand injury.

Disability
Disability, the next level of physical-functional effect, influences the person's ability to perform his or her normal personal, vocational, and recreational tasks or activities. A

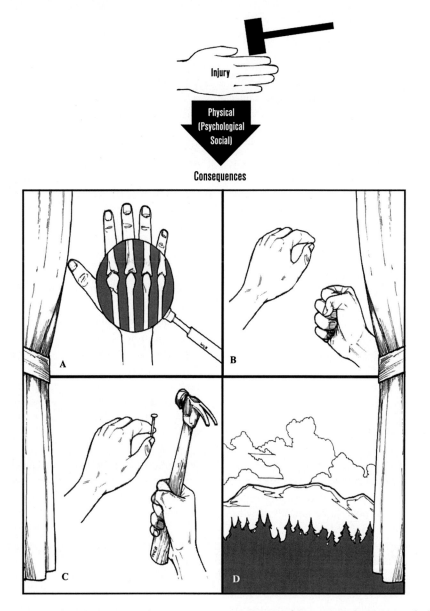

Figure 98-2.   A multidimensional perspective: consequences of a traumatic hand injury. **A,** The wound-healing response. **B,** The impact on cell/tissue/organ/system function: impairment. **C,** The impact on the person's task/activity function: disablement. **D,** The impact on the person's life role function: handicap.

traumatic hand injury may influence such normal functional abilities as hair combing, holding a racquet, playing a guitar, or throwing a ball (Figure 98-2, *C*). Hand therapists develop an understanding of the injured person's normal personal, vocational, and recreational tasks and activity functional demands and help the person recover the ability to perform daily tasks and activities.

Handicap

Handicap, the final level of physical-functional effect, is external to the person and influences the person's ability to perform the normal roles in life. A traumatic hand injury may influence a person's ability to be a spouse, a parent, a carpenter, or a musician (Figure 98-2, *D*). Hand therapists develop an

understanding of the injured person's functional demands in his or her normal life environment and give support to that person in the performance of his or her normal life roles.

DISABLEMENT: THE NEGATIVE IMPACT OF THE INJURY ON THE PERSON'S FUNCTIONAL ABILITIES

The nature and severity of the functional impairment, disability, and handicap associated with any traumatic hand injury tends to correlate with the nature and severity of the injury-healing process. However, this correlation is imperfect. A seemingly minor injury in some individuals can have a devastating effect on their functional abilities, whereas in other individuals a seemingly devastating injury may have a minor functional impact.

The negative impact of the injury-healing process on the functional abilities of the person is called *disablement*.[94] Disablement is a dynamic process that constantly changes over time and is influenced by any number of potential factors or mediators along the way. Some of the potential mediators come from within the person, such as the influence of his or her own health, attitudes, behaviors, and healing responses. However, the vast majority of mediators come from outside the person, with specific medical and rehabilitation interventions acting as only one potential mediating force[87] (Figure 98-3, *A*).

No one person or professional domain possesses all the necessary knowledge, skills, and abilities for the total management of a patient with a traumatic hand injury. The challenge for individual clinicians is to keep a multidimensional focus on the entire "disablement" process. It is easier to see how each of the domains of clinical practice fit nicely together as parts of a continuum of care. The knowledge and skills of individual clinicians are likely to have a maximal impact only if those clinicians keep focused on the total rehabilitative needs of the hand-injured patient.

THERAPEUTIC EVALUATIONS

The purpose of an initial therapeutic evaluation is to develop an understanding of the current status of the injury and wound-healing response and the various levels of functional impact on the patient. It is then possible to identify specific problems that can be addressed with therapeutic interventions. All therapeutic evaluations would ideally allow therapists to evaluate how the status of the patient changes over time and to critically evaluate how specific therapeutic interventions may have influenced these changes.

All therapeutic evaluations would ideally lead to a multilevel understanding of the current status of the patient (Figure 98-3, *B*). In reality, it is often not possible or practical for individual clinicians to spend the time and effort required to measure all aspects of a patient's current status. A common clinical dilemma is "If I can't evaluate everything, then how much should I evaluate?" The key to solving this dilemma is a coordinated team effort, or "interdisciplinary care,"[21] that includes the patient as an active and central team member in so-called *patient-centered management*.[75]

An interdisciplinary management focus ensures that no one clinician or clinical discipline needs to take on the responsibility for the total management of a hand-injured person. If each clinician or clinical discipline can contribute a different view or level of understanding to a composite picture, then everyone involved in patient management, including the patient, can develop a more complete understanding of the problems. A patient-centered focus allows the individual clinician to first assess the situation and to identify specific problem areas he or she can address given his or her area of expertise. The clinician then identifies priorities for specific evaluation and treatment based on what the patient perceives as most important.

LEVELS OF CLINICAL EVALUATIONS

Injury-Healing Response Level

Evaluations at the injury-healing response level involve taking a close, often microscopic look at the traumatized hand to define and diagnose the nature of the specific injury, biologic problem, or healing status (see Figure 98-2, *A*). Clinicians with this level of understanding can plan interventions directed primarily toward managing the specific injury, biologic problem, or healing status. Clinical evaluations and interventions at this level have traditionally fallen within the physician's domain of clinical practice.

Tissue/Hand Dysfunction Level

Evaluations at the tissue/hand dysfunction level define specific functional limitations of the affected tissues and/or the hand and determine the underlying cause for each limitation (see Figure 98-2, *B*). Clinicians with this level of understanding can plan interventions directed primarily at maximizing the normal structure and functional potential of the specific tissues or hand dysfunction. Clinical evaluations and interventions at this level have traditionally fallen within the physical therapy domain of clinical practice.

Task/Activity Dysfunction Level

Evaluations at the task/activity dysfunction level define a person's limited capacity to perform specific tasks or activities related to his or her normal personal, vocational, and recreational functional demands and identify specific causes for nonsuccessful performance (see Figure 98-2, *C*). Clinicians with this level of understanding can plan interventions directed primarily at maximizing the person's ability to perform specific tasks/activities. Clinical evaluations and interventions at this level have traditionally fallen in the occupational therapist's domain of clinical practice.

Life Role Dysfunction Level

Evaluations at the life role dysfunction level define a person's limited capacity to perform his or her normal life roles and identify specific reasons for nonsuccessful performance of these roles (see Figure 98-2, *D*). Clinicians with this level of understanding can direct their efforts toward supporting an individual in his or her ability to perform the various roles in life. Clinical evaluations and interventions at this level have traditionally been overlooked by all domains of clinical/medical practice, yet this level of functioning is of primary importance to the patient.

GOALS OF HAND THERAPY

The ultimate goal of all therapeutic interventions, given the disablement/recovery process after a traumatic hand injury, is

CHAPTER 98 Therapeutic Management of Hand Trauma 1709

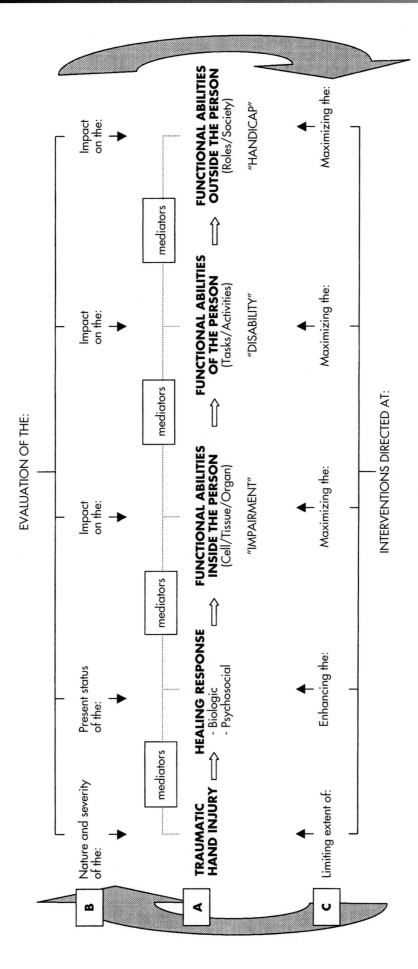

Figure 98-3. The process of hand therapy. Therapeutic management of traumatic hand injuries involves understanding the relationship between **(A)** the disablement process, **(B)** the ongoing need to (re)evaluate, and **(C)** development of interventions directed at minimizing the negative functional impact of the injury-healing response on the hand-injured person.

to limit the degree of disablement associated with the injury. Generally speaking, this can be achieved by aiming to do the following (Figure 98-3, C):
- Enhance the healing potential of the injured tissues
- Maximize the potential for recovery to a normal structure and function of the affected tissues
- Maximize the potential for recovery of the person's ability to perform normal tasks and activities of daily living
- Maximize the potential for the individual to return to his or her normal daily roles

Specific treatment goals within each of these general categories need to be clearly delineated for each patient. Individual treatment goals and priorities are defined in consultation with the patient and should be explicitly stated in terms of a measurable criterion or variable that is achievable. The goals should also be clearly defined in terms of time frames and circumstances for achievement.

PRINCIPLES OF TREATMENT

General management principles based on the general treatment goals stated above can be categorized into two areas: wound-healing principles and early graduated reactivation.

Wound-Healing Principles
Specific therapeutic management strategies are chosen based on the likelihood that they will positively influence the biologic status of the tissues at the specific time of intervention.[37] The principles will vary depending on the stage of connective tissue healing.

INFLAMMATORY STAGE (3 TO 5 DAYS AFTER WOUNDING). *Principle:* Minimize physical intervention by providing adequate and appropriate support (AAS) to the healing tissues to allow them an opportunity to respond naturally to the traumatic injury. Direct therapeutic interventions during the first few days should only occur if there is a problem.

FIBROBLASTIC STAGE (5 TO 21 DAYS AFTER WOUNDING). *Principle:* Manage the behavior of the fibroblast[36] by avoiding unnecessary immobilization or stress deprivation and find ways to introduce early controlled normal physiologic stresses to the healing tissues[9,10] by early graduated reactivation.

EARLY MATURATION/REMODELING STAGE (21 DAYS TO 3 MONTHS AFTER WOUNDING). *Principle:* Direct the collagen remodeling process through gentle persistent persuasion. Therapy should not attempt to physically tear or break the healing scar. Instead therapy should be directed toward frequent daily sessions of repetitive normal physiologic loading of the healing tissues.[9] These stresses should be graduated both in intensity and duration as the healing tissue's strength and tolerance to stresses increase.

LATE MATURATION/REMODELING STAGE (MORE THAN 6 MONTHS AFTER WOUNDING). *Principle:* Aim for a permanent structural and/or a functional adaptive change in the mature connective tissue. This is achieved through consistently and patiently, over a long duration, increasing the *specific* functional demands on the mature connective tissue. This concept is called *specificity of loading.* If the aim is to get a permanent adaptive lengthening in the tissue, then a consistent low load (gentle stretch) and long duration (in hours and over the course of weeks) end-range functional stretch must be applied. If the aim is to get a permanent adaptive increase in the tissue's capacity to withstand repetitive loads, then a graduated increase in various forms of repetitive stresses should be applied.

Early Graduated Reactivation
Principle: Whenever possible, and as early as possible, provide an opportunity for a safe, appropriate, and graduated reactivation of the following:
- The healing tissue's normal functions (i.e., tendons need to act like tendons, bones need to act like bones)
- The person back to his or her normal personal, vocational, and recreational tasks and activities
- The person back to his or her normal daily life roles

THERAPEUTIC TOOLS

A wise adage states that a scalpel is just a knife until it is placed in the hands of a skilled surgeon. What makes the scalpel a beneficial tool is its appropriate use by a trained and thoughtful surgeon. Likewise, therapy tools require good clinical decision making because inappropriate or thoughtless use of "therapeutic tools" can lead to ineffective or even detrimental outcomes. Therapists have many potential tools available to use; however, discussion will be limited to the three most commonly used hand therapy tools: splints, modalities, and exercise and functional reactivation programs.

Splinting
PROBLEM-ORIENTED SPLINTING. A simple functional definition of a splint is a device applied to or around a body part for a specific purpose or goal. The general goals or purposes for a splint are summarized as follows:
- To provide support and/or protection to vulnerable or healing tissues (Figure 98-4, *A;* see Figure 98-6, *B*)
- To facilitate function at the tissue or organ level (see Figures 98-7, *B* and 98-13, *A*)
- To facilitate performance of an individual's task/activity or life role functional abilities (Figure 98-4, *B;* see Figure 98-11, *C* and *D*)

WHAT MATERIALS CAN BE USED TO MAKE A SPLINT? Essentially any material that helps the therapist achieve the stated purpose or goal can be used for a splint. Most hand-therapy clinics use low-temperature thermoplastic mate-

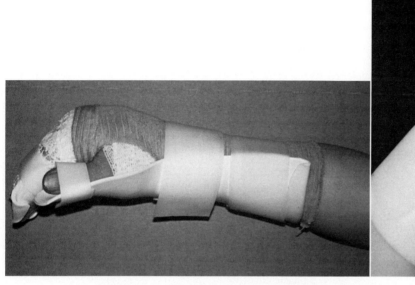
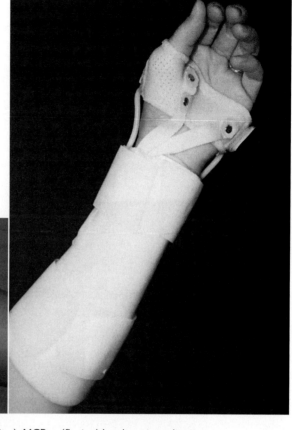

Figure 98-4. **A,** A volar thumb (neutral), IP$_{2-5}$ (extension), MCP$_{2-5}$ (flexion) hand-resting splint in the "position of function." **B,** A limited-motion wrist splint (extension, radial-ulnar deviation, midcarpal supination). This splint can be used in the rehabilitation of patients with healing scapholunate ligament and scaphoid fractures.

rials to fabricate commonly used hand splints. The properties of thermoplastic materials vary. Some are more rigid, others are more easily conformed, and still others have greater "memory" or elastic properties. This versatility, however, comes at a price, because thermoplastic materials are expensive. Other materials commonly used for hand and forearm splints are various metals (aluminum, copper, steel), leather, plaster, various cloth materials (cotton and wet suit material), adhesive straps, and athletic tape.

THE ART AND SCIENCE OF SPLINT FABRICATION. Once the therapist has mastered the "art" of handling and using the various materials available to fabricate splints, he or she is left with the universal challenge of designing the right splint for the right purpose at the right time—"the science." The appropriate splint that meets the defined goals and purpose of a patient with a defined problem at one point in time will change with time as the underlying problem changes.[64] The same splint may *not* be appropriate for a different patient with the identical problem at the same time. Splints are not designed to fit a specific diagnosis, but rather to fit a specific patient. The underlying principle, as with all other therapeutic interventions, is to

design a splint based on a clearly defined purpose or goal for its use.

MODALITIES

Therapeutic modalities used in hand therapy can be categorized based on their physiologic or physical effects, such as changing tissue temperature by either cooling or heating, mechanical tissue or cell disruption, nerve or muscle tissue stimulation, and other tissue stimulation techniques (e.g., ultrasound or laser therapy, or continuous passive motion units). There are many different modalities available to hand therapists around the world. Table 98-1 provides a summary of the commonly used modalities and their proposed physiologic and physical effects.*

Indications for the Use of Modalities

The thoughtful and judicious use of expensive modalities is important because many cannot be taken home with the patient. The time-limited effects of the modality are therefore

---

*References 23, 34, 57, 70, 77, 96.

Table 98-1.

Proposed Physiologic and Physical Effects of Commonly Used Therapeutic Modalities

PROPOSED PHYSIOLOGIC/PHYSICAL EFFECT	MODALITY
TISSUE COOLING	
Cryotherapy	Local "slush" immersion, ice packs, ice towels, ice massage, evaporation sprays, cold-compression pumps
TISSUE HEATING AND COOLING	Contrast baths
TISSUE HEATING	
Superficial	
Conduction heating	Local "hot" immersion, paraffin, hot packs, hot water bottles, electric heating pads
Convection heating	Whirlpool, fluidotherapy, hair dryer
Conversion heating (nonionizing radiate energy)	Infrared
Deep Conversion Heating	
Chemical energy	Metabolic activity
Mechanical energy	Continuous ultrasound (1 MHz)
Electromagnetic energy	Shortwave diathermy, microwave diathermy
MUSCLE AND NERVE STIMULATION/ACTIVITY	
Denervated muscle	Direct current: low-voltage galvanic
Innervated muscle stimulation ("muscle stim")	High-voltage pulsed galvanic; long duration, low frequency: Faradic (monophasic and biphasic currents); medium frequency: Faradic (interferential, Russian currents)
Muscle activity	Surface: EMG units, biofeedback
Sensory nerve stimulation "TENS"	Short duration, low frequency: Faradic (monophasic and biphasic currents)
Nerve conduction	Surface nerve conduction units
OTHER CELL/TISSUE STIMULATION	
Mechanical: connective tissue	Pulsed ultrasound (1 MHz)
Wound/tissue healing	
Mechanical	Pulsed ultrasound (1 and 3 MHz)
Visible/infrared	Medium power laser (therapeutic), low-dose infrared
Electromagnetic	Pulsed short wave, pulsed microwave, high-voltage pulsed galvanic
Ultraviolet	Low-dose ultraviolet
ALTERED TISSUE FLUID DYNAMICS	
External compression	Compression pump units, compression wraps
Increased/decreased vascular	See heating/cooling
Muscle pump	See muscle stimulation
Mechanical streaming	Pulsed ultrasound (1 MHz)
Electrical streaming	Direct current: low and high voltage; interferential currents; pulsed shortwave; pulsed microwave
OTHER EFFECTS	
Passive tissue mobilization	Continuous passive motion units
Medication transmission	
Electrical current transmission	Iontophoresis (direct current: galvanic)
Mechanical transmission	Phonophoresis (ultrasound)
Cellular/tissue destruction	
"Freezing"	See cooling: <5° C
"Cooking"	See heating: >45° C
Bacterial infection	High-dose ultraviolet
Mechanical destruction	Medium-power laser (eye): therapeutic, High-power laser: industrial and surgical Static ultrasound: cavitation and standing waves

Data from references 23, 34, 56, 70, 77, and 96.

location specific and confined to the limits of the hand-therapy clinic. An important consideration before the use of any modality or therapeutic intervention is this: does the specific beneficial effect derived from use of this modality outweigh the costs in relation to the expense, time spent in application, and increased patient dependence on hands-on therapy? If the answer to this question is yes, it is then necessary to select an appropriate modality for a clearly defined treatment goal or objective.

Purposeful Use of Modalities

Micholivitz[70] suggests that there are three primary purposes for modality use: to modulate pain, to facilitate healing, and to improve tissue mobility.

Pain modulation modalities vary from simple heat or ice packs and contrast baths to more sophisticated electrophysical modalities such as transcutaneous electrical nerve stimulation (TENS) devices, iontophoresis, biofeedback, high-voltage pulsed currents, and interferential currents.[57,70,96] If the modality is meant to modulate a patient's perception of pain, then it is essential to measure pain parameters both before and after modality application to ensure that the desired effect has occurred. The effectiveness of pain-modulating modalities in modifying a patient's pain symptom is related to an appropriate match of the right modality for the specific pain trigger, which is the underlying source or cause for the pain.

Facilitated tissue healing in wounds that are slow to heal has also been suggested to occur with various modalities such as ultrasound,[23] high-voltage pulsed currents,[77] and medium power laser.[34] The studies that make these claims, however, do not tend to meet the rigors of critical scientific review,[38,80] nor do they clearly substantiate the underlying physiologic mechanisms for these claims. The use of modalities to facilitate tissue healing is therefore still within the realm of clinical anecdotal evidence, leaving plenty of room for future basic science and clinical research. The use of cold to reduce pain perception and the initial vascular inflammatory reactions, the use of heat to improve tissue circulation, compression pumps and wraps to reduce tissue edema, and whirlpool baths to help clean and debride dirty wounds are all valid therapeutic modalities that support normal tissue wound healing.[57,70,96]

Therapists also frequently use modalities as adjunctive treatment to improve tissue mobility. The primary underlying physiologic reaction is related to the heating effects of the various modalities. Increased tissue temperature improves regional tissue circulation and facilitates muscle tissue relaxation.[57,70,96] It also reduces the viscosity of tissue fluids and improves the potential for connective tissue stretch.[95,101] This heating effect, combined with a low-load, long-duration stretch applied at the extreme of collagen tissue extensibility permits better overall connective tissue elongation.[81] For this effect to occur, however, the tissues need to be heated to the extremes of safe therapeutic levels in the range of 42° C to 45° C.[57,70,96] Most hand tissues can be heated to therapeutic ranges with superficial heat applications such as paraffin, hot water, hot packs, and fluidotherapy. Heating deeper tissues can

be achieved with continuous ultrasound and short wave and microwave diathermy.[57,70,96]

Long-term increased connective tissue extensibility can be facilitated by the additional use of splints to maintain the elongated position, as well as specific exercises and/or functional use at the extremes of the tissue extensibility. This type of therapy may be termed "use it or lose it" therapy. Other modalities may be useful in improving general tissue mobility. Continuous passive-motion devices, for example, may be helpful in maintaining the mobility of noncontractile restrictive tissues, whereas direct muscle stimulation and biofeedback may facilitate a stronger active muscle contraction leading to better tendon glide and active joint mobility.[14]

EXERCISE AND FUNCTIONAL REACTIVATION PROGRAMS

Exercise prescription and functional reactivation programs, like splint application and modality use, need to be designed specifically for each problem presented. It is not appropriate for clinicians to provide a generic exercise program based on a diagnosis. The concept of tailoring individual exercise programs to address specific tissues or hand or individual dysfunction is called *specificity of exercise*. Two individuals, one who does heavy manual labor and the other a concert violinist, can both sustain a laceration and repair of a flexor tendon in the index finger of the left hand. Both individuals will require very different exercise and functional reactivation programs to help them achieve their maximal individual tissue, hand, task/activity, and life role functional potential. Those two people may share common tissue goals, such as maximizing motion of the affected muscle or tendon unit, and be assigned some common exercises, but they will also be given very different and specific exercises directed toward maximizing their individual functional potential. The laborer, for example, may require a progressive exercise and functional activity program with increased intensity and duration directed at improving his capacity to grasp, hold, lift, and carry materials of varying size and weight and to improve his tolerance to cold, vibration, and impact stresses. The concert violinist, on the other hand, may need to work more specifically on improving his inner range active finger "tuck" flexion, independent index fingertip pinch strength, and overall finger and hand endurance and coordination.

A key clinical concept to remember is that functional or adaptive changes take time; exercise and functional reactivation programs can take weeks or months. Strength gains are achieved by progressively increasing resistance or load over a minimum duration of 6 weeks.[48] Measures of gains in pinch and grip strength with maximal voluntary effort are commonly assessed using isometric grip or pinch dynamometers. Endurance, or the ability to perform repeatedly over time, is improved by using a moderate load and increasing the number of repetitions or sets performed until the point of fatigue, defined as more than a 30% decrease in power.[86]

Endurance gains can be measured by timed task or activity performance or isokinetic constant speed measures of "percent lost over time."

The clinician and patient should understand the exact problem as it relates to specific tissue, hand, and individual task/activity and life role dysfunction. It is then much easier to design exercise and functional reactivation programs around improving these specific functional losses. It is also important to remember that affected tissues, hands, and individuals all have varied and complex functional demands. The upper extremity is subjected to many different and repeated functional stresses throughout a person's normal day.

Comprehensive exercise and functional reactivation programs must address *all* areas of potential dysfunction. An individual with a diagnosis of tendinitis of the extensor carpi radialis brevis/longus (ECRB/L) muscle tendon (MT) units, for example, may need to modify or adapt to certain functional tasks and activities to reduce the specific stresses on the affected MT units. An exercise program should also aim to restore *all* of the affected MT units' daily functional demands if the individual is to function in a pain-free manner during all of his or her daily activities. The ECRB/L MT units, for example, need to be able to act as a wrist-joint stabilizer (lifting a grocery bag from the trunk of the car), contract strongly in either a concentric (wringing a washcloth) or eccentric (playing tennis) fashion during wrist-joint motion, function in a stretched (wrist flexion, elbow extension) or shortened (wrist extension, elbow flexion) position, function in a skilled or coordinated fashion (writing, drawing, brushing teeth), and finally function repeatedly (endurance) throughout the day.

SPECIFIC MANAGEMENT STRATEGIES

Management of Primary Tendon Repairs

TENDON STRUCTURE. The primary structural component of tendon is water, which accounts for two thirds of tendon's overall mass and collagen. Collagen constitutes approximately three fourths of the tendon's dry mass.[92] The remaining portion of the tendon tissue matrix is composed of a few cells, primarily tenocytes, and other tissue proteins such as elastin fibers, glycosaminoglycans, glycoproteins, and lipoproteins.[6]

The collagen fibers run in a parallel fashion throughout the tendon's length and are bound together with strong intrafiber and interfiber chemical bonds or crosslinks. The collagen fibers are densely packed and organized in a hierarchical fashion. The respective layers of tendon tissue fibers are the primary tendon fiber, tendon fascicle, and the whole tendon, with each fiber layer contained respectively by the endotenon, peritenon, and epitenon sheaths.[6,71] Tendon tissue not found within a fibroosseous tunnel is surrounded by an additional less dense and randomly organized connective tissue sheath called the *mesotendon.* Tendon tissue lying within a fibroosseous tunnel, which acts as a mechanical pulley, is surrounded by a specialized synovial sheath (Figure 98-5).[6,20] The mesotendon layer within the fibroosseous tunnels of the digital flexor system also forms a protective sheath around small specialized vascular channels referred to as *vincula* (not shown in diagram).[98]

TENDON FUNCTION. Tendons function as part of an MT unit (see Figure 98-5). The bone-muscle-tendon/pulley-bone kinetic chain is a dynamic, contractile, multilinked mechanical system that provides motor control to the musculoskeletal

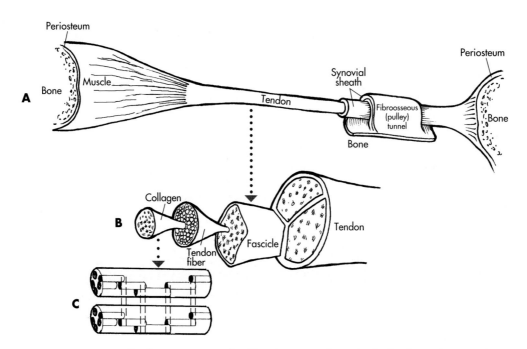

Figure 98-5. Tendon structure. **A,** The bone-muscle-tendon/pulley-bone kinetic chain. **B,** Tendon tissue hierarchical organization. **C,** Intrafiber and interfiber tendon crosslinks.

system. The primary function of tendon within this mechanical system is to transmit tensile forces. The parallel arrangement of densely accumulated collagen fibers within the tendon fulfills this functional demand.[11]

Human tendons have the ability to withstand large tensile forces without any structural dysfunction. Human tendons have a normal tensile strength (rupture stress = tensile load/cross-sectional area) of 50 to 100 N/mm^2, depending on the rate of elongation or strain. The tensile strength of human tendon is roughly equivalent to that of hemp rope or cast aluminum materials.[33] The inherent strength of tendon permits a significant safety margin to rupture even when the tendon is subjected to the very large tensile loads that can occur with maximal eccentric loading (i.e., full passive composite MT-unit stretch combined with maximal active-resisted muscle contraction).

TENDON NUTRITION. Nutritional support for the tendon tissue comes from two sources: vascular perfusion and synovial diffusion. There are a series of fine vascular arcades within the tendon tissue connected in a segmental fashion to the extrinsic vascular network. The extrinsic segmental vessels that perfuse the tendon tissue come from the surrounding muscle, bone, or periosteal tissues, or from vessels traveling within the mesotendon layer.[6,24] Vascular perfusion is the dominant nutrition source for tendon tissue not contained within a synovial sheath.

Tendon tissue surrounded by a synovial sheath has access to an additional nutritional pathway. The synovial fluid that bathes the tendon tissue serves not only to reduce surface friction but also provides important nutritional support to the regional tendon tissue. Synovial fluid nutrition is a dynamic process in which the fluid is diffused in and out of the tissue with the intermittent shear, compression, and tension forces that occur with MT-unit motion.[65,98]

TENDON HEALING. Tendon healing is still not fully understood[47,56]; however, it has been shown that lacerated and primarily repaired tendons have the capacity to heal through an intrinsic and/or extrinsic tissue-repair process. Intrinsic healing within the tendon itself is more likely to occur when the healing tendon tissue has adequate nutritional support and is protected from structurally deforming tensile forces during the early postoperative healing phase. Controlled motion applied to a healing tendon during this early postoperative phase has been shown to enhance synovial fluid diffusion,[65] early tensile strength gains,[27] and normal tendon tissue morphology.[3,47,49]

Extrinsic healing by tissues surrounding the tendon is more likely to occur in situations of compromised nutritional status and/or with excessive disruption or irritation during early tendon healing. The normal tendon structure has a limited vascular supply can be compromised during the original and/or surgical traumas.[88] Therefore it is not uncommon for the intrinsic healing mechanisms of a tendon to be secondary to an ingrowth of granulation tissue from more vascular connective tissues in the region. The unfortunate consequence

of this extrinsic healing process is an inevitable tethering of the healing tendon to the surrounding connective tissue structures to create healing success, but a functional failure.

AIMS OF TREATMENT. The general aims of therapeutic management after primary tendon repair are to support the intrinsic healing process of the tendon, to maximize the functional potential of the total MT unit, to maximize the injured person's ability to use the affected hand and upper extremity for his or her normal daily tasks and activities, and to support the injured person in his or her return to a normal life role.

PRINCIPLES OF TREATMENT. The general treatment principles for primary tendon injuries can be summarized as follows:

1. Support the intrinsic healing process within the tendon by finding safe and effective ways to apply early controlled or limited stresses to the healing tendon.
2. Strive to maximize the functional potential of the entire MT unit, not just the tendons. A ruptured tendon is not functional; however, a well-healed, structurally intact tendon does not necessarily mean there will be excellent MT-unit function. A normal functioning MT unit must be structurally intact, with a functioning motor nerve supply. It must be able to glide freely throughout its full length. It should have adequate length and flexibility to allow full range of motion of the joints it crosses. It should have adequate strength to withstand a maximal eccentric load and should have endurance to withstand the ongoing tensile, shear, and compression forces generated during normal daily use.
3. Gradually reactivate the patient back into his or her normal daily tasks, activities, and life roles as early as is safely possible.

GENERAL MANAGEMENT STRATEGIES. The therapeutic management of patients after primary tendon repair can be divided into five phases:

1. Immediate postoperative management (0 to 3 days)
2. The early postoperative or protected phase (3-5 days to 3-4 weeks)
3. The graduated active mobilization phase (3 to 6-8 weeks)
4. The graduated strengthening/stretching phase (6 to 10-12 weeks)
5. The unrestricted phase (>12 weeks)

These phases correlate with expected increases in tensile strength that occur with normal connective tissue healing[66] and can be applied equally to flexor and extensor tendon repairs. The most important clinical factor is the thoughtful application of general therapy principles, through a critical evaluation of specific management strategies and appropriate modification of these strategies for each individual patient.

Immediate Postoperative Phase (Day 0 to 3). The inflammatory phase of wound healing occurs during the first 3 to 5 days after injury. Hand therapy does not appear to offer a theoretical advantage to connective tissue healing during this time.[50] It therefore seems appropriate to allow the healing tendon and secondary soft tissue to recover from the original and surgical traumas by letting them rest in a shortened position with AAS. In support of this concept, Hakilis et al[39] recently demonstrated in an experimental study on surgically traumatized chicken flexor tendons that the work of flexion, defined as the force required to flex the digit, was increased significantly when measured on the seventh postoperative day in those tendons allowed immediate mobilization when compared with those tendons mobilized after the third postoperative day.

Early Postoperative or Protected Phase (3 Days to 3-5 Weeks). Starting at about day 3 when the fibroblastic activity is increasing and the inflammatory process is decreasing, it is time to begin asking a healing tendon to start acting like a tendon. There are four general approaches to providing early controlled stress to a healing tendon (Figures 98-6 and 98-7):

1. *Motion-assisted splinting:* This technique uses a splint designed to limit the potential for composite stretch of the repaired tendon. It adds some form of motion assistance such as elastic traction to the affected tendon. If the repaired tendon is a flexor tendon, the motion assistance is into flexion[67] (Figure 98-6, *A*), with motion assistance in extension for extensor-tendon repairs[78] (Figure 98-7, *A*).

2. *Controlled passive motion:* This technique involves teaching the patient limited passive joint exercises in conjunction with a protective splint[15] (Figure 98-6, *B*). The patient is asked to perform passive joint exercises frequently throughout the day while the splint prevents placing excessive tension on the tendon.

3. *Controlled tenodesis:* This technique uses normal tissue tension or the passive tenodesis effect that occurs during composite hand and wrist flexion and extension motions (i.e., wrist flexion causes passive finger extension, wrist extension causes passive finger flexion). This strategy is used more commonly in the rehabilitation of replanted digits when both the flexor and extensor tendons have been repaired[84]; however, it has also been used to mobilize digital flexor tendon repairs[16] (Figure 98-6, *C*).

4. *Controlled active motion:* The use of early controlled active mobilization has only recently been reintroduced as an acceptable clinical method.[85] Early active tendon mobilization can be accomplished by having the patient perform a limited isotonic muscle contraction to produce a limited arc of motion[26,85] (Figures 98-6, *D* and 98-7, *C*), or by having the patient passively place the joint(s) at a specific angle and then maintain this position with a limited-force isometric muscle contraction[16] (Figures 98-6, *C* and 98-7, *D*).

Graduated Active Mobilization Phase (3 to 6-8 Weeks). The healing tendon has enough tensile strength during this time frame to withstand a full active isotonic muscle contraction, but not enough to withstand a passive composite stretch or a resisted active contraction. Therapy during this time frame should be directed toward restoring both full composite and differential muscle-tendon excursion (Figure 98-8, *A* and *B*). If the person cannot get a full active composite lengthening of the repaired MT unit, then some form of protective splinting should be continued at night and during functional use to prevent the repaired tendon from being inadvertently stretched. The person's functional activities should also be restricted to activities that will not put a direct resistance or stretch on the repaired tendon.

Graduated Stretching/Strengthening Phase (6-8 Weeks to 10-12 Weeks). The healing tendon has enough strength during this time frame to withstand a resisted muscle contraction or a composite passive stretch, but not both at the same time (eccentric loading). If joint mobility and tendon excursion are still not full, these areas should become a high priority. The therapeutic techniques that can be used to help achieve these ends include serial splinting, dynamic splinting, and resisted exercise. Therapy should be directed toward maximizing the person's strength, endurance, and functional abilities when full joint mobility and tendon excursion are restored. The individual should be able to return to most household, work, and recreational activities by 8 to 10 weeks without fear of tendon rupture. Contact sports, skiing in snow or water, golf, and heavy resisted fingertip pinch tasks should still be avoided with digital flexor-tendon injuries because they can produce large eccentric loads on the repaired tendon.

Unrestricted Phase (>12 Weeks). The healed tendon scar should be able to withstand eccentric loading or maximal active contraction combined with a passive composite stretch by 12 weeks. This means that there should be no further restrictions on the person's functional activities or on the therapeutic techniques available to therapists. Unfortunately, any restrictive scars that are present are also as strong as the healing tendon scar, meaning that the potential effectiveness in influencing the remodeling of these restrictive scars may be limited. The individual's focus during this time frame should therefore be directed at maximizing his or her strength, endurance, and functional abilities. Further increases in tendon excursion and joint mobility will be slow,[83] but can be improved with persistent and appropriate stretching (low load, long duration) and frequent daily attempts at maximal active effort inner range composite excursion exercises.

Management of Closed Proximal Interphalangeal Joint Injuries

PROXIMAL INTERPHALANGEAL JOINT ANATOMY. The PIP joint is composed of complex multiple tissue structures that contain bony elements (distal P1 and proximal P2), articular cartilage, synovial membrane and fluid, capsular/ligamentous structures, and neurovascular tissues.[4,7,54] The flexor and extensor tendons also cross the PIP joint, and the whole joint is encased in an additional soft tissue sleeve consisting of the skin and subcutaneous structures. Any one or all of these tissues can be involved in a closed traumatic injury of the PIP joint (Figure 98-9, *A* and *B*).

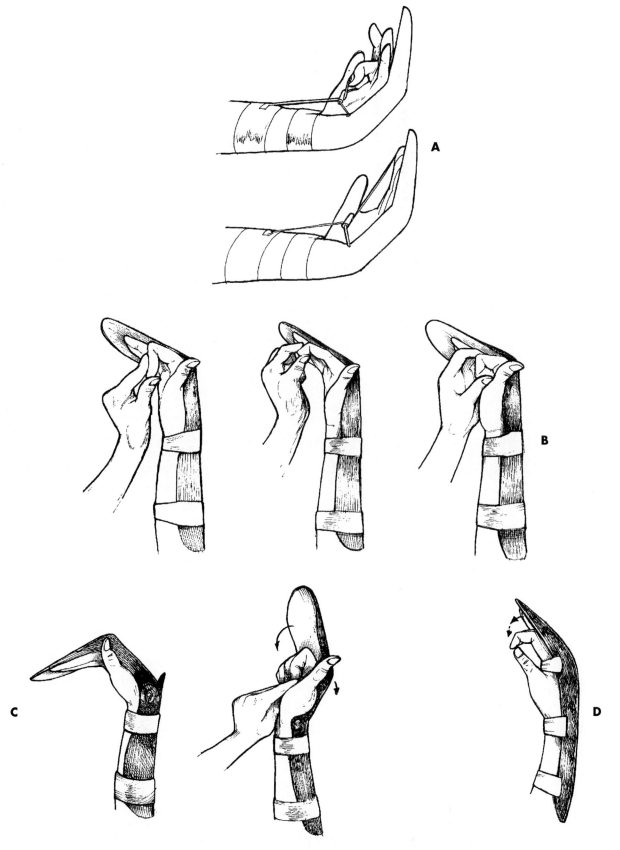

Figure 98-6. Early controlled mobilization options for zone 2 flexor tendon repairs. **A,** Dynamic flexion: motion-assisted splinting. **B,** Passive flexion and extension mobilization. **C,** Passive tenodesis and/or place and hold active mobilization. **D,** Limited arc active motion.

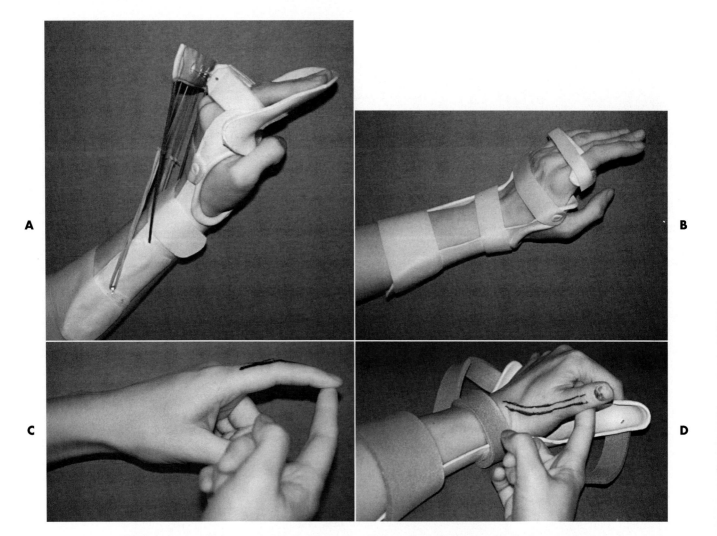

Figure 98-7. Early controlled mobilization options used for extensor tendon repairs. **A,** Dynamic extension: motion-assisted splint for zone 5 injuries. **B,** Active-assisted extension: motion-assisted splint for zone 5 injuries. **C,** Limited arc active motion for zone 3 injuries. Often a small volar finger splint is used as a motion-controlling template to ensure that the patient does not flex beyond a certain joint angle when doing therapeutic exercises. **D,** Place and hold active motion for extensor pollicis longus injuries.

PROXIMAL INTERPHALANGEAL JOINT MOBILITY. The PIP joint is traditionally classified as a simple hinge joint that allows approximately 100 degrees of flexion and extension motion.[54] Leibovic and Bowers[54] call the PIP joint a "sloppy hinge" joint and remind us that PIP-joint motion really occurs in three planes with six degrees of freedom of motion (Figure 98-9, *C*). The primary motions of flexion and extension are volitional and occur in the sagittal plane around a frontal axis. However, there is also some involuntary supination/pronation that occurs throughout the arc of flexion and extension around a longitudinal axis, as well as some involuntary radial/ulnar deviation in the frontal plane around a transverse axis.[22,54] The three-dimensional change in the relationship of the proximal and middle phalangeal bones to each other is referred to as *osteokinematics*.[41] Movement of the PIP joint also produces a certain degree of roll, slide, and spin that occurs between the two articular surfaces. The change in the relationship of the two articular surfaces is also involuntary and is referred to as *PIP-joint arthokinematics.*[41]

Normal PIP-joint mobility only occurs when the MT units that control the volitional motions are innervated, structurally intact, and free to glide along their total kinematic chain. The PIP joint and its surrounding tissues must also be structurally intact, be of normal size and shape, and be free to move in relation to each other.

PROXIMAL INTERPHALANGEAL JOINT STABILITY. The PIP joint is a small joint compared with the rest of the joints in the human body. However, because it is part of the functionally active hand, the PIP joint is continuously subjected to compression, torsion, and various other deviating stresses. The varied and continuous functional demands placed on the PIP joint require that it not only have enough mobility to meet these functional demands but also to have enough

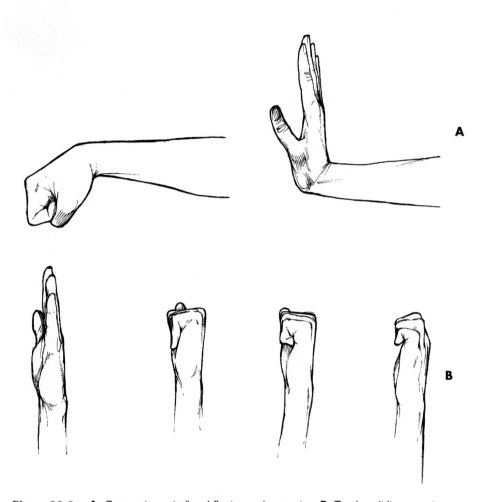

Figure 98-8. **A,** Composite wrist/hand flexion and extension. **B,** Tendon gliding exercises.

static and dynamic stability to withstand the deforming forces that also occur with functional use.

The degree to which both the voluntary and involuntary motions do or do not occur is dependent on (1) selective soft tissue tension, (2) the shape of the articular surfaces, and (3) the degree of articular surface/bony congruity during joint motion. The three primary static soft tissue restraints to excessive PIP-joint mobility are the volar plate and the two collateral ligament complexes, which are divided into the true collateral ligaments (TCLs) and accessory collateral ligaments (ACLs).[54] Bowers[7] has described these three structures as functioning as a three-sided stabilizing box, all inserting to some degree on the lateral tubercle on the volar aspect of the base of the middle phalanx. Bowers refers to this common insertion as the *critical corner* because disruption here is likely to affect two sides of this three-sided box and potentially cause some joint instability (see Figure 98-9, *A*).

The soft tissues around the joint generally allow unrestricted flexion and extension throughout the normal 0-to 100-degree range of motion. However, as the extremes of motion are reached, selective tension in the various supporting tissues begins to limit mobility. The greatest potential for

accessory joint mobility occurs between ~30 to 70 degrees because the soft tissues are under the least tension in this range. The limit of extension is determined primarily by the very strong volar plate complex. Flexion is normally limited by bone-on-bone approximation. Lateral stability in the PIP joint is greatest at the extremes of flexion and extension. Lateral stability between 0 to 30 degrees is caused by tension in the ACLs, whereas lateral stability between 70 to 100 degrees is caused primarily by tension within the TCLs. Lateral stability between 30 to 70 degrees in a nonloaded joint occurs because of bone-on-bone approximation. Compression or axial loading of the PIP joint occurs with active muscle contraction, which creates tension in the tendons in an open kinetic chain (a free distal element). Compression loading increases in a closed kinetic chain (a fixed or resisted distal element) as additional compression forces are transmitted through the bony elements of the finger. Compression loading provides even greater joint stability because of improved articular congruity.

SPECTRUM OF JOINT INJURY: THE 4 × 4 RULE. The ability to predict a likely pattern or spectrum of potential tissue injury is a valuable tool in planning management strategies for

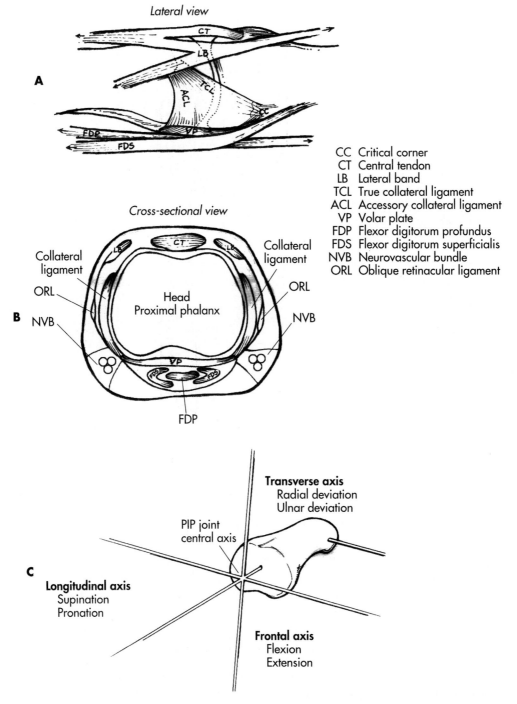

Figure 98-9. PIP-joint anatomy. **A,** Lateral view. **B,** Cross-sectional view. **C,** Joint motion axes and associated degrees of freedom. NOTE: The central PIP-joint axis is located in the head of the proximal phalanx.

closed PIP-joint injuries. Predicting the likely spectrum of injury is helped by breaking down the pattern of force transmission through the joint into four potential component forces—(1) radial/ulnar deviation, (2) flexion/extension, (3) supination/pronation, and (4) compression/traction—and by thinking in terms of four potential layers of tissue injury: (1) bone/cartilage, (2) capsule/ligament, (3) tendon, and (4) skin/subcutaneous (Figure 98-10). We call this the *4 × 4*

rule. Rarely will a closed PIP-joint injury occur in only one plane of motion, or result in only one tissue layer injury.

An excessive flexion-compression-radial deviation force is likely to produce a very different pattern of tissue injury than is a flexion-traction-pronation injury. The 4 × 4 rule helps the clinician to think in terms of the "total" spectrum of potential injury and to develop thoughtful and complete evaluation and management strategies.

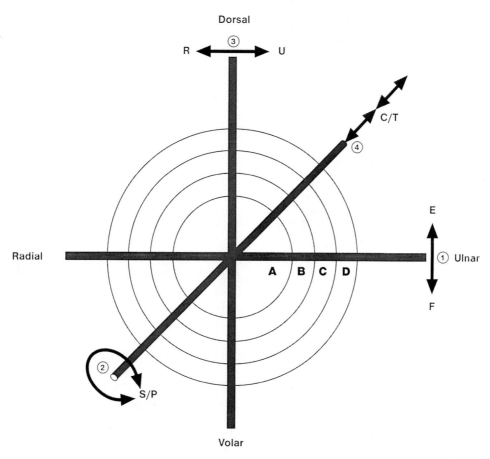

Figure 98-10. Spectrum of joint injury: the 4 × 4 rule. The four component forces include *1*, flexion/extension; *2*, supination/ pronation; *3*, radial/ulnar deviation; *4*, compression/tension. The four layers of tissues include **(A)** bone/cartilage, **(B)** capsule/ ligaments, **(C)** tendon/muscle, and **(D)** skin/subcutaneous tissues.

THERAPEUTIC EVALUATIONS. The purpose of a therapeutic evaluation after a closed PIP-joint injury is to be able to evaluate the structural integrity and function of all the potentially involved tissues, to determine how the tissue dysfunction is affecting the volitional and accessory joint mobility, and to determine how the tissue dysfunction is affecting the static and dynamic joint stability. Therapeutic evaluation of a traumatic joint injury includes taking a history, reviewing and discussing radiographs and operating room reports with the referring physician, and a visual examination for abnormalities in finger and/or joint alignment. The therapist should palpate the digit for specific point tenderness and selectively evaluate the quality and quantity of volitional joint mobility. Selective capsular and ligamentous stress testing should be performed when indicated and the quality and quantity of accessory joint motions determined. The status and function of the digital tendons should be noted. It is important to stress, however, that the specific direction of each individual patient evaluation will vary depending on the pattern and severity of injury, the timing of therapeutic evaluation and treatment, and the extent of previous medical and/or surgical interventions.

GENERAL MANAGEMENT PRINCIPLES. The general aims of therapeutic management of closed traumatic PIP-joint injuries are to maintain the structural integrity and function of the injured and noninjured tissues, to establish and/or maintain maximal volitional and accessory joint mobility and maximal static and dynamic joint stability, and to return patients to their normal daily task, activity, and life role functions. These aims can generally be achieved by following these management principles:

- Protect the injured tissues with AAS to allow tissue healing. The PIP joint should be immobilized in as close to 0 degrees of extension as possible.
- Avoid unnecessary functional restrictions to the uninjured tissues in the involved PIP joint and finger.[40]
- Gradually reactivate the injured tissues as early as possible by reintroducing normal physiologic stresses to the joint in *a pattern opposite to the pattern of injury.* If, for example, the primary injury was an extension-compression-radial deviation, then start early reactivation with flexion and gradually reintroduce the injured joint to extension-compression-radial deviation stresses as tolerated.
- Selectively reactivate the patient back to normal daily tasks, activities, and life roles by providing the necessary support or

protection to the PIP joint during functional use, and by modifying and/or avoiding specific tasks and activities as indicated. If, for example, the primary tissue injury occurred from a compression force, then teach the patient to avoid, limit, or modify pinching and other closed kinetic chain activities that are likely to aggravate the sensitive healing tissues.

A Simple Clinical Solution: Variations of the "Figure-Of-Eight" Splint. It is not possible to outline specific therapeutic management strategies for all potential PIP-joint injuries. However, we have included some clinical variations for a practical and functional finger-based PIP joint "figure-of-8" splint[51] that we have found useful (Figure 98-11). This splint can be easily modified to either allow or restrict various degrees of extension and/or flexion and radial/ulnar deviation. Unfortunately, this practical little splint does not protect the joint from torsion or compression forces, so the patient should also be instructed on how to limit these forces during functional use while the injured tissues are healing.

MANAGEMENT OF HAND FRACTURES

Strong hard bones make useful limbs, useful limbs maintain strong hard bones.

Hancox[35]

The ultimate goal of fracture management is to restore normal bone tissue structure and function without compromising the functional abilities of the surrounding tissues or the injured person's ability to use the affected area for performance of his or her normal daily tasks, activities, and life roles. This goal can be difficult to achieve when managing hand fractures.

The limited volume and multiple-tissue layers in the hand result in restricted tolerance for swelling, callus formation, and the diminished normal tissue stresses associated with immobilization necessary for fracture healing. Trauma sufficient to cause a fracture is also likely to cause regional soft tissue injury, which can be further compounded by the addition of planned surgical trauma. The challenge for the therapist is to effectively rehabilitate both the affected tissues and the individual, without compromising the bone-healing process. The clinical key to remember is that specific management strategies will depend on the stability of the healing fracture. This stability is directly related to both the method of fracture fixation and the timing of intervention (Figure 98-12).

Fracture Healing

All fractures ultimately heal by primary or secondary bone regeneration. The healing process is considered a failure if stable bony union does not occur. The fracture site in normal healing may pass through an initial fibro-cartilage-callus healing phase, depending on the method of fracture fixation chosen. Primary bone healing occurs by direct regeneration of bone cells across a gap of less than 1 mm when

the two fracture surfaces are compressed and held firmly together. Primary fracture healing will only occur with open reduction and internal fixation (ORIF) rigid fracture fixation.[17] Secondary bone healing occurs when the soft fibrocartilage callus produced in the reparative phase between the bone ends is slowly converted by ossification to immature and finally to mature bone tissue. Secondary healing is more likely to occur when there is a large fracture gap and/or regional fracture mobility.[17]

Fracture Fixation: Closed Versus Open

Healing fractures like compression forces, but not shear, torsion, or tensile forces. Adequate fracture fixation after reduction is therefore the key to the ultimate structural and functional potential of the healed bone tissue. Fracture fixation can be achieved by closed and/or open methods (see Figure 98-12). Additional support for a fracture after a closed reduction can be provided by externally applied casts, splints, nails, pins, and/or external fixators. The fracture will ultimately heal by secondary healing with this method of fixation. Excessive motion at the fracture site can adversely affect this biologic sequence, resulting in a delayed union or nonunion.[61]

An open reduction requires some degree of surgical exposure for direct fracture visualization, reduction, and fixation. The surgeon uses some form of internal fracture stabilization using plates, pins, screws, or wires to compress the two fracture surfaces together. A successful ORIF should provide enough intrinsic stabilization to facilitate direct or primary bone healing and eliminate fracture mobility as a potential mediating factor in rehabilitation.[45]

Therapeutic Management Strategies

All healing fractures require AAS during the first 3 to 5 days in the inflammatory phase to allow the tissues the opportunity to recover from the shock of the trauma. The AAS should be continued during the next 2 to 3 weeks of the proliferation phase, especially when a fracture is potentially unstable. Care should be taken, however, to ensure that "overimmobilization" is avoided because this can lead to diminished soft tissue mobility and function or "fracture disease," a fracture healing success but a soft tissue functional failure.

The complications associated with fracture immobilization can occur by immobilizing more joints than are necessary on either side of the fracture and/or by immobilization for a prolonged period of time. The duration of immobilization should be limited to prevent regional tendons, ligaments, and nerves from being encased in the external fracture callus[17] and to limit the dynamic vascular changes that can occur as the tissues become dependent on external tissue pressure rather than the internal muscle pump.[8]

A thoughtful fabrication of casts and splints that immobilizes only those joints necessary to secure fracture stabilization and that keeps skin creases cleared for moving parts will help limit the complications associated with fracture immobilization.

Early active motion during the first 2 to 3 weeks is an

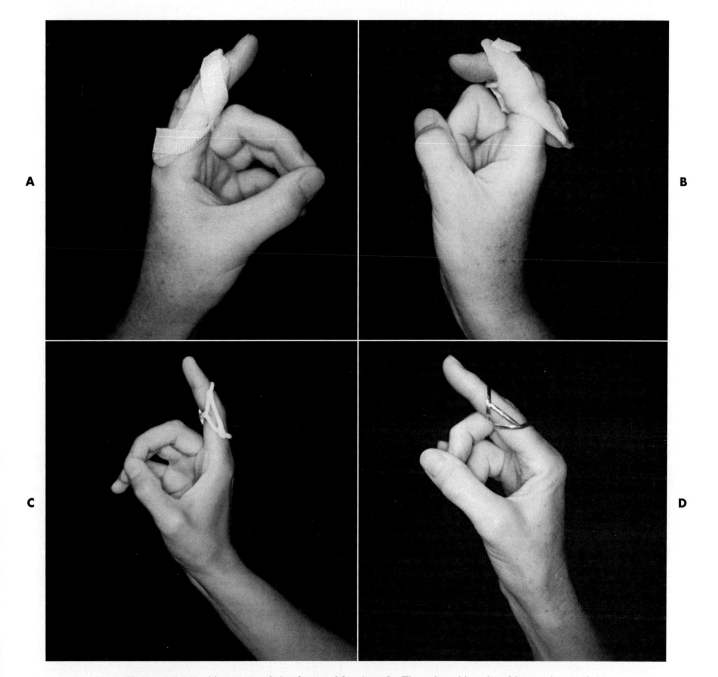

Figure 98-11. Variations of the figure-of-8 splint. **A,** This adjustable splint fabricated out of low-temperature thermoplastic material can be used in acute injuries to the volar plate (with or without an avulsion) and/or the accessory collateral ligament. The joint is usually blocked in ~30 degrees of extension. **B,** This adjustable splint fabricated from a low-temperature thermoplastic splinting material can be used in acute injuries to both the true and accessory collateral ligaments. The joint is blocked in ~30 degrees of extension, with an additional flexion block at ~70 degrees. **C,** This fixed splint fabricated out of low-temperature thermoplastic material can be used in subacute injuries to the volar plate and collateral ligaments and for longer-term sports protection for the same injuries. This splint can protect the PIP joint from hyperextension and radial/ulnar deviation forces. **D,** This fixed splint, similar to the thermoplastic splint in **C,** is fabricated out of sterling silver (Cygnet Orthotics, Vancouver, British Columbia). This splint is intended for the long-term support of chronic hyperextension and/or lateral joint instability.

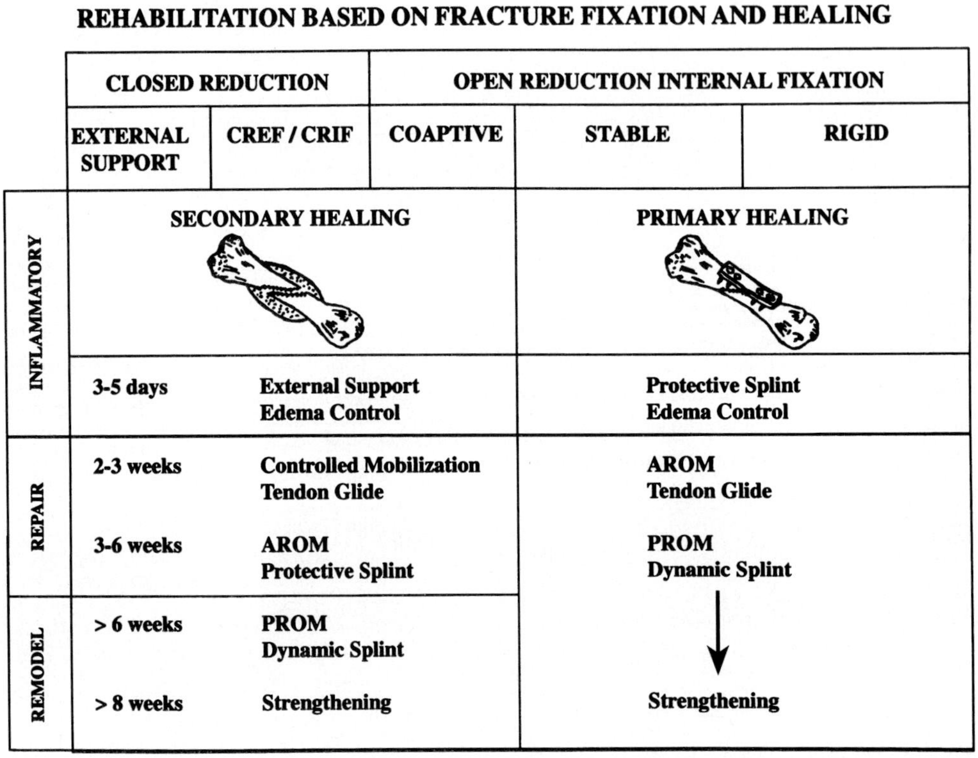

REHABILITATION BASED ON FRACTURE FIXATION AND HEALING

	CLOSED REDUCTION		OPEN REDUCTION INTERNAL FIXATION		
	EXTERNAL SUPPORT	CREF / CRIF	COAPTIVE	STABLE	RIGID
INFLAMMATORY	SECONDARY HEALING		PRIMARY HEALING		
INFLAMMATORY	3-5 days	External Support Edema Control	Protective Splint Edema Control		
REPAIR	2-3 weeks	Controlled Mobilization Tendon Glide	AROM Tendon Glide		
REPAIR	3-6 weeks	AROM Protective Splint	PROM Dynamic Splint		
REMODEL	> 6 weeks	PROM Dynamic Splint			
REMODEL	> 8 weeks	Strengthening	Strengthening		

Figure 98-12. Progression of therapy depends on the type of "fracture healing," which in turn is dependent on the type of fracture fixation used.

acceptable rehabilitation technique after an ORIF with stable, rigid fracture fixation. A protective splint, however, may still be necessary between exercise sessions to protect the healing tissues. Therapists should work together with the surgeon during this same time frame in patients with a less stable fracture fixation to find safe and effective ways to provide some form of early controlled or protected motion. This concept is especially important after an ORIF. It is of little value to open and fix a fracture and then not move it.[17]

Direct visualization is advantageous in fracture reduction, but there is a price to pay for this approach. The surgical intervention causes an additional soft tissue injury, leading to more fibroblasts and the formation of scar tissue that ultimately must be remodeled.

Fractures managed with rigid and stable fracture fixation should be able to tolerate dynamic splinting and progressive passive stretching exercises at approximately 3 weeks after surgery. Fractures managed by secondary healing techniques have only enough "clinical" stability to tolerate gentle controlled active mobilization, with supportive splinting continued between exercise sessions.[99] Immobilization of the injured finger to an adjoining digit with buddy straps may also be used to assist with alignment and promote active motion. Recalcitrant edema, stiffness, and hypersensitivity should also be addressed, and the patients' fears should be alleviated. It has been shown that therapy costs are reduced and return to work expedited when these "red flags" of fracture disease are addressed early in the course of treatment[31] (Box 98-1).

Box 98-1.
Red Flags in Early Fracture Management*

Pain
Swelling
Stiffness
Dissatisfaction
Loss of AROM

From Gardener D, Goodwill C, Bridges P: J Occup Med 10(3):114-117, 1968.
*These factors may lead to increased therapy costs if ignored.

Early bony union is likely to occur in fractures managed with secondary healing techniques at about 6 weeks. The healing fracture should then be able to tolerate the forces that occur with dynamic splinting and progressive passive stretching. Resisted functional activities and strengthening exercises, however, should be avoided until 8 weeks after surgery, when stable bony union is evident.

Studies of patients with long-bone fractures managed by rigid internal fixation suggest that periosteal blood flow is compromised and osteopenia with local plate and pin resorption is evident.[93] Rigid implants also shield the fracture site from normal physical stresses that contribute to tensile strength gains.[17] These concerns have not specifically been addressed in the healing of small-bone fractures managed with rigid fixation. It still seems prudent, however, despite the lack of evidence to the contrary, to delay the introduction of resisted functional activities and strengthening exercises until 8 weeks after injury in hand fractures managed with stable and rigid fixation.

Caveats of Therapy

Certain general clinical principles of hand fracture management are summarized here for brevity:

- Fracture rehabilitation is based on the method of fixation and the stage of healing.
- Splints and casts used for tissue immobilization should include only the necessary joints. Leave skin creases free for moving parts, and strive for the position of function (metacarpophalangeal [MCP]–joint flexion, interphalangeal [IP]–joint extension). The position of MCP flexion and IP extension will also relax the interossei, reducing their deforming pull on finger fractures.
- Therapy progression in patients with multiple fractures must be paced to accommodate the weakest form of fixation.
- The most important early active range-of-motion (AROM) exercises in patients with finger fractures are flexor digitorum profundus (FDP) glide to prevent adherence of the deep flexor and central slip glide for PIP extension. This is especially relevant in P1 fractures because of the intimacy of central clip, lateral bands, and flexor tendons to the underlying bone. Burkhalter[10] has coined the term *no-man's-land fractures* for P1 fractures. Adherence of these tendon structures to P1 fractures causes excessive motion at the MCP joint and diminished motion at the PIP joint. This limited motion presents as a loss in the extremes of active extension (Figure 98-13, *A*) and flexion (Figure 98-13, *B*). Blocking MCP-joint extension during IP-joint flexion exercises (not shown), and blocking MCP-joint flexion during IP-joint extension exercises (Figure 98-13, *C*) is important in treating patients with P1 fractures. Blocking motion in the proximal MCP joint directs the active forces to the distal PIP joint, facilitating tendon gliding.
- Fractures close to the MCP joint often result in a clawlike posture, limiting the potential for MCP flexion. In this situation, a finger-based gutter splint (not shown) that immobilizes the PIP and DIP joints during exercises will redirect the active motion forces more proximally to the MCP joint.

MANAGEMENT OF COMPRESSION/TENSION NEUROPATHY

Nerve compression is a nerve injury in slow motion. Compressed nerves cry out with a language all their own. It is the clinician's responsibility to learn this language and interpret these signals correctly before they are silenced by axonal death.

Early Compression/Tension Neuropathy

Intermittent or low-level compressive/tension forces applied to peripheral nerves compromise venous and lymphatic return in the epineural vascular system, leaving intrinsic blood flow unaffected.[58] Mildly compressed nerves are nonsymptomatic unless provoked by specific arm postures or functional activities that further reduce an already compromised blood supply.[12] Just as choking signals impaired air flow, intermittent paresthesias signal impaired blood flow to peripheral nerves. Neural ischemia that results from selective extremity postures is the basis of provocative neural tension/compression testing.[62] An upper-extremity battery of provocative tests is listed on the form depicted in Figure 98-14. Provocative tests that elicit patient symptoms in less than 1 minute are considered positive. These easily administered tests are early indicators of a temporary local conduction block, secondary to regional ischemia.

Ongoing or Chronic Compression/Tension Neuropathy

Ongoing compression/tension will ultimately lead to regional demyelination and internal peripheral nerve scarring.[59] These structural changes, combined with internal capillary obstruction in the deeper endoneural layers, lead to internal edema.[90] Increased tissue fluid pressure, or an internal compartment syndrome, creates further compression on the remaining viable intrinsic blood vessels. The patient with a peripheral nerve in this state will have symptoms of persistent peripheral nerve dysfunction (e.g., paresthesia, pain, weakness, fatigue, incoordination). The persistent symptoms may be more motor or sensory in origin, depending on the internal topography of the peripheral nerve. Patients with median nerve compression at the wrist (carpal tunnel syndrome) tend to present with diminished vibratory sensibility before the development of thenar atrophy,[73] whereas patients with radial or ulnar nerve entrapments at the elbow often initially present with both motor and sensory symptoms.[53]

A helpful clinical rule suggested by McComas[60] is to look at the "last innervated-first affected muscles" for symptoms of early peripheral nerve motor dysfunction. Abrams[1] outlines the specific muscles to examine for early motor dysfunction. They are the abductor pollicis brevis (APB) for the median nerve, the first dorsal interossei for the ulnar nerve, and the extensor pollicis longus (EPL) for the radial nerve.

Therapeutic Management Strategies

It is important to obtain baseline measurements before beginning any therapeutic treatment if therapists want to be able to assess the efficacy of therapeutic interventions in altering the patients' symptoms. Comprehensive motor and sensory nerve function tests should be performed at the initial evaluation, as well as documenting the type, frequency, and duration of specific symptoms occurring throughout their daily life. Failure to improve after a comprehensive conservative management program is suggestive of a significant peripheral nerve functional and/or structural problem. Surgical intervention directed at reducing local structural impingement

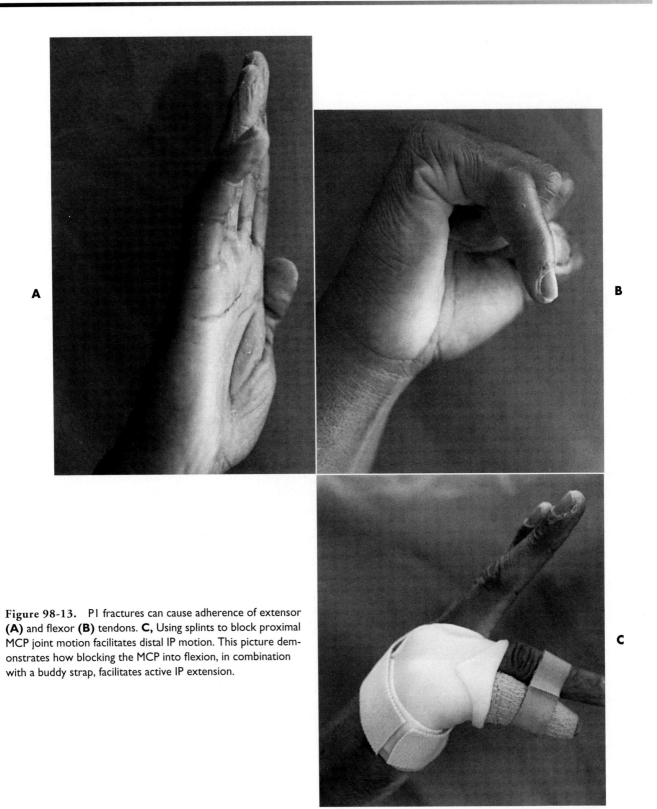

Figure 98-13. P1 fractures can cause adherence of extensor (**A**) and flexor (**B**) tendons. **C,** Using splints to block proximal MCP joint motion facilitates distal IP motion. This picture demonstrates how blocking the MCP into flexion, in combination with a buddy strap, facilitates active IP extension.

is indicated in this situation to prevent permanent nerve dysfunction.

In the early or initial stage, before excessive myelin damage, various conservative management strategies have been shown to be successful in reducing patient symptoms. These strategies can include local injections, iontophoresis, splinting, and posture and task/activity modification.[5,32,72] However, the elimination of symptoms using nonsurgical methods can be slow, often taking months. Seror[82] reported improved conduction velocities and diminished symptoms in patients with cubital tunnel syndrome who wore elbow splints regularly at night for 6 months.

A slow change in the patient's symptoms with long-term interventions requires exceptional patient compliance. Two

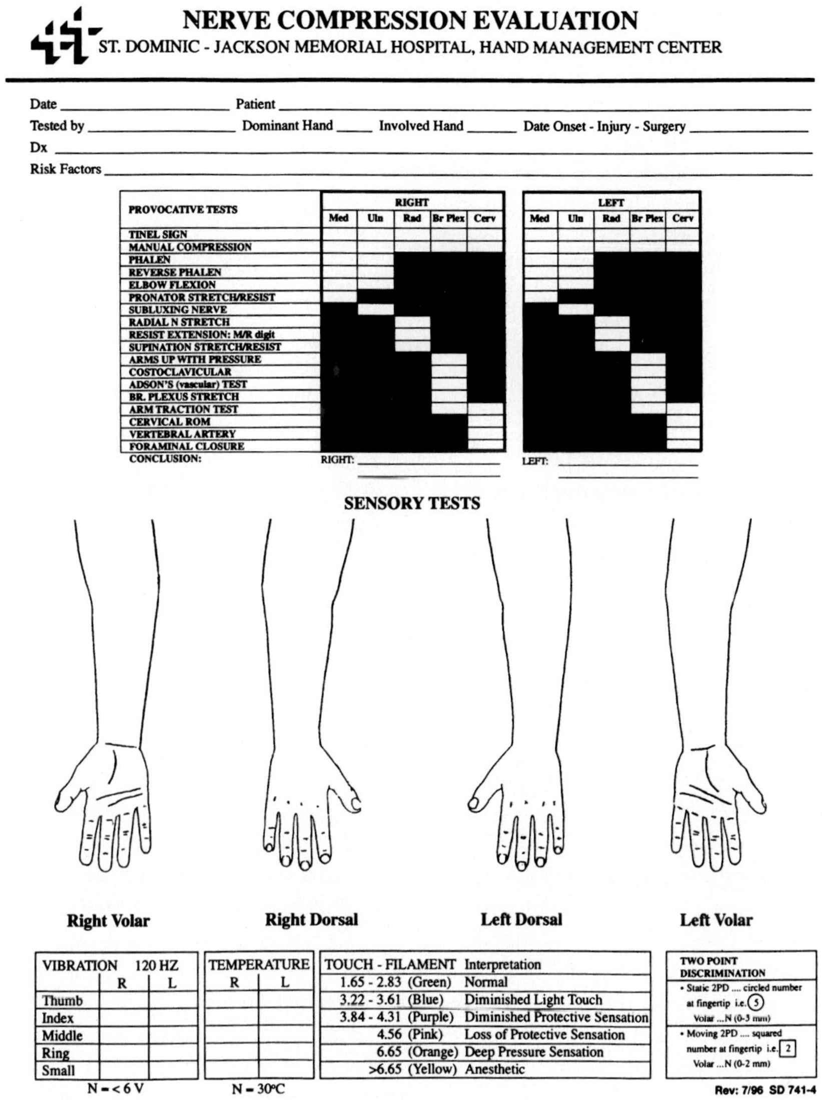

NERVE COMPRESSION EVALUATION
ST. DOMINIC - JACKSON MEMORIAL HOSPITAL, HAND MANAGEMENT CENTER

Date _____ Patient _____
Tested by _____ Dominant Hand _____ Involved Hand _____ Date Onset - Injury - Surgery _____
Dx _____
Risk Factors _____

PROVOCATIVE TESTS	RIGHT					LEFT				
	Med	Uln	Rad	Br Plex	Cerv	Med	Uln	Rad	Br Plex	Cerv
TINEL SIGN										
MANUAL COMPRESSION										
PHALEN										
REVERSE PHALEN										
ELBOW FLEXION										
PRONATOR STRETCH/RESIST										
SUBLUXING NERVE										
RADIAL N STRETCH										
RESIST EXTENSION: M/R digit										
SUPINATION STRETCH/RESIST										
ARMS UP WITH PRESSURE										
COSTOCLAVICULAR										
ADSON'S (vascular) TEST										
BR. PLEXUS STRETCH										
ARM TRACTION TEST										
CERVICAL ROM										
VERTEBRAL ARTERY										
FORAMINAL CLOSURE										
CONCLUSION:	RIGHT: _____					LEFT: _____				

SENSORY TESTS

Right Volar   Right Dorsal   Left Dorsal   Left Volar

VIBRATION 120 HZ			TEMPERATURE		TOUCH - FILAMENT	Interpretation
	R	L	R	L	1.65 - 2.83 (Green)	Normal
Thumb					3.22 - 3.61 (Blue)	Diminished Light Touch
Index					3.84 - 4.31 (Purple)	Diminished Protective Sensation
Middle					4.56 (Pink)	Loss of Protective Sensation
Ring					6.65 (Orange)	Deep Pressure Sensation
Small					>6.65 (Yellow)	Anesthetic
N = < 6 V			N = 30°C			

TWO POINT DISCRIMINATION
• Static 2PD .... circled number at fingertip i.e. ⑤
  Volar ...N (0-3 mm)
• Moving 2PD .... squared number at fingertip i.e. ☐2
  Volar ...N (0-2 mm)

Rev: 7/96 SD 741-4

Figure 98-14. A nerve compression evaluation form outlining common sensory and provocative tests used in the evaluation of patients with upper-extremity compression.

thirds of patients are either noncompliant or minimally compliant when following medical advice,[68] which suggests the therapist must take an active role in supporting patients in their ongoing efforts to make significant changes in their lives.

A client-centered approach that respects the patient's needs and desires can be helpful in improving an individual's commitment or compliance with a program. One-on-one patient education sessions that clearly outline the expected duration of treatment, expected treatment outcome, reasons for each specific exercise, splint, and task/activity modification, and causes for symptom recurrence are also essential.[30,68] Other strategies for improving patient compliance include providing patients with clear written and/or picture instructions for home programs, asking them to demonstrate exercises and splint application, educating their family members and co-workers, and providing "real-life situation" assistance in changing or modifying specific physical barriers in their daily lives. For example, on-site job analysis and training may prove to be more effective in overcoming job-specific physical barriers because patients have been shown to have difficulty in transferring proper body mechanics techniques learned in the clinic to the job situation.[13]

Therapeutic management strategies for compression neuropathy often occur in conjunction with ongoing medical interventions (interdisciplinary care). Antiinflammatory medications or local injections are often used to help resolve any inflammatory component that is thought to be contributing to a nerve compression. Management of peripheral compression neuropathy is also likely to be unsuccessful without medical management of coexisting medical conditions such as diabetes, kidney dysfunction, and thyroid conditions, which are suspected to be contributing to the problem. Mackinnon and Novak,[63] in their commentary on upper quadrant cumulative pain syndromes and in support of the concept of managing the whole patient/problem with multidimensional, multidirectional care, stated, "simple, single diagnosis and treatment plans when applied to problems having multiple components will fail to show symptom resolution."

Single-level medical interventions, such as cortisone injections or medications or therapy alone, are unlikely to be successful. Providing a patient with only a splint for treatment of carpal tunnel syndrome is also a single-level intervention and does not address the total picture. Therapeutic management strategies for compression neuropathies in the upper extremity need to be multifaceted to improve the likelihood of success. The scope of potential nonsurgical and postsurgical therapeutic management strategies is listed below.

NONSURGICAL THERAPEUTIC MANAGEMENT STRATEGIES

- Posture (dynamic and static) correction
- Splints to rest joints and muscles in positions that reduce compression or stretch on a nerve
- Stretching exercises to lengthen shortened muscles that may be contributing to altered postures and nerve compression (e.g., neck flexors, pectoralis minor, pronators, wrist and finger flexors, interossei)
- Strengthening exercises for weak or overstretched muscles, with specific emphasis on the proximal cervical, scapular, and glenohumeral stabilizers
- Nerve and tendon gliding exercises, to maintain normal mobility and flexibility of the involved MT units and nerves
- Personal, recreational, and vocational task/activity modifications (e.g., no forced overtime, job task and/or station rotation, lowered production speed or quotas, avoidance of repetitive movements, avoidance of extreme and/or specific postures, limited cold and vibration exposure, and ergonomic modifications of work station and tools)

POSTSURGICAL THERAPEUTIC MANAGEMENT STRATEGIES: EARLY INTERVENTION

- Wound care
- AAS of healing tissues
  - Rigid night splints to place the involved tissues at rest and allow them time to heal and recover
  - Flexible, nonconstrictive, motion-controlling splints during the day to protect the healing tissues by preventing extremes and/or specific directions of motion
- Antiswelling measures such as elevation, active exercises, light compression garments, or dressings
- Early postoperative nerve and tendon gliding exercises
- Graduated reactivation of affected regional tissue functions, including progressive range of motion (ROM), stretching/flexibility, strengthening, and endurance exercises
- Graduated and modified reactivation of the patient's normal daily task/activity and life role capabilities

POSTSURGICAL THERAPEUTIC MANAGEMENT STRATEGIES: LATE INTERVENTION

- Scar remodeling with conformers; desensitization therapy using contrast baths and massage; progressive texture, vibration, and pressure tolerance; TENS; functional activities

- Management of residual joint contractures with splinting, heat, and passive stretching and active/resisted end-range exercises and functional activities
- All strategies listed in nonsurgical therapeutic management strategies

Carpal Tunnel Clinical Outcomes

DeStafano,[18] in a comprehensive follow-up study of 425 patients diagnosed with carpal tunnel syndrome, reported that more patients are being treated with initial conservative methods today compared to 20 years ago. He suggested that this may be due to an earlier presentation with less severe symptoms. The average time for symptom resolution in the nonoperative patients in this study was 6 to 9 months, regardless of the nerve conduction velocity (NCV) test results. Splinting and oral antiinflammatory drugs were the management of choice, and work issues were not addressed. Nerve decompression in patients who failed conservative treatment performed within 3 years of the onset of symptoms was six times more likely to be successful. This study also suggested that patients who were likely to experience successful symptom resolution would do so within 6 to 12 months.

Other studies have suggested that grip and pinch strength in most patients will return to normal by 3 months after carpal tunnel surgery.[102] Higgs[42] found a higher percentage of patients who were employed in light-load, low-repetition jobs had resolution of symptoms after surgery, whereas those patients with severe NCV abnormalities before surgery were less likely to be symptom free after surgery.

Levine et al[55] developed a disease-specific patient questionnaire in 1993 that measures the symptom severity and functional status of patients with carpal tunnel syndrome. Amadio et al[2] compared the use of this disease-specific questionnaire with physical measures such as pinch and grip strength, ROM, dexterity and sensibility, and generic (SF-36[97]) and arthritis (AIMS2[69]) health status questionnaires in 22 postoperative carpal tunnel patients. All three questionnaire assessments in this study were able to measure significant changes in a patient's perception of reduced symptoms and improved functional abilities 3 months after surgery. These patients had improved dexterity at 3 months, but other physical measures were not significantly different when compared with preoperative values. This finding suggests that functional status or health-related quality of life measurements may be a more sensitive way to evaluate treatment efficacy in patients with upper-extremity compression syndromes in which symptoms are vague and difficult to measure using physical measurements of specific tissue dysfunction.

OUTCOMES

The term *outcome* implies completion. Therapeutic outcomes are therefore "something" at the completion or after the process of therapy. What makes any measurement a measure of outcome is the timing of the measurement, not the type of measurement taken.

MEANINGFUL OUTCOME MEASUREMENT

Therapists are encouraged to measure outcomes. However, measuring something for the sake of measurement can be a meaningless endeavor if we don't first have a goal in mind. Before measuring, clinicians should consider these questions:

What are we trying to measure?

Why are we trying to measure it?

How are we going to measure it?

Is it reasonable and practical to measure it?

What Therapeutic Outcomes Are We Trying to Measure?

There are two general measurement categories that can be assessed after the completion of therapy:

1. Evaluation of some aspect of an individual's or population's status
2. Evaluation of certain aspects of the therapeutic process

There are several types of measures within each category. Meaningful outcome measurement often involves taking a number of different measures related to both the process of therapy and the status of the patient/population. Impairment ratings,[19] functional status (FS) measures,[44,46,52] satisfaction measures,[43] and health-related quality of life measures are examples of individual/population status measures.[69,97] Financial, efficiency, and goal-attainment[74] measures are examples of measures of the therapeutic process.

Why Are We Trying to Measure Therapeutic Outcomes?

The reason for measuring outcomes will depend on the motivations or perspectives of the persons measuring. Policy makers, payers, employers, physicians, therapists, and patients will all have very a different perspective of what may be a meaningful or useful measure of therapeutic outcome. There are at least three areas from a therapist's perspective that justify therapeutic outcome measurement:

1. *Clinical responsibility:* Therapeutic outcome measurement can help therapists understand the implications of their specific management strategies for the individual patient and patient populations they treat.[91]
2. *Professional responsibility:* Therapists who want nontherapist groups to consider and critically evaluate the effect or importance of therapy need to define which specific measurements and evaluations these groups should consider.[25,76]
3. *Scientific responsibility:* Critically measuring therapeutic outcomes can offer scientific support or nonsupport for the efficacy of specific clinical interventions. This concept, called *evidence-based practice,*[80] can help therapists make clinical decisions based on a critical evaluation of the scientific evidence available.

How Are We Trying to Measure Therapeutic Outcomes?

The art of meaningful outcome measurement is selecting the right measurement tools. What makes a therapeutic outcome measurement scientifically and clinically useful is not what we measure or why we measure it, but how we go about measuring it. Measurement is a process of quantification of a specific concept. Quantification of a clinical concept is a complex process and falls within the domain of measurement theory.[28,29,79] The first step in determining how to measure or quantify a specific clinical outcome is to clearly define or operationalize the clinical concept to be measured. The second step is to then select an appropriate tool or instrument for measurement of the concept as defined.

Traditionally, the level of measurement of therapeutic outcomes has been at the cell/tissue/organ/system or impairment level. This level of measurement is perhaps the easiest because we already have many measurement tools readily available to help us measure impairment level clinical concepts such as joint mobility, muscle strength, and digital sensibility. An impairment level outcome measure is the physical impairment rating scales[19] used by insurance companies as a way to measure a permanent physical impairment associated with an injury.

The question is, how meaningful are physical impairment level measures for the clinicians and the patients involved? Impairment level measures do not consider the impact of the injury at the task/activity level (disability) or life role functioning level (handicap), nor do they measure the psychosocial impact of the trauma. Perhaps a multidimensional measurement of these concepts would provide a more meaningful measure of the total impact of a traumatic hand injury on the individual affected. Multidimensional measurement tools are commonly referred to as *functional status* or *health-related quality of life* measurement instruments.

Numerous functional status and health-related quality of life questionnaires have been developed to measure a person's own perception of his or her symptoms, functional abilities, behavior, and feelings within specific domains or defined content areas.[89] Generic instruments have been designed to measure more global aspects of a person's overall ability to function and are generally believed to be less sensitive to regional or disease-specific dysfunction. Regional or disease-specific instruments have also been developed and are more sensitive to specific areas of dysfunction but are not believed to capture a person's perception of his or her overall functional abilities.

There are many excellent multidimensional outcome-measurement questionnaires or tools that have been or are currently being developed and tested for validity and reliability in many patient populations. Most of these questionnaires are simple and do not take a great deal of time and effort to complete. The most commonly used generic multidimensional clinical outcome tool used in the upper extremity literature to date is the SF-36 Medical Outcomes Study (MOS) 36-item short-form health survey.[97] Box 98-2, borrowed directly from Stock et al,[89] provides an overview of many of the currently

Box 98-2.
Functional Status Measures for the Neck and Upper Limb

1. General Musculoskeletal Measures
   Disability Rating Index (DRI) (Salen et al, 1994)
   Pain Disability Index (PDI) (Tait et al, 1987)
2. Neck and Upper Limb Measure
   Neck and Upper Limb functional status Index (NULI-20; NULI-35) (Stock et al, 1995, 1996)
3. Upper Limb Measures
   Disabilities of the Arm, Shoulder, and Hand (DASH) (IWH/AAOS; Hudak et al, 1996)
   St. Michael's Upper Extremity Reconstructive Service Patient Self-Evaluation Form (Beaton and Richards, 1996)
   Toronto Extremity Salvage Score (TESS) (Davis, 1996)
   Adapted CTS Severity and Functional Status Scale (Pransky, Katz, in press)
4. Neck and Shoulder Measure
   Neck and Shoulder Disability Questionnaire (Viikari-Juntura et al, 1988)
5. Neck Measures
   Neck Disability Index (Vernon and Mior, 1991)
   Northwick Park Neck Pain Questionnaire (Leak et al, 1994)
   Échelle Fonctionnelle Cervicale (Fortin, 1996)
   AAOS Cervical Spine Instrument
6. Shoulder Measures
   American Shoulder and Elbow Surgeons Evaluation Form (ASES) (Richards et al, 1994)
   Simple Shoulder Test (Lippitt et al, 1993)
   Shoulder Pain and Disability Index (SPADI) (Roach et al, 1991)
   Shoulder Severity Index (Algofunctional Index) Patte, 1987)
   Subjective Shoulder Rating Scale (Kohn et al, 1992)
   Croft Shoulder Questionnaire (Croft et al, 1994)
   UCLA Shoulder Rating Scale (Ellman et al, 1986, 1991)
   Constant Score (Constant and Murley, 1987)
   University of Pennsylvania Shoulder Outcome Evaluation Form (Leggin)
7. Elbow Measure
   Elbow Disability Question (Akermark et al, 1995)
8. Wrist/Carpal Tunnel Syndrome Measures
   Carpal Tunnel Symptom Severity Scale and Functional Status Scale (Levine et al, 1991)
   Wrist Pain and Disability Patient Rating Scale (MacDermid, 1996)
   Carpal Tunnel Functional Status Instrument (Rossignol et al, 1996)

From Stock SR, Katz J, Beaton D: Measuring severity and disability in neck and upper extremity disorders: summary of a critical review of existing instruments. In *Proceedings of the consensus conference on case definitions of upper extremity musculoskeletal disorders, Nov. 15-16, 1996,* Baltimore, 1997, Center for VDT and Health Research, Johns Hopkins University. Please see original publication for cited references.

available instruments that may be useful for an upper extremity–injured population.

We need to remember, as clinicians and critical consumers, that no one tool or instrument will measure all clinical concepts in all clinical situations. Therefore before we measure, we need to always consider using a number of different tools or instruments. The art of clinically meaningful outcome measurement is selecting the right tools for the job. It is our responsibility, as clinicians, to first clearly determine exactly what concepts we are trying to measure and in what specific patient population. Secondly, it is then essential to critically evaluate which tools may be potentially useful for our specific use. It is not appropriate to use or develop a tool for measurement without first examining the validity, reliability, and sensitivity of the measurement tool or instrument.

Is It Reasonable and Practical to Measure Therapeutic Outcomes?

It is possible to define what concepts or outcome variables we would like to measure to justify why we want to measure them and to feel confident that we have scientific and clinically appropriate instruments to measure the given concepts or variables, but in many instances it is still not practical for therapists to measure them. The process of outcome measurement itself can be a complicated, time-consuming, and expensive endeavor, and most therapists do not have the necessary resources or infrastructure to measure outcomes efficiently and effectively.

The decision of what to measure is often determined by the practicality of finance, whether the people and institutions involved can reasonably afford the time and effort that goes into measuring therapeutic outcomes. Therapists are supportive of the concept of outcome measurement and are spending the time and effort to learn more about the what, why, and how of therapeutic outcome measurement. Unfortunately, for most therapists the institutional support and finances are still not available for them to pursue meaningful outcome measurement. Our biggest hurdle at present is communicating to insurers and payors the value of meaningful therapeutic outcome measurement.

ACKNOWLEDGMENTS

The authors would like to thank Robin Parish, MA, OTR for allowing us to adapt Figure 98-1 from her graduate thesis presentation; Julianne Howell, MS, PT, CHT for thoughts on the red flags in fracture management; Suzanne Greer, OTR for her artistic input; Graham Coultard, Communication Services, WCB of British Columbia, for his help in illustration production; and Gregory Feehan, PhD for his editorial input.

REFERENCES

1. Abrams RA, Ziets RJ, Lieber RL, et al: Anatomy of the radial nerve motor branches in the forearm, *J Hand Surg [Am]* 22(2):232-237, 1997.

2. Amadio PC, Silverstein MD, Ilstrup DM, et al: Outcome assessment for carpal tunnel surgery: the relative responsiveness of generic, arthritis-specific, disease-specific, and physical examination measures, *J Hand Surg [Am]* 21:338-346, 1996.

3. Aoki M, Kubotz H, Pruitt DL, et al: Biomechanical and histologic characteristics of canine flexor tendon repair using early postoperative mobilization, *J Hand Surg [Am]* 22(1):107-114, 1997.

4. Baille DS, Benson LS, Marymont JV: Proximal interphalangeal joint injuries of the hand. Part I. Anatomy and diagnosis, *Am J Orthop* 10:474-477, 1996.

5. Banta C: A prospective nonrandomized study of iontophoresis, wrist splinting, and antiinflammatory medication in the treatment of early mild carpal tunnel syndrome, *J Occup Med* 36(2):166-168, 1994.

6. Benjamin M, Ralphs JR: Tendons and ligaments: an overview, *Histol Histopathol* 12(4):1135-1144, 1997.

7. Bowers W (editor): *The interpahalangeal joints,* New York, 1987, Churchill Livingstone.

8. Brand P: Postoperative stiffness and adhesions. In *Clinical mechanics of the hand,* St. Louis, 1985, Mosby.

9. Buckwalter JA: Effects of early motion on healing of musculoskeletal tissues, *Hand Clin* 12(1):13-24, 1996.

10. Burkhalter W, Reyes F: Closed treatment of fractures of the hand, *Bull Hosp Jt Dis Orthop Inst* 44:145-162, 1984.

11. Butler DL, Grood ES, Noyes F: Biomechanics of ligaments and tendons, *Ex Sport Sci Rev* 6:125-181, 1978.

12. Butler DS: *Mobilization of the nervous system,* New York, 1991, Churchill Livingstone.

13. Carlton R: The effects of body mechanics instruction on work performance, *Am J Occup Ther* 41(1):16-20, 1987.

14. Cannon N, Mullins P: Modalities in upper extremity rehabilitation. In Makick M, Kasch M (editors): *Manual on management of specific hand problems,* Pittsburgh, 1984, AREN Publishers.

15. Cannon NM, Strickland JW: Therapy following flexor tendon surgery, *Hand Clin* 1:147-164, 1985.

16. Cannon N: Post flexor tendon repair motion protocol, *The Indiana Hand Center Newsletter* 1(1):13-18, 1993.

17. Chapman M, Woo S: Principles of fracture healing. In Chapman M, Moison M (editors): *Operative orthopedics,* Philadelphia, 1988, JB Lippincott.

18. DeStefano F, Nordstrom D, Vierkant R: Long-term symptom outcomes of carpal tunnel syndrome and its treatment, *J Hand Surg [Am]* 22:200-210, 1997.

19. Doege T (editor): *Guides to the evaluation of permanent impairment,* ed 4, Chicago, 1994, American Medical Association.

20. Doyle JR: Anatomy of the finger flexor tendon sheath and pulley system, *J Hand Surg [Am]* 13(4):473-484, 1988.

21. Ducanis AJ, Golin AK: *The interdisciplinary health care team: a handbook,* Germantown, Md, 1979, Aspen Systems Corp.

22. Dubousset JF: Finger rotation during prehension. In Tubiana R (editor): *The hand,* vol 1, Toronto, 1981, WB Saunders, pp 202-206.

23. Dyson M, Pond JB, Joseph J, Warwick R: The stimulation of tissue regeneration by means of ultrasound, *Clin Sci* 35:271-285, 1968.

24. Edwards DAW: The blood supply and lymphatic drainage of tendon, *J Anat* 80:147-152, 1946.

25. Ellenberg AB: Outcomes research: the history, debate, and implications for the field of occupational therapy, *Am J Occup Ther* 50(6):435-441, 1996.

26. Evans RB, Thompson DE: An analysis of factors that support early active short arc motion of the central slip, *J Hand Ther* 5:187-201, 1992.

27. Feehan LM, Beauchene JG: Early tensile properties of healing chicken flexor tendons: early controlled passive motion verses postoperative immobilization, *J Hand Surg [Am]* 15:140-147, 1990.

28. Fisher AG: Functional measures, part 1: what is function, what should we measure, and how should we measure it? *Am J Occup Ther* 46(2):183-185, 1992.

29. Fisher AG: Measurement-related problems in functional assessment, *Am J Occup Ther* 47(4):331-338, 1993.

30. Furth H, Holm M, James A: Reinjury prevention follow-through for clients with cumulative trauma disorders, *Am J Occup Ther* 48(10):890-899, 1994.

31. Gardener D, Goodwill C, Bridges P: Cost of incapacity due to fractures of the wrist and hand, *J Occup Med* 10(3):114-117, 1968.

32. Gelberman R, Aronson D, Weismor H: Carpal tunnel syndrome: results of prospective trial of steroid injection and splinting, *J Bone Joint Surg* 62A:1181-1184, 1980.

33. Gordon JE: *Structures: or why things don't fall down,* New York, 1978, Penguin Books.

34. Hall G, Anneroth G, Schennings T, et al: Effect of low level energy laser irradiation on wound healing: an experimental study in rats, *Swed Dent J* 18:29-34, 1994.

35. Hancox N: *Biology of bone,* London, 1972, Cambridge University Press.

36. Hardy M: Preserving function in the inflamed and acutely injured hand, *Clin Phys Ther* 9:1-15, 1986.

37. Hardy M: The biology of scar formation, *Phys Ther* 69:1014, 1989.

38. Harris SR: How should treatment be critiqued for scientific merit? *Phys Ther* 76(2):175-181, 1996.

39. Hakilis MN, Manske PR, Kubota H, et al: Effect of immobilization, immediate mobilization, and delayed mobilization on the resistance to digital flexion using a tendon injury model, *J Hand Surg [Am]* 22(3):464-472, 1997.

40. Hernandez MA, Corley FG: Finger joint injury: intervene early to minimize dysfunction, *J Musculoskeletal Med* 12(8):66-76, 1995.

41. Hertling D, Kessler RM: *Management of common musculoskeletal disorders: physical therapy principles and methods,* ed 2, New York, 1990, JB Lippincott.

42. Higgs P, Edwards DF, Martin DS, Weeks PM: Relation of preoperative nerve conduction values to outcome in workers with surgically treated carpal tunnel syndrome, *J Hand Surg [Am]* 22:201-205, 1997.

43. Hsieh MO, Kagle JD: Understanding patient satisfaction and dissatisfaction with health care, *Health Soc Work* 16(4):281-289, 1991.

44. Hudek PL, Amadio PC, Bombardier C, et al: Development of an upper extremity outcome measure: the DASH, *Am J Induct Med* 29:602-608, 1996.

45. Jabaley M: *Internal fixation of the hand*, ASPRS, Plastic Surgery Education Foundation videoconference, EF Teleplast Series, 1997.

46. Jette AM: Using health-related quality of life measures in physical therapy outcomes research, *Phys Ther* 73(8):528-537, 1993.

47. Khan U, Edwards JCW, McGrouther DA: Patterns of cellular activation after tendon injury, *J Hand Surg [Br]* 21(6):813-820, 1996.

48. Kisner C, Colby L: Introduction to therapeutic exercise. In *Therapeutic exercise: foundation and techniques,* Philadelphia, 1985, FA Davis Co.

49. Kubota H, Manske PR, Aoki M, et al: Effect of motion and tension in injured flexor tendons in chickens, *J Hand Surg [Am]* 21(3):456-463, 1996.

50. Lane JM, Black J, Bora FW: Gliding function following flexor-tendon injury, *J Bone Joint Surg* 58A:985-989, 1976.

51. Laporte JM, Berrettone MD, Seitz WH, et al: The figure-of-eight splint for proximal interphalangeal joint volar plate injuries, *Orthop Rev* 21(4):457-462, 1992.

52. Law M, Baptiste S, Carswell A, et al: *Canadian occupational performance measure,* ed 2, Toronto, 1994, CAOT Publications ACE.

53. Lawrence T, Mobbs P, Fortems Y, Stanley JK: Radial tunnel syndrome: a retrospective review of 30 decompressions of the radial nerve, *J Hand Surg [Br]* 20(4):454-459, 1995.

54. Leibovic SJ, Bowers WH: Anatomy of the proximal interphalangeal joint, *Hand Clin* 10(2):169-178, 1994.

55. Levine DW, Simmons BP, Koris MJ, et al: A self-administered questionnaire for the assessment of severity of symptoms and functional status in carpal tunnel syndrome, *J Bone Joint Surg* 75A:1585-1592, 1993.

56. Liu SH, Yang RS, al Shaikh R, Lane JM: Collagen in tendon, ligament, and bone healing; as current review, *Clin Orthop* 318:265-278, 1995.

57. Low J, Reed A: *Electrotherapy explained: principles and practice,* Toronto, 1991, Butterworth-Heinemann Ltd.

58. Lundborg G: Structure and function of the intraneural microvessels as related to trauma, edema formation, and nerve function, *J Bone Joint Surg* 57:938-948, 1975.

59. Lundborg G, Dahlin L: The pathophysiology of nerve compression, *Hand Clin* 8(2):215-227, 1992.

60. McComas AJ: *Neuromuscular function and disorders,* Boston, 1977, Butterworth.

61. McFarland E, Young M: Biomechanical principles in rehabilitation of fractures, *Phys Med Rehab* 9(1):269-283, 1995.

62. Mackinnon S, Dellon A: Experimental study of chronic nerve compression, *Hand Clin* 2(4):639-650, 1986.

63. Mackinnon S, Novak C: Clinical commentary: pathogenesis of cumulative trauma disorder, *J Hand Surg [Am]* 19(15):813-823, 1994.

64. Maddy L, Meyerderks E: Dynamic extensor assist splinting of acute central slip lacerations, *J Hand Ther* 10(2):206-212, 1997.

65. Manske PR, Lexker PA: Flexor tendon nutrition, *Hand Clin* 1(1):13-24, 1985.

66. Mason M, Allen H: The rate of healing tendons: an experimental study of tensile strength, *Ann Surg* 113:424, 1941.

67. May EJ, Silfverskiöld KL, Sollerman CJ: Controlled mobilization after flexor tendon repair in zone II: a prospective comparison of three methods, *J Hand Surg [Am]* 17:942-952, 1992.

68. Mayo N: Patient compliance: practical implications for physical therapist, *Phys Ther* 58(9):1083-1090, 1978.

69. Meenan RF, Mason JH, Anderson JJ, et al: AIMS2: the content and properties of a revised and expanded arthritis impact measurement scales health status questionnaire, *Arthritis Rheum* 35:1-10, 1992.

70. Micholovitz S: *Thermal agents in rehabilitation,* Philadelphia, 1986, FA Davis Co.

71. Nimni MB: Structure, function and metabolism in normal and fibrotic tissue, *Sem Arth Rheum* 13:1-86, 1981.

72. Novak C, Mackinnon S: Thoracic outlet syndrome, *Ortho Clin North Am* 27(4):747-762, 1996.

73. Omer G: Median nerve compression at the wrist, *Hand Clin* 8(2):317-324, 1992.

74. Ottenbacher KJ, Cusick A: Goal attainment scaling as a method of clinical service evaluation, *Am J Occup Ther* 44(6):519-525, 1990.

75. Pollock N: Client-centered assessment, *Am J Occup Ther* 47(4):298-301, 1993.

76. Pransky G, Himmelstein J: Outcomes research: implications for occupational health, *Am J Ind Med* 29:573-583, 1996.

77. Reed B: Peripheral vascular effects of electrical stimulation. In Currier D, Nelson R: *Dynamics of human biologic tissues,* Philadelphia, 1992, FA Davis Co.

78. Rosenblum NI, Robinson SJ: Advances in flexor and extensor tendon management, *Clin Phys Ther* 9:17-44, 1986.

79. Rothstein JM: Measurement and clinical practice: theory and application, *Clin Phys Ther* 7:11-46, 1985.

80. Sackett D: Rules of evidence and clinical recommendations on the use of antithrombotic agents, *Chest* 95:2S-3S, 1989.

81. Sapega A, et al: Biophysiologic factors in range of motion exercises, *Physician Sportsmed* 9(12):57-65, 1981.

82. Seror P: Treatment of ulnar nerve palsy at the elbow with a night splint, *J Bone Joint Surg* 75B(2):322, 1993.

83. Silfverskiöld KL, May EJ, Törnvall AH: Flexor digitorum profundus tendon excursions during controlled motion after flexor tendon repair in zone II: a prospective clinical study, *J Hand Surg [Am]* 17:122-131, 1992.

84. Silverman PM, Willette-Green V, Petrille J: Early protected motion in digital revascularization and replantation, *J Hand Ther* 2:84-95, 1989.

85. Small JO, Brennen MD, Colville J: Early active mobilization following flexor tendon repair in zone 2, *J Hand Surg [Br]* 14(4):383-391, 1989.

86. Sparto P, Parmianpour M, Feinsel T, et al: The effect of fatigue on multijoint kinematics, coordination, and postural stability during a repetitive lifting test, *J Ortho Sports Phys Ther* 25(1):3-12, 1997.

87. Steins SA, Haselkorn JK, Peters DJ, et al: Rehabilitation intervention for patients with upper extremity dysfunction: challenges of outcome evaluation, *Am J Indust Med* 29:590-601, 1996.

88. Strickland JW: Flexor tendon surgery, part 1, primary flexor tendon repair, *J Hand Surg [Am]* 14(3):261-272, 1989.

89. Stock SR, Katz J, Beaton D: Measuring severity and disability in neck and upper extremity disorders: summary of a critical review of existing instruments. In *Proceedings of the Consensus Conference on Case Definitions of Upper Extremity Musculoskeletal Disorders,* Nov 15-16, 1996, Baltimore, 1997, Center for VDT and Health Research, Johns Hopkins University, 1997.

90. Sunderland S: *Regeneration of the axon and associated changes in nerve and nerve injury,* Edinburgh, 1978, Churchill Livingstone.

91. Testa MA, Simonson DC: Current concepts: assessment of quality-of-life outcomes, *N Engl J Med* 334(13):835-840, 1996.

92. Tsuzaki M, Yamauchi M, Banes AJ: Tendon collagens: extracellular matrix composition in shear stress and tensile components of flexor tendons, *Connect Tissue Res* 29(2):141-152, 1993.

93. Uhthoff H, Goto S, Cerckel P: Influence of stable fixation on trabecular bone healing: a morphologic assessment in dogs, *J Ortho Res* 5:14-22, 1987.

94. Verbrugge LM, Jette AM: The disablement process, *Soc Sci Med* 38(1):1-14, 1994.

95. Viidik A: Functional properties of collagenous tissues, *Int Rev Conn Tiss Res* 2:127-215, 1973.

96. Wadsworth H, Chanmugan APP: *Electrophysical agents in physiotherapy: therapeutic and diagnostic use,* ed 2, Marrickville, NSW, 1983, Science Press.

97. Ware JE, Snow KK, Kosinski M, Gandak B: *SF-36 health survey: manual and interpretation guide,* Boston, 1993, The Health Institute, Nimrod Press.

98. Weber ER: Nutritional pathways for flexor tendons in the digital theca. In Hunter JM, Schneider LH, Mackin EJ (editors): *Tendon surgery in the hand,* St. Louis, 1987, Mosby.

99. Wilson R, Carter M: Management of hand fractures. In Hunter JM, Schneider LH, Mackin EJ, Callahan AD (editors): *Rehabilitation of the hand,* ed 3, St. Louis, 1990, Mosby.

100. World Health Organization: *International classification of impairments, disabilities and handicaps,* Geneva, 1993, WHO.

101. Wright W, Jones RJ: Quantitative and qualitative analgesia of joint stiffness in normal subjects and in patients with connective tissue diseases, *Ann Rheum Dis* 20:36-46, 1961.

102. Young V, Logan SE, Fernando B, et al: Grip strength before and after carpal tunnel decompression, *South Med J* 85(9):897-900, 1992.

CHAPTER

Congenital Anomalies of the Hand

Donald R. Laub, Jr.
Amy L. Ladd
Vincent R. Hentz

INTRODUCTION

Almost every parent marvels at the perfection of his or her newborn's hands, but when a congenital malformation occurs this wonder is replaced with dismay. Upper limb malformations in the United States occur in 0.16% to 0.18% of live births, but those figures may be higher in certain populations.[17] Only a few of these patients have significant functional or cosmetic problems.[11] Because of this rarity and the great variety of deformity, most patients with congenital malformations are referred to an academic hand surgeon or pediatric orthopedic surgeon. Prenatal diagnosis has now been described and this will only further increase the numbers of referrals.[19]

There are a great diversity and variety of congenital hand deformities, with each case being a unique situation with its own abnormal anatomy. The subject can only be approached with a firm knowledge of general surgical principles, which can then be adapted to each individual circumstance. Many classification schemes for congenital hand deformities have been devised. Some were too general to differentiate between various malformations, whereas others were too detailed to be functional. The current scheme has been agreed on by the American Society of Surgery of the Hand and the International Federation of Societies for Surgery of the Hand and was published by Swanson in the very first issue of the *Journal of Hand Surgery*.[27] It groups congenital malformations into seven groups based on abnormalities that occur during embryologic events (Box 99-1). Each group, of course, will have varying degrees of severity. The deformities addressed in this chapter are grouped for ease of discussion by these classifications and then subdivided by type of malformation.

INDICATIONS

ABNORMAL ANATOMY

Flatt[13] introduced an anatomic classification scheme that gives a broad overview of the range of deformities (Box 99-2). Many other books written on the subject of congenital limb malformations provide more detailed information. Only the general guidelines for treating some of the more commonly encountered conditions are discussed here.

Parents are understandably distressed by the appearance of a child's anomalous hand, and they may be hoping that surgery can create a "normal hand." They need to be reminded that children with congenital anomalies view themselves as "normal." Children, in contrast to the adult who suffers a traumatic injury, know only the hand they possess. They develop their own methods of manipulating objects and are usually not self-conscious of their appearance until they become school aged. The parent, however, may still be grieving the loss of an anticipated "perfect" child. The pediatrician, geneticist, and in some cases, psychologist can play a very key role in counseling the parents of these children. The hand surgeon should have at least a basic working knowledge of the incidence, inheritance patterns, and the growth potential of the malformation, in addition to explaining the role surgery can play to improve hand function and appearance.

Informed consent for treatment of congenital anomalies of the hand must be tailored to the individual case, but general potential complications exist and are discussed here by way of introduction. These risks include infection, hemorrhage, and potential complications related to anesthesia. Scarring and functional recovery should also be addressed.

Preoperative evaluation should include an appropriate evaluation for associated problems, such as blood dyscrasias in children with radial aplasia, or other congenital malformations

---

Box 99-1.
International Federation of Societies for Surgery of the Hand Classification of Congenital Hand Anomalies

   I. Failure of formation of parts
  II. Failure of differentiation of parts
 III. Duplication
 IV. Overgrowth
  V. Undergrowth
 VI. Constriction ring syndrome
VII. General skeletal abnormalities

Data from Swanson AB: *J Hand Surg [Am]* 1:8-22, 1976.

Box 99-2.
Flatt's Classification, Based on Abnormal Anatomy

THE THUMB
Inadequate thumb
Absent thumb
Extra thumbs

THE FINGERS
Small and absent fingers
Crooked fingers
Webbed fingers
Constriction ring syndrome
Extra fingers
Large fingers

THE HAND
Central defects
Radial defects
Ulnar defects

Data from Flatt AE: *The care of congenital hand anomalies,* St. Louis, 1994, Quality Medical Publishers.

Box 99-3.
Bayne's Classification of Radial Ray Deficiency

Type   I   Short distal radius
Type II   Hypoplastic radius
Type III Partial absence of the radius
Type IV Radial agenesis

Data from Bayne LG, Lovell WW, Marks TW: *J Bone Joint Surg* 52A:1065, 1970.

---

that are more common in children with congenital hand malformations. Specialized pediatric anesthesia may be needed for some children. Other operative procedures may be coordinated with additional treating physicians so the child undergoes anesthesia only once.

OPERATIONS

The type of incision, bony fixation, periods of immobilization, and the sutures used are points of individual preference. We indicate our preferred techniques and, where appropriate, other alternatives. We routinely administer preoperative prophylactic antibiotics. The tourniquet is also routinely used,

and additional exsanguination in the young child can be gained by wrapping and clamping an esmarch bandage around the distal arm. The goal is to achieve a pressure slightly above arterial pressure, thereby excluding the periosteal feeders of the distal humerus. The surgeon uses loupe magnification for all procedures. Kirschner wires (K wires) will suffice for fixation in the younger child, whereas in the adolescent or adult rigid internal fixation may be required.

Fast-absorbing, plain gut sutures are used whenever possible in the skin because this obviates the need for the frequently unpleasant task of suture removal. K wires used for fixation are left outside the skin to facilitate removal. A wrist block of 0.25% bupivacaine at the end of the procedure can provide long-lasting pain relief. The toxic dose of 3 mg/kg is easily reached in small children, and must be remembered. Almost all young children are dressed with a bulky hand dressing and a well-padded fiberglass cast. If the elbow is bent slightly greater than 90 degrees and supracondylar flattening is performed, even the most active child cannot wriggle out of the dressing. The older, cooperative patient may be placed in a short arm cast or splint. Immobilization should be maintained for 2 weeks after a predominantly soft tissue procedure, but longer in bone procedures involving an osteotomy (e.g., 4 to 6 weeks). Guarded early mobilization may be used in cases with rigid internal fixation.

FAILURE OF FORMATION OF PARTS

Longitudinal Arrest: Radial Ray Deficiency

Radial ray deficiency is also called *preaxial hypoplasia* or *radial club hand.* A child with this malformation may have other associated anomalies such as blood dyscrasias, cardiac defects, or VATER syndrome (vertebral anomalies, tracheoesophageal [TE] fistula, renal agenesis).[12] There may commonly be more distal anomalies of the affected limb, such as an absent or hypoplastic thumb and/or scaphoid bone. A fusion flexion contracture of the elbow is also common.

Bayne[3] classified radial ray deficiencies into four types based on the radiologic appearance (Box 99-3). He found type IV (radial agenesis) to be the most common. When the radius is absent, the hand deviates quite severely radially because of lack of support. Surgical correction may provide a stable wrist and improve appearance, but will not improve the growth potential of the forearm. Surgery for both hands is contraindicated in patients with bilateral radial aplasia and stiff elbows because the child will be unable to bring either hand to his mouth.[13]

Preoperative splinting should begin at birth. The ideal time to operate on the child is at approximately 6 to 18 months of age, if other medical conditions are stable and the parents are prepared for surgery.

Centralization of the carpus on the ulna provides a stable hand after the constricting radial soft tissue is released. A tendon transfer or tendon imbrication is performed, and the skeleton is stabilized on the distal ulna. Buck-Gramcko[7] prefers radialization of the ulna by placing the radial carpus and second metacarpal over the center of the ulna, increasing the ulnar positioning of the hand. Corticotomy and distraction lengthening methods show promise, but will require research before gaining popular acceptance.

We prefer centralization, based on the method of Bayne[3] (Figure 99-1). The ulnar side of the wrist is approached through a zigzag incision. The ulnocarpal capsule is released. The structures on the radial side of the wrist are identified through a separate radial incision. The radial sensory branch is usually absent. The flexor carpi radialis (FCR), brachioradialis, and radial wrist extensors may be present, however, and available for transfer. Centralization of the carpus on the ulna is accomplished by fully releasing the wrist capsule. The cartilaginous distal ulnar epiphysis may be contoured to allow acceptance of the carpus, but the physis must be carefully preserved with its blood supply. If the ulna is extremely bowed, an osteotomy secured simply with a K wire or pin can straighten the forearm. A pilot hole is drilled first, then the drill is removed and holes are drilled through the carpus and third metacarpal. The ideal skin exit would be just proximal to the physis of the third metacarpal head. The carpus is then reduced and the pin is driven retrograde into the pilot hole in the ulna. The capsule on the radial side is shortened, and the radial tendons, if present, are transferred to the extensor carpi ulnaris (ECU). Bayne recommends also transferring the flexor carpi ulnaris (FCU) to the ECU.[3]

Bayne removes the pin in 6 to 8 weeks, but we have had better success keeping the pin in several months or longer, removing it only when it protrudes or otherwise becomes symptomatic. A night splint should be continued until the skeleton is mature. The pin is more easily removed from the distal metacarpal side. We have had a pin fracture in one child, but the retained pin has not been a problem.

Revision or secondary surgery is not uncommon. A second pin may be inserted if deformity recurs, particularly after an early pin removal. Revision centralization or osteotomy may be needed, particularly in complete absence of the radius (for which multiple osteotomies, including both opening and closing wedges, may be required). We have utilized secondary muscle tendon transfers to better balance the centralized hand. The abductor digiti minimi (ADM) is mobilized from its origin by an osteotomy of the pisiform and reattached to the dorsal-ulnar aspect of the ulna, making this muscle an ulnar deviator and extensor of the wrist. Wrist motion is most desirable, but fusion may be a salvage procedure if the deformity recurs and a better cosmetic appearance is desired. Fusion may be indicated early in severe cases in which complete correction is almost impossible. Procedures may be performed as early as 3 to 6 months after centralization in patients with a hypoplastic thumb.

Longitudinal Arrest: Central Ray Deficiency

A central deficiency denotes complete or partial absence of the third ray and is divided into typical and atypical varieties. The typical variety consists of bilateral absence of the third finger, and syndactyly of the first and sometimes fourth web may be present. Central ray deficiency is inherited as an autosomal dominant trait and is associated with other musculoskeletal and organ-system abnormalities. The atypical form is sporadic in inheritance and presents unilaterally with a deeply cleft hand. Complete or partial absence of the second, third, or fourth rays is seen, and the hand may have bizarre skeletal aberrations, such as transverse phalangeal or metacarpal bars. The child with a central ray deficiency typically has good hand function but may not want to use the hands because of their appearance. Flatt describes this deformity as a "functional triumph and a social disaster."[13] Surgical correction is therefore indicated to correct the syndactyly where this exists and to improve the appearance by closing the cleft. More complex deformities have been repaired with either the Snow-Littler[25] or the Miura-Komada[24] technique, both of which are termed reverse pollicization. Both techniques transfer the index ray to the base of the third metacarpal, but the two techniques differ in their design of skin flaps for creation of the first web space.

The Miura-Komada technique uses a linear incision carried out in the cleft from the ulnar border of the ring finger to the radial border of the index finger and continued dorsally in a V across the index finger (Figure 99-2). A volar incision is made at the base of the index finger, carefully preserving the neurovascular structures. The bases of the second and third metacarpals are exposed, and a dorsal rectangular flap is developed with an additional incision angled over the second metacarpal. The fascia over the first dorsal interosseous muscle is released. The origin of this muscle and of the adductor pollicis is also released from the base of the thumb metacarpal. The adductor pollicis may be absent or anomalous. An osteotomy of the proximal index metacarpal is performed, and the ray is transferred to the base of the third metacarpal. We prefer an oblique osteotomy, which allows some lengthening of the transferred digit if needed. If the third metacarpal is absent or rudimentary, the index metacarpal is positioned somewhat more toward the ulnar side of the hand and slightly angulated that way. K-wire fixation is adequate in children. The dorsal skin flap is transferred to the radial border of the transferred index finger.

The functional outcome in the treatment of children with a cleft hand associated with first web-space syndactyly depends on the outcome of the first web-space correction. The intermetacarpal ligament should be reconstructed to stabilize the second through the fourth digits and a new web space should be created, which is placed at the correct proximal-distal location. Secondary procedures, such as skin grafts or flaps, stabilization with tendon transfers, or procedures for thumb hypoplasia, may be needed.

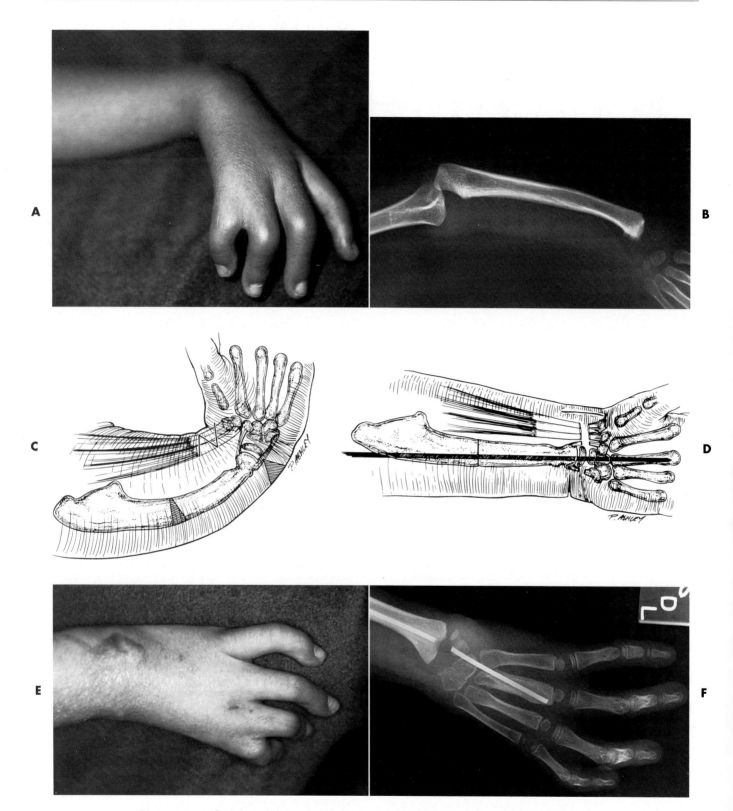

Figure 99-1.   Radial ray deficiency. **A,** A 2-year-old child with left radial ray deficiency (note that this is the left hand of the patient whose right hand is seen in Figure 99-7). **B,** Radiograph of the limb, with the radius completely absent. **C,** Diagram of the deformity and the operative plan. **D,** Diagram of the completed operative procedure. **E,** Patient's hand after surgery. **F,** Postoperative radiograph taken 3 months after surgery. The fractured pin was left in place and the retained fragments have not been a problem. (From Herndon J: *Surgical reconstruction of the upper extremity,* Stamford, Conn, 1999, Appleton & Lange, pp 895-921.)

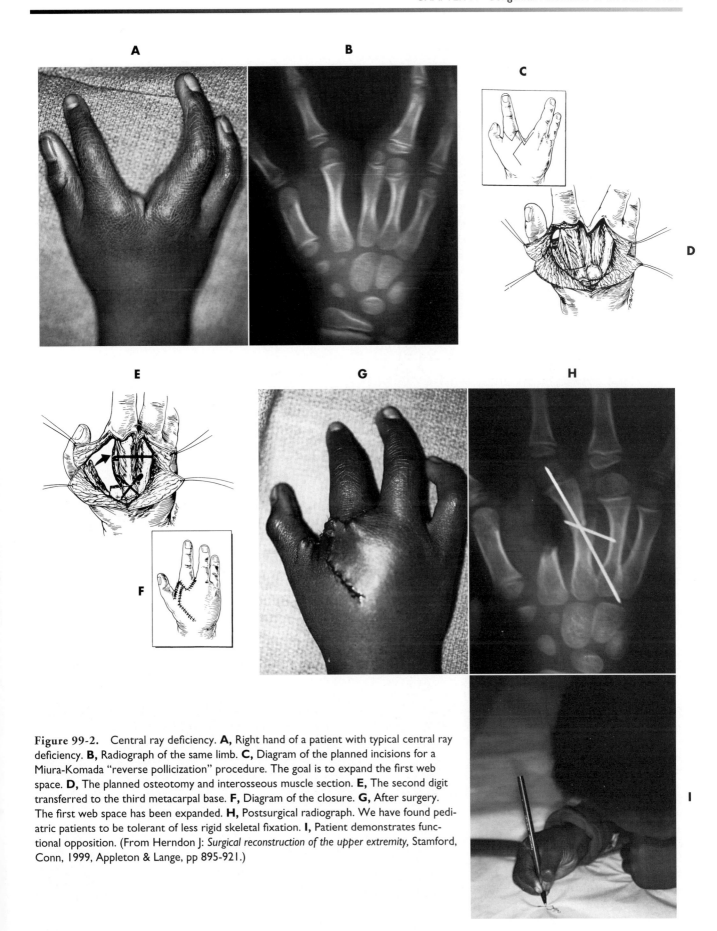

Figure 99-2. Central ray deficiency. **A,** Right hand of a patient with typical central ray deficiency. **B,** Radiograph of the same limb. **C,** Diagram of the planned incisions for a Miura-Komada "reverse pollicization" procedure. The goal is to expand the first web space. **D,** The planned osteotomy and interosseous muscle section. **E,** The second digit transferred to the third metacarpal base. **F,** Diagram of the closure. **G,** After surgery. The first web space has been expanded. **H,** Postsurgical radiograph. We have found pediatric patients to be tolerant of less rigid skeletal fixation. **I,** Patient demonstrates functional opposition. (From Herndon J: *Surgical reconstruction of the upper extremity,* Stamford, Conn, 1999, Appleton & Lange, pp 895-921.)

FAILURE OF DIFFERENTIATION OF PARTS

Syndactyly

Patients with a failure of part differentiation may be subdivided into those with only soft tissue involvement, termed *simple syndactyly,* and those with skeletal involvement, or *complex syndactyly.* Syndactyly involving the entire length of two adjacent digits is termed *complete,* whereas those with only a partial length involved are termed *incomplete.* Syndactyly is one of the most common congenital anomalies, occurring in 1 in every 2000 births.[10,17] Simple syndactyly most commonly affects the third web space (between the third and fourth fingers), followed by the fourth, second, and rarely the first web space.[13] Isolated syndactyly is common bilaterally, may be inherited as an autosomal dominant trait, and is rare in patients of African descent.

Syndactyly release is usually performed around 12 to 18 months of age, depending on the surgeon's experience and the family's concerns. Flatt recommends waiting until 2 to 4 years of age for the common third web-space simple syndactyly because he experienced fewer complications, and growth of the digits was unaffected.[13] Earlier surgery is recommended in border digits or in patients with compound syndactyly because growth may be affected.

Only one side of any given digit should be operated on at one time to prevent vascular compromise if one digital vessel is absent or divided. Full-thickness skin grafts are usually required to close the web space and are preferred over split-thickness grafts, which are more prone to contract. Syndactyly release is based on using opposing zigzag incisions (Figure 99-3).[1] These flaps can be designed to provide an equal amount of skin to each digit, which we prefer, or more skin can

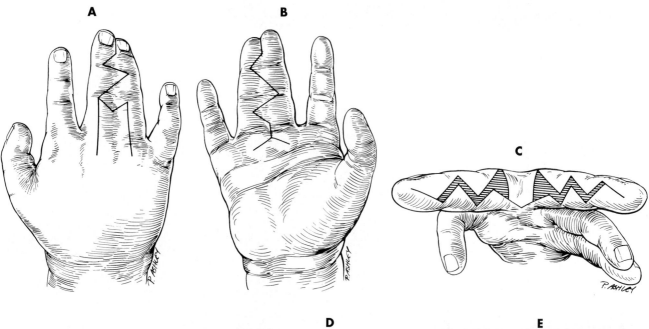

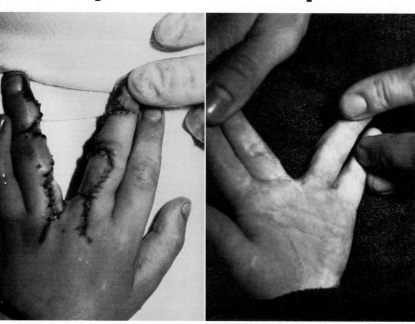

Figure 99-3. Simple syndactyly. **A,** Dorsal view of a planned separation of a third and fourth finger simple syndactyly. **B,** Palmar view of the planned separation of a third and fourth finger simple syndactyly. **C,** Diagram of the planned closure. It is important that the web space be primarily closed. The shaded areas cannot be closed without undue tension, and skin grafts must be used. **D,** Wound appearance after closure. **E,** Web space has been preserved. (From Herndon J: *Surgical reconstruction of the upper extremity,* Stamford, Conn, 1999, Appleton & Lange, pp 895-991.)

be allotted to one digit over the other, leaving only one digit requiring skin grafts. The fingertip is divided longitudinally, to avoid damage to the nail bed. The web space is lined with a dorsal rectangular flap based proximal to the metacarpophalangeal (MCP) joint and extending sometimes as distal as the proximal interphalangeal (PIP) joint. This is the most critical determinant for successful surgery. Every effort should be made to bring the tip of the flap into the palm, rather than only to the edge of the web. Lost flaps or grafts, or poorly positioned flaps can result in scarring that will create deforming forces producing angulation of the digits. Correction of this problem should wait for full scar maturity. Dorsal flap necroses at the tip will create a web space that is cleft-shaped rather than smooth. Upton[29] has described many useful procedures to correct this problem. Judicious defatting may be performed when dissecting the flaps, but dorsal veins should be preserved. The palmar flap is usually not incised until the neurovascular bundles are identified and the dorsal flap inset is measured. The most proximal dissection of the web division is the bifurcation of the common digital artery because the common digital nerve bifurcates more proximally and is rarely a problem. The tourniquet is released once the flaps are defatted and inset. Hemostasis is ensured, and a template is made of the remaining skin required to close the defect with a graft.

A full-thickness skin graft is harvested from the groin. If the lateral side of either nail fold is deficient, a graft of glabrous skin from the hypothenar eminence or lateral aspect of the great toe gives a more natural appearance to the fingertip.[26] We currently use simple bulky dressings and a cast, rather than complicated bolster dressings. Occasionally a digit will have postoperative axial rotation, particularly the little or ring fingers. This can be corrected by a secondary osteotomy. Again, it is best to defer secondary surgery, such as correction of a flap or graft loss, until the scars are fully matured.

Functional improvement is often more important than the cosmetic appearance in patients with complex syndactyly, such as acrocephalosyndactyly (Apert's disease) (Figure 99-4). Staged reconstruction follows the principles of simple syndactyly, but requires osteotomies of the synostoses and more liberal use of skin grafts. Occasionally, in patients with more complex hands, it is best to reconstruct a hand with only three fingers and a thumb. The surgeon should counsel the family about the limited functional potential of rudimentary digits if this procedure is needed.

DUPLICATION

Polydactyly: Preaxial, Central, and Postaxial

Preaxial, central, and postaxial polydactyly are common deformities, in some series more common than syndactyly.[8] Preaxial polydactyly of the thumb is the most common congenital deformity seen by the hand surgeon. Postaxial fifth-finger polydactyly is more common, but it is usually a

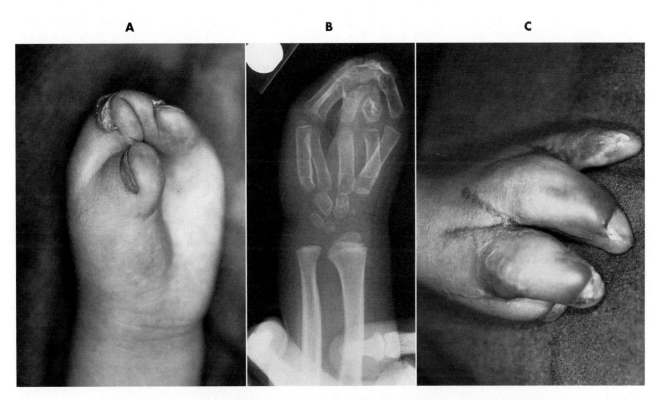

Figure 99-4. Complex syndactyly. **A,** Photograph of a child's hand with Apert's acrocephalosyndactyly. This appearance has been likened to a "rosebud." **B,** Radiograph of this hand, showing the distal bone fusion. **C,** The patient's hand after surgery, showing a simplified four-digit hand. We have found this to be much more successful than attempting complex procedures for preserving five digits. (From Herndon J: *Surgical reconstruction of the upper extremity,* Stamford, Conn, 1999, Appleton & Lange, pp 895-991.)

rudimentary tag and is most often removed by the pediatrician by tying it off while the newborn is in the hospital nursery. If we are consulted for these rudimentary "nubbins," we will often remove them in the clinic or at the site of consultation under local anesthesia.

Some forms of polydactyly are best described as a "polysyndactyly," especially the rare central polydactyly, because the supernumerary digits are rarely complete and functional and present with features of complex syndactyly.

Skin incisions should be planned as indicated by the level and site of duplication and should allow ablation of central, less well-innervated skin (Figure 99-5). The collateral ligaments and attached periosteum are preserved and sutured to the remaining digit to preserve joint stability, and split tendons can also be preserved and transferred. A common phalanx or metacarpal that is too large can have the condyle pared to match the more distal phalanx.

Care must be taken to preserve the physis of the metacarpal head if the duplication occurs at the MCP-joint level. This is less of a concern in more distal duplications because the physis is at the proximal end of the more distal bones. A closing wedge osteotomy can be performed if there is clinodactyly or other angulation deformity. K-wire fixation is sufficient in children.

Thumb polydactyly was classified by Wassel (Figure 99-5, D).[30] The most common level is duplication of the proximal and distal phalanges (type IV). Thumb polydactyly occurs sporadically and unilaterally, whereas thumb triphalangia (Wassel type VII) may be hereditary and associated with great-toe polydactyly. The ulnar digit is usually more developed in thumb polydactyly and is therefore preserved. We do not recommend the central ablation technique of Bilhaut.[4]

Revision surgery may be necessary if angulation or clinodactyly recurs. Reconstruction of the collateral ligaments may suffice for patients with mild angulation, but for more advanced deformity, a cartilage fusion using the chondrosis technique described by Kowalski and Manske may be required.[16] The articular cartilage of both sides of the joint is carefully shaved until the ossification center is exposed. The growth center is preserved, and stability is obtained without halting growth.

Patients with postaxial or fifth finger polydactyly usually present a less complicated reconstruction. Delta phalanges and irregular epiphyses may need to be excised in more complicated symbrachydactyly cases.

UNDERGROWTH

Hypoplasia of Fingers and Thumb

Hypoplastic fingers may also be classified as a symbrachydactyly because most are usually short and webbed. This malformation bridges several categories in the classification scheme and may be classified either as a failure of formation (i.e., longitudinal arrest, hypoplasia) or a failure of differentiation. Short fingers with intact phalanges may be treated with a syndactyly release as described previously.

Digits with absent phalanges but with a skin envelope present can be reconstructed with a composite graft including toe phalanx, joint, and possibly tendon[14] (Figure 99-6). A dorsal zigzag incision is made on the finger, and a pocket is developed to receive the graft. Fibrous bands may need to be resected. The size of the pocket and a preoperative radiograph dictate which toe phalanx is used. The toe phalanx is harvested through a dorsal longitudinal incision. Slips of tendon may be taken if a joint ligament reconstruction is required. The grafted phalanx is secured with simple K-wire fixation.

The hypoplastic thumb may be classified as a radial longitudinal failure of formation. Hypoplasia of the thumb has been classified in five types by Blauth (Box 99-4).[2] No treatment is required in patients with type I thumbs. Patients with types II and III thumbs with stable carpometacarpal (CMC) joints (type IIIA) are candidates for reconstruction. The techniques used include deepening of the first web space with transposition flaps, or a four-flap Z-plasty, stabilization of the MCP joint, correction of any extrinsic tendon abnormalities, and/or an opponensplasty usually using the Huber technique of transferring the ADM.[15] We prefer the modification of the ADM transfer described by Manske and McCarroll.[22,23] This muscle transfer gives bulk to the thenar eminence, whereas transfer of a tendon, such as the superficialis, does not. The ADM is exposed through a curvilinear incision starting on the ulnar side of the proximal phalanx of the fifth digit, curving radially proximal to the MCP joint to cross the wrist radial to the pisiform. Care is taken to avoid much dissection on the proximal and radial side of the ADM muscle where the neurovascular structures enter. A second incision is made over the MCP joint of the thumb, and a subcutaneous tunnel is developed between the two incisions. It is important that the muscle not be constricted in this tunnel. Some fibers of the ADM may need to be freed from the ulnar side of the pisiform to obtain adequate length, however complete detachment is not necessary and may expose the neurovascular bundle to the risk of overstretching, with resultant ischemia and paralysis of the transferred muscle.

The method for inserting the transferred tendon depends on the patient's deformity.[18,20,22] The MCP joint can be partially stabilized by suturing the transferred ADM tendon to the joint capsule or collateral ligament. Two additional transfers are indicated in patients with type III thumbs for whom reconstruction is attempted. The extensor indicis proprius (EIP) is transferred for thumb extension, and the ring finger flexor digitorum superficialis (FDS) is used as an adductor transfer. One slip of the FDS is attached to the extensor mechanism and the other to both the ulnar base of the proximal phalanx and the metacarpal head.

Types IIIB, IV, and V hypoplastic thumbs are best reconstructed by pollicization of the index finger. The technique of pollicization was first described by Littler[21] and later modified by Buck-Gramcko.[6] The index digit is shortened by removing almost all of the metacarpal except for the metacarpal head, which assumes the function of the trapezium

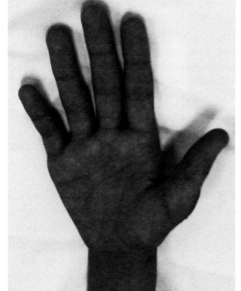

Figure 99-5. Preaxial polydactyly. **A,** Photograph of a patient's hand with a Wassel type IV duplication of the thumb. The first dorsal interosseous and adductor pollicis are atrophied. **B,** Radiograph of the hand. **C,** Schematic excision of a Wassel type II duplication. **D,** The Wassel thumb duplication classification. **E,** Postoperative view. (Figures 99-5, *A-D* from Herndon J: *Surgical reconstruction of the upper extremity,* Stamford, Conn, 1999, Appleton & Lange, pp 895-921.)

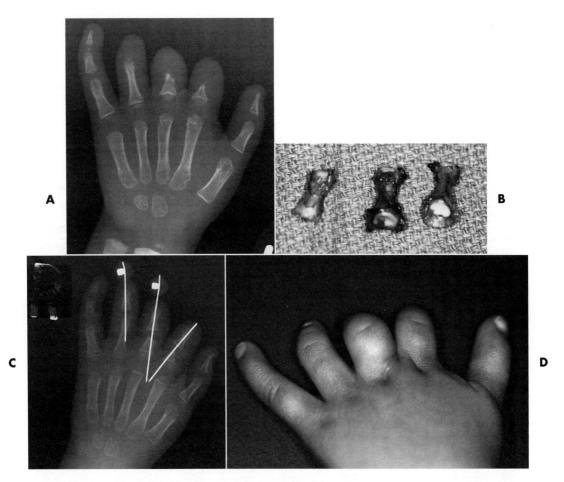

Figure 99-6. Hypoplasia of fingers: composite joint grafts. **A,** Radiograph of a patient's hand with a transverse deficiency at the level of the proximal phalanges. **B,** Composite graft of toe phalanges with articular cartilage, harvested in the method of Goldberg and Watson.[14] **C,** Radiograph of the grafts secured with longitudinal K wires. **D,** Postsurgical appearance. Skin creases indicate motion in the newly created joints. (From Herndon J: *Surgical reconstruction of the upper extremity,* Stamford, Conn, 1999, Appleton & Lange, pp 895-921.)

Box 99-4.
Hypoplasia of the Thumb,
Blauth Classification

Type I	Minimal shortening or narrowing
Type II	Narrow first web space
	Intrinsic thenar muscle hypoplasia
	MCP joint instability
Type III	Narrow first web space
	Intrinsic thenar muscle hypoplasia
	MCP joint instability
	Extrinsic tendon abnormalities
	Metacarpal hypoplasia with CMC joint stable (type IIIA)
	Metacarpal hypoplasia with CMC joint unstable (type IIIB)
Type IV	Rudimentary phalanges
	Thumb attached by skin bridge
Type V	Aplastic thumb

Data from Wassel HD: *Clin Orthop* 64:175-193, 1969.

(Figure 99-7). The finger is dissected as an island flap on its flexor and extensor tendons, the two neurovascular pedicles, and dorsal veins and nerves. The finger is pronated 140 to 160 degrees and fixated into the correct axis of the thumb. Hyperextension of the index MCP joint is prevented by fixing the metacarpal head in full extension, as described by Buck-Gramcko. The first dorsal interosseous (DI) assumes the function of the abductor pollicis brevis (APB); likewise the first palmar interosseous (PI) serves as the adductor pollicis (AP), the extensor digitorum communis (EDC) to the index functions as the abductor pollicis longus (APL), and the EIP is the extensor pollicis longus (EPL).

The operation is begun on the palmar side of the hand. A gentle S-shaped incision is placed over the index metacarpal. This must be placed sufficiently radial to prevent an adducted first web space. Flaps are developed, and the neurovascular pedicle to the index and long fingers is identified volar to the intermetacarpal ligament. The artery to the radial side of the long finger is divided, and the common digital nerve is dissected proximally, separating the fascicles of the index and long fingers as far as is needed. The next incision is made dorsally over the

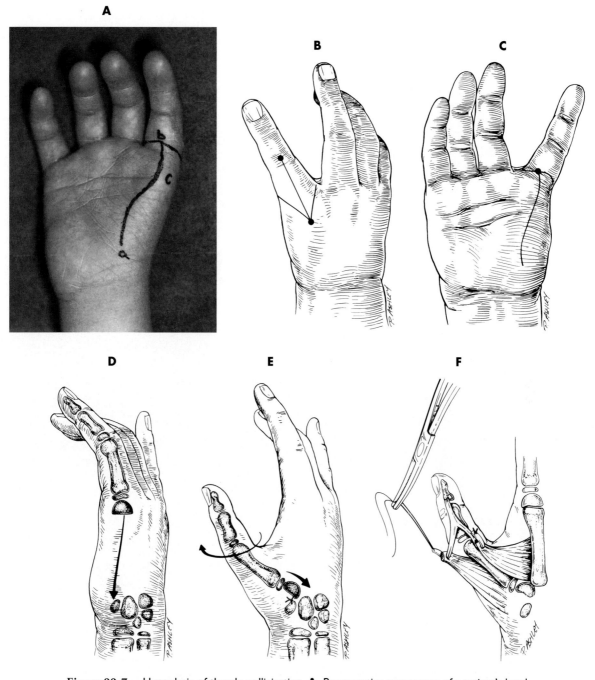

Figure 99-7. Hypoplasia of thumb: pollicization. **A,** Preoperative appearance of a patient's hand, with complete agenesis of the thumb. This is the right hand of the patient shown in Figure 99-1. **B,** Dorsal diagram of the planned incisions. **C,** Palmar diagram of the planned incisions. **D,** Diagram of the second metacarpal resection. **E,** Diagram showing proximal transposition, pronation, and hyperextension of the MCP joint. **F,** Diagram showing the first dorsal interosseous muscle taking the role of the abductor pollicis brevis, with the first palmar interosseous becoming the adductor pollicis.
Continued

proximal phalanx, shaped in a V at the MCP joint and extending circumferentially around the index finger. The flaps are designed to inset into the new thumb position as illustrated. Dorsal flaps are elevated, carefully preserving dorsal veins and the radial nerve or artery contributions to the finger, if present.

The flexor tendons must then be released by dividing the

A1 and, if needed, the A2 pulleys. The palmar and dorsal interossei are dissected from the shaft of the index metacarpal subperiosteally through both a palmar and a dorsal approach. The insertion of the first dorsal interosseous is divided just distal to the musculotendinous junction, preserving the lateral band contribution to the extensor mechanism as a wing for future reattachment. The EDC and the EIP are identified

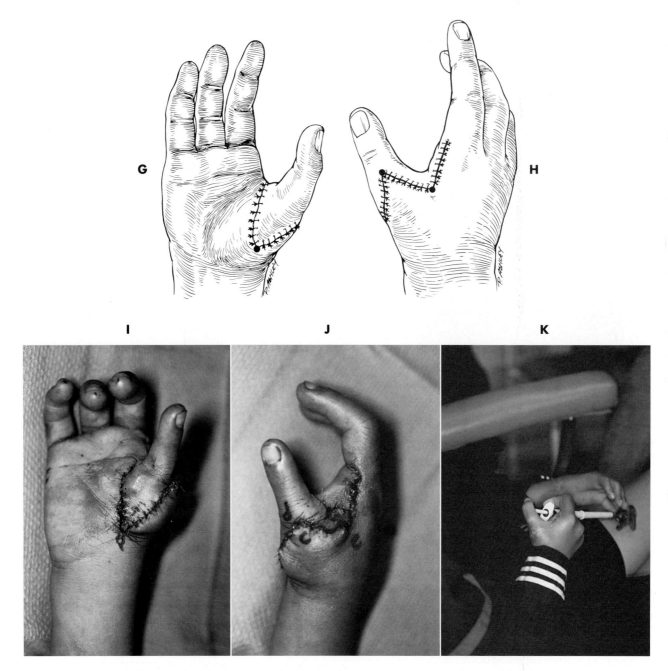

Figure 99-7, cont'd. G, Palmar diagram of the planned closure. **H,** Dorsal diagram of the planned closure. **I,** Palmar appearance of the closure. **J,** Dorsal appearance of the closure. **K,** Patient demonstrates functional opposition. (From Herndon J: *Surgical reconstruction of the upper extremity,* Stamford, Conn, 1999, Appleton & Lange, pp 895-921.)

proximally, and the EDC is divided at the MCP level. The shaft of the metacarpal is removed, including the physis. Only the base and the epiphysis are preserved.

The index metacarpal is fixed in the proper thumb axis by K wires or heavy suture to the residual second metacarpal base. Extensor tendons are appropriately shortened, but flexor tendons are not because they achieve better results in our hands if allowed to equilibrate over time. Some surgeons, however, prefer to shorten the flexor tendons.[18]

OUTCOMES

It is difficult to evaluate postoperative functional improvement in young children. Specific measurements such as pinch strength will improve with growth even without surgical intervention. The cooperation of younger children is often erratic. Children can also perform functional "trick" compensations for many deficiencies. Consequently, postoperative functional evaluation is expressed in qualitative, not quantitative terms.

We have recently reviewed our experience with the complex brachysyndactylies of Apert's syndrome in 10 patients.[8] We found a good outcome with functional hands and patient and parent satisfaction with simple surgeries that did not require distant flaps or revision surgery.

COMPLICATIONS

None of the congenital limb malformations are life threatening, and few are even limb threatening. Therefore reconstruction should be planned in such a way that any threats to the patient's life or limb are minimized. Practically speaking, this means recognizing the limitations of the anesthesiology department and timing surgical procedures accordingly. No rigid surgical schedule should take precedence over the patient's health when, for example, respiratory infection or other major anomalies are present.[12]

The complication of tissue loss very occasionally may occur as a result of the anomaly itself, such as with very severe constrictive band syndrome, but more often is caused by the surgical procedure itself. Poor skin flap vascularity may result in skin necrosis or infection, and this may be prevented by placement of skin grafts when excessive tension is created during skin closure. An island pedicled flap, such as the index finger during an index pollicization, can be at risk for vascular compromise secondary to excessive traction, twisting, or kinking of the pedicle, or even vasospasm. When this occurs, the cause must be sought and immediately corrected, or the transferred tissue must be returned to its preoperative position. Sometimes, however, even a minor repositioning is sufficient to restore normal blood flow.

Neurological complications may occur from congenital inadequacy, surgical damage, or circulatory deficiency. The last may be the most troublesome because it leads to a dysesthetic, autonomically impaired digit. Scrupulous attention to details during surgery is the best prophylaxis to prevent these problems.

Hypertrophic scars may develop, particularly in black or Asian patients.[9] Postsurgical stiffness of digits is common but improves with time and usage.

The most common complications in reconstruction of the upper limb are skeletal in nature. Bone complications are rare compared with those of joints, which may be stiff, unstable, or have persistent or recurrent angulation. Persistent deviation may be secondary to angulation of the joint surface, which may be secondary to uneven growth of the physis. Another cause, however, may be persistent deviating forces from unrecognized, and thus untreated, abnormal insertions of the flexor or extensor tendons. This can be improved by closing wedge osteotomies and reinsertion of the offending tendons. Severely deviated or unstable joints can be corrected by arthrodesis or chondroses. A joint that had motion before surgery but loses it after surgery may be caused by adherence of the unrecog-

nized limb of a bifid tendon, which may require surgical correction.[12]

FUNCTIONAL AND PSYCHOLOGIC OUTCOME

Bradbury et al[5] in Leeds, England reviewed both the functional and psychological outcomes in a series of 14 children who underwent microvascular toe transfer for congenital hand anomalies. Both the patients, their families, and an independent professional panel participated. It was found that all of the children experienced significant functional and aesthetic improvement after surgery. The level of psychosocial adjustment of the parents was found to be the most important predictor of psychosocial outcome and satisfaction for the patients.

Townsend et al[28] in Hawaii reviewed 65 cases of supernumerary thumb excision with an average of 9 years follow-up. They found half of the 49 patients treated by excision, with or without ligamentous reconstruction, experienced unacceptable results. The most common unacceptable results were joint deviation, instability, and bony prominence. The complications in this group were surgically salvageable. Five patients, however, had a central wedge excision procedure and all of the patients had unacceptable, short, fat, and stiff thumbs with nail deformities.[4] These unacceptable thumbs were not surgically salvageable.

FUTURE INVESTIGATION

It is hard to design outcome research for congenital hand anomalies. Children are ever-changing and adaptable, and they are very inventive at making their own hands functional. In some congenital deformities, such as aplasia of the thumb, creation of an opposable digit by index pollicization yields such an obvious functional improvement that few children remain untreated and an outcome study is not generally deemed necessary. The results are less apparent with other anomalies, such as surgical correction of central ray deficiency. Most patient series are small, and treatments tend to be individualized, making comparison studies difficult. Careful long-term longitudinal studies with defined goals, comparing one treatment plan with another, will be required to justify one approach over another and provide outcome data.

SUMMARY

Surgical correction of congenital hand anomalies is a demanding challenge, but it offers a chance to significantly improve the extremity function and cosmetic appearance in children who will use the affected extremity for the rest of their lives. The diversity of these anomalies provides a challenge even to those surgeons who devote a lifetime to the correction of these problems.

REFERENCES

1. Bauer TB, Tondra JM, Trusler HM: Technical modification in repair of syndactylism, *Plast Reconstr Surg* 17:385-391, 1956.

2. Blauth W, Schneider-Sicker F: *Congenital deformities of the hand,* New York, 1976, Springer-Verlag.

3. Bayne LG, Lovell WW, Marks TW: The radial club hand, *J Bone Joint Surg* 52A:1065, 1970.

4. Bilhaut M: Guerison d'un pouce bifide per un nouveau procede operaire, *Congr Fr Chir* 4:576, 1890.

5. Bradbury ET, Kay SP, Hewison J: The psychological impact of microvascular free toe transfer for children and their parents, *J Hand Surg* 19B:689-695, 1994.

6. Buck-Gramcko D: Pollicization of the index finger, *J Bone Joint Surg* 53:1605-1617, 1971.

7. Buck-Gramcko D: Radialization as a new treatment for radial club hand, *J Hand Surg [Am]* 10:964-968, 1985.

8. Chang J, Laub DR Jr, Ladd AL, Hentz VR: A simplified approach in the surgery of brachysyndactyly in Apert's syndrome. Submitted to *J Hand Surg,* not yet published.

9. Chen DS: Reconstruction of first web space of hand: followup analysis of 40 cases, *Chines J Surg* 30:515-517, 1992.

10. Cheng JC, Chow SK, Leung PC: Classification of 578 cases of congenital upper limb anomalies with IFFS system: 10 years experience, *J Hand Surg [Am]* 12:1055-1060, 1987.

11. Conway H, Bowe J: Congenital deformities of the hands, *Plast Reconstr Surg* 18:286-290, 1956.

12. Doboyns JH: Problems and complications in the management of upper limb anomalies, *Hand Clin* 2(2):373-381, 1986.

13. Flatt AE: *The care of congenital hand anomalies,* St. Louis, 1994, Quality Medical Publishers.

14. Goldberg NH, Watson HK: Composite toe (phalanx and epiphysis) transfers in the reconstruction of the aphalangic hand, *J Hand Surg [Am]* 7:454-459, 1982.

15. Huber E: Hilfsoperation bei median uslahmung, *Dtsch Arch Klin Med* 136:271, 1921.

16. Kowalski MF, Manske PR: Arthrodesis of digital joints in children, *J Hand Surg [Am]* 13:874-879, 1988.

17. Lamb DW, Wynne-Davies R, Soto L: An estimate of the population frequency of congenital malformations of the upper limb, *J Hand Surg [Am]* 7:557-562, 1982.

18. Latimer J, Shah M, Kay LS: Abductor digiti minimi transfer for the restoration of opposition in children, *J Hand Surg [Br]* 19:653-658, 1994.

19. Leung KY, MacLachlan NA, Sepulveda W: Prenatal diagnosis of the "lobster claw" anomaly (ultrasound), *Obstet Gynecol* 6(6):443-446, 1995.

20. Lister G: Pollex abductus in hypoplasia and duplication of the thumb, *J Hand Surg [Am]* 16:626-633, 1991.

21. Littler JW: Neurovascular pedicle method of digital transposition for reconstruction of the thumb, *Plast Reconstr Surg* 12:303, 1953.

22. Manske PR, McCarroll HR Jr: Abductor digiti minimi opponensplasty in congenital radial dysplasia, *J Hand Surg [Am]* 3:552-559, 1978.

23. Manske PR, McCarroll HR Jr: Index finger pollicization of the congenitally absent or nonfunctioning thumb, *J Hand Surg [Am]* 10:606, 1985.

24. Miura T, Komada T: Simple method for reconstruction of the cleft hand with adducted thumb, *Plast Reconstr Surg* 64:65-67, 1979.

25. Snow JW, Littler JW: *Surgical treatment of cleft hand: transcript of the International Society of Plastic and Reconstructive Surgeons, fourth congress,* Rome, 1967, Exerpta Medical Foundation, p 888.

26. Sommerkamp TG, Ezaki M, Carter PR, Hentz VR: The pulp plasty: a composite graft for complete syndactyly fingertip separations, *J Hand Surg [Am]* 17:15-20, 1992.

27. Swanson AB: A classification for congenital limb malformations, *J Hand Surg [Am]* 1:8-22, 1976.

28. Townsend DJ, Lipp EB Jr, Chun K, et al: Thumb duplication, 66 years experience: a review of surgical complications, *J Hand Surg [Am]* 19:973-976, 1994.

29. Upton J: Congenital anomalies of the hand and forearm. In McCarthy JG (editor): *Plastic surgery,* ed 3, Philadelphia, 1990, WB Saunders.

30. Wassel HD: The results of surgery for polydactyly of the thumb: a review, *Clin Orthop* 64:175-193, 1969.

PART II

SOFT TISSUE REPAIR

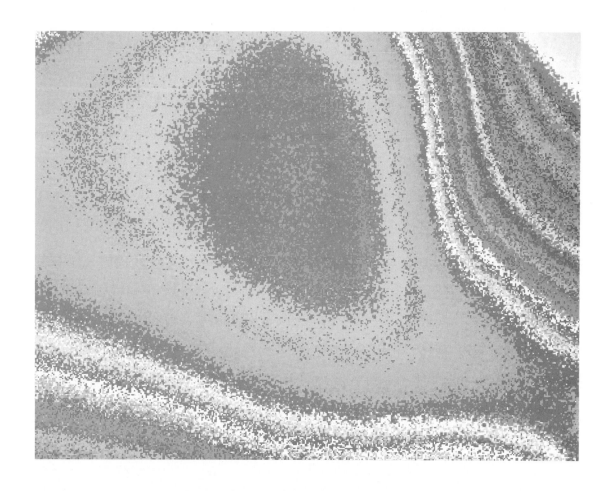

Fingernails

100

Michael W. Neumeister
Elvin G. Zook

INTRODUCTION

Human fingernails, located on the dorsal aspect of the terminal 40% of the distal phalanx of each finger, are dynamic and physiologically important organs of the hand.

Trauma to the fingertip and nail unit remains the most common of all hand injuries. The fingertip is one of the last anatomical structures to be pulled away after closing doors or using saws, machines, chains, or hammers.[20,70] The long finger is most commonly involved in these injuries, followed by the ring, index, and little fingers and the thumb.[70] The distal phalanx provides bony support for the nail bed and is fractured in 50% of fingertip injuries. Loss of nail-bed integrity can produce a permanent and significantly dysfunctional deformity of the fingernail. Thus it is imperative to respect the fingernail unit and to provide primary anatomical repair of nail-bed injuries whenever possible.

The nail bed lies protected between the nail plate and the distal phalanx. Blunt or sharp trauma to the nail compresses the nail bed and can result in lacerations and more complex crush injuries. Avulsion injuries are common and usually signify a greater level of trauma. Regrowth of the nail plate after an injury is influenced by the integrity of the nail bed and the nail folds. A smooth nail bed is essential for the regrowth of a nail with a normal appearance. Inadequate or unrepaired nail-bed lacerations may form granulation tissue or scar, which results in an area of nonadherence or other nail-plate deformities. Damage to the germinal matrix can result in absent or poor nail formation, a split-nail deformity, or synechial adhesions of the nail fold to the nail bed. A comprehensive awareness of fingernail anatomy, the dynamics of nail regeneration and adhesive properties, and the unfortunate sequelae of inadequate initial management sets the stage for the appropriate treatment of nail-bed injuries.

ANATOMY AND PHYSIOLOGY

The fingernail aids the hand in manipulating and grasping fine objects. Loss of the nail results in a measurable decrease in fingertip sensitivity.[6,19,59,70] The two-point discrimination of the fingertip is enhanced by the counter-force or buttress effect of the nail plate on the distal finger pad. The rigid nail also protects the vulnerable distal fingertip and distal phalanx from trauma. The entire fingernail unit or perionychium consists of the nail plate, the proximal nail fold (eponychium), the lateral nail fold (paronychium), the nail bed/skin junction under the distal edge of the nail plate (hyponychium), and the germinal and sterile matrices (Figure 100-1).[11,19,67,69,72] The nail plate itself is a multilayered, stacked sheet of cornified cells derived from anucleate onychocytes that arise from the germinal matrix epithelium of the nail bed.[25,37,60,62] The eponychial fold covers the softer and less cornified proximal nail plate (Figure 100-2). The cells of this proximal plate are not completely anucleate and project a white color because of nuclear parakeratosis, which occurs only at the level of the germinal matrix (Figure 100-3).[17,19,25,62] The lunula, a white semicircle just distal to the eponychial fold,[13,66] represents the parakeratotic proximal nail plate where the germinal matrix extends just beyond the nail fold. The sterile matrix epithelium does not undergo parakeratosis and therefore the nail plate takes on color that corresponds to the underlying well-vascularized nail bed.

The epithelium of the germinal matrix, sterile matrix, and eponychial fold contribute to the production of the nail plate through three modes of keratinization (Figure 100-4). The germinal matrix epithelium undergoes onychokeratinization, forming the main substance of the hardened nail plate, which is composed of stratified layers of cornified onychocytes.[18,19] The sterile matrix epithelium produces a semirigid keratin through a process known as *onycholemmal keratinization*. This semirigid keratin, sometimes referred to as the *horny solehorn*, increases the overall thickness of the nail and also acts as a "super glue" adhesive that enables the nail plate to maintain its adherence to the nail bed.[19,68] The external sheen of the healthy nail plate is a product of epidermoid keratinization from the dorsal roof of the eponychial fold. The cuticle, hyponychium, and lateral nail folds also contribute slightly to the surface epidermoid keratinization of the nail plate.[19]

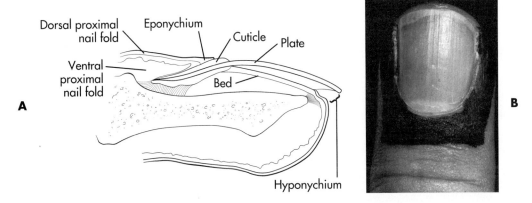

Figure 100-1. **A,** Anatomy of the fingertip. **B,** The darkened area (paronychium) and the nail bed and plate make up the perionychium.

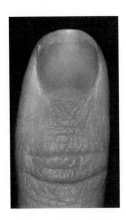

Figure 100-2. The eponychium is the proximal nail fold and adheres strongly to the nail plate. The cuticle represents the "nail vest" of the eponychium.

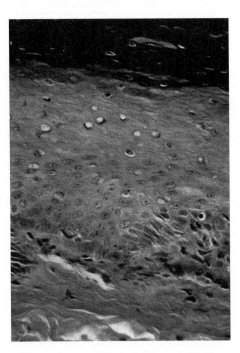

Figure 100-3. The nuclear parakeratosis of the germinal matrix cells is unique to this site. Nuclear enlargement and degeneration progress as the cells migrate dorsally.

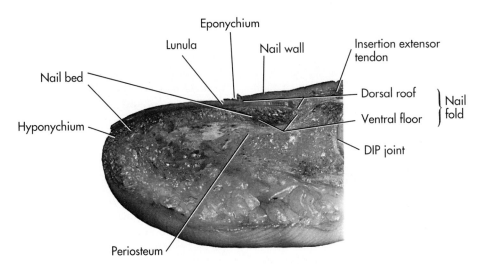

Figure 100-4. Sagittal view of the perionychium. The germinal matrix contributes as much as 90% of the nail-plate's substance by means of onychokeratinization. The sterile matrix contributes approximately 9% of the nail-plate structure by means of onycholemmal keratinization. The eponychium, lateral nail folds, and hyponychium add to the nail plate by means of epidermoid keratinization.

The hyponychium represents the junction of the terminal nail bed and the glabrous skin of the fingertip (Figure 100-5). The nail plate becomes nonadherent at this level and extends for a variable distance over the tip of the finger. A build-up of keratin, polymorphonuclear cells, lymphocytes, and debris

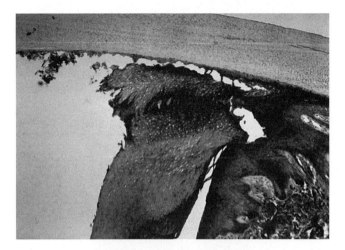

Figure 100-5. The hyponychium contains a build-up of keratin, polymorphonucleocytes, lymphocytes, and debris.

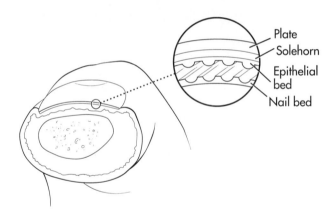

Figure 100-6. Coronal section of the nail plate and nail bed. The interdigitating ridges between the two structures offer a strong cohesiveness.

occurs under the surface of the distal nail at this transition from nail bed to fingertip skin.[35,44,65,72] The hyponychium therefore serves as a mechanical and important immunologic protective barrier at the distal end of the nail bed. The importance of the hyponychium cannot be overstated because of the variety of potentially contaminated areas that the fingertip comes in contact with during activities of normal daily living.

The nail bed is an extremely vascular, longitudinally ridged structure (Figure 100-6).[66] The most superficial layer of the nail bed is derived from the germinal matrix and glides as a unit with the nail plate as it grows distally.[27,28,30,64] The remarkable adherence of the nail plate to the nail bed is the result of the adhesive properties of the solehorn layer and the parallel ridging on the undersurface of the nail plate that interdigitates with the ridges of the underlying nail bed, which is itself intimately attached to the periosteum of the distal phalanx.[17,19,64] The nail bed is intimately anchored directly to the periosteum of the tuft of the distal phalanx. Retaining ligaments attach the nail bed to the bone at the proximal nail fold and distal nail grove respectively.[55] The nail bed itself consists of fibroconnective tissue and is devoid of adnexa structures.

The nail bed receives its vascularity from the ulnar and radial digital arteries. Branches of these vessels course around the distal phalanx and penetrate fibrous septa to form a proximal and distal anastomotic arcade within the basal layer of the nail bed (Figure 100-7).[46,53,61] A superficial arcade traverses the germinal matrix distal to the termination of the extensor tendon on the distal phalanx. Multiple arteriovenous anastomoses and myoneural glomus units are present within the nail bed.[22] Capillaries are abundant in the germinal matrix. The distal arborizing arcade of vessels in the distal nail bed communicate with a similar arcade from the volar pulp vessels. Venous drainage of the nail bed follows the arteries.[54] Two large venous channels emerge from the lateral aspect of the nail bed and proceed dorsally to converge with the dorsal venous drainage system of the finger just distal to the distal interphalangeal (DIP) joint. The lymphatic vessels follow the same route and have a similar network. The nerve supply to the nail bed is from the radial and ulnar digital nerves, which parallel the course of the arterial supply to the nail bed.

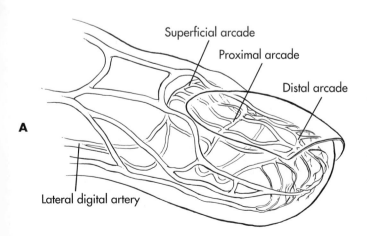

A

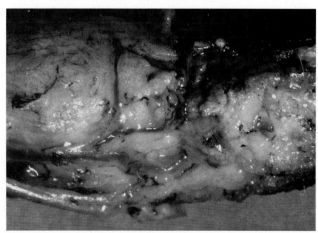

B

Figure 100-7. **A,** The vascular arcades of the vessels feeding the nail bed. **B,** A dye injection study of the fingertip vessels.

Box 100-1.
Factors That Can Affect the Rate of Nail Growth

FACTORS THAT SPEED GROWTH
Male gender
Location on dominant hand
Location on long fingers (compared with little fingers)
Summer (growth is slower during winter)
Age between 10 and 20 years
Daytime (growth is slower at night)
Nail biting
Location on fingers (growth of toenails is slower)
Pregnancy
Psoriasis

FACTORS THAT RETARD GROWTH
Paralysis or immobilization
Poor nutrition
Poor vascularity (local or systemic)
Lactation
Acute infections
Chemotherapy
Yellow nail syndrome

The thickness of the nail plate is approximately 0.5 mm in females and 0.6 mm in males and tends to increase with age. The nail grows of a rate of approximately 1.8 to 4.5 mm per month,[23] or 0.1 mm per day; thus the average nail can regrow completely in 6 to 9 months.[65,68] A number of factors can affect the rate of nail growth (Box 100-1).* Periods of stress or illness can detrimentally inhibit nail growth, and biting or trimming of the nail can accentuate growth. The hardness of the nail is dependent on its onychocyte bands, matrix proteins, and hydration level.[2] The water content of fingernails varies from 10% to 30%.[56] Brittle nail plates have a lower water content.

The hand surgeon acquainted with the anatomy and physiology of the perionychium understands the predictable pattern of nail-plate regeneration after injury.[5,10,58] A traumatic nail-plate avulsion exposes the underlying nail bed, making it susceptible to harsh environmental conditions. Blood and plasma exudate create a scab over of this exposed nail bed.[63] The surface epithelium and keratinous solehorn invariably remain adherent to the avulsed nail plate. The lateral nail folds and hyponychium provide the reparative epidermis that migrates under the scab to cover the nail bed.[10,27] This new layer is hyperplastic and somewhat hyperkeratotic but provides protection to the bed.[63] The vast neural and vascular supply to the nail bed makes this freshly exposed area somewhat hypersensitive after initial avulsion of the nail plate. A new nail plate begins to regenerate within 2 to 3 weeks. This delay produces a proximal thickening or *rolling front* of the advancing nail plate (Figure 100-8). Replacement of the reparative epidermis with bed epithelium immediately precedes, or is synchronous with, the progression of the new nail plate. Both the epithelium and nail plate are products of the germinal matrix.[25,37,46,63] The nail plate conforms to the constraints of the lateral nail folds, eponychium, and the contours of the nail bed on the distal phalanx. These structures are important to the ultimate shape of the nail plate.[3,30,41] The proximal lateral nail migrates to the level of the hyponychium and at this point no longer adheres to the nail bed.

*References 9, 16, 21, 23, 26, 33, 39, 65, 68.

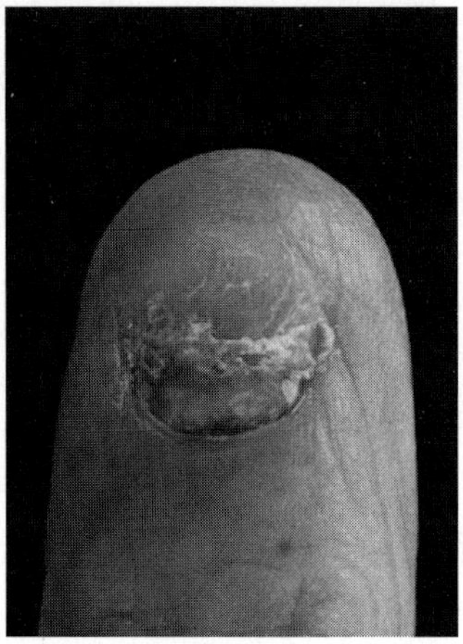

Figure 100-8. The regenerating nail is confined by the nail folds and the contour of the underlying nail bed and phalanx. A "rolling front" of the nail plate is commonly seen until the nail reaches the hyponychium.

INDICATIONS AND OPERATIONS

TRAUMATIC NAIL DEFORMITIES

It is easier to appropriately manage the nail-bed wound at the time of the initial injury than to reconstruct secondary nail deformities. The importance of anatomical alignment of the nail bed after injury cannot be overstated or underestimated. A poorly coapted nail-bed laceration that heals with significant scar tissue cannot maintain the adherence of the regenerating nail.[31,59,67,70] The result is a loss of continuity between the nail plate and the nail bed at the level of the scarring. The nail continues to grow away from the nail bed at this level and can become problematic by catching on clothing and other objects. The fingertip is repeatedly traumatized as a consequence.

Nail-bed injuries should be treated with the respect that all other hand injuries demand. An appropriate patient history and physical examination should be performed. A knowledge of the mechanism of injury helps the surgeon identify other

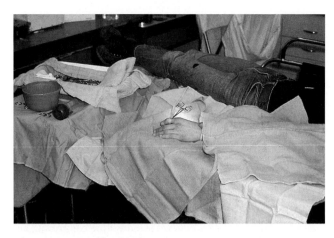

Figure 100-9. The hand is prepared with a sterilizing solution and draped to allow easy manipulation of the fingers. The digital tourniquet (Penrose) provides a bloodless field to appropriately visualize the nail-bed repair.

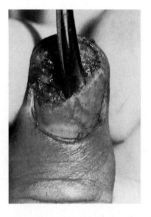

Figure 100-10. The nail plate is elevated with an elevator or sharp scissors. The lateral and proximal nail folds must be elevated to prevent traumatic removal of the nail plate.

potential injuries to the finger or hand. Radiographs are obtained because distal phalanx fractures are an extremely common finding in patients with fingertip injuries. Most of these injuries can be managed in an emergency department. The patient is placed in the supine position and the whole hand is prepared with a sterilizing solution and properly draped. The draping should allow for easy manipulation of the entire hand while maintaining complete sterility. Digital block anesthesia is used and the finger is exsanguinated with a Penrose drain, in much the same way that an esmarch is used for other upper extremity injuries (Figure 100-9). Loupe magnification is required to appropriately visualize the nail bed and to anatomically repair lacerations.

The nail plate or remnant of nail is removed with careful dissection, using a Freer periosteal elevator or curved sharp-point scissors. The instrument is placed between the nail plate and nail bed and gently swept from side to side to release the plate from the nail bed and lateral nail folds (Figure 100-10). The eponychial fold is elevated off the nail plate in a similar

fashion. The surface under the removed nail plate is cleaned of any solehorn layer and debris. The nail plate, when present, is placed in a sterile saline and is replaced into the nail fold at the end of the procedure. Subsequently the exact nature and extent of the injury to the nail bed can be visualized and appropriately managed surgically.

SUBUNGUAL HEMATOMA

A subungual hematoma is the result of an injury to the sterile or germinal matrix that causes bleeding beneath the nail plate and the subsequent separation of the nail plate from the nail bed. The hematoma puts pressure on the nail bed and causes a marked throbbing after injury.

Some degree of nail-bed injury is necessary to cause subungual bleeding. It is important to determine when the degree of injury warrants removal of the nail plate and repair of the nail matrix. We have advocated removal of the nail plate and examination of the nail matrix when 50% or more of the visible nail is undermined by hematoma.[67] Other authors in a small series demonstrated a low incidence of late nail deformity when contained subungual hematomas were treated by observation alone. If the hematoma has been decompressed by disruption of the hyponychium, paronychium, or eponychium, removal of the nail plate and repair of the matrix is warranted. The method of repair should be chosen based on each patient's particular circumstances. Aggressive treatment by exploration and primary nail-bed repair should yield an excellent result but may delay the return of normal activity. A properly treated acute nail-bed wound provides results that are much better and more cost effective than a secondary reconstruction.

Subungual hematomas involving less than 50% of the visible nail are often treated conservatively with simple hand elevation.[48] Intense pain or throbbing warrants evacuation of the hematoma. A small opening in the nail plate over the hematoma allows release of the blood that is trapped under pressure. The finger is prepared with a sterile solution. The hole in the nail plate is made with a hand-held disposable cautery, a heated paper clip, or a #11 scalpel blade. After the instrument penetrates the nail plate, the hematoma is ejected from the hole. Care is taken not to project the instrument into the extremely sensitive nail bed. The wound may continue to "ooze" for some time. A light dressing is applied for 24 to 48 hours; subsequently the wound may be left open. Residual subungual hematomas migrate distally for 4 to 9 weeks as the nail grows.

SIMPLE AND STELLATE LACERATIONS

These two types of injuries are classified together because their treatment is essentially identical. Simple and stellate lacerations of the nail bed typically result from a localized blow to the fingernail. The nail bed is lacerated or crushed between the nail plate and the distal phalanx.[15] If a relatively localized force strikes the nail, it causes a linear compression of the nail bed and a relatively straight laceration. A stellate laceration is cre-

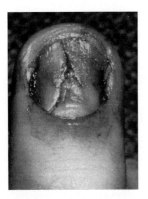

Figure 100-11. Simple laceration of the nail bed. The matrix injury should be repaired with a 7.0 chromic suture under loupe magnification. The nail plate is returned to its anatomic location under the eponychial fold.

ated by a greater force over a wider area, which causes more compression of the nail bed between the nail and the bone and results in an exploding type of injury.[20,70]

The nail bed must be irrigated thoroughly, and devitalized tissue must be carefully debrided. The irregular edges should be approximated as accurately as possible, with minimal trimming, to prevent tension on the repair. A nail bed repaired under tension promotes scarring and poor adhesion of the nail plate as it regenerates. The nail bed may need to be undermined approximately 1 to 2 mm on each side of the wound edges to achieve accurate coaptation.[67] The 7-0 chromic suture on a small needle is minimally traumatic to the nail bed yet offers appropriate strength for the repair (Figure 100-11). Repair of a stellate laceration can be somewhat more time consuming because of the diffuse nature of the laceration; however, because there is no loss of nail bed substance, meticulous attention to detail can render excellent results both functionally and cosmetically (Figure 100-12). After the nail bed has been repaired, the previously removed nail plate is used as a compressive

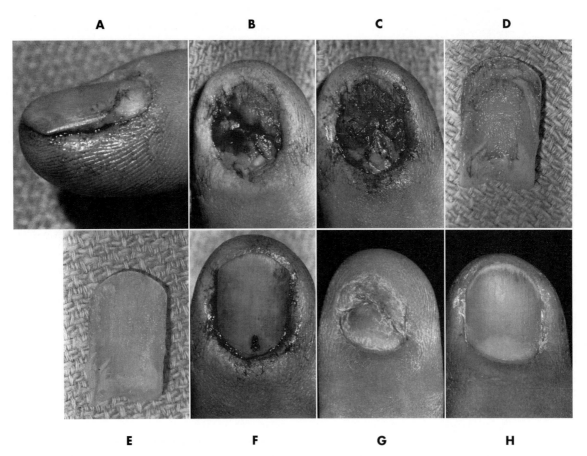

Figure 100-12. **A,** Avulsion of the proximal nail from the nail fold. **B,** Stellate laceration of the nail bed is visible only after the nail has been removed. **C,** The lacerations of the nail bed are approximated with 7-0 chromic sutures and magnification. **D,** The undersurface of the nail after it has been removed from the nail bed. **E,** The undersurface of the nail is shown after it has been scraped clean. **F,** A hole has been burned through the nail to allow drainage in an area that is not over the repair. **G,** Two months after the injury, the nail is progressing from the nail fold. **H,** One year after the injury.

dressing and also is used to hold the eponychial fold open. A hole is drilled or burned through the plate in an area that is not over the laceration to allow plasma and blood to drain when the tourniquet is released. The nail is replaced into the eponychial fold and a distal 5-0 nylon suture is used to secure the replaced plate to the distal skin of the fingertip. Replacement of the nail plate serves a number of functions. It helps to mold the edges of the nail-bed laceration, assists in holding distal phalangeal fractures in a reduced position, maintains the integrity of the eponychial fold, protects the nail-bed repair, and makes the fingertip more comfortable for the patient while the new nail regenerates. Occasionally, the nail plate is avulsed and lost at the scene of the accident. A 0.02-sheet of silicone or nonadherent lubricated gauze can be placed over the nail bed and into the eponychial fold in place of the original nail plate (Figure 100-13). Failure to follow the appropriate principles of nail-bed

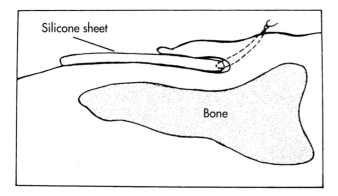

Figure 100-13. A silicone sheet is placed under the eponychial fold. The distal or proximal end is sutured in place to maintain its position.

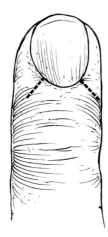

Figure 100-14. Incisions made at a right angle to the eponychial fold allow easy access to the germinal matrix.

repair often results in greater bed scarring and ultimately in the loss of nail-plate adherence, as well as longitudinal splitting of the nail or nail contour irregularities.

Lacerations that involve the germinal matrix of the nail bed require a similar repair. Access to the germinal matrix is achieved through two incisions made at right angles at the junction of the lateral paronychium and the proximal eponychium (Figure 100-14).[68,70] Incisions made at angles other than 90 degrees in this area can lead to consequential synechial adhesions of the eponychium to the nail bed or to eponychial fold deformities secondary to scar contracture. The nail pate or silicone sheet is placed in the eponychial fold to prevent synechial adhesions between the germinal matrix and the roof of the eponychial fold. A 6-0 monofilament suture is used to close lacerations or access incisions in the eponychial fold. Lacerations involving the germinal matrix of the dorsal roof and ventral floor must be repaired separately and with great care. The knots of the sutures should be placed in the nail fold and not within the substance of the nail bed because the latter may promote scarring or poor coaptation.

The entire fingertip is dressed with a nonadherent gauze such as Adaptic or Xeroform, antibiotic ointment, and a bulky wrap. A finger cap splint is used to protect the distal end of the finger. In 5 to 7 days the finger is examined for signs of seroma, hematoma, and infection, and the nylon suture in the nail plate is removed. The old nail plate often adheres for 1 to 3 months before it is displaced by the new regenerating nail.

CRUSH INJURIES

Crush injuries portend a poorer prognosis than simple or stellate lacerations.[20] These nail-bed injuries are caused by a wider and more forceful area of trauma to the nail plate. The nail bed is in multiple fragments, and some may remain attached to the undersurface of the nail plate. The nail plate should be explored carefully for these fragments. The avulsed nail bed can be removed from the nail plate and replaced with free grafts. In cases of severe crush injuries, all of the fragments of the nail bed must be approximated as accurately as possible to minimize scarring. Larger severely crushed areas of the nail bed may not be salvageable and are best treated with a split sterile matrix graft. A tension-free, anatomical repair of the nail bed should be performed to optimize the final result.

Associated distal phalanx fractures are extremely common in patients with crush injuries. The larger displaced fragments of the distal phalanx can be held in appropriate reduction by a longitudinal 0.028 to 0.035 g Kirschner (K) wire (Figure 100-15). Smaller tuft fractures do not require pin fixation; replacement of the nail plate after repair may suffice. The nail plate acts as an external splint because of its contoured shape and proximity to the periosteum. The fingertip, including the DIP joint, should be splinted for 4 to 6 weeks.

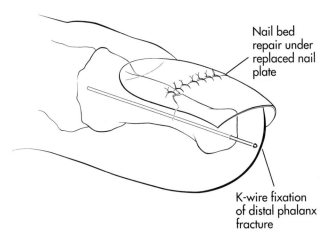

Figure 100-15. A K-wire fixation of the phalanx fracture. The nail bed is subsequently repaired.

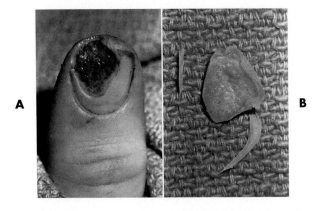

Figure 100-16. **A,** A dorsal amputation injury with loss of nail plate, nail bed, and hyponychium. Fragments of the avulsed nail bed often adhere to the nail plate. **B,** The nail bed should be removed from the segment of nail plate, returned to its anatomic position on the finger, and sutured in place.

AVULSION INJURIES

Avulsion injuries may result in partial or total loss of the nail bed and thus exposure of the dorsal distal phalanx. Such trauma causes the most serious nail-bed injuries and the highest incidence of long-term nail deformities. Fragments of the avulsed nail bed often maintain their adherence to the undersurface of the nail plate (Figure 100-16). These fragments must be carefully removed, accurately replaced, and sutured in place on the nail bed with 7-0 chromic sutures. Occasionally, the proximal nail bed—including the germinal matrix—is avulsed, but the distal end continues to adhere. The nail bed must be returned under the eponychial fold and maintained in place with sutures (Figure 100-17). In some cases there is complete loss of a segment of nail bed. Composite avulsions of the nail bed and eponychium should be sutured back in place (Figure 100-18) because reconstruction of the eponychium as a secondary procedure is often difficult.

Avulsion defects of the sterile matrix nail bed should be managed acutely for the best result.[45,47,67] Split-thickness sterile matrix grafts can be harvested from uninjured areas of the involved fingers if there is a large enough donor site available to accommodate the defect (Figure 100-19).[34,49,52,67] Great-toe donor nail-bed grafts may be warranted for larger defects.[67] The toe, like the hand, must be prepared and draped. Defects in the germinal matrix must be treated with full-thickness grafts from a toe. Harvesting a portion of the germinal matrix of the toe renders that portion of the donor toe unable to regenerate a nail plate. Thus obliteration of the toe's remaining germinal matrix is often recommended to eliminate toenail remnants. A germinal matrix defect requires a full-thickness graft to support regeneration of the nail plate, but a sterile matrix defect requires only a split-thickness graft to function.[67] The graft can be placed directly on the exposed cortex of the distal phalanx, sutured to the surrounding nail bed, and appropriately dressed.

Harvesting of a split-thickness nail-bed graft is performed

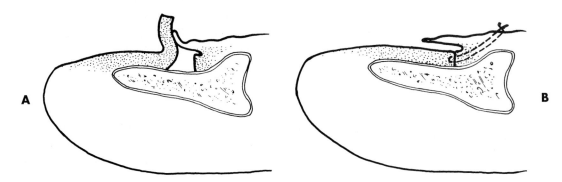

Figure 100-17. **A,** The germinal matrix has been torn from the proximal portion of the nail fold and is loosened from the periosteum, causing it to emerge from the nail fold. **B,** The germinal matrix (ventral floor of the nail fold) has been replaced and is secured with horizontal mattress sutures. (Copyright SIU School of Medicine.)

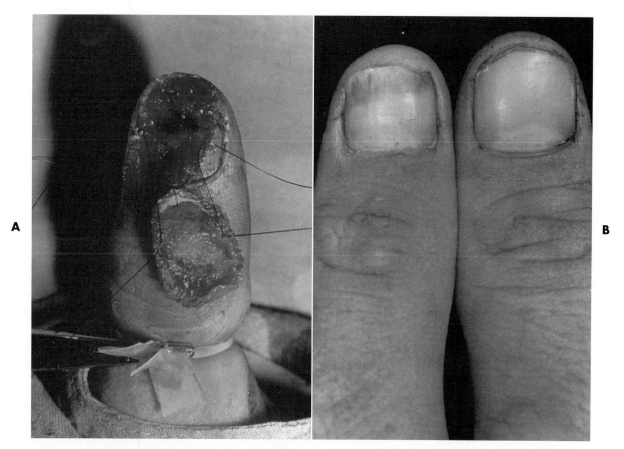

Figure 100-18. **A,** An avulsion of approximately 80% of the nail plate, nail bed, hyponychium, and eponychium. The nail plate was removed and an anatomic repair was performed. **B,** The regenerated nail 1 year later, compared with the normal side.

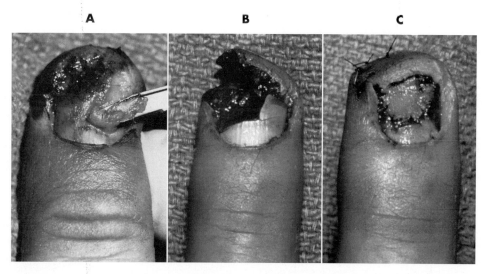

Figure 100-19. **A,** A fingertip injury with an avulsed segment of nail bed. Small defects can be repaired with split-thickness nail-bed grafts from the adjacent, uninjured area of the nail bed. **B,** A large nail-bed avulsion defect required split-thickness nail-bed grafts from the great toe. **C,** The nail-bed grafts are sutured in place with 7.0 chromic suture.

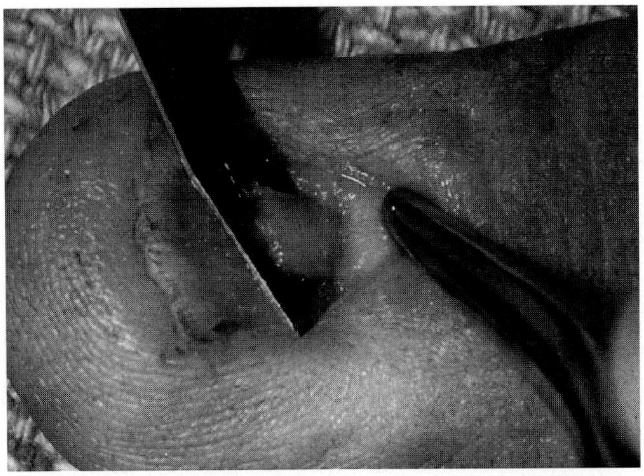

Figure 100-20. The nail-bed graft is harvested with a #15 blade scalpel; the blade can be seen through the graft at all times. A graft that is 8/1000 of an inch thick can be obtained with this technique.

with a #15 scalpel blade (Figure 100-20). A graft that is 8/1000 of an inch can be elevated with the aid of loupe magnification and a jeweler forceps. The feathered edge of the scalpel blade should be seen through the graft as it is being elevated. Removal of a graft that is too thick may result in a donor-site deformity. The curve of the nail bed is followed with gentle sweeping movements of the scalpel blade during elevation of the split-thickness nail-bed graft. It is better to take a slightly larger graft and trim this to fit the fingernail defect than to harvest an inadequate graft and attempt to close the recipient site under tension.

Reconstruction of a nail-bed defect with a split sterile matrix graft optimizes nail adherence and minimizes subsequent deformity. Other options, such as the use of a split-thickness skin graft or a dermal graft, do not allow adherence of the regenerating nail plate. These tissues should be used only if there are no other donor sites available. Bipedicled (germinal or sterile) or transposition matrix flaps have been described but may result in secondary deformities to the donor and recipient sites. These flaps require undermining of the matrix and a lateral incision to allow transposition of the tissue to close the defect. The donor area is closed either primarily or with a skin graft. Shepard[51] has obtained good results with bipedicled germinal matrix flaps in patients with germinal matrix defects.

COMPOSITE GRAFTS

The role of composite tissue grafts warrants special attention.[12,14] Segments of the distal nail bed and the distal glabrous skin of the fingertip are often avulsed in continuity. The avulsed tissue contains two unique anatomic structures: the hyponychium and the nail bed. The hyponychium cannot be reconstructed with local tissue transfers or grafts; thus it is prudent to preserve this avulsed composite tissue, if possible.[43] Composite tip amputations distal to the lunula can be replaced as a composite graft in children younger than 10 years of age. The composite tissue amputation is gently trimmed of

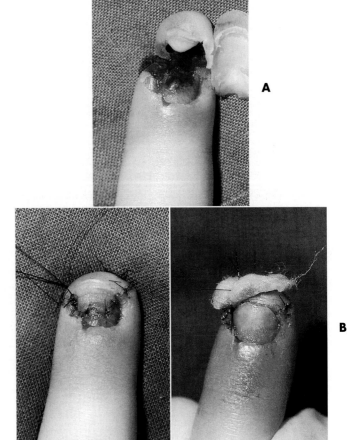

Figure 100-21. Avulsion injury caused when 7-year-old child caught his finger in the car door. **A,** The avulsion injury to the fingertip involved a composite of nail bed, hyponychium, and glabrous volar skin. **B,** The composite graft is sutured in place without defatting. The skin is closed with 5.0 nylon, and the nail bed is sutured with 7.0 chromic suture. **C,** A tie-over bolster dressing stabilizes the composite graft.

devitalized or contaminated tissue, preserving the nail bed, glabrous skin, fat, and sensitive distal tuft (Figure 100-21). The nail bed is anatomically aligned and sutured with 7-0 chromic sutures and the skin is closed with nonabsorbable sutures. The ends of the nonabsorbable sutures are kept long and are used with wet cotton to make a tie-over bolster dressing. It is essential to treat this composite graft with complete upper-limb immobilization after surgery to improve the chances of graft survival. For children, a long-arm cast with the elbow flexed more than 90 degrees is used to encompass a bulky hand dressing. This is the safest way to keep the fingertip immobilized for the next 7 to 10 days. The child's parents should be informed of the potential for composite graft failure and the possible need for further procedures to obtain definitive coverage.

Composite fingertip amputation in adults and children older than 10 years of age should be treated by converting the amputated tip to a full-thickness skin graft. The tissue is

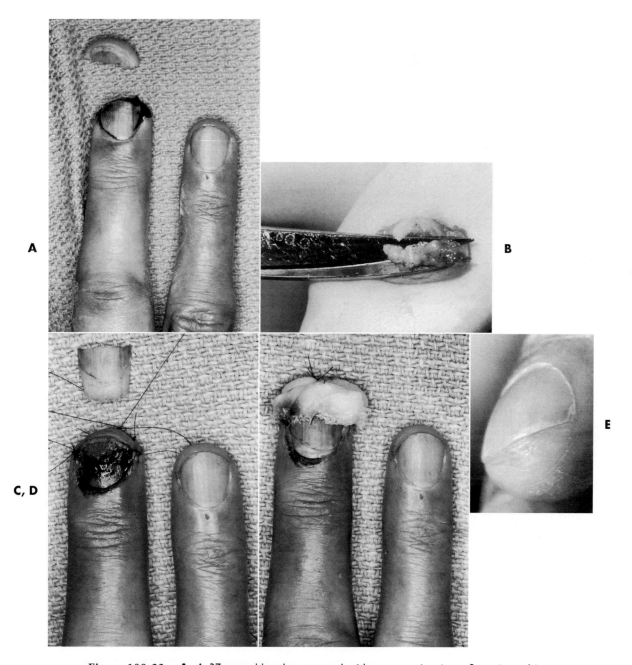

Figure 100-22. **A,** A 37-year-old male presented with a composite tissue fingertip avulsion. **B,** The composite tissue is defatted with curved scissors. **C,** The skin of the composite graft is sutured in place with 5.0 nylon suture. The nail bed is coapted with 7.0 chromic suture. **C,** A tie-over bolster dressing is secured over the graft to ensure stability. **E,** The 2-year follow-up of the composite graft to the fingertip.

defatted to the level of the dermis, and the nail bed is preserved (Figure 100-22). The distal phalanx is shortened just below the remaining pulp soft tissue, and the full-thickness graft is applied and secured with a stent dressing. The pulp in the fingertip is deficient after healing, but the hyponychium and the nail bed are restored. Reconstruction of the tip with a true composite graft has a very low survival rate among adults and wastes valuable time. Dressings are removed from patients with full-thickness skin grafts in 7 to 10 days. The fingertip is washed and redressed on a daily basis, and a protective dressing is required for 2 to 3 weeks.

RECONSTRUCTION

Secondary reconstruction procedures for the nail are always less effective than appropriate and meticulous acute care of a nail-bed injury.[6,29,59,67,71] The appearance and shape of a nail improve during the first year after an injury; thus attempts at reconstruction of the nail bed should be postponed for at least 1 year. Typical nail deformities that require reconstruction include nonadherent nails, split-nail deformities, irregular contours, hook nail, and loss of the eponychium with synechiae.

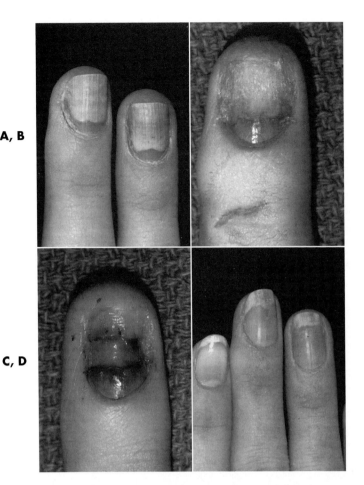

A, B

C, D

Figure 100-23. **A,** The nail plate on the ring finger does not adhere beyond the level of the nail-bed scar. **B,** The nail plate is removed and the keratinous material is shaved off the nonadherent area. **C,** A split-thickness nail-bed graft from the great toe is sutured in place at the site of the nail-bed defect. **D,** One year after grafting.

THE NONADHERENT NAIL

The most common deformity of the nail plate after injury is nonadherence. The etiology is usually partial avulsion of the nail bed, with increased keratosis or scarring of the sterile matrix, which prevents intimate attachment of the nail plate to the nail bed. The regenerating nail progresses to the site of scar tissue and loses its adherence. The nail continues to grow distally in a more dorsal direction, leaving an upwardly deviated nonadherent nail. This is problematic because the nail continuously catches on clothing and other articles, which can cause significant trauma to the area under the nail. The deformity is unsightly and is often a source of dissatisfaction to the patient.

Treatment of the nonadherent nail involves trimming the nail back to normal sterile matrix.[71] The scar in the nail bed is excised and the defect is closed primarily or with split matrix grafts. Primary closure may be obtained with minimal undermining of the nail bed if the defect is less than 1 to 2 mm. The nail plate should adhere to the graft (Figure 100-23). Occasionally, hyperkeratosis of the nail bed is the cause of plate nonadherence. This is treated by removing the nail proximal to the area of nonadherence and scraping the sterile matrix with the edge of the scalpel blade to remove the hyperkeratosis to the level of the normal nail bed. The nail subsequently grows out and completely or partially adheres to the nail bed. The procedure may be repeated if total adherence is not achieved.

SPLIT NAIL

A longitudinal split in the nail is often caused by an underlying axial scar that begins in the germinal matrix of the nail bed.[7,38] The scar divides the nail plate during formation and does not allow the nail plate to adhere to the sterile matrix. This area of nail plate is significantly weakened because of the differential forces on either side of the underlying scar. The nail plate subsequently grows out as two distinct plates (Figure 100-24).[52]

A	B	C	D	E

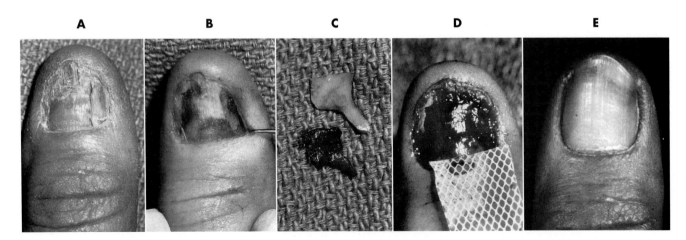

Figure 100-24. **A,** A split and nonadherent nail deformity secondary to trauma. **B,** Removal of the nail plate reveals scarring that extends proximally toward the eponychial fold. **C,** The scarred area excised. **D,** The defect is closed with a split nail-bed graft, and a silicone sheet is used in the eponychial fold. **E,** One year later, the nail plate is smooth and adherent.

Scarring between the dorsal roof and the ventral floor of the eponychial fold also may cause a diversion of the nail as it grows out from the germinal matrix. This usually indicates a more severe injury to the nail bed, the eponychium, and possibly the germinal matrix. A third possible cause of a split nail plate is related to the presence of a defect in the germinal matrix; in

such cases the nail plate forms on either side of the defect. It is important to understand and recognize the etiology of a split nail because the treatment is determined by the underlying pathology.

Longitudinal scars on the sterile matrix of the nail bed are usually amenable to excision and primary closure.[67] Occasionally small Z-plasties (2 mm in length) are used to alter the direction of the scar. Larger scars require a split-thickness nail-bed graft after excision. Loss of the central portion of the germinal matrix requires placement of a full-thickness germinal matrix graft from the toe (Figure 100-25). Synechial adhesions between the dorsal roof and the nail bed are treated by removing the nail plate and dividing the synechia transversely to recreate a nail fold (Figure 100-26). Upward traction on the open portion of the nail fold should allow visualization for performing the transverse incision. The germinal matrix is carefully inspected for scar tissue. The scar tissue must be resected, and a germinal matrix graft must be applied. Simple excision of the germinal matrix scar with primary approximation is less effective. Scar tissue should be removed from the dorsal roof of the eponychium and a split-thickness sterile matrix graft from the finger or the toe should be applied and sutured in place with a 7.0 chromic suture. Reconstruction of the dorsal roof of the eponychium restores normal sheen to the regenerating nail. A silicone sheet is placed in the nail fold to maintain the integrity of the eponychial fold until the grafts have obtained appropriate vascularity. It is worth emphasizing that the judicious use of sterile matrix grafts or germinal matrix grafts offers the best reconstructive results.

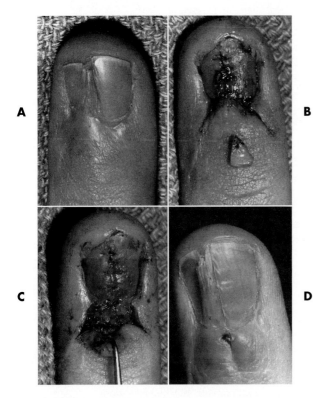

Figure 100-25. **A,** A severely split nail; no hard nail is produced in the germinal matrix. **B,** A part of the scar has been removed from the matrix and a fragment of germinal matrix from a second toe is ready to replace the missing germinal matrix. **C,** The fragment of germinal matrix is sutured in place. **D,** Several months after grafting, hard nail can be seen growing from the nail fold.

THE HOOK NAIL

The hook-nail deformity typically is caused by a fingertip amputation with loss or partial loss of the supporting tuft of the distal phalanx and loss of the distal nail bed and fingertip soft tissue. The regenerating nail plate follows the contour of

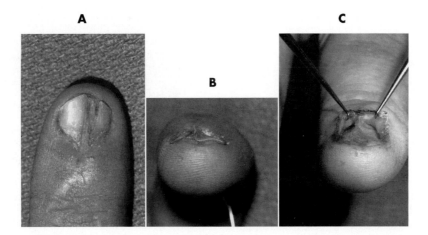

Figure 100-26. **A,** A split in a nail believed to be caused by the nail fold synechia. **B,** The elevated, disrupted portion of the nail produces a functional problem. **C,** The synechia between the dorsal roof and the ventral fold. *Continued*

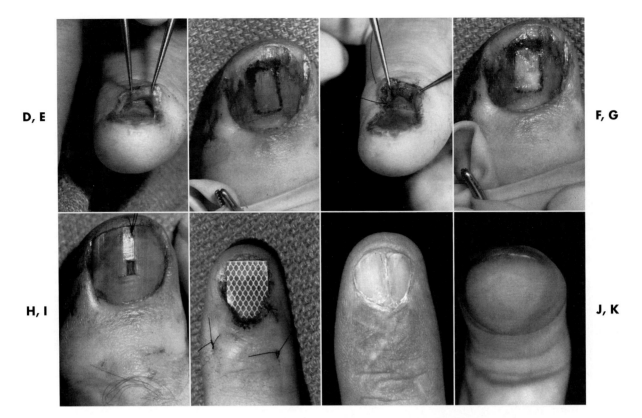

Figure 100-26, cont'd. **D,** The synechia between the dorsal roof and the ventral fold has been sharply divided; little normal matrix remains on the dorsal roof. **E,** The large toenail has been removed and an area of sterile matrix has been marked for replacement of the dorsal roof. **F,** The split-thickness sterile matrix graft has been removed. **G,** The graft of sterile matrix is sutured raw side up on the dorsal roof. **H,** The toenail is placed into the nail fold and is secured with a suture. **I,** A piece of 0.021 silicone reinforced sheet is placed to keep the nail fold open. **J,** Despite some deformity, the nail irregularity is much smaller and is essentially asymptomatic. **K,** The protrusion and roughness of the nail is much improved after surgery.

the repaired fingertip amputation, angling in a dorsal-to-volar direction (Figure 100-27). Amputated fingertips that heal by secondary intention create cicatricial forces on the nail bed over the tip, forcing the overlying nail plate volarly to produce the hook-nail deformity. The hook-nail deformity causes more than cosmetic disfigurement. The tip of the finger is often tender and chronically irritated, and the sensation on the tip of the finger may be compromised. The patient also may have difficulty grasping fine objects. Occasionally the nail may catch on clothing or other objects and consequently undergo trauma.[32]

Correction of a hook-nail deformity can be somewhat difficult because of the inability to recreate sufficient bony and soft tissue support.[1] Appropriate management of the acute injury may prevent the development of a hook-nail deformity by placement of bony support and flap coverage. Secondary reconstruction is centered on recreating the initial defect and restoring bony and/or soft tissue support. Soft tissue support on the volar aspect of the finger can be accomplished with V to Y Atasoy/Kleinert flaps, lateral Kutler flaps, a cross-finger flap, or a thenar crease flap (Figure 100-28). Split nail-bed grafts are applied directly to the volar flaps, and the proximal edge is sutured to the native nail bed. Restoration of bony support is

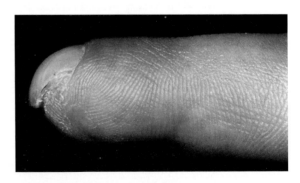

Figure 100-27. The hook-nail deformity results from poor nail-bed support, typically from amputation of the tuft of the distal phalanx. (Copyright SIU School of Medicine.)

less predictable. Distraction osteogenesis, bone grafting, and step cutting in the distal phalanx are likely to lead to a high rate of resorption. Microvascular composite flaps composed of nail bed, bone, and soft tissue from the toe have been used with

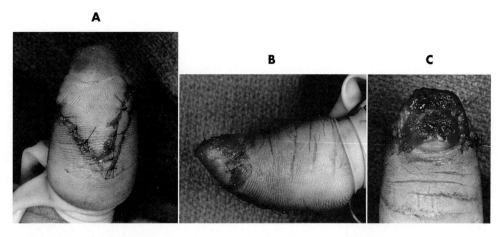

Figure 100-28. **A,** Local V-Y flap advancement provides support for the nail bed. **B,** The volar skin is advanced to the distal edge of the nail bed. **C,** The nail bed repair and flap support should help prevent hook-nail deformities.

excellent results.[36] A high level of microsurgical expertise is required for this procedure, and the patient must be willing to sacrifice a toe. Composite tissue grafts from the toe have a limited role because only a small amount of tissue can be used for this procedure; grafts of the local flaps previously mentioned are more easily and reliably performed.

Revision amputation is an alternative to reconstructing a problematic hook-nail deformity. The nail bed is resected to the level of the remaining bony support to help prevent growth of the nail plate over the tip of the finger.

LINEAR RIDGING

A linear ridging deformity of the nail that occurs after trauma is often associated with an underlying bone or soft tissue abnormality (Figure 100-29). The ridging typically represents more of a cosmetic deformity than a functional problem. Incongruities or irregularities of the distal phalanx cortex can displace the nail bed dorsally. The nail plate maintains its adherence unless overlying scar tissue is present. Significant scar tissue or foreign bodies underneath the nail bed overlying the distal phalanx also may result in ridging of the nail plate. Radiographs, tomograms, or computed tomography (CT) scans may help delineate the exact etiology but these imaging techniques are rarely indicated because the management of this deformity is similar to that of the split nail deformity.

The nail plate must be removed, and the sterile matrix must be visualized. An incision is made over the ridge in a longitudinal fashion. The sterile nail bed is elevated both radially and ulnarly to expose the underlying tissue. Scar tissue, foreign bodies, or bony exostoses are removed. The nail bed is redraped and sutured with 7-0 chromic sutures. Excessive scarring of the sterile matrix warrants excision and replacement with a split-thickness nail bed graft. The nail plate or silicone sheeting is subsequently placed over the repair and under the eponychial fold.

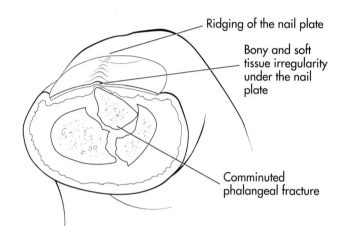

Ridging of the nail plate

Bony and soft tissue irregularity under the nail plate

Comminuted phalangeal fracture

Figure 100-29. Linear ridging of the nail plate is the result of underlying soft tissue or bony incongruities.

RECONSTRUCTION OF THE EPONYCHIUM

Loss of the eponychium is most commonly caused by burns. Friction avulsions and crush and complex lacerations also may contribute to loss of the eponychium. The eponychium contributes to the epidermoid keratinization of the nail, providing the characteristic sheen on the dorsal nail plate. Loss of the eponychium typically results in an unsightly nail or a notched deformity that occasionally can be a source of tenderness for the patient (Figure 100-30).

The reconstructive options for correcting this deformity have varied.[4,24,71] Composite grafts can be obtained from the large or second toe. These composite grafts include the dorsal roof of the eponychial fold as well as the dorsal skin. It is often necessary to remove the nail plate entirely to appropriately visualize the remaining edges of the proximal nail fold. The composite graft is subsequently sutured in place with 7-0 chromic and 6-0 nylon sutures and the nail plate is replaced. The surgical site is covered with sterile gauze and dressed as

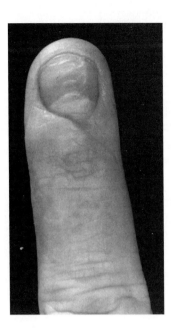

Figure 100-30. Full-thickness loss of the eponychium causes deformity and roughness of the nail surface.

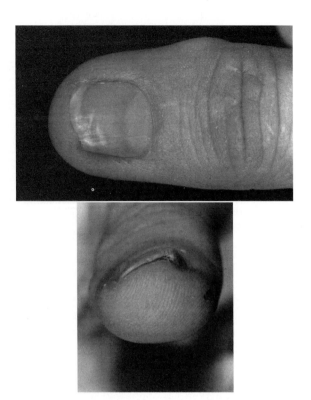

Figure 100-31. The pincer nail deformity results from loss of lateral support of the nail bed.

previously described. The survival of the grafts may be somewhat precarious; thus meticulous attention after immobilization is necessary.

Occasionally the skin on the dorsum of the fingers may be rotated or transposed for use as local flaps for reconstruction of the eponychium. A split sterile matrix graft is sutured to the undersurface of the flap to restore the dorsal roof bed. The donor site of the flap is closed primarily or covered with a split-thickness skin graft.

PINCER NAIL DEFORMITY

The nail plate has a biconvex shape, with less convexity in the proximal to distal plane and a greater convexity in the ulnar to radial plane (Figure 100-31). Proximal nail folds, lateral nail folds, and the contour of the distal phalanx are major contributors to the overall shape of the nail plate.[3,30,41] These forces define the nail's path and configuration as it grows or regenerates, unless other masses or tumors alter the nail's course. A pincer nail deformity represents a loss of the normal convex shape of the nail plate. The lateral edges of the nail plate have a marked convexity, characterized by an acute volar turn that takes on the distinctive shape of an "omega" sign when viewed head on at the distal phalanx. The exact etiology of this deformity is somewhat

obscure but may be related to a loss of the lateral integrity of the distal phalanx, which allows a greater curvature of the nail plate. A pincer nail may manifest itself as an unsightly deformity of the nail or occasionally as an ingrown nail that penetrates the lateral paronychium. Paronychial infections may be more common in patients with this type of nail irregularity.[57]

Restoration of the normal contour and shape of the nail plate is achieved with the aid of dermal grafts under the lateral edges of the nail bed (Figure 100-32). The nail plate is removed, and an oblique incision is made in the pulp of the distal fingertip just distal to the end of the lateral nail folds. A Freer periosteal elevator is introduced into the wound and passed proximally, elevating the nail bed off the distal phalanx. A tunnel 2 to 3 mm wide is created, which extends the full distance of the nail bed (including the germinal matrix). The surgeon must take care not to damage or buttonhole the overlying nail bed. Nylon sutures (5-0) are placed through the dorsal skin into the tunnel created between the distal phalanx and the lateral bed. The suture is carried out of the wound to capture the proximal end of a dermal graft. The suture subsequently is passed back through the tunnel and out of the dorsal skin, exiting near the entrance of the previous suture. The surgeon advances the dermal graft through the tunnel by pulling on the sutures. A suture is tied securely to the dermal graft in the tunnel. The excess length of the dermal graft is excised

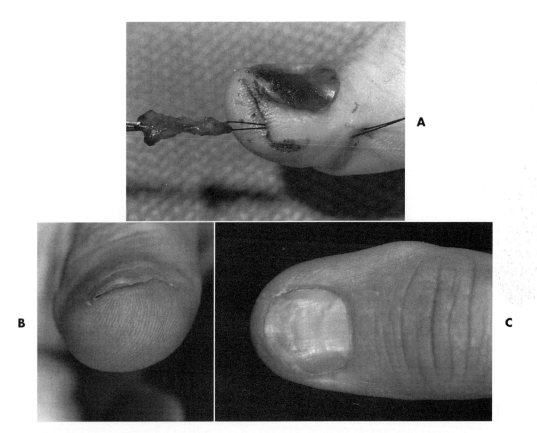

Figure 100-32. Correction of the pincer nail deformity. **A,** The nail plate is removed and oblique incisions are made at the distal end of the lateral nail folds. A dermal graft is introduced into a tunnel created between the nail bed and the distal phalanx. **B** and **C,** The results 1 year after surgery.

and the wound is closed with a single nylon suture. The identical procedure is performed on the opposite side of the nail plate, and a silastic sheet is introduced into the eponychial fold. The sheeting is removed after approximately 10 days. The procedure has had excellent results in restoring the natural contours of the nail plate.

OUTCOMES

True outcome studies of nail-bed injuries have not been performed. The results of repair are typically evaluated in comparison with the patient's other fingernails. The importance of meticulous, immediate repair of nail-bed injuries cannot be overstated.[52,59,67] The results of initial repairs far exceed those of reconstructive attempts. The severity and nature of the inciting trauma play a significant role in the functional and cosmetic outcome of the nail.[20,60,67,70] Simple or stellate lacerations that are amenable to an anatomic repair render superb results, typically providing the patient with a nail that appears normal. Severe crush injuries, or nail beds with a secondary deformity that requires reconstruction have a less predictable outcome and may result in ribbing, coarseness,

longitudinal ridging, nonadherence, eponychial synechiae, or split-nail deformity.[20,67]

Tuft or more proximal distal phalanx fractures are commonly associated with nail-bed injuries. Zook found that approximately 50% of nail-bed injuries were associated with distal phalanx fractures.[67] Nail-plate surface irregularities are more common after distal phalanx fractures but adherence may not be affected. This underscores the need for appropriate anatomical reduction of bony fragments and possible K-wire fixation during the treatment of a nail-bed or fingertip injury.[52,70] Adjacent soft tissue injuries do not significantly affect nail regeneration unless the trauma involves the eponychial or lateral nail folds.[20]

The lack of nail-plate adherence creates problems that are more functional than cosmetic when more than one third of the distal nail is nonadherent.[40,67] Nail roughness or dorsal deviation of the nail results in snagging and catching on various objects. The fingertip may become hypersensitive and uncomfortable with continued trauma to the fingertip. Dirt and other debris gather underneath the nonadherent nail and cause further irritation. Adherence of more than two thirds of the nail bed rarely results in a functional impairment.[67]

Infections of the nail bed after repair are uncommon. In a series of 184 repairs, Zook reported two cases of infection that had poor results, but 90% of the patients had good results, with the regenerated nails of the injured fingers being identical to the patients' uninjured nails.[71] Patients with crush or avulsion injuries had worse results than those with stellate or simple lacerations.[20,71] Patients with a combination of nail-fold and nail-bed injuries had poor results.

Split-thickness sterile matrix grafts are required for areas of nail-bed loss.[50-52,59,67,70] The excellent results obtained from split grafting nail-bed defects have made this procedure common practice for most hand surgeons. The donor site heals without difficulty, and most authors report no residual deformities secondary to graft harvesting.[52,67] Orientation of the split graft on the recipient bed does not affect adherence or nail-plate morphology. Shepard[52] observed good results in 75 of 84 patients with split sterile matrix grafts. The other nine patients had some nail-plate irregularity (linear ridging or distal nonadherence), which was noted exclusively at the site of avulsion and not at the site of donor harvesting. However, germinal matrix defects must be treated with full-thickness germinal matrix grafts. Zook et al[70] report good results with this technique.

The type of material placed in the eponychial fold does not appear to influence the outcome or the appearance of the re-generating nail plate.[20] Nail plate, sterile nonadherent gauze, and silicone sheet can be used interchangeably.

Soft tissue loss from the distal finger pulp in conjunction with a nail-bed injury indicates a more severe injury. Local or regional flaps have been used in conjunction with nail-bed grafts to reconstitute the integrity of the distal fingertip and nail bed. A minor hooking of the nail commonly occurs after this repair, and results generally are not as satisfactory as those associated with the repair of simple nail-bed lacerations. Some authors have had excellent results using microsurgical free transfers to reconstitute the nail and distal finger, with or without the presence of bone.[36] These composite toe flaps require advanced technical expertise but can restore nail bed, finger pulp, and bony support. Microneural repair restores sensation to the fingertip. Composite ear cartilage grafts,[42] reverse dermal grafts,[8] and split-thickness skin grafts[24] have been used for peronychial reconstruction with moderately successful results.

Meticulous anatomical coaptation of the injured nail bed renders better results. Ultimately, careful initial repair results in a better outcome than does secondary reconstructive surgery.

REFERENCES

1. Atasoy E, Godfrey A, Kalisman M: The "antenna" procedure for the "hook nail" deformity, *J Hand Surg* 8:55, 1983.
2. Baden HP, Goldsmith LA, Fleming B: A comparative study of physiochemical properties of human keratinized tissue, *Biochem Biophys Acta* 322:269, 1973.
3. Baran R: Pincer and trumpet nails, *Arch Dermatol* 110:639, 1974.
4. Barfod B: Reconstruction of the nail fold, *Hand* 4:85-87, 1972.
5. Bean WB: Nail growth: 30 years of observation, *Arch Intern Med* 134:497, 1974.
6. Bunke HJ, Gonzalez RI: Fingernail reconstruction, *J Plast Reconstr Surg* 30:452-461, 1962.
7. Carter WW: Treatment for split finger nails, *JAMA* 90:1619-1620, 1928.
8. Clayburgh RH, Wood MB, Cooney WP: Nail bed repairs and reconstruction with reverse dermal grafts, *J Hand Surg* 8:594-599, 1983.
9. Dawber R: Fingernail growth in normal and psoriatic subjects, *Br J Dermatol* 82:454, 1970.
10. Dawber R, Baran R: Nail growth, *Cutis* 39:99, 1987.
11. Ditre CM, Howe NR: Surgical anatomy of the nail unit, *J Dermatol Surg Oncol* 18:665, 1992.
12. Douglas B: Successful replacement of completely avulsed portions of fingers as composite grafts, *Plast Reconstr Surg* 23:213-225, 1959.
13. Drapne JL, Wolfram-Gabel R, Idy-Perett I, et al: The lunula: a magnetic resonance imaging approach to the subnail matrix area, *J Invest Dermatol* 106:1081, 1996.
14. Elsahy NI: When to replant a fingertip after its complete amputation? *Plast Reconstr Surg* 60:14-21, 1977.
15. Flatt AE: Nail bed injuries, *Br J Plast Surg* 8:38-43, 1955.
16. Geoghegan B, Roberts DF, Sampford MR: Possible climatic effect on nail growth, *J Appl Physiol* 13:135, 1958.
17. Germann H, Barran W, Plewig G: Morphology of corneocytes from human plates, *J Invest Derm* 74:115, 1980.
18. Gonzalez-Serva A: Onycholemmal keratinization: ensheathing and fastening of the nail plate (abstract), *J Invest Dermatol* 98:582, 1992.
19. Gonzalez-Serva A: Structure and function. In: *Nails, therapy, diagnosis, surgery,* ed 2, Philadelphia, 1997, WB Saunders, pp 12-31.
20. Guy RJ: The etiologies and mechanism of nail bed injuries, *Hand Clin* 1:9-19, 1990.
21. Halban J, Spitzer MZ: Uber das gesteigerte washstum der nagel in der schwangerscharf Monatsschrift fur *Geburtschulfe and Gynakologie* 82:25, 1929.
22. Hale AR, Burch GE: The arteriovenous anastomoses and blood vessels of the human finger, *Medicine* 39:191, 1960.
23. Hamilton JB, Terada H, Mestier GE: Studies of growth throughout the lifespan in Japanese: growth and size of nails and their relationship to age, heredity and other factors, *J Gerontol* 10:401, 1955.
24. Hanrahan EM: The split thickness skin graft as a cover following removal of a finger nail, *Surg* 20:398-400, 1946.
25. Hashimoto K: Ultrastructure of the human toenail. II. Keratinization and formation of the marginal band, *J Ultrastruct Res* 36:391-410, 1971.
26. Head H, Sherren J: The consequence of injury to the peripheral nerves in man, *Brain* 28:263 1908.
27. Johnson M, Comaish JS, Shuster S: Nail is produced by the normal nail bed: a controversy, *Br J Dermatol* 125:27, 1991.
28. Johnson M, Shuster S: Continuous formation of nail along the bed, *Br J Dermatol* 128:227, 1993.
29. Johnson RK: Nailplasty, *Plast Reconstr Surg* 47:275-276, 1971.

30. Kiligman AM: Why do nails grow out instead of up? *Arch Dermatol* 84:313-315, 1961.

31. Kleinert HB, Putcha S, Ashbell TS, et al: The deformed fingernail: a frequent result of failure to repair nail bed injuries, *J Traumatol* 7:177-190, 1967.

32. Kosima I, Morihuchi T, Umeda N, Yameda A: Trimmed second toetip transfer for reconstruction of claw nail deformity of the fingers, *Brit J Plast Surg* 45:591-594, 1992.

33. LeGros-Clark WE, Buxton LHD: Studies in nail growth, *Br J Dermatol* 50:221, 1938.

34. McCash CR: Free nail grafting, *Br J Plast Surg* 8:19-33, 1956.

35. McGinley KJ, Larson EL, Leyden JJ: Composition and density of microflora in the subungual space of the hand, *J Clin Microbiol* 26:950-953, 1988.

36. Morrison WA: Microvascular nail transfer, *Hand Clin* 6(1):9-76, 1990.

37. Norton LA: Incorporation of thymidinemethyl H^3 and glycine 2-H^3 in the nail matrix and bed of humans, *J Invest Derm* 56:61, 1971.

38. Ogo K: Split nails, *Plast Reconstr Surg* 86(6):1190-1193, 1990.

39. Orentreich N, Monkofsky J, Vogelman JH: The effect of aging on the rate of linear nail growth, *J Invest Dermotol* 73:126, 1979.

40. O'Shaughnessy M, McCann J, O'Connor TP, Condon KC: Nail re-growth in fingertip injuries, *Irish Med J* 83(4):136-137, 1990.

41. Parrinello JF, Japour CJ, et al: Incurvated nail. Does the phalanx determine nail plate shape? *J Am Podiatr Med Assoc* 85:696, 1995.

42. Rose EH: Nailplasty utilizing a free composite graft from the helical rim of the ear, *J Plast Reconstr Surg* 66:23-29, 1980.

43. Rose EH, Norris MS, Lucos A, et al: The cap technique: non-surgical attachment of finger tip amputation, *J Hand Surg* 14:513-518, 1989.

44. Runne U, Orfanos CE: The human nail, *Curr Probl Dermatol* 9:102, 1981.

45. Saita A, Suzuki Y, Fujino K, et al: Free nail bed graft for treatment of nail bed injuries of the hand, *J Hand Surg* 8:171-178, 1983.

46. Sammon PD: The human toe nail: its genesis and blood supply, *Br J Dermatol* 71:296, 1959.

47. Schiller C: Nail replacement in finger tip injuries, *Plast Reconstr Surg* 19:521-530, 1957.

48. Seaberg DC, Angelos WJ, Paris PM: Treatment of subungual hematomas with nail trephination: a prospective study, *Am J Emerg Med* 9(3):209-210, 1991.

49. Shepard GH: Treatment of nail bed avulsions with split-thickness nail bed grafts, *J Hand Surg* 8:49-54, 1983.

50. Shepard GH: The use of split-thickness nail bed graft for the correction of the chronically deformed nail, *Orthop Trans* 13(1):6, 1989.

51. Shepard GH: Management of acute nail bed avulsion, *Hand Clin* 6(1):39-56, 1990.

52. Shepard GH: Nail grafts for reconstruction, *Hand Clin* 6(1):79-101, 1990.

53. Smith DO, Oura C, Kimura C, Toshimori K: Artery anatomy and tortuosity in the distal finger, *J Hand Surg [Am]* 16:297, 1991.

54. Smith DO, Oura C, Kimura C, Toshimori K: The distal venous anatomy of the finger, *J Hand Surg [Am]* 16:303, 1991.

55. Soon PS, Arnold MA, Tracey DJ: Paraterminal ligaments of the distal phalanx, *Acta Anat [Basel]* 142:339, 1991.

56. Spruit D: Measurement of water vapor loss through human nail in vivo, *J Invest Dermatol* 56:359, 1971.

57. Suzuki K, Yagi I, Kondo M: Surgical treatment of pincer nail syndrome, *Plast Reconstr Surg* 63:570, 1979.

58. Swanker WA: Reconstructive surgery of the injured nail, *Am J Surg* 74:341-345, 1947.

59. VanBeek AL, Kasson MA, Adson MH, Dal V: Management of acute fingernail injuries, *Hand Clin* 6(1):23-35, 1990.

60. Veller OD: Composition of human nail substance, *Am J lin Nutr* 23:1272, 1970.

61. Wolfram-Gabel R, Sick H: Vascular networks of the periphery of the fingernail, *J Hand Surg [Br]* 20:488, 1995.

62. Zais N: Embryology of the human nail, *Arch Dermatol* 87:77, 1963.

63. Zais N: The regeneration of the primate nail: studies of the squirrel monkey, *Saimiri J Invest Derm* 44:107, 1965.

64. Zais N: The movement of the nail bed, *J Invest Derm* 48:402, 1967.

65. Zais N: *The nail in health and disease*, ed 2, Norwalk, Conn, 1990, Appleton and Lange, pp 1-255.

66. Zook EG: The perionychium: anatomy, physiology, and care of injuries, *Clin Plast Surg* 8:21-31, 1981.

67. Zook EG: Nail bed injuries, *Hand Clin* 1:701-716, 1985.

68. Zook, EG: Anatomy and physiology of the perionychium, *Hand Clin* 6(1):1-7, 1990.

69. Zook EG, Brown RE: The perionychium. In Green, DP (editor): *Operative hand surgery*, ed 4, New York, 1999, Churchill Livingstone.

70. Zook EG, Guy RJ, Russell RC: A study of nail bed injuries: causes, treatment, prognosis, *J Hand Surg* 9A:247-252, 1984.

71. Zook EG, Russell RC: Reconstruction of a functional and esthetic nail, *Hand Clin* 6(1):59-68, 1990.

72. Zook EG, Van Beek AL, Russell RC, Beatty ME: Anatomy and physiology of the perionychium: a review of the literature and anatomic study, *J Hand Surg* 5:528-536, 1980.

CHAPTER

Management of Fingertip Injuries

101

Sean Lille
Arian Mowlavi
Robert C. Russell

INTRODUCTION

The human hand serves a unique function and separates man from the rest of the animal kingdom. A hand can be strong and powerful, yet delicate and precise. The physical characteristics of the hand often adapt to an individual's pattern of function or occupation. The thick, calloused hands of a manual laborer have hypertrophied muscles that are adapted for functions involving power and grasp. The hands of a concert pianist or an artist are supple and have increased sensibility. A blind patient requires a two-point discrimination of 2 mm to read Braille (the normal two-point discrimination of 5 mm can be improved by practice). The use of the hand clearly influences its level of function. For this reason, the anticipated function of a patient's hand must be considered after injury to determine the best method of repair and rehabilitation.

The fingertip is a highly specialized end-organ that is adapted for touch. It is richly supplied with special sensory receptors that enable the hand to "see" by relaying the shape, texture, and temperature of manipulated objects.[26,91] The special sensory receptors cannot be replaced when tissue with nonglabrous skin is used for reconstruction. Surgical management after injury should attempt to restore this special sensibility by using glabrous skin and subcutaneous tissue whenever possible for reconstruction. Successful repair of a fingertip injury requires a knowledge of anatomy and the techniques available for reconstruction, as well as sound surgical judgment.

ANATOMY

Glabrous skin consists of stratified squamous epithelium, which forms a series of ridges that create a nonslip surface and provide the characteristics of a distinctive fingerprint.[5] The volar skin, which is specially adapted for pinch and grasp functions, is stabilized by numerous fibrous septa, including Cleland's and Grayson's ligaments (Figure 101-1), which anchor the skin to the underlying bone and flexor tendon sheath. The distal pulp is divided by radial fibrous septa, which

create a multipyramidal structure of fibroadipose tissue compartments. This arrangement provides the fingertip with stability during pinch and grip functions.[78]

The axial digital nerves and arteries, respectively, traverse the subcutaneous tissue between Grayson's ligaments volarly and Cleland's ligaments dorsally, arborizing into many small branches within the pulp of the fingertip (see Figure 101-1). The digital nerves trifurcate near the distal interphalangeal (DIP) joint, sending one dorsal branch to the paronychium, one branch to the fingertip, and a third branch to the volar pulp.[120] A dorsal sensory branch of each digital nerve originates at the level of the mid-proximal phalanx and innervates the skin over the middle and distal phalanx (Figure 101-2). The digital nerves lie volar to the arteries in the digit, but in the palm they are dorsal to the common digital arteries. The skin on the dorsum of the hand is thinner than skin covering other parts of the hand, is loosely adherent, and has little subcutaneous tissue. The skin and subcutaneous tissue of the finger contain special sensory receptor sites in the form of Pacinian and Meissner corpuscles, which exist only in the glabrous skin of the hands and feet, and Merkel cell neurite discs, which are present throughout the body.[18]

The fingernail is an epidermal structure that originates from the germinal matrix at the base of the nail fold.[125] It allows prehension of small objects and enhances the stabilization of grip. The nail originates from the germinal matrix within the nail fold, which compresses the growth of the expanding cell mass into a smooth, flat, plate structure as it extends distally over the sterile matrix. Nail growth occurs at a rate of 0.1 mm per day, but is halted for 21 days after a traumatic injury.[66] The undersurface of the nail bed closely adheres to the periosteum of the tuft of the distal phalanx. The entire nail bed actively contributes to the generation of the nail plate, which thickens as it grows distally toward the hyponychium. The hyponychium is the mass of keratin found between the distal end of the nail plate and the fingertip. It contains the greatest density of lymphatics in the body and serves as a barrier to bacterial infiltration underneath the nail plate.[47] The nail plate adheres to the nail bed by a series of longitudinal ridges. The lunula is the white semicircle at the base of the

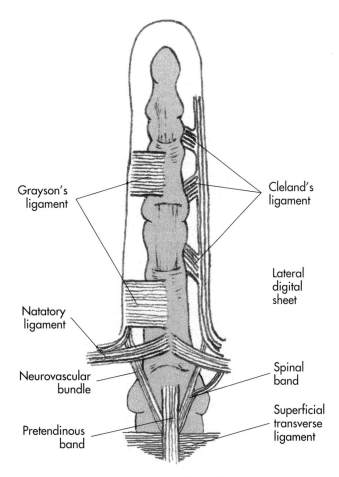

Figure 101-1. Finger anatomy. Cleland's ligaments are dorsal and Grayson's ligaments are volar to the bilateral digital arteries and nerves, which course into the fingertip and arborize into many small branches. The arteries are volar to the nerves in the palm but reverse at the distal palmar crease and are dorsal in the digits. (Modified from McFarlane RM: *Plast Reconstr Surg* 54:31, 1974.)

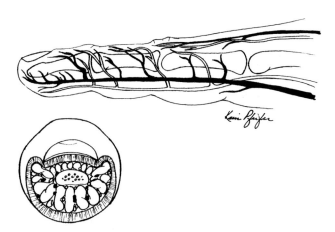

Figure 101-2. Fingertip anatomy. The fingernail originates from the germinal matrix in the base of the nail fold. The deep surface of the nail bed is closely adherent to the periosteum of the distal phalanx. Numerous fibrous septa connect the volar digital skin to the underlying bone. Bilateral digital arteries and nerves send branches dorsally to supply the skin over the middle and distal phalanges.

nail, just distal to the eponychium or cuticle. The paronychia is the skin surrounding the nail plate, and the paronychium includes the germinal and sterile nail bed, the surrounding paronychia, the distal hyponychium, and the nail plate.

GENERAL PRINCIPLES OF MANAGEMENT

The fingertip is the most distal portion of the upper extremity and is the part of the hand that is most frequently injured. Nail-bed and fingertip injuries usually result in time lost from work and, if improperly repaired, can be permanently disabling. Ideal fingertip reconstruction should attempt to maintain length, prevent joint contracture, preserve nail function, and provide sensate soft tissue coverage that enables pain-free use of the finger. A thorough patient history and examination of the injured finger must be completed before treatment is initiated. The etiology and time of injury, as well as the patient's age, gender, occupation, and hand dominance should be documented. The relative importance of each finger to overall hand function also must be considered. An injury to the tip of the nondominant small finger sustained by a mechanic (who crushed the finger in a machine) most likely would be managed by completion of the amputation. A cleanly cut soft tissue amputation of the dominant index fingertip of a professional musician would clearly warrant pulp reconstruction.

Most patients with fingertip injuries can be treated in an emergency department as outpatients and with the use of digital block anesthesia. Most injuries have varying degrees of soft tissue damage to the fingertip or nail bed that can be treated by careful primary repair.[45,56,80] More severe injuries that require flap coverage or extensive bone fixation are best repaired in the operating room under regional block or general anesthesia. Preoperative radiographs should be taken to identify phalangeal fractures or retained foreign bodies. Nondisplaced fractures can be effectively splinted after soft tissue repair and/or reconstruction. Displaced fractures require reduction and, if unstable, fixation with Kirschner wires (K wires) before soft tissue reconstruction.[122,126]

Fingertip injuries associated with loss of soft tissue should be examined to determine the level and angle of soft tissue loss, the amount of remaining nail bed and supporting distal phalanx, and the presence or absence of exposed bone (Figure 101-3).

Special attention must be given to the extent of soft tissue damage and the angle of amputation because these factors often dictate the optimum treatment plan. Superficial tip wounds without exposed bone may be allowed to heal by secondary intention or may be closed with a skin graft (line A). Transverse amputations through the middle of the nail bed are best treated by primary closure using local advancement flaps (line C). Pulp amputations with exposed bone that are angled volarly usually require regional or distant flap coverage (line B). Amputations that are directed dorsally, with less than one quarter of the nail bed remaining, typically should be treated by ablation of the nail bed and completion of the amputation by primary closure or by the use of local advancement flaps (line D).

Digital block anesthesia for patients treated in an emergency department is administered by injecting 4 to 5 ml of 1%

lidocaine without epinephrine, using a small 25- to 27-gauge needle in a ring around the base of the proximal phalanx (Figure 101-4). The addition of sodium bicarbonate (44 mEq/L) to Xylocaine in a 1:9 ratio raises the pH to near normal tissue range, results in a decrease in the duration of onset, but reduces the discomfort of injection for the patient. The entire hand and distal forearm are prepared with a surgical soap and solution, then draped using sterile technique and placed on an arm board (Figure 101-5). A 1-inch Penrose drain is placed around the base of the injured finger and held flat with a hemostat to provide even pressure and a blood-free surgical field.[38,118] The wound should be thoroughly irrigated with normal saline, under tourniquet control, and inspected before the initiation of treatment. Irrigation can be accomplished with a 5- to 10-ml

syringe or a sterilized plastic spray bottle.[125] All nonviable soft tissue is debrided, and the selected fingertip closure is completed. The fingertip is dressed with nonadherent gauze and a sterile dressing before the tourniquet is released. A metal or plastic splint is incorporated into the last layer of the dressing to protect the repair and to prevent painful tactile stimulation. All patients should be given tetanus prophylaxis.

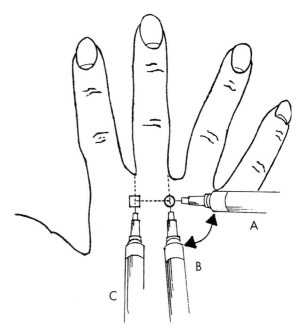

Figure 101-4. Digital block anesthesia can be used to treat most fingertip injuries by injecting 4 to 5 ml of 1% xylocaine around the base of the finger.

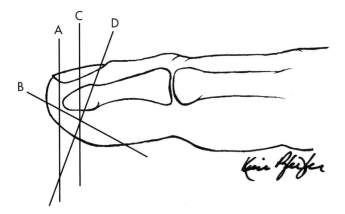

Figure 101-3. Angle and level of amputation. **A,** Loss of skin only, without exposed bone. **B,** Volarly directed amputation. **C,** Transversely directed amputation. **D,** Dorsally directed amputation.

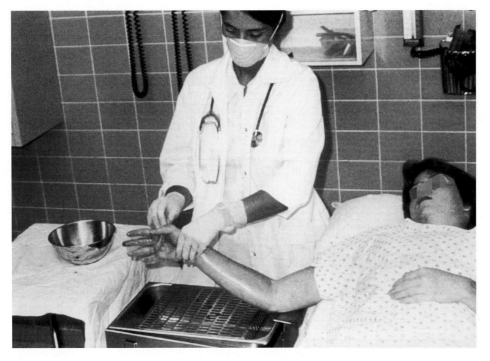

Figure 101-5. The entire hand and forearm are washed with surgical soap and solution and draped in a sterile fashion on an arm board.

NAIL-BED INJURIES

INDICATIONS

Significant nail-bed lacerations should always be repaired to prevent subsequent nail deformity.[124] Blunt trauma, direct lacerations, or distal phalanx fractures can lacerate the nail bed. A subungual hematoma is evidence of nail-bed trauma. These hematomas can vary in size; some may be imperceptible, whereas others may compromise nail-bed survival. Small subungual hematomas do not require treatment, but larger hematomas require trephination therapy to relieve pain.* If a subungual hematoma involves more than 25% of the nail plate, the plate should be removed and the nail-bed laceration repaired.[3,69,113,123] Subungual hematomas often are associated with distal phalangeal fractures, which should be evaluated radiographically. Small fractures of the distal tuft do not require treatment. More proximal distal phalanx fractures through the nail or base of the distal phalanx should be reduced and may require pin fixation, usually with a single longitudinal K wire or with crossed K wires (0.028 to 0.035 inches) placed across the DIP joint (Figure 101-6).[20,47,69,104]

Persistent nail deformity can result if the nail bed is not anatomically repaired.[3,123] The status of the nail bed should be determined by removing the entire nail plate with the tip of hemostat of a Freer elevator. Matrix lacerations should be repaired under direct observation, using loupe magnification and 7-0 chromic sutures. The nail plate is replaced in the

eponychial fold as a stent to prevent scarring of the underlying bed matrix to the nail-fold roof. Nonadherent gauze or a silicon sheet can be used to hold the nail fold open if the nail plate is missing. New nail growth displaces the replaced nail plate after the nail bed is healed. Split nail-bed grafts from the adjacent intact matrix[102] or full- or split-thickness toenail matrix grafts from the foot[67,97,102] should be used at the time of injury to replace areas of avulsed nail matrix, as described in Chapter 100.

NONOPERATIVE TREATMENT

Fingertip injuries with no evidence of exposed bone and with skin loss equal to or less than 1 cm in diameter can be allowed to heal by secondary intention (Figure 101-7).* The wound is cleansed two or three times daily with mild soap and water and is dressed with nonadherent gauze and antibiotic ointment such as Neosporin or Bacitracin. Healing occurs by contraction and epithelialization and is usually complete by 3 to 6 weeks, depending on the size of the defect.

Some authors prefer nonoperative treatment to the use of skin grafts or local flaps.[9,49] Das[24] postulated that some degree of soft tissue regeneration occurs in children after loss of soft tissue associated with a fingertip injury and recommends nonoperative treatment in most cases. However, the nonoperative method may not provide the best functional or aesthetic out-

*References 69, 86, 100, 109, 119.

*References 10, 19, 24, 31, 52, 63, 95, 116, 121.

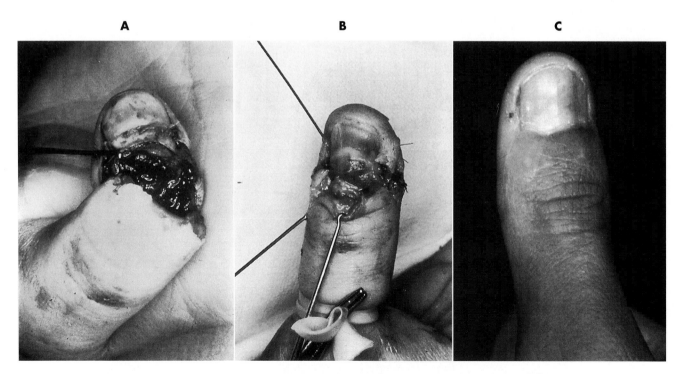

Figure 101-6. **A,** A proximal nail-bed laceration with an open fracture of the distal phalanx in a yourn woman whose thumb was caught in the reins of a horse. **B,** The fracture was reduced and pinned and the nail bed was repaired with fine chromic sutures under tourniquet control using loupe magnification. The nail plate was replaced in the eponychial fold to prevent scarring. **C,** The thumb has a normal appearance and function after treatment.

come.[63] Loss of volume, pulp firmness, cold intolerance, and hypersensitivity have been reported after nonoperative treatment.[49,63,110] However, although as many as one third of patients initially may complain of cold intolerance, symptoms tend to subside with time.[42] Joint stiffness and hypersensitivity, as well as dysesthesia, also tend to be transient.[66] A desensitization program is often helpful after the wound is stable.[109]

OPERATIONS

Primary Closure With or Without Bone Shortening

Primary closure ensures the preservation of glabrous pulp skin and special sensory receptor sites.[9,109,110] Therefore all viable local soft tissue should be used to close fingertip wounds whenever possible for the best functional result (Figure 101-8). A limited amount of bone shortening of the distal phalanx may

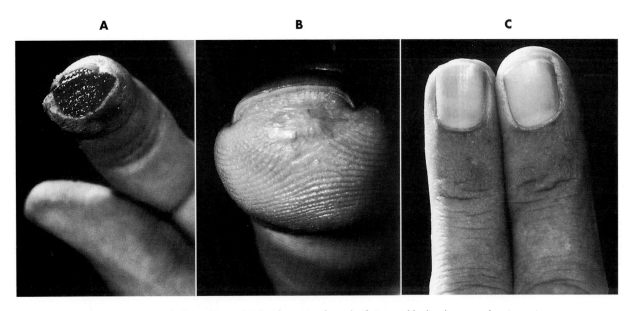

Figure 101-7. **A,** Partial loss of index fingertip after a knife injury. Healing by secondary intention produced very little dorsal **(B)** or volar **(C)** deformity.

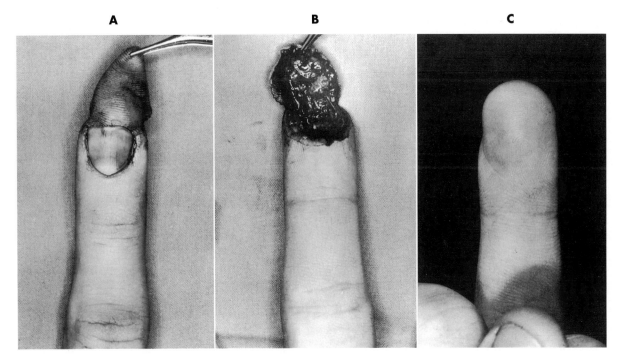

Figure 101-8. **A,** and **B,** Incompletely amputated long fingertip from a car-door injury. **C,** The distally based volar flap is closed primarily, producing good results 2 years later.

be necessary to achieve primary closure without tension. Partially devascularized skin flaps should be handled carefully and closed loosely to prevent necrosis.[66] The viability of local tissue must be determined after debridement, with the tourniquet released. If soft tissue loss to the fingertip is asymmetrical, a fillet flap can be used after bone shortening to obtain primary closure. Amputations through the lunula can be closed with local tissue after bone shortening and the excision of residual nail fold germinal matrix. Inadequate germinal matrix resection can produce an irritating cutaneous nail horn, often necessitating a secondary surgical revision.

Skin-Graft Coverage

A fingertip pulp injury that does not expose bone can be closed using a split- or full-thickness skin graft,* which contracts during healing and decreases the size of the original defect (Figure 101-9). Split-thickness grafts contract more than full-thickness grafts and are desirable in some cases; however, the return of sensation appears to be better with thicker grafts.[50,79,88,89,105]

Sharply amputated soft tissue that has not been crushed can be defatted and replaced as a full-thickness skin graft. The skin, hyponychium, and distal sterile matrix can be replaced as a unit.[103] All skin grafts should be immobilized with a stent dressing and an external digital splint for 7 days. The graft is sutured in place with 5-0 nylon sutures, which are left long and are tied over a moist cotton stent dressing using nonadherent gauze between the grafts and cotton stent. If the amputated part is too severely injured or is not available, a split- or full-thickness skin graft from the hypothenar eminence can be used.[87,99] The ulnar side of the hypothenar eminence is an excellent graft donor site for fingertip injuries and leaves an inconspicuous donor site scar. Nonglabrous skin from the forearm or groin is less desirable because of poor color match, a donor site scar, and the lack of special sensory receptor sites.[14-16,93,99] Split-thickness grafts can be excised in an emergency department with a hand-held Weck knife, using a 0.10- to 0.25-inch guard. The donor site from smaller full-thickness grafts excised in an ellipse can be closed primarily. Newly grafted skin should be protected for at least 2 weeks with an external cap splint.

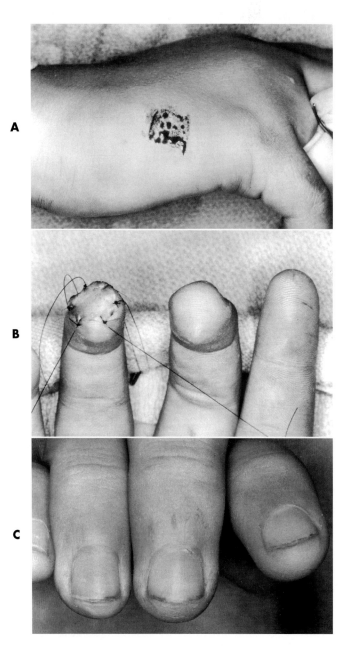

Figure 101-9. **A,** The donor site of a split-thickness skin graft harvested from the hypothenar eminence using local anesthetic. **B,** The graft is sutured into position before placement of a stent dressing. **C,** 18 months later, the fingertip has healed without nail deformity.

COMPOSITE AMPUTATIONS

INDICATIONS

In patients younger than 6 years of age, a complete guillotine amputation of the fingertip distal to the lunula can be replaced with a composite graft. The finger stump and the amputated tip are thoroughly irrigated and minimally debrided. The fractured distal phalanx is then pinned with a single longitudinal K wire (0.028 inches). The skin is closed with fine chromic suture, and the entire extremity is immobilized in a bulky hand dressing and an above-elbow cast for 10 to 14 days. Composite fingertip grafts in adults are unreliable and should not be attempted. In adults, distal finger pulp amputations that do not expose bone can be replaced as full-thickness skin grafts. Replantation in cases of fingertip amputation at the level of the DIP joint can yield good functional and aesthetic results and is worthwhile in young patients.[111]

---

*References 7, 13, 34, 43, 65, 70, 84, 92, 98.

OPERATIONS

Local Flap Reconstruction

A variety of local advancement flaps have been used to cover digital-tip amputation stumps with exposed bone. Closure techniques that preserve length and provide local soft tissue coverage with normal glabrous skin offer significant benefits. However, such flaps may be contraindicated in patients with marginal peripheral circulation from previous trauma or severe peripheral vascular disease.

Kutler Lateral V-Y Flaps

Small lateral V-Y advancement flaps cut from both sides of the amputated fingertip were first described by Kutler.[58] These flaps are used for transverse or slightly volar amputations at the mid-nail level. Before flap elevation and mobilization, the skin and subcutaneous tissue of the amputated stump are carefully debrided and any exposed bone is trimmed. Triangular skin flaps are drawn bilaterally along the lateral aspect of the remaining distal phalanx. The base of each triangle is placed along the cut edge of the amputation stump (Figure 101-10), with the tip of the flap at the DIP-joint flexion crease. The skin is carefully incised with a scalpel, preserving the terminal branches of the digital arteries and nerves, and the fibrous septa in the subcutaneous tissue are gently spread with a sharp-

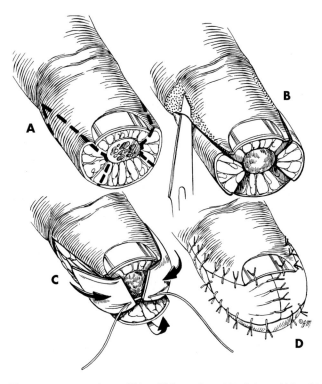

Figure 101-10. Lateral V to Y flaps. **A** and **B,** Bilateral V to Y advancement flaps cut from the sides of the injured finger and gently advanced over the tip by dividing the fibrous septa from the underlying bone. **C,** The volar skin corners can be trimmed to improve tip contour. **D,** The flaps are sutured together in the midline over the tip and the donor sites are closed in a Y.

pointed scissors. The flaps are mobilized by dividing the septal connections to the distal phalanx at the level of the periosteum with the tip of the scissors. Gentle skinhook traction is used to advance the flaps over the amputated fingertip. The flaps must be mobilized sufficiently to allow closure without tension. The donor defect is closed in a Y fashion, and the distal edge of the nail bed is sutured to the edge of the advanced flaps. The remaining volar skin may need to be trimmed distally to contour the tip closure. It is best to release the digital tourniquet before applying the dressing to assess the viability of the flaps. Although such flaps look good in illustrations, we have found that they are small, difficult to dissect safely, and often provide limited advancement (Figure 101-11).[36,42,46,66]

Volar V-Y Flaps

Another local flap technique that provides coverage of transverse mid-nail or dorsally directed fingertip amputations was described by Tranquilli-Leali[112] and Atasoy et al.[4] This technique involves a single V-shaped volar flap drawn on the remaining distal phalanx, with the tip of the flap at the DIP-joint flexion crease (Figure 101-12). The skin is incised with a scalpel, preserving the neurovascular bundles in the flap. The fibrous septa in the subcutaneous tissue are gently freed from the underlying distal phalanx and tendon sheath with an iris scissor. Careful skinhook traction is used to advance the flap over the amputated fingertip, and the flap is sutured to the distal edge of the nail bed while the donor defect is closed in a Y fashion. Tension-free closure is mandatory to prevent necrosis or the development of a curved-nail deformity. The flap should always be advanced distally as far as possible to support the cut edge of the nail bed, which helps prevent a curved-nail deformity. However, a flattened appearance of the tip remains a common disadvantage of this flap.[66]

Several modifications of the volar V-Y flap may reduce this problem. Furlow described a larger volar skin flap that extends proximally to the proximal interphalangeal (PIP)–joint crease (Figure 101-13). Parallel mid-lateral incisions are extended proximally onto the middle phalanx and the V portion of the flap is cut, with its apex at the PIP-joint flexion crease. The entire volar skin flap, including the neurovascular bundles, is elevated off the flexor-tendon sheath. The distal flap edges are sutured to each other, creating a more natural rounded tip, which is advanced distally over the tip defect; the donor site is closed in a Y over the middle phalanx.[42] This technique creates a more normal-looking tip but requires more dissection of the finger.

Volar Neurovascular Advancement Flaps

A technique first described by Moberg,[74] and later popularized by O'Brien and Snow,[82,108] illustrates how the entire volar surface of an injured digit can be advanced distally as a neurovascular flap to reconstruct an amputated fingertip (Figure 101-14). The procedure has been described for all digits of the hand but is ideally suited for transverse distal thumb-tip amputations. The amputation stump is debrided and the flap is outlined bilaterally in the mid-axial line along the distal and

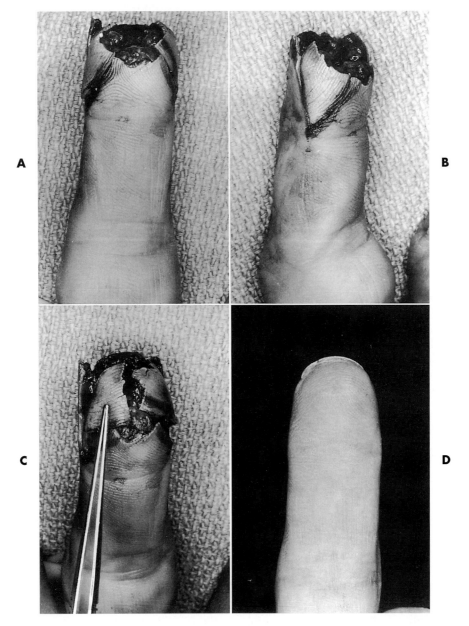

Figure 101-11. **A** and **B**, Transverse mid-nail fingertip amputation sustained by a 26-year-old man. Bilateral triangular flaps designed along the lateral aspects of the remaining distal phalanx, which do not cross the interphalangeal flexion crease. **C**, The flaps are mobilized at the level of the periosteum and advanced over the amputated fingertip. **D**, The healed fingertip has good sensation and contour.

Figure 101-12. Volar V-to-Y flap. **A**, A single volar flap is cut from the remaining distal phalanx skin to close the site of a distal transverse fingertip amputation. **B** and **C**, The fibrous septa are divided from the underlying distal phalanx and the bone is shortened to permit flap advancement without tension. **D**, The flap is sutured to the distal nail bed and the donor defect is closed in a Y.

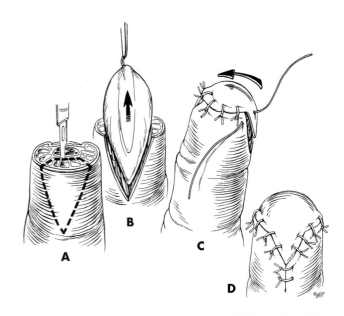

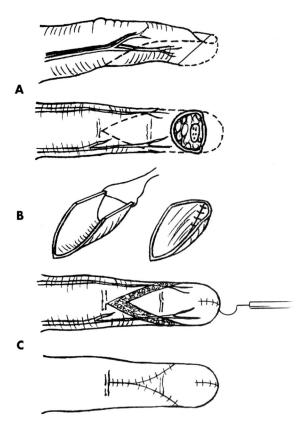

Figure 101-13. A, The Furlow modification of the V-Y advancement flap elevates a volar flap off the middle phalanx on both neurovascular bundles. **B,** The leading edge of the flap is sutured together to improve the finger pulp contour. **C,** The cupped flap is advanced distally with a skin hook and the donor site over the middle phalanx is closed in a Y.

proximal phalanx. The skin is incised, and the entire volar skin and subcutaneous tissue of the digit, including both neurovascular bundles, is elevated at the level of the flexor tendon sheath. The branches of the digital nerve and artery that course dorsally at the base of the proximal phalanx should be preserved to maintain the dorsal digital nerve and blood supply. Care should be taken to avoid injury to the dorsal arterial branches off the digital arteries, which can lead to dorsal skin necrosis.[66] The thumb is flexed and the flap is advanced distally approximately 1 cm to permit closure of the amputation stump, O'Brien[82] modified this technique to gain further advancement of the flap by connecting the lateral incisions at the base of the digit, creating a neurovascular island flap. He closed the proximal flap donor site with a split-thickness skin graft.*

When further flap advancement is necessary to preserve length in the thumb, we prefer to create a large V-Y advancement flap across the metacarpophalangeal (MCP) joint, using a method similar to that described by Furlow to close digital-tip amputations. The proximal neurovascular bundles can be dissected to increase flap mobility, and the primary donor

---

*References 33, 36, 51, 55, 60, 82, 94.

site may be closed in a Y configuration. The volar neurovascular flap technique supplies glabrous skin with near-normal sensation but requires extensive soft tissue dissection. Vascular compromise to the pedicle's digital arteries can occur from compression, tension, or kinking; however, such compromise may be prevented with careful dissection and flap advancement without tension.[16,108] Patients begin active extension exercises and passive stretching in 10 to 14 days to regain full extension, which is usually accomplished without difficulty.

Regional Flaps

Volarly directed fingertip amputations or digits with extensive soft tissue trauma and exposed tendon, bone, or joint surfaces that cannot be closed with local flaps can be closed with regional flaps from adjacent uninjured digits.

Standard Cross-Finger Flaps

Transfer of a delayed skin flap using dorsal skin and subcutaneous tissue from the middle phalanx of an adjacent finger was first described by Gurdii and Pangman in 1950[44]; more extensive reports by other authors followed.[21,22,58] The procedure offers one method for preserving length, particularly in patients with volarly directed fingertip amputations with significant pulp loss. The procedure is usually performed under regional anesthesia in the operating room, with proximal tourniquet control. The wound is extensively irrigated, debrided of devitalized tissue, and the dimensions of the tip defect are determined. A pattern of the tip defect is made and a flap of adequate length and orientation is drawn over the middle or proximal phalanx of an adjacent donor finger (Figure 101-15). The flap is based laterally along the mid-lateral line and elevated above the level of the peritenon, which is preserved over the extensor system. The dorsal flap is raised, beginning with a mid-lateral incision and elevating the flap toward the opposite lateral border of the digit. Some of the overlying dorsal veins must be divided during elevation of the flap, but as many as possible toward the base of the flap should be preserved. To mobilize the flap, Clelland's cutaneous ligaments should be divided near the base of the flap. After the flap is completely elevated, the tourniquet is released and hemostasis is obtained. The injured finger is flexed, and the flap is sutured over the volar tip defect. A nylon anchor suture should be placed from the proximal edge of the tip defect of the injured finger to the proximal corner of the donor defect. This suture holds the fingers together and prevents tension on the flap.

The donor site is closed with a full-thickness skin graft from the antecubital fossa, medial arm, or groin, and the digits are immobilized with a plaster splint. Children may require a long-arm cast with the elbow flexed at 90 degrees for additional immobilization. Two to three weeks after the initial surgery, the flap is divided and inset, and any remaining base is replaced on the donor finger. Immediate active and passive range-of-motion exercises are initiated for all digits to prevent stiffness. Complications associated with the placement of cross-finger flaps include donor-site depression, skin-graft hyperpigmentation, digital stiffness, and cold intolerance. Cross-finger flaps

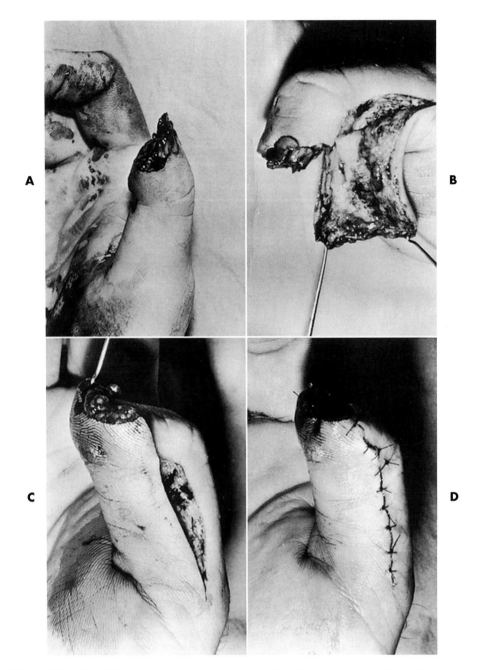

Figure 101-14. Volar neurovascular advancement flap. **A,** A transverse thumb-tip amputa-tion can be closed with a volar neurovascular advancement flap cut bilaterally in the mid-lateral line along the sides of the thumb. **B,** The flap is elevated at the level of the flexor-tendon sheath; it includes both neurovascular bundles and is advanced by flexing the interphalangeal joint. **C,** Further advancement can be achieved by extending the flap as a V into the palm and closing it as a Y **(D).**

appear to regain sensation and some two-point discrimina-tion.[53,57] Multiple fingertip amputations can be closed at the same time with flaps from adjacent digits (Figure 101-16). Cross-finger flaps also can be deepithelialized and turned upside down over a dorsal digit defect as described in Chapter 102.

A modification of the cross-finger flap uses one or both dorsal branches off the proper digital nerves that course

dorsally on both sides of the PIP joint to innervate the dorsal skin of the middle phalanx. The dorsal nerve branch along the cut edge of the innervated flap is identified and isolated a short distance proximally. The nerve is divided and after the flap is turned over, the nerve in the flap is joined to the distal end of the digital nerve, which is identified in the edge of the pulp defect of the injured finger. When the cross-finger flap is divided, a second nerve repair using the oppo-

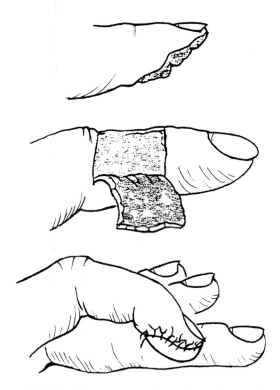

Figure 101-15. Standard cross-finger flap. A volar fingertip pulp amputation is best covered with a standard cross-finger flap elevated from the dorsal surface of the middle phalanx of an adjoining digit. The flap is elevated superficial to the peritenon of the extensor tendon and turned over like the page of a book. The injured finger is flexed and the flap is sutured over the tip defect. The donor site is closed with a skin graft.

site dorsal nerve branch can be done to the remaining digital nerve.

Side Cross-Finger Flaps

A proximally based side cross-finger flap that is well suited for thumb-tip amputations was first described by Russell et al.[96] This flap is centered just above the mid-axial line, preferably on the nondominant ulnar side of the proximal phalanx of the index or long finger (Figure 101-17).

The amputated thumb tip is debrided and flexed into the palm to a position beneath the donor digit (see Figure 101-14). The dimensions of the flap are drawn slightly larger than those of the thumb tip defect. A proximally based flap is elevated from the side of the finger at the level of the extensor peritenon and volarly along the neurovascular bundle, which is left intact. The flap is subsequently turned 90 degrees and sutured over the amputated thumb tip. The flap donor site can be closed primarily or covered with a skin graft. The flap is divided in 2 to 3 weeks, and immediate active range-of-motion exercises are begun. A donor defect on the ulnar side of the finger is not visible during most hand use. Fingertip amputations also can be closed with this technique in children or in young adults with supple digits. However, prolonged finger immobilization in a flexed position is not recommended for most adults.

Thenar Metacarpophalangeal Flexion Crease Flaps

In 1926 Gatewood was the first to describe a flap elevated from the soft tissue over the thenar eminence[40]; various modifications were described later by other authors.[6,73,107] An often tender and unappealing donor site scar on the palm led to modifications of the thenar flap that permit primary donor-site closure to help reduce this morbidity. Russell et al[96] described a radially based flap elevated from the thumb MCP joint flexion crease that can be made 1 to 2 cm wide. The flap easily reaches the tip of the index and long fingers; in some patients, even ring and small fingertip injuries and the donor site can be closed primarily by flexing the thumb (Figure 101-18). Injury to the underlying flexor tendon and the neurovascular structures (especially the radial digital nerve of the thumb) must be avoided during flap elevation. The injured digit and thumb are splinted in less flexion after flap inset (compared with splinting after standard palmar flap procedures). The flap is divided and inset is 2 to 3 weeks later. Active range-of-motion exercises are initiated immediately after division of the flap to minimize residual stiffness. A flap from the thenar MCP-joint flexion crease is ideally suited to close small fingertip amputations. Moreover, such a flap produces very little donor-site deformity and no loss of thumb motion. Relative contraindications include patients prone to arthritis or joint stiffness[109] and larger defects in which the skin of the MCP joint may be inadequate for closure.

Neurovascular Island Flaps for Thumb Reconstruction

Large volar thumb defects are best reconstructed with a sensate flap because loss of sensation to the thumb pad can cause a significant functional deficit. A neurovascular island pedicle flap from the long or ring finger was first proposed by Moberg[74] and later performed by Littler.[62] Several similar procedures also have been reported.[8,17]

The skin and subcutaneous tissue from the nondominant ulnar side of the long or ring finger is elevated as an island flap on the digital nerve and artery and transposed across the palm on the neurovascular bundle to close the thumb defect (Figure 101-19). The digital nerve fascicles must be dissected from the common digital nerve in the palm and the proper digital artery to the adjacent digit must be sacrificed to move the flap on the common digital neurovascular bundle. A generous cuff of subcutaneous tissue around the pedicle is necessary to preserve venous drainage. The patency of the digital arteries remaining in the donor and adjacent digit must be determined with a digital Allen's test before flap elevation to ensure there is blood supply to those digits after transfer. The donor finger loses sensation in the tip, and the donor defect, even when covered with a full-thickness skin graft, can result in contractures and a noticeable deformity. Cortical reorientation is better when the flap is harvested from the long finger because it lies within the distribution of the median nerve, but adult patients never completely relocalize digital flap sensation to the thumb. This has led some authors to recommend delayed flap

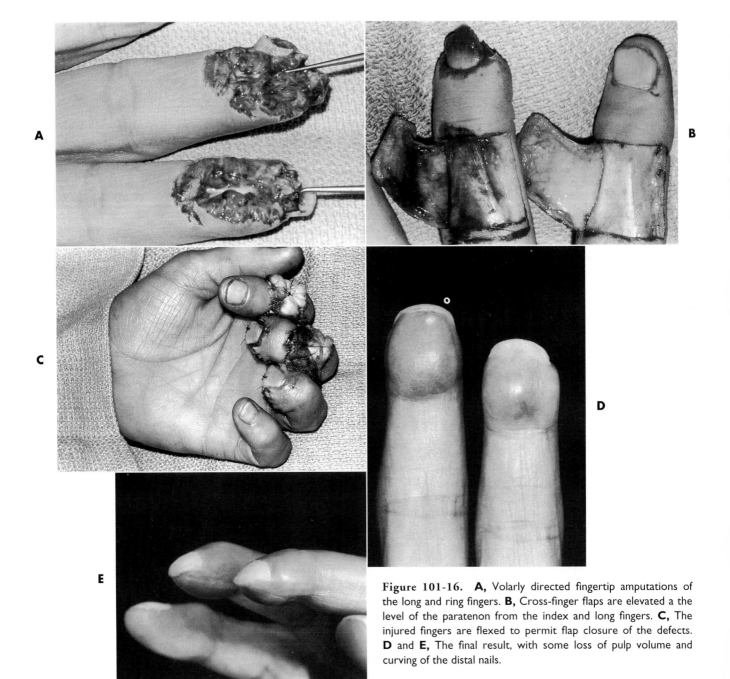

Figure 101-16. A, Volarly directed fingertip amputations of the long and ring fingers. **B,** Cross-finger flaps are elevated a the level of the paratenon from the index and long fingers. **C,** The injured fingers are flexed to permit flap closure of the defects. **D** and **E,** The final result, with some loss of pulp volume and curving of the distal nails.

nerve transection and repair to the cut ulnar digital nerve of the thumb.

We prefer to use a neurotized flap elevated from the dorsal surface of the index finger as a cross-finger or pedicled flap to reconstruct large volar thumb defects. This cross-finger flap uses the skin and subcutaneous tissue over the proximal phalanx of the index finger, which is innervated by superficial branches of the radial nerve. The flap can be elevated as a standard cross-finger flap from the dorsum of the index finger and turned over to cover the volar thumb defect.[1,11,41,48] The dorsal branches of the radial nerve entering the flap are preserved and dissected proximally by means of a separate inci-

sion. The nerve is transposed through a connecting dorsal ulnar incision to the ulnar side of the thumb during the initial procedure, or is later transected and connected to the ulnar digital nerve of the thumb when the flap is divided and inset.

Kite Flap

The *kite flap,* described by Foucher[35,36] and later remodified by others, is a more elegant flap modification based on the first dorsal metacarpal artery (Figure 101-20). The dimensions of the volar thumb defect are drawn on the dorsal surface of the index finger over the radial side of the proximal phalanx. The

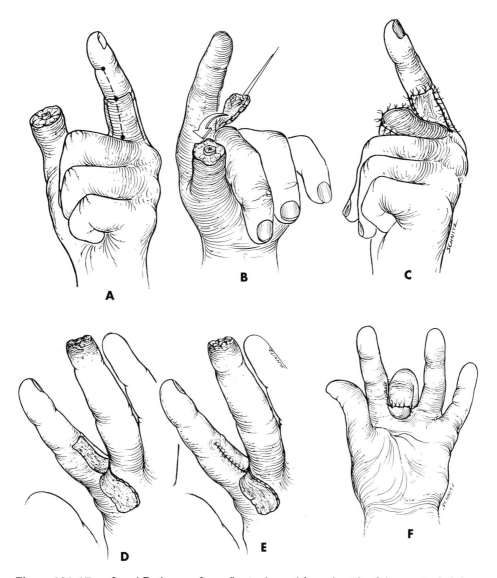

Figure 101-17. **A** and **D,** A cross-finger flap is elevated from the side of the proximal phalanx of the donor finger and is centered on the mid-lateral line. The neurovascular bundles are left intact. **B** and **E,** The flap is rotated 90 degrees to cover a thumb tip defect and can be used for fingertip amputations in young patients. **C** and **F,** The donor site is closed primarily or is skin grafted.

flap can be elevated distally up to the PIP-joint flexion crease and proximally to include skin and subcutaneous tissue over the MCP joint. A curvilinear incision is drawn on the dorsum of the hand from the proximal flap edge toward the base of the first and second metacarpals to expose the neurovascular pedicle. The skin edges of this proximal incision are elevated at the level of the dermis, preserving the subcutaneous tissue, which contains the neurovascular pedicle. The distal edge of the flap is elevated superficial to the level of the extensor peritenon. The dissection is continued proximally to include a cuff of subcutaneous tissue that contains the superficial venous plexus and fascia overlying the first

dorsal interosseous muscle. This subcutaneous tissue also contains the first dorsal metacarpal artery and branches of the radial nerve.

The flap is transposed on the vascular pedicle and may be tunneled beneath the remaining dorsal or ulnar thumb skin into the volar defect or placed, under direct observation, through an incision that connects to the thumb defect. The donor site on the dorsum of the index finger is covered with a skin graft, and the incisions are closed primarily (Figure 101-21). It is important to relieve tension on the neurovascular pedicle, which can be facilitated by flexing and adducting the thumb. Cortical misrepresentation and

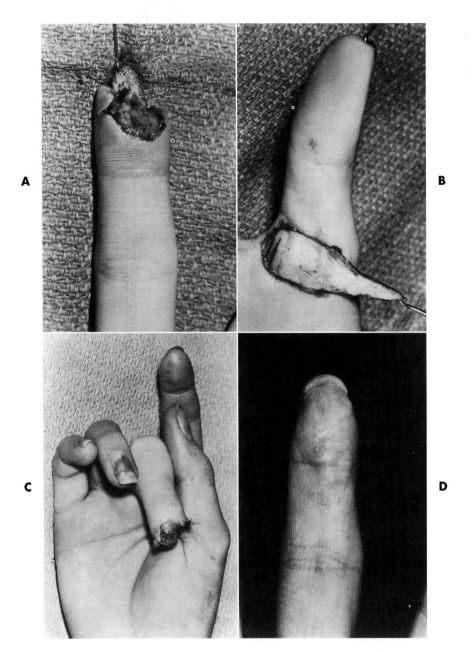

Figure 101-18. **A,** Volarly directed mid-nail amputation of the long fingertip sustained by a 16-year-old girl. **B,** A thenar-crease flap is radially based and elevated at the level of the flexor tendon sheath, leaving the neurovascular bundles intact. **C,** The flap is sutured to the long finger nail bed, and the volar skin defect and the donor site on the thumb are closed primarily. **D,** 6 months later, the long fingertip exhibits full range of motion.

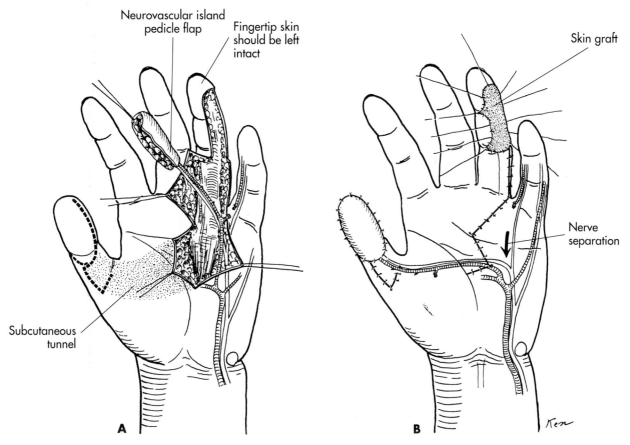

Figure 101-19. Littler flap. **A** and **B,** Neurovascular island flap is elevated from the side of the donor finger on a single neurovascular pedicle and transferred across the palm to close a volar thumb defect. The donor site is skin grafted.

donor-site morbidity are less of a problem with this flap than with the Littler neurovascular island flap from the long or ring fingers.

The skin over the proximal phalanx of the index finger can be used to resurface the thumb pad as a standard cross-finger flap based on the radial side of the index finger. The dorsal sensory branches of the radial nerve supplying the skin can be connected to the digital nerves of the thumb. At the initial procedure the ulnar branch of the dorsal radial nerve is sutured to the radial digital nerve of the thumb. When the flap is divided 2 weeks later, the radial dorsal branch of the radial nerve is sutured to the ulnar digital nerve of the thumb.[41,117]

Distant Flap Coverage

The use of local flaps is often restricted by the size of the digital defect. Attempts to advance a local flap more than 2 cm can result in a tight closure, which may cause paresthesia from stretched nerves, a painful tip, or partial or complete flap necrosis.[75] A large digital soft tissue avulsion injury, a degloving injury, or loss of tissue from

multiple adjacent digits may require coverage with a distant flap when local tissue is inadequate or unavailable. Distant pedicle flaps from the chest,[17] abdomen,[71] and groin[68] have been used to reconstruct digital soft tissue defects (Chapter 102); however, these flaps often are bulky on the hand, have poor color match, and lack sensation. Furthermore, hand immobilization in a dependent position after elevation of the pedicle flap can result in swelling and joint stiffness, which make this reconstructive option less desirable than the use of local flaps. Free tissue transfers from the opposite forearm,[30,106] dorsal foot, or lateral arm, or temporoparietal fascial flaps do not have the disadvantages associated with prolonged dependent immobilization, but cannot match the contour, bulk, and return of sensation that is possible with local glabrous skin flaps (Chapter 122).[23,83,127]

Toe Transfers

Complete or partial toe transfers can be used in special circumstances to reconstruct fingertip defects in patients who have sustained thumb avulsion injuries or the loss of multiple digits; such transfers also may be used for cosmetic

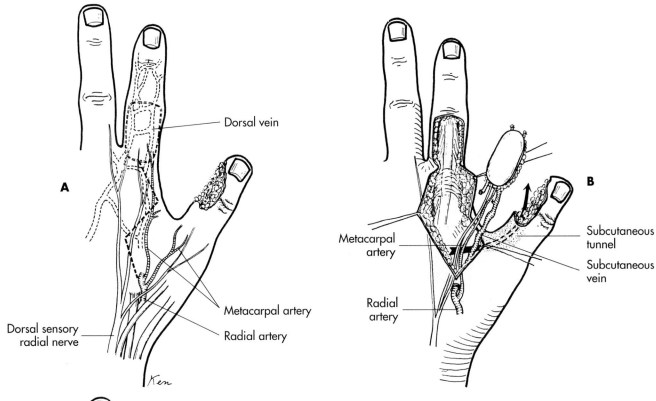

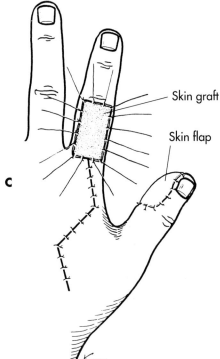

Figure 101-20. A-C, The first dorsal metacarpal artery flap is elevated off the proximal phalanx of the index finger as a neurovascular island flap, including cutaneous branches of the radial nerve. The donor site is closed with a skin graft.

concerns—typically in women patients (Chapters 122 and 125). Functional deformity of the donor site is minimal when the transferred tissue is distal to the metatarsophalangeal joint.[75]

The modified toe transfer, or *wrap-around* flap, was first described by Morrison and has gained popularity for subtotal amputations distal to the MCP joint. Portions of a toe currently may be used to reconstruct digital tip defects with or without a nail bed.* The advantages of this type of flap include less donor-site morbidity, an improved cosmetic appearance of the reconstructed thumb or digit, and the ability to obtain reinnervated glabrous skin for the fingertip after repair of the digital nerve[24] in the toe flap to those in the reconstructed digit.

---

*References 27-29, 59, 61, 76, 77, 115.

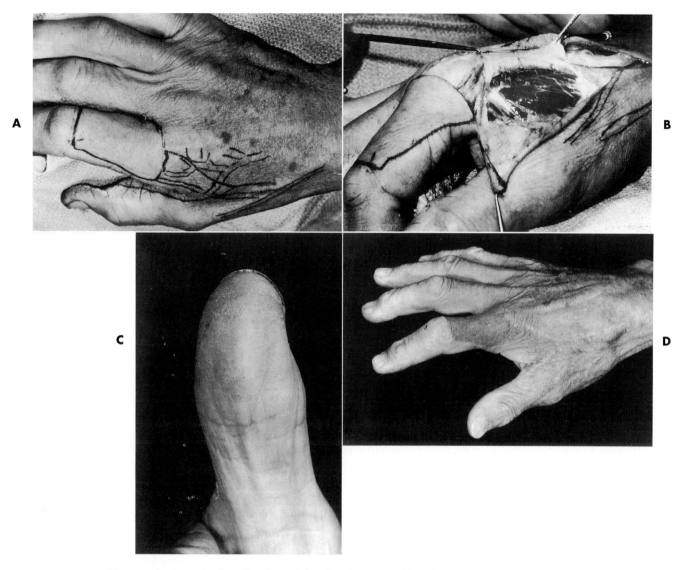

Figure 101-21. **A,** Complete loss of thumb pulp sustained by a 56-year-old man after a crush injury. A neurovascular island pedicle flap is drawn over the index proximal phalanx and is supplied by superficial branches of the radial nerve and the first dorsal metacarpal artery. **B,** The flap is elevated on a neurovascular pedicle, which includes the fascia over the first dorsal interosseous muscle, and is transposed to the thumb defect. **C,** 2 years later, the thumb has a stable soft tissue cover and has retained sensation. **D,** The donor site exhibits some depression and hyperpigmentation.

OUTCOMES

The ultimate goal of fingertip reconstructive procedures is to obtain a functional and aesthetically pleasing hand for the injured patient. Functional evaluation involves objective and subjective criteria, including motion, two-point discrimination, complaints of hyperesthesias, cold intolerance, and the time required for healing (i.e., how soon the patient can return to work or daily living activities). Overall, patient satisfaction depends on these functional factors as well as the aesthetic result of a chosen treatment.

Primary closure and skin grafting are acceptable options when minimal soft tissue loss has occurred and no critical underlying structures are exposed. A retrospective analysis of 52 cases compared primary closure after minimal shortening with the use of split-thickness skin grafts from the hypothenar area, and found no difference in two-point discrimination, paresthesia, or cold intolerance during early or late follow-up.[12] However, the investigators noted that the group of patients who had split-thickness skin grafts returned to work an average of 6 days earlier.[12] Use of a full-thickness rather than a split-thickness skin graft has been advocated to improve functional results by including all layers of the dermis, producing more durable wound coverage.[42] Full-thickness skin grafts from the hypothenar eminence provide particularly satisfying results because they replace the special sensory receptor sites of the glabrous skin.[42] Full-thickness skin grafts from the hypothenar area were used to cover tip defects in 25 patients who underwent follow-up evaluation an average of 9.5 months after surgery.[99] All grafts healed primarily without subsequent breakdown or patient complaints of hypersensitivity or cold intolerance. A two-point discrimination of 10 mm or less was obtained by 86% of patients, and 100% were able to differentiate coarse from smooth touch.[99]

Management of fingertip injuries with serial dressing changes and healing by secondary intention yields excellent results, especially for defects that measure less than 1 cm and do not involve exposed tendon or bone. Larger skin defects in children have been managed effectively with dressing changes.[12] A review of patients with tip defects that were smaller than 8 mm and were allowed to heal by secondary intention resulted in a patient satisfaction rate of 90%, with a low percentage of complaints regarding decreased sensation.[42] One prospective randomized study involving 60 children compared nonoperative management with the use of a split-thickness skin graft and local V-Y advancement flap coverage. Nonoperative management yielded the best results, with an average two-point discrimination of 3.5 mm and no loss of school days. However, dressing changes were required for more than 5 weeks. Children treated with split-thickness skin grafts had an average two-point discrimination of 7.5 mm and an average loss of 3 to 9 days of school; this group required dressing changes for 2.6 weeks. Children with local advancement flap coverage had an average two-point discrimination of 4.5 mm and no loss of school days; these children required dressing changes for 5 weeks.[24]

A volar V-Y advancement flap remains the best option for covering defects with exposed bone when there is sufficient local glabrous tissue present. Acceptable two-point discrimination, ranging from 4 to 9 mm, has been obtained consistently by investigators and in most cases patients are able to return to work within 1 month after injury.[24,42] Several series using this method of closure, which included a total of 134 thumb and fingertip repairs, have demonstrated the restoration of normal sensation or two-point discrimination to be within 2 mm of the contralateral, noninjured digit in the majority of cases.* Potential complications include dorsal skin necrosis, cold intolerance, dysesthesia, and flexion contractures. Dorsal thumb skin or flap necrosis is a rare occurrence as long as the vascular plexus supplying these areas is preserved during dissection. There were no cases of dorsal skin or flap necrosis in one study involving 69 digits.[64] Dysesthesia has not been a universal finding but cold intolerance has been reported consistently (in one study the latter was reported by 7 of 25 patients).[2] However, cold intolerance typically decreases with time. Clinically significant flexion contracture has not been reported; Maclit and Watson demonstrated full range of

motion in digits that were normal before surgery.[64] Two limitations associated with the use of neurovascular flaps confined to volar pulp tissue distal to the DIP-joint crease included limited advancement and coverage of transverse amputations only. One investigator modified the flap by extending it over the middle phalanx and down to the PIP joint to increase mobility of the tip pulp.[39] The reported complications associated with this modification included cold intolerance in 13% of patients, hyperesthesia in 7% of patients, and hook-nail deformities in 9% of patients[39]; these complications were similar to those associated with the original method.[32] The average time lost from work with this method was 56 days.[64] A study that assessed patients with lateral Kutler V-Y flaps reported an average of 61 days lost from work[37]; 50% of patients experienced cold intolerance and hypersensitivity, which subsided over time.

A well-designed cross-finger flap with a full-thickness skin graft donor-site closure provides a satisfactory aesthetic result, especially in light-skinned patients who do not experience the changes in pigment seen in darker-skinned patients. Hyperesthesia rarely occurs after this procedure, but restoration of normal sensation and full joint mobility may not be possible.

Cross-finger flaps without innervation usually provide a return of protective sensation, with an average two-point discrimination of 8 to 9 mm; however, some studies have indicated a significant rate of associated cold intolerance and donor-site morbidity.[81] Return of sensation has been most satisfactory in patients younger than 20 years of age; a higher rate of finger stiffness, donor site tenderness, and cold intolerance occurs in patients older than 40 years of age.[57] One study of six patients who received radially innervated cross-finger flaps for thumb reconstruction reported two-point discrimination of 8 to 12 mm after 6 months, which was not significantly different from the results of standard cross-finger flaps.[117] A larger series of patients must be followed for a longer period to determine whether there is a difference in the quality of sensory return.[41]

Thenar flaps may produce increased donor-site morbidity and a tendency for digital stiffness. One prospective study of 32 patients reported that 30 out of 32 patients were satisfied and had good recipient skin quality; however, 20 of these patients complained of donor-site problems such as scarring, with and without hyperesthesia. Interestingly, this study also showed that patients with work-related injuries returned to work 8 weeks or more after injury, compared with 3.7 weeks among those whose injuries were not work-related.[73] Technique modifications, such as elevating the flap from the MCP joint flexion crease, help decrease donor-site morbidity and the potential for stiffness.[6,107]

Neurovascular island flaps elevated from an adjacent, unaffected finger (such as the kite flap or flag flap) transfer an innervated skin island that is nourished by a dorsal metacarpal artery.[35,42] These flaps are elevated from more proximal areas on the dorsal surface of the hand and have been criticized for achieving less than optimal two-point discrimination. One study of kite flaps reported two-point discrimination ranging from 12 to 15 mm, which provides only protective sensation.[35]

---

*References 25, 54, 64, 72, 85, 90.

SUMMARY

Fingertip injuries are among the most common injuries seen in the emergency room and require precise wound closure for optimal results. The glabrous skin of the fingertip contains special sensory receptor sites that are uniquely adapted for digital proprioception and should be preserved whenever possible. Important factors such as the cause of injury; the patient's age; the level, angle, and type of tip amputation; and the patient's anticipated hand use must be considered when the type of wound closure is chosen. The method of repair should be individualized to provide optional hand function for each patient.

REFERENCES

1. Adamson JE, Horton CE, Crawford HH: Sensory rehabilitation of the injured thumb, *Plast Reconstr Surg* 40:53, 1967.

2. Adani R, Busa R, Castagnetti C, et al: Homodigital neurovascular island flaps with "direct flow" vascularization, *Ann Plast Surg* 38:36, 1997.

3. Ashbell TS, Kleinert HE, Putcha SM, Kutz JE: The deformed fingernail, a frequent result of failure to repair nail bed injuries, *J Trauma* 7:177, 1967.

4. Atasoy E, Ioakimidis E, Kasdan ML, et al: Reconstruction of the amputated finger tip with a triangular volar flap: a new surgical procedure, *J Bone Joint Surg* 52(5):921, 1970.

5. Barron JN: The structure and function of the skin of the hand, *Hand* 2:93, 1970.

6. Barton NJ: A modified thenar flap, *Hand* 7:150, 1975.

7. Beasley RW: Principles and techniques of resurfacing operations for hand surgery, *Surg Clin North Am* 47:389, 1967.

8. Berger A, Meissl G: Reestablishment of sensation in the distal phalanges using innervated flaps or grafts, *Handchirurgie* 7(4):169,1975.

9. Bojsen-Moller J, Pers M, Schmidt A: Fingertip injuries: late results, *Acta Clin Scand* 122:177, 1961.

10. Bossley CJ: Conservative treatment of digit amputations, *NZ Med J* 82:379, 1975.

11. Bralliar F, Horner RL: Sensory cross-finger pedicle graft, *J Bone Joint Surg* 51(7):1264, 1969.

12. Braun M, Horton RC, Snelling CFT: Fingertip amputation: review of 100 digits, *Can J Surg* 28(1):72, 1985.

13. Brown FE: V-Y Closure of fingertip injuries. In Blair WF (editor): *Techniques in hand surgery,* Baltimore, 1996, Williams and Wilkins.

14. Browne EZ: Skin grafts. In Green DP (editor): *Operative hand surgery,* ed 2. New York, 1988, Churchill Livingstone.

15. Browne EZ: Vascular anomalies. In Young JR, et al (editors): *Peripheral vascular diseases,* St. Louis, 1991, Mosby.

16. Browne EZ: Complications of fingertip injuries, *Hand Clin* 10(1):125, 1994.

17. Chase RA: Early salvage in acute hand injuries with a primary island flap, *Plast Reconstr Surg* 48;521, 1971.

18. Chase RA: *Atlas of hand surgery,* Philadelphia, 1973, WB Saunders.

19. Chow SP, Ho E: Open treatment of fingertip injuries in adults, *J Hand Surgery* 7:470, 1982.

20. Coyle M, Leddy J: Injuries of the distal finger, *Primary Care* 7:245, 1980.

21. Cronin TD: The cross-finger flap: a new method of repair, *Am Surg* 17:419, 1951.

22. Curtis RM: Cross-finger pedicle flip in hand surgery, *Ann Surg* 145:650, 1957.

23. Daniel RK, Terzis J, Midgley R: Restoration of sensation to an anesthetic hand by a free neurovascular flap from the foot, *Plast Reconstr Surg* 57:275, 1976.

24. Das SK, Brown HG: Management of lost fingertips in children, *Hand* 10:16, 1978.

25. De Smet L, Kinnen L, Moermans JP, et al: Fingertip amputations: distal or advancement flaps, *Acta Orthop Belg* 55:177, 1989.

26. Dellon AL: *Evaluation of sensibility and reduction of sensation in the hand,* Baltimore, 1981, Williams and Wilkins.

27. Doi K: Microsurgical thumb reconstruction: report of six cases with a wrap around flap from the big toe and iliac bone graft, *Ann Acad Med Singapore* 11:225, 1982.

28. Doi K, Hatori S, Kawai S, et al: A new procedure on making a thumb: one stage reconstruction with free neurovascular flaps and iliac bone graft, *J Hand Surg* 6:346, 1981.

29. Doi K, Kawata N, Kawai S: Reconstruction of the thumb with a wrap around flap and an iliac bone graft, *J Bone Joint Surg* 67(3):439, 1985.

30. Dolich BH, Olshanskv Kj, Barbar AH: Use of a cross forearm neurocutaneous flap to provide sensation and coverage in hand reconstruction, *Plast Reconstr Surg* 62:550, 1978.

31. Douglas BS: Conservative management of guillotine amputation of the finger in children, *Aust Paediatr* 8:86, 1972.

32. Elliot D, Moiemen S, Jigjinni VS: The neurovascular Tranquilli-Leali flap, *J Hand Surgery* 20B:815, 1995.

33. Elliot D, Wilson Y: V-Y advancement of the entire volar tissue of the thumb in distal reconstruction, *J Hand Surg* 18B:399, 1993.

34. Flatt AE: *The care of minor hand injuries,* ed 3, St. Louis, 1972, CV Mosby, pp 137.

35. Foucher G, Braun JB: A new island flap transfer from the dorsum of the index to the thumb, *Plast Reconstr Surg* 63:344, 1979.

36. Foucher G, Jay Boulas H, Braga Da Silva J: The use of flaps in the treatment of fingertip injuries, *World J Surg* 15:458, 1991.

37. Frandsen PA: A V to Y plasty as treatment of fingertip amputations, *Acta Orthop Scand* 49(3):255, 1978.

38. Frykman GK: Iatrogenic digital nerve compression, American Society for Surgery of the Hand Correspondence (club newsletter), November 1, 1979.

39. Furlow LT: V-Y "cup" flap for volar oblique amputation of fingers, *J Hand Surg [Br]* 9:253, 1984.

40. Gatewood: A plastic repair of finger defects without hospitalization, *JAMA* 87:1479, 1926.

41. Gaul JS: Radial innervated cross-finger flap from index to provide sensory pulp to injured thumb, *J Bone Joint Surg* 51A:1257, 1969.

42. Goitz RJ, Wetkaemper JG, Tomaino MM, et al: Soft-tissue defects of the digits: coverage considerations, *Hand Clin* 13:189, 1997.

43. Graham WP: Incisions, amputations and skin grafting in the hand, *Orthop Clin North Am* 1:213, 1970.

44. Gurdin M, Pangmait WJ: The repair of surface defects of fingers by transdigital flaps, *Plast Reconstr Surg* 5:368, 1955.

45. Guy R: The etiologies and mechanism of nail bed injuries, *Hand Clin North Am* 6:9, 1990.

46. Haddad RJ: The Kotler repair of fingertip amputations, *South Med J* 61:1264, 1968.

47. Hart RG, Kleinert HE: Fingertip and nail bed injuries, *The Hand in Emergency Medicine* 11:755, 1993.

48. Holevich J: A new method of restoring sensibility to the thumb, *J Bone Joint Surg* 45B:496, 1963.

49. Holrn A, Zachariae L: Finger tip lesions: an evaluation of conservative treatment versus free skin grafting, *Acta Orthop Scand* 45:382, 1974.

50. Hutchinson J, Tough JS, Wyburn GM: Regeneration of sensation in grafted skin, *Br J Plast Surg* 2:82, 1949.

51. Hynes DE: Neurovascular pedicle and advancement flaps for palmar thumb defects, *Hand Clin* 13:207, 1997.

52. Illingworth CM: Trapped fingers and amputated fingertips in children, *J Pediatic Surg* 9:853, 1974.

53. Johnson RK, Iverson RE: Cross-finger pedicle flaps in the hand, *J Bone Joint Surg* 53A:913, 1971.

54. Keim HA, Grantham SA: Volar flap advancement for thumb and fingertip injuries, *Clin Orthop* 66:109, 1969.

55. Kinoshita Y, Kojima T, Matsuura S, et al: Extending the use of the palmar advancement flap with V-Y closure, *J Hand Surg* 22B: 212, 1997.

56. Kleinert HE: Fingertip injuries and their management, *Am Surg* 25:41, 1959.

57. Kleinert HE, McAlister CG, MacDonald CJ, et al: A critical evaluation of cross finger flaps, *J Trauma* 14;756, 1974.

58. Kutler W: A new method for fingertip amputations, *JAMA* 133:29, 1947.

59. Landi A, Morrison W, Soragni: The wrap around technique. In Land A (editor): *Reconstruction of the thumb,* London, 1989, Chapman and Hall.

60. Lanzetta M, St-Laurent J-Y: Pulp neurovascular island flap for finger amputation, *J Hand Surg* 21A:918, 1996.

61. Leung PC, Ma F: Digital reconstruction using the toe flap: report of 10 cases, *J Hand Surg* 7:366, 1982.

62. Littler JW: Neurovascular pedicle transfer of tissue in reconstructive surgery of the hand, *J Bone Joint Surg* 38A:917, 1956.

63. Louis D, Palmer A, Burney R: Open treatment of digital tip injuries, *JAMA* 244:697, 1980.

64. Macht SD, Watson HK The Moberg volar advancement flap for digital reconstruction, *J Hand Surg* 5:372, 1980.

65. Mandal AC: Thiersch grafts for lesions of the fingertip, *Acta Chirg Scand* 129:325, 1965.

66. Martin C, Gonzalez del Pino J: Controversies in the treatment of fingertip amputations, *Clin Orthop* 353:63, 1998.

67. McCash CB: Free nail grafting, *Br J Plast Surg* 8:19, 1955.

68. McGregor IA, Jackson IT: The groin flap, *Br J Plast Surg* 25:3, 1972.

69. Melone C, Grad J: Primary care of fingernail injuries, *Emerg Med Clin North Am* 2:255, 1985.

70. Micks JE, Wilson JN: Full thickness of sole-skin grafts for resurfacing the hand, *J Bone Joint Surg* 49A:1128, 1967.

71. Milford L: The hand. In Crenshaw EH (editor): *Campbell's operative orthopaedics,* St. Louis, 1971, CV Mosby.

72. Millender LH, Albin RE, Nalebulf EA: Delayed volar advancement flap for thumb tip injuries, *Plast Reconstr Surg* 52:635, 1973.

73. Miller AJ: Single fingertip injuries treated by thenar flap, *Hand* 6:311, 1974.

74. Moberg E: Aspects of sensation in reconstructive surgery of the upper extremity, *J Bone Joint Surg* 46A:817, 1964.

75. Morrison WA: Thumb and fingertip reconstruction by composite microvascular tissue from the toes, *Hand Clin* 8:537, 1992.

76. Morrison WA, O'Brien BM, MacLeod AM: Thumb reconstruction with a free neurovascular wrap around flap from the toe, *J Hand Surg* 5:575, 1980.

77. Morrison WA, O'Brien BM, MacLeod AM: Experience with thumb reconstruction, *J Hand Surg* 9B:223, 1984.

78. Murai M, Lau HK, Pereira BP, Pho RW: A cadaver study on volume and surface area of the fingertip, *J Hand Surg* 22A:935-941, 1997.

79. Napier JR: The return of pain sensibility in full thickness skin grafts, *Brain* 75:147, 1952.

80. Newmeyer W, Kilgore E: Common injuries of the fingernail and nail bed, *Am Fam Physician* 6:93, 1977.

81. Nicolai JPA, Hentenaar G: Sensation in cross-finger flaps, *Hand* 13:12, 1981.

82. O'Brien B: Neurovascular island pedicle flaps for terminal amputations and digital scars, *Br J Plast Surg* 21:258, 1968.

83. Ohmori K, Harii K: Free dorsalis pedis sensory flap to the hand with microneurovascular anastomoses, *Plast Reconstr Surg* 58:546, 1976.

84. O'Malley TS: Full thickness skin grafts in finger amputations, *Wis Med J* 33:337, 1934.

85. Pakiam AI: The reversed dermis flap, *Br J Plast Surg* 31:131, 1978.

86. Palamarchuk HJ, Kerzner M: An improved approach to evacuation of subungual hematoma, *J Am Podiatr Med Assoc* 11:566, 1989.

87. Patton HS: Split-skin grafts from the hypothenar area for fingertip avulsions, *Plast Reconstr Surg* 43:426, 1969.

88. Ponten B: Grafted skin, observations on innervation and other qualities, *Acta Chir Scand* 257:1, 1960.

89. Porter RW: Functional assessment of transplanted skin in volar defects of the digits: a comparison between free grafts and flaps, *J Bone Joint Surg* 5OA:955, 1968.

90. Posner MA, Smith RJ: The advancement pedicle for thumb injuries, *J Bone Joint Surg* 53A:1618, 1971.

91. Quilliam TA, Ridley A: The receptor community in the finger tip, *J Physiol* 216:15P, 1971.

92. Reed V, Harcourt AK: Immediate full thickness grafts to finger tips, *Surg Gynecol Obstet* 68:925, 1939.

93. Ridley A: A biopsy study of the innervation of forearm skin grafted to the finger tip, *Brain* 93:547, 1970.

94. Rohrich RJ, Antrobus SD: Volar advancement flaps. In Blair WF (editor): *Techniques in hand surgery,* Baltimore, 1996, Williams and Wilkins.

95. Rosenthal LJ, Reiner MA, Bleicher MA: Nonoperative management of distal fingertip amputations in children, *Pediatrics* 64:1, 1979.

96. Russell RC, Van Beek AL, Wavak P, et al: Alternative hand flaps for amputations and digital defects, *J Hand Surg* 6:399, 1981.

97. Saito H, Suzuki Y, Fujno K, Tajima T: Free nail bed graft for treatment of nail bed injuries of the hand, *J Hand Surg* 8:171, 1983.

98. Schenck RR: Full thickness skin grafts to the hand, In Blair WF (editor): *Techniques in hand surgery,* Baltimore, 1996, Williams and Wilkins.

99. Schenck RR, Cheema TA: Hypothenar skin grafts for fingertip reconstruction, *J Hand Surg* 9A:750, 1984.

100. Seaberg DC, Angelos WJ, Paris PM: Treatment of subungual hematomas with nail trephination: a prospective study, *Am J Emerg Med* 9:209, 1991.

101. Shaw MH: Neurovascular island pedicled flaps for terminal digital scars: a hazard, *Br J Plast Surg* 24:161, 1971.

102. Shepard GH: Treatment of nail bed avulsions with split-thickness nail bed grafts, *J Hand Surg* 8:49, 1983.

103. Showalter JT: Results of replacement of fingertip tissue, *Int Surg* 50:306, 1968.

104. Siegle R, Swanson N: Nail surgery: a review, *J Dermatol Surg Oncol* 8:659, 1982.

105. Sintoni-Rugiu P: An experimental study on the reinnervation of free skin grafts and pedicle flaps, *Plast Reconstr Surg* 38:98, 1966.

106. Smith RC, Furnas DW: The hand sandwich: adjacent flaps from opposing body surfaces, *Plast Reconstr Surg* 57:351, 1976.

107. Smith Rj, Albin R: Thenar "H-flap" for fingertip injuries, *J Trauma* 16:778, 1976.

108. Snow JW: The use of a volar flap for repair of fingertip amputation: a preliminary report, *Plast Reconstr Surg* 40:163, 1967.

109. Stevenson T: Fingertip and nail bed injuries, *Orthop Clin North Am* 23:149, 1992.

110. Sturman Mj, Duran RJ: Late results of fingertip injuries, *J Bone Joint Surg* 45A:289, 1963.

111. Suzuki K, Matsuda M: Digital replantations distal to the distal interphalangeal joint, *J Reconstr Microsurg* 3:291, 1987.

112. Tranquilli-Laeli E: Ricostruzioiie dell 'apice delle falangi ungtieali mediante autoplastica volare pedui, colata per scorrimento, *Infort Traum Lavoro* 1:186, 1935.

113. Tubiana R: Fingertip injuries. In Tubiana R (editor): *The Hand,* vol 1, Philadelphia, 1981, WB Saunders.

114. Tupper J, Miller G: Sensibility following volar V-Y plasty for fingertip amputations, *J Hand Surg* 10B:183, 1985.

115. Urbaniak JR: Wrap-around procedure for thumb reconstruction, *Hand Clin* 1:259, 1985.

116. Verdan CE, Egloff DV: Fingertip injuries, *Surg Clin North Am* 61:237, 1981.

117. Walker MA, Hurley CB, May JW: Radial nerve cross-finger flap differential nerve contribution in thumb reconstruction, *J Hand Surg [Am]* 11(6):888,1986.

118. Wavak P, Zook EG: A simple method of exsanguinating the finger prior to surgery, *J Am Coll Emerg Phyicians* 7:124, 1978.

119. Webb H: New trephine for subungual hematoma, *Lancet* 2:424, 1965.

120. Wilgis EFS, Maxwell GP: Distal digital nerve grafts: clinical and anatomical studies, *J Hand Surg* 4:439, 1979.

121. Young WA, Andrassy RJ: Conservative management of fingertip amputations in children, *Tex Med* 79:58, 1983.

122. Zacher JB: Management of injuries of the distal phalanx, *Surg Clin North Am* 64:747, 1984.

123. Zook EG: Injuries of the fingernail. In Green D (editor): *Operative hand surg,* New York, 1988, Churchill Livingstone.

124. Zook EG, Guy Rj, Russell RC: A study of nail bed injuries: causes, treatment, and prognosis, *J Hand Surg* 9:247, 1984.

125. Zook EG, Miller M, Van Beek AL, et al: Successful treatment protocol for canine fang injuries, *J Trauma* 20:243, 1980.

126. Zook EG, Van Beek AL, Russell RC, et al: Anatomy and physiology of the perionychium: a review of the literature and anatomic study, *J Hand Surg* 5:528, 1980.

127. Zuker RM, Manktelow RT: The dorsalis pedis free flap: technique of elevation, foot closure, and flap application, *Plast Reconstr Surg* 77:93, 1986.

CHAPTER

Pedicled Flaps and Grafts

102

Robert L. Walton
Michael W. Neumeister

INTRODUCTION

The restoration of normal hand function and appearance after a severe injury is one of the most challenging endeavors in reconstructive surgery. Management must include obtaining a stable bony skeleton; repairing muscles, tendons, vessels, and nerves; and providing stable wound coverage. A spectrum of reconstructive efforts may be required to reach a successful conclusion, but all are contingent on the magnitude of injury. Adequate skin and soft tissue coverage of the hand is important to ensure the protection and function of the underlying structures. It also represents that portion of the repair most readily apparent to the patient. Even without deeper levels of hand injury, loss of the integument may limit mobility, impair sensibility, and compromise pinch and grasp function. Loss of normal skin elasticity impairs flexion and extension. Disruption of the tactile surface greatly impairs fine motor control and touch. Exposure of tendons, bone, or neurovascular structures may lead to desiccation, subsequent necrosis, infection, vessel thrombosis, and/or amputation.

The patient's occupation, overall health, and personal goals must be carefully weighed and discussed with the patient to arrive at the most appropriate surgical approach for each situation. Hands, in particular, are an important aspect of body image. They are highly visible in both public and private situations and may be viewed as a measure of one's strength, beauty, health, wealth, and normalcy. Minor aesthetic deformities of the hand may have pervasive consequences in both professional and private life. This chapter will focus on the restoration of skin and soft tissue defects of the hand utilizing skin grafts and local flaps.

ANATOMY

The types of skin on the volar and dorsal surfaces of the hand are markedly different.[43] The distinct functional characteristics of the missing integument must be considered when planning a reconstructive effort. The palmar glabrous skin is thicker and more adherent than the dorsal hand skin. The glabrous skin is specially adapted for pinch and grasp functions. This skin also contains special sensory receptor sites, including Pacinian and Meissner corpuscles, that are not present in nonglabrous skin.[58] These receptor sites provide extraordinary tactile sensitivity to the palm of the hand and fingertips. The palmar skin surface contains numerous papillary ridges, or fingerprints, which create a pattern unique to each individual finger. Palmar skin is also populated with eccrine sweat glands, which, together with the papillary ridges, improve the friction coefficient of palmar skin, facilitating prehensile grip. The palmar skin is anchored to the underlying palmar fascia and digital tendon sheaths by numerous fibrous septa that serve to stabilize the skin against shear forces during prehension and, again, improve the friction coefficient. The palmar skin is well padded with compartments of subcutaneous fat between the fibrous septa.

The palmar skin is extremely vascular. It is supplied by multiple capillaries arising from the superficial palmar arches and the common and proper digital arteries. The dorsum of the hand receives its blood supply from the dorsal and palmar vascular arcades. The dorsal branch of the radial artery passes through the anatomic snuff box and then bifurcates. The more radial branch travels between the first and second metacarpals to form part of the deep palmar arch. The ulnar branch forms the dorsal radiocarpal arch, which gives rise to the first, second, third, and fourth dorsal metacarpal arteries. The dorsal metacarpal arteries usually course between the extensor tendons within the fascia over the dorsal interosseous muscles and are accompanied by venae comitantes. Branches from these arteries supply the overlying dorsal skin and subcutaneous tissue. Communicating palmar perforating vessels emerge from between the metacarpal necks to anastomose with the dorsal metacarpal arteries. Branches from the volar digital vessels supply the dorsum of the fingers.

The skin on the dorsum of the hand is nonglabrous, thin, and very mobile to accommodate the flexion and extension arcs of the wrist and digits. Because it is structured for mobility and not stability, the dorsal subcutaneous tissue does not contain the same fibrous septa found on the palmar surface and is therefore more susceptible to avulsion or traction injuries. Small wounds of the volar surface may be allowed to heal by secondary intention with very little adverse consequences or loss of digital range of motion. Dorsal wounds treated in a similar fashion may cause functional impairment because of failure of the dorsal skin envelope to accommodate the tension imposed on it by joint flexion.

TREATMENT OPTIONS AND INFORMED CONSENT

Treatment options for the resurfacing of hand injuries with loss of soft tissue include nonoperative wound care; primary closure; skin grafts; local, regional, or distant pedicle flaps; or free flaps.

Direct approximation of the skin edges should be attempted whenever possible. Larger wounds require skin grafts or tissue flaps. Skin grafts survive initially by plasma imbibition, inosculation, and vascular in-growth from the recipient bed, which occurs within 2 to 5 days after surgery. Use of skin grafts is therefore restricted to wounds with an excellent blood supply. Hand wounds with exposed tendons or bones cannot be closed with a skin graft. Skin flaps provide their own blood supply and offer a more stable, protective covering. Flaps can also be used with more extensive injuries to re-establish proper contour. However, flaps are often limited in size or in their ability to be advanced, transposed, or rotated into a defect. Both flaps and grafts necessitate a donor site, which can create a noticeable deformity.[74] This must be clearly explained to the patient before surgery.

Informed consent is vital to the successful use of skin grafts and flaps in the hand. The size and location of the donor wounds and any anticipated functional losses should be explained to the patient before surgery. The patient should also be told that debridement of the wound may cause enlargement of the existing defect. The surgeon should discuss both surgical and nonsurgical treatment options based on the size of the deformity and the patient's hand dominance, occupation, age, expectations, and desires. Patient education allows a better understanding of the issues that must be considered for surgical reconstruction and subsequently offers realistic expectation of the outcome and, ultimately, a greater overall patient satisfaction.

NONOPERATIVE TREATMENT OF WOUNDS

Occasionally wounds are allowed to heal by secondary intention.[1,5,7,29] This may take 6 to 12 weeks to obtain definitive closure. Meticulous dressing changes are required on these areas that are often painful. The normal process of wound contraction should be anticipated in any wound left open for more than 4 to 5 days. This can lead to undesirable and potentially unstable scars.[6,20,51,58,59] Once this process has begun, it is not altered significantly by subsequent wound closure because of the enhanced local proinflammatory milieu.[20] Accordingly, designing a treatment plan to incorporate secondary healing along with subsequent surgical revision will not only delay recovery but may lead to a suboptimal result because of contraction and scarring. The decision to allow a wound to heal by secondary intention therefore should be based on variables such as ultimate function and scarring, time and cost constraints, work status, and the need for revision surgeries.

Significant advancements have been made over the last century in soft tissue coverage of the hand. Wolf (full thickness) and Thiersch (split thickness) skin grafts were popularized in the late 1800s. World War I saw the development of distant tube pedicle flaps for soft tissue coverage. The majority of local hand flaps, such as volar and neurovascular island flaps, were described in the 1950s.* The unique soft tissues in the hand offer the best tissue for reconstruction but the amount available is often limited. Large or complex injuries can now be closed using free tissue transfers by microsurgical technique, but these flaps usually lack the special characteristics of normal hand skin and soft tissue. Healthy composite tissue can be microsurgically transferred from areas remote from the zone of injury. Salvageable components of an extensive hand wound, such as skin, nerves, nail bed, tendons, and/or bones may be employed as spare parts in treatment of traumatic injuries.

OPERATIONS

SKIN GRAFTS

Skin grafts are tangentially harvested portions of the integument that include all of the epidermis and either all or part of the dermis.[9,62] Skin-graft closure of wounds on the hand can often provide the simplest and best means for wound closure (Figure 102-1). Skin grafts conform nicely to irregular surfaces, have a relatively unlimited donor-site availability, and provide minimal bulk (Figure 102-2). They do not, however, provide vascular, stable coverage of exposed vital structures such as bone or tendon. The skin graft viability ultimately depends on the quality of the recipient bed and proper immobilization. Common causes of graft failure include inadequate debridement of devitalized tissue of the recipient bed, hematoma, shear forces, and infection. Debridement and closure of the wound before the fifth postinjury day diminishes the incidence of wound contraction.[20] The longer the delay before wound closure, the greater the secondary contraction.

It is essential that traumatic wounds undergo meticulous debridement of all devitalized tissue. Hemostasis must be secured, and the wound should be copiously irrigated. Heavily

---

*References 3, 4, 8, 10, 17, 24, 37, 41, 46, 57, 65, 66.

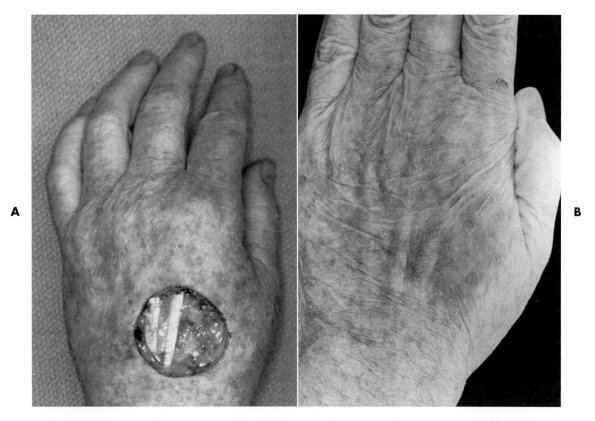

Figure 102-1. **A,** A 3 × 3 cm defect is created on the dorsum of the hand after excision of a squamous cell carcinoma. The paratenon is preserved. **B,** The late result of the skin-grafted site.

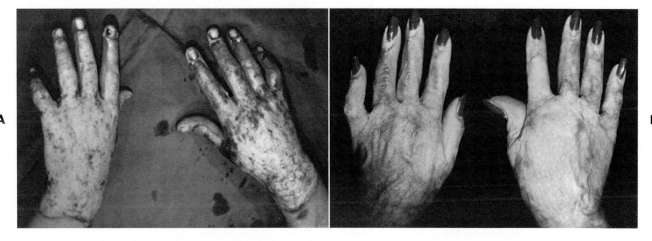

Figure 102-2. **A,** Burns to the dorsum of the hand necessitated debridement. **B,** Sheet grafts were applied with good late results.

contaminated wounds may require a "second look" procedure in which the affected area is dressed with a saline or temporary biologic dressing (such as xenograft or homograft) for 24 hours, followed by another surgical debridement. This attempts to ensure an appropriate vascular recipient bed devoid of contaminants and debris. A well-applied split-thickness or full-thickness skin graft may fail if equal attention is not paid to placement of the dressing. The skin graft is sutured in place over the defect. A nonadherent dressing layer, such as a Xeroform or Adaptic, covers the skin graft, and a tie-over

bolster dressing of cotton or polyurethane foam is used to optimize immobilization and promote adherence and subsequent vascularization. A bulky hand dressing and splint are required to prevent further mobility of the hand. The dressings are left in place for 5 to 7 days, unless drainage or odor dictates earlier examination. Meshing or pie-crusting of grafts may allow expansion of the graft and a greater ability for it to contour but do not provide an adequate conduit for egress of seroma or hematoma because these small interstices fill with fibrin and are sealed within a short time after application.

Additionally, the interstices heal by secondary intention, with resultant contracture and a poor aesthetic result. Therefore meshed skin grafts are rarely employed in the hand.

There is ongoing debate over the optimal type of skin graft for wound coverage in the hand. Split-thickness skin grafts may offer a better take but they are inferior to full-thickness grafts in their stability and pliability because of the lack of the full complement of dermis in split grafts.[12,16] We favor full-thickness grafts when possible because they are thicker, more pliable, and provide a more aesthetic outcome. Additionally, the specialized sense organs present in the glabrous skin of full-thickness grafts may provide a better recovery of sensibility.[23]

Split-Thickness Skin Grafts

A split-thickness skin graft is more likely to "take" than a full-thickness skin graft. There is also greater donor-site availability with split-thickness grafts. The thinner the graft the more secondary wound contraction occurs.[64] This contraction may be desirable on areas such as the fingertip and back of the hand.

Skin thickness and quality vary with the patient's sex, age, and body location. The epidermis in infancy is very thin, becoming thicker in puberty and subsequently thinning markedly to infantile levels during older age. The dermis demonstrates a similar pattern and is markedly thicker in males. Skin thickness may therefore vary markedly (0.020 to 0.10 inches), but generally speaking most grafts have a maximum thickness of 0.040 (female) to 0.060 (male) inches. Split-thickness skin grafts are typically harvested at thin levels from 8 to 14 thousandths of an inch or thick levels from 16 to 20 thousandths of an inch. We try to keep split-thickness grafts under 0.010 inches in infants and the elderly. Grafting from thicker areas such as the thigh, buttocks, or trunk diminishes the risk for full-thickness injury and facilitates rapid re-epithelialization. All split-thickness donor sites are prone to pigmentation change and hypertrophic scarring, with the severity depending on the age of the patient, the location of the donor site, and secondary healing problems such as infection.

Split-thickness grafts may be harvested free hand with a gentle gliding action of the knife blade tangential to the skin surface. This method requires a certain degree of technical precision. A Weck or Goulian blade with preset depth gauges is a more predictable method to harvest free hand. A number of commercial dermatomes are available to harvest skin of preset width and depth (Figure 102-3). The harvesting of skin from donor sites is facilitated by the application of a lubricating substance such as mineral oil. Uniform traction on the skin and pressure on the dermatome helps avoid "skip areas" or grafts of irregular thicknesses. Infiltration of large volumes of saline or epinephrine solution tumesces the donor site and may aid in harvesting the graft in thin patients or from donor-site locations that have an uneven contour. The tumescent technique has an added benefit of minimizing blood loss. Substantial blood loss from donor sites can be minimized by applying an epinephrine and peroxide–soaked gauze pad to the donor site.

Split-thickness graft donor sites heal by re-epithelialization. Epithelial cells migrate from the skin appendages, hair follicles, sweat glands, and sebaceous glands. The greater the concentration of skin appendages, the faster the re-epithelization. The donor site may be dressed with a sterile, semipermeable, biooclusive dressing such as Op-Site or Tegaderm. Application of this dressing is relatively pain free but the dressing may accumulate serosanguinous fluid under it. A small suction drain made from a 19-gauge butterfly catheter attached to a red-top blood vial outside the Op-Site dressing may allow evacuation of the drainage. Open gauze dressings, such as Xeroform, Adaptic, or scarlet red, that dry to form an artificial scab result in more painful donor-site treatment and are prone to early infection and subsequent conversion to a deeper dermal injury. There may also be delayed healing. This method, however, may be preferable in large donor areas in which the use of occlusive dressings is impractical.

Full-Thickness Skin Grafts

Full-thickness skin grafts offer specialized sensory organs for reinnervation, improved color and texture, and less secondary contraction, and are an optimal alternative to split-thickness

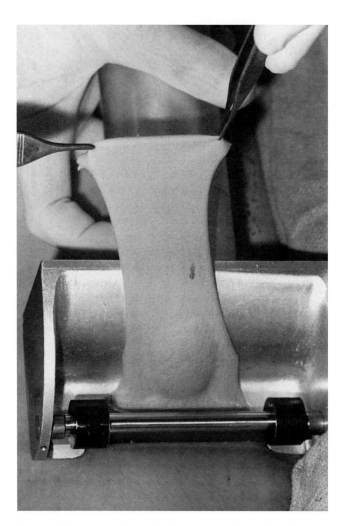

Figure 102-3. A skin graft is harvested with the aid of a Paget dermatome.

grafts for coverage of defects on the digits or hands.[23,38,39,72] Small volar defects, such as fingertip injuries, are easily closed with full-thickness skin grafts from the hypothenar or thenar eminence, which are ideal donor sites because they contribute glabrous skin. This type of skin is often superior to skin from distant donor sites. Larger donor sites of full-thickness skin grafts are limited. Glabrous plantar skin from the instep of the foot has an enormous density of specialized sensory organs and can provide a generous source of full-thickness skin for palmar or volar digital resurfacing. However, this donor site itself may need to be skin grafted if segments wider than 2 to 3 cm are harvested.

Alternative full-thickness donor sites for resurfacing dorsal or other large hand defects include the wrist, inguinal region, medial arm, or forearm. The volar wrist crease provides good quality skin with excellent color match. The resemblance of this donor site scar to the wrist lacerations associated with suicide attempts makes this donor site less desirable. The lateral inguinal region provides an inconspicuous donor site to obtain a large area of good-quality, hairless skin. The poor color match of the groin skin to that of the hand makes this site less optimal. We do not shave the groin before skin graft harvest so that the more hirsute areas can be excluded from the harvest. A full-thickness graft exhibits significant primary contraction immediately after the harvest because of its dermal elasticity. A template of the defect should be fashioned using a glove paper or a foil suture package to ensure the graft is of appropriate size and configuration. This maneuver economizes graft harvest and facilitates closure of the donor site. Full-thickness grafts must be trimmed of all fat and subcutaneous tissue. The rich dermal vascular bed of the graft is more easily revascularized than is the poorly vascularized subcutaneous tissue and fat. Meticulous immobilization of the recipient bed facilitates vascularization and take of the graft.

FLAPS

Flaps are vascular composites of skin, fat, fascia, muscle, or bone that obtain their blood supply from a single vascular pedicle in an axial pattern or through the base of the flap in a random fashion. The size and configuration of a particular flap is both defined and limited by the vascular anatomy. Failure to appreciate the anatomic vascular configuration of each flap territory can lead to an unreliable design and result in partial or complete flap necrosis.[30,34,57] The size of a given flap may be extended by performing surgical delays. This strategy, however, necessitates an extra operation and an additional 7- to 10-day period before wound closure, and may result in prolonged edema and loss of pliability, complicating the mechanics of the flap transfer.

The flap can provide immediate and reliable wound-coverage protection of vital structures and can facilitate the gliding of tendons and nerves. Many flap donor sites in the hand and wrist can be closed primarily, but some may require skin grafting or secondary flap coverage, which must be discussed with the patient. Additionally, a flap may be

undesirably bulky or have a poor color or texture match compared with the surrounding skin on the hand.[70] This may require secondary debulking or revision surgery. Flaps may be transferred from adjacent tissues or moved from remote sites by microsurgical technique and are defined not only by their vascular anatomy but by the type and direction of movement employed to position the flap into a given defect. Alternatively, flaps may be described in terms of their overall composition of varying tissue types. Box 102-1 illustrates the various means of classifying flaps.

Local Flaps
The term *local flap,* by definition, indicates that the flap is being elevated from tissue immediately adjacent to the wound to be covered.

Advancement Flaps
Advancement flaps also achieve wound closure by elevation and movement of the skin and subcutaneous tissue adjacent to the defect into the defect itself. The advancement is achieved by utilizing the native extensibility of the skin by geometric configuration and accommodation (Figure 102-4). The majority of advancement flaps depend on contributions from both random and direct axial blood flow for their vascularity. The type of advancement flap and its size, location, and extent of advancement determine the size of the donor defect. Tension on the skin and subsequent vascular compromise are the usual limitations to movement of these flaps. However, the donor site for most advancement flaps can be closed primarily. There

---

Box 102-1.
Classifications of Flaps Used in Hand Surgery

COMPOSITION
Fasciocutaneous
Musculocutaneous
Osseocutaneous
Fascial
Muscle
Osseous

VASCULARITY
Random pattern
Axial pattern
Antegrade/retrograde
Island flap
Free flap

MOVEMENT
Advancement
Transposition
Rotation
Interpolation

LOCAL
Local
Regional
Distant

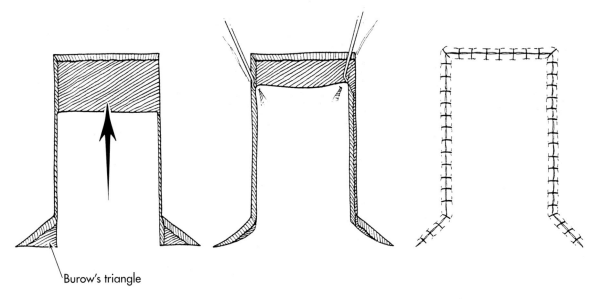

Burow's triangle

Figure 102-4. A flap can be designed to advance into a defect by exploiting the elastic properties of skin.

are various types of advancement flaps used on the dorsum of the hand, such as direct advancement or V-Y flaps.

Transposition Flaps

Transposition flaps are designed to move skin and subcutaneous tissue into an adjacent defect. The donor defect created is closed primarily with a skin graft, an advancement flap, or another transposition flap. The pivot point of the transposition flap is at its base farthest away from the defect (Figure 102-5). The rhomboid flap is a transposition flap classically designed with equal and parallel limbs oriented at 60 and 120 degrees as a parallelogram (Figure 102-6).[18,19] The flap is moved by a combination of advancement and transposition into the defect, which is also configured in a rhomboid shape. The donor site created is equal in size to the original defect. The point of closure of the donor site is the area under the greatest tension. As a result, a slight indentation (indenting cone) may be seen at this site, whereas a slight redundancy of skin may be noted at the opposite side of the flap's base, forming a dog ear (standing cone) (Figure 102-7).

The orientation of the donor site should be designed to permit easy primary donor-site closure by approximation of adjacent tissues. Various modifications of this flap have altered the standard angles of the rhomboid. The Duformontel flap is often employed for larger, more square defects (Figure 102-8). Curving the corners of the Limberg flap can be done to cover defects that are oval rather than rhomboid in sape.[55] Rhomboid flaps provide an aesthetic result because they transfer a relatively large amount of like tissue and permit primary donor-site closure. The limbs of the flap are straight and less prone to producing a late biscuit or trap-door appearance that results from centrifugal contraction in flaps

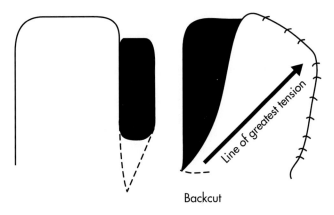

Backcut

Line of greatest tension

Figure 102-5. A transposition flap pivots on its base at the point farthest from the defect (direction of movement). Occasionally, back cuts at this point can gain distance in flap movement.

that have an oval design. Transposition flaps are commonly employed for the release of scar contractures involving the volar digits or web space. They can be easily designed on the dorsum of the hand after excision of tumors, for closure of traumatic defects, and for coverage of forearm and elbow defects (Figure 102-9).

The classic Limberg (rhomboid) flap is designed so all sides of the flap are of equal length. The surgical defect is cut into a rhomboid shape. The flap is designed from adjacent tissue beginning at the 120-degree angle of the defect (Figure 102-10). One limb is incised parallel to the defect and a second limb extends away from the 120-degree corner of the defect. This classic rhomboid flap therefore has four differ-

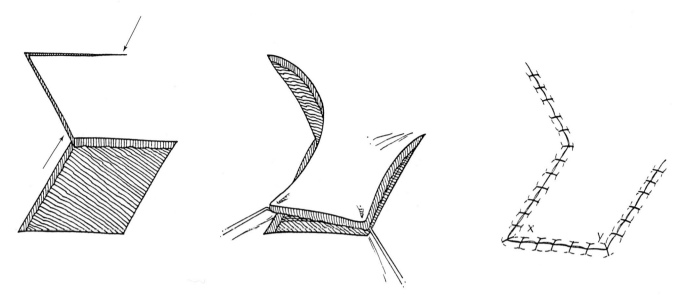

Figure 102-6. The donor site is closed by local tissue undermining as the flap is transposed into place.

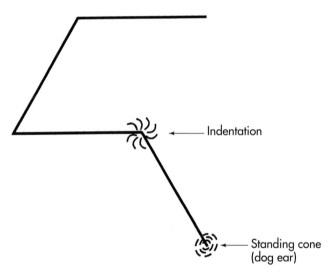

Figure 102-7. Tension at the point of donor-site closure may result in a slight indentation of the tissue. The base of the leading edge of the flap has little tension and a dog ear (standing cone) may arise.

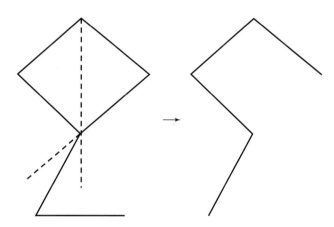

Figure 102-8. The Duformontel flap is a modification of the Limberg flap. Lines are extrapolated from the superior angle of the flap through the inferior angle. A line is also extrapolated from the leading edge of the flap. These two lines are bisected to form the second limb of the flap. The remaining limb of the flap is marked parallel to the other horizontal border of the flap.

ent flaps that can be created using this design from tissue adjacent to the defect. A further variation of the Limberg flap design uses multiple flaps based on a hexagonal defect (Figure 102-11).

A Cuono flap incorporates multiple transposition flaps for closure of diamond-shaped defects (Figure 102-12).[18,19] This flap is essentially two side-by-side Z-plasties on either side of the defect.

Z-Plasty

The Z-plasty remains widely employed as an important method in the treatment of linear scar, tissue contracture, and skin deficiencies in the hand.[63] Conceptually, a Z-plasty represents the movement of two adjacent triangular flaps into juxtaposition such that the flaps interchange their positions. The Z-plasty acts to break up and redistribute scar tissue and alters tension along a given line that is subsequently lengthened by the transposition of full-thickness skin flaps across its axis. A Z-plasty gains length at the expense of width. This technique is commonly used to release volar contractures after trauma or in patients with Dupuytren's disease. Alternatively, Z-plasties have been used to create or deepen a web space between digits. Ideally, the length of each lateral limb should be equal of that of the central

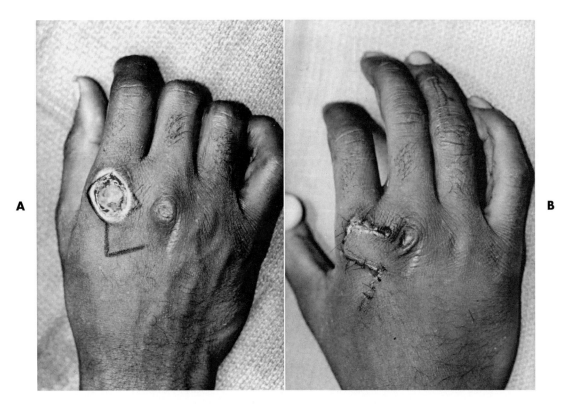

Figure 102-9. **A,** The defect on the dorsum of the hand is fashioned into a rhomboid shape. The flap extends from the obtuse angle. **B,** The flap is transposed into the defect and the donor site is closed with local undermining.

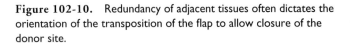

Figure 102-10. Redundancy of adjacent tissues often dictates the orientation of the transposition of the flap to allow closure of the donor site.

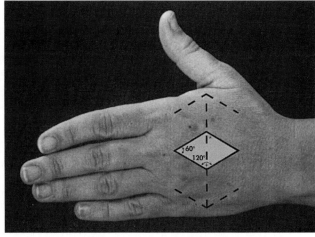

limb. The angle chosen between the central limb and the lateral limbs determines the potential gain in length obtained by transposing the flaps (Table 102-1). Unfortunately, the tissue on the hand is different from the theoretical mathematic models. Increasing the angle between the central and lateral limb results in a greater amount of tension required to transpose the flaps and can result in increased tension on wound closure, with dehiscence and possible flap necrosis. The correct orientation of the limbs of the Z-plasty should align with the lines of minimal tension (Figure 102-13). A longitudinal scar contracture on the volar surface

of a digit can be corrected by excising the central scar and planning the flaps with their bases on a digital flexion crease. Transposition of the flaps not only releases the scar contracture but orients the central limb of the scar within a natural phalangeal flexion skin crease (Figure 102-14). Several modifications of Z-plasty flaps have been designed that alter the angles, the number of flaps, or the orientation of the flaps.[63]

Appropriate flap design is clearly a balance of the reconstructive needs, the tissue available, and the ability to close the donor site. The larger the Z-plasty flap angles off the

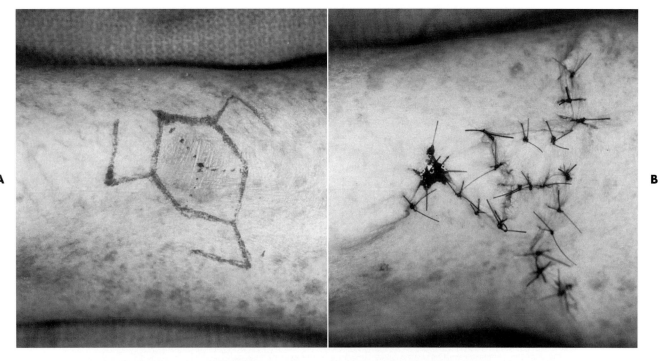

Figure 102-11. **A,** Multiple Limberg flaps can be used together to close wounds in which the local tissue has limited mobility. **B,** The defect is closed by transposing the flaps together.

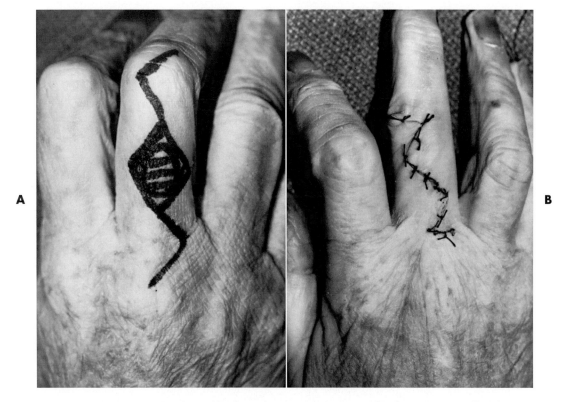

Figure 102-12. **A,** The Cuono flap is designed around a diamond-shaped defect. The Z-plasties at opposing sides of the defect allow closure in areas of limited mobility. **B,** The flaps are interdigitated to close the wound.

Table 102-1.
Z-Plasty Angles and Theoretical Gain
in Length of the Central Limb

ANGLE LATERAL LIMB (degrees)	GAIN
30	25
45	50
60	75
75	100
90	120

From Rohrich RJ, Zbar RIS: *Plast Reconstr Surg*, 103(5):1513-1517, 1999.

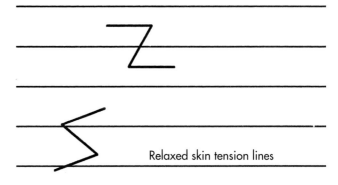

Figure 102-13. The Z-plasty should be aligned in the lines of relaxed skin tension to decrease conspicuous scars.

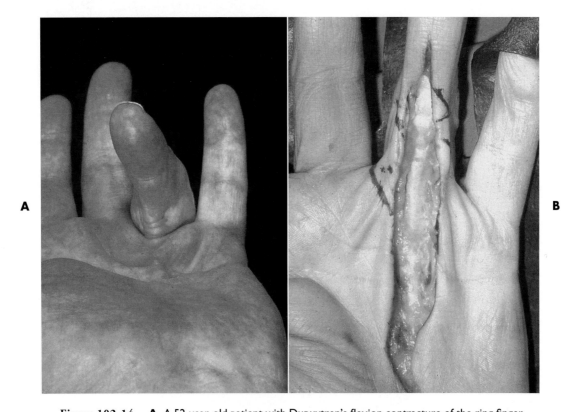

Figure 102-14. **A,** A 52-year-old patient with Dupuytren's flexion contracture of the ring finger at the MCP joint. **B,** The central scar was resected and Z-plasties were planned to release the contracted skin. *Continued*

central limb, the greater the gain in length but the more difficult it is to transpose the flaps. Smaller flaps may produce a better aesthetic result, but may inadequately release the tension or be vascularly compromised by virtue of their small size. Multiple Z-plasties in a line can be used to achieve the length gain that would occur with a single 90-degree angled Z-plasty and they do not produce excessive tension after transposition.

Alternatively, a four-flap Z-plasty designed with two 90-degree angled flaps that are each divided into two 45-degree flaps is especially useful to release and deepen an adducted first web space. The four flaps created in this design are then interdigitated (Figure 102-15). A well-designed Z-plasty dissected appropriately to its base will almost transpose itself into its new juxtaposed position. The "jumping man" flap uses the principles of opposing Z-plasties and central advancement

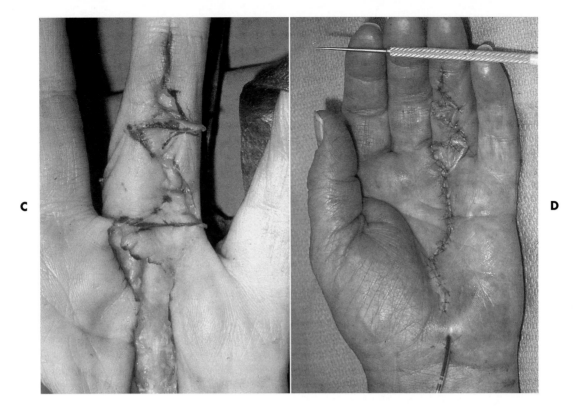

Figure 102-14, cont'd. C, The limbs of the Z-plasty flaps are of equal lengths and are designed to fall with their central limb at the MCP and PIP joint flexion creases. **D,** The Z-plasties are transposed to accomplish lengthening and natural crease alignment, allowing full extension of the digit.

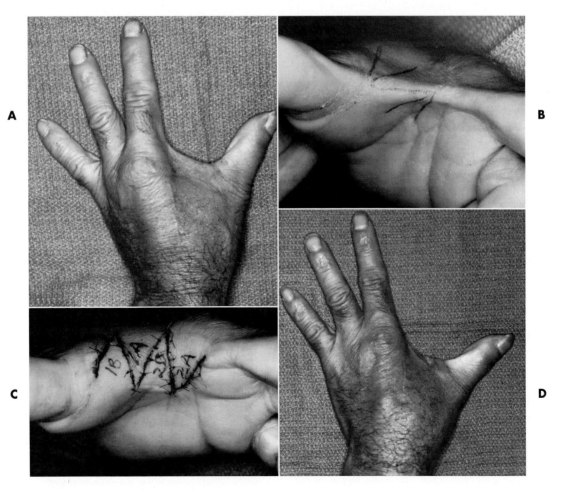

Figure 102-15. A, A first web arch-space contracture impairs the ability to grasp. **B,** A four-flap Z-plasty is designed with two 90-degree angled flaps, each subsequently divided into two 45-degree angled flaps. **C,** Transposition of the flaps deepens the web space and extends the distance between the first and second metacarpal. **D,** The late result of the four-flap Z-plasty, illustrating the preservation of the deepened first web space.

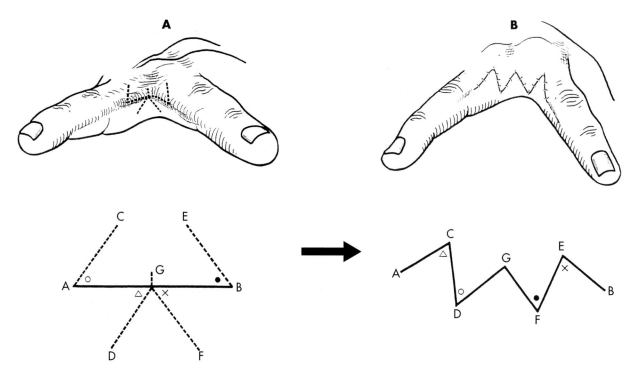

Figure 102-16. **A,** The "jumping man" flap uses opposing Z-plasties and a central advancement to elongate and deepen the web space. **B,** Transposition and advancement of the flaps breaks up the cicatricial contracture.

of one of the flaps (Figure 102-16). This design is especially useful in areas that have a natural "saddle" shape, such as the first web space.[28]

Flaps for Smaller Volar Defects

Defects on the volar surface of the fingers are often allowed to heal by secondary intention. Vital structures such as tendons, bone, or vascular bundles require vascularized tissue coverage. Local tissue from the involved finger can be designed as random or axial pattern flaps from either the dorsal lateral surface[32] or the midlateral aspect of the digit.[49] Random flaps are generally obliquely oriented and proximally based toward the dorsolateral aspect of the finger (Figure 102-17).[35,40,50,71] These flaps should have a 1.0- to 1.5-cm base and be no longer then 2 cm in length to remain viable. The digital neurovascular bundle is not incorporated within the flap. The flap is transposed and inset into the defect. The donor site is closed with a split-thickness or full-thickness skin graft. A bolster tie-over dressing is employed over the graft to promote graft take.

Axial pattern flaps in the fingers are based on the midlateral aspect of the digit to incorporate a digital artery. These flaps can extend the entire length of the finger and are usually 1 to 2 cm in width (Figure 102-18). Before flap elevation, the patency of both digital arteries on the affected finger must be tested with a digital Allen's test or Doppler signal to verify adequate two-vessel perfusion. Harvesting one digital artery with the flap when the contralateral vessel is not patent will render the distal finger ischemic. The skin, subcutaneous

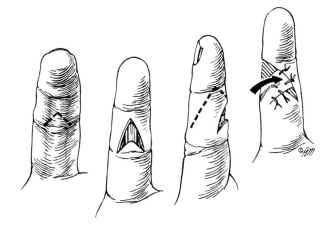

Figure 102-17. Small local flaps on the finger are usually random pattern and obliquely oriented to close volar or dorsal defects on the finger. The donor site is closed with a small skin graft or allowed to heal by secondary intention.

tissue, and digital fascia are incised to visualize the neurovascular bundle. It is often easier to isolate, ligate, and transect the digital artery at the distal end of the flap first, and then proceed with the flap elevation in a proximal direction. This ensures the vessel is incorporated within the flap. The digital nerve remains in situ by gentle dissection under loupe or microscopic visualization. Care must be taken not to disturb the branches of the digital artery that feed the overlying skin. The flap can be transposed easily into a volar or dorsal defect. Back cuts in the

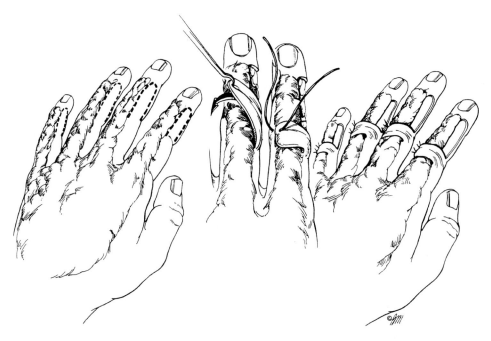

Figure 102-18. Axial pattern flaps incorporate one digital artery, are usually 1 to 2 cm in diameter, and can extend the entire length of the finger to cover volar or dorsal defects with exposed bone or tendon.

base of the flap to facilitate movement are safe as long as the axial vessel is preserved.

Axial flaps are more commonly employed with antegrade arterial inflow. Retrograde inflow can supply a distally based axial flap to cover more distal defects on a finger.[61] Such flaps also require adequate contralateral digital artery patency to foster enough backflow in the flap's axial vessel to perfuse its skin paddle. This backflow is a direct result of the arcuate anastomoses between the two digital arteries at the level of the proximal and distal interphalangeal (IP) joints.

Wider skin paddles of up to 4 cm have been harvested based on one digital vessel to cover large defects on adjacent digits (C-ring) (Figure 102-19).[31,60] Another modification to the digital axial flap involves incorporating the digital nerve to obtain a sensate flap. This, of course, is at a cost of rendering the distal finger insensate. This is generally unnecessary and should not be widely employed.

Neurovascular Island Flap

The ulnar volar aspect of the long or ring finger or the radial volar surface of the small finger may be used to resurface large volar thumb defects. First described by Littler,[46] this procedure requires that an island of skin is elevated based on a single neurovascular bundle and is dissected proximally to the common digital artery bifurcation just proximal to the web space. The proper volar digital artery to the adjoining digit is ligated. Dissection of the pedicle is continued in a proximal direction on the common digital artery to extend the flap's arc of rotation. The nerve is dissected in a similar fashion, except

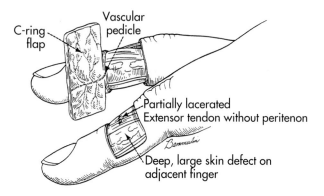

Figure 102-19. The C-ring flap involves principles of the cross-finger flap and the axial digital artery flaps. Flaps up to 4 cm in width can be mobilized on a single digital vessel. (From Atosoy E, O'Neill WL Jr: Local flap coverage about the hand. In Levin LS, Germann G: *Atlas of the hand clinics,* Philadelphia, WB Saunders.)

the digital nerve to the adjacent digit must be preserved. An intrafascicular dissection of the common digital nerve is required to gain added pedicle length. An Allen's test of both the donor and the adjacent finger is necessary before surgery to verify the patency of all the digital vessels. The ends of these fingers will have only one digital artery after the transfer. A subcutaneous tunnel is dissected across the palm to the thumb defect, and the skin island and pedicle are passed into the thumb defect. Care must be taken to avoid undue tension or twisting of the neurovascular pedicle.

Some surgeons prefer to connect the palmar donor-site incision to the thumb defect with a second zig-zag incision to transfer the flap pedicle under direct vision. The donor site on the finger requires a skin graft for closure. The ulnar border of the long finger, which has a long neurovascular bundle, is not required for pinch. It is therefore the preferred site for the neurovascular island harvest. The ring-finger donor site, innervated by the ulnar nerve, is preferred to resurface index or thumb defects in patients with a median nerve injury (Figure 102-20). A major criticism of the neurovascular island flap is the palmar scarring and the neurovascular deficit created in the donor finger. Another major disadvantage of this neurovascular island flap is the inability in adults to retrain the cerebral cortex to localize different sensory stimuli from the thumb. The cerebral cortex in children is more plastic and with time they can often retrain their brain to interpret flap stimulation as thumb sensation. Modifications of the Littler neurovascular island flap have included the distal phalanx, nail bed, or larger amounts of the distal soft tissue. This unique adaptation utilizes the "spare parts" concept in trauma patients with injury to several digits in which the proximal donor finger is not salvageable but the distal tissue is viable on its neurovascular bundle (Figure 102-21). All or part of the viable distal tissue can be transferred on a neurovascular pedicle to reconstruct distal defects of adjoining digits or the thumb.

First Dorsal Metacarpal Artery Flap

The first dorsal metacarpal artery flap is an axial flap that includes the skin and subcutaneous tissue over the dorsal proximal index finger. The dominant branch of the radial

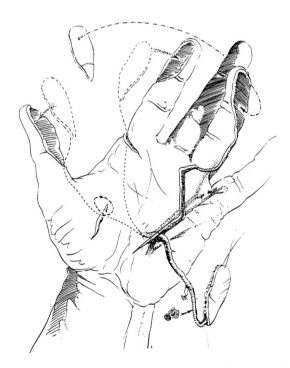

Figure 102-20. The Littler neurovascular island flap is based on a digital nerve and artery from the ulnar ring or long finger. The pedicle is dissected back into the palm to gain adequate length to reach the thumb. (From Littler W: Principles of reconstructive surgery of the hand. In Converse JM [editor]: *Reconstructive plastic surgery,* vol 4, Philadelphia, 1967, WB Saunders.)

artery at the wrist travels in the base of the anatomic snuff box before giving off terminal branches to the dorsal carpal arch and the first dorsal metacarpal artery. The first dorsal metacarpal artery courses within the fascia and occasionally within the belly of the first dorsal interosseous muscle adjacent to the second metacarpal bone.[14,21] There is an anastomotic communication within the first web space with the palmar vessels. Superficial veins course in a more superficial plane above the dorsal metacarpal artery. Venae comitantes, however, are present in close continuity with the artery. Multiple branches from these vessels supply the overlying fascia, subcutaneous tissue, and skin.

The first dorsal metacarpal artery flap can be raised as an antegrade, proximally based, fasciocutaneous flap (Figure 102-22).[22,25,26] Alternatively, it can also be raised as a reverse flow, distally based, fasciocutaneous or fascial flap. Unique variations of this flap have been performed, utilizing it as a flow-through flap and as a free tissue transfer.

Similar flaps based on the second and third dorsal metacarpal arteries can be elevated. The third metacarpal artery has a small caliber, and the reliability of the skin paddle may be questionable. The vessels in these flaps can be dissected back to the level of the distal carpus, where the arteries arise from the dorsal carpal arch. These flaps can be transposed to cover exposed tendons or bone over the metacarpophalangeal (MCP) joint on adjacent fingers.

Retrograde dorsal metacarpal artery flaps are based on the communicating web-space perforators that penetrate from the palmar arches through to the dorsal surface of the hand at the level of the metacarpal necks.[52] These palmar perforators anastomose with the dorsal metacarpal arteries located above the fascia of the dorsal interosseous muscle between each of the metacarpals. The skin paddles of the retrograde dorsal metacarpal artery flaps are centered between the bases of the metacarpals on the dorsum of the hand (Figure 102-23, *A*). The skin paddle that can measure 2 to 3 cm in diameter becomes unreliable proximal to the wrist. The proximal edge of the flap is dissected down to the fascia of the interosseous muscle. The dorsal metacarpal artery is ligated proximally and the flap is elevated in a retrograde fashion. The pedicle can be dissected back to the level of the metacarpal necks where the palmar communicating perforators emerge from the volar surface between the metacarpals (Figure 102-23, *B*). The pedicle should be dissected with a safe cuff of investing fascia to ensure patency. The flap can then be inset by direct transposition or tunneling under an intact skin bridge (Figure 102-23, *C*). The arc of rotation allows this flap to be used to cover defects up to the level of the proximal interphalangeal (PIP) joint. The donor site can usually be closed primarily. Larger donor defects may require a skin graft for definitive closure. Therefore it is important not to disrupt the paratenon over the extensor tendons during the dissection.

Reverse Radial Forearm Flap

The radial artery arises in the proximal forearm as one of the terminal branches of the brachial artery. The radial artery travels in a plane above the flexor digitorum superficialis (FDS)

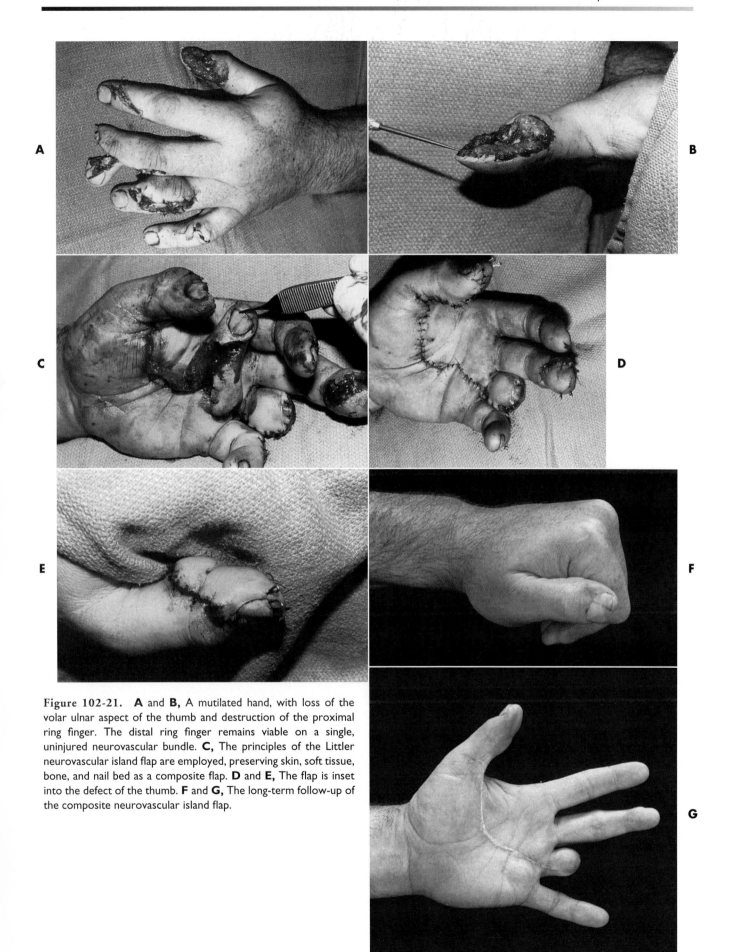

Figure 102-21. A and **B,** A mutilated hand, with loss of the volar ulnar aspect of the thumb and destruction of the proximal ring finger. The distal ring finger remains viable on a single, uninjured neurovascular bundle. **C,** The principles of the Littler neurovascular island flap are employed, preserving skin, soft tissue, bone, and nail bed as a composite flap. **D** and **E,** The flap is inset into the defect of the thumb. **F** and **G,** The long-term follow-up of the composite neurovascular island flap.

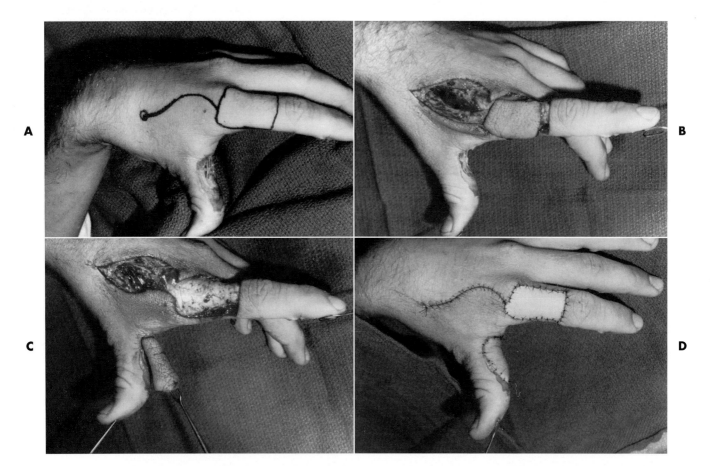

Figure 102-22. **A,** The first dorsal metacarpal artery flap is designed with the skin paddle over the dorsal proximal phalanx of the index finger. **B,** The skin paddle is elevated at a level above the paratenon. The pedicle lies within the fascia of the first dorsal interosseous muscle. The fascia must be harvested with the pedicle to ensure viability. **C,** The flap is tunneled under a skin bridge to the defect on the thumb. **D,** The donor site is closed with a skin graft.

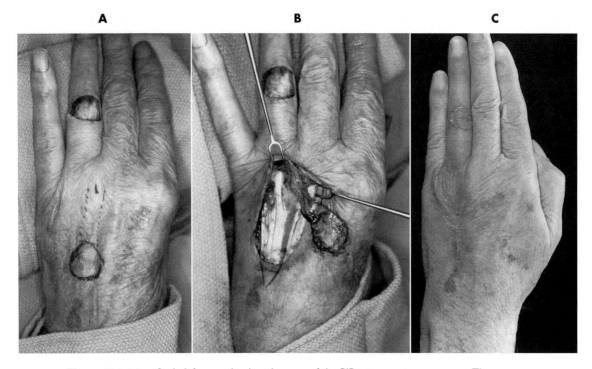

Figure 102-23. **A,** A defect on the dorsal aspect of the PIP joint requires coverage. The reverse dorsal metacarpal artery flap is designed with a skin paddle just distal to the wrist and centered between the metacarpal bases. **B,** The flap is based on the communicating perforators from the palmar arch to the dorsal arterial system. **C,** The flap is tunneled under a skin bridge and inset. Coverage is stable with preserved range of motion.

muscle and is sandwiched between the flexor carpi radialis (FCR) and brachioradialis muscles, becoming more superficial in the distal third of the forearm. The radial artery bifurcates just proximal to the wrist. The larger branch courses dorsoradially under the abductor pollicis longus (APL) and extensor pollicis brevis (EPB) tendons through the base of the anatomic snuff box, exiting under the extensor pollicis longus (EPL) tendon. This branch itself bifurcates to supply the dorsal arch and dorsal metacarpal arteries. The large branch pierces the first web space between the heads of the adductor pollicis (AP) muscle to communicate with the ulnar artery through the deep palmar vascular arch. The second terminal branch of the radial artery continues volarly through the base of the thenar muscles to communicate with the superficial palmar vascular arch. Perforating vessels that arise from the main radial artery in the forearm travel in a fascial mesentery between the FCR and brachioradialis muscles to supply the forearm fascia, subcutaneous tissue, and skin.[68] There are a greater number of perforators in the proximal and distal forearm, leaving the middle forearm relatively devoid of perforators. The entire forearm skin can survive on the perforators that arise from the radial artery. The venous drainage of this skin is derived from both the superficial system (cephalic and basilic veins) and the deep system (venae comitantes). Adequate drainage can be accomplished by either system. A radial forearm flap elevated on the distal radial artery must drain the flap in a retrograde fashion. Venous congestion is not usually a problem. This lack of venous congestion, in most cases, has been explained by the presence of multiple communications between the two venae comitantes,[45] vein denervation,[68] increased venous pressures that promote valve incompetence,[69] and venous filling by the capillary communications from the radial artery.[73] Performing an anastomosis from a vein at the proximal edge of the flap to a recipient vein in the hand to allow antegrade venous return may alleviate fears of congestion if the concern arises.

FLAP PLANNING AND ELEVATION

The blood supply of the reverse radial forearm flap relies on flow from the ulnar artery through an intact palmar arch to the radial artery. Survival has been reported on corollary communications with the ulnar artery in the absence of an intact palmar arch.[75] The flap can be harvested as a fasciocutaneous or fascial flap.

The vascularity of the hand is tested with the Allen's test[2] to assess the patency and integrity of the radial and ulnar arteries and the palmar vascular arches. The flap is designed on the volar proximal forearm centered over the radial artery. A larger caliber superficial vein, often the cephalic, is incorporated within the flap to anastomose in the hand if venous congestion is a problem. The skin is incised around the flap and the dissection is carried deep through the antebrachial fascia. The flap is then elevated from its lateral and medial edge to the brachioradialis and FCR muscles, respectively. Each muscle is retracted to expose the radial artery, its venae comitantes, and the perforating branches that course within the investing fascia around the vessels. Care must be taken not

to injure the radial artery or its fascial septum containing the perforators because they supply the fascia and skin of the flap.

A curvilinear incision is made from the distal end of the flap to a pivot point approximately 2 to 3 cm proximal to the wrist. The subcutaneous tissue is dissected through the antebrachial fascia to isolate the radial artery and venae comitantes in continuity with the proximal skin paddle. Ligaclips are used to ligate deep branches from the radial artery. The flap is elevated from proximal to distal after proximally ligating and dividing the radial artery, venae comitantes, and the superficial veins. The flap is then transposed distally and inset into the hand defect (Figure 102-24). Composite flaps including tendons (FCR and palmaris longus [PL]) and bone have been described (Figure 102-25).[27,76] Fascia alone can be harvested, with the advantage of maintaining the overlying skin on the forearm. A distally based fasciocutaneous flap can occasionally be based solely on perforators at the wrist level. This flap can be elevated to close smaller hand defects and to preserve the radial artery in the forearm.[75] The large arc of rotation is more difficult to achieve without compromising the blood supply to the flap.

The forearm donor site can be closed primarily if the flap dimensions are less than 5 to 6 cm in width.[67] A split-thickness skin graft, however, is usually required to close the donor site.

The Posterior Interosseous Forearm Flap

ANATOMY. The posterior interosseous artery arises from the common interosseous artery or the ulnar artery just distal to the antecubital fossa.[11] It pierces the interosseous membrane under the supinator muscle and courses on the APL muscle in close proximity to the posterior interosseous nerve. At the distal end of the supinator, the posterior interosseous artery divides into descending and ascending recurrent branches. The ascending branch courses in a retrograde fashion to anastomose with the posterior radial collateral artery just distal to the elbow. The descending branch of the posterior interosseous artery travels on the dorsal surface of the forearm over the AP muscle within the intermuscular septum between the extensor carpi ulnaris (ECU) and the extensor digiti quinti (EDQ) muscles.[53,54] The posterior interosseous artery terminates at the wrist, where it anastomoses with the dorsal arterial arch of the carpus and perforating anterior interosseous artery. Multiple septocutaneous perforators (7 to 14) arise from the posterior interosseous artery to service the dorsal forearm skin.[42] The largest and most constant perforator arises just distal to the supinator muscle.

OPERATIONS. The surface marking for the course of the posterior interosseous artery corresponds to a line drawn from the lateral epicondyle to the distal radioulnar joint (DRUJ). A Doppler is used to mark skin perforators along this line. The large proximal perforator, which should be included in the skin paddle, is usually located just distal to the juncture of the proximal one third and distal two thirds of the axis of the posterior interosseous artery. This may vary from 5 to 11 cm from the radial humoral condyle. This skin island can be 6 to 8 cm in width and should be centered over the posterior interosseous artery (Figure 102-26, *A*). The radial side of the flap is incised through the skin, subcutaneous

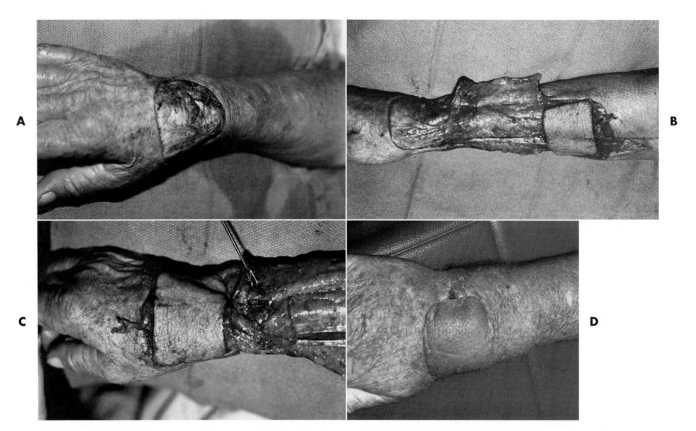

Figure 102-24. **A,** The defect on the dorsum of the wrist has exposed tendons. **B,** A reverse radial forearm flap is based on the retrograde flow from the radial artery supplied by the ulnar artery through an intact palm vascular arch. **C,** The flap is transposed into the defect. The donor site often requires skin grafting for closure. **D,** The late result of the transposed reverse radial artery forearm flap.

tissue, and dorsal antebrachial fascia. A curvilinear incision is extended distally from the skin island to the wrist. The anastomosis between the posterior interosseous artery and the communicating perforators of the anterior interosseous artery should be visualized at this level. The extensor digitorum communis (EDC) and the EDQ are retracted radially, exposing the supinator muscle. The posterior interosseous artery can be seen emerging from the distal edge of the supinator with the posterior interosseous nerve adjacent to the APL muscle. The perforating vessels to the skin can be seen in the septum investing the pedicle. The proximal posterior interosseous artery is isolated from the posterior interosseous nerve and divided.

The ulnar side of the flap is now dissected down through the antebrachial fascia. The flap is elevated in a proximal to distal direction. The ECU is retracted ulnarly and the EDC, EDQ, and the extensor indices proprius (EIP) are retracted radially. The flap is mobilized into the defect and then inset (Figure 102-26, *B*). The donor site can be closed primarily if the defect is less than 5 cm in width. Larger defects require closure with a split-thickness skin graft. The posterior interosseous flap has been elevated as an osteocutaneous flap, incorporating a small segment of proximal ulna.[15] The blood supply to this segment of bone, however, is variable and unreliable.

Reverse Ulnar Artery Flap

ANATOMY. The ulnar artery flap is analogous to the radial forearm flap. The ulnar-volar aspect of the forearm provides thinner, less hirsute skin in comparison to its radial artery counterpart. Although many surgeons hesitate to sacrifice the hand's presumed dominant blood supply, it has nonetheless been demonstrated that this flap can be safely harvested.[33,36,44,47,48] The ulnar vascular pedicle lies within a fascial septum between the flexor carpi ulnaris (FCU) and FDS muscles distal to the take off of the common interosseous branch. The flap is rendered sensate by inclusion of the medial antebrachial cutaneous nerve, which can be anastomosed to a recipient nerve. The reverse ulnar artery flap was originally described as a fasciocutaneous flap but may also incorporate the FCU muscle and the PL tendon. The reverse ulnar artery flap has a superficial and deep venous drainage. The basilic vein is the major superficial drainage of the medial forearm, and the two venae comitantes provide the deep drainage.

OPERATIONS. Much of the forearm skin can be elevated on the distally based ulnar artery. The skin island is designed proximal enough to follow a gentle arc of rotation into the defect on the hand. The borders of the flap are incised down through the antebrachial fascia. The medial and lateral edges

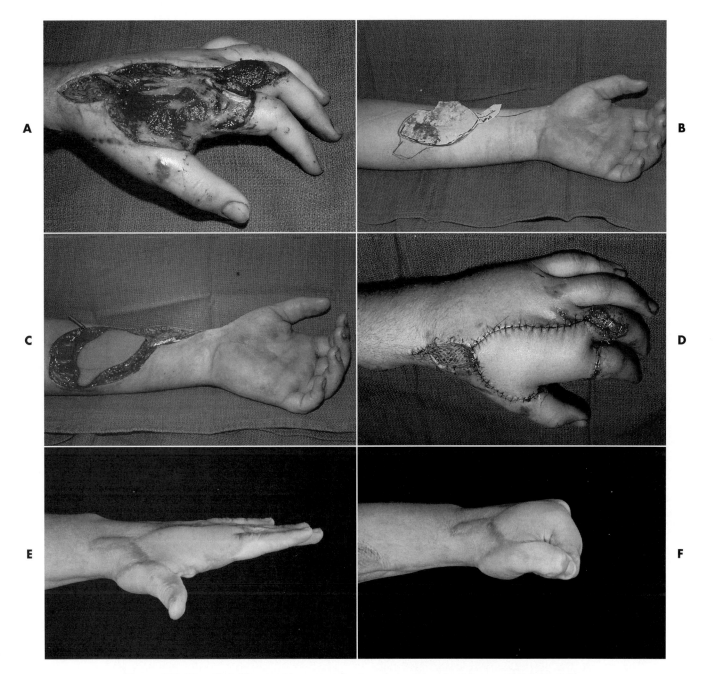

Figure 102-25.   **A,** A 23-year-old man sustained a soft tissue avulsion injury to the left hand. The metacarpals were exposed and the extensor tendon to the index finger had a segmental defect. **B,** A template of the defect was placed on the volar forearm over the radial artery. **C,** The reverse radial forearm flap was elevated, including the palmaris longus tendon. **D,** The flap was transposed into the defect on the dorsum of the hand. The extensor tendon was reconstructed with the vascularized palmaris longus tendon included within the flap. **E** and **F,** The 2-year follow-up visit illustrates stable soft tissue coverage and excellent range of digital motion.

of the flap are elevated to the septum between the FCU and the FDS. The perforators to the overlying skin can be seen in the septum. The proximal ulnar artery, its venae comitantes, and the superficial veins are isolated and ligated and the flap is elevated in a proximal to distal direction. A Ligaclip is used to ligate deep branches from the ulnar artery. Venous congestion may occasionally be noticed with this reverse flap, as it is with the reverse radial forearm flap. Anastomosis of the superficial vein with a recipient vein on

the hand should alleviate this congestion. The ulnar artery flap donor site is believed to be aesthetically more favorable than the radial artery flap deformity and may be closed primarily or with a skin graft, depending on the size of the defect.

Distant Flaps

Local or regional tissue occasionally is not suitable for coverage of open wounds of the hand. The use of pedicle flaps

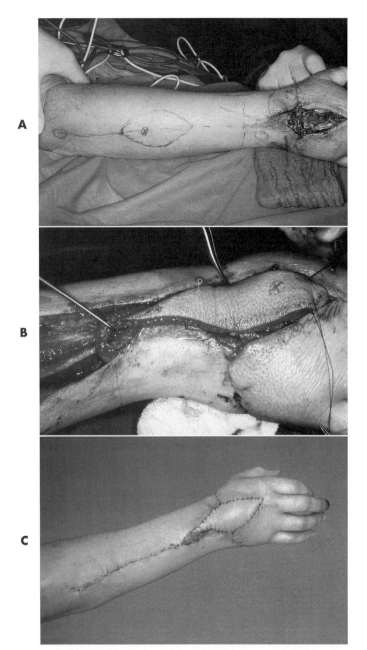

Figure 102-26. **A,** A 26-year-old patient sustained a soft tissue injury to the dorsum of his left hand. Extensor tendons were exposed. The reverse posterior interosseous artery flap was designed to cover the defect. The artery travels in a line drawn from the lateral epicondyle to the distal radioulnar joint. **B,** The perforator vessels are visualized at the distal wrist as the posterior interosseous artery is elevated within the intermuscular system. **C,** The flap is inset and the donor site is closed primarily. (Courtesy Gunter Germann, PhD.)

from the trunk or opposite extremity has been tempered by the advent of free tissue transfers. There are, however, occasional indications that call for a thoracoepigastric, anterior abdominal, groin, or contralateral extremity flap. These flaps offer the advantages of an easy dissection, decreased operative time, and good reliability. The disadvantages that often supersede the advantages include maintaining the hand in a constant, immobile position for 2 to 3 weeks.

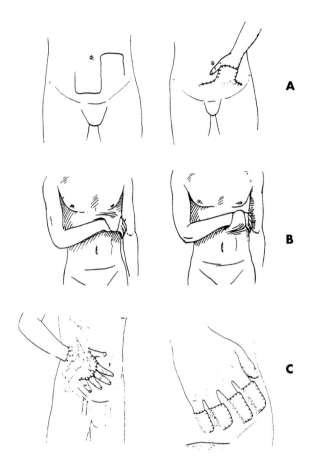

Figure 102-27. Various thoracoepigastric and abdominal wall flaps have been designed to provide vascularized tissue coverage for defects on the hand. (**A** redrawn from Groner JP, Weeks PM: Skin and soft tissue replacement in the hand. In Smith JW, Aston SJ [editors]: *Grabb & Smith's plastic surgery*, ed 4, Philadelphia, 1991, Little, Brown & Co. **B** redrawn from Kats RG, White WL: Anterior chest wall skin flaps to the forearm and hand. In Converse JM [editor]: *Grabb's encyclopedia of flaps: upper extremities*, ed 2, Philadelphia, 1998, Lippincott-Raven.)

Stiffness and limb edema may be increased during this period of immobilization.

ANATOMY. The cutaneous blood supply to the anterior trunk comes from a variety of anatomic angiosomes. Direct cutaneous and perforating musculocutaneous branches arise from the thoracoacromial, superficial, and lateral thoracic arteries; internal mammary arteries; and intercostal arteries to supply the upper torso. The deep and superficial epigastric vessels, the intercostals, and the superficial circumflex iliac arteries (SCIA) contribute blood supply to the anterior trunk from the pubis to the xiphoid. Flaps elevated on the thoracoepigastric axis are random pattern.

OPERATIONS. A number of thoracoepigastric and/or abdominal wall flaps have been described to facilitate closure of skin defects on the hand. Figure 102-27 illustrates a number of flap designs. A template is made of the defect on the finger or hand. If possible, it is helpful to design the flap to maintain the

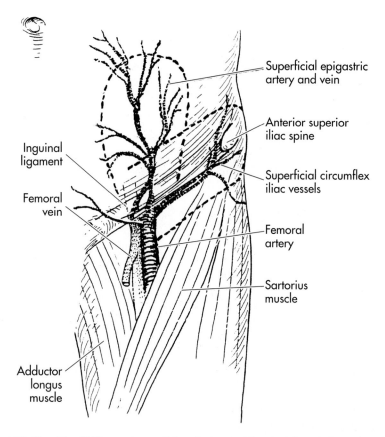

Figure 102-28. The SCIA travels parallel to the inguinal ligament 3 cm below a line drawn from the anterior superior iliac spine to the pubic tubercle. The flap is centered over the vessel.

hand in a comfortable and slightly elevated position to prevent further edema.

The skin and subcutaneous tissue are incised down to the fascia, and the flap is elevated at this plane to a point that will allow complete coverage of the wound. The flap is inset, and the donor site is closed primarily or with a split-thickness skin graft.

Pedicle Groin Flap

The groin flap has been successfully utilized to cover soft tissue defects on the hand measuring up to 17 × 30 cm.[13,56] The flap is supplied by the superficial circumflex iliac vessels, which branch from the femoral vessels and course laterally just inferior and parallel to the inguinal ligament. This flap can be easily and quickly raised and the donor site can usually be closed primarily, placing the scar in line with the inguinal ligament. A major drawback to utilizing the groin flap for hand defects is the necessity to keep the hand immobilized in a dependent position for 2 to 3 weeks before dividing and insetting the flap. This may have deleterious effects on eventual functional outcome because of increased edema and stiffness of the hand.

ANATOMY. This axial flap supplied by the SCIA usually arises from the femoral artery at a point approximately 3 cm below the mid-inguinal point. Variations in the point of origin, size,

and branches of this vessel have been described.[56] The SCIA lies below the deep fascia as it courses laterally and superiorly 2 to 3 cm below and parallel to the inguinal ligament. The vessel progresses laterally to a point 2 to 5 cm medial to the sartorius muscle, where it pierces the deep fascia and travels in the subcutaneous plane as a deep and superficial branch. The superficial branch further divides to an upper and lower branch just beyond the anterior superior iliac spine.

OPERATIONS. The flap should be designed intraoperatively with the aid of a Doppler flow probe. A line is drawn from the anterior superior iliac spine to the pubic tubercle, marking the course of the inguinal ligament. The superficial circumflex iliac vessels are identified approximately 3 cm below this line with a Doppler flow probe and traced laterally past the anterior superior iliac spine (Figure 102-28). The flap is centered over the marked course of the vessel and can be extended 5 to 10 cm past the anterior superior iliac spine. The length of the flap is variable but can extend 5 cm or more beyond the anterior superior iliac spine. The flap is elevated from a lateral to medial direction. It can be raised in a subcutaneous plane lateral to the border of the sartorius muscle to provide thin flap coverage for the hand. The deep fascia is incised at the lateral border of the sartorius and the dissection is carried medially in a plane below the deep fascia to incorporate the SCIA. The fascia must also be incised at the border of the inguinal ligament. The flap may be

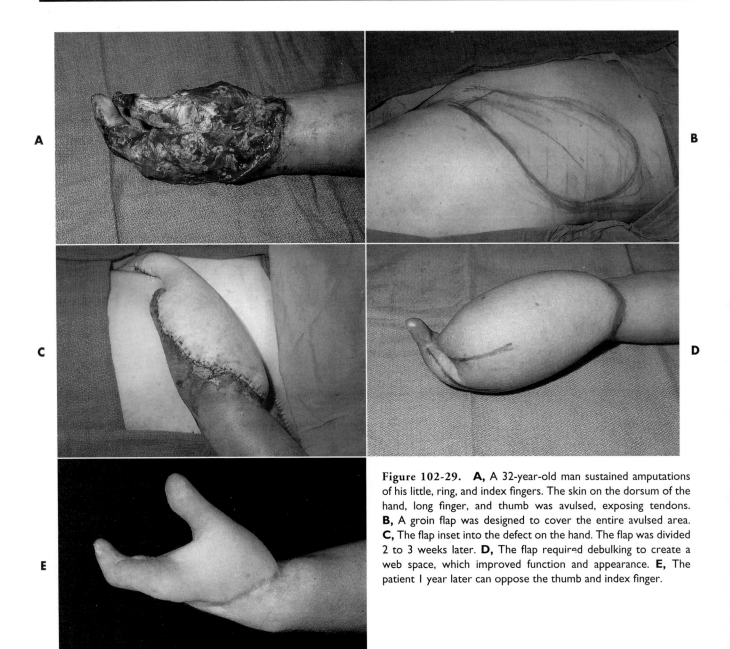

Figure 102-29. **A,** A 32-year-old man sustained amputations of his little, ring, and index fingers. The skin on the dorsum of the hand, long finger, and thumb was avulsed, exposing tendons. **B,** A groin flap was designed to cover the entire avulsed area. **C,** The flap inset into the defect on the hand. The flap was divided 2 to 3 weeks later. **D,** The flap required debulking to create a web space, which improved function and appearance. **E,** The patient 1 year later can oppose the thumb and index finger.

dissected medially to the point of origin of the SCIA from the femoral artery. Direct closure of the donor site can usually be accomplished if the flap width is 10 cm or less. The flap is inset into the defect on the hand (Figure 102-29). The pedicle can be safely divided in 2 to 3 weeks and the flap definitively inset.

considered a pivotal adjunct toward the achievement of an optimal reconstruction. Nature's economy of design has bestowed critical function to each structure in the hand, including the integument, and therefore severely limits the local reconstructive options. The clever and frugal employment of adjacent tissues, however, can yield solutions that are both efficient and desirable.

OUTCOMES

Successful hand reconstruction must confer both satisfactory functional and aesthetic results. Utilization of local tissues to achieve color and texture match and restore useful sensibility is

FUNCTIONAL OUTCOMES

Postoperative function must be assessed from objective parameters as well as from the patient's own perspective. The impact of any given injury must be considered in relation to the patient's occupation and preinjury level of function. In addition to grasp and pinch, maintenance of appropriate wrist position constitutes the minimal elements of a "functional hand." These requisites would be adequate for a lawyer, yet devastating for a guitarist or a surgeon. The definition of a "functional outcome" in hand reconstruction is therefore quite variable.

Anatomic Considerations

A number of pedicled and local reconstructive options have been detailed in the preceding text. The appropriate application of each procedure to a given defect must take into account patient-related and anatomic/physiologic factors. Adequate debridement and wound preparation is the key to success of any wound closure procedure. The anatomic considerations clearly encompass the differing qualities of flap tissue. The palmar skin is glabrous, thick, adherent, intensely sensate, and firmly secured to the underlying tissues, thus preventing slippage or rotation in power grip and grasp. In contrast, dorsal skin is hirsute, thin, mobile, and pliable, allowing for joint excursion with minimal bulk.

A treatment approach to soft tissue injuries of the hand is based on the location and size of the defect. This strategy serves only as a general guideline because the appropriateness of utilizing a specific procedure must be individualized after evaluating and considering the unique circumstances of each soft tissue defect, including associated injuries, patient variables, and surgeon preferences.

Regardless of the technical precision of execution, an unsatisfactory result will invariably occur if the wrong reconstructive option is exercised. In general, the choice between a flap or graft is relatively straightforward. This decision is based on the depth of injury, the compromise of vital structures, the quality of the exposed tissues, and the vascularity of local and regional tissues. If the recipient bed is suitable, coverage with a skin graft may not only be the most straightforward option, but the best surgical solution. Clearly, denuded artery, nerve, bone, or tendon require flap coverage. Compromised wound beds from trauma, infiltration injury, radiation, or collagen vascular disease may heal most favorably with flap coverage. Cigarette smoking, with its pervasive effect on wound healing and flap vascularity, poses a problematic situation that should be a caution to overly creative or optimistic flap design. We favor the use of hardy, axial-based flaps in these patients and preferentially employ free tissue transfer when appropriate. Recently it has been suggested that postoperative smoking is most devastating to skin flaps and therefore we try to strictly enforce postoperative abstinence.[10] In elective reconstructive efforts we begin patients who smoke on low-dose calcium channel-blocking agents (nifedipine 10 mg by mouth twice a day) for a minimum of 2 weeks preoperatively for the vasodilatory effects. This is usually well tolerated, although systemic flushing and postural hypotension are side effects that some patients find troublesome.

Patient Satisfaction

The decision to use a given surgical intervention on a compromised hand must be based on the surgeon's belief that the procedure is the one best suited to overall patient well-being. This includes awareness and consideration of the economic aspect of the injury, which may confer an enormous lifestyle change. Hand injuries constitute one of the most common causes of emergency room visits, affecting hundreds of thousands of patients annually. The resultant cost from surgical therapy, time lost from work, and decreased productivity are enormous. The type of treatment prescribed may have resounding consequences. For example, the decision to allow a wound to heal by secondary intention should be based not only on the physiologic and anatomic factors, such as wound location and size, that will determine the aesthetic and functional result but also on the realistic length of time this will take to occur and how this may affect the patient's ability and desire to earn a living in the interim.

In addition to the functional and aesthetic outcome of each therapeutic intervention, postoperative patient satisfaction and psychologic level of function are most closely linked to their premorbid status. Informed consent, in which patients are educated to the realistic surgical options available and expected outcomes and allowed to participate in the decision-making process, facilitates satisfaction and compliance. In most circumstances, there will be a donor site to contend with, and patients must be advised of the consequences of this as well. Patients should be made aware of the length and type of disability, the anticipated time for healing and therapy, and the importance of their commitment to the reconstructive process. They should be encouraged to avoid dwelling on the inevitable comparisons to their premorbid function and appearance and focus their energies on optimizing their current status. Early psychologic intervention and counseling is encouraged in devastating injuries and when indicated by any patient. Psychologic testing suggests that the negative impact of both the aesthetic and functional aspects of injury are most severe early after injury, and that the severity lessens with time.

REFERENCES

1. Allan MJ: Conservative management of fingertip amputations in children, *Hand* 12:257-265, 1980.
2. Allen EV: Thromboangiitis obliterans: methods of diagnosis of chronic occlusive arterial lesions distal to the wrist, with illustrative cases, *Am J Med Sci* 178:237-244, 1929.
3. Atasoy E, Ioakimidis E, Kasdan ML, et al: Reconstruction of the amputated fingertip with a triangular volar flap: a new surgical procedure, *J Bone Joint Surg* 51A:921-926, 1970.
4. Barton NJ: A modified thenar flap, *Hand* 7:150, 1975.
5. Bate JT: Second and third intention of finger amputations: a salvage procedure, *Clin Orthop* 57:151-155, 1966.
6. Baur PS, Larson DL, Stacey TR: The observation of myofibroblasts in hypertropic scars, *Surg Gynecol Obstet* 141:22-26, 1975.
7. Beasley RW: Principles and techniques of resurfacing operations for hand surgery, *Surg Clin North Am* 47:389-413, 1967.
8. Beasley RW: Reconstruction of amputated fingertips, *Plast Reconstr Surg* 44:349, 1969.

9.   Blair VP, Brown JB: Use and uses of large split skin grafts of intermediate thickness, *Surg Gynecol Obstet* 49:82-97, 1929.

10. Broadbent TR, Woolf RM: Thumb reconstruction with contiguous skin-bone pedicle graft, *Plast Reconstr Surg* 26:494-499, 1960.

11. Buchler U, Frey H-P: Retrograde posterior interosseous flap, *J Hand Surg [Am]* 16:283-292, 1991.

12. Chang LD, Bunke G, Slezak S, Bunke HJ: Cigarette smoking, plastic surgery and microsurgery, *J Reconstr Microsurg* 12:467-474, 1996.

13. Chuang DCC, Colony LH, Chen HC, Wei FC: Groin flap design and versatility, *Plast Reconstr Surg* 84:100-107, 1989.

14. Cormack GC, Lamberty BGH: *The arterial anatomy of skin flaps,* ed 2, Edinburgh, 1994, Churchill Livingstone.

15. Corps BVM: The effect of graft thickness, donor site and graft bed on graft shrinkage in the hooded rat, *Br J Plast Surg* 22:125-133, 1969.

16. Costa H, Soutar DS: The distally based island posterior interosseous flap, *Br J Plast Surg* 41, 221-227, 1988.

17. Cronin TD: The cross-finger flap: a new method of repair, *Am J Surg* 17:419, 1951.

18. Cuono CB: Double Z-plasty repair of large and small rhombic defects: the double-Z rhomboid, *Plast Reconstr Surg* 71:658-667, 1983.

19. Cuono CB: Double Z-rhombic repair of both large and small defects of the upper extremity, *J Hand Surg [Am]* 9(2):197-202, 1984.

20. Donoff RB, Grillo HC: The effects of skin grafting on healing open wounds in rabbits, *J Surg Res* 19:163-165, 1975.

21. Earley MJ: The arterial supply of the thumb first web space and index finger and its surgical application, *J Hand Surg [Br]* 11:163-170, 1986.

22. Earley MJ, Milner RH: Dorsal metacarpal flaps, *Br J Plast Surg* 40:333-337, 1987.

23. Fitzgerald MJT, Martin F, Paletta FX: Innervation of skin grafts, *Surg Gynecol Obstet* 124:808-811, 1967.

24. Flatt AE: The thenar flap, *J Bone Joint Surg* 39B:80-85, 1957.

25. Foucher G, Bishop A: Island flaps based on the first and second dorsal metacarpal arteries. In Levin E, Germann G (editors): *Local flaps about the hand: atlas of the Hand Clinics,* Philadelphia, 1998, WB Saunders.

26. Foucher G, Braun JB: A new island flap transfer from the dorsum of the index to the thumb, *Plast Reconstr Surg* 63:344-349, 1979.

27. Foucher G, Van Genechten F, Merle M, et al: A compound radial artery forearm flap in hand surgery: an original modification of the Chinese forearm flap, *Br J Plast Surg* 37:139-148, 1984.

28. Fraulin FO, Thomson HG: First web space deepening: comparing the four flap and five flap Z-plasty: which gives the most gain, *Plast Reconstr Surg* 104(1):120-128, 1999.

29. Gatewood A: A plastic repair of finger defects without hospitalization, *JAMA* 87:1479, 1926.

30. Germann G: Principles of flap design for surgery of the hand. In Levin E, Germann G: *Local flaps about the hand: atlas of the Hand Clinics,* Philadelphia, 1998, WB Saunders.

31. Germann G, Mandy S, Kania N, Ruff T: The reverse pedicle heterodigital cross-finger island flap, *J Hand Surg [Br]* 22:25-29, 1997.

32. Gibraiel EA: A local finger flap to treat post-traumatic flexion contractures of a finger at the MP joint, *Plast Reconstr Surg* 30:134, 1979.

33. Glasson DW, Lovie MJ: The ulnar island flap in hand and forearm reconstruction, *Br J Plast Surg* 41:349-353, 1988.

34. Grad JB, Beasley RW: Fingertip reconstruction, *Hand Clin* 1:667-681, 1985.

35. Green DP, Dominguez OJ: A transpositional skin flap for release of volar contractures of a finger at the MP joint, *Plast Reconstr Surg* 64:516-519, 1979.

36. Guimerteau JC, et al: The reverse ulnar artery forearm island flap in hand surgery: 54 cases, *Plast Reconstr Surg* 81:925-930, 1988.

37. Gurdin M, Pangman WJ: The repair of surface deficits of fingers by transdigital flaps, *Plast Reconstr Surg* 5:368-371, 1950.

38. Holm A, Zachariae L: Fingertip lesions: an evaluation of conservative treatment versus free skin grafting, *Acta Orthop Scand* 1974;45:382, 1974.

39. Illingworth CM: Trapped fingers and amputated fingertips in children, *J Ped Surg* 9:853, 1974.

40. Joshi BB: Dorsolateral flap from the same finger to relieve flexion contracture, *Plast Reconstr Surg* 49:186-189, 1972.

41. Kutler W: A new method for fingertip amputations, *JAMA* 133:29-30, 1947.

42. Lai CS, et al: The adipofascial turn-over flap for complicated dorsal skin defects of the hand and finger, *Br J Plast Surg* 44:165-172, 1991.

43. Lever WF: Histology of the skin. In Lever WF, Shaumberg-Lever G (editors): *Histopathology of the skin,* ed 5, Philadelphia, 1975, JB Lippincott.

44. Li Z, Liu K, Cao Y: The reverse flow ulnar artery island flap: 42 clinical cases, *Br J Plast Surg* 42:256-259, 1989.

45. Lin S-D, Lai C-S, Chiu C-C: Venous drainage in the reverse forearm flap, *Plast Reconstr Surg* 74:508-512, 1984.

46. Littler JW: Neurovascular pedicle transfer of tissue in reconstructive surgery of the hand (abstract), *J Bone Joint Surg* 38A:917, 1956.

47. Lovie MJ, Duncan GM, Glasson DW: The ulnar artery forearm free flap, *Br J Plast Surg* 37:446-492, 1984.

48. Lovie MJ, Duncan GM, Glasson DW: The ulnar artery forearm free flap, *Br J Plast Surg* 41:349-354, 1988.

49. Lueders HW, Shapiro RL: Rotation finger flaps in reconstruction of burned hands, *Plast Reconstr Surg* 47:176-185, 1971.

50. MacDougal B, Wray CR, Weeks PM: Lateral-volar finger flap for the treatment of burn syndactyly, *Plast Reconstr Surg* 57:167-175, 1976.

51. Madden JW: On "the contractile fibroblast," *Plast Reconstr Surg* 52:291-292, 1973.

52. Maruyama Y: The reverse dorsal metacarpal flap, *Br J Plast Surg* 43:24-27, 1990.

53. Masquelet AC, Penteado CV: Le lambeau interosseux posterieur, *Ann Chir Main* 6:131-139, 1987.

54. Mazzer N, Barbieri CH, Cortez M: The posterior interosseous forearm island flap for skin defects in the hand and elbow, *J Hand Surg [Br]* 21:237-243, 1996.

55. McGeorge BC: Modified rhombic flap for closure of circular or irregular defects, *J Cutan Med Surg* 3(2):74-78, 1998.

56. McGregor IA, Jackson IT: The groin flap, *Br J Plast Surg* 25:3-16, 1972.

57. Moberg E: Aspects of sensation in reconstructive surgery of the upper extremity, *J Bone Joint Surg* 46A:817-825, 1964.

58. Montagna W: Morphology of cutaneous sensory receptors, *J Invest Dermatol* 69:4-7, 1977.

59. Morton D, Madden JW, Peacock EE: Effect of a local smooth muscle antagonist on wound contraction, *Surg Forum* 23:511-512, 1972.

60. Mutaf M, Sensoz O, Ustuner ET: A new design of the cross-finger flap: the C-ring flap, *Br J Plast Surg* 46:97-104, 1993.

61. Niranjan NS, Armstrong JR: A homodigital reverse pedicle island flap in soft tissue reconstruction of the finger and the thumb, *J Hand Surg [Am]* 193:135-141, 1994.

62. Reverdin JL: De la Greffe epidermique, *Arch Gen Med* 276:555-702, 1872.

63. Rohrich RJ, Zbar RI: A simplified algorithm for the use of Z-plasty, *Plast Reconstr Surg* 103(5):1513-1517, 1990.

64. Rudolph R, Gruber S, Suzuki M, Woodward M: Control of contractile fibroblasts by skin grafts, *Surg Forum* 28:524-525, 1977.

65. Smith RJ, Albin R: Thenar H-flap for fingertip injuries, *J Trauma* 16:778, 1976.

66. Snow JW: The use of a volar flap for repair of fingertip amputations: a preliminary report, *Plast Reconstr Surg* 40:163, 1967.

67. Swanson E, Boyd JB, Manktekow RT: The radial forearm flap: reconstructive applications and donor site defects in 35 consecutive patients, *Plast Reconstr Surg* 85:258-262, 1990.

68. Timmons MJ: The vascular basis of the radial forearm flap, *Plast Reconstr Surg* 77:80-92, 1986.

69. Torii S, Namiki Y, Mori R: Reverse-flow island flap: clinical report and venous drainage, *Plast Reconstr Surg* 79:600-609, 1987.

70. Verdan C, Egloff D: Fingertip injuries, *Surg Clin North Am* 61:237-252, 1981.

71. Vilain R, Dupus JF: Use of the flap for coverage of a small area on a finger or the palm: 20 years experience, *Plast Reconstr Surg* 51:397-403, 1973.

72. Wavak P: Reverse cross finger flap, *Orthop Rev* 8:43, 1979.

73. Wee JT: Reversed venous flow in the distally pedicled radial forearm flap: surgical implications, *Hand Chir Microsurg Chir Plast Chir* May 20(3):119-123, 1988.

74. Weeks PM, Wray CR: *Management of acute hand injuries,* St. Louis, 1973, Mosby, p 141.

75. Weinweig N, Chen L, Chen ZW: The distally based radial forearm fasciocutaneous flap with preservation of the radial artery: an anatomic and clinical approach, *Plast Reconstr Surg* 94(5):675-684, 1994.

76. Yajima H, Inada Y, Shono M, et al: Radial forearm flap with vascularized tendons for hand reconstruction, *Plast Reconstr Surg* 98:328-333, 1996.

Compartment Syndrome

103

William A. Zamboni
Elizabeth M. Kiraly

INDICATIONS

DEFINITION

A *compartment syndrome* is defined as increased tissue pressure within a limited or closed space that compromises circulation, initiating subcritical perfusion to the tissues within the compartment.[13] Different terms exist in the literature to define this syndrome or its sequelae (chronic or recurrent, acute and subacute). This chapter focuses on acute compartment syndrome and concentrates on the diagnosis, treatment, and outcomes associated with this condition.

ETIOLOGY

Numerous etiologies of an acute compartment syndrome have been described in the literature, the most common of which results from a fracture or bony injury. Most etiologies fit into two categories of the anatomic development of a compartment syndrome: those that decrease the size of the compartment or those that increase the fluid content within the compartment.[15] The former group includes constrictive dressings, casts or splints, closure of fascial defects, and thermal injuries. Sources of increased compartmental fluid include bleeding from vascular or muscular injury, electrical injury, anticoagulation or thrombolytic therapy,[24] congenital or acquired bleeding disorders, edema from crush, reperfusion after ischemia, venipuncture or intravenous (IV) fluid infiltration, and infection.[20]

It is important from a treatment perspective to make a distinction between a subfascial versus a subcutaneous etiology for a compartment syndrome. An escharotomy, for instance, may be all that is necessary to treat a patient with a subcutaneous compartment syndrome of the hand secondary to a thermal injury. A crush injury to the hand, with muscle injury and subfascial compartment syndrome, will require intrinsic fasciotomies. It is also useful when evaluating a patient for an upper-extremity compartment syndrome to separate extrinsic forearm and arm compartments from intrinsic hand involvement because one may exist without the other.

DIAGNOSIS

Clinical examination remains the best method to diagnose an acute compartment syndrome.[8] As with any medical condition, a good history is always helpful to establish a diagnosis. A recent history of trauma to an extremity, arterial or venous cannulation, or revascularization by thrombectomy or embolectomy to a limb should all raise suspicion that a compartment syndrome could have occurred.[8] Careful and serial clinical examinations should be performed in these patients. If the patient is unconscious or unable to communicate and no history can be obtained, more reliance is placed on the physical examination.

The clinical symptom most consistent with a compartment syndrome is pain. The pain is usually out of proportion to the examination. Passive movement or stretching of the affected muscles using the passive stretch test produces exquisite pain that is unrelieved by analgesia or immobilization and becomes progressive.[15] Decreased sensation or paresthesia is a later finding and is a reflection of neuronal ischemia in the affected compartment. Additional findings associated with a compartment syndrome include progressive muscle weakness, excessive swelling, and palpable firmness of the compartment. The latter sign may occasionally be masked by subcutaneous edema.[12] It is important to note the resting position of the extremity. Forearm supination, wrist and interphalangeal (IP) joint flexion, and metacarpophalangeal (MCP) joint extension are indicative of a compartment syndrome (Figure 103-1, *A* and *B*).

The examination should *not* rely on loss of distal perfusion, which is a late sign. Arterial blood pressure is usually higher than the intracompartmental pressure. The peripheral and digital arterial circulation may therefore be intact when neuromuscular tissue is compromised.

Direct measurement of the compartment pressure may be indicated if the clinical examination is unreliable or equivocal. These tests should not dissuade the clinician from the diagnosis of a compartment syndrome based on the clinical examination findings.

The infusion technique described in Whitesides et al[26] provides a simple but indirect measure of the compartment pressure by using a 20-ml syringe attached to a three-way

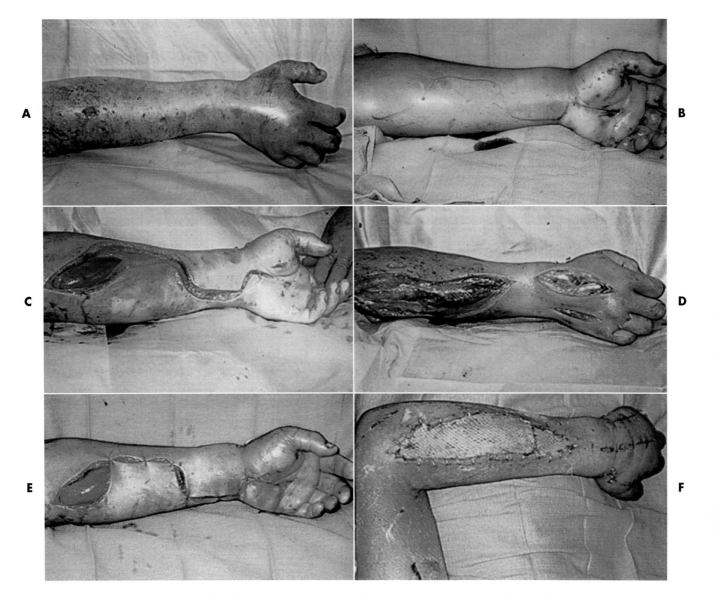

Figure 103-1. **A,** Preoperative appearance of compartment syndrome after crush injury. **B,** Volar markings for incision including carpal tunnel release. **C,** Fasciotomy demonstrating muscle bulging after volar compartment release. **D,** Dorsal forearm and intrinsic fasciotomies were required. **E,** The skin edges of the volar incision were loosely approximated with widely placed sutures. **F,** Skin grafting was required for the dorsal incision.

stopcock with two sets of IV tubing connected to an 18-gauge needle inserted into the compartment and attached to a mercury manometer. A small amount of saline is slowly injected into the arm. The pressure needed to overcome the tissue pressure is recorded on the manometer.

Mubarak and colleagues[16] directly measure compartment pressures with the Wick catheter. The catheter is filled with saline and is zero calibrated and then connected to a transducer and recorder. A 14-gauge needle introduces the catheter 2 to 3 cm into the muscle. The outer cannula is removed, leaving the Wick catheter, which is a piece of unraveled Dexon suture in a polyethylene catheter, in the compartment. The catheter equilibrates immediately, providing an accurate tissue pressure measurement.

We prefer to use the Stryker device because it is the simplest and quickest way to measure compartment pressure. The device is self-contained and requires only local anesthesia and sterile saline. An 18-gauge needle is inserted after calibration directly into the volar forearm. Equilibration is achieved within 1 minute, and a digital readout displays the pressure.

Thresholds for performing fasciotomy based on measured compartment pressure vary among different authors. Matsen[13] recommends fasciotomy at 45 mm Hg, whereas Whitesides[26] recommends 20 mm Hg below diastolic pressure. Mubarak and Hargens[15] use 30 mm Hg for 8 hours or when associated with a clinical picture of compartment syndrome. We use the criteria of 50 mm Hg as an absolute indication for fasciotomy. Pressures between 30 to 50 mm Hg must be correlated with

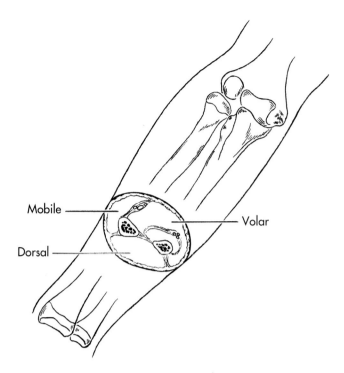

Figure 103-2. Cross section through the mid forearm showing the volar and dorsal compartments and the mobile wad.

the patient's clinical condition. If by examination a compartment syndrome is not apparent, then hourly serial examinations are carried out for up to 8 hours until there is resolution of pressure; if the pressure is not resolved, a fasciotomy is performed. An extremity with a pressure measurement of less than 30 mm Hg can generally be treated with elevation and conservative management.

ANATOMY

The forearm is invested by the antebrachial fascia, a dense fibrous tissue that envelops each compartment and muscle. Vertical septa pass between muscles, some originating as deep as the periosteum. Transverse septa separate the deep and superficial muscles. The fascia is thicker posteriorly and in the distal forearm.[17]

Three compartments exist in the forearm: (1) the volar (flexor), (2) the dorsal, and (3) the mobile wad (radial) (Figure 103-2). These compartments, unlike those in the leg, are interconnected.[5] These interconnections provide a method for release of all three compartments by release of the volar compartment. Decompression of the volar compartment should include both the superficial and deep muscles.[2] If after the release of the volar compartment, the dorsal compartment remains tight by examination or measurement, then it should also be decompressed. This will also release the mobile wad.

The hand contains 10 separate noncommunicating compartments, each of which must be considered in a compartment syndrome.[7] The compartments consist of four dorsal interossei, three volar interossei, the hypothenar and thenar

muscles, and a separate compartment for the adductor pollicis. Each of these compartments must be released separately by fasciotomy. The fascia surrounding the interosseous muscles is strong and inelastic, providing resistance to expansion of injured muscles. Halpern et al[6] believe radially oriented muscles are more prone to develop a compartment syndrome because they depend more on the volar metacarpal arteries, which are end arteries.

The intrinsic compartments are tested by passively abducting and adducting the fingers while keeping the proximal interphalangeal (PIP) joints flexed and the MCP joints in extension. Palmar abduction stretches the adductor muscles, radial abduction of the thumb stretches the thenar muscles, and extension and adduction of the small finger tests the hypothenar muscles.

The finger is invested by tight fascia, including Cleland's and Grayson's ligaments, and numerous fibrous septa that anchor the volar glabrous skin to the underlying bone and tendon sheath. This skin anchoring causes a localized compartment syndrome with subcutaneous swelling because the skin is unable to stretch. The diagnosis of a subcutaneous digital compartment syndrome can be made by palpation. If the digit is taut and noncompressible, decompression should be performed.

PATHOPHYSIOLOGY

Normal fluid homeostasis between the intravascular and extravascular spaces of the tissue within a compartment is maintained by capillary and tissue hydrostatic and osmotic pressures. Cells, fibers, fluids, gels, and matrices also contribute to intracompartmental pressure.[12] The baseline pathophysiology in a compartment syndrome is a disturbance in the arteriovenous (AV) gradient as described by Matsen and Rorabeck.[14]

An increased compartment pressure produces a concomitant increase in venous pressure in the postcapillary venules, increasing the hydrostatic fluid shift to the extracellular space. The increased venous pressure lowers the local AV gradients, decreasing capillary blood flow and resulting in muscle and nerve tissue ischemia. Concomitant decreased arterial perfusion from direct injury, hypovolemia, or shock further decreases the AV gradient. When the compartment pressure exceeds venous pressure, there is no perfusion. Restoration of blood flow after a global ischemic event can result in a reperfusion injury with free radical–induced accelerated tissue damage.[29] The edema and interstitial hemorrhage associated with an ischemia reperfusion injury is likely to perpetuate and exacerbate a further increase in tissue pressure.

FUNCTION AND SEQUELAE

A Volkmann's ischemic contracture is the end state of an untreated compartment syndrome. The classic picture of a forearm contracture described by Volkmann[25] in 1881 is the result of muscle necrosis, fibrosis, and shortening causing contracture of the wrist and digits. Tendon transfers are possible to restore function only if only one compartment has been injured. A free muscle transfer must also be considered in severe cases.[10]

Limb loss is the most devastating sequelae. This can occur acutely in patients with severe burns or crush injuries, but a delayed amputation may be necessary if a nonfunctional limb results from a compartment syndrome.

INFORMED CONSENT

Once the diagnosis of a compartment syndrome is made, surgical decompression should be performed and the operating room is rapidly prepared. Emergency fasciotomy is the surgical treatment for this condition. The patient must be informed of the consequences of not undergoing decompression, which include the development of a Volkmann's contracture, a nonfunctioning arm or hand, and possibly limb amputation. The risks of the procedure should also be explained, including bleeding, infection, and possible limb amputation. The necessity of future surgery should also be explained at this time, including the possibility of further exploration and debridement if progressive muscle necrosis occurs and the potential for delayed wound closure, either primarily or with skin grafts.

OPERATIONS

NONINVASIVE/PREVENTATIVE TREATMENT

Noninvasive intervention has no place in the treatment of a full-blown compartment syndrome. However, several nonsurgical measures can be instituted in an early developing compartment syndrome to prevent the need for a later fasciotomy.

1. *Elevation* of limbs with posttraumatic injuries should be standard practice. The most effective method of elevation is to place the extremity in a stockinette suspended from a pole used to hang bags of IV fluids. A reduction of the dependent edema in an injured extremity can help reduce the compartment pressure.

2. *Splinting* of the extremities after all fractures have been reduced is critical. The hand should be immobilized in the safe position with the wrist in extension, the MCP joints in flexion, and the IP joints in neutral while the extremity is elevated to minimize joint edema and potential subsequent contracture.

3. *Enzymatic debridement* is a useful method to prevent surgical intervention in certain situations. Several products have been developed that can potentially eliminate the need for escharotomy in patients with near or completely circumferential partial-thickness extremity burns.[11] These agents can be used when compartment pressures are elevated but there is not yet a clear indication for escharotomy. Travase was the most popular compound

used for enzymatic debridement, but its production and use were recently discontinued. The most common agent used at our institution is Accuzyme,[1] a hydrophilic ointment base containing papain and urea. Accuzyme is a potent digestant of nonviable protein matter but is harmless to viable tissue. Its optimal pH range of activity is 3 to 12, and it can be inactivated by salts of heavy metals such as lead, silver, and mercury. The wound is cleansed with saline, and the eschar is crosshatched with a #15 blade to allow deeper penetration of the ointment, which is applied directly to the wound. Reapplication is carried out every 8 to 12 hours and is discontinued after 48 to 72 hours. Concomitant use of peroxide or Silvadene should be avoided because these agents inactivate the papain.

Collagenase (Santyl) ointment[19] can also be employed early in the care of a burn wound. The collagenase enzyme, derived from *Clostridium histolyticum,* is carried in a petrolatum base and has the ability to digest native and denatured collagen in necrotic tissue. Its optimal pH range is 6 to 8, and it is adversely affected by detergents and heavy metal ions. It is applied once daily unless the dressing is soiled. The method of application is the same as Accuzyme, and care should be taken to avoid spreading ointment outside the wound area. Collagenase does not contain any antibacterial properties, and therefore the addition of a topical antibiotic powder may be indicated if the wound is contaminated.

Use of these substrates requires careful clinical serial observation and examination of the extremity. Escharotomy and/or fasciotomy is indicated if compartment pressures continue to rise and a compartment syndrome develops.

INVASIVE TREATMENT

The surgical treatment of an acute compartment syndrome is urgent decompression by fasciotomy. If the compartment syndrome is caused by constricted burned skin after a thermal injury, then an escharotomy with or without a deeper fasciotomy is indicated. The surgeon must consider the systemic manifestations of a compartment syndrome, including skeletal muscle cell death with rhabdomyolysis and the release of myoglobin, which can cause renal failure. Fluid resuscitation is initiated to maintain a high urine output that is monitored hourly after catheterization with a Foley catheter. The urine is checked for myoglobin and, if present, intervention to prevent renal compromise should be instituted. The patient's urine output should be maintained to a level of at least 1 ml/kg per hour and the urine pH should be kept above 7 by alkalization with systemic IV sodium bicarbonate, adding 50 mg to each liter of IV fluid. If the urine output falls in spite of adequate fluid resuscitation, a diuretic such a mannitol should be given.

Patients who develop a compartment syndrome caused by anticoagulant or thrombolytic therapy should be immediately evaluated to determine if these medications can be discontinued. Thrombolytic agents should be stopped immediately;

however, heparin reversal with protamine is not always indicated because heparin has a very short half-life. Patients who are receiving Coumadin therapy must be evaluated often in consultation with their treating physician to determine if stopping their anticoagulation poses a medical risk.

Fluid resuscitation of patients in shock from trauma should be initiated during transport to the hospital and should be considered in surgery. Patients who are too unstable for transport may require fasciotomy at the bedside.

METHOD OF FASCIOTOMY

General anesthesia is preferred over regional blocks when performing a fasciotomy. An axillary block may place increased fluid pressure on the nerve sheaths, and Bier block anesthesia requires extremity exsanguination, which could increase pressure within the compartments. The patient is placed in the supine position and the arm is supported on an arm board. A tourniquet is placed when possible, and the extremity is then prepped and draped. A sterile tourniquet is preferred if the proximal extremity requires fasciotomy. The extremity is elevated without exsanguination before inflating the tourniquet. This allows visualization of the subcutaneous veins during the fasciotomy, allowing the veins to be cauterized. Several incisions have been described for fasciotomy, and the surgeon must consider the anatomical location of the compartment to be released when planning the incisions. This requires a separate evaluation of the compartments within the upper arm, forearm, and hand.

A volar forearm fasciotomy should include release of the carpal tunnel, especially in patients with an electrical injury. The incision is begun with a standard carpal tunnel incision in the palm, carried proximally toward the ulnar border of the distal forearm, and then curved centrally at the level of the musculocutaneous junction (Figure 103-3, *A*; see Figure 103-1, *B*). The releasing incision can be continued proximally with a zigzag incision across the antecubital fossa to prevent a future flexion contracture at the elbow. An ulnar location of the fasciotomy in the distal forearm avoids injury to the radial artery and the median nerve and retains a radially-based skin flap, which provides coverage of the distal forearm flexor tendons. The curvilinear proximal forearm incision allows good exposure to the volar forearm and avoids a longitudinal incision that can result in a scar contracture. The antebrachial fascia over the flexor mass is incised longitudinally with a scalpel, and the fasciotomy is extended using scissors with a pushing technique.

Fasciotomies of the forearm muscles should be systematic and complete. Superficial, intermediate, and deep compartments should be examined. Release of the superficial compartment containing the pronator teres (PT), flexor carpi ulnaris (FCU), flexor carpi radialis (FCR), and palmaris longus (PL) muscles decompresses all of the flexor compartments in most cases. The compartments containing the flexor digitorum profundus (FDP), flexor pollicis longus (FPL), and the pronator quadratus (PQ) must be evaluated and released if

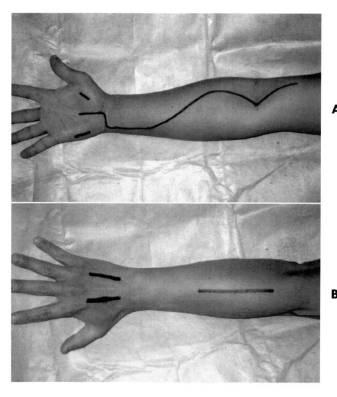

Figure 103-3. **A,** Volar incisions for hand and forearm fasciotomy. A carpal tunnel incision is extended along the ulnar distal forearm. The incision then curves centrally at the musculocutaneous junction. A zigzag incision is used at the antecubital fossa. Incisions are made over the thenar and hypothenar muscle groups. **B,** Dorsal incision to release the mobile wad and dorsal compartments. Incisions over the second and fourth metacarpals allow intrinsic release of dorsal/volar interosseii muscles.

necessary.[23] Fasciotomy of the deeper compartments may be necessary in some cases, especially in patients with electrical burns in which muscle injury is usually most severe in the compartments adjacent to bone. An epimysiotomy should be performed on any compartment muscle that is tense and bulging after fasciotomy is performed (see Figure 103-1, *C*). Repair of associated injuries such as bone fixation and nerve, artery, or tendon repair can be completed after adequate decompression by fasciotomy.

A complete release of the volar compartment will generally also decompress the mobile wad and the dorsal compartment. If the mobile wad and dorsal compartment remain tense after a complete release of the volar compartment, then dorsal fasciotomies through a longitudinal incision on the dorsum of the forearm should be performed (see Figures 103-1, *D* and 103-3, *B*). Release of the intrinsic muscles of the hand should include the interosseous compartments as well as the thenar and hypothenar muscle groups. Release of the interosseous compartments can be carried out through two longitudinal incisions on the dorsum of the hand along the axis of the second and fourth metacarpals (Figures 103-3, *B* and 103-4). Fasciotomies on the radial side of the second metacarpal and the ulnar side of the fourth metacarpal will release the dorsal and volar interosseous compartments. The thenar and

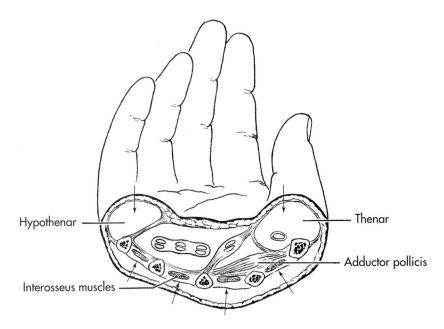

Figure 103-4. Intrinsic compartments of the palm. Arrows indicate location of fasciotomies.

hypothenar muscle groups can be decompressed through small longitudinal incisions as shown in Figure 103-3, *A* and 103-4.

The tourniquet is deflated after complete release of all fascial compartments and hemostasis is achieved. All decompressed muscles are then inspected for viability. The skin edges are loosely approximated with widely-spaced sutures or staples if excessive edema is not present (see Figure 103-1, *E*). The skin incisions are left open if there is nonviable muscle, and the incisions are covered with topical antimicrobial dressings. It is sometimes difficult to assess muscle viability at the initial decompression and debridement in patients with an electrical injury. Obviously nonviable, gray-appearing muscle should be debrided, but any questionable muscle should be left alone and evaluated again during subsequent serial debridements. An anatomic debridement with identification of each individual muscle group helps the surgeon formulate a long-term plan to determine which muscle groups remain viable and are available for use as motor units.

Digital decompression is indicated when swelling in the subcutaneous compartment creates pressures that compromise the blood supply to the digits; this is most commonly seen in patients with circumferential thermal injury (Figure 103-5). The skin incisions should be made in the midaxial line at the most dorsal point of the flexion crease at the PIP and distal interphalangeal (DIP) joints. These incisions are made on the ulnar side of the index, long, and ring fingers and along the radial side of the thumb and small finger.

POSTOPERATIVE MANAGEMENT

A sterile dressing should be applied in the operating room after surgery, with a volar forearm splint to hold the hand in the safe position. The arm is elevated at all times by suspension in a stockinette on an IV pole, as described earlier. Elevation on pillows is usually not adequate because the arm position cannot be maintained while the patient is sleeping. IV antibiotics should be administered for contaminated wounds on an individual basis considering intraoperative wound cultures. Finger perfusion should be assessed on an hourly basis by examination of the fingertip/nail bed capillary refill. Mild postoperative pain is expected but should be controllable with routine analgesics. If the patient complains of severe pain, it is then important to check the passive movement of the extremity to rule out the possibility of a persistent compartment syndrome. The frequency of the dressing changes should be based on the individual requirements of the wound. Saline gauze dressings are appropriate for clean wounds. Topical antimicrobial agents such as Sulfamylon, Silvadene, or Bacitracin ointment are necessary for contaminated extremity wounds, especially when there is muscle necrosis as is commonly seen in patients with an electrical injury. Hyperbaric oxygen therapy should be considered after surgery for patients who have experienced a prolonged compartment syndrome in which muscle may have been ischemic for more than 4 hours. A reperfusion injury occurs from release of oxygen free radicals in such cases when perfusion is

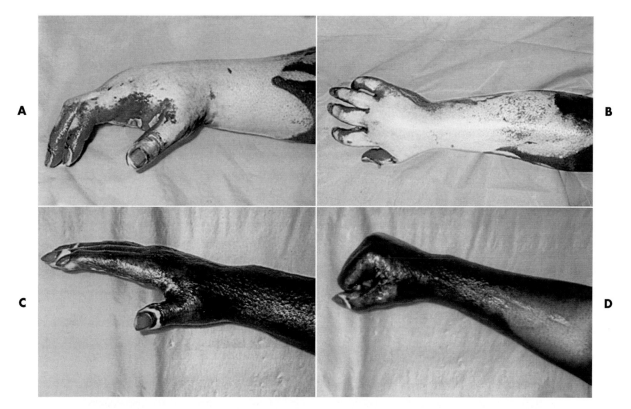

Figure 103-5. **A** and **B,** Subcutaneous and intrinsic compartment syndrome from a full-thickness burn. Patient required emergent escharotomies and intrinsic fasciotomies followed by tangential excision and split-thickness skin grafting 4 days later. **C** and **D,** Final range of motion 6 months after injury.

re-established by fasciotomy. Hyperbaric oxygen administered soon after reperfusion has been shown to be effective in experimental compartment syndrome models and in other situations resulting in an ischemic reperfusion injury.[22,27,28,29,30] Hyperbaric oxygen therapy should follow protocols outlined by the UHMS Hyperbaric Oxygen Committee Report.

SECONDARY PROCEDURES

The necessity and extent of subsequent surgical procedures depends largely on the condition of the wound after the first operation. Most patients can have their wounds closed primarily after resolution of edema, usually in 7 to 10 days. Intraoperative skin stretching devices and a layered skin closure reduce tension and help approximate the skin edges.[9] Skin grafting is employed when primary closure is not feasible (see Figure 103-1, *F*). Skin grafts adherent to muscle can restrict muscle contracture and may be released by serial excision of the graft and advancement of the skin edges. Tissue expanders can be placed adjacent to the graft to expand the normal skin, which can then be advanced to close the defect after graft excision. Functional muscle or free muscle transfers may be required in patients with severe neuromuscular loss or damage.

OUTCOMES

STATISTICS AND FUNCTIONAL OUTCOME

A fasciotomy performed in a timely fashion by an experienced surgeon familiar with upper-extremity anatomy should have a high success rate in relieving a compartment syndrome. Sheridan and Martin[21] reported that patients who had a fasciotomy done within 12 hours from the onset of increased compartment pressure had normal function in 68% of cases, but when surgery was performed after 12 hours only 8% of patients had normal function. Peters and Scott[18] reported children had a full functional recovery when fasciotomy was done within 24 hours of injury.

The functional outcome after a fasciotomy is based on two factors: the amount of viable muscle and the etiology of the compartment syndrome. The sequelae of a compartment syndrome, such as myoglobinuria and renal failure, should also be considered in evaluating the long-term results. Muscle recovery is largely dependent on the length of time it was ischemic before fasciotomy. Early recognition and prompt intervention provide the best chance for full functional recovery (see Figure 103-5).

The presence of associated injuries and the etiology of a compartment syndrome greatly influence the degree of functional recovery. Crush injuries have the poorest functional results,[4] whereas complex fractures and/or nerve involvement can also impair recovery and decrease final limb function.[3] Brostrom, Stark, and Svartengren[3] noted median nerve involvement was present in all 16 patients in their study, and eight had ulnar nerve symptoms. All median nerves recovered, but persistent neuropathy was noted in two ulnar nerves.

Physical therapy and rehabilitation contribute significantly to a successful outcome and must be aggressive and initiated early for maximum recovery. Appropriate splinting, methods of edema control, and active and passive range of motion exercises are all important therapeutic modalities. Myonecrosis and subsequent fibrosis resulting in functional impairment may require surgical rehabilitation by tissue and tendon transfers. Limb loss is an uncommon end-stage sequelae that can be managed by early prosthetic fitting and functional rehabilitation.

ECONOMIC ISSUES

Information relative to the cost to society for treating patients with a compartment syndrome is sparse. Financial considerations include the initial operating room expenses, the surgeon's fee, and the hospital stay, which varies according to the patient's condition and the degree of associated injuries. Long-term costs include those associated with secondary reconstructive procedures to restore limb function and an aesthetic result.

Rehabilitation by physical therapy should be included in computing the cost impact. Minimal therapy requirements are generally three times a week for 6 weeks and can range from $2000 to $5000 depending on the geographic location. The economic impact of long-term disability is more difficult to assess. A patient with a nonfunctional limb can have a lifetime loss of wages plus the social cost of supporting the person on disability. Insurance payments and legal liability suits also figure strongly into economic issues.

REFERENCES

1. Accuzyme ointment, Healthpoint Medical, San Antonio, Texas 78215.
2. Allen MJ, Barnes MR: Chronic compartment syndrome of the flexor muscles in the forearm: a case report, *J Hand Surgery [Br]* 14(1):47-48, 1989.
3. Brostrom LA, Stark A, Svartengren G: Acute compartment syndrome in forearm fractures, *Acta Ortho Scan* 61(3):50, 1990.
4. Gelberman RH, Garfin SR, Hergenroeder PT, et al: Compartment syndromes of the forearm: diagnosis and treatment, *Clin Orthop* 161:252-261, 1980.
5. Gelberman RH, Zakaib GS, Mubarak SJ, et al: Decompression of forearm compartment syndrome, *Clin Orthop* 161:252-261, 1981.
6. Halpern AA, Greene R, Nichols T, et al: Compartment syndrome of the interosseus muscles, *Clin Orthop* 140:23-25, 1979.
7. Halpern AA, Mochizuki RM: Compartment syndrome of the interosseus muscles of hand: a clinical and anatomic review, *Orthop Rev* 9:121-127, 1980.
8. Holden CEA: The pathology and prevention of Volkmann's ischemic contracture, *J Bone Joint Surgery* 61B:296-300, 1979.
9. Hussman J, Kucan JO, Zamboni WA: Elevated compartmental pressures after closure of a forearm burn wound with a skin-stretching device, *Burns* 23(2):154-156, 1997.
10. Krimmer H, Hahn P, Lanz U: Free gracilis muscle transplantation for hand reconstruction, *Clin Orthop* 314:13-18, 1995.
11. Kucan JO, Smoot EC, Fallon P: Combined treatment of the burn wound with Travase, biobrane, 5% Mafenide acetate solution. In American Burn Association meeting abstract, Washington, DC 1987.
12. Mabee JR: Compartment syndrome: a complication of acute extremity trauma, *J Emerg Med* 12(5):651-656, 1994.
13. Matsen FA, et al: Diagnosis and management of compartmental syndromes, *J Bone Joint Surg* 62A:286-291, 1980.
14. Matsen FA III, Rorabeck CH: Compartment syndromes, *AAOS Instr Course Lecture* 38:463-472, 1989.
15. Mubarak SJ, Hargens AR: Acute compartment syndromes, *Surg Clin North Am* 63:539-565, 1983.
16. Mubarak SJ, Owens CA, Hargens AR, et al: Acute compartment syndromes: diagnosis and treatment with the aid of the Wick catheter, *J Bone Joint Surg* 60A:1091-1095, 1978.
17. Naidu SH, Heppenstall RB: Compartment syndrome of the forearm and hand, *Hand Clin* 10(1):13-27, 1994.
18. Peters CL, Scott SM: Compartment syndrome in the forearm following fractures of the radial head or neck in children, *J Bone Joint Surg* (7):1070-1074, 1995.
19. Santyl Ointment, manufactured by Advance Biofactures Corp., 35 Wilbur Street, Lynbrook, NY 11563. Distributed by Knoll Pharmaceuticals, 30 N. Jefferson Rd, Whippany, NJ 07981.
20. Schnall SB, Holtom PD, Silva E: Compartment syndrome associated with infection of the upper extremity, *Clin Orthop* Sep(306):128-131, 1994.
21. Sheridan GW, Martin FA: Fasciotomy in treatment of the acute compartment syndrome, *J Bone Joint Surg* 58A:112, 1976.
22. Strauss MB, Hargens AR, Gershuni DH, et al: Reduction of skeletal muscle necrosis using intermittent hyperbaric oxygen in a model compartment syndrome, *J Bone Joint Surg* 65(A):656, 1983.
23. Summerfield SL, Folberg CR, Weiss APC: Compartment syndrome of the pronator quadratus: a case report, *J Hand Surg* 22A:266-268, 1997.
24. Thomas WO, Harris CN, D'Amore TF, Parry SW: Bilateral forearm and hand compartment syndrome following thrombolysis for acute myocardial infarction: a case report, *J Emerg Med* 12(4):467-472, 1994.
25. Volkmann R: Die ischaemisschen Muskallahmangen und Kontnakturen, *Zentralbl Chir* 8:801-803, 1881.
26. Whitesides TE, Harvey TC, Morimoto K, et al: Tissue pressure measurement as a determinant for the need of fasciotomy, *Clin Orthop* 113:43, 1975.

27. Wong HP, Zamboni WA, Stephenson LL: Effect of hyperbaric oxygen on skeletal muscle necrosis following primary and secondary ischemia in a rat model, *Surg Forum* 47:705-707, 1996.

28. Zamboni WA: The microcirculation and ischemia reperfusion: basic mechanisms of hyperbaric oxygen. In Kindwall EP, Larson DL (editors): *Hyperbaric medicine practice,* Flagstaff, Ariz, 1994, Best Publishing Company, 1994.

29. Zamboni WA: Applications of hyperbaric oxygen therapy in plastic surgery. In Orani G, Maroni A, Wattel F (editors): *Handbook on hyperbaric medicine,* 1996, Springer-Verlag, Italia SRL.

30. Zamboni WA, Roth AC, Russell RC, et al: Morphologic analysis of the microcirculation during reperfusion of ischemic skeletal muscle and the effect of hyperbaric oxygen, *Plast Reconstr Surg* 91:1110-1123, 1993.

PART III

FRACTURES AND DISLOCATIONS

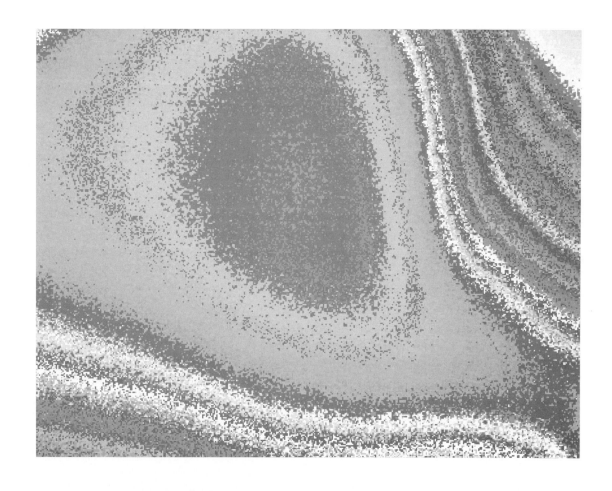

CHAPTER

Amputations

104

Gregory J. Adamson
Ronald E. Palmer

The beauty and strength of the mechanical construction lie not in one part or in another, but in the harmonious concatenation which all the parts, soft and hard, rigid and flexible, tension bearing and pressure-bearing, make up together.

Sir D-Arcy Wentworth Thompson[57]

INTRODUCTION

Before embarking on a discussion of hand amputations, it is important to review the primary functions of the hand. The primary motor functions of the hand include prehension (grasp) and pinch. *Grasp* describes holding an object in the palm. The acts of carrying an attaché or climbing a rope are examples of grasping function. The action of the ulnar three digits is pivotal to the performance of power grasp in a normal hand.[5,47] Grasp requires a minimum of one mobile digit.[47] *Pinch* describes holding an object between the opposed thumb pad and the fingers, usually the index and long fingertips. Manipulating a zipper, a toothpick, or a writing instrument are examples of pinch. Pinch requires a minimum of the thumb and a single digit, or their functional substitute.[58]

Another primary function of the hand is that of a sensory organ.[8,27,35] The property of tactile gnosis allows the normal hand to "see."[35] This is obvious to anyone who has carefully watched small children playing, and yet this is a function that most take for granted daily. Loss of any of these three primary functions of prehension, pinch, and sensibility truly disables the hand.

In the past 3 decades there has been an explosion in our understanding and application of microvascular techniques for replantation of amputated limbs and digits.[65] Not all devascularized parts, however, can be revascularized, and in many patients completion of the amputation remains the best surgical option. The hand surgeon who performs a digital or hand amputation must have a thorough knowledge of anatomy and should attempt to preserve as much function as possible.

Treatment begins by obtaining a thorough medical and social history. Many factors may influence the physician's assessment and treatment recommendation, including the patient's age, general medical condition, nicotine use, occupation and functional demands of the hand, and the presence of associated injuries.[25] The mechanism of injury should be documented. Clearly, crush and avulsion injuries have a poorer prognosis than do sharp injuries. A thorough examination of the hand and upper extremity is then performed. This includes testing light touch, two-point discrimination, and pinprick sensibility, as well as tests of soft tissue viability, such as capillary refill and tissue turgor. A preliminary check for tendon function is performed if possible. Adequate radiographs should be obtained before transporting the patient to surgery.

A complete assessment is sometimes not possible in the emergency room and must be completed in surgery after the patient has been adequately anesthetized.[4,26] The surgeon must have a complete armamentarium of reconstructive and amputation techniques and exercise sound surgical judgment after assessing the degree of injury to determine the best surgical course of action. It should be understood and conveyed to the patient that the severity of the injury will usually correlate with the final outcome.[29] The surgeon should thoroughly discuss and obtain informed consent from the patient for all proposed and possible procedures that may be anticipated. We favor a frank discussion with the patient or family, not erring on the side of unreasonable expectations nor extinguishing the hope for a functionally acceptable limb. The physician should be realistic in his approach when explaining the surgical possibilities but remain compassionate and caring to the concerned patient and/or family. Failure to foster patient trust and understanding in this situation may lead to legal consequences, despite superlative surgery.

The advantages of a judicious amputation should be understood by both the surgeon and patient. These include a short convalescence, an early return of hand function and return to work,[22] and a low probability of further surgery. In our experience, these advantages have sometimes led not only to patient acceptance but the desire to proceed with an amputation instead of an advanced reconstructive procedure.

Important goals after an amputation include patient and

family acceptance of the altered limb and a return to the community and the work place.[33] It is not uncommon, however, for such an injury to lead to depression. An emotional progression similar to the Kubler-Ross[24] description of the response to death and dying is often noted in amputees. The patient experiences initial shock and denial, followed by anger, bargaining, depression, grief, and finally a peaceful acceptance. A team approach is often helpful, with support offered by a surgeon, therapists, a psychiatrist or psychologist, hospital staff, clergy, family, and friends.[33,64] Finally, in selected patients, an accomplished prosthetist may provide important prosthetic care.

DIGITAL AMPUTATIONS

INDICATIONS

The most common indication for digital amputation continues to be complex, nonsalvageable, traumatic injuries (Figure 104-1).[22] Additional indications include significant vascular disorders, necrosis, infections, tumors, congenital anomalies, and minimally functional/dysesthetic digits (Figure 104-2). A single-digit amputation, proximal to the flexor digitorum superficialis (FDS) tendon insertion, remains a relative indication for primary closure, even when the finger is replantable (Figures 104-3 and 104-4).[60]

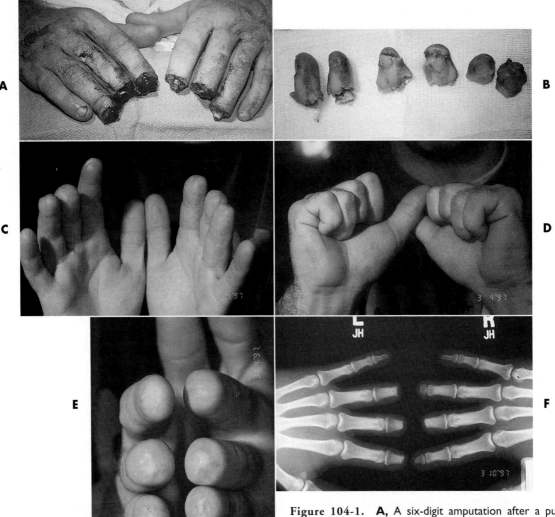

Figure 104-1. A, A six-digit amputation after a punch-press injury. **B,** Crushed fingertips, not suitable for replantation. Note red-line sign of long fingertips. **C,** Very functional digits after an amputation. The patient returned to work 8 weeks after surgery. **D,** The hands have excellent grip. **E,** Good quality digital tip skin, with near normal sensibility. **F,** Note the uniformity of soft tissue coverage in all digits.

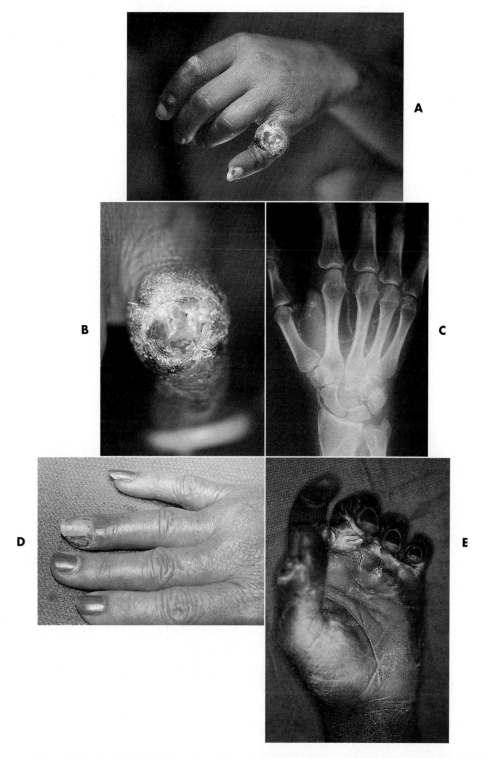

Figure 104-2. **A,** A diabetic patient with a chronic dorsal ulcer of the fifth finger. **B,** The PIP joint is exposed. **C,** A plain-film radiograph shows advanced arterial disease with vessel calcification. **D,** Another diabetic patient with full-thickness, radial, nail-fold necrosis and underlying exposed and necrotic bone. **E,** A frostbite injury, with mummified fingers, in an unfortunate alcoholic patient. The level of soft tissue demarcation is now evident.

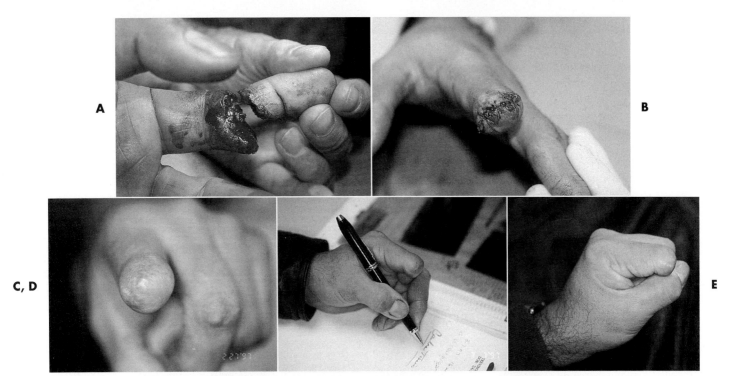

Figure 104-3. **A,** Patient with an industrial press injury to the left index finger. The only structure in continuity was the radial digital nerve. **B,** A loose primary closure using available ulnar skin. **C,** A healed amputation stump with good skin cover and excellent sensibility. **D,** The patient has "crossed-over" pinch function to the long finger. **E,** There is excellent motion, with the injured finger clearly aiding in grasp function. The patient returned to manual labor 6 weeks after surgery.

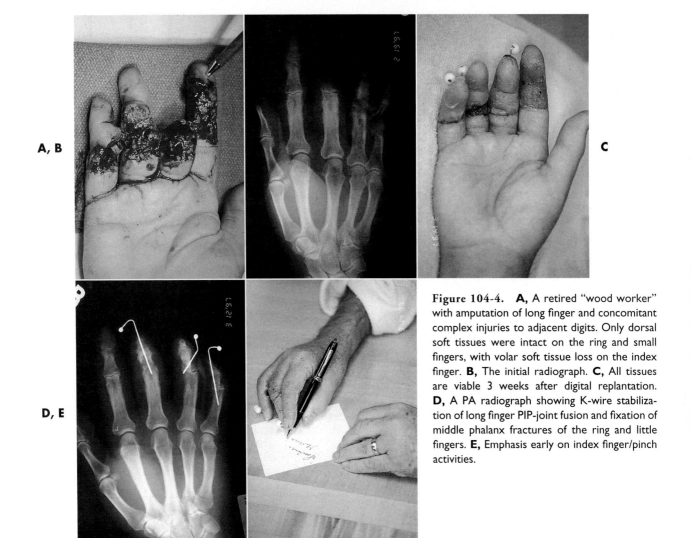

Figure 104-4. **A,** A retired "wood worker" with amputation of long finger and concomitant complex injuries to adjacent digits. Only dorsal soft tissues were intact on the ring and small fingers, with volar soft tissue loss on the index finger. **B,** The initial radiograph. **C,** All tissues are viable 3 weeks after digital replantation. **D,** A PA radiograph showing K-wire stabilization of long finger PIP-joint fusion and fixation of middle phalanx fractures of the ring and little fingers. **E,** Emphasis early on index finger/pinch activities.

OPERATIONS

The goals of digital amputation include stump coverage with adequate and sensate skin, preservation of length, and maintenance of the FDS insertion whenever possible.[20] Loss of FDS function will diminish grip strength and active digital flexion, with complete loss at the proximal interphalangeal (PIP) joint and approximately 50% loss at the metacarpophalangeal (MCP) joint.[31] Several techniques to close digital amputations have been advanced. They differ primarily in the manner in which soft tissue coverage is obtained. The techniques include healing by secondary intention alone,[25,30,34] skeletal shortening and closure, skin-graft coverage, local and distant pedicle flap coverage,[2,6,21] replantation, and microvascular flap coverage techniques.

We favor the simplest appropriate and reliable form of coverage available to the treating physician, understanding that there is clear variability in training, microvascular skill, and philosophy among practicing hand surgeons today. We treat the majority of patients in whom amputation is indicated by minimal skeletal shortening and loose soft tissue closure. The advantages are numerous and include minimal additional trauma to the injured digit and a simple and short one-stage surgical procedure that usually provides an excellent functional result. Primary amputation closure permits earlier motion and return to work compared with complex reconstructive procedures, such as replantation or free tissue transfer.

TECHNIQUE

After adequate anesthesia, gross wound contamination is removed with saline-soaked sponges. Grease and dirt are then removed with a mechanical soap cleansing. The limb is then surgically prepped and draped in a standard fashion. We presently use Techni-Care scrub solution, which combines excellent antimicrobial action with minimal tissue toxicity.[55] The wound, under tourniquet control, is then copiously irrigated with sterile saline. A mechanical pulsatile system is used when there is evidence of gross contamination. A short period should be spent identifying pertinent anatomical structures before beginning the surgical debridement. Nonviable, marginally viable, and remaining grossly contaminated tissues are excised. The soft tissue envelope is assessed. Palmar skin is best suited for distal stump coverage because it is durable and has good sensibility. We will, however, use any available distal skin to facilitate a primary closure and maximize length (see Figure 104-3).

In a traumatic guillotine-type amputation, we fashion somewhat abbreviated fishmouth flaps. The bone is shortened as needed to a point approximately 4 mm proximal to the soft tissue envelope. The distal end of the bone should be contoured to remove any bony prominences. This prevents a bulbous appearance of the stump,[40] and allows for a more even distribution of forces across the newly reconstructed stump tip. The flexor tendon or tendons are then extracted from the retinacular sheath with the aid of a small clamp,

examined carefully for any evidence of gross contamination, then transected and allowed to retract back into the retinacular sheath. Any protruding remnants of the extensor mechanism are trimmed just proximal to the level of the final bone cut. The digital flexors and extensors should not be sutured to each other over the end of the stump. Suturing them together may limit the excursion of both the flexor and extensor mechanisms, resulting in Quadrigia syndrome.[39,61]

We also do not recommend selective reattachment of the flexors or extensors to bone. Selective reattachment may cause a significant imbalance of digital motion in the injured as well as in the uninjured fingers. Retraction of the profundus after division over the middle phalanx can, however, create pull on the lumbrical muscle and produce a lumbrical plus deformity. The digital arteries are then identified and cauterized or ligated. The digital nerves are identified, distracted distally approximately 1 to 1.5 cm from the amputation site, and transected. This allows the remaining nerve ends to retract into healthy soft tissues and decreases the incidence of symptomatic neuroma formation. Sometimes it is necessary to gently and circumferentially dissect a digital nerve proximally to permit adequate advancement before transection. All visible vessels are cauterized, and the tourniquet is then released. A meticulous final hemostasis is then performed. Soft tissue closure is then carried out using interrupted nonabsorbable suture (Figure 104-5).

Skin flaps should be reapproximated with little or no tension. It is not uncommon for small areas of the skin closure to be without epithelium (see Figure 104-3), although in these areas there should be adequate subcutaneous coverage of bone. In our experience, these areas epithelialize within 1 to 2 weeks of surgery. This method of closure is advocated to maximize bone length. For near transverse amputations where any further shortening would result in loss of the insertion of the FDS, we favor the use of a V-Y volar advancement flap,[2] cross-finger flap,[21] or thenar flap[6,56] over further bone shortening. A cross-finger or distant pedicle flap, such as a thoracoabdominal, upper inner arm, or groin flap is utilized for more oblique amputations with significant volar soft tissue loss. We have not employed a full length volar advancement flap[49] for such a defect in a digit because of the possibility of disruption of the dorsal soft tissue arterial supply and subsequent dorsal vascular embarrassment.[25]

A bulky and mildly compressive dressing is applied, followed by plaster splints. Gentle range of motion exercises are begun at 3 to 5 days after surgery. We recommend elevation and rest of the limb between periods of exercise to reduce inflammation. A large percentage of our patients are placed on antiinflammatory agents at approximately 1 week after surgery to facilitate recovery.

OUTCOMES

Hand function after digital amputation can be quite good. A simple amputation may indeed result in better overall function than a complicated reconstruction or replantation.[1,60]

Several complications of digital amputation have been

observed. The most common complication is that of a symptomatic neuroma. Prevention, by facilitating the transected nerve ends to retract into healthy tissues, cannot be overemphasized (see Figure 104-5, *D*). Another preventative measure is the early return to vigorous hand use by the patient. Fisher found that with rapid return to work, only four of 144 patients developed a painful neuroma, two of which required surgery.[14] Desensitization therapy results in adequate resolution in the majority of patients with symptomatic neuromas.[32] Several surgical treatment alternatives have been advanced for patients with recalcitrant digital neuromas.[17,23,54] We favor relocation of the painful neuroma into an adequate soft tissue bed, where it is less likely to be disturbed.[19] Others have inserted the neuromas into drill holes in the bone or placed the cut nerve end into a vein graft, which is used to direct the regenerating axons away from the amputation stump.

St. Laurent and Duclos[52] advocate an interesting technique to avoid painful neuroma formation. They cite as their inspiration the island pedicle flap technique of Littler. The digital nerves are kept in continuity with a small region of the finger pulp, which is used as an acral skin graft for the resultant stump. Neuroma formation is avoided because the nerves are never truly cut.

Tethering of a transected profundus tendon in the surrounding soft tissues can lead to Quadrigia syndrome.[39,61] The muscle bellies of the profundus tendons have numerous connections and function like a single muscle unit. Diminished excursion of a tethered profundus tendon during flexion

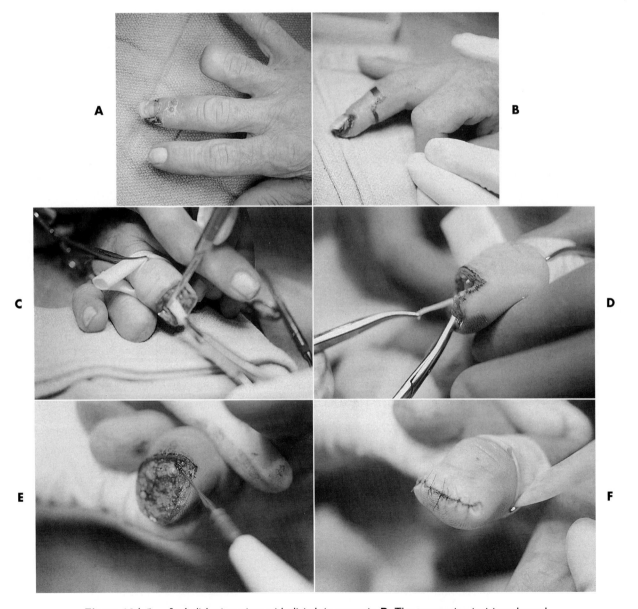

Figure 104-5. **A,** A diabetic patient with digital tip necrosis. **B,** The amputation incision planned with a longer volar flap. **C,** Distraction and transection of the profundus tendon. **D,** Distraction and transection of the digital nerves. **E,** Meticulous hemostasis obtained with the tourniquet temporarily removed. **F,** Closure almost complete. Suture line has been brought dorsal, maximizing use of the palmar skin for the new tip.

limits the excursion of the neighboring digital profundus tendons because of these connections. Early motion to limit adhesions helps to prevent this problem. Diminished motion of the neighboring distal interphalangeal (DIP) joints is the indication for surgical release of the tethered profundus tendon.[39]

The lumbrical plus finger[42] is another potential complication of digital amputation. The lumbrical muscle originates on the profundus tendon and inserts into the radial lateral band of the extensor mechanism. Proximal migration of a severed profundus tendon with an intact lumbrical can cause increased tension on the extensor mechanism. This can lead to paradoxical extension of the PIP joint of the affected finger during grasp. This problem rarely occurs and is effectively treated by incision or partial excision of the lumbrical apparatus.[48]

Two common problems after a digital amputation are cold intolerance and dysesthesia. Herndon[18] has found dysesthesia to be much more common after V-Y or full-length volar advancement flap coverage of amputation stumps. He also reported decreased sensibility in patients with volar V-Y flaps compared with other stump-closure methods.[18,59] Backman et al[3] reported the incidence of cold intolerance after amputation

to be equivalent to patients with replanted digits. Fortunately, cold intolerance and dysesthesia will usually progressively resolve for up to 2 years after injury.

THUMB AMPUTATIONS

Grasp function after loss of a digit can be nearly normal. Thumb amputation proximal to the midportion of the proximal phalanx, however, results in loss of pinch function. This fact should heighten our awareness when treating a patient with a thumb amputation in which adequate preservation of length for pinch is vital to hand function.

Thumb amputation continues to be a good indication of replantation, although amputations distal to the mid-proximal phalanx are well treated by revision amputation. Distal thumb amputations have function equivalent to replanted thumbs (Figure 104-6).[16] Surgical treatment of these injuries is similar

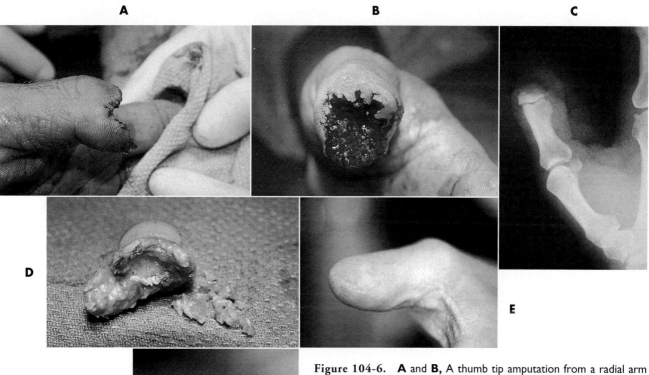

Figure 104-6. **A** and **B,** A thumb tip amputation from a radial arm saw. **C,** An oblique radiograph, with amputation through the base of the distal phalanx. **D,** No vessels were available in the amputated thumb. **E** and **F,** The appearance and function of the thumb 4 months after surgery. The patient resumed work as a carpenter 4 weeks after surgery.

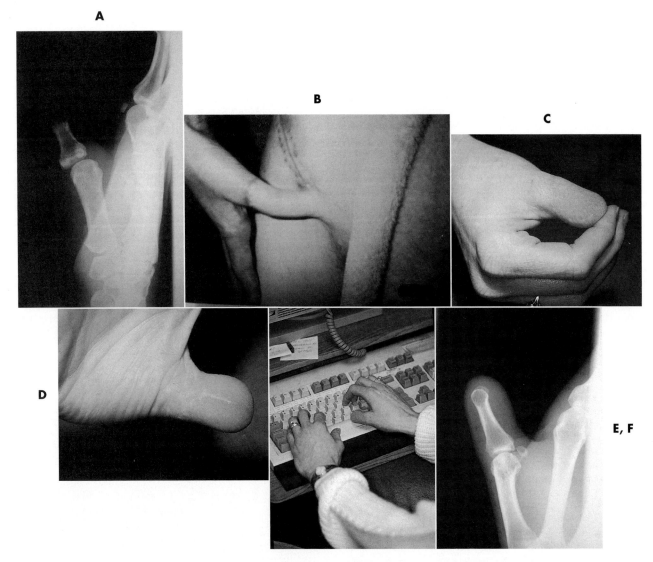

Figure 104-7. A, A patient with a thumb avulsion injury. Note loss of soft tissue distal to the MCP joint. **B,** The skeletonized thumb is covered with a tubed groin flap. **C** and **D,** The appearance of the thumb 20 months after surgery. The digit has poor sensibility, with a two-point discrimination of approximately 20 mm. **E,** The patient is employed as an office administrator and wishes no reconstructive surgery to improve sensibility. **F,** There is excellent soft tissue coverage of the proximal phalanx.

to that for digital amputation, with a few notable exceptions. We sometimes use a full-length volar advancement flap for coverage to preserve length.[35] A midlateral incision from the amputation stump is made along the proximal phalanx and cut in a V at the MCP flexion crease. Dorsal branches of the digital arteries and nerves should be dissected but preserved. The volar soft tissue is elevated off the flexor tendon sheath and advanced distally. The IP joint, if it remains, can also be flexed.[7,25,41] The maximum volar advancement of this flap is approximately 1 cm. Early, active range-of-motion exercises are indicated to straighten the thumb and prevent flexion contractures.

When larger soft tissue defects are present, a distant pedicle flap or a cross-finger flap are required for closure (Figure 104-7). Thumb amputations proximal to the midproximal phalanx would require some form of reconstruction, which is detailed in Chapters 125 and 126. If future microvascular

thumb reconstruction is contemplated, the digital nerves in the proximal stump should not be shortened at the time of primary wound closure.

METACARPAL-LEVEL AMPUTATIONS

Amputations at the MCP joint and distal metacarpal level are treated much the same way we treat digital amputations. Rotation flaps, pedicle flaps, and free flaps are sometimes necessary to obtain coverage. We often favor a trial period of at least 6 months for patients with traumatic amputations before any further reconstructive surgery. This allows the patient to

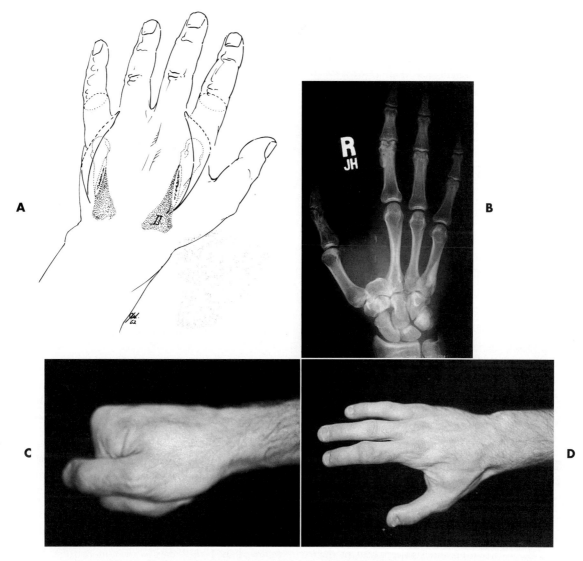

Figure 104-8. **A,** Schematic of second and fifth ray amputation. **B,** Radiograph of a patient's hand 2 years after second-ray amputation. **C** and **D,** There is improved hand appearance and excellent function. (**A** courtesy J.W. Littler.)

more fully understand his or her functional limitations. Patients with amputation at the MCP level may benefit from a subsequent ray amputation or border digit to central ray translocation.

INDEX RAY AMPUTATION

The prominent second metacarpal stump that results from an index MCP disarticulation or distal metacarpal-level amputation may act as an obstruction within the widened first web.[10] This is particularly true for patients such as artisans who depend on precision pinch for their employment. Some patients are equally disturbed with the appearance of their hand, which is improved by an index ray amputation.

OPERATIONS

The technique of ray amputation has been described in detail.[10,37] A racquet-shaped incision is made with a proximal extension over the dorsal surface of the second metacarpal. The extensor tendons are divided proximally, and the second metacarpal is exposed in a subperiosteal plane. The proximal metaphyseal osteotomy should preserve the insertions of the flexor carpi radialis and the extensor carpi radialis longus and brevis tendons. The digital flexor tendons are distracted and then transected. The neurovascular bundles are transected, and the distal ends of the digital nerves are carefully placed between the remaining first and second dorsal interosseous muscles. Skin flaps are trimmed as needed, and the wound is closed. We do not suture the first dorsal interosseous tendon to the second dorsal interosseous tendon because this may create a radial abduction deformity.[37] Motion is begun approximately 1 week after surgery (Figure 104-8).

OUTCOMES

Murray et al[37] reported a 20% decrease in grip strength after an index ray amputation. Garcia-Moral et al[15] reported a 14% loss in grip strength. It is our belief that a metacarpal amputation should not decrease grip strength any more than a previous MCP disarticulation. All ray amputations, however, do narrow the palm. This will destabilize grasp somewhat, particularly during concomitant forearm rotation. Murray et al[37] report a 50% decrease in pronation strength subsequent to index ray amputation, compared with the normal limb. Tender neuromas in the new widened first web space have also been reported.[13,37]

FIFTH RAY AMPUTATION

The indication for a fifth ray amputation is primarily that of an improved cosmetic appearance. Ironically, this can sometimes also lead to increased limb function because the patient conceals the hand less often. The technique and results are similar to those described for index ray amputation.

THIRD OR FOURTH RAY AMPUTATION

Patients who have had a previous amputation of the ring or long finger may sometimes drop small objects held in their palm through the widened central "web space." In addition, amputations proximal to the transverse intermetacarpal ligament can lead to instability and volar prominence of the metacarpal, with resultant discomfort.[44] There is also an obvious cosmetic deformity.

OPERATIONS

Alternatives for the patient desirous of functional and cosmetic improvement include simple metacarpal excision with distal interspace narrowing or border ray translocation to a central ray position. We favor the latter procedure. We particularly see the benefit of the index to long ray translocation, given that pinch activities are facilitated with two parallel digits. These procedures have been well described in the literature.[9,44,45]

A dorsal longitudinal and volar zig-zag incision is planned to excise a wedge of soft tissue both dorsally and volarly between the index and long metacarpals for an index to long ray translocation or between the little and ring metacarpals for a little to ring ray translocation. The skin incisions distally can be fashioned to avoid entering the web space.[43] The central

metacarpal is removed after a proximal metaphyseal osteotomy is performed. The two interosseous muscles associated with this ray are also excised. The border metacarpal is then sectioned and translocated to a central position. A careful check of alignment, with emphasis on rotation, is performed before stabilization with Kirschner wires (K wires) proximally and distally. The deep intermetacarpal ligament is repaired. Guarded motion is begun approximately 2 weeks after surgery.

OUTCOMES

The results of simple metacarpal excision with distal interspace narrowing compared with ray translocation are comparable.[50] Steichen and Idler[51] reported their results of metacarpal excision and distal interspace narrowing. They found a 26% diminished grip strength of the affected hand. There was no diminution of motion. Colen et al,[12] reporting on border metacarpal to central metacarpal translocations, noted a 20% decrease in grip strength and a 9% loss of motion, compared with the unaffected hand.

COMPLEX HAND AMPUTATIONS

The primary functions of prehension, pinch, and sensibility must be considered, and appropriate reconstructive procedures employed when treating patients who have had multiple digits and/or large parts of the hand injured. Chase's concepts of conservation of usable parts are of great value.[11] When tissue viability is in doubt, a judicious initial debridement can be followed in 1 to 2 days with a more formal procedure. It should also be remembered that it is sometimes best to expeditiously refer such a patient to a more experienced hand surgeon.

Rose and Bunke[46] have emphasized the need to focus reconstructive efforts on the thumb and central rays. Amputated digits can be redistributed as needed to maximize function. The importance of an opposable thumb cannot be overemphasized. Pinch and modified grasp are possible with a thumb and palm alone (Figure 104-9). First web space deepening, toe to thumb transfer, pollicization, distraction osteogenesis, and other reconstructive techniques can be used to achieve this end. (Please refer to Chapters 125 and 126 for a thorough description of these techniques.) There have been a wide variety of reconstructive techniques developed to treat patients with mangling hand injuries with loss of all digits, the thumb, and sometimes the entire hand, when replantation is not possible or fails. The Krukenberg procedure[38,53] has been shown to be quite effective, allowing modified grasp and pinch between the distal ulnar and radial stumps. Microvascular surgeons have restored pinch and grasp function in patients with hand and forearm amputations by the transfer of toes and contralateral fingers to the remaining stump.[36,62,63] The varied

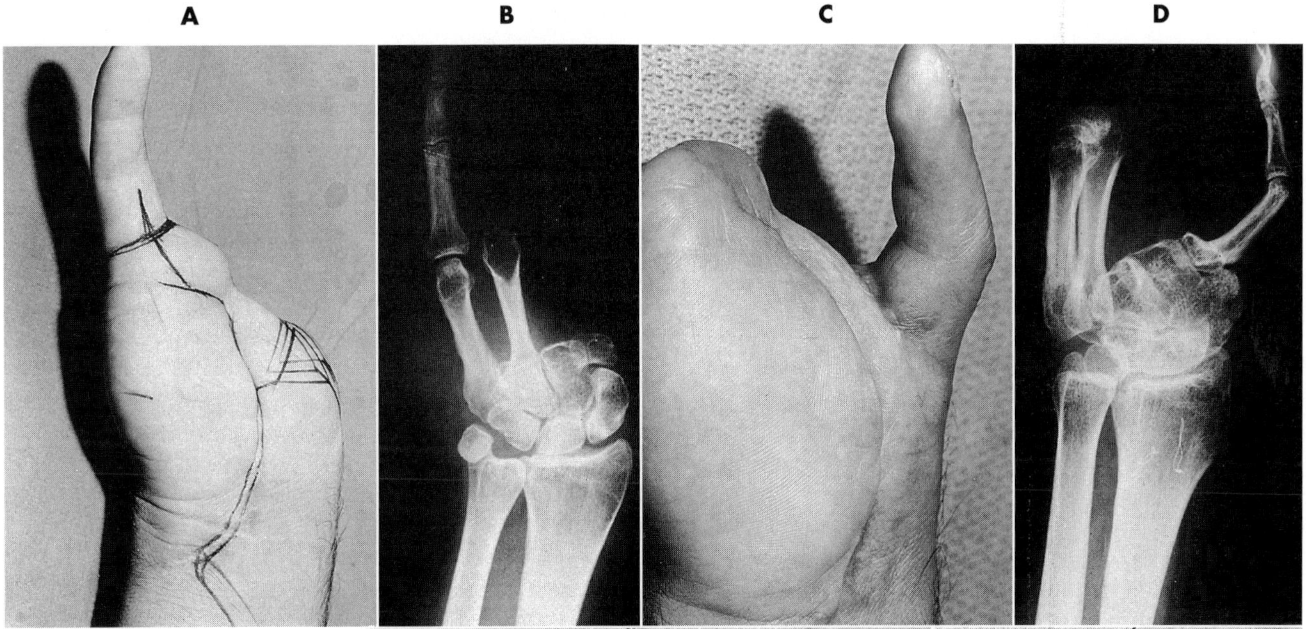

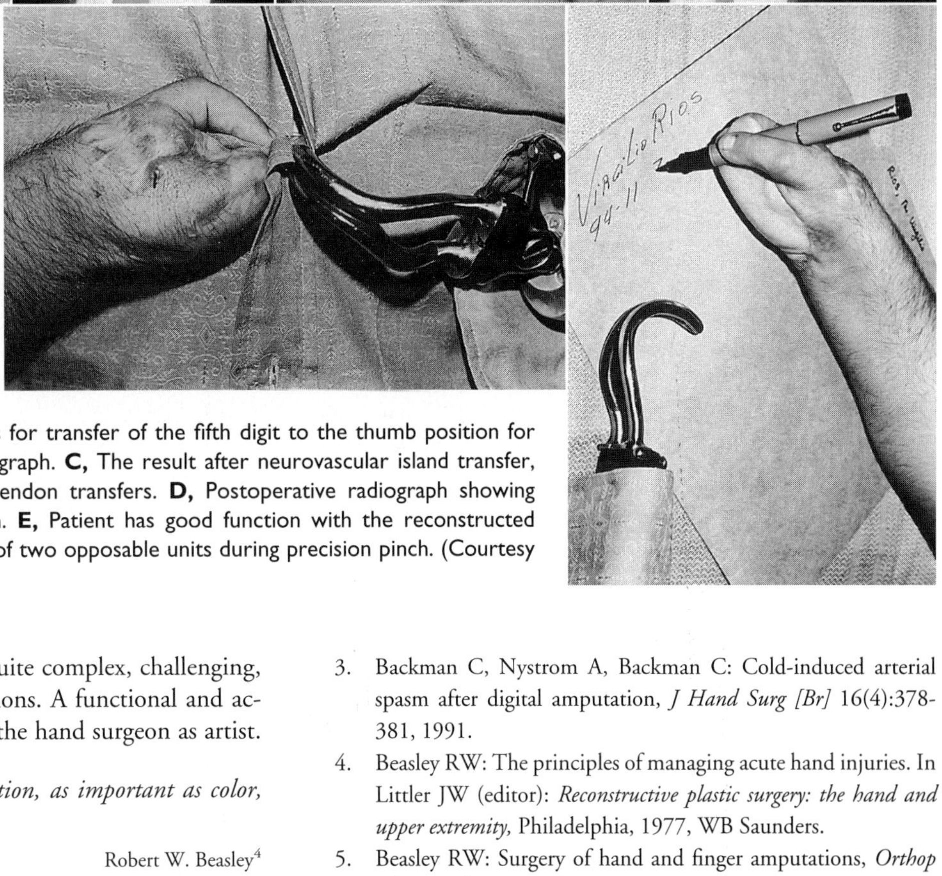

Figure 104-9. A, Planned incisions for transfer of the fifth digit to the thumb position for opposition. **B,** Preoperative AP radiograph. **C,** The result after neurovascular island transfer, with separate flexor and extensor tendon transfers. **D,** Postoperative radiograph showing proximal phalanx to trapezoid fusion. **E,** Patient has good function with the reconstructed hand. **F,** Note the excellent position of two opposable units during precision pinch. (Courtesy J.W. Littler.)

nature of these injuries has led to quite complex, challenging, and innovative reconstructive solutions. A functional and acceptable outcome truly exemplifies the hand surgeon as artist.

There is an aesthetic quality in function, as important as color, number, and form.

Robert W. Beasley[4]

REFERENCES

1. Arnaud JP, Mallet T, Pecout C, et al: Isolated complex injuries to the index: the place of amputation, *J Chir Paris* 123:321-325, 1986.

2. Atasoy E, Ioqkimidis E, Kasdan D, et al: Reconstruction of the amputated fingertip with triangular volar flap: a new surgical procedure, *J Bone Joint Surg* 52A:921-926, 1970.

3. Backman C, Nystrom A, Backman C: Cold-induced arterial spasm after digital amputation, *J Hand Surg [Br]* 16(4):378-381, 1991.

4. Beasley RW: The principles of managing acute hand injuries. In Littler JW (editor): *Reconstructive plastic surgery: the hand and upper extremity,* Philadelphia, 1977, WB Saunders.

5. Beasley RW: Surgery of hand and finger amputations, *Orthop Clin North Am* 12:763, 1981.

6. Beasley RW: Principles of soft tissue replacement for the hand, *J Hand Surg* 8:781-784, 1983.

7. Brunelli F, Brunelli G, Vigasio A: Dorsocubital flap of the thumb: an anatomical study with clinical applications (apropos of 22 cases) *Ann Chir Plast Esthet* 41(3):259-268, 1996.

8. Bunnell S: *Surgery of the hand,* Philadelphia, 1944, JB Lippincott.

9. Carroll RE: Transposition of the index finger to replace the middle finger, *Clin Orthop* 13:27, 1959.

10. Chase RA: The damaged index digit: a source of components to restore the crippled hand, *J Bone Joint Surg* 50A:1152, 1968.

11. Chase RA: Conservation of usable structures in injured hands. In Littler JW (editor): *Reconstructive plastic surgery: the hand and upper extremity,* Philadelphia, 1977, WB Saunders.

12. Colen L, Bunkis J, Gordon L, et al: Functional assessment of ray transfer for central digital loss, *J Hand Surg [Am]* 10:232, 1985.

13. Fisher EG, Goldner JL: Index ray deletion: complication and sequel, *J Bone Joint Surg* 54A:898, 1971.

14. Fisher GT, Boswick JA Jr: Neuroma formation following digital amputations, *J Trauma* 23(2):136-142, 1983.

15. Garcia-Moral CA, Putman J, Taylor PA, et al: 9-Ray resection of the index finger, *Orthop Trans* 15:71, 1991.

16. Goldner RD, Nunley JA, Belding NR, et al: 111 thumb amputations (replantation versus revision), *Microsurg* 11:243, 1990.

17. Gorkish K, Boese-Landgraf J, Vaubel E: Treatment and prevention of amputation neuromas and hand surgery, *Plast Reconstr Surg* 73(2):293-299, 1984.

18. Herndon JH: Amputations of the hand. In Evasts CM (editor): *Surgery of the musculoskeletal system,* ed 2, New York, 1990, Churchill Livingstone.

19. Herndon JH, Eaton RG, Littler JW: Management of painful neuromas in the hand, *J Bone Joint Surg* 58A:369, 1976.

20. Herndon JH, Littler JW, Watson JW, Eaton RC: Traumatic amputation of the thumb and three fingers: treatment by distal pollicitization, *J Bone Joint Surg* 57A:708-709, 1975.

21. Kappelda DA, Burech JG: Cross finger flaps: an established reconstructive procedure, *Hand Clin* 1:677-684, 1985.

22. Kleinert J: Amputation and prosthetics. In Manske P (editor): *Hand surgery update,* 1996, American Academy of Orthopaedic Surgeons.

23. Kon M, Bleom JJ: The treatment of amputation neuromas and fingers with a centrocentral nerve union, *Ann Plast Surg* 18(6):506-510, 1987.

24. Kubler-Ross E: *Questions and answers on death and dying,* New York, 1974, McMillan.

25. Leclercq C, Brunelli F: Treatment of finger tip amputations. In Peimer C (editor): *Surgery of the hand and upper extremity,* New York, 1996, McGraw-Hill.

26. Littler JW: Neurovascular pedicle transfer of tissue in reconstructive surgery, *J Bone Joint Surg* 38A:917, 1956.

27. Littler JW: Principles of reconstructive surgery of the hand. In Littler JW (editor): *Reconstructive plastic surgery of the hand and upper extremity,* Philadelphia, 1977, WB Saunders.

28. Littler JW: Surgery of the hand: introduction. In Littler JW (editor): *Reconstructive plastic surgery of the hand and upper extremity,* Philadelphia, 1977, WB Saunders.

29. Littler JW, Herndon JH, Thompson JS: Examination of the hand. In Littler JW (editor): *Reconstructive plastic surgery: the hand and upper extremity,* Philadelphia, 1977, WB Saunders.

30. Louis DS, Palmer AR, Burney R: Open treatment of digital tip injuries, *JAMA* 244:697-698, 1980.

31. Louis DS: Amputations. In Green DP (editor): *Operative hand surgery,* ed 3, New York, 1993, Churchill Livingstone.

32. Mackinnon SE, Dellon AL: *Surgery of the peripheral nerve,* New York, 1988, Thieme Medical Publishers.

33. Mendelsohn RL, Burech JG, Polack EP, et al: The psychological impact of traumatic amputations: a team approach (physician, therapist, and psychologist): *Hand Clin* 2:577-583, 1986.

34. Mennen U, Wiese A: Fingertip injuries management with semi-occlusive dressing, *J Hand Surg [Br]* 18:416, 1993.

35. Moberg E: Aspects of sensation and reconstructive surgery of the upper extremity, *J Bone Joint Surg* 46A:817-825, 1964.

36. Morrison WA, O'Brien BM, MacLeon AM: Ring finger transfer and reconstruction of transmetacarpal amputations, *J Hand Surg [Am]* 9:4-11, 1984.

37. Murray JF, Carman W, MacKenzie JK: Transmetacarpal amputation of the index finger: clinical assessment of hand strength and complications, *J Hand Surg [Am]* 2:471, 1977.

38. Nathan PA, Trung NB: The Krukenberg operation: a modified technique avoiding skin grafts, *J Hand Surg [Am]* 2(2):127-130, 1977.

39. Neu BR, Murray JF, Mackenzie JK: Profundus tendon blockage: quadriga and finger amputations, *J Hand Surg [Am]* 10:878-883, 1985.

40. Omer G: Upper extremity amputation. In Jupiter JB (editor): *Flynn's hand surgery,* Baltimore, 1991, Williams & Wilkins.

41. Omokawa S, Mizumoto S, Iwai M, et al: Innervated radial thenar flap for sensory reconstruction of fingers, *J Hand Surg [Am]* 21(3):373-380, 1996.

42. Parkes A: The "lumbrical plus" finger, *J Bone Joint Surg* 53B:236, 1971.

43. Plasschaert MJ, Hage JJ: A web-saving incision for amputation of the third or fourth ray of the hand, *J Hand Surg [Br]* 13(3):340-341, 1988.

44. Posner MA: Transposition of the index ray. In Blair WF (editor): *Techniques in hand surgery,* Baltimore, 1996, Williams & Wilkins.

45. Posner MA: Transposition of the small ray. In Blair WF (editor): *Techniques in hand surgery,* Baltimore, 1996, Williams & Wilkins.

46. Rose EH, Bunke HJ: Selective finger transposition and primary metacarpal ray resection in multi-digit amputations of the hand, *J Hand Surg [Am]* 8:178, 1983.

47. Slocum DB: Amputations of fingers and the hand, *Clin Orthop* 15:35-59, 1959.

48. Smith RJ: Intrinsic contracture. In Green DP (editor): *Operative hand surgery,* ed 3, New York, 1993, Churchill Livingstone.

49. Snow JW: The use of a volar flap for repair finger tip amputations: a preliminary report, *Plastic Reconstr Surg* 52:299, 1973.

50. Sotereanes DG, Schmidt CC: Hand and digital amputations. In Peimer C (editor): *Surgery of the hand and upper extremity,* New York, 1996, McGraw-Hill.

51. Steichen JB, Idler RS: Results of central ray resection without bony transposition, *J Hand Surg [Am]* 11:466, 1986.

52. St. Laurent JY, Duclos L: Prevention of neuroma in elective digital amputations by utilization of neuro-vascular island flap, *Ann Chir Main Memb Super* 15(1):50-54, 1996.

53. Swanson AB: The Krukenberg procedure in the juvenile amputee, *J Bone Joint Surg* 46A:1540, 1964.

54. Tada K, Nakashima H, Yoshida T, et al: A new treatment of painful amputation neuroma: a preliminary report, *J Hand Surg [Br]* 12(2):273-276, 1987.

55. *Techni-Care Technical Bulletin,* Care-Tech Laboratories, St. Louis, 1991.

56. Teissier J, Gomis R, Ginoves P, et al: Thenar and hypothenar flaps for covering distal and dorsal digital amputations, *Ann Chir Plast Esthet* 31(3):214-218, 1986.

57. Thompson Sir DW: *On growth and form,* Cambridge, England, 1917, University Press.

58. Tubiana R, Stack G, Hakstian RW: Restoration of prehension after severe mutilations of the hand, *J Bone Joint Surg* 48B:455, 1966.

59. Tupper J, Miller G: Sensitivity following volar V-Y plasty for fingertip amputations, *J Hand Surg [Br]* 10:183, 1985.

60. Urbaniak JR, Roth JH, Nunley JA, et al: The results of replantation after amputation of a single finger, *J Bone Joint Surg* 67A:611, 1985.

61. Verdan CE: Syndrome of the Quadrigia, *Surg Clin North Am* 40:425, 1960.

62. Vilkki SK: A technique for toe-to-stump transplantation after wrist amputation: a modern alternative to the Krukenberg operation, *Hand Chir* 17:92-97, 1985.

63. Wei FC, el-Gammal TA, Lin CH, et al: Metacarpal hand: classification and guidelines for microsurgical reconstruction with toe transfers, *Plas Reconstr Surg* 99(1):122-128, 1997.

64. Wilson RL, Carter-Wilson MS: Rehabilitation after amputations in the hand, *Orthop Clin North Am* 14(4):851-872, 1983.

65. Yim KK, Wei FC: Free tissue transplantation in the 90s, *Int Angiol* 14(3):327-331, 1995.

CHAPTER 105

Metacarpal and Phalangeal Fractures

Alan E. Freeland
Peter J. Lund

INDICATIONS

THE PROBLEM: INSTABILITY

Instability is the primary problem of metacarpal and phalangeal fractures that lead to surgical intervention. Instability is hallmarked by the tendency of the fracture to displace or remain displaced. Displacement is defined by the deformity it creates. Deformity can occur as angulation, shortening, rotation, or combinations of these. Each component of deformity can be measured. Rotation and angulation are measured in degrees. Shortening is measured in millimeters. Rotational deformity and lateral angulation are poorly tolerated because just a small amount can cause finger impingement or overlap during flexion. Even though shortening has an effect on the muscle length-tension curve, the hand most easily accommodates this component of deformity. Metacarpal fractures can tolerate up to 4 mm of shortening; phalangeal fractures tolerate somewhat less. The hand can functionally adjust to dorsal angulation in the metacarpal equal to its motion at the carpometacarpal (CMC) joint plus approximately 10 degrees, or volar angulation of the proximal phalanx of up to 25 degrees.[6]

ABNORMAL ANATOMY AND PATHOPHYSIOLOGY

A fracture is unstable if it cannot be reduced or maintained in an anatomic or nearly anatomic position without fixation when the hand is placed in the "safe" or functional position. The three principle determinants of fracture stability or instability are fracture configuration, periosteal and surrounding soft tissue sleeve integrity or loss, and muscle balance or imbalance. Transverse fractures have a stabile configuration, whereas spiral, oblique, and comminuted fractures, including those with bone loss, are unstable. The amount of initial fracture displacement, up to and including open fractures, is an indicator of the periosteal sleeve disruption, potential fracture instability, and fracture severity. Muscle imbalance causes dorsal angulation in unstable metacarpal fractures (Figure 105-1, *A*) and volar angulation in unstable phalangeal fractures (Figure 105-1, *B*).[31] It also can cause a rotational deformity,

especially in oblique fractures. Muscle contraction causes bone shortening.

TREATMENT GOALS

The goals of fracture management are anatomic or near-anatomic reduction and stability, using techniques that are as atraumatic or minimally traumatic as possible, with early, active, pain-free or minimally painful digital motion (Figure 105-2).[19,21,26] Function follows form. Early fracture reduction and stability give the injured patient the optimal opportunity for the best outcome. The more stable the fracture, the better the pain control, especially during therapy. Stable fracture fixation allows therapy to advance more rapidly and intensely.

The intangibles of judgment and the individual surgeon's education, background, training, experience, comfort, familiarity, and skills with particular approaches, methodologies, and implants are equally important and sometimes paramount in choosing a particular treatment. The information presented in this chapter reflects our personal preferences. It is for educational purposes only and is not intended to represent the only, nor necessarily the best, methods or procedures appropriate for the situations discussed. Rather, our intent is to present an approach, view, statement, or opinion that may be helpful or of interest to other practitioners.

TREATMENT ALTERNATIVES

Simple undisplaced or minimally displaced fractures are often stable regardless of configuration because the undamaged or minimally disrupted periosteum satisfactorily holds them in a proper position while the "safe" or functional hand position prevents muscle imbalance from deforming them. Some simple transverse and short oblique fractures that are displaced are stable after closed manipulative reduction because of the combination of stable fracture configuration, interlocking of bony interstices, and the restoration of the soft tissue envelope and muscle balance. These fractures can be treated by static or functional splinting, bracing, or casting techniques.[5] Fractures

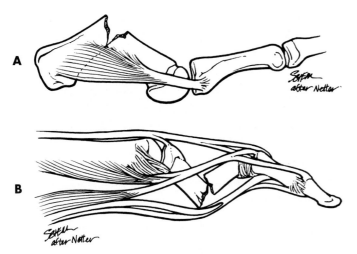

Figure 105-1. **A,** The intrinsic muscles are unopposed volar to the center of rotation of the fractured metacarpal, creating dorsal angulation at the fracture site. **B,** The intrinsic muscles flex the proximal fragment and the extrinsic extensor tendons extend the distal fragment, causing volar angulation of the fractured proximal phalanx.

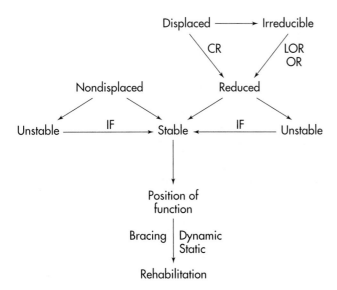

Figure 105-2. Fracture management algorithm. *CR,* Closed reduction; *IF,* internal fixation; *LOR,* limited open reduction; *OR,* open reduction. (From Freeland AE, Sennett BJ: Phalangeal fractures. In Peimer CA [editor]: *Surgery of the hand and upper extremity,* New York, 1996, McGraw Hill.)

that lose their reduction during treatment should be considered for some type of percutaneous or even open stabilization.

Fractures that most frequently require some type of implant stabilization include articular, periarticular, spiral, oblique, comminuted, and open fractures. Stability is especially important in open fractures with comminution, bone loss, or tendon injury. Multiple fractures in the same digit, ray, or hand often cause more than ordinary composite instability and should be given special consideration for firm fixation. Fixation of hand fractures can be particularly important in restoring polytraumatized patients to activities of daily living and helping them to

perform transfers and use assistive devices, including crutches, canes, and walkers. Noncompliant patients are good candidates for internal fixation of unstable fractures.[25]

COMPLICATIONS

Inadequately reduced or stabilized fractures are subject to delayed healing, nonunion, pseudarthrosis, union with deformity, a higher than normal incidence of tendon adhesions, joint contracture, and ankylosis. Without fracture stability and early motion, all of the tissues included within the zone of injury heal as a single unit with pervasive scar. Operative complications include, but are not limited to, failure of the procedure; implant failure, including breakage and pullout; infection; problems with the incision, wound, and bone healing; stiffness; deformity; loss of strength, power, and endurance; injury to deep structures, such as tendons, arteries, and nerves; chronic pain syndromes that can be caused by nerve injury, scar, or decreased vascularity; and, rarely, amputation.

INFORMED CONSENT

As part of obtaining an informed consent, patients are counseled individually before surgery regarding their diagnosis, the treatment goals and options, and the potential benefits and risks or complications of the procedure. We counsel patients about all of the risks outlined above. When we think a particular treatment option is clearly superior, we inform the patient. If no treatment option is superior, we outline the choices. Although we cannot guarantee procedures, we can explain reasonable expectations, guarantee that we will do our best, and relay our optimism that we are guiding the patient toward his or her best chance for an optimal result.

OPERATIONS

CLOSED REDUCTION AND INTERNAL FIXATION

Percutaneous Kirschner-Wire Techniques

When surgery is necessary, many closed, simple fractures can be adequately stabilized for a sufficient period of time by percutaneous Kirschner-wire (K-wire) fixation. C-arm fluoroscopy is extremely helpful to monitor both percutaneous and open techniques. Intraoperative fluoroscopy helps to minimize operative dissection, increase the accuracy of implant placement, and decrease operating time.

Percutaneous fracture fixation using K wires is an effective method for maintaining the reduction of unstable, closed, simple, extraarticular metacarpal fractures (Figure 105-3). Bosworth introduced this method for displaced metacarpal head (boxer's) fractures in 1937.[3] Percutaneous K wires control rotation better than intramedullary wires. These pins should be inserted with the fracture reduced and the metacarpophalangeal (MCP) joint flexed at 70 to 90 degrees to avoid

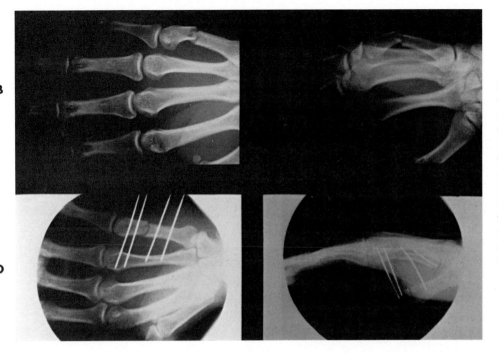

A, B

C, D

Figure 105-3. **A** and **B,** A closed transverse, dorsally angulated, metacarpal, distal diaphyseal fracture can be reduced but is *not* stable. **C** and **D,** Two transverse K wires transfix the reduced fracture proximally and distally. A single wire on either side of the fracture would be unprotected against rotational forces. Wires are inserted proximal to the fracture in the fourth and fifth metacarpals because of their flexible CMC joints.

Figure 105-4. **A** and **B,** Closed, transverse, volarly angulated, extraarticular fractures of the proximal phalanges of the middle and ring fingers are difficult to control individually because of their severe displacement and periosteal disruption and collectively because there are two of them. **C** and **D,** The problem is solved by closed reduction and internal fixation with two intramedullary K wires for each fracture.

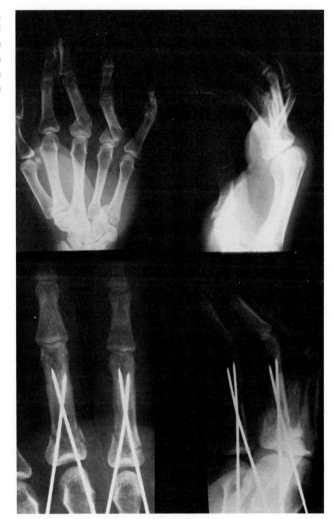

A, B

C, D

MCP-joint extension contracture. MCP-joint flexion aids in reducing the fracture and helps to control both angulation and rotation during closed reduction of a metacarpal fracture.

VomSaal[44] in 1952 was an early advocate of percutaneous intramedullary K-wire fixation for phalangeal fractures. One or more percutaneous intramedullary wires are particularly useful for splinting transverse and short, oblique phalangeal fractures (Figure 105-4).[2,24] Rotation is controlled by manually compressing and interlocking the fracture interstices during manipulative reduction and wire insertion. We prefer using two wires. The wires are started on the lateral edges of the proximal condyles and then guided through the medullary canal, across the fracture, and into the medullary canal of the distal fragment, where they should engage or penetrate cortical bone. This avoids perforation and potential injury to the extensor mechanism and articular cartilage at the MCP joint that can occur by driving a single wire across the metacarpal head. It also avoids the potential risk of developing a fatigue fracture of the K wire at the MCP joint.

Closed, displaced spiral and oblique diaphyseal phalangeal fractures are reliably treated by closed reduction and internal fixation using two or more transfixing K wires or percutaneous screws (Figures 105-5 and 105-6).[2,16,20,24] Closed condylar

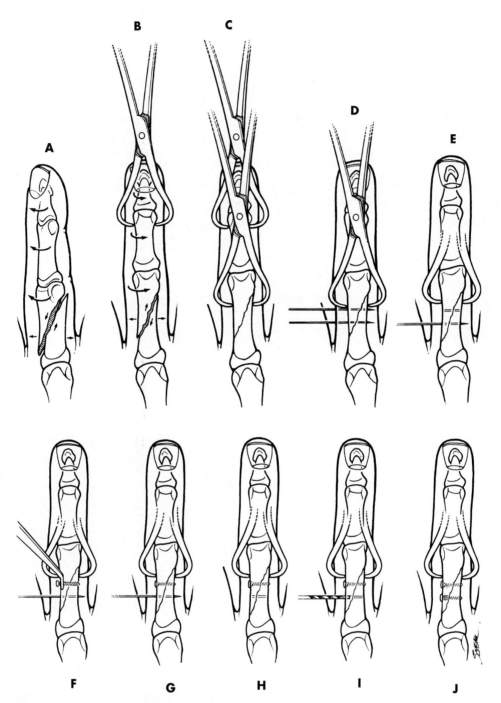

Figure 105-5. A, A spiral, oblique, proximal phalangeal diaphyseal fracture is shortened, rotated, and angulated. **B,** Traction and manipulation help the periosteum to guide the fracture toward reduction. **C,** Using fluoroscopy, the reduction is completed with a tenacular clamp. **D,** Stabilization is completed with two parallel transcutaneous K wires at the junctures of each third of the fracture. The wires then can be cut and capped above the skin. **E,** The distal (or proximal) K wire is removed. **F,** The proper screw length is selected using a depth gauge, or as shown here, by holding the screw over the core hole and verifying the length visually using C-arm fluoroscopy. This avoids disengaging the fracture reduction with the depth gauge. There are very small tolerances for forces at the fracture site. **G,** A self-tapping mini screw is inserted without drilling a gliding hole to avoid disruption of the fracture reduction. This is a "fixation" screw (i.e., there is no compression). **H,** The second K wire is removed. **I,** A gliding hole (same diameter as the thread diameter of the screw) is drilled in the near cortex. **J,** A mini lag (compression) screw is inserted. (From Freeland AE, Sennett BJ: Phalangeal fractures. In Peimer CA: *Surgery of the hand and upper extremity,* New York, 1996, McGraw Hill.)

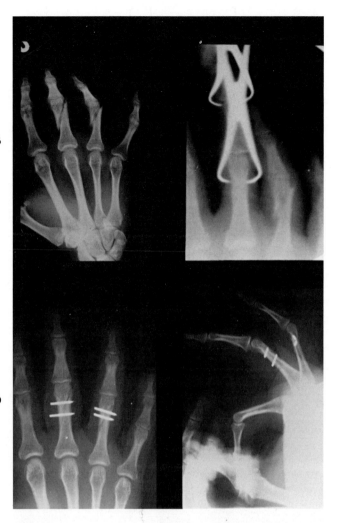

A, B

, D

Figure 105-6. A, Closed, displaced, unstable, spiral, oblique, proximal phalangeal fractures of the middle and ring fingers. **B,** Reduction. **C** and **D,** Pinning is performed using the technique shown in Figure 105-5, *A-D.* (From Freeland AE, Sennett BJ: *Phalangeal fractures.* In Peimer CA: *Surgery of the hand and upper extremity,* New York, 1996, McGraw Hill.)

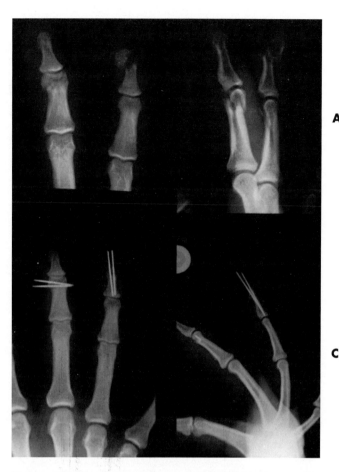

A, B

C, D

Figure 105-7. A and **B,** A closed, displaced, unstable, unicondylar fracture of the middle phalanx of the middle finger and a displaced, unstable, short, oblique fracture of the distal phalanx of the ring finger. **C** and **D,** Two transverse K wires stabilize the reduced unicondylar fracture, similar to the technique shown in Figure 105-5, *A-D.* Two intramedullary K wires stabilize the short, oblique, distal phalangeal fracture of the ring finger.

metacarpal and phalangeal fractures can be treated by similar techniques (Figure 105-7).[34,46] If these fractures have to be opened, it is extremely important to preserve the blood supply of the major articular fragment, not only for fracture healing but also to prevent avascular necrosis and subsequent arthrosis.

Closed intracondylar metacarpal and phalangeal fractures with major fragments can be treated with percutaneous wire fixation if they can be manipulated into a reduced position. The "rule of the majority" or "vassal rule" is applied.[19,26] The major fragments are restored. Smaller or "vassal" fragments follow the major fragments into position or can be ignored. Again, if open reduction is necessary, preservation of the blood supply to all fracture fragments is of paramount importance (Figures 105-8 to 105-11).

Percutaneous Screw Techniques

Mini screws and plates with sizes proportional to the small bones of the hand were developed in 1973 by Mathyes.[26] Currently, several manufacturers provide modern, refined mini and micro screws and plates that are low profile, sufficiently strong, and biologically inert. Mini and micro screws can be thought of as K wires with a head and threads. They offer substantially more stability than K wires and can, in some cases, be inserted percutaneously. Mini and micro self-tapping screws are now universally available. This speeds and simplifies the process of insertion. Oblique and spiral diaphyseal fractures (Figure 105-12) and unicondylar phalangeal fractures with a large fragment are most suitable for this technique (Figures 105-13 to 105-15). A 45 thousandths

Text continued on p. 1854

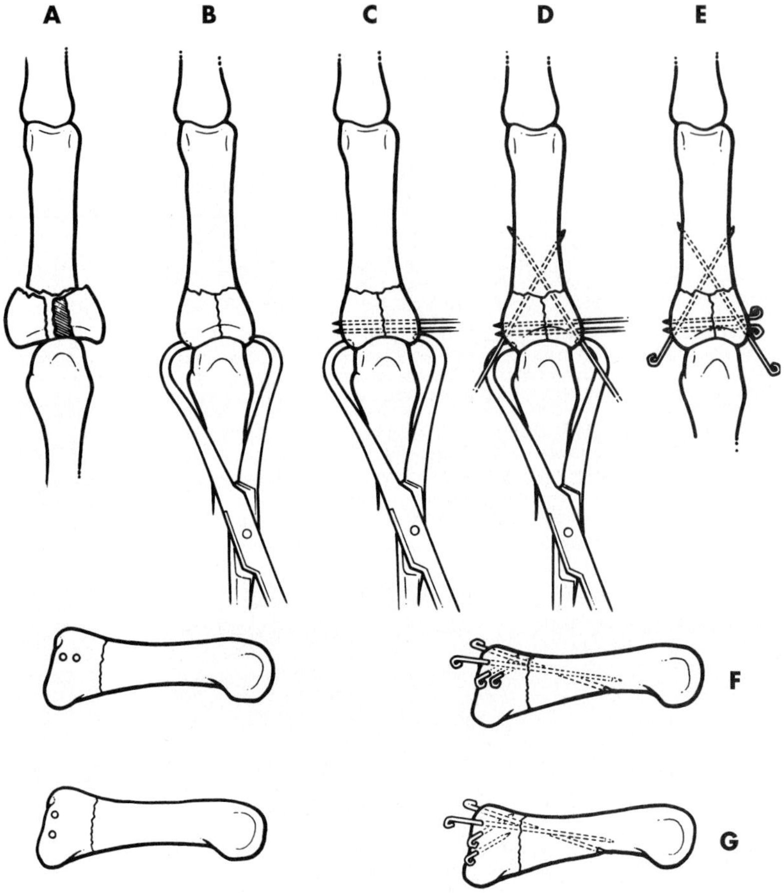

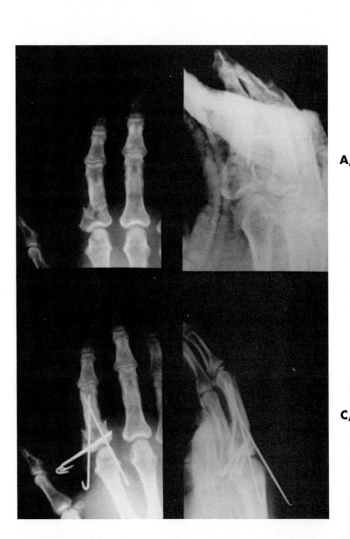

A,

C,

Figure 105-8. A closed, displaced, intraarticular, split fracture of the base of the proximal phalanx **(A)** is reduced with traction and a percutaneous tenacular clamp **(B)**. **C,** The large metaphyseal fragments are stabilized by two parallel K wires, restoring joint congruity. **D,** The repaired metaphysis is fixed to the diaphysis with crossed percutaneous K wires. **E,** The wires are cut above the skin and bent or capped. The metaphyseal wires may be placed horizontally **(F)** or vertically **(G)**.

Figure 105-9. **A** and **B,** A closed, displaced, intraarticular, split fracture cannot be controlled by closed technique. **C** and **D,** The technique used in Figure 105-8, *A* stabilizes the fracture.

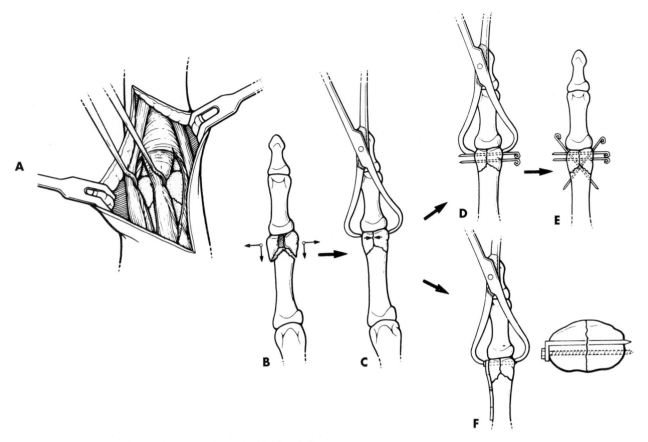

Figure 105-10.   **A** and **B,** A displaced bicondylar fracture is exposed through a dorsal incision. **C,** The fracture is reduced by traction and closed manipulation if possible or, if not, by open reduction. **D,** A distally eccentric tenacular clamp stabilizes the reduction while the condylar fragments are stabilized by parallel K wires. **E,** The restored condyles are fixed to the diaphysis with crossed K wires. **F,** When the fracture must be opened to achieve reduction and the condylar fragments are large (at least 5 mm in smallest diameter), they can be stabilized with a laterally applied minicondylar plate, sometimes through a mid-axial rather than a dorsal incision. (From Freeland AE, Benoist LA: *Hand Clin,* 10:239-250, 1994).

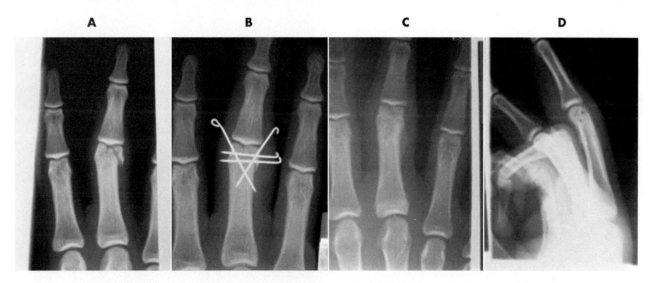

Figure 105-11.   A displaced bicondylar fracture **(A)** is treated by the technique described in Figure 105-10 **(B).** The fracture healed **(C** and **D)** with nearly full functional recovery **(E** and **F).** (From Freeland AE, Sennett BJ: Phalangeal fractures. In Peimer CA: *Surgery of the hand and upper extremity,* New York, 1996, McGraw Hill.)   *Continued*

E

F

Figure 105-11, cont'd. For legend see p. 1851.

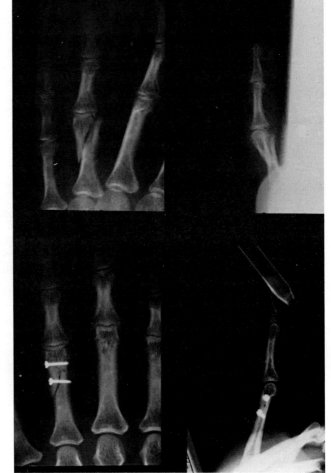

A,

C,

Figure 105-12. **A** and **B,** This spiral, oblique, proximal phalangeal fracture is shortened, rotated, and unstable. **C** and **D,** The fracture was reduced and stabilized using the technique in Figure 105-5.

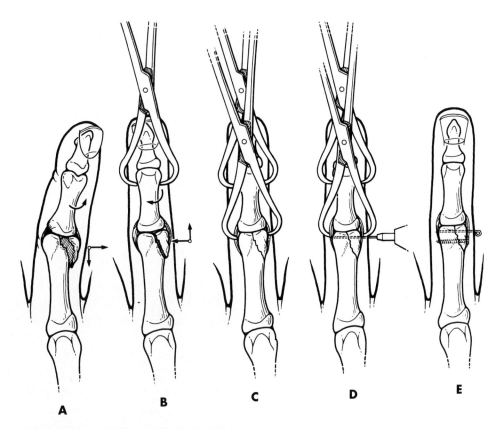

Figure 105-13. The sequential reduction and fixation of a displaced unicondylar fracture of the proximal phalanx. **A,** A displaced unicondylar fracture results in angulation, shortening, and rotation of the finger at the PIP joint. **B,** A tenacular clamp applied to the distal portion of the middle phalanx corrects shortening, angulation, and rotation while improving the position of the fractured condyle. **C,** A second tenacular clamp applied transcutaneously at the fracture site completes and compresses the reduction. **D,** The fracture is provisionally fixed by a distally eccentric small-gauge K wire placed in subchondral bone. **E,** A maxillofacial or mini fragment lag screw is placed centrally in the fracture fragment to provide compression and definitive fixation. If screw fixation is secure, the K wire may be removed at the time of surgery. The K wire may be retained for 2 to 4 weeks at the discretion of the surgeon to provide additional stability, especially against rotary forces. Depending on the size of the fracture fragment and the judgment of the surgeon, combinations of two K wires, two screws, or a screw and a K wire may be used. (From Freeland AE, Benoist LA: *Hand Clin* 10:239-250, 1994.)

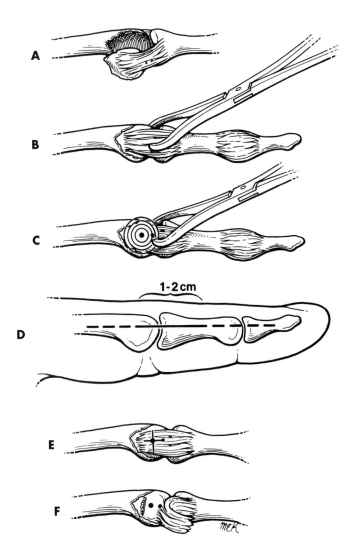

Figure 105-14. **A,** A displaced unicondylar fracture is viewed laterally. **B,** Reduction is achieved with a tenacular clamp. **C,** The concept of targeting is used to select an eccentric subchondral position for provisional K-wire fixation. Different combinations of K wires and screws can be chosen by the surgeon. **D,** The fracture is approached through a limited portion of the mid-axial incision. Use of fluoroscopy is very helpful. **E,** An incision is made in the origin of the collateral ligament so that the screw head can be recessed beneath it. **F,** Occasionally, the proximal portion of the collateral ligament may be reflected for exposure. (From Freeland AE, Benoist LA: *Hand Clin* 10:239-250, 1994.)

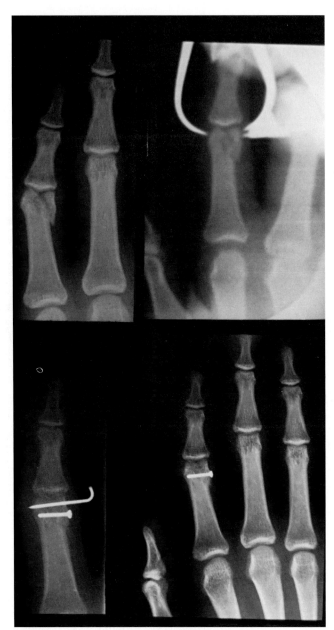

Figure 105-15. **A,** A closed, displaced, unstable, unicondylar fracture results in angulation, shortening, and rotation of the index finger at the level of the PIP joint. **B,** Reduction is completed by the percutaneous application of a tenacular clamp. A K wire is poised for insertion in the cannulated barrel of the clamp. **C,** The fracture has been reduced and fixed with a combination of a small-gauge K wire and a mini screw. **D,** The K wire can be removed at any time (usually not later than 4 weeks). The wire provides the screw with additional protection from bending and rotational forces. A firmly applied lag screw can be used alone in cancellous metaphyseal bone where it is often adequately protected by the interlocking bony interstices. The surgeon must decide on the right combination. (From Freeland AE, Benoist LA: *Hand Clin* 10:239-250, 1994.)

(1.1 mm)– diameter K wire is used. This is the same diameter as the core of the 1.5-mm mini screw. One K wire can be removed while the other provisionally holds the reduction. A 1.5-mm, self-tapping mini screw can then be directly inserted. The remaining K wire can then be removed and replaced with a lag screw.[15,18] The original screw can optionally be replaced in the lag mode for maximum stability. We rarely find this to be necessary. We believe the risks of stripping the screw hole in the bone or having other technical difficulties outweigh the advantages of the increased strength in most cases. We now use this method in preference to percutaneous pinning whenever we believe we can do it without getting into technical difficulty. Revision to percutaneous K wires or open reduction are the contingencies. Table 105-1 lists the commonly available K-wire

diameters in both inches and millimeters so that the surgeon can correlate them with available screw core and thread diameters from any vendor. For example, if a 0.062 thousandths inch (1.5 mm)–diameter Kirschner wire were used, or if the surgeon needed to salvage a stripped 1.5-mm screw hole, he

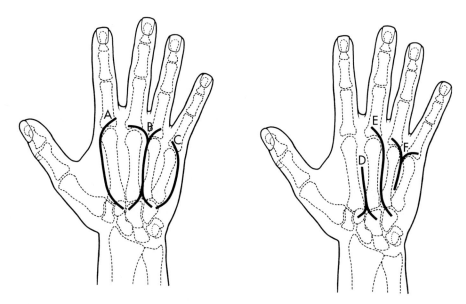

Figure 105-16. **A,** Incision offset radially for second metacarpal exposure. **B,** Incision between the third and fourth metacarpals can be used to approach either or both. **C,** Incision offset ulnarly for fifth metacarpal exposure. **D,** Incision can be curved proximally over one or both metacarpals. **E,** S-shaped incision approaches one metacarpal proximally and the other distally through a single incision. **F,** Incision can be curved distally over one or both adjacent metacarpals. (From Freeland AE, Geissler WB: Plate fixation of metacarpal shaft fractures. In Blair WF, Steyers CM [editors]: *Techniques in hand surgery,* Baltimore, 1996, Williams & Wilkins.)

Table 105-1.
Conversion Tables for Screw and K-wire Diameters (values closely approximated)

METRIC (mm)	ENGLISH (inches)
0.7	0.028
0.8	0.035
1.1	0.045
1.3	0.054
1.5	0.065
2.0	0.080
2.7	0.10

or she would use a 2.0-mm thread–diameter screw that has a 1.5-mm core diameter.

OPEN REDUCTION AND INTERNAL FIXATION

When fractures are open or require surgery for reduction, fixation, or both, the surgeon will usually select the strongest implant available that is appropriate to satisfy the mechanical requirements for fracture stability. This is where mini and micro screws and plates have their most important role. Open

and complex fractures require increased stability for optimal healing and functional recovery. Small fragments, comminution, and poorly mineralized bone may not hold implants well and may have to be splinted or bypassed by K wires, plates, external fixators, or traction.

Anatomy and Approaches

Peacock[37] described the concept of "one wound, one scar." All tissues in the zone of injury tend to heal in one confluent scar. This can be mediated to some extent by the choice of incision placement and by secure fracture fixation. Incisions for metacarpal fractures should be offset from the metacarpal and its extensor tendon (Figure 105-16).[17] The fracture can be approached subperiosteally with an effort to protect the integrity of the gliding tissue between the skin and the extensor tendon and between the extensor tendon and the bone. A single incision can be used to approach adjacent fractured metacarpals.

Pratt[38] described the classic dorsal approach to the proximal phalanx in 1959 (Figure 105-17). This is a very utilitarian approach and can be moved so that it is centered over the fracture.[15,35] Its disadvantage is that it creates a zone of injury dorsally that encompasses skin, extensor tendon, and bone. It may be slightly less traumatic to incise between the lateral band and the central extensor tendon than splitting the central extensor tendon.

An even better alternative, when possible, is a mid-axial approach (Figure 105-18).[12,33] The proximal phalanx and interphalangeal (IP) joint are surrounded by collagenous structures that undergo a proliferative fibroplasia when stimulated by injury. By placing the incision in the mid-axial line, it

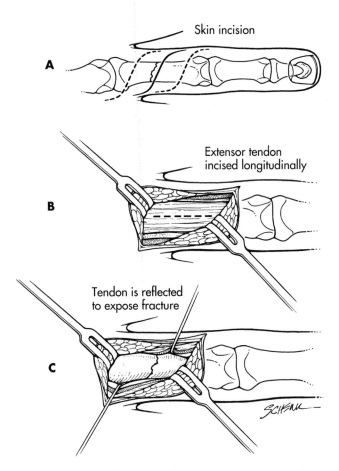

Figure 105-17. A, A dorsal incision can be placed to correspond to the fracture site. It is offset to avoid direct alignment with the extensor tendon **(B),** which can be incised in its mid-portion or along either edge **(C)** to expose the fracture. (Modified from Pratt DR: *Clin Orthop* 15:22, 1959).

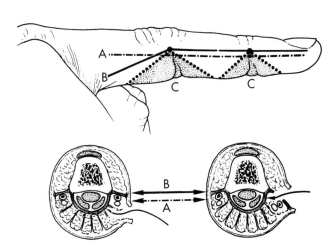

Figure 105-18. The midlateral line **(A)** and mid-axial incision and approach **(B)** are demonstrated both in profile and in cross section. (From Littler JW, Cramer LM, Smith JW [editors]: *Symposium on reconstruction surgery,* St. Louis, 1974, Mosby.)

theoretically does not move during flexion and extension of the finger. Tension is thus neutralized as a stimulus to scar formation. Additionally, the zone of injury is moved from the dorsum of the finger to a more innocuous area. The lateral band can be retracted for screw or plate application, or if necessary, resected so that it does not rub or form scar over the implants. Plate bulk does not interfere with extensor tendon excursion in either flexion or extension.

Open Screw Fixation

Spiral and oblique metacarpal (Figure 105-19) and phalangeal diaphyseal fractures may be stabilized by screws alone when the fracture length is twice or more the bone diameter in the region of the fracture. A single screw should not be used alone to secure a shaft fracture because it will not tolerate the bending or rotational forces generated during normal use. A neutralization screw in the case of long oblique or spiral fractures that are more than twice the bone diameter, or a neutralization plate in the case of short oblique or spiral fractures (less than twice the bone diameter) must be used to counter the bending and rotational forces (Figures 105-20 and 105-21). A single neutralization screw is placed first, with the remaining screws placed perpendicular to the fracture plane as they follow its curve. The number and position of screws that can safely be used to secure a given fracture can be determined by dividing the fracture length by the bone diameter. One or two mini screws can be used to stabilize large condylar fractures. The criteria and principles are otherwise the same when using open-fracture exposure as they are for percutaneous screws. The principle fracture fragment should be at least three times larger than the diameter of the screw used to secure it so it does not fragment.

Mini Plates

The main concern in using mini plates on the metacarpals, and especially the phalanges, has been the amount of scar-generating subperiosteal dissection that is necessary for their application. These plates are most suitable for treatment of open fractures in which the wound has already created all or most of the exposure necessary for their application, or when open fracture reduction is necessary for stabilization. Plates are indicated for nonunion reconstructions, corrective osteotomies, fractures with comminution or bone loss, multiple phalangeal or metacarpal fractures, severely displaced or unstable fractures (especially border metacarpals), fractures of the thumb, and in unreliable patients. The substantially greater stability of plate fixation in these situations provides the best opportunity for a favorable functional outcome. Maximum discretion must be exercised by the surgeon when choosing plate fixation of phalangeal fractures.

Another concern of plate fixation for metacarpal and phalangeal fractures has been that the plate bulk can cause extensor lag and prevent full flexion, especially when it is applied in its most accessible and stable dorsal position. The closer a plate approaches a joint, the more this is likely to happen. The central slip is also vulnerable to attenuation or damage in the distal portion of the proximal phalanx, which can create a secondary boutonniere deformity.

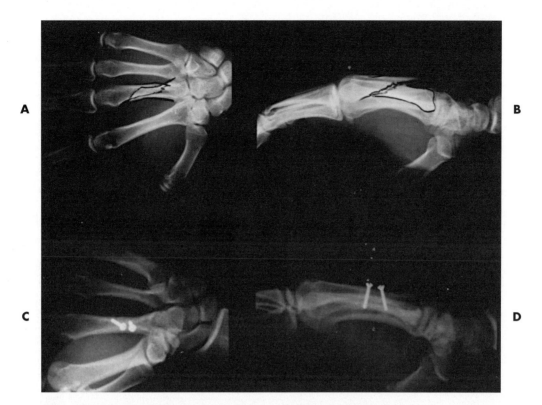

Figure 105-19. **A** and **B,** A closed, displaced, unstable, long, spiral, oblique fracture of the third metacarpal could not be reduced by closed manipulation. **C** and **D,** A precise open reduction was stabilized by two compression screws placed perpendicular to a spiraling fracture plane at the junctures of each third of the fracture. A screw placed perpendicular to the fracture plane has maximum compression. One of the screws was also perpendicular to the long axis of the bone, providing maximum protection against axial shorting caused by shear forces.

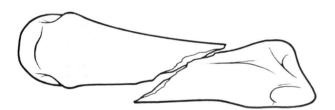

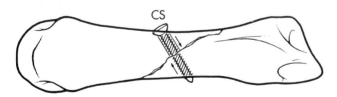

Figure 105-20. An interfragmentary mini lag screw compresses an anatomically reduced fracture and is then protected from bending and rotational stresses by a neutralization mini plate. The sequence of screw application is shown by the numbers adjacent to each screw site. (From Freeland AE, Jabaley M: Management of hand fractures by stable fixation. In Habal MB [editor]: *Advances in plastic and reconstructive surgery,* Chicago, 1986, Year-Book Medical Publishers Inc.)

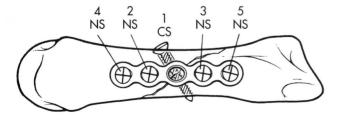

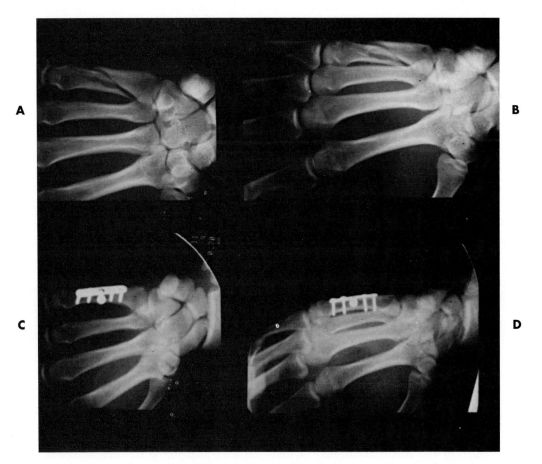

Figure 105-21. A closed, displaced, unstable, short, oblique midshaft metacarpal fracture (**A** and **B**) is fixed by the technique shown in Figure 105-20 (**C** and **D**).

The most recent generation of plates features lower-profile versions of previous designs to address this problem and to slightly decrease the dissection needed for their application and allow faster bone revascularization. Newly designed plates, such as the mini condylar plate,[4,36] have vastly improved our ability to stabilize metaphyseal fractures because they are both lower profile and can be applied laterally as well as dorsally. Maxillofacial micro plates have also been used effectively for fixation of phalangeal fractures.[40] Interosseous or tension band wiring provides a nearly comparable alternative, especially when combined with one or more K wires.[22,30,32] Restriction of motion and irritation from the ends of the wires are the potential complaints.

The final serious objection to plate fixation in metacarpals and phalanges is the need for a second operation for removal. The lower profile of modern plates makes it much less likely that they will cause irritation because of prominence under the skin or deep structures. Titanium is a nonallergenic and non-inflammatory material and it is replacing stainless steel as the metal of choice for fixation devices. Application with unicortical screws, when feasible, lessens bone trauma from drilling and heat. Resorbable plates and screws for use with simple metacarpal fractures are in the developmental stage.[39] Plates, screws, or combinations that adequately stabilize reduced fractures until

they heal, support functional recovery, and then disappear without a trace or a problem have distinct appeal. Cyanoacrylic glue or marine-derived adhesive may replace screws for some, if not all, plate applications.[1]

Fixation plates have two names: an anatomic name and a physiologic or functional name. Anatomic names refer to the design, such as straight, T, angular, tubular, mini condylar, H, and low profile. Compression, neutralization, and buttressing are functions performed by plates. A bridging plate is a type of neutralization plate. Plates are selected on the basis of their anatomy or design, their physiology or function, and their versatility of application for either the dorsal or mid-axial approach.

Straight compression plates are used to stabilize transverse, unstable, midshaft metacarpal fractures (Figures 105-22 and 105-23),[18] whereas mini condylar plates adapt to similar fractures at either the proximal or distal metaphyseal diaphyseal junction (Figure 105-24).[4,36] Figures 105-20 and 105-21 demonstrate a straight neutralization plate.[18] A mini condylar plate could be used in the same fashion at the metaphyseal diaphyseal junction.[4,36] Buttressing is used exclusively to support metaphyseal fractures (Figure 105-25). Mini condylar plates are usually preferred,[4,36] although T, L, and oblique angled plates are an option.

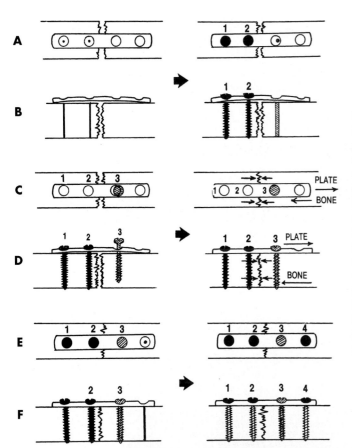

Figure 105-22. **A,** This diagram demonstrates a transverse fracture that has been reduced. The gap in the illustration represents a gap of less than 1 mm. Two neutral (centered) holes are drilled on the left side of the fracture. Note that the plate has a very slight bend of 5 degrees. **B,** Two neutral screws are placed on the left side of the fracture site. A drill hole is placed eccentrically away from the fracture site on the right side of the fracture. **C,** A mini screw is started in the eccentric drill hole on the right side of the plate. **D,** As the mini screw tightens, the screw head engages the plate and causes translation of the bone and the mini plate in opposite directions, compressing the fracture. The slight bend in the plate allows uniform compression across the entire fracture. **E,** After compression is obtained, a neutral drill hole is centered in the remaining plate hole. **F,** A neutral screw is then inserted, completing the construct. (From Freeland AE, Jabaley ME: Management of hand fractures by stable fixation. In Habal MB [editor]: *Advances in plastic and reconstructive surgery,* Chicago, 1986, Year-Book Medical Publishers Inc.)

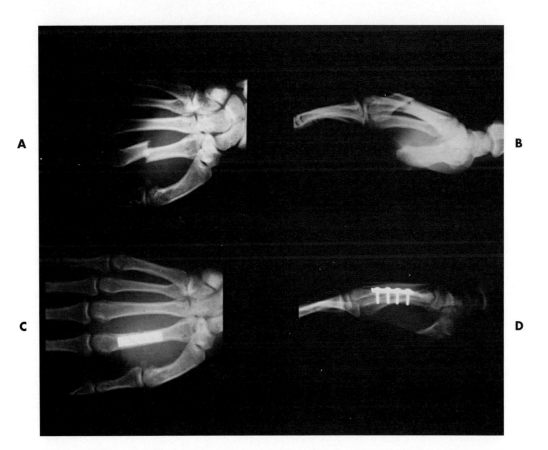

Figure 105-23. A displaced, shortened, irreducible, midshaft, transverse fracture of the second metacarpal **(A** and **B)** is treated by open reduction and internal fixation using a four-hole, limited-contact, straight, mini compression plate **(C** and **D)** by the technique shown in Figure 105-22.

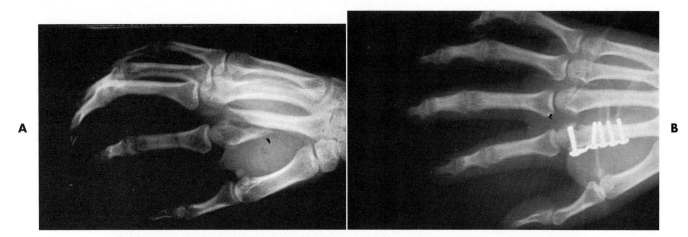

Figure 105-24. A completely displaced, shortened, irreducible, subcapital (boxer's) fracture of the fifth metacarpal **(A)** is treated by open reduction and internal fixation **(B)** using a mini condylar plate in the compression mode as shown in Figure 105-22.

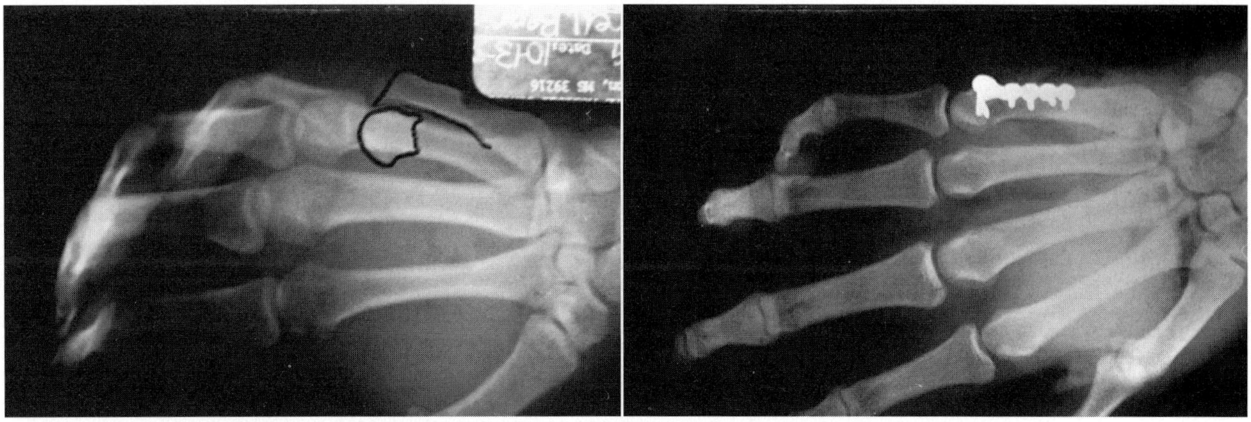

Figure 105-25. A closed, displaced, oblique fracture at the distal diaphyseal metaphyseal junction of the index metacarpal **(A)** is treated by open reduction and internal fixation **(B)** with a mini condylar plate applied in the buttress (supporting) mode.

POSTOPERATIVE MANAGEMENT

After surgery, the patient's hand is placed in a soft, sterile, conforming dressing in the "safe" or functional position. Extra padding is placed over bony prominences and in areas of superficial neurovascular structures. Circumferentially applied dressing materials, such as gauze and elastic bandages, should be *laid* on as they are applied, rather than pulled and stretched. This will minimize the risk of a tight dressing when postoperative swelling occurs. The dressing and hand position are supported by a short arm plaster splint.

The dressing is split on one side from top to bottom and rewrapped in the recovery room just before discharge for outpatients and within 24 hours for most inpatients. The patient is then instructed on how to loosen and rewrap the dressing should it become too tight. The patient is provided with a sling and instructions for the use of ice, elevation, digital motion, and overall activity. A prescription and instructions for pain medicine are provided.

Because there are no fibroblasts in the wound for 48 hours after injury and no fibrin of any strength for 4 to 5 days, it is not essential to start motion *immediately (within 24 hours)* after injury. The hand can be immobilized for 2 or 3 days to reduce swelling and inflammation. Early mid-range motion resulting in about 5 mm of tendon excursion can then be initiated, which is gradually increased as healing progresses and pain and swelling subside. This should prevent serious scar adhesions in most cases, especially in simple, closed fractures treated by closed or percutaneous methods, just as it does for tendon lacerations and repair.[11] Early motion after surgery is particularly important for phalangeal fractures that occur in "no person's land," just as it is in flexor tendon lacerations.

Motion is clearly the most important component of rehabilitation. Once motion is ensured, strength, power, and endurance follow. Activities of daily and independent living are integrated within the patient's pain and functional tolerance. Work and recreation are resumed when the patient's capabilities meet or exceed those of his job. Skilled workers and athletes may need special strengthening and conditioning programs.

SECONDARY PROCEDURES

Operations to Gain Skeletal Union

Nonunion of hand fractures occurs at a rate of less than 1% in closed fractures.[29] Traumatic or operative devascularization, displacement, distraction, soft tissue interposition, persistent motion at the fracture site, bone loss, or infection may be causative or contributing factors. The most common cause of nonunion is inadequate or improper K-wire stabilization of comminuted fractures. A persistent or expanding radiolucent line, sclerosis of the fracture margins, submarginal cyst formation, medullary sealing, osteopenia, rounding or mushrooming of the fracture ends, or a lack of bony reaction may appear on radiographs. Nonunions are unstable to manual stress testing. This often can be demonstrated on stress radiographs.

A nonunion may be intraarticular or extraarticular, displaced or nondisplaced. Intraarticular nonunions should be restored and secured when the joint is reparable. Arthroplasty or arthrodesis must be considered if the joint has irreparable damage. If the nonunion is extraarticular, reduction is performed when necessary, and secure fixation is applied. The application of compression through plating may be sufficient to heal the aligned hypertrophic or oligotrophic nonunion. The potential for healing with compression alone may be demonstrated preoperatively by the increased uptake of radioactive isotope at the nonunion site on bone scan. Bone grafting is used for defects and to replace atrophic bone.

Corrective Osteotomy

Malunion occurs when a fracture heals with enough deformity to interfere with hand or digital function. Because fingers diverge when extended and converge when flexed, it is often only possible to appreciate functional deformities during flexion. When deformity is mild, the patient is pain free, and hand function is normal or nearly so, the potential risks of surgery, including subsequent adhesions and joint contractures, may far outweigh any potential advantages. This is particularly true in the fingers, especially in flexor tendon zone II. A corrective osteotomy should be considered when the deformity is sufficient to cause pain or a functional deficit. Wedge osteotomy corrects angulation, whereas derotation corrects a rotational deformity. These techniques can be used individually or in concert. The goals of treatment simulate those of the initial fracture treatment: to correct the deformity, achieve bony union, and to recover as much lost function as possible. Again, stable fixation is essential because corrective osteotomy requires substantial soft tissue dissection and is destabilizing. Bone grafting is used for defects or to ensure healing. Intramedullary bone pegs can be useful in some cases.

Capsulectomy and Tenolysis

Digital scarring and loss of motion can be caused by the initial injury, inadequate treatment, operative dissection, or a failure to initiate early digital motion. Contracture or ankylosis of the MCP joint and extensor tendon adhesions over the dorsum of the hand that do not respond adequately to therapy and dynamic splinting may be fairly reliably addressed by operative release of the cord portion of the collateral ligaments and by tenolysis, respectively.[23] This also affords an opportunity for implant removal.

Flexion contracture of the proximal interphalangeal (PIP) joint that occurs after treatment is common with fractures of and about the proximal phalanx and the PIP joint and is much more difficult to treat than its metacarpal counterpart. Operative release of the volar plate checkrein ligaments is indicated for PIP-joint flexion contracture greater or equal to 30 degrees, which occurs after a simple low-energy fracture and persists after adequate splinting and hand therapy.[45] Contractures present after injuries of higher energy and greater complexity, such as a crush or open injury, and are best treated by a dorsal incision to first approach the collateral ligaments, which are then excised. If this is not successful, the insertion of the volar plate is divided. One or both of these procedures will relieve most PIP-joint contractures.[23]

The prognosis for improvement is poor when there are extensor tendon adhesions over the proximal phalanx. Tenolysis in this area has not proven very successful. If the lateral bands are not involved in the scarring, an alternative treatment is to excise the scarred central extrinsic extensor tendon, sparing at least the proximal 4 to 6 mm of the central slip to avoid a boutonniere deformity. This dissociates the intrinsic and extrinsic extensor tendons and allows the intrinsic extensor tendons to independently straighten the PIP joint. This seems to work better than tenolysis, but is still not entirely reliable. Joint contracture secondary to flexor tendon adhesions alone can be treated by tenolysis and/or volar plate release. When there is severe joint injury or secondary ankylosis, especially in open crush injuries, tenolysis and joint capsulotomy are less successful in restoring normal motion.

OUTCOMES

OUTCOME MEASUREMENTS

Outcome studies for patients who have undergone treatment of metacarpal and phalangeal fractures have traditionally been measured in relation to the total active digital range of motion (TAM). The End Result Committee of the American Society for Surgery of the Hand standardized the TAM values (Table 105-2). Previous published investigators have not always used the Clinical Assessment Committee's TAM criteria but often chose criteria that closely approximated it. We have taken the editorial privilege of extrapolating their TAM results to correspond to the ASSH End Result Committee's criteria. This was done to facilitate comparisons. Any errors that have occurred as a result of this effort are ours and are unintentional. The obverse of the functional motion recovery is stiffness, which is the most common and serious complication of

Table 105-2.
Digital Functional Assessment Chart*

	TOTAL ACTIVE MOTION (TAM)		
RESULT	PERCENT	FINGERS	THUMB
Excellent	85-100	220-260	119-140
Good	70-84	180-219	98-118
Fair	50-60	130-179	70-97
Poor	<50	<130	<70

*The End Result Committee report of 1976 is available from the American Society for Surgery of the Hand, 6060 Greenwood Plaza Blvd, #100, Englewood, CO, 80111-4801.

hand-fracture management. Outcomes instruments that assess socioeconomic factors are currently being created for patients with upper-extremity injury. These instruments would assess cost of treatment, the number and consequence of secondary procedures, time off work, lost income, and subjective patient satisfaction criteria.

OUTCOME DETERMINANTS

Patient Factors
The return of active digital motion is influenced by several factors, including age, systemic disease, and patient compliance. Strickland et al[42] reported an average 20% decrease in digital TAM in patients over 50 years of age with nonarticular phalangeal fractures. Swanson et al[43] found the infection rate in open fractures was 25% in patients with systemic illness and 2.1% in healthy patients.

Fracture Factors
Factors that influence the final functional TAM include the anatomic location of the fracture, its configuration, the amount of displacement, and stability after reduction. Strickland et al[42] noted the average TAM functional recovery after simple transverse phalangeal fractures was 76%, but it was only 62% in comminuted phalangeal fractures. They also noted an 88% return in TAM with nondisplaced, extraarticular phalangeal fractures without tendon injuries, which decreased to 80% in minimally displaced fractures and to 74% in markedly displaced fractures. Huffaker et al[27] reported an average recovery of 220 degrees TAM in extraarticular fractures in a large series of patients with finger fractures. The average TAM recovery in patients with joint involvement was only 175 degrees.[27] Simple extraarticular fractures recovered 256 degrees TAM, which decreased to 224 degrees with joint involvement. Extraarticular crush injuries recovered 206 degrees TAM, whereas fingers with intraarticular fractures regained only 150 degrees. James reported flexion contractures of the PIP joint in

58 of 75 digits with unstable proximal phalangeal fractures, whereas only 17 fingers recovered full motion.[28]

Management Factors
Many factors influence the final result of a phalangeal or metacarpal fracture, including recognition and diagnosis, timing and adequacy of reduction and stabilization, type of implants, condition and management of soft tissues, operative incisions and approaches, and rehabilitation. The surgeon can affect the final outcome by his or her actions or nonaction in all of these areas.

The most controversial area by far in hand-fracture management is implant selection. Dissection in the hand increases the amount of scar, which translates into loss of motion. Generally, the surgeon wants to select an implant that will reliably secure the reduced fracture until it heals adequately enough to sustain unrestricted active motion. The disadvantage of open reduction and internal fixation is scar-generating dissection. The advantages are ease and accuracy of anatomic reduction and implant insertion and maximizing functional recovery by creating stability secure enough to control pain and allow early active, unrestricted motion. Early pain-free, active range of motion can offset the disadvantages of scar-generating dissection in some, and perhaps many, instances, but probably not all.[7-10,13,14,41]

Green and Anderson[24] obtained a full range of motion in 18 of 21 patients with 26 closed, simple, extraarticular, proximal phalangeal fractures treated with either intramedullary or transverse percutaneous pinning. Belsky et al,[2] in a similar prospective series of 100 consecutive fractures in 95 patients, achieved 61 excellent, 29 good, and 10 poor results. Forty-five transverse or short oblique fractures were treated with one or more intramedullary wires, and 55 long spiral or oblique fractures were transfixed with two or more K wires. Diwaker and Stothard[9] reported only 68% good or excellent results treating closed, displaced, unstable metacarpal and phalangeal fractures with K wires. Widgerow et al[47] had 1 excellent, 21 good, and 1 poor result in 23 simple, extraarticular phalangeal fractures treated with open reduction and K-wire fixation. Opening the fractures in their series led to a slight decrease in TAM compared with patients with similar fractures treated by percutaneous technique. They had four good results and one with like treatment of articular fractures. Lister[32] obtained an average TAM of 192 degrees (74%) in 24 digits with articular fractures and 210 degrees (81%) in 23 nonarticular fractures using open interosseous wiring techniques.

McElfresh and Dobyns[34] in 1984 verified that anatomic reduction, stability, and early motion were the critical determinants of outcome in articular fractures of the metacarpal head. Weiss and Hastings[46] provided an excellent review in 1993 of the configurations of unicondylar phalangeal fractures, their methods of reduction and stabilization, and their results. A single wire did not provide rotational stability, requiring a second wire or a screw in this group of patients.

Crawford[7] treated 20 closed, displaced, unstable hand fractures, including three unicondylar; ten long, spiral, oblique, proximal phalangeal fractures; and seven Bennett fractures, with open reduction and internal mini screw fixation. All achieved excellent results and 19 had full range of motion. Diwaker and Stothard[9] reported 93% good or excellent results treating simple closed, displaced, unstable metacarpal and phalangeal fractures with open screw fixation. These results were better than they achieved with comparable fractures using K wires. Ford et al[13] reported 90% good or excellent results in a group of patients with simple displaced, unstable fractures of the proximal and middle phalanges, all treated with screw fixation. Fifteen of the 38 digits were open injuries.[13]

Ford et al[14] also treated 22 patients with 26 simple metacarpal fractures by open screw fixation and reported 75% excellent and 17% good results. Fourteen digits had full range of motion.[14] Intraarticular metacarpal head fractures, or those open fractures with extensor tendon injury, all regained less than 220 degrees of TAM. Dabezies and Schutte[8] treated a mixed group of 52 closed, simple, unstable metacarpal and phalangeal fractures with plates and screws, with a majority of digits regaining excellent results in all fracture categories. Only two fractured digits in their series, one metacarpal and one phalangeal, appeared to result in serious digital stiffness and a poor result. Puckett et al[40] successfully treated 113 of 115 hand fractures with maxillofacial mini and micro plates. "Success" was not defined by TAM, but the authors indicated that bone healing and functional recovery were realized. They attributed part of their success to the low profile of the plate, which allowed them to protect extensor tendon gliding by suturing the periosteum over the plate. Stern et al[41] noted that approximately 10% of metacarpal fractures in their series treated with plates had significant adhesions and restriction of motion.

Strickland et al[42] contrasted an average TAM recovery rate of 75% to 80% of normal when mobilization was started in any of the 4 weeks immediately after injury, but only 66% if started after 4 weeks. Interestingly, prolonged immobilization more dramatically influenced the final results of functional motion recovery in undisplaced and minimally displaced fractures than in markedly displaced fractures. Nondisplaced fractures mobilized within 4 weeks recovered 90% of normal motion, while those immobilized more than 4 weeks precipitously fell to 65%. Minimally displaced fractures gradually declined from 98% recovery when mobilized in the first week to 74% when motion was initiated after 4 weeks. Markedly displaced fractures regained about 75% of motion if mobilized within the first 4 weeks, but only 61% after 4 weeks.

SUMMARY

Inadequate fracture reduction, instability after fixation, excessive operative dissection, and prolonged immobilization can all result in potentially stiffening scar formation. This is particularly true of fractures to the proximal phalanx and/or IP joint in "no person's land." Both the flexor and extensor tendons are

closely adherent to the bone and require very little scar to restrict motion. The best results are possible when metacarpal and phalangeal fractures can be placed in anatomic or near anatomic reduction and held with sufficient stability to allow early, active digital motion without loss of position until fracture healing has occurred. When internal fixation is necessary, an implant and approach should be selected that provide reliable stability with the least amount of operative trauma. Results with screw fixation equal or exceed those with K-wire fixation for comparable fractures. Plates should be used with discretion, especially on phalangeal fractures.

REFERENCES

1. Ahn DK, Sims CD, Randolf MA, et al: Craniofacial skeletal fixation using biodegradable plates and cyanoacrylic glue, *Plast Reconstr Surg* 99:1508-1517, 1997.
2. Belsky MR, Eaton RG, Lane LB: Closed reduction and internal fixation of proximal phalangeal fractures, *J Hand Surg [Am]* 9:725-729, 1984.
3. Bosworth DM: Internal splinting of fractures of the fifth metacarpal, *J Bone Joint Surg* 19A:826-827, 1937.
4. Buchler U, Fisher T: Use of a minicondylar plate for metacarpal and phalangeal periarticular injuries, *Clin Orthop* 214:53-58, 1987.
5. Burkhalter WE: Closed treatment of hand fractures, *J Hand Surg [Am]* 14:390-393, 1989.
6. Coonrad RW, Pohlman MH: Impacted fractures in the proximal portions of the proximal phalanx of the finger, *J Bone Joint Surg* 51A:1291-1296, 1969.
7. Crawford GP: Screw fixation for certain fractures of the phalanges and metacarpals, *J Bone Joint Surg* 58A:487-492, 1976.
8. Dabezies EJ, Schutte JP: Fixation of metacarpal and phalangeal fractures with miniature plate and screws, *J Hand Surg [Am]* 11:283-288, 1986.
9. Diwaker HN, Stothard J: The role of internal fixation in closed fractures of the proximal phalanges and metacarpals in adults, *J Hand Surg [Br]* 11B:103-108, 1986.
10. Duncan RW, Freeland AE, Jabaley ME, Meydrech EF: Open hand fractures: an analysis of the recovery of active motion and of complications, *J Hand Surg [Am]* 18:387-394, 1993.
11. Duran RJ, Houser RG: Controlled passive motion following flexor tendon repair in zone two and three. In: *AAOS symposium on tendon surgery in the hand,* St. Louis, 1975, Mosby.
12. Field LD, Freeland AE, Jabaley ME: Midaxial approach to the proximal phalanx for fracture fixation, *Contemp Orthop* 25:133-137, 1992.
13. Ford DJ, El-Hadidi S, Lunn PG, et al: Fractures of the metacarpals: treatment by AO screw and plate fixation, *J Hand Surg [Br]* 12:34-37, 1987.
14. Ford DJ, El-Hadidi S, Lunn PG, et al: Fractures of the phalanges: results of internal fixation using 1.5 mm and 2 mm AO screws, *J Hand Surg [Br]* 12:28-33, 1987.
15. Freeland AE, Benoist LA: Open reduction and internal fixation method for fractures at the proximal interphalangeal joint, *Hand Clin* 10:239-250, 1994.

16. Freeland AE, Benoist LA, Melancon KP: Parallel miniature screw fixation of spiral and long oblique hand phalangeal fractures, *Orthopaedics* 17:199-200, 1994.

17. Freeland AE, Geissler WB: Plate fixation of metacarpal shaft fractures. In Blair WF, Steyers CM (editors): *Techniques in hand surgery,* Baltimore, 1996, Williams & Wilkins.

18. Freeland AE, Jabaley ME: Management of fractures by stable fixation, *Adv Plast Reconstr Surg* 2:79-121, 1986.

19. Freeland AE, Jabaley ME, Hughes JL: *Stable fixation of the hand and wrist,* New York, 1986, Springer-Verlag.

20. Freeland AE, Roberts TS: Percutaneous screw treatment of spiral oblique finger proximal phalangeal fractures, *Orthopaedics* 14:384-388, 1991.

21. Freeland AE, Sennett BJ: Phalangeal fractures. In Peimer CA (editor): *Surgery of the hand and upper extremity,* New York, 1996, McGraw Hill.

22. Gingrass RP, Fehring BHT, Matloub HS: Intraosseous wiring of complex hand fractures, *Plast Reconstr Surg* 66:383-394, 1980.

23. Gould JS, Nicholson BG: Capsulectomy of the metacarpophalangeal and proximal interphalangeal joints, *J Hand Surg [Am]* 4:482-486, 1979.

24. Green DP, Anderson JR: Closed reduction and percutaneous pin fixation of fractures phalanges, *J Bone Joint Surg* 55A:1651-1653, 1973.

25. Hall Jr RF: Treatment of metacarpal and phalangeal fractures in noncompliant patients, *Clin Orthop* 214:31-36, 1987.

26. Heim U, Pfeiffer KM: *Internal fixation of small fractures,* Berlin, 1989, Springer-Verlag.

27. Huffaker WH, Wray Jr RC, Weeks PM: Factors Influencing final range of motion in the fingers after fractures of the hand, *Plast Reconstr Surg* 63:82-87, 1979.

28. James JIP, Wright TA: Fractures of metacarpals and proximal and middle phalanges of the finger, *J Bone Joint Surg* 48B:181-182, 1966.

29. Jupiter JB, Koniuch MP, Smith RS: The management of delayed union and nonunion of the metacarpals and phalanges, *J Hand Surg [Am]* 10:457-466, 1985.

30. Jupiter JB, Sheppard JE: Tension wire fixation of avulsion fractures in the hand, *Clin Orthop* 214:113-120, 1987.

31. Lampe EW: Surgical anatomy of the hand, *Ciba-Geigy Clinical Symposia* 40:28, 1988.

32. Lister G: Intraosseous wiring of the digital skeleton, *J Hand Surg [Am]* 3:427-435, 1978.

33. Littler JW: Hand, wrist and forearm incisions. In Littler JW (editor): *Symposium on reconstructive surgery,* St. Louis, 1974, Mosby.

34. McElfresh EC, Dobyns JH: Intra-articular metacarpal head fractures, *J Hand Surg [Am]* 8:383-393, 1983.

35. O'Brien ET: Fractures of the metacarpal and phalanges. In Green DP (editor): *Operative hand surgery,* New York, 1982, Churchill Livingstone.

36. Ouellette EA, Freeland AE: Use of the minicondylar plate in metacarpal and phalangeal fractures, *Clin Orthop* 237:38-46, 1996.

37. Peacock EE, VanWinkle W: *Surgery and biology of wound repair,* Philadelphia, 1970, WB Saunders.

38. Pratt DR: Exposing fractures of the proximal phalanx of the finger longitudinally through the dorsa extensor apparatus, *Clin Orthop* 15:22-36, 1959.

39. Prevel CD, Eppley BL, Ge J, et al: A comparative biomechanical analysis of resorbable rigid fixation versus titanium rigid fixation of metacarpal fractures, *Ann Plast Surg* 37:377-385, 1996.

40. Puckett CL, Welsh CF, Croll GH, et al: Application of maxillofacial miniplating and microplating systems to the hand, *Plast Reconstr Surg* 92:699-709, 1993.

41. Stern PJ, Wieser MJ, Reilly DG: Complications of plate fixation in the hand skeleton, *Clin Orthop* 214:59-65, 1987.

42. Strickland JW, Steichen JB, Kleinman WB, et al: Phalangeal fractures: factors influencing performance, *Orthop Rev* 1:39-50, 1982.

43. Swanson TV, Szabo RM, Anderson DD: Open hand fractures: prognosis and classification, *J Hand Surg [Am]* 16:101-107, 1991.

44. VomSaal FH: Intramedullary fixation in fractures of the hand and fingers, *J Bone Joint Surg* 35A:5-16, 1953.

45. Watson HK, Light TR, Johnson TR: Checkrein resection for flexion contractures of the middle joint, *J Hand Surg* 4:67-71, 1979.

46. Weiss APC, Hastings H II: Distal unicondylar fractures of the proximal phalanx, *J Hand Surg [Am]* 18:594-599, 1993.

47. Widgrow AD, Edinburg M, Biddulph SL: An analysis of proximal phalangeal fractures, *J Hand Surg [Am]* 12:134-139, 1987.

Phalangeal Dislocations and Ligamentous Injuries

106

Tracy E. McCall
Richard E. Brown

THE PROXIMAL INTERPHALANGEAL JOINT

ANATOMY

The wide adaptability and function of the hand relies in a large part on the range of motion and stability of the proximal interphalangeal (PIP) joint. The normal range of motion of the PIP joint is from full extension (0 degrees) to 110 degrees of flexion while allowing only 7 to 8 degrees of lateral motion.[9] The PIP joint is a ginglymus, or hinge-type joint, having two condyles on the proximal phalanx articulating with two corresponding facets on the middle phalanx. A median ridge on the middle phalanx articulates with the intercondylar groove on the proximal phalanx, creating a tongue-in-groove arrangement, stabilizing the joint against lateral and rotational deforming forces.[13]

The fingertips must alter their alignment during movement. In extension they are essentially parallel to the palm and separate from one another, and in flexion the fingertips converge to oppose the thumb. Convergence of the fingertips occurs through slight asymmetry in all the finger joints. Three points of asymmetry in the PIP joint work to create convergence of the fingertips. Examination of the heads of the proximal phalanges in the transaxial plane illustrates two of these points well. The condyles of each joint are of different heights and have a slightly different radius of curvature. The radial condyle of the index and middle fingers, and the ulnar condyle of the small finger are higher dorsally so that a line drawn across their dorsal margins will slope toward the ring finger (Figure 106-1, *A*). In the coronal plane, the PIP joints angle away from the second web space (Figure 106-1, *B*). This results in a greater distal protrusion of the ulnar condyle of the index finger and of the radial condyle of the long, ring, and small fingers. In addition, a small amount of rotation occurs at each PIP joint during flexion of the finger. The index finger

middle phalanx supinates during flexion,[23,28] and in the ring and small fingers the middle phalanx pronates.[23]

The ligamentous support structures of the PIP joint form a three-sided box that resembles a wheelbarrow. The collateral ligaments make up the sides of the box, and the volar plate forms the floor (Figure 106-1, *C*). The collateral ligaments are composed of two parts: the proper (PCL) and accessory (ACL) collateral ligaments. The PCL is the thicker portion of the collateral ligament and provides most of the lateral joint stability. The PCL originates from the dorsolateral sides of the head of the proximal phalanx and then fans out to attach along the lateral margin of the middle phalanx, blending with the periosteum for a distance of several millimeters. The PCL's volar-most portion blends with the volar plate in an area termed the *critical corner* for its significant contribution to joint stability. The ACL functions as a suspensory ligament for the volar plate and flexor tendon sheath. Its fibers originate with the PCL on the proximal phalanx and attach to the volar plate and also to the middle phalanx at the critical corners. The ACL prevents the flexor tendon sheath from moving away from the PIP joint during flexion.[9,13,23]

The volar plate is a thick ligament on the volar surface of the joint that prevents hyperextension. The volar plate grossly resembles a swallow's tail. It originates just inside the second annular (A2) pulley by two laterally located extensions. The space between these extensions allows passage of the vincular vessels (Figure 106-1, *D*). Distally, the volar plate blends with the volar periosteum of the middle phalanx, with the strongest attachments located laterally. Microscopically the volar plate consists of three layers. The most dorsal layer is divided into a proximal membranous portion and a distal meniscoid extension. The second layer contains fibers that run parallel to the finger and form the checkrein ligament. The third layer contains fibers that are

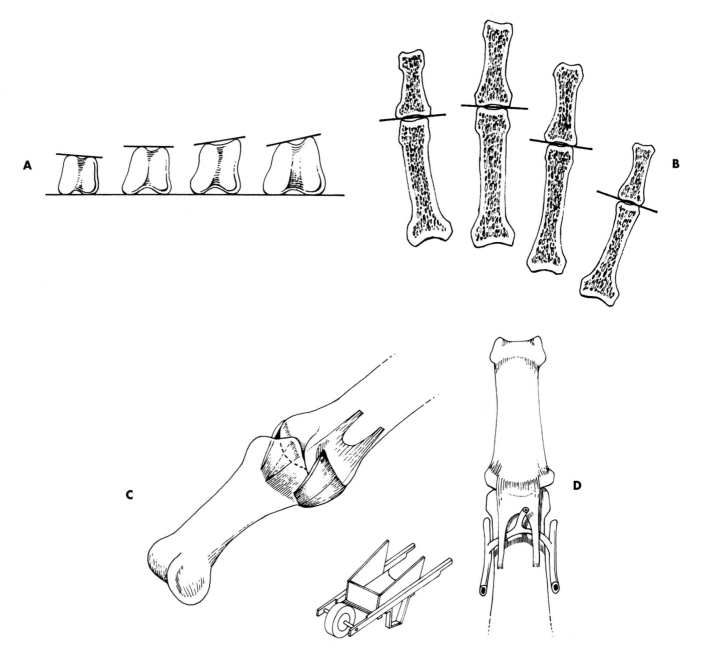

Figure 106-1. Anatomy of the PIP joint. **A,** The heads of the proximal phalanges are viewed in the transaxial plane. The radial condyle of the index and long fingers is larger than the ulnar condyle, whereas the opposite is true of the small finger. This gives a dorsal slant toward the ring finger. **B,** The PIP joint is shown in the coronal plane. A line drawn through the joints will slant away from the second web space. **C,** The PIP joint can be compared to a wheelbarrow. The volar plate forms the floor of the wheelbarrow, and the collateral ligaments form the sides. This creates a three-dimensional box that is resistant to dorsally and laterally deviating forces while allowing volar flexion. **D,** The volar plate is shown from the volar side, illustrating its swallow's tail configuration. The vincular vessel is supplied by two branches from the digital arteries, which pass between the volar plate and the bone. (Illustrations by Ed Stewart.)

oriented transversely and anchor the flexor tendon sheath to the volar plate.[42] There is a small recess separating the meniscoid portion from the middle phalanx that allows the volar plate to hinge open with flexion of the PIP joint.[8,9,13] Dorsal joint stability is provided by the central tendon slip of the extensor digitorum communis (EDC) tendon. A dorsal plate has been recently identified on the volar aspect of the central slip. It is a fibrocartilaginous structure with a biconcave shape that stabilizes the extensor tendon at the PIP joint.[35]

HYPEREXTENSION INJURIES TO THE PROXIMAL INTERPHALANGEAL JOINT

INDICATIONS

Ligamentous injuries to the PIP joint may occur dorsally, volarly, or laterally. Hyperextension injuries are the most common, particularly in association with ball handling sports.[10] The ligaments are only partially torn in sprains, and the patient usually gives a history of trauma and complains of a swollen and tender joint. On physical examination there is tenderness of the involved ligament with stress testing but no significant joint laxity. The finger should be anesthetized and examined for both active and passive stability to adequately differentiate sprains from the more serious subluxations and dislocations. The patient moves the anesthetized finger through its normal range of motion to assess active stability. Full range of motion without displacement indicates the presence of adequate ligamentous stability. To assess passive stability, the examiner gently stresses the ligaments of the anesthetized injured finger and compares these with the uninjured side.[14]

Several subluxation and dislocation classification schemes have been proposed. The most commonly used is that of Dray and Eaton.[12] Type I hyperextension injuries result from volar plate avulsion, usually at its distal end.[7] The articular surfaces remain in contact, but the joint may be locked in extreme hyperextension if the injury is severe (Figure 106-2, *A*). The finger will be unstable in extension because of the loss of palmar stabilization. Type II injuries are characterized by dorsal dislocation of the middle phalanx, in which the middle phalanx is displaced dorsal to the condyles of the proximal phalanx in a bayonet alignment. The volar plate is disrupted and the collateral ligaments are split bilaterally (Figure 106-2, *B*). Type III injuries are fracture dislocations in which the volar plate remains attached and a fracture occurs through the base of the middle phalanx. The fracture is an avulsion injury and involves a portion of the articular surface (Figure 106-2, *C*). Type III injuries are divided into stable injuries—in which the avulsed fragment involves less than 40% of the total articular surface—and unstable injuries, in which the fragment involves more than 40% of the joint surface. A fracture involving less than 40% of the joint surface of the middle phalanx is stable because the dorsal portion of the collateral ligament system remains attached to the middle phalanx.[12] Accurate closed reduction may be possible in such cases.

Schenck[33] proposed further subdivision of type III fracture dislocations. He graded type III articular fractures by the percent involvement of the joint surface. Grade I fractures involve less than 10% of the joint surface, grade II between 11% and 20%, grade III between 21% and 40%, and grade IV greater than 40%. The dislocation or subluxation is then graded by percent. Grade A injuries are less than 25%, grade B are 25% to 50%, grade C are greater than 50%, and grade D injuries are totally dislocated. The authors have found it difficult to be this accurate in estimating the grade of fracture

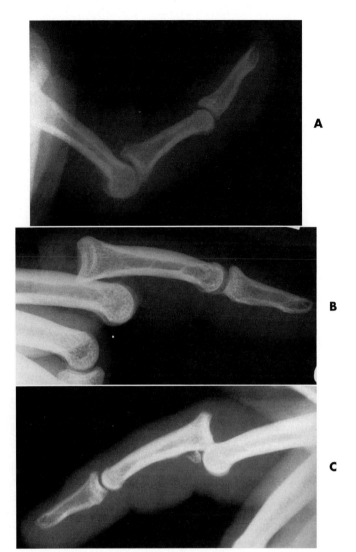

Figure 106-2. Hyperextension injury of the PIP joint. **A,** Type I hyperextension injury of the PIP joint. The articular surfaces are in contact, but the joint is locked in hyperextension. **B,** A bayonet alignment of the proximal and middle phalanges indicates a type II hyperextension injury of the PIP joint. **C,** Type III hyperextension injuries have a bayonet alignment, but also have an avulsion of the insertion of the volar plate. A small avulsion fragment is present in this radiograph. The fragment involves less than 40% of the articular surface; therefore this is a stable type III fracture dislocation.

fragments, and do not feel this classification is useful in guiding treatment.

OPERATIONS

Protective extension block splinting in 20 to 30 degrees of flexion for 7 to 14 days is usually sufficient for healing of stable injuries, including sprains and types I, II, and III stable hyperextension injuries.[12] Gentle active and passive motion should be instituted once splinting is discontinued, although buddy taping is indicated for added protection during

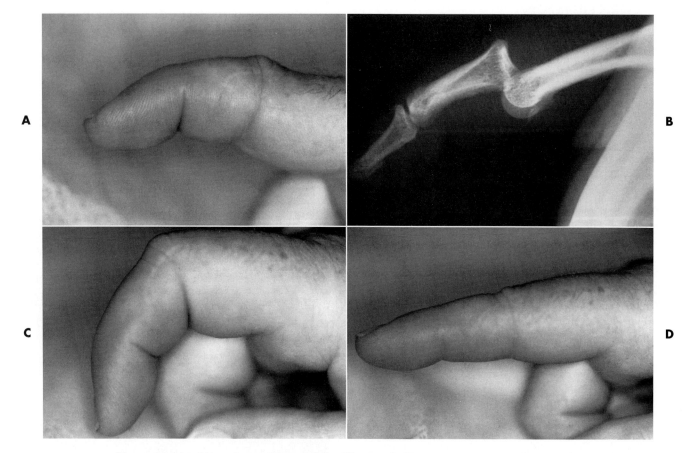

Figure 106-3. Hyperextension injury of the PIP joint. **A,** This patient presented with an acute type III stable dislocation of the right index finger. Clinically the dorsal dislocation of the middle phalanx is apparent. **B,** The dislocation is much more obvious radiographically. **C,** The patient has good flexion after closed reduction. **D,** He does not redislocate on extension. This injury may be successfully treated with splinting.

activities in which reinjury is possible. The authors' preferred method is to buddy tape stable injuries for a total of 3 to 4 weeks, with radiographic examination at 1 and 3 weeks after injury. This encourages active range of motion of the injured joint while providing protective support, thus avoiding secondary flexion contractures (Figure 106-3).

Treatment of unstable type III fracture dislocations is more difficult, and a variety of methods have been proposed. Open dorsal PIP-joint injuries are not common but can have serious ramifications despite their relatively benign appearance. The palmar skin is torn over the PIP joint in these injuries (Figure 106-4).[47] They should be treated in the operating room with intravenous (IV) antibiotics and copious joint irrigation.[39] The dislocation should be reduced and the volar plate repaired. Some authors do not repair the volar plate, fearing increased adhesions. Commonly, despite the radiographic appearance, the volar fragment is actually a comminuted mass of smaller bone fragments. The PIP joint requires precise reduction or cartilaginous degeneration and subsequent arthritis will result. Some authors recommend closed reduction and splinting when there is severe comminution of the fracture.[26] A variation on this is the *doorstop procedure,* in which the reduced finger is placed in full flexion at the PIP joint and a smooth

Kirschner wire (K wire) is placed into the head of the proximal phalanx. The protruding wire then acts as an extension-blocking splint, with the PIP joint blocked at approximately 45 degrees of flexion.[40]

The operative treatment of unstable type III joint injuries follows one of three basic methods: open reduction and internal fixation, dynamic skeletal traction, or volar plate arthroplasty. Open reduction with internal fixation is most successful in fractures with a single large fragment. A volar approach to the PIP joint is recommended.[12,41] The joint is approached through a standard Brunner-type incision, and the portion of flexor sheath between the distal A2 and proximal A4 pulleys is elevated and hinged on its radial border. The joint can be reduced by gently applying longitudinal traction and flexing the finger. A dorsal blocking K wire is then placed into the head of the proximal phalanx, preferably as described above in the doorstop procedure. If a dorsal blocking K wire does not maintain the reduction, the PIP joint must be transfixed. Reduction must be radiographically confirmed before proceeding. The fracture fragment may then be held with either a 1.5 mm screw, or crossed 0.028 K wires applied from the volar side and drawn in a retrograde fashion so that their tips do not protrude past the volar edge of the fracture fragment. Limited

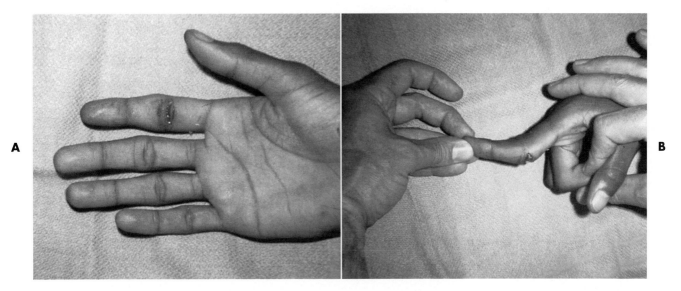

Figure 106-4. Hyperextension injury of the PIP joint. **A,** A volar skin tear over the PIP joint indicates a likely volar plate injury. **B,** A hyperextension of the PIP joint resulting in a complete rupture of the volar plate. This is an open injury, which requires operative irrigation and debridement. (Copyright SIU School of Medicine.)

motion is begun in 10 days if a dorsal blocking (doorstop) pin is present. The dorsal blocking pin is removed at 4 weeks, and the crossed K wires are removed at 6 weeks. The joint may then be protected by buddy taping. Active assisted and passive range-of-motion exercises are added at 8 weeks. Dynamic orthoses such as the joint jack can be added at 10 weeks to improve the range of motion.[41] A variation on this procedure is the cerclage fixation of the fracture dislocation, which has been reported to also work for multiple fracture fragments. One drawback to cerclage fixation is the increased mass beneath the volar plate, which can require excision of a portion of the volar plate.[43]

Volar plate arthroplasty is preferable to open reduction and internal fixation when multiple comminuted fragments are present (Figure 106-5). The joint is approached by a similar volar Brunner incision. The flexor sheath between the A2 and A4 pulleys is excised. The remaining collateral ligament attachments to the middle phalanx are excised, with the exception of the most volar remnants. The joint may then be hyperextended to afford a complete exposure of the joint surfaces. The loose bone is debrided. The volar plate is freed from its collateral ligament attachments and advanced 4 to 6 mm into the defect. The volar plate is attached to the bone by a pull-out suture. Great care must be taken during placement of the pull-out suture to avoid impaling the lateral bands with the suture by placing the DIP joint in flexion. The collateral ligaments are then reattached to the lateral margins of the volar plate, and the joint is held in 30 degrees of flexion for 2 weeks by K-wire fixation. After removal of the K wire, flexion using a dorsal extension-blocking splint is instituted. This splint is removed at 4 weeks. Dynamic extension splinting is begun at 5 weeks if full active extension is not present.[12]

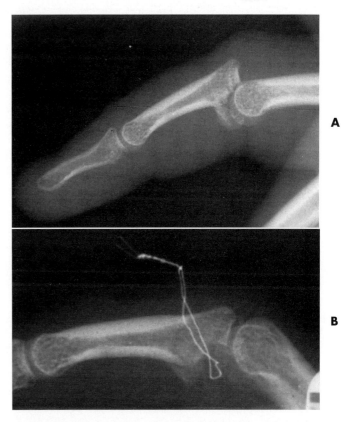

Figure 106-5. Fracture dislocation of the PIP joint. **A,** This Type III unstable fracture dislocation of the PIP joint was treated by excision of the multiple fracture fragments and advancement of the volar plate. **B,** Postoperatively, the pull-out wire shows the positioning of the volar plate in the defect left after debridement of the fracture fragments.

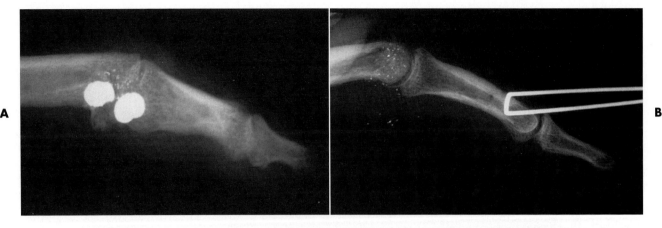

Figure 106-6. Fracture dislocation of the PIP joint. **A,** A type III unstable fracture dislocation of the PIP joint sustained in a gunshot injury was treated by debridement and dynamic traction. **B,** The final outcome shows a smooth articular surface, although there is some loss of the joint space.

The third alternative for type III unstable injuries is dynamic traction. Several methods have been proposed, all of which provide a combination of distal dynamic traction and joint movement (Figure 106-6). Once applied, the splint is maintained for 6 to 8 weeks. Although these devices can be somewhat difficult to apply and may require parts not available in all hospitals, they afford a particular advantage in the type III unstable injury with multiple fragments. The surgeon must use great care not to impale the lateral bands with any of these techniques.

Schenck's arcuate splint combines distal dynamic traction and early passive movement (Figure 106-7, *A*). A 0.045 K wire is drilled transversely through the distal head of the middle phalanx. The wrist and MCP joints are splinted in a safe position, and a large 10½-inch ring is secured to the splint, with its axis centered directly on the axis of the PIP joint. Rubber bands then attach the K wire to a shuttle on the ring. By moving the shuttle around the ring, the PIP joint may be put through its range of motion while maintaining distally based longitudinal traction. The range of motion may be limited by blocking the motion of the shuttle on the ring.[32] A smaller, spring-based apparatus has been proposed by Inanami (Figure 106-7, *B*). K wires are inserted transversely through the head of the proximal phalanx and the distal and middle parts of the middle phalanx. A rhomboid-shaped spring fitted over the proximal and distal pins provides the longitudinal distraction force. A two-armed spring is then placed over the central pin so that the arms rest volarly on the proximal and distal pins. This spring provides a volarly distracting force on the displaced middle phalanx. This double-spring arrangement is placed on both sides of the finger. Movement at the PIP joint is not obstructed because the apparatus may rotate about the axis of the proximal pin.[18] The force couple splint (Figure 106-7, *C*) can provide good reduction of a dorsal dislocation and allow joint motion; however, it does not provide any longitudinal traction. A 0.045 K wire is inserted transversely through the proximal portion of the middle phalanx, and a second K wire is placed

transversely through the head of the proximal phalanx at the axis of rotation of the PIP joint. A threaded 0.062 K wire is placed as a dorsal post distal to the initial K wire. The distal 0.045 K wire is then bent at 90 degrees on both sides of the finger so that its ends pass volar to the proximal K wire. A second 90-degree bend is made in the K wire just proximal to its passage beneath the proximal K wire. By connecting the dorsally protruding ends of the bent K wire with the dorsal post, the proximal K wire can be used as a fulcrum to hold the PIP joint in reduction.[2] A commercially available PIP hinge is also available from Smith & Nephew Richards Inc. (Figure 106-7, *D*).

OUTCOMES

Mild sprains will heal with virtually no long-term complications. Severe sprains can require a minimum of 18 months for the joint to reach its maximum improvement, and the joint may have some permanent residual enlargement.

The results of operative treatment of type III unstable fracture dislocations correlate with active range of motion, which decreases with the severity of the initial injury. Very few patients regain full pain-free range of motion after open reduction with internal fixation of type III unstable fracture dislocations.[41] Volar plate arthroplasty is a difficult technique, and failures include recurrent dislocation, angulation, flexion contractures, and DIP-joint stiffness from lateral band scarring when caught in the pull-out suture. Volar plate arthroplasty, in addition, does not function as well when a large percentage of the articular surface must be removed.[12] Similarly, a good outcome with dynamic traction methods may be difficult to achieve because of the accuracy required in K-wire placement and the cumbersome nature of the apparatus. The key to these methods is patient compliance with passive range-of-motion exercises. To date, no large studies have been done comparing the results of these methods.

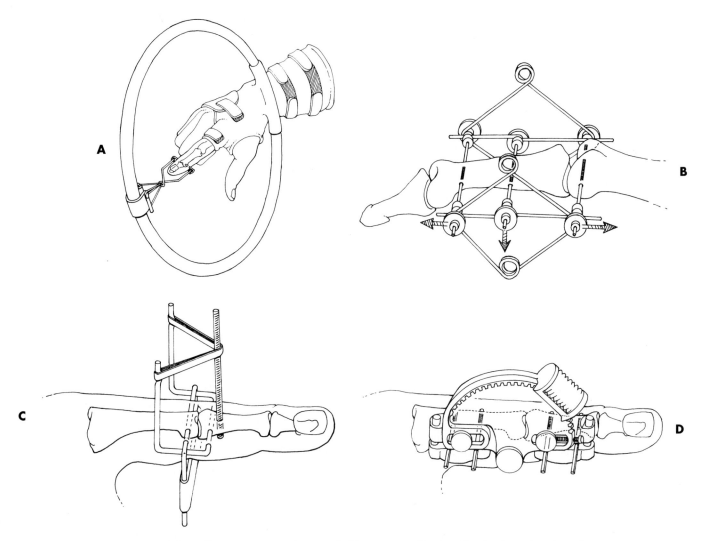

Figure 106-7. Dynamic traction devices. **A,** The arcuate splint provides distal traction through rubber bands connecting a pin in the middle phalanx to the splint's ring. The PIP joint is at the axis of this ring, allowing the patient to perform passive range of motion exercises by sliding the shuttlecock around the ring. Distal traction can be maintained at all times. **B,** Two rhomboid springs provide distal traction in this splint. The center leaf spring provides a volar force to prevent dorsal dislocations. The apparatus will rotate about the proximal pin during PIP joint flexion. **C,** The force couple splint can provide good relocation of the dorsal dislocation; however, it does not provide any joint distraction. **D,** A commercially available PIP-joint hinge provides distal traction and both active and passive range of motion. The hinge will maintain a reduction, but does not provide any relocating force intrinsic to its design. (Illustrations by Ed Stewart.)

CHRONIC FRACTURE DISLOCATION OF THE PROXIMAL INTERPHALANGEAL JOINT

Chronic PIP-joint fracture dislocations that are older than 4 weeks can be very difficult to manage. The patient often presents with considerable pain and stiffness. These injuries may be treated by any of the above methods used for acute fracture dislocations. Open reduction of the joint can be complicated, however, by significant soft tissue adhesions and malunion of the fracture fragments. Donaldson recommends open reduction with a simple capsulotomy and reduction of the joint, stressing in particular release of the adhesions between the meniscoid portion of the volar plate and the middle phalanx. Adhesions between the volar plate and the middle phalanx keep the middle phalanx from gliding around the head of the proximal phalanx during flexion and lead to redisplacement.[11] Zemel[46] pins the joint in approximately 30 degrees of flexion, then performs an osteotomy of the base of the middle phalanx so that the volar lip of the middle phalanx can be tilted to embrace the volar aspect of the proximal phalanx. This restores the volar buttress to the middle phalanx to prevent repeat dislocation. In some cases a bone graft was required to support the fracture fragments.[46] Secondary chronic hyperextension of the PIP joint may be corrected with a sublimis tenodesis. The radial slip of the sublimis tendon is divided proximally and sutured to the proximal phalanx by means of an interosseous wire or suture, with the joint placed in approximately 10 to 20 degrees of flexion. The tendon slip acts as a checkrein to prevent PIP-joint hyperextension.

The results of treatment for chronic injuries remain inferior to the treatment in acute injuries, regardless of the method used. Two major problems develop in the chronic PIP-joint fracture dislocation: repeated joint instability secondary to the loss of ligamentous support and degenerative disease secondary to the initial joint injury.

COLLATERAL LIGAMENT INJURY AT THE PROXIMAL INTERPHALANGEAL JOINT

INDICATIONS

Collateral ligament injuries usually result from laterally deviating forces, often combined with rotational stress, such as a sudden jerk from a dog leash wrapped around the fingers. The radial side of the digit is more commonly injured than the ulnar side.[3] Lateral instability of greater than 20 degrees indicates a complete tear of the collateral ligament[21] and the possibility of a Stener-type lesion where the ligament becomes entrapped in the joint.[3,38] In these cases, a slight joint incongruity may be seen on plain radiographs. Stress radiographs of the anesthetized finger should be obtained to adequately evaluate the degree of lateral instability. Operative intervention is indicated for injuries with greater than 20 degrees of lateral instability and joint incongruity demonstrated radiographically.

OPERATIONS

Most partial tears of the collateral ligament can be treated by splinting or buddy taping to the finger on the injured side for approximately 3 weeks. Instability is usually due to a ligament rupture proximally or an avulsion fracture of the middle phalanx at the insertion of the ligament. A distal tear of the volar plate may also occur, particularly when a lateral dislocation is present.

The joint is approached through a midlateral incision. Ligament ruptures may be repaired by direct suture if sufficient tissue remains, or by fixation to the bone with an interosseous wire or suture anchor. Avulsion fractures are treated by wire fixation with a figure-of-eight wire, which is passed first through the distal ligament or bony fragment and then through a hole drilled distally in the middle phalanx. Reduction is obtained by tightening the wire.[6,21]

Incomplete collateral ligament ruptures, with less than 20 degrees of lateral instability, can be safely treated without surgery. Buddy taping for 3 to 4 weeks is usually sufficient in most cases.

OUTCOMES

Most PIP-joint collateral ligament injuries heal without difficulty. Residual lateral instability is less of a problem than PIP-joint stiffness. Nonoperative intervention is therefore indicated for all but a very specific subset of lateral PIP-joint injuries (i.e., those with greater than 20 degrees of lateral instability and joint incongruity on x-ray examination). Early motion is again the key to obtaining optimal results. Currently, no outcome studies exist on this specific problem.

VOLAR DISLOCATIONS

INDICATIONS

Volar dislocations of the PIP joint are much less common than dorsal or lateral injuries.[12] Volar dislocations result from rotational and longitudinal compression in a partially flexed finger. Several variations of this injury are possible. A pure volar dislocation may occur with rupture of the central slip and some involvement of the collateral ligaments. If significant rotational force is present, a unilateral dislocation of the PIP joint may occur with rupture of one collateral ligament and a distal tear in the volar plate. The ipsilateral proximal phalangeal condyle herniates through the extensor mechanism and becomes trapped between the extensor tendon and the lateral band, creating an irreducible dislocation.

OPERATIONS

Closed reduction should be attempted in all volar PIP-joint dislocations. Reduction should be attempted using gentle distal traction with the metacarpophalangeal (MCP) and PIP joints flexed.[12] This relaxes the lateral bands. Usually full active extension will be present after reduction. Lack of active extension and/or incongruous reduction on lateral radiographs indicates possible entrapment of ligament, tendon, or joint capsule, which requires open reduction through a midlateral incision. The joint can be easily reduced after removing the entrapped structures. The lateral band may be ruptured and can be repaired if it has not been severely traumatized.[12] The PIP joint is immobilized in extension for 5 to 7 days after reduction. The finger is then placed in a dynamic extension splint for another 2 to 3 weeks.

OUTCOMES

Irreducible volar PIP-joint dislocations may have a better prognosis than reducible volar dislocations because the extensor mechanism is more likely to be intact in an irreducible dislocation.[19] Most patients do well after adequate reduction. Fibrosis of the joint after any type of dislocation may occur up to 1 year after the injury.[12]

THE DISTAL INTERPHALANGEAL JOINT

ANATOMY

The distal interphalangeal (DIP) joint is very similar anatomically to the PIP joint. The arc of motion of the DIP joint is more limited than the PIP joint, with approximately 80 degrees of flexion to 10 to 20 degrees of hyperextension, but the positioning of this joint is much more precise. Each DIP joint has a slightly different angulation to facilitate pinch contact with the thumb. During flexion the distal phalanx of the index finger deviates ulnarly, whereas the distal phalanx of the ring and small fingers deviates slightly radially.[9] No rotation occurs in the long-finger DIP joint. The ligamentous structures of the DIP joint are similar to the PIP joint in that both have a volar plate and collateral ligaments. In addition to its ligaments, support is provided by the insertions of the flexor and extensor tendons and also the snug overlying skin.[9,13] Dislocation of the DIP joint is therefore much less common than the PIP joint because of this added support. In addition, the distal phalanx has a relatively short lever arm, and the DIP joint has the ability to hyperextend.[9]

INDICATIONS

Dorsal DIP-joint dislocations occur more commonly than volar dislocations, and irreducible dislocations rarely occur. There are several mechanisms that can prevent closed reduction of the dorsal DIP-joint dislocation. Dorsal dislocation of the flexor digitorum profundus (FDP) tendon behind a condyle of the middle phalanx[1] or a volar plate avulsion with interposition into the joint can often require open reduction to replace the disrupted anatomy. Buttonhole tears of the volar plate, which occasionally involve the FDP tendon, can entrap the distal end of the middle phalanx like a noose.[15] Volar plate avulsion in a dorsal DIP-joint dislocation is more likely to be proximal, and the joint is more likely to be open (Figure 106-8).

OPERATIONS

Dorsal dislocations of the DIP joint are reduced, and the joint is immobilized in slight flexion for 10 to 21 days. Most closed DIP-joint dislocations are stable after reduction. Palmar dislocations are splinted in extension after reduction, also for 10 to 21 days. Antibiotics and copious irrigation are indicated when an open dislocation is present. Irreducible dislocations should be opened through any open wounds, if present. Gentle retraction of the involved structures will usually free the joint.

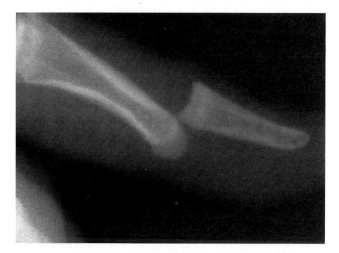

Figure 106-8. Dorsal dislocation of the DIP joint.

The joint may then be treated as in a closed reduction. Chronic dislocations, those present for more than 4 weeks, usually are not reducible without surgery. The soft tissues undergo contraction and hold the dislocated distal phalanx in its abnormal position. Open reduction is carried out through a volar incision. The volar aspects of the collateral ligaments often must be released, and occasionally a dorsal capsulotomy is necessary to reduce the joint. If the reduction is not stable, the joint should be fixed with a K wire. When a dislocation has been present for several months and has caused subsequent degeneration of the articular surfaces, a primary joint fusion is indicated.[24]

OUTCOMES

Full range of motion of the DIP joint can be regained without difficulty if the joint is splinted no longer than 4 weeks. Splinting may be required for periods of high stress activity, such as athletic events, for several months. K-wire fixation of the DIP joint may occasionally cause nail-bed deformity, and care must be used when placing these wires across the joint.

THE METACARPOPHALANGEAL JOINT

ANATOMY

The mobility of the MCP joint is unique among finger joints. The MCP joint allows a significant amount of lateral movement when held in extension, whereas in flexion it becomes much more stable, with little lateral movement possible. The articular surface is a condyle shape when viewed from a lateral position.[12] The head of the metacarpal is trapezoidal when viewed end-on, with its volar surface nearly twice as wide as its dorsal surface.[13] The MCP joint contributes to convergence of the fingers during grasp by a slight ulnar rotation of the index finger metacarpal head and slight radial rotation of the ring and small finger metacarpal heads.[9] The MCP-joint capsule extends from the neck of the metacarpal to the base of the proximal phalanx. The volar plate is firmly attached to the proximal phalanx, but has only a loose membranous attachment to the neck of the metacarpal proximally.[45] This loose proximal attachment allows 30 degrees of hyperextension at the MCP joint. The volar plates of the MCP joints are also stabilized by the deep transverse metacarpal ligament, which interconnects the lateral sides of the neighboring plates.[9] The collateral ligaments originate dorsal to the axis of rotation on the metacarpal head and insert volarly on the base of the proximal phalanx. The ACLs insert into the volar plate. The shape of the metacarpal head and the dorsal origin of the collateral ligaments combine to keep the ligaments taut in joint flexion and lax in extension. The ligaments must stretch over the condyle during flexion. The MCP joint should be splinted in some flexion to keep the collateral ligaments from contracting and limiting joint motion.

INDICATIONS

Dislocation of the MCP joint is a rare injury. Both volar and dorsal dislocations have been reported, the latter being more common. Dorsal dislocations result from forced hyperextension of the joint and are most commonly seen in the border digits, with index dislocation more common than that of the small finger. Dislocation of the central digits is infrequent and is almost always associated with dislocation of the adjoining small or index finger.[12] Volar dislocations may be produced by flexion of the MCP joint, with a subsequent force applied perpendicular to the proximal phalanx (as in a fight),[44] or by hyperextension.[5] Hyperextension most commonly will result in MCP-joint subluxation, an incomplete dislocation, or dorsal dislocation. Both subluxation and dislocation of the MCP joint entail a proximal rupture of the volar plate. However, with a subluxation the volar plate remains draped over the volar surface of the metacarpal head, whereas the volar plate is drawn up and folded into the joint in the dislocated finger. A finger subluxation is characterized by marked hyperextension (60 to 80 degrees) of the MCP joint, and the articular surfaces remain in partial contact.[12] The base of the proximal phalanx is located dorsal to the metacarpal head in a dorsal dislocation. Dorsal dislocations present with slight hyperextension at the MCP joint and slight flexion of the distal joints. The finger angulates toward and partially overlaps the adjacent central digit. An area of puckered skin in the palm is evident over a palpable firmness of the metacarpal head (Figure 106-9).[12,20] A dorsal dislocation of the MCP joint is usually irreducible by closed methods because the volar soft tissues form a noose around the neck of the metacarpal and prevent reduction. In the index finger, these structures are the flexor tendons ulnarly and the lumbrical muscle radially.[12,20] In the small-finger dislocation the flexor tendons and lumbrical are located radially, and the abductor digiti quinti and flexor digiti minimi are found ulnarly.

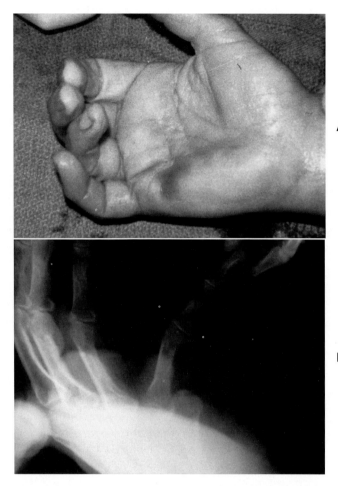

Figure 106-9. Metacarpal joint of the finger. **A,** Clinical appearance of a small-finger MCP-joint dorsal dislocation. Note the slight extension of the MCP joint and the area of fullness over the metacarpal head. **B,** Radiograph showing the bayonet alignment of the same small finger MCP-joint dorsal dislocation. (Copyright SIU School of Medicine.)

OPERATIONS

Closed reduction should be attempted in all cases under anesthesia. When closed reduction is unsuccessful, open reduction is best performed through a dorsal approach. The dorsal capsule, volar plate, or collateral ligaments may be found interposed inside the joint. The volar plate may be avulsed either proximally or distally.[5,44] The joint should be cleared and the ligaments repaired.

Dorsal subluxation may be treated with closed reduction. Longitudinal traction and hyperextension should not be used because either may draw the volar plate into the joint and convert the injury to a complete dislocation. To appropriately reduce an MCP-joint dorsal subluxation, the wrist is flexed to relax the flexor tendons. The examiner then applies pressure dorsally over the base of the proximal phalanx in a distal and volar direction. This pushes the base of the proximal phalanx off the dorsum of the metacarpal and back into position. The finger should then be placed in an extension-blocking splint for 2 to 3 weeks.

A dorsal dislocation of the MCP joint should be approached through a palmar incision, either just distal to the palmar crease or using a Brunner-type incision over the metacarpal head. The neurovascular bundle on the radial side of the index or ulnar side of the small finger may be stretched over the metacarpal head and can easily be divided during exposure of the joint. Release of the A1 pulley gives greater laxity of the flexor tendons and allows the head of the metacarpal to be reduced.[12] The MCP joint should be immobilized in 30 degrees of flexion for no more than 2 weeks in a volar splint. A dorsal extension-blocking splint is then used for another 2 weeks to block MCP-joint hyperextension while facilitating flexion of the IP joints.

OUTCOMES

Acute MCP-joint dislocations and subluxations can respond well to appropriate treatment, with return of full range of motion.[17] Occasionally, the range of motion may be reduced, although improvement may be noted for as long as 8 months after injury. McLaughlin[27] found that prolonged immobilization led to a decrease in the final range of motion, and he recommended immobilization of the MCP joint for only a few days or not at all. Degenerative arthritis results from trauma or devascularization of the articular cartilage. This may occur with late reduction, repeated attempts at closed reduction, or with traumatic handling of the joint during open reduction. Physeal closure has been reported as a complication of MCP-joint dislocation in children secondary to devascularization of the metacarpal head.[25] Digital nerve damage may occur when the nerve is positioned over the metacarpal head.[12]

INDICATIONS

Collateral ligament injury at the MCP-joint level is an uncommon injury. It is most often seen in the middle, ring, and small fingers, and is caused by sudden deviation of the digit, usually in an ulnar direction with the MCP joint flexed.[12,45]

OPERATIONS

Most MCP-joint collateral ligament injuries represent sprains and may be treated by splinting the joint in moderate flexion (30 degrees) for 3 weeks, followed by buddy taping to the radial adjacent digit for another 2 to 3 weeks.[12] This conservative treatment may also be effective with a complete ligamentous rupture; however, eventual surgical repair may also be required. Gross instability to laterally deviating forces may be demonstrated when the joint is in full flexion if the collateral ligament has been completely disrupted. Radiographic evaluation may demonstrate an avulsion fracture. Surgical treatment is performed through a dorsal incision. The ligament is reattached using a pull-out suture, and the joint is held in flexion.[34,45] Gentle protected range-of-motion exercises are begun after 3 weeks of immobilization.

OUTCOMES

Full recovery from sprains may take up to 18 months, with significant tenderness present for many months.[45] Operative treatment of a complete ligamentous disruption usually results in correction of instability and return of full pain-free range of motion.[34] Schubiner and Mass[34] reported that 8 of 10 patients regained full range of motion after operative treatment of complete MCP-joint collateral ligament ruptures.

THE LOCKED METACARPOPHALANGEAL JOINT

INDICATIONS

Locking of a digital MCP joint is characterized by rigid loss of extension with little loss of flexion. Locking often occurs suddenly.[45] It is an unusual condition often confused with trigger finger. The two may be differentiated by the free extension allowed at the PIP and DIP joints in the locked finger. Locking may be divided into degenerative and spontaneous groups. Degenerative cases are generally in patients over the age of 50, most commonly involve the long finger, and have degenerative changes on radiographic examination. Locking in the degenerative group is caused by osteophytes or degenerative changes in the joint capsule.[30] Spontaneous cases are found in patients younger than 50, are most common in the index finger, and usually present with no radiographic findings. Causes of spontaneous joint locking include abnormal bands or membranes within the joint, capsular tears, irregular articular surfaces, and entrapped sesamoids or loose bodies.[30]

OPERATIONS

Occasionally an intraarticular injection of an anesthetic can by used to distend the joint capsule and free the locking joint. This method can be used in either degenerative or spontaneous cases.[30] More commonly, joint exploration must be performed to free the joint.[45] The joint is generally approached through a volar incision. The joint is explored, and the offending structure excised.[30]

OUTCOMES

Active range-of-motion exercises may be started immediately after surgery. Full function is usually recovered quickly, and recurrences are uncommon.[30]

METACARPOPHALANGEAL-JOINT INJURIES OF THE THUMB

In contrast to the finger MCP joint, stability of the thumb MCP joint is of paramount importance for both power grip and precision grasp. Range of motion in the thumb MCP joint is less than that of the fingers and varies greatly between individuals. Total range of motion may vary from 5 to 100 degrees of flexion.[13] Several differences between the MCP joints of the thumb and fingers give the thumb increased stability. The metacarpal head is wider in the thumb than in the fingers.[4,31] The radial and ulnar sesamoid bones are incorporated into the lateral margins of the distal palmar plate (Figure 106-10).[4,37] The flexor pollicis brevis and the adductor

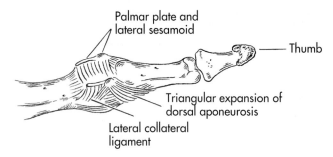

Figure 106-10. The volar aspect of the thumb MCP joint is shown with the incorporation of the sesamoid bones into the volar plate.

pollicis tendons partially insert into the sesamoid bones and provide additional support to the joint.[4,37] The joint is further supported by the surrounding tendons—the extensor pollicis longus and brevis dorsally, the flexor pollicis longus volarly, the adductor pollicis with its aponeurosis medially, and the flexor pollicis brevis and abductor pollicis brevis laterally (Figure 106-11).[4]

INDICATIONS

Dislocation of the thumb MCP joint usually occurs as a result of a hyperextension force. Dislocations of the MCP joint are much more common in the thumb than in the fingers because of its exposed position.[13] Commonly, the volar plate ruptures proximal to the sesamoid bones. Entrapment of the metacarpal head does not occur because the thumb lacks a lumbrical. These dislocations are therefore usually amenable to closed reduction. Open reduction is indicated when closed reduction cannot be achieved secondary to interposition of the volar plate, sesamoid bones, or flexor pollicis longus tendon (Figure 106-12).[12]

OPERATIONS

Closed reduction of a dorsally dislocated thumb MCP joint is performed by flexing the metacarpal into the palm and applying longitudinal traction. The MCP joint is then flexed, maintaining distal traction, to relocate the base of the proximal

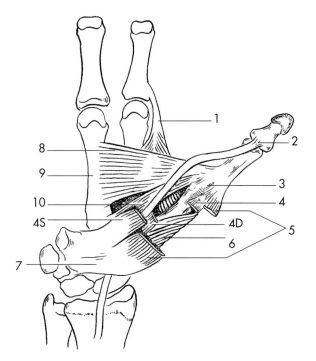

1. First dorsal interosseous muscle
2. Flexor pollicis longus
3. Volar plate
4. Flexor pollicis brevis
4S. Flexor pollicis brevis superficial head
4D. Flexor pollicis brevis deep head
5. Abductor pollicis brevis
6. Opponens pollicis
7. Flexor retinaculum
8. Adductor pollicis transverse head
9. Third metacarpal
10. Adductor pollicis oblique head

Figure 106-11. Anatomy of the thumb.

phalanx. A post-reduction radiograph should be obtained to confirm joint reduction. Splinting in slight flexion for 3 to 4 weeks is sufficient.[12,13]

Open reduction is best performed through a palmar incision. Reduction of the anatomic structures is usually sufficient,[31] however some authors recommend volar plate repair. Occasionally the sesamoid bones may be fractured and the fragments displaced. This indicates a disruption of the tendons associated with the sesamoids. A circumferential suture can be used to hold the sesamoid fragments in approximation,[37] or the sesamoid fragments can be removed and the tendon repaired.

Volar dislocation of the thumb MCP joint is much less common than dorsal dislocation but has been reported.[29] Closed reduction should be attempted with appropriate anesthesia. Volar dislocations may require open reduction when interposition of the dorsal capsule or extensor pollicis longus or extensor pollicis brevis tendons is involved.[29]

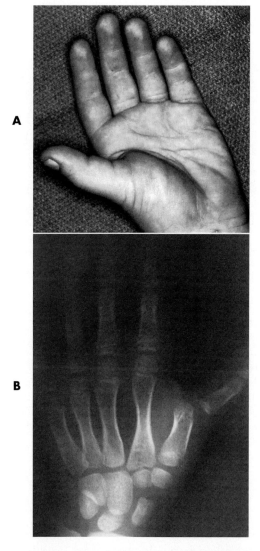

Figure 106-12. Dorsal dislocation of the MCP joint of the thumb. **A,** Clinical appearance of a dorsally dislocated thumb MCP joint. Note the hyperextension of the joint and the bulge of the metacarpal head. **B,** Radiographic appearance of the dorsally dislocated thumb MCP joint.

COLLATERAL LIGAMENT INJURIES IN THE THUMB METACARPOPHALANGEAL JOINT

INDICATIONS

As in the finger, the collateral ligament system of the thumb MCP joint consists of proper (PCL) and accessory (ACL) collateral ligaments. The PCLs are taut in flexion and relaxed in extension, whereas the opposite is true of the ACLs.[4] Although the ulnar collateral ligament is stronger than the radial collateral ligament,[22] the ulnar collateral ligament is more commonly injured.[12] Disruption of the thumb ulnar collateral ligament is known as *gamekeeper's thumb* or *skier's thumb* and occurs as a result of an acute or chronic radially deviating force on the thumb. Associated injuries include avulsion fractures at the insertion of the collateral ligament, injuries to the joint capsule and volar plate, and tearing of the adductor aponeurosis.[12] Most commonly, the collateral ligament ruptures distally.

Stener[36] described the pathologic anatomy associated with a complete rupture of the ulnar collateral ligament. The Stener lesion occurs when the adductor aponeurosis becomes interposed between the free ends of a completely ruptured ulnar collateral ligament (Figure 106-13). The radially deviating forces that cause the collateral ligament to tear also cause the adductor aponeurosis to slide distally—past the point of collateral ligament rupture. As the thumb returns to its normal position, the adductor aponeurosis slides beneath the free end of the ruptured ulnar collateral ligament and sweeps it proximally. Adequate healing cannot occur with the ends of the ulnar collateral ligament separated by the adductor aponeurosis.

The diagnosis of a Stener lesion is made on the basis of the clinical examination. The presence of significant ecchymosis, edema, and point tenderness should raise suspicion of a complete ligamentous rupture. A rotational deformity may also be present.[12] Lateral stress testing in a complete ligament injury will show 30 degrees or more of radial deviation of the proximal phalanx from the metacarpal in comparison with the normal side. Controversy exists on the appropriate position of the joint for lateral stress testing. As the PCL of the MCP joint is lax in extension, stress testing of the joint in this position may give false positive results. The examiner must use care when testing the joint in 30 degrees of flexion because rotation of the thumb at the basilar joint can give the appearance of MCP joint laxity.[31] Examination in both positions and comparison with the normal side is recommended. PA and lateral radiographs of the thumb should be obtained to look for bony avulsions. The treatment of thumb MCP-joint collateral ligament tears depends on the severity of the injury. A complete tear of the ligament, and possible Stener lesion, is present when more than 30 degrees of motion is found on lateral stress testing. Partial ligament injuries are divided into two groups on the basis of their severity: grade 1 injuries have a stable joint and a clear endpoint on lateral stress testing; grade 2 injuries are slightly more severe, and the endpoint on lateral stress testing is less definite.[31]

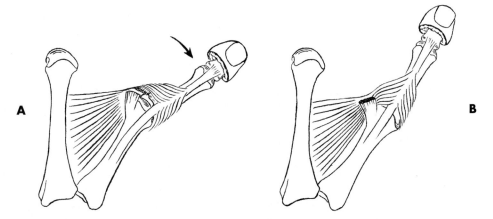

Figure 106-13. Stener lesion. **A,** A radially deviating force ruptures the ulnar collateral ligament of the thumb MCP joint. The deviating force causes the thumb to shift so that the adductor aponeurosis slides distal to the rupture in the ulnar collateral ligament. **B,** When the thumb returns to its normal orientation the free end of the ulnar collateral ligament is swept above the adductor aponeurosis.

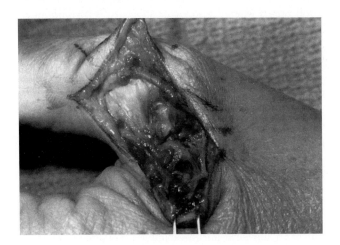

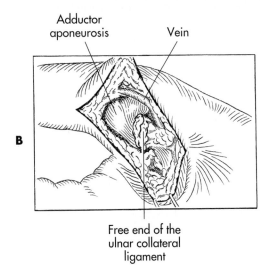

Figure 106-14. Stener lesion. **A,** An acute rupture of the ulnar collateral ligament of the thumb with a Stener lesion. The ligament can be seen folded proximally and superficial to the adductor aponeurosis. **B,** The same Stener lesion seen in an illustration. (**A** copyright SIU School of Medicine.)

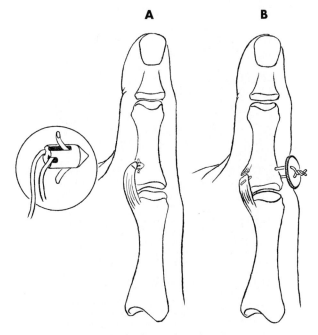

Figure 106-15. Operative repair of the Stener lesion. **A,** The ulnar collateral ligament may be reattached using a suture anchor. **B,** Pull-out wires have been used to secure the ulnar collateral ligament for many years. They may be more time consuming than the more recent suture anchor; however, they will provide similar results.

OPERATIONS

Ulnar collateral ligament injury is more common, but the treatment of both the ulnar and radial collateral ligaments is similar. Partial ligament injuries (grades 1 and 2) may be treated with splinting. A thumb spica splint should be formed using great care to deviate the MCP joint toward the side of injury.[12] Grade 1 injuries should be splinted for 7 to 10 days, and grade 2 injuries splinted for 3 to 4 weeks.[16,31] Avulsion fractures with

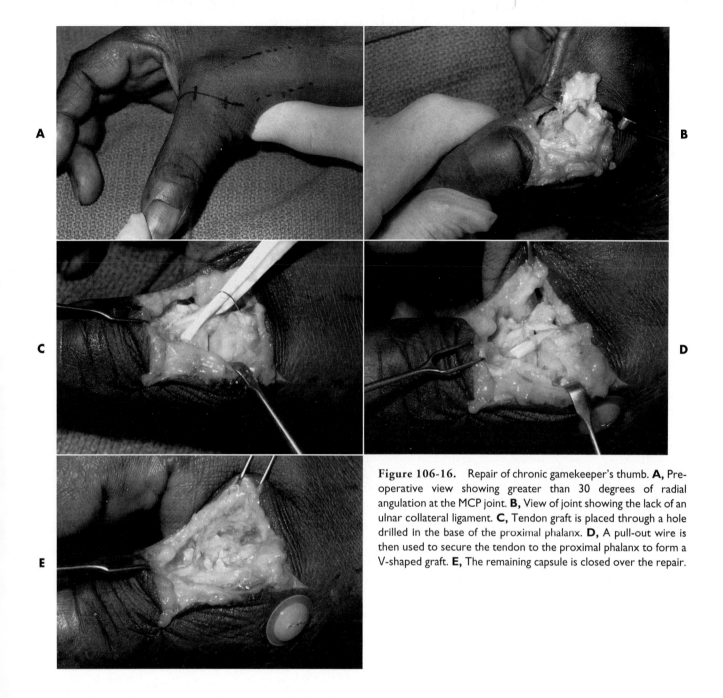

Figure 106-16. Repair of chronic gamekeeper's thumb. **A,** Preoperative view showing greater than 30 degrees of radial angulation at the MCP joint. **B,** View of joint showing the lack of an ulnar collateral ligament. **C,** Tendon graft is placed through a hole drilled in the base of the proximal phalanx. **D,** A pull-out wire is then used to secure the tendon to the proximal phalanx to form a V-shaped graft. **E,** The remaining capsule is closed over the repair.

greater than 2 mm of displacement are suspicious for complete ligamentous rupture. Complete tears of the ulnar collateral ligament should be treated surgically.[16,36] A trial of splinting is not indicated because a delay in the repair of the ligament may reduce the success of the repair.

Surgical repair of the ulnar collateral ligament may be undertaken through a chevron incision,[16] an oblique dorsal incision,[12] or a curved dorsal incision.[31] The sensory branches of the radial nerve should be protected. When a Stener lesion is present, the ulnar collateral ligament can be seen overlying the normally sharp and clear edge of the adductor aponeurosis (Figure 106-14). The adductor aponeurosis should be divided parallel to the extensor tendon, leaving a small rim of aponeurosis attached to the extensor tendon to facilitate repair. A primary repair of the collateral ligament can be performed in

acute cases. The collateral ligament is gently teased back into its appropriate alignment and reattached using a suture anchor, pull-out wire, or periosteal bone flap. When a bony avulsion fragment is present, the fragment may be reattached using a 1.5 mm minifragment screw in the case of a very large fragment, or a pull-out wire in the case of smaller or multiple fragments. The fragment may also be excised, and the ligament reattached as described above. The adductor aponeurosis and wound are then closed, and a protective splint is applied (Figure 106-15).

It is unlikely that the ligament can be restored to its full length in chronic injuries. The ligament must be reconstructed with either a tendon transfer or a tendon graft in these cases (Figure 106-16). Tendon transfers have been reported using the extensor indicis proprius, abductor pollicis longus, adduc-

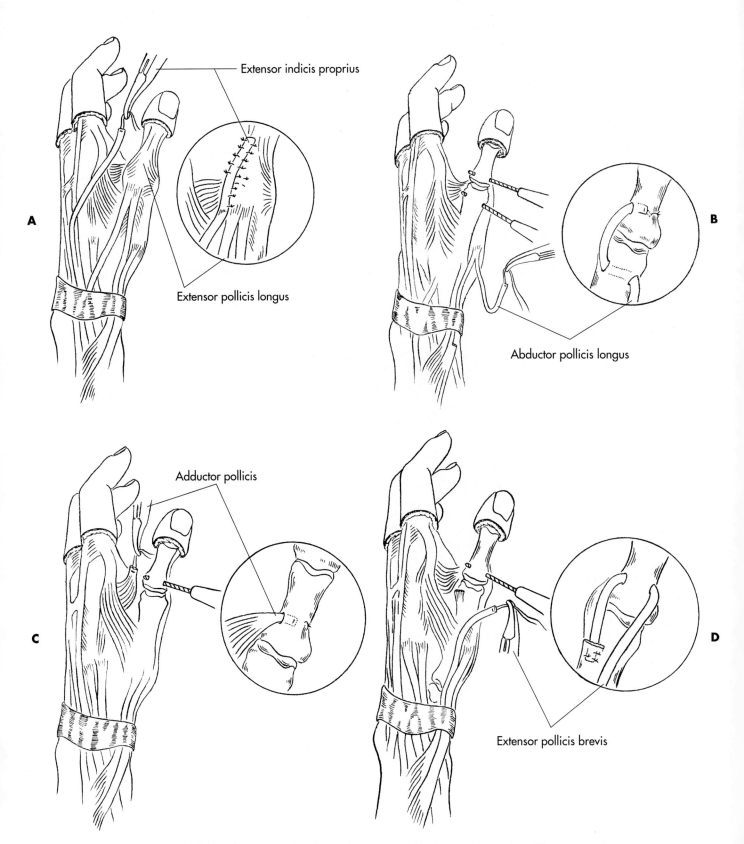

Figure 106-17. Repair of a chronic gamekeeper's thumb using tendon transfers. These methods have been previously described; however, they are no longer used frequently. **A,** The extensor indicis proprius tendon may be divided distally and transferred to the thumb. The tendon is sutured both proximal and distal to the joint, providing a sturdy replacement for the ulnar collateral ligament. **B,** The abductor pollicis longus tendon may be split lengthwise. Half of the tendon is then divided proximally, woven through a transversely drilled hole in the metacarpal and inserted into the ulnar side of the proximal phalanx. **C,** The adductor pollicis may be freed from the aponeurosis and inserted directly into the proximal phalanx. **D,** The extensor pollicis brevis transfer is performed using half of the tendon, which is divided distally. A drill hole is made through the metacarpal at an angle of 45 degrees dorsal to medial. The tendon is passed through this hole and inserted into the base of the proximal phalanx.

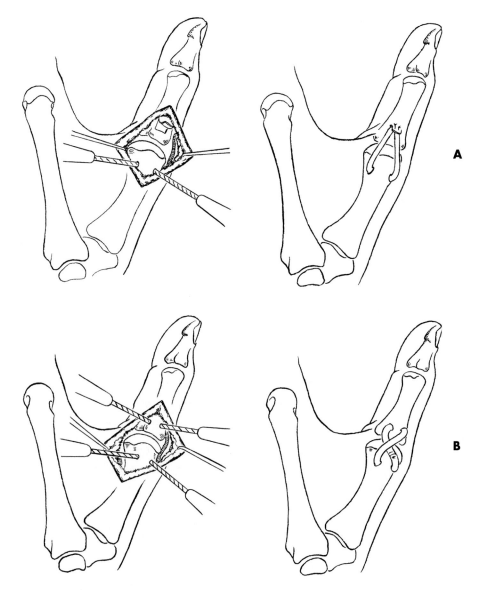

Figure 106-18. Tendon grafts to reconstruct the ulnar collateral ligament. Two basic weaves have been described for tendon graft fixation of the ruptured ulnar collateral ligament. **A,** A hole is drilled across the ulnar side of the metacarpal. The tendon is passed through this hole, then both ends are inserted into a periosteal window elevated on the proximal phalanx. **B,** Two holes are drilled, one across the ulnar side of the metacarpal and one across the ulnar side of the proximal phalanx. The tendon is passed through the holes in a figure-of-eight fashion, then sutured to itself or the remaining periosteum.

tor pollicis, and extensor pollicis brevis (Figure 106-17). If the transferred tendon is weak, it should be attached to both the proximal phalanx and the metacarpal so that it also functions as a checkrein. A tendon graft, most commonly the palmaris longus, may be woven across the ulnar side of the joint to reconstruct the ligament. Several weave methods have been described (Figure 106-18).[31]

strengthening exercises begin after 6 weeks. The joint should be protected from radially deviating forces during stressful activities for 3 to 4 months after surgery. Discomfort may be expected for up to 1 year. Less favorable results are found in patients with chronic ligament injuries. Often, secondary articular degeneration has occurred, and fusion of the joint should be considered if arthritic pain is the main symptom.

OUTCOMES

Most patients do well after an acute collateral ligament repair. Casting is recommended for a full 4 weeks after surgery, followed by 2 weeks of protective splinting. Range of motion and

REFERENCES

1. Abouzahr MK, Poblete JVP: Irreducible dorsal dislocation of the distal interphalangeal joint: case report and literature review, *J Trauma* 42:743-745, 1997.

2. Agee JM: Unstable fracture dislocations of the proximal interphalangeal joint: treatment with the force couple splint, *Clin Orthop* 214:101-112, 1987.

3. Ali MS: Complete disruption of collateral mechanism of proximal interphalangeal joint of fingers, *J Hand Surg [Br]* 9:191-193, 1984.

4. Barmakian JT: Anatomy of the joints of the thumb, *Hand Clin* 8(4):683-691, 1992.

5. Betz RR, Browne EZ, Perry GB, Resnick EJ: The complex volar metacarpophalangeal joint dislocation: a case report and review of the literature, *J Bone Joint Surg* 64A:1374-1375, 1982.

6. Bischoff R, Buechler U, De Roche R, Jupiter J: Clinical results of tension band fixation of avulsion fractures of the hand, *J Hand Surg [Am]* 19:1019-1026, 1994.

7. Bowers WH: The proximal interphalangeal joint volar plate. II. A clinical study of hyperextension injury, *J Hand Surg [Am]* 6:77-81, 1981.

8. Bowers WH, Wolf Jr JW, Nehil JL, Bittinger S: The proximal interphalangeal joint volar plate. I. An anatomical and biomechanical study, *J Hand Surg [Am]* 5:79-88, 1980.

9. Craig SM: Anatomy of the joints of the fingers, *Hand Clin* 8(4):693-700, 1992.

10. Dawson WJ: The spectrum of sports-related interphalangeal joint injuries, *Hand Clin* 10(2):315-326, 1994.

11. Donaldson WR, Millender LH: Chronic fracture-subluxation of the proximal interphalangeal joint, *J Hand Surg [Am]* 3:149-153, 1978.

12. Dray GJ, Eaton RG: Dislocations and ligament injuries in the digits. In Green DP (editor): *Operative hand surgery,* New York, 1993, Churchill Livingstone.

13. Eaton RG: *Joint injuries of the hand,* Springfield, Ill, 1971, Charles C. Thomas.

14. Eaton RG, Littler JW: Joint injuries and their sequelae, *Clin Plast Surg* 3:85-98, 1976.

15. Ghobadi F, Anapolle DM: Irreducible distal interphalangeal joint dislocation of the finger: a new cause, *J Hand Surg [Am]* 19:196-198, 1994.

16. Husband JB, McPherson SA: Bony skier's thumb injuries, *Clin Orthop* 327:79-84, 1996.

17. Idler S: Irreducible dorsal dislocations of the metacarpophalangeal joint. In Blair WF (editor): *Techniques in hand surgery,* Baltimore, 1996, Williams & Wilkins.

18. Inanami H, Ninomiya S, Okutsu I, et al: Dynamic external finger fixator for fracture dislocation of the proximal interphalangeal joint, *J Hand Surg [Am]* 18:160-164, 1993.

19. Inoue G, Noboru M: Irreducible palmar dislocation of the proximal interphalangeal joint of the finger, *J Hand Surg [Am]* 15:301-304, 1990.

20. Kaplan EB: Dorsal dislocation of the metacarpophalangeal joint of the index finger, *J Bone Joint Surg* 39A:1081-1086, 1957.

21. Kiefhaber TR, Stern PJ, Grood ES: Lateral stability of the proximal interphalangeal joint, *J Hand Surg [Am]* 11:661-669, 1986.

22. Kraemer BA, Gilula LA: Anatomy affecting the metacarpal and phalangeal bones of the hand. In Gulula LA (editor): *The traumatized hand and wrist,* Philadelphia, 1992, WB Saunders.

23. Leibovic SJ, Bowers WH: Anatomy of the proximal interphalangeal joint, *Hand Clin* 10(2):169-178, 1994.

24. Lenzo SR: Distal joint injuries of the thumb and fingers, *Hand Clin* 8(4):769-775, 1992.

25. Light TR, Ogden JA: Complex dislocation of the index metacarpophalangeal joint in children, *J Pediatr Orthop* 8:300-305, 1988.

26. McElfresh EC, Dobyns JH, O'Brien ET: Management of fracture-dislocation of the proximal interphalangeal joints by extension-block splinting, *J Bone Joint Surg* 54A:1705-1711, 1972.

27. McLaughlin HL: Complex "locked" dislocation of the metacarpophalangeal joints, *J Trauma* 5(6):683-688, 1963.

28. Minamikawa Y, Horri E, Amadio PC, et al: Stability and constraint of the proximal interphalangeal joint, *J Hand Surg [Am]* 18:198-204, 1993.

29. Miyamoto M, Hirayama T, Uchida M: Volar dislocation of the metacarpophalangeal joint of the thumb: a case report, *J Hand Surg [Br]* 11:51-54, 1986.

30. Posner MA, Langa V, Green SM: The locked metacarpophalangeal joint: diagnosis and treatment, *J Hand Surg [Am]* 11:249-253, 1986.

31. Posner MA, Retaillaud JL: Metacarpophalangeal joint injuries of the thumb, *Hand Clin* 8(4):713-732, 1992.

32. Schenck RR: Dynamic traction and early passive movement for fractures of the proximal interphalangeal joint, *J Hand Surg [Am]* 11:850-858, 1986.

33. Schenck RR: Classification of fractures and dislocations of the proximal interphalangeal joint, *Hand Clin* 10(2):179-185, 1994.

34. Schubiner JM, Mass DP: Operation for collateral ligament ruptures of the metacarpophalangeal joints of the fingers, *J Bone Joint Surg* 71B:388-389, 1989.

35. Slattery PG: The dorsal plate of the proximal interphalangeal joint, *J Hand Surg [Br]* 15:68-73,1990.

36. Stener B: Displacement of the ruptured ulnar collateral ligament of the metacarpophalangeal joint of the thumb, *J Bone Joint Surg* 44B:869-879,1962.

37. Stener B: Hyperextension injuries to the metacarpophalangeal joint of the thumb: rupture of ligaments, fracture of sesamoid bones, rupture of flexor pollicis brevis, *Acta Chir Scand* 125:275-293, 1963.

38. Stern PJ: Stener lesion after lateral dislocation of the proximal interphalangeal joint: indication for open reduction, *J Hand Surg [Am]* 6:602-604, 1981.

39. Stern PJ, Lee AF: Open dorsal dislocations of the proximal interphalangeal joint, *J Hand Surg [Am]* 10:364-370, 1985.

40. Twyman RS, David HG: The doorstop procedure: a technique for treating unstable fracture dislocations of the proximal interphalangeal joint, *J Hand Surg [Br]* 18:714-715, 1993.

41. Uhl RL, Blair WF: Open reduction and internal fixation of proximal interphalangeal joint fracture dislocations. In Blair WF (editor): *Techniques in hand surgery,* Baltimore, 1996, Williams & Wilkins.

42. Watanabe H, Hashizume H, Inoue H, Ogura T: Collagen framework of the volar plate of human proximal interphalangeal joint, *Acta Med Okayama* 48(2):101-108, 1994.

43. Weiss APC: Cerclage fixation for fracture dislocation of the proximal interphalangeal joint, *Clin Orthop* 327:21-28, 1996.

44. Wood MB, Dobyns JH: Chronic, complex volar dislocation of the metacarpophalangeal joint: report of three cases, *J Hand Surg [Am]* 6:73-76, 1981.

45. Zemel NP: Metacarpophalangeal joint injuries in fingers, *Hand Clin* 8(4):745-754, 1992.

46. Zemel NP, Startk HH, Ashworth CR, et al: Chronic fracture dislocation of the proximal interphalangeal joint: treatment by osteotomy and bone graft, *J Hand Surg [Am]* 6:447-455, 1981.

47. Zook EG, Van Beek AL, Wavak P: Transverse volar skin laceration of the finger: a sign of volar plate injury, *The Hand* 11(2):213-216, 1979.

Fractures and Dislocations of the Carpus

107

Julia A. Katarincic

FRACTURES OF THE SCAPHOID

INDICATIONS

All fractures and potential fractures of the scaphoid should be treated cautiously with a high level of clinical suspicion that provides adequate initial treatment. The majority of scaphoid fractures are seen in young adult males. The typical mechanism is a fall that creates a sudden stress on a dorsiflexed (95 to 100 degrees), radially deviated wrist.[49] Typically, twice the energy is required to fracture a scaphoid compared with that of a Colles' fracture. Because of the high-energy mechanism of injury and precarious blood supply, avascular necrosis or nonunion of scaphoid fractures are common.

Most patients present clinically with pain in their anatomic snuffbox. Alternatively, they may be extremely tender over the scaphoid tubercle. Initial radiographs should be taken on all patients. These include anteroposterior (AP), lateral, and scaphoid views centered on the wrist. If radiographic findings are negative but clinical suspicion is high, the patient should be placed in a short arm thumb spica splint. A scaphoid fracture may not be seen radiographically for 10 to 21 days after the injury but should be treated appropriately from the initial presentation. The patient should be rechecked at 7 to 10 days with new radiographs. If repeat radiographs are negative but clinical suspicion remains high, a bone scan is most helpful in confirming the diagnosis (Figure 107-1). Technetium bone scans have a false positive rate of 6% to 16%, but no false negatives have been reported.[17]

If a fracture is seen on the initial radiographs, the appropriate treatment should be initiated. According to Russe,[41] the majority of scaphoid fractures are either transverse (60%) or horizontal oblique (35%). These fracture patterns tend to be stable. Vertical oblique fractures (5%) are more prone to displacement because of the shear forces across the fracture site (Figure 107-2). A more detailed classification of scaphoid fractures has been proposed by Herbert and Fischer.[25] Type A fractures are stable, and type B are unstable displaced fractures. Type C is a delayed union, and type D is an established nonunion (Figure 107-3). Only type A fractures in this classification are considered stable and amenable to operative treatment.

Treatment of a nondisplaced, stable scaphoid fracture should consist of cast immobilization. A fractured scaphoid will take approximately 8 to 12 weeks to heal and should be immobilized for 12 weeks. There has been some debate whether short or long arm immobilization is preferable. A randomized prospective trial has shown an increased rate of healing after 6 weeks of long arm thumb spica casting followed by 6 weeks of short arm thumb spica casting, and this is our recommended method of treatment.[15] During the initial 4 weeks of treatment, radiographs should be repeated and scrutinized for evidence of displacement. If there is any doubt about fracture alignment on the initial or follow-up films, tomograms should be obtained. Union rates after closed splinting, despite appropriate treatment, are only 90%. A high degree of clinical suspicion, initiation of appropriate initial treatment, and close scrutiny of radiographs during the early treatment period are essential to increase the chance of obtaining fracture union.

An unstable scaphoid fracture is first suspected after review of the initial radiographs. There may be evidence of displacement—including rotation—or extensive comminution. There may be obvious displacement on the AP view, or the distal scaphoid may appear flexed. The lateral view may reveal excessive flexion of the distal pole. The lateral radiograph is also helpful for determining signs of instability (Figure 107-4). One should be suspicious if there is a dorsal intercalated segment instability (DISI) deformity or some degree of scaphoid shortening and therefore probable fracture comminution. Those cases should be treated operatively with the use of a bone graft through a volar approach to restore scaphoid length. There may also be evidence on the lateral radiograph of an increased intrascaphoid angle (Figure 107-5).[3] A normal intrascaphoid angle is approximately 24 degrees, and any sign that this is significantly increased should again be treated with operative intervention utilizing a bone graft through a volar approach. Trispiral tomograms are frequently helpful in evaluating a scaphoid fracture that may be unstable to further identify any comminution to the fracture pattern, evidence of an increased intrascaphoid angle, or any associated rotatory deformity through the fracture.

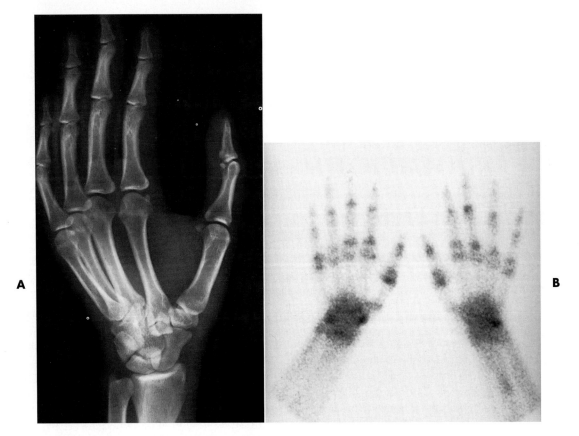

Figure 107-1. **A,** Radiograph of a patient 1 week after a scaphoid fracture without a visible fracture line. **B,** Positive bone scan 8 days after the scaphoid fracture.

Horizontal oblique   Vertical oblique   Transverse

Figure 107-2. Russe's classification of scaphoid fractures. (Copyright Mayo, 1997.)

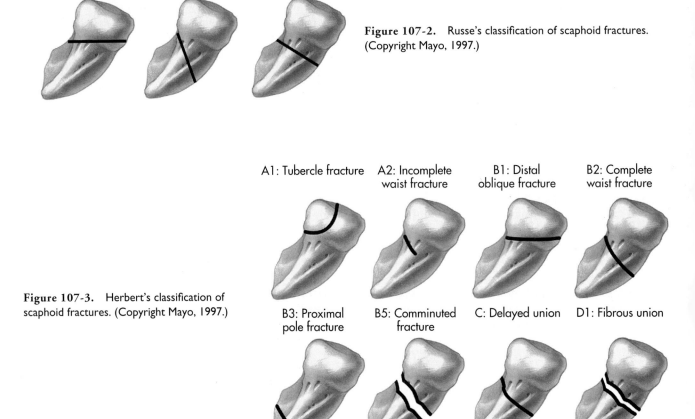

A1: Tubercle fracture   A2: Incomplete waist fracture   B1: Distal oblique fracture   B2: Complete waist fracture

Figure 107-3. Herbert's classification of scaphoid fractures. (Copyright Mayo, 1997.)

B3: Proximal pole fracture   B5: Comminuted fracture   C: Delayed union   D1: Fibrous union

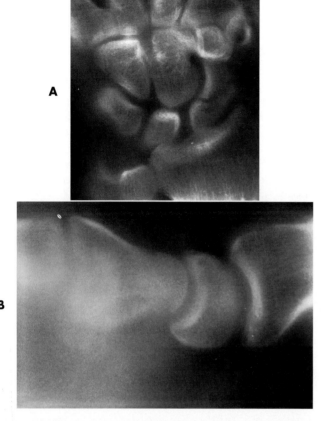

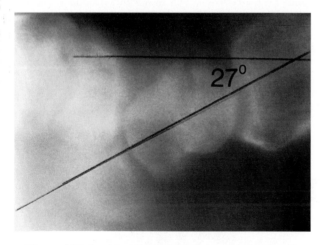

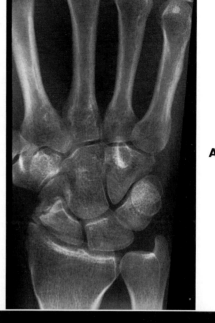

Figure 107-4. Scaphoid wrist fracture (A) and a DISI deformity visible on lateral tomogram (B).

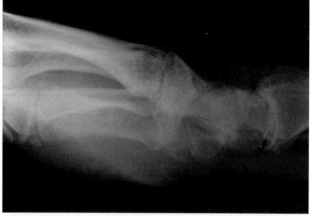

Figure 107-6. Radiographs of a long-standing scaphoid non-union with midcarpal degenerative changes. The injury was treated by scaphoid excision and fusion of the capitate-hamate-lunate-triquetrum.

Figure 107-5. Measurement of the intrascaphoid angle.

Nonunion is the most common complication of a scaphoid fracture. Nonunion has been reported to occur in up to 30% of scaphoid waste fractures and up to 100% of proximal pole fractures. The reason for this high nonunion rate is the anatomy of the blood supply to the scaphoid bone, which has been described by Taleisnik and Kelly[43] and later by Gelberman and Menon.[21] The primary blood supply is from the radial artery through one dorsal and one volar vascular pedicle. From 70% to 80% of the blood supply comes in along the dorsal ridge. Both vascular pedicles, however, enter in the distal half of the scaphoid. This puts the proximal portion of the bone at risk of avascular necrosis, with fractures of the proximal scaphoid at risk of developing a nonunion. If there is no evidence of a scaphoid fracture union by 4 to 6 months, it should be considered a nonunion. A small group of patients with nondisplaced fractures that have remained unhealed after splinting have been able to heal by electrical stimulation with early but satisfactory results.[17] The majority of these patients, however, require operative treatment.

Observation of a scaphoid nonunion is not indicated. Studies have shown that scaphoid nonunions progress to a predictable pattern of arthrosis. The time frame for these degenerative changes to occur ranges from 7 to 31 years.[33,40] Salvage procedures for the treatment of established scaphoid nonunions result in much greater morbidity (with loss of motion) than when scaphoid nonunions are treated before this arthritic pattern has occurred (Figure 107-6).

The surgical treatment method for a scaphoid nonunion varies if there is evidence of carpal instability. A nondisplaced scaphoid nonunion with no carpal collapse is best treated using a Russe bone graft, which has been shown to provide union rates of approximately 85%.[41] When a nonunion has evidence of carpal instability, a volar wedge graft from the iliac crest—combined with internal fixation—will restore carpal height and provide union rates of 85% to 90%.[13]

More attention has been recently paid to the use of vascularized bone grafts in the treatment of proximal pole nonunions. The early reported results are encouraging using the dorsal supraretinacular vessel of the first dorsal compartment as described by Zaidemberg et al.[51] Sheetz et al[42] have recently described a more elaborate blood supply anatomy to the dorsal radius, with more potential donor sites for a vascularized bone graft to the carpus (Figure 107-7). Union

rates of up to 90% have been reported using a dorsal approach and vascularized bone grafts.[51]

OPERATIONS

The most common approach to the scaphoid is from a volar incision. Russe first popularized this approach, which has been adapted by most surgeons. This approach can be used to treat all but the most proximal pole fractures or nonunions. A dorsal approach is favored for these patients, not only to ensure better fixation of the proximal pole but to also provide the opportunity to use a vascularized bone graft. The advantage of using a volar approach for most fractures is that visualization is much better. However, the radioscaphocapitate ligament is divided in this approach, and this must be meticulously repaired to prevent any long-term radiocarpal instability. An advantage to the dorsal approach is that the radioscaphocapitate ligament is not divided; however, one needs to pay attention to the dorsal blood supply, which can usually be visualized entering the dorsal ridge.

The volar approach can be used for acute fractures, fractures and nonunions requiring a volar inlay graft as described by Russe, or fractures requiring a large, volar, iliac crest wedge graft.

The carpus is approached volarly through a longitudinal incision over the flexor carpi radialis sheath angling radially at the wrist crease. The sheath is opened, the tendon is retracted radially, and the floor of the sheath is opened. Once the floor is divided, one must take care to identify the radioscaphocapitate ligament (Figure 107-8). This ligament is essential to prevent-

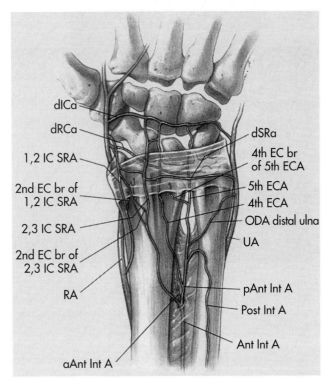

Figure 107-7. Potential sources of vascularized bone graft from the distal radius. *aAnt Int A,* Anterior division of the anterior interosseous artery; *Ant Int A,* anterior interosseous artery; *dICa,* dorsal intercarpal arch; *dRCa,* dorsal radiocarpal arch; *dSRa,* dorsal supraretinacular arch; *ODA distal ulna,* oblique dorsal artery of the distal ulna; *pAnt Int A,* posterior division of the anterior interosseous artery; *Post Ant A,* posterior interosseous artery; *RA,* radial artery; *UA,* ulnar artery; *1,2 IC SRA,* 1,2 intercompartmental supraretinacular artery; *2nd EC br of 1,2 IC SRA,* second extensor compartment branch of 1,2 intercompartmental supraretinacular artery; *2,3 IC SRA,* 2,3 intercompartmental supraretinacular artery; *2nd EC br of 2,3 IC SRA,* second extensor compartment branch of 2,3 intercompartmental supraretinacular artery; *4th ECA,* fourth extensor compartment artery; *4th EC br of 5th ECA,* fourth extensor compartment branch of fifth extensor compartment artery; *5th ECA,* fifth extensor compartment artery. (From *J Hand Surg [Am]* 20:906, 1995.)

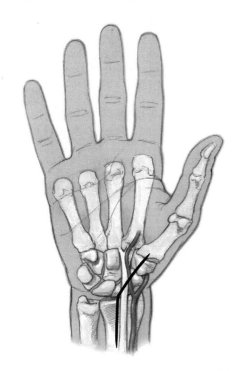

Figure 107-8. The volar approach to the scaphoid through the FCR tendon sheath. (Copyright Mayo, 1997.)

ing ulnar translocation of the carpus and should be either elevated off the radial styloid or divided in a way that it can be repaired. The scaphoid is visible deep to the radioscaphocapitate ligament. Kirschner wires (K wires) in the proximal and distal poles can be used as joy sticks to reduce the fracture. If reduction and fixation alone are sufficient, multiple K wires, a Herbert screw, or an Accutrax screw can be passed across the fracture site. The compressive screws provide better fixation, but if their passage or the use of the compression drill guide will displace the fracture, K wires should be used.

A nondisplaced, stable nonunion should be treated with an additional graft as described by Russe. The same volar approach to the carpus is used. Any fibrous tissue or necrotic bone should be removed from the nonunion site with hand-powered instruments. This debridement should be carried back to bleeding bone in the proximal and distal poles. Two pieces of unicortical bone graft are harvested from the iliac crest and placed in the nonunion site, with the cancellous surfaces opposed (Figure 107-9). Internal fixation that will provide stability but not displace the graft should be utilized.

The same approach is used for a fracture or nonunion requiring a dorsal wedge graft to increase the scaphoid length. A radiograph of the opposite wrist is helpful to determine how large of a graft will be needed. Joy sticks are useful to manipulate the fracture fragments. If a nonunion is present, the debridement should proceed as previously described. The bicortical piece of iliac crest graft is placed between the proximal and distal scaphoid poles and held with internal fixation (Figure 107-10). A screw may potentially displace a dorsal graft volarly, and therefore K wires may be a better choice for fixation.

A dorsal approach is used for either a displaced proximal pole fracture or a nonunion (Figure 107-11). The interval between the first and second compartments is used to approach the dorsal scaphoid. Care should be taken to avoid injuring the radial sensory nerve, the radial artery, and the dorsal ridge vessels to the scaphoid. The surgeon can gain better fixation of a small proximal pole fragment, or potentially use a vascularized bone graft as described by Zaidemberg et al[52] or Sheetz et al[42] through this approach.

All surgically treated patients are placed in a long arm cast for approximately 6 weeks, after which tomograms are obtained to evaluate fracture healing. We change the patient to a short arm cast for an additional 6 weeks if there is evidence of bone healing. If there is no evidence of healing, we continue to immobilize the fracture in a long arm cast for an additional month. The progress of healing is assessed at monthly intervals with new radiographs. Tomograms are obtained for confirmation when union is suspected. Immobilization should be continued until there is evidence of union on either tomograms or a computed tomography (CT) scan. The K wires are typically removed after 3 months because of loosening or skin problems, but when necessary they are continued longer if there are no complications. After the cast is removed, an Orthoplast splint is used until the patient regains protective strength and range of motion.

The most important component in preparing patients for this operation is to explain to them the complexity of a scaphoid fracture and the time required for healing. Patients need to be informed of the problems with the blood supply to the proximal bone and the subsequent difficulties this can cause in bone healing. They should typically be told to expect an average of 3 months of casting for an acute fracture and 4 to 6 months in the cast for treatment of a nonunion. Preoperative education is essential because compliance decreases as time from the operation increases in some patients, especially young males.

The advantage of operating on these patients early is that the salvage procedures usually result in a decreased range of wrist motion. A patient with a nonunion who is seen before the onset of arthritic changes should have an open reduction and fixation with a bone graft because, if left untreated, the progression to osteoarthritis is well documented. A wrist denervation procedure may be performed in a patient who responds well to a diagnostic anesthetic injection of the anterior and posterior interosseous nerve.[10] This procedure may greatly decrease pain while sparing motion but will not alter the progression of the arthritic changes. Isolated radial styloidectomy can be minimally successful in certain patients with low-demand hand use by limiting the pain experienced on radial deviation. The salvage procedure options for patients with a painful arthritic scaphoid include either a scaphoid excision and a four-corner fusion (capitate, hamate, triquetrum, lunate) or a proximal row carpectomy.[28,31] The choice depends on the surgeon's preference, as well as the status of the proximal capitate articular surface. A proximal row carpectomy should be considered only if the proximal articular surface of the capitate is in good condition. Both salvage procedures typically result in wrist motion of approximately 50% of normal. If there is significant advanced

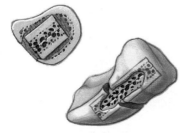

Figure 107-9. Russe's technique of placing an iliac crest bone graft across a scaphoid fracture. (Copyright Mayo, 1997.)

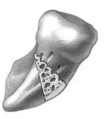

Figure 107-10. A volar wedge graft for a scaphoid fracture or nonunion with collapse. (From Sheets KK, Bishop AT, Berger RA: J Hand Surg [Am] 20:902-914, 1995.)

intercarpal and/or radiocarpal arthritis, the only salvage procedure option is a total wrist fusion. The use of a dorsal wrist fusion plate provides excellent stability and a high union rate in patients with advanced osteoarthritis.[50]

OUTCOMES

Overall union rates after closed treatment of nondisplaced scaphoid fractures range from 90% to 95%, whereas those for open treatment of nonunions are in the range of 85% to 90%.[13,22,25,41] All efforts should be made to try to gain primary scaphoid union because of the significant morbidity associated with salvage procedures. Patients have the best potential to regain full wrist motion and strength after a primary scaphoid union that maintains carpal alignment.

From all standpoints, a scaphoid fracture is a difficult fracture to treat. Even in the best of circumstances, patients are typically immobilized for 3 months, during which time they need to avoid any heavy lifting and must be closely followed. This certainly will have a short-term economic

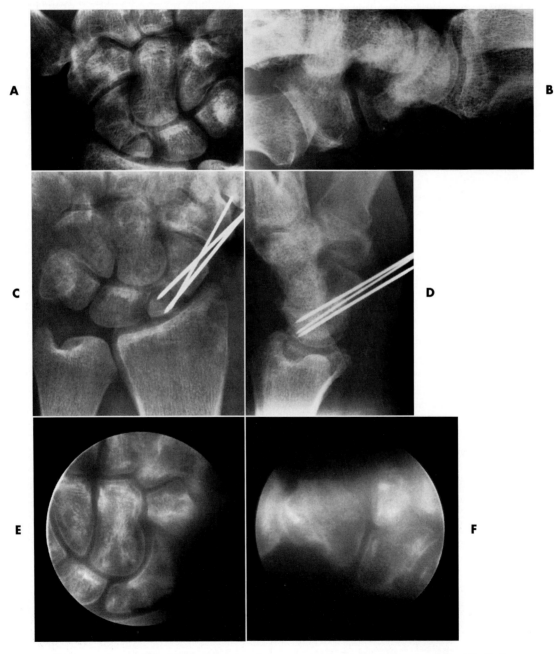

Figure 107-11. **A** and **B,** Radiographs of a proximal pole scaphoid nonunion. **C** and **D,** Radiographs show an operative reduction and internal fixation of the proximal pole scaphoid nonunion with a vascularized distal radius bone graft. **E** and **F,** Tomograms of the wrist 12 weeks after surgery.

impact on the patient. The 4 to 6 months of immobilization typically required to treat nonunions will have an even greater impact.

FRACTURES OF THE TRIQUETRUM

INDICATIONS, OPERATIONS, AND OUTCOMES

Triquetral fractures are the second most common carpal bone fracture. They typically result from a fall on a dorsal- or palmar-flexed wrist. There are two theories about the mechanism of injury. One is that there is a shear force created by the impingement of the ulnar styloid on the dorsal triquetrum during extreme wrist hyperextension. The second theory is that during a forced volar flexion injury there is an avulsion of the radiotriquetral ligament.[18] Patients with this type of fracture describe point tenderness dorsally over the triquetrum on physical examination. The stability of the lunotriquetral joint should be checked in all patients.

Radiographs in AP, lateral, and oblique planes are usually sufficient to identify the fracture. If the radiographs show a dorsal avulsion fracture, one should also check the lateral view for any evidence of a volar intercalated segment instability (VISI) deformity and the AP view for a break in Gilula's lines (Figure 107-12).[6] A lunotriquetral injury should be confirmed and treated appropriately. Patients with an isolated dorsal avulsion fracture of the triquetrum can be treated by approximately 4 weeks of immobilization in a short arm cast with no significant long-term morbidity.

A vertical body fracture can occur as part of a greater perilunate injury. This has to be recognized not as an isolated triquetral fracture, but as a component of the greater perilunate injury and needs to be treated accordingly as discussed later in this chapter.

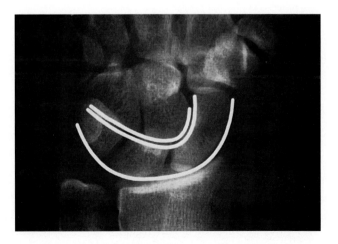

Figure 107-12. Radiograph demonstrating Gilula's lines.

FRACTURES OF THE PISIFORM

INDICATIONS

Pisiform fractures are usually caused by direct trauma to the ulnar side of the wrist, and patients typically present with ulnar-sided wrist pain.[15] The pain is exacerbated by palpation of the pisiform, compression of the pisotriquetral joint, and occasionally resisted wrist-palmar flexion. Typically, AP, lateral, and oblique radiographs and a carpal tunnel view are sufficient to make the diagnosis, but tomograms may be helpful to confirm a clinical suspicion when routine radiographs are negative. Lateral tomograms may also help to differentiate between a pisiform fracture and pisotriquetral arthritis. One should remember in reviewing plain films that there may be multiple ossification centers in the pisiform, and clinical correlation is necessary to diagnose a fracture.

All acute pisiform fractures can be treated closed. Patients should be placed in a short arm cast in about 30 degrees of wrist flexion and some ulnar deviation. Splint treatment is an alternative, but there is more of a delay before patients can return to their normal activities. Surgery is only indicated with the development of pisotriquetral arthritis.

OPERATIONS

Surgical treatment of a fractured pisiform is rarely indicated and is reserved for late cases that develop pisotriquetral arthrosis. Excision should be reserved as a salvage operation, even in cases with severe comminution. The preferred method of pisiform excision is through a volar Bruner incision centered between the flexor carpi ulnaris and the hamate hook. The flexor carpi ulnaris is retracted ulnarly, and the pisiform is identified. The ulnar neurovascular bundle sits just radial to the pisiform, and it should be identified and protected. The pisiform is then excised. The patient is kept in a short arm splint for 4 weeks after surgery.

OUTCOMES

Most patients will regain full, pain-free wrist motion after closed treatment. Secondary arthritis should first be treated by pisotriquetral steroid injections to relieve pain, and only if this fails should the pisiform be excised. Pisiform excision is a well-tolerated procedure. Most patients have satisfactory pain relief and are able to return to normal activities.

FRACTURES OF THE HAMATE

INDICATIONS

A hamate bone fracture is a very uncommon injury. Fractures can be divided into either those of the body or those of the hamate hook. Both injuries require a high degree of clinical

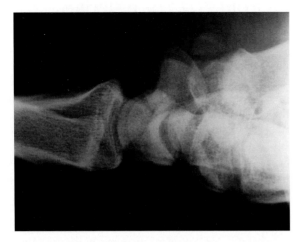

Figure 107-13. The lateral radiograph of a patient with a fracture of the tip of the hamate hook.

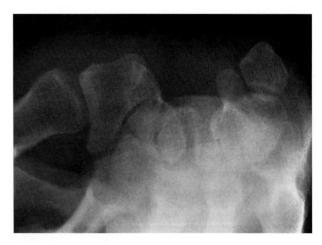

Figure 107-14. A carpal tunnel view of a wrist with a fracture through the base of the hamate hook.

suspicion to make the diagnosis.[9] A hook fracture is a more common injury and may occur through the base or the tip of the hook (Figure 107-13). The mechanism is usually direct trauma to the volar aspect of the hand, which often occurs during a sporting activity such as golf, baseball, or tennis. The other mechanism is an avulsion by the transverse carpal ligament caused by a fall onto an outstretched hand. Patients with a hamate hook fracture usually complain of either dorsal or volar wrist pain over the hamate. They may also have pain with flexion of the fourth and fifth fingers caused by either a tenosynovitis or partial rupture of the ulnar profundus tendons.

The diagnosis of a hamate hook fracture is made from plain radiographs, including a carpal tunnel view in most cases (Figure 107-14). A bone scan or tomograms, however, may be required to make the diagnosis in patients with negative plain-film radiographs and in injuries for which the physician has a high degree of clinical suspicion (Figure 107-15).

Treatment of a nondisplaced hamate hook fracture consists of a short arm cast, including the fourth and fifth fingers to lower the risk of profundus rupture, for 5 or 6 weeks. A displaced acute fracture should be treated with open reduction and internal fixation or excision using a volar approach. A chronic hamate hook nonunion is probably best treated by excision of the fragment.

Hamate body fractures are typically associated either with carpometacarpal fracture dislocations or perilunate injuries. Typically, these injuries are unstable and require closed surgical reduction and fixation.

It is important to try to preserve the hamate hook if possible because it acts as a fulcrum for the profundus tendons of the fourth and fifth fingers, which are necessary for power grip. There is a high nonunion rate when hamate hook fractures are not treated appropriately, which causes pain and weakness of grip. The surgeon should therefore maintain a high degree of clinical suspicion in symptomatic patients and should order appropriate radiographic studies to make the diagnosis.

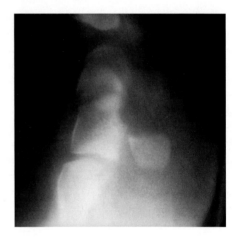

Figure 107-15. Tomogram of a hamate hook fracture.

OPERATIONS

Hamate hook fractures have historically been treated closed, resulting in a high incidence of nonunion. Surgeons have now become more aggressive, especially in treating open fractures. More surgeons are now attempting open reduction and internal fixation of hamate fractures. Hamate hook fractures are approached utilizing a volar incision over the hook (Figure 107-16). The topographic anatomy on the ulnar side of the wrist is well described, and this knowledge is helpful in approaching the hamate.[11] Care must be taken early in the dissection to protect the ulnar neurovascular bundle, which is dorsal and ulnar to the hook of the hamate. The transverse carpal ligament, once identified, is taken down and the fracture visualized. The hook must be anatomically reduced and held with either K wires or a minifragment screw. The flexor tendons of the fourth and fifth fingers should be checked for synovitis or attenuation. The transverse carpal ligament should be reattached to its insertion on the ulnar carpus during closure.

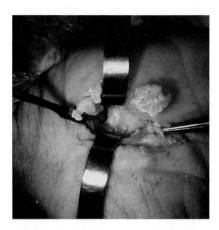

Figure 107-16. A volar approach is preferred for open reduction and internal fixation of a hamate hook fracture or excision of the distal fragment.

Hamate body fractures are typically approached dorsally. A straight longitudinal incision over the palpable hamate is utilized to expose not only the fracture site but also, if needed, the carpometacarpal (CMC) joint. The fracture should be anatomically reduced and held with either K wires or a minifragment screw.

The postoperative immobilization for hamate hook fractures is longer than one would think. There are multiple forces acting on the hook, and therefore the hand should be immobilized until there is evidence of union, either on tomograms or CT scan. This typically requires 8 weeks of immobilization. The cast and K wires are removed after evidence of union, and patients are slowly allowed to increase their activities. Hamate body fractures tend to heal somewhat more quickly. The pins can usually be removed by 6 weeks, an Orthoplast splint can be applied, and the patient can begin range-of-motion exercises. Typically, no formal therapy is required other than instructions in improving wrist range of motion and strengthening.

There is some controversy about the treatment of hamate hook nonunions. Historically, excision through a volar approach has been preferred because of excellent pain relief. Some recent authors, however, have stressed the anatomic importance of the hook for the profundus tendons of the fourth and fifth fingers in maintaining grip strength. They have therefore advocated open reduction and internal fixation of hamate hook nonunions with bone grafts. No large studies have yet compared the results of both treatments, though excision is more accepted in the literature.

OUTCOMES

The overall satisfaction rate of patients treated for hamate hook fractures is approximately 90%. Some patients have reported residual symptoms, including painful grasp, weakness of grasp, or ulnar sensory nerve symptoms. However, functional recovery in most patients is good. Most of the patients returned to work and almost all returned to their sporting activities, which may need to be modified to some extent. There should be no loss of wrist or finger function.

Hamate body or hook fractures are quite uncommon. A high clinical suspicion is warranted and a diagnosis should be pursued aggressively with appropriate radiographic tests. Nondisplaced fractures should all be treated closed. Displaced fractures should be treated by open reduction and fixation, and nonunions of the hook should be excised. Overall patient satisfaction is quite high, although patients may have some residual problems with slightly reduced grip strength.

TRAPEZIAL FRACTURES

INDICATIONS

Trapezial fractures represent about 5% of carpal bone injuries. The fractures can be either through the body or the trapezial ridge.

Fractures of the trapezial ridge are typically caused by a fall on an outstretched hand. The mechanism of injury is either a direct blow to the bony prominence or an avulsion through the transverse carpal ligament. On clinical examination the patient describes volar point tenderness along the trapezium and also may have some tenderness along the flexor carpi radialis tendon sheath. Plain radiographs, including a carpal tunnel view, help make the diagnosis.

Trapezial ridge fractures have been classified by Palmer[37] into type I and type II. Type I fractures are through the base of the ridge and heal well with immobilization. Type II fractures are through the tip of the trapezium and have a higher incidence of nonunion (Figure 107-17). Both types, however, should be treated conservatively in a short arm thumb spica cast, immobilizing the thumb CMC joint for 4 to 6 weeks.

Trapezial body fractures may be associated with a blow to the dorsum of the hand, a first CMC-joint dislocation, or a fall on the outstretched hand, with the hand being forced into radial deviation. Nondisplaced fractures can also be treated closed in a thumb spica cast for 6 weeks. Displaced intraarticular fractures should be treated by open reduction and internal fixation (Figure 107-18).

Anatomic healing of these fractures is important because the trapezial ridge is the origin of the transverse carpal ligament. Intraarticular trapezial fractures that are not anatomically reduced may develop long-term degenerative changes that cause pain and decrease function.

OPERATIONS

Most trapezoid fractures can be treated closed. Fractures of the trapezial ridge or intraarticular or displaced fractures should be approached from a volar direction. A Gedda-Moberg incision at the base of the hand can be made and the thenar muscles elevated. The capsule of the CMC joint is incised, and one can see the ridge as well as the articular surface. The ridge piece can be excised if it is small (type 2). Next, the intraarticular component can be reduced and fixed, typically with K wires. The transverse carpal ligament should be repaired if it has been elevated to visualize the fracture.

Patients are immobilized in a thumb spica cast for 6 weeks after surgery.

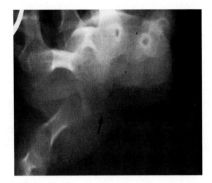

Figure 107-17. A type II trapezial ridge fracture.

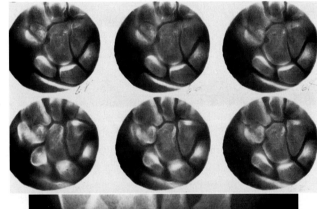

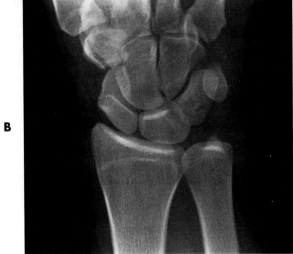

Figure 107-18. Trapezial fracture treated by open reduction and internal fixation.

OUTCOME

Most patients do well after reduction of a trapezial fracture. The range of motion and pinch strength improve once immobilization is discontinued.

FRACTURES OF THE LUNATE

INDICATIONS, OPERATIONS, AND OUTCOMES

Fractures of the lunate are also quite uncommon. There are two patterns seen with isolated fractures. The first is an impaction fracture resulting from an axial load and compression on the lunate between the capitate and the distal radius. The second type are dorsal avulsion or impaction fractures caused by impingement of the lunate on the dorsal edge of the radius.

Patients with lunate fractures complain of middorsal wrist pain, typically after a fall on an outstretched wrist. Standard AP, lateral, and oblique radiographs of the wrist will usually identify the fracture. The lunate can be difficult to visualize on the lateral radiograph, and therefore tomograms or a CT scan may be useful in selected cases.

Some authors believe that fractures of the lunate may predispose the patient to the late development of Kienböck's disease. The more accepted theory, however, is that secondary lunate fractures may develop as Kienböck's disease progresses.

Nondisplaced lunate fractures can be treated closed and with cast immobilization. The lunate is the keystone of the wrist and is the insertion site of the long and short radiolunate ligaments. Anatomic reduction of displaced fractures is therefore imperative. Open reduction through a dorsal approach is preferred, if possible, because it avoids disruption of the important volar radiocarpal ligaments.

FRACTURE OF THE CAPITATE

INDICATIONS

Isolated fractures of the capitate are quite rare. They are classified by whether the fracture is isolated or part of a perilunate injury. Capitate fractures are usually sustained by the transmission of a force down the shaft of the third metacarpal directly to the capitate bone.[39] A dorsal capitate fracture can be associated with a CMC fracture/dislocation. Nondisplaced fractures can be treated closed with a short arm cast immobilization, whereas displaced fractures require operative treatment.

Capitate fractures are more commonly associated with perilunate dislocation injuries. The greater arc of a perilunate dislocation injury typically results in a fracture through the waist of the capitate. In certain instances, when a perilunate dislocation is reduced, the capitate fragment will be rotated 180 degrees so that the proximal articular surface is now facing distally. This is known as the *scaphocapitate syndrome* and implies a significant soft tissue injury. Any displaced capitate fracture or fracture associated with a metacarpal injury requiring open reduction should be treated operatively.

The proximal articular surface of the capitate is essential to midcarpal motion, which accounts for about 50% of wrist motion. It is therefore imperative that displaced capitate fractures be anatomically reduced to prevent reduced wrist motion.

OPERATIONS

Surgical reduction of the capitate should be performed through a dorsal wrist approach. The fragments can be reduced and are typically held with a K wire or compression screw (Figure 107-19). Bone grafting should be considered if there is a significant amount of comminution, to prevent any significant capitate shortening that could interfere with midcarpal motion.

Capitate fractures should be immobilized for 6 to 8 weeks after surgery. The cast should include the second and third metacarpophalangeal (MCP) joints. The K wires can be removed when radiographs reveal evidence of fracture consolidation and motion has begun. A longer immobilization is required for perilunate injuries.

OUTCOMES

Little is written regarding the follow-up of capitate fractures. A patient with an isolated extraarticular fracture that heals normally should not develop a limited range of wrist motion. Anatomic reduction, as with any intraarticular fracture, is important. Nonunions are uncommon; however, to obtain the best results, early diagnosis and treatment should be performed.

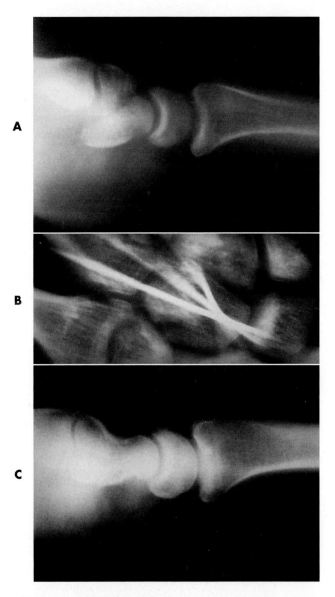

Figure 107-19. **A** and **B,** Tomograms of a capitate fracture treated by open reduction and internal fixation. **C,** Tomogram of a healed capitate fracture.

AVASCULAR NECROSIS OF THE CARPUS

The lunate is the most common site for avascular necrosis in the carpus. Kienböck's disease was first described in 1843 by Peste, who believed that a traumatic event lead to collapse of the lunate. In 1910 Kienböck,[30] a Viennese radiologist, was able to correlate the clinical and radiographic examination and described a vascular injury to the lunate. A number of anatomic variables are thought to predispose a patient to abnormalities in Kienböck's disease. Ulnar variance, lunate fossa inclination, lunate vascularity, and lunate geometry combined with the right mechanism of injury may predispose a patient to develop Kienböck's disease. Ulnar variance was noted by Hulten[27] in 1928 to be present in 78% of patients with Kienböck's disease. Similar findings were noted by Gelberman et al,[21] who believed this variance was statistically significant but not a primary etiologic factor. Poor intraosseous vascularity has also been implicated in Kienböck's disease. The majority of lunate bones have a **Y** or **I** configuration to the intraosseous vessel and are at risk of losing the dorsal or palmar blood flow after a traumatic event.[19] A triangular-shaped lunate, compared with one that is more trapezoidal in shape, concentrates the shear stresses from the capitate and may also increase the chances of microfractures within the lunate.

The typical patient with avascular necrosis of the carpus is a young male laborer who presents with a history of dorsal wrist pain that is aggravated by activity. Only half of all patients with Kienböck's disease recall a specific traumatic event. Patients experience a decreased range of wrist motion, especially palmar flexion, and their grip strength is diminished. Median nerve symptoms are present in a small number of patients.[5] Standard PA and lateral radiographs should be taken, ensuring that the forearm is in neutral rotation on the PA film. The radiographs should be reviewed for fragmentation or shortening of the lunate, hypodensity of the lunate, evidence of lunate fossa flattening, or a decrease in carpal height (Figure 107-20). To help stage the disease, tomograms or a CT scan with overlapping cuts are obtained. These studies can better visualize the lunate on the lateral views and identify any collapse or fragmentation.

If there is still a question of the diagnosis, a magnetic resonance imaging (MRI) scan can be obtained but needs to be evaluated in three planes to prevent overreading (Figure 107-21).

Lichtman and Degnan[32] have classified Kienböck's disease into five groups radiographically. The radiographs of patients with stage I disease are normal, but tomograms or a CT scan may show a linear fracture of the lunate. The lunate is sclerotic in stage 2, but the height is maintained. In stage 3A there is collapse without a fixed scaphoid deformity, and in 3B a fixed deformity of the scaphoid is present. Degenerative changes within the carpus are seen in stage 4. This classification, combined with a review of the anatomy of the radiolunate joint, will influence treatment.

The options for treatment are conservative therapy, a joint-leveling procedure, a revascularization procedure, or a salvage procedure. The stage of disease, the presence of negative ulnar variance, and the individual patient will help guide the treatment decisions. Patients with early stage 1 disease can have the area immobilized for a short period, but if no symptomatic improvement is seen in approximately 3 months, a more aggressive approach should be taken. Treatment for patients with late stage 1, 2, or 3A disease depends on the ulnar variance. If there is a negative ulnar variance, a radial-lengthening or ulnar-shortening procedure can be performed.[4,50] Patients with a neutral or positive ulnar variance can get improvement by using a pedicled distal radial bone graft.[42] Capitate shortening has also been described by Almquist[2] in those patients with a neutral ulnar variance, with good early results. Alternative procedures in this group include an opening or closing wedge radial osteotomy. Measurements of the altered joint forces in clinical cases contradict those obtained from cadaver laboratory studies, so the preferred direction of the radial wedge osteotomy is not yet known.[47,51]

The recommended treatment for patients with stage 3B disease is a limited intercarpal fusion. Scaphoid-trapezium-trapezoid (STT),[48] scaphocapitate (Figure 107-22),[38] or capitohamate fusion have all been recommended. Laboratory studies show a scaphocapitate fusion or a capitate shortening produces the greatest decrease in forces across the

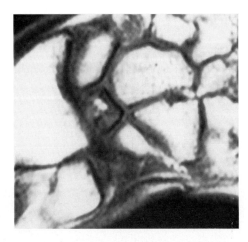

Figure 107-21. MRI of a patient with Kienböck's disease.

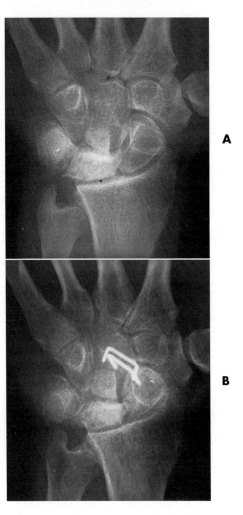

Figure 107-22. Stage IIIB Kienböck's disease treated with a scaphocapitate fusion.

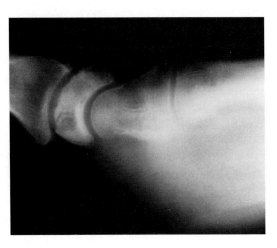

Figure 107-20. Lateral tomogram showing collapse of the lunate in a patient with Kienböck's disease.

lunate.[26,44,46] Patients with stage 4 disease may benefit from a proximal row carpectomy if the lunate fossa and proximal capitate articular surfaces are still intact. Patients with severe degenerative changes in the radiocarpal joint are best treated by a total wrist fusion, which is the recommended salvage procedure.

OPERATIONS

Joint-Leveling Procedures

A radial-shortening or an ulnar-lengthening procedure can be performed on the same group of patients, but a radial-shortening osteotomy is preferred because it has a higher union rate.

A dorsal midline incision is utilized, and the fourth extensor compartment is entered. The sensory branch of the posterior interosseous nerve is resected. A 2-to 3-mm segment of metaphyseal radius is removed as determined preoperatively by radiographic measurement of the amount of variance. Two saw blades can be used, keeping one in the first osteotomy site while the second cut is being made, to help keep the cuts parallel. A compressive plate is applied, the wound is closed, and a short arm cast is worn until there is evidence of union. An ulnar lengthening is performed by a direct incision through the subcutaneous border of the ulna. The dorsal sensory branch of the ulnar nerve should be protected in the dissection. Two distal drill holes of a 3.5 dorsal compression plate (DCP) are placed before making the osteotomy. The ulna is lengthened the desired amount to correct the variance, and a tricortical piece of iliac crest graft is placed in the bone deficit and held with the compression plate. The wound is closed, and a long arm cast is applied until there is evidence of union.

Intercarpal Fusions

A similar approach to the dorsum of the wrist is made through a dorsal midline incision for any of the intercarpal fusion procedures. Dissection is carried through the fourth dorsal compartment, resecting the distal sensory branch of the posterior interosseous nerve. The carpus is exposed through a lateral V capsulotomy based between the radiotriquetral and dorsal intercarpal ligaments.[7] The appropriate joints are decorticated, and a bone graft from the distal radius is obtained. Fixation is provided by K wires, compressive screws, or staples. A meticulous closure of the wrist capsule should be performed, after which patients are placed in a short arm cast until there is evidence of a solid fusion.

Revascularization

The standard dorsal midline incision to the wrist is used. The supraretinacular vessels should be identified and protected before the retinaculum is divided. The fourth compartment is entered, and care is taken to protect the posterior interosseous artery. A capsulotomy is performed, and a drill hole is made in the dorsal lunate. All necrotic bone is debrided carefully by hand, and the lunate is opened like a piece of pita bread. The vascularized segment of radius is elevated on its vascular pedicle, and cancellous bone is harvested from the same donor site. The cancellous bone is packed into the lunate and covered by the vascularized bone flap. No fixation of the graft is needed, but an external fixator is applied across the wrist for 2 months to unload the lunate.

OUTCOMES

The best results from joint-leveling procedures for patients with Kienböck's disease have been reported with radial shortening. Weiss et al[50] reported on 29 patients undergoing a radial-shortening osteotomy, with 87% having good pain relief with an average increase in motion of 33%. Armistead et al[4] reported good pain relief in 18 of 20 patients undergoing an ulnar-lengthening procedure, but there were three patients with nonunions that required reoperation.[4] A radial-shortening osteotomy provides good pain relief with few complications.

Weiss et al[50] also reported good results with intercarpal fusions. Pisano reported good pain relief in 10 of 17 patients treated with a scaphocapitate fusion, but with reductions in postoperative range of motion. Watson described good to excellent results in 16 of 16 patients treated with STT fusions, but four did require late reoperation.

Almquist reported immediate pain relief and a postoperative grip strength of 80% of the unoperated side in patients with an ulnar neutral variance who underwent capitate shortening. He had no cases of avascular necrosis, however this is a concern with this procedure.

The results after revascularization procedures are preliminary. Mazur et al[35] reported early results showing decreased pain in nine patients undergoing a vascularized graft from the distal radius.

AVASCULAR NECROSIS OF OTHER CARPAL BONES

INDICATIONS, OPERATIONS, AND OUTCOMES

Avascular necrosis of the remainder of the carpus is rare. Preiser's disease, or avascular necrosis of the scaphoid, was first described after trauma.[14] During trauma, the scaphoid is at risk for vascular compromise because of its vascular anatomy. Failing conservative immobilization, surgical procedures include revascularization or partial wrist fusion. Revascularization using a pedicled distal radius graft as previously described by Sheetz et al[42] for Kienböck's disease is an option if no arthritic changes have occurred. After the development of degenerative changes, a scaphoid excision and four-corner fusion (capitate, hamate, triquetrum, lunate) provides pain relief and leaves the patient with radiocarpal motion.

Avascular necrosis of the hamate and capitate have been described in case reports only. These patients have presented with dorsal wrist pain and the avascular necrosis is documented by MRI.

DISLOCATIONS OF THE CARPUS

INDICATIONS

Dislocations of the carpus, either volar or dorsal, are an injury created by a high amount of energy. Typically there is a substantial dorsal and volar soft tissue injury, as well as occasional bony injuries. In 1980 Mayfield et al[34] described a sequence of ligamentous injury of the wrist, citing four stages beginning at the radial side of the wrist and moving circumferentially around the lunate (Figure 107-23). The direction of injury in the classification by Mayfield et al[34] is the wrist being forced into progressive dorsiflexion, ulnar deviation, and intercarpal supination. There is an injury to the scapholunate ligament in stage I. Progressing toward the ulna in stage II, there has been associated disruption of the capitolunate joint. Stage III continues to progress ulnarly around the lunate to include disruption of the lunotriquetral joint. There is a dorsal perilunate dislocation at this point. There is disruption of the dorsal radiocarpal ligament in stage IV, resulting in a volar dislocation of the lunate.

This spectrum of injury described by Mayfield et al can be either a bony or soft tissue injury. Johnston and Tonkin[29] divided the categories into greater-arc and lesser-arc injuries (Figure 107-24). The lesser-arc injuries in their description were only ligamentous, whereas the greater-arc injuries were bony.

Patients sustaining a perilunate or lunate dislocation present with a history of high-energy trauma. Forced dorsiflexion is a typical injury that patients will describe. There is usually significant soft tissue swelling, but if seen early only a mild dinner-fork deformity may be present. Before any treatment is undertaken, obtaining AP and lateral radiographs is imperative. A lateral film is often the most helpful to distinguish a lunate from a perilunate dislocation and the direction of the dislocation. The lunate fossa is empty with a volar lunate dislocation, and the lunate is visualized volarly (Figure 107-25). The remainder of the carpus is colinear with the radius. In the volar or dorsal perilunate dislocation, the lunate remains in the lunate fossa of the radius, and the remainder of the carpus is displaced.

When seen acutely, these dislocations should be reduced. A volar lunate or dorsal perilunate dislocation is reduced by applying a distraction force across the carpus. The carpus is next extended and then flexed, maintaining volar pressure on the lunate to bring the remainder of the carpus back to its normal position. The maneuver is reversed for a palmar perilunate dislocation. After the dislocation is reduced, AP and lateral radiographs should again be taken. One must closely assess the radiographs for any evidence of intercarpal instability patterns. The scapholunate as well as the lunacapitate angle should be assessed on the lateral view. On the AP, one should evaluate Gilula's lines for any evidence of a break in the proximal or distal carpal rows (see Figure 107-12).

Much has been written about the closed versus open treatment of these injuries. Adkinson and Chapman[1] have shown that only 33% of their patients undergoing closed treatment had good or excellent results. It is known from observations made during open treatment that perilunate dislocations have significant dorsal and ulnar soft tissue injury, and open treatment has resulted in good to excellent results in 80% to 90% of cases.[12,24,36,45] There are significant

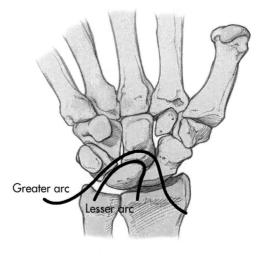

Figure 107-24. Greater (bony) and lesser (ligamentous) arc injuries. (Copyright Mayo, 1997.)

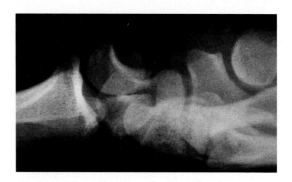

Figure 107-25. Lateral radiograph of an acute lunate dislocation.

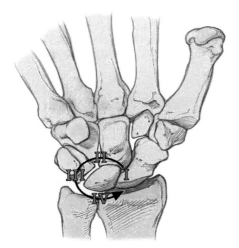

Figure 107-23. Mayfield's four stages of perilunar instability. (Copyright Mayo, 1997.)

ligamentous injuries associated with these dislocations that should be treated aggressively and surgically repaired.

A better understanding of the treatment principles for these injuries can be obtained by knowing the anatomy of the intrinsic and extrinsic ligaments that contribute to carpal stability or instability.[8] The volar radiocarpal ligaments, the

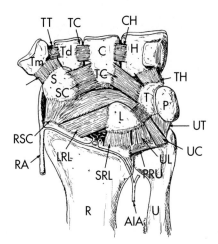

Figure 107-26. Anatomy of the volar carpal ligaments. *AIA,* Anterior interosseus artery; *C,* capitate; *CH,* capitate hamate; *H,* hamate; *LRL,* lateral radial lunate; *P,* pisiform; *PRU,* palmar radioulnar; *R,* radius; *RA,* radial artery; *RSC,* radial scaphoid capitate; *S,* scaphoid; *SC,* scaphoid capitate ligament; *SRL,* superior radial lunate; *T,* triquetral; *TC,* trapezoid capitate; *TC,* triquetral capitate; *Td,* trapezoid bone; *TH,* triquetral hamate; *TM,* trapezium; *TT,* trapezium trapezoid; *U,* ulna; *UC,* ulna collateral; *UL,* ulna lunate; *UT,* ulna triquetral. (From *Hand Clin* 13:68, 1997.)

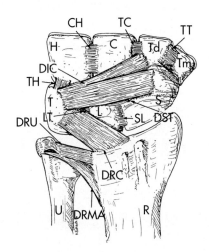

Figure 107-27. Anatomy of dorsal carpal ligaments. *C,* Capitate; *CH,* capitate hamate ligament; *DIC,* dorsal intercarpal ligament; *DRC,* dorsal radio carpal ligament; *DRMA,* dorsal radial metaphyseal arcuate ligament; *DRU,* dorsal radio ulnar ligament; *DST,* dorsal scaphoid triquetral; *H,* hamate; *L,* lunate; *LT,* lunate triquetral; *R,* radius; *S,* scaphoid; *SL,* scaphoid lunate ligament; *T,* triquetral; *TC,* trapezoid capitate ligament; *Td,* trapezoid bone; *TH,* triquetral hamate; *Tm,* trapezium bone; *TT,* trapezoid trapezium ligament; *U,* ulna. (From *Hand Clin* 13:75, 1997.)

radioscaphocapitate, and long and short radiolunate ligaments, are the primary stabilizers of the wrist (Figure 107-26). The ulnolunate and ulnotriquetral ligaments on the volar side of the wrist are involved. There is very little ligamentous support volarly under the proximal capitate. This is known as the *space of Poirier,* which is disrupted in stage II perilunate injuries. The dorsal ligaments are less stout (Figure 107-27). The radiotriquetral is the extrinsic component and the dorsal intercarpal the intrinsic component. Both are usually injured in these dislocations.

A carpal dislocation is a devastating injury. All patients need to be counseled that they are going to lose a significant degree of wrist function. Anatomic reduction of the osseous structures and ligamentous repair will afford patients the best potential for long-term wrist function.

OPERATIONS

There has been much written in the literature about the advantages of a dorsal or volar surgical approach to carpal dislocations. It has been shown, however, that combining the dorsal and volar approach does lead to a slightly improved outcome, and this is our preferred surgical technique.

Surgery should be delayed after an adequate closed reduction until the soft tissues are in a condition to undergo surgical treatment. The exception to this rule is in cases where the dislocation cannot be reduced, or in a patient with an acute, persistent carpal tunnel. A dorsal approach is first made through the fourth dorsal compartment. The posterior interosseous nerve is resected to decrease the chances of long-term wrist pain. The extensor tendons are retracted, and a significant amount of dorsal soft tissue disruption is usually seen. It is common that the radiotriquetral ligament is avulsed off the proximal radius. The carpus is reduced through this dorsal approach. The lunate is the keystone of the wrist, and we often find that reducing the lunate to the radius and then reversing the pattern of injury starting with the triquetrum and moving radially over to the scaphoid provides the easiest mechanism of reconstruction. The scapholunate and lunotriquetral ligaments are repaired after bony reduction and fixation with K wires.

A second, volar incision is made next. The carpal tunnel is released and the flexor tendons are retracted, revealing a transverse rent across the entire radiocarpal joint, which is repaired with a running suture (Figures 107-28 to 107-30).

After surgery, the wrist is elevated and placed in a bulky compressive dressing. We do not cast postoperative wrists until the swelling is resolved, which can take up to 2 weeks. At that point, we place them in a short arm thumb spica cast. The recommended immobilization time has increased with knowledge of ligamentous healing, and typically the pin fixation is continued for 10 to 12 weeks. The K wires are then removed, and gentle wrist range-of-motion exercises are initiated. The wrist is supported in a removable Orthoplast splint until strength and protective motion have returned. This is a

Figure 107-28. Intraoperative view of a volar capsular tear in a patient with a perilunate dislocation.

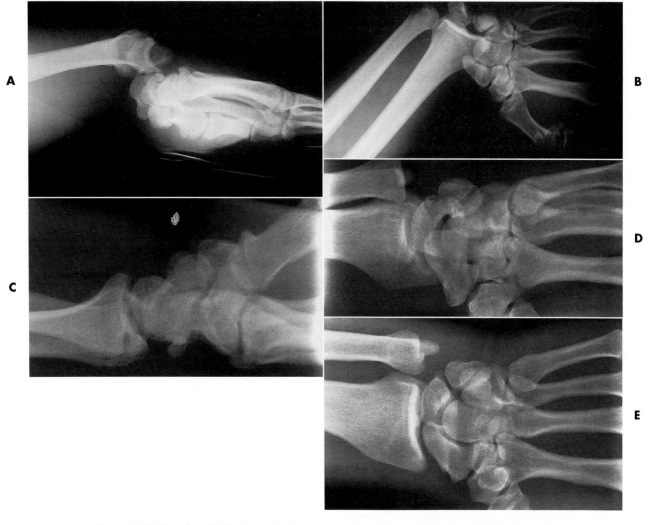

Figure 107-29. **A** and **B,** Radiographs of an acute volar perilunate dislocation. **C-E,** Radiographs after a closed reduction showing evidence of carpal instability.

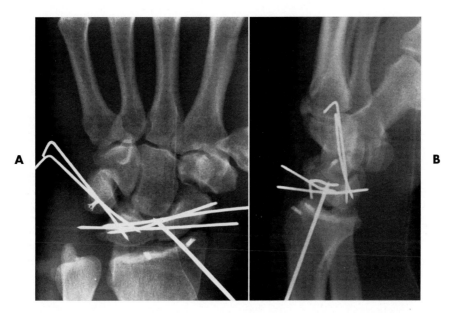

Figure 107-30. Open reduction and internal fixation of the perilunate dislocation.

devastating injury and the patient should be counseled preoperatively to this effect.

A greater-arc injury, with an associated scaphoid-capitate-triquetrum-ulnar styloid fracture, will often have less of a ligamentous injury. Open reduction and fixation of all fractures should be performed. The scaphoid is approached volarly, then if needed the capitate and triquetrum are reduced dorsally. An associated ulnar styloid fracture should be treated by open reduction and internal fixation because it is a component of the instability pattern. Reduced fractures should be immobilized until healing is demonstrated either on radiographs, tomograms or CT scan, usually in 8 to 12 weeks.

Patients with carpal dislocation that is not treated surgically often present late with advanced intercarpal arthritis. Salvage procedures typically are not useful at that point, and the procedure of choice for treatment is a total wrist fusion.

OUTCOMES

Cooney et al[12] have reported 80% to 90% good to excellent results in patients after a dorsal and volar reduction/fixation technique. Early anatomic restoration of carpal anatomy with attention to the bony and soft tissue structures will provide the best chance for these patients to regain wrist motion. Unfortunately, stiffness is a problem, but the immobilization required to allow ligamentous healing predisposes most patients to this result. The severity of the injury often keeps patients from returning to their occupation for 9 to 12 months. Many patients cannot return to heavy labor activity that they may have done before injury. All patients should work diligently on antiedema and finger range-of-motion exercises while they are in the cast.

A thorough knowledge of the wrist ligamentous anatomy is important to ensure anatomic reconstruction of the soft tissues. Combined dorsal and volar approaches have been found to provide the best long-term results.

REFERENCES

1. Adkinson JW, Chapman MW: Treatment of acute, lunate, and perilunate dislocations, *Clin Orthop* 164:199-207, 1982.
2. Almquist EE: Capitate shortening in the treatment of Kienböck's disease, *Hand Clin* 9:505-512, 1993.
3. Amadio PC, Berquist TH, Smith DK: Scaphoid malunion, *J Hand Surg [Am]* 14:679-687, 1989.
4. Armistead RB, Linscheid RL, Dobyns JH, Beckenbaugh RD: Ulnar lengthening in the treatment of Kienböck's disease, *J Bone Joint Surg* 64A:170-178, 1982.
5. Beckenbaugh RD, Shives TC, Dobyns JH, Linscheid RL: Kienböck's disease: the natural history of Kienböck's disease and consideration of lunate fractures, *Clin Orthop* 149:98-106, 1980.
6. Bellinghausen HW, Gilula LA, Young LV, Weeks PM: Post-traumatic palmar carpal subluxation: report of two cases, *J Bone Joint Surg* 65A:999, 1983.
7. Berger RA, Bishop AT, Bettinger PC: New dorsal capsulotomy for the surgical exposure of the wrist, *Ann Plast Surg* 35:54-59, 1995.
8. Berger RA, Landsmeer JMF: The palmar radiocarpal ligaments: a study of adult and fetal human wrist joints, *J Hand Surg [Am]* 15:847-854, 1990.
9. Bishop AT, Beckenbaugh RD: Fractures of the hamate hook, *J Hand Surg [Am]* 13:135-139, 1988.
10. Buck-Gramcko D: Wrist denervation procedures in the treatment of Kienböck's disease, *Hand Clin* 9:517-520, 1993.

11. Cobb TC, Cooney WP, An KN: Clinical location of hook of hamate: a technical note for endoscopic carpal tunnel release, *J Hand Surg [Am]* 19:516-518, 1994.

12. Cooney WP, Bussey R, Dobyns JH, Linscheid RL: Difficult wrist fractures: perilunate fracture-dislocations of the wrist, *Clin Orthop* 214:136-147, 1987.

13. Cooney WP, Linscheid RL, Dobyns JH, Wood MB: Scaphoid nonunions: role of interior interpositional bone grafts, *J Hand Surg [Am]* 13:635-650, 1988.

14. Ferlic DC, Morin P: Idiopathic avascular necrosis of the scaphoid: Preiser's disease? *J Hand Surg [Am]* 14:13-16, 1989.

15. Fleege MA, Jebson PJ, Renfrew DL, et al: Pisiform fractures, *Skel Radiol* 20:169-172, 1991.

16. Frykman GK, Taleisnik J, Peters G, et al: Treatment of nonunited scaphoid fractures by pulsed electromagnetic field and cast, *J Hand Surg [Am]* 11:344-349, 1986.

17. Ganel A, Engel J, Oster Z, Farine J: Bone scanning in the assessment of fractures of the scaphoid, *J Hand Surg [Am]* 4:540-543, 1979.

18. Garcia-Elias M: Dorsal fractures of the triquetrum: avulsion or compression fractures? *J Hand Surg [Am]* 12:266-268, 1987.

19. Gelberman RH, Bauman TD, Menon J, Akeson WH: The vascularity of the lunate bone and Kienböck's disease, *J Hand Surg [Am]* 5:272-278, 1980.

20. Gelberman RH, Menon J: The vascularity of the scaphoid bone, *J Hand Surg [Am]* 5:508-513, 1980.

21. Gelberman RH, Salamon PB, Jurist JM, Posch JL: Ulnar variance in Kienböck's disease, *J Bone Joint Surg* 57A:674-676, 1975.

22. Gelberman RH, Wolock BS, Siegel DB: Fractures and nonunions of the carpal scaphoid, *J Bone Joint Surg* 71A:1560-1565, 1989.

23. Gellman H, Caputo RJ, Carter V, et al: Comparison of short and long thumb-spica casts for nondisplaced fractures of the carpal scaphoid, *J Bone Joint Surg* 71A:354-357, 1989.

24. Green DP, O'Brien ET: Open reduction of carpal dislocations: indications and operative techniques, *J Hand Surg [Am]* 3:250-265, 1978.

25. Herbert TJ, Fischer WE: Management of the fractured scaphoid using a new bone screw, *J Bone Joint Surg* 66B:114-123, 1984.

26. Horii E, Garcia-Elias M, Bishop AT, et al: Effect on force transmission across the carpus in procedures used to treat Kienböck's disease, *J Hand Surg [Am]* 15:393-400, 1990.

27. Hultén O: Über anatomische variationen der handgelenk-knochen, *Acta Radiol Scand* 9:155-168, 1928.

28. Imbriglia JE, Broudy AS, Hagberg WC, McKernan D: Proximal row carpectomy: clinical evaluation, *J Hand Surg [Am]* 15:426-430, 1990.

29. Johnston GH, Tonkin MA: Excision of pisiform in pisotriquetral arthritis, *Clin Orthop* 210:137-142, 1986.

30. Kienböck R: Üe des mondbeins und kompression fracturen, *Fortschr Roentgenstrahlen* 16:77-103, 1910-1911.

31. Krakauer JD, Bishop AT, Cooney WP: Surgical treatment of scapholunate advanced collapse, *J Hand Surg [Am]* 19:751-759, 1994.

32. Lichtman DM, Degnan GG: Staging and its use in the determination of treatment modalities for Kienböck's disease, *Hand Clin* 9(3):409-416, 1993.

33. Mack GR, Bosse MJ, Gelberman RH: The natural history of scaphoid nonunion, *J Bone Joint Surg* 66A:504-509, 1984.

34. Mayfield JK, Johnson RP, Kilcoyne RK: Carpal dislocations: pathomechanics and progressive perilunar instability, *J Hand Surg [Am]* 5:226-241, 1980.

35. Mazur KU, Bishop AT, Berger RA: *Vascularized bone grafting for Kienböck's disease: methods and results of retrograde-flow metaphyseal grafts and comparison with cortical graft site.* Presented at the American Society for Surgery of the Hand Annual Meeting, Nashville, Tenn, 1996.

36. Moneim MS, Hofammann KE III, Omer GE: Transcaphoid perilunate fracture-dislocation: results of open reduction and pin fixation, *Clin Orthop* 190:227-235, 1984.

37. Palmer A: Trapezial ridge fractures, *J Hand Surg [Am]* 6:561-564, 1981.

38. Pisano SM, Peimer CA, Wheeler DR, Sherwin F: Scaphocapitate intercarpal arthrodesis, *J Hand Surg [Am]* 16:328-333, 1991.

39. Rand JA, Linscheid RL, Dobyns JH: Capitate fractures: a long term follow-up, *Clin Orthop* 165:209-216, 1982.

40. Ruby LK, Belsky MR: The natural history of scaphoid nonunion: a review of fifty-five cases, *J Bone Joint Surg* 67A:428-432, 1985.

41. Russe O: Fracture of the carpal navicular: diagnosis, nonoperative treatment and operative treatment, *J Bone Joint Surg* 42A:428-432, 1985.

42. Sheetz KK, Bishop AT, Berger RA: The arterial blood supply of the distal radius and ulna and its potential use in vascularized pedicled bone grafts, *J Hand Surg [Am]* 20:902-914, 1995.

43. Taleisnik J, Kelly PJ: The extraosseous and intraosseous blood supply of the scaphoid bone, *J Bone Joint Surg* 48A:1125-1137, 1966.

44. Trumble T, Glisson RR, Seaber AV, Urbaniak JR: A biomechanical comparison of the methods for treating Kienböck's disease, *J Hand Surg [Am]* 11:88-93, 1986.

45. Viegas DF, Bean JW, Schram RA: Transscaphoid fracture/dislocations treated with open reduction and Herbert screw internal fixation, *J Hand Surg [Am]* 12:992-999, 1987.

46. Viegas SF, Patterson RM, Peterson PD, et al: Evaluation of the biomechanical efficacy of limited intercarpal fusions for the treatment of scapholunate dissociation, *J Hand Surg [Am]* 15:120-128, 1990.

47. Watanabe K, Nakamura R, Horii E, Miura T: Biomechanical analysis of radial wedge osteotomy for the treatment of Kienböck's disease, *J Hand Surg [Am]* 18:686-690, 1993.

48. Watson HK, Ryu J, Dibella A: An approach to Kienböck's disease: triscaphe arthrodesis, *J Hand Surg [Am]* 10:179-187, 1985.

49. Weber E, Chao E: An experimental approach to the mechanism of scaphoid waist fractures, *J Hand Surg [Am]* 3:142-148, 1978.

50. Weiss AP, Weiland AJ, Moore JR, Wilgis EF: Radial shortening for Kienböck's disease, *J Bone Joint Surg* 73A:384-391, 1991.

51. Werner FW, Palmer AK, Utter RG: Distal radial osteotomy for treatment of Kienböck's disease: a biomechanical study, *Orthop Trans* 12:486-487, 1988.

52. Zaidemberg C, Siebert JW, Angrigani C: A new vascularized bone graft for scaphoid nonunion, *J Hand Surg [Am]* 16:474-478, 1991.

PART IV

THE WRIST

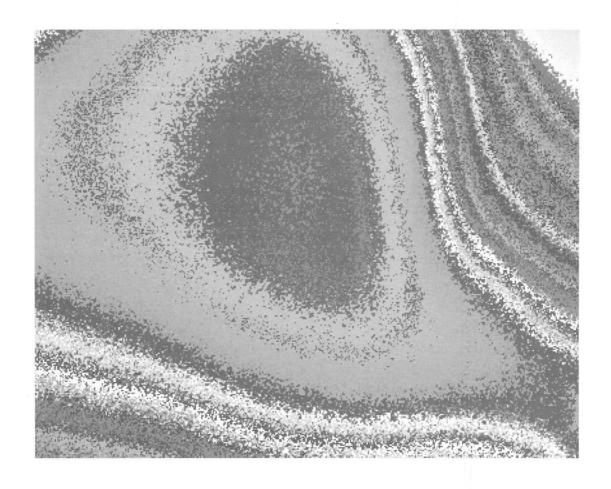

CHAPTER

Fractures of the Distal Radius and Ulna

108

David Ring
Jesse B. Jupiter

INTRODUCTION

The management of distal radius fractures was for many years considered relatively straightforward.[7,11] This attitude was generally ascribed to a combination of the predictability of solid union and the often limited functional demands of the elderly, osteoporotic individuals who most commonly sustain this injury. Dissatisfaction with the results of cast treatment of distal radius fractures has inspired a number of investigators to study the relationship between the functional result and the accuracy of restoration of anatomy.* It is now recognized from these studies that failure to restore the extraarticular anatomy of the distal radius can lead to disturbed wrist and hand kinematics, radiocarpal arthrosis, ulnocarpal abutment, and distal radioulnar joint incongruity. Patients with low functional demands continue to be well treated with closed reduction and cast immobilization, but more invasive techniques are often necessary to ensure restoration of distal radial anatomy in active older patients and young adults.

INDICATIONS

EPIDEMIOLOGY

Fractures of the distal radius are extremely common, accounting for nearly one sixth of all fractures seen in emergency rooms.[50] The incidence of adult injuries peaks in the seventh decade of life, at which time females outnumber males by as much as sevenfold.[2] Fracture of the distal radius is clearly associated with osteoporosis, and the majority of fractures occur as a result of relatively low-energy falls from a standing height. As many as 45% of patients with a distal radius fracture may have associated osteoporosis-related fractures, most commonly involving the hip or proximal humerus.[6] The possibility that the fall that caused the fracture in an elderly patient was related to an associated medical illness, side effects from

medication, or an unsafe home environment should also be considered.

Some observations suggest that the prevalence patterns for distal radius fractures may be related as much to the epidemiology of falls as to weakened bone. The predominance of injuries in females may be at least partially explained by the fact that late middle-aged women fall more often than do men of the same age.[15] The decreased prevalence of fractures in the very old may be a result of their decreased reaction times, resulting in falls directly onto the hip rather than onto an outstretched hand.[13]

Distal radius fracture in younger adults is usually the result of a high-energy traumatic injury such as a motor vehicle accident or a fall from a height. In this situation, it is important to perform a thorough trauma evaluation and to remain vigilant for the possibility of a an open wound or other soft tissue injury, a forearm compartment syndrome, or an acute carpal tunnel syndrome. Associated injuries, particularly of the carpus, forearm, or elbow, are also not uncommon after such high-energy injuries.

ANATOMY

Familiarity with wrist anatomy is important for describing and classifying injury to the distal radius and ulna and is essential when considering treatment. The distal radius appears in the evolution of the human upper extremity to have gradually assumed a role as the foundation of the wrist joint, whereas the ulna has receded from the carpus to increase forearm rotation and wrist mobility.[35,38] There is relatively little osseous or articular constraint at the radiocarpal articulation, permitting circumduction through a substantial range of both dorsal and palmar flexion, as well as ulnar and radial deviation. This wrist mobility is important to the normal functioning of the upper extremity because a wide range of wrist positioning is necessary to optimize the mechanical advantage of the extrinsic hand musculature for object manipulation and tool use.[58]

The distal radioulnar joint is an integral part of the forearm articulation, which serves to provide supination and pronation to the upper extremity. This rotational motion was an

---

*References 4, 5, 8, 14, 17, 19-21, 25, 26, 33, 36, 39, 41, 65.

important evolutionary development that, along with a prehensile thumb and a large cerebral cortex, determines the unmatched ability of humans to manipulate their environment.[35,38] It facilitates tool use by greatly expanding the variety of positions in which the hand can be placed in space. Incongruity or instability of the distal radioulnar joint can compromise the function of the entire forearm complex.

Ligaments assume the primary role for stability in the wrist and distal radioulnar joint. The volar radiocarpal ligaments are the most important stabilizers of the radiocarpal articulation, with the dorsal radiocarpal ligaments playing a relatively limited role (Figure 108-1).[42] The radioscaphocapitate and radiolunotriquetral ligaments arise from the radial styloid such that radial styloid fractures are often associated with carpal instability.[57] The radioscapholunate ligament arises from the ulnar aspect of the volar articular rim. Avulsion fractures of the radial styloid and volar articular rim are encountered in radiocarpal fractures/dislocations.[22]

The triangular fibrocartilage complex also plays a role in providing both distal radioulnar and ulnocarpal stability.[51,52] This complex consists of several named anatomic structures that are confluent. The volar and dorsal radioulnar ligaments represent the peripheral portions of the triangular fibrocartilage, the central portion of which acts primarily as a cushion between the carpus and ulnar head. The triangular fibrocartilage arises from the base of the ulnar styloid and inserts onto the ulnar rim of the distal radial articular surface. The meniscus homologue, the ulnar collateral ligament, and the sheath of the extensor carpi ulnaris contribute to both ulnocarpal and distal radioulnar stability. The ulnotriquetral and ulnolunate ligaments arise from the triangular fibrocartilage and contribute to ulnocarpal stability (see Figure 108-1, B).

The articular surface is divided into scaphoid and lunate facets by a well-defined ridge. Both facets are concave and congruent with the rounded articular surfaces of the carpal bones. Mechanical studies have suggested that approximately 80% of axial compressive loads pass through the radiocarpal articulation with the wrist in neutral position, and the remaining 20% pass through the ulnocarpal articulation and the triangular fibrocartilage complex (see Figure 108-1, B).[51,52]

The sigmoid notch on the ulnar aspect of the distal radius articulates with the distal ulna. The hyaline cartilage covering this notch is continuous with that of the radiocarpal articular surface. The sigmoid notch is roughly cylindrical in shape, with a slight conicity that varies in degree and direction according to the ulnar variance of the individual (Figure 108-2).[35] Motion between the distal ulna and radius occurs through a mixture of translation and rotation.

The articular end of the radius slopes in an ulnar and palmar direction. Radiographic measurements quantifying this

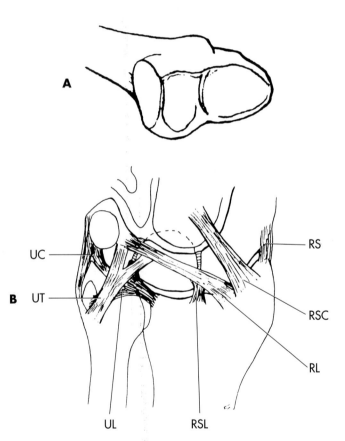

Figure 108-1. **A** and **B,** The complex articulation between the distal radius, distal ulna, and carpus allows a wide range of motion while relying on ligaments for stability. The distal radius presents a continuous articular surface, which is divided into three distinct facets: the scaphoid and lunate facets for articulation with the carpus and the sigmoid notch for articulation with the ulnar head. Stout volar radiocarpal and ulnocarpal ligaments maintain normal kinematics. *RL,* Radiolunate ligament; *RS,* radioscaphoid ligament; *RSC,* radioscaphocapitate ligament; *RSL,* radioscapholunate ligament; *UC,* ulnar capsule; *UL,* ulnolunate ligament; *UT,* ulnotriquetral ligament. (From Fernandez DL, Jupiter JB: *Fractures of the distal radius: a practical approach to management,* New York, 1995, Springer-Verlag.)

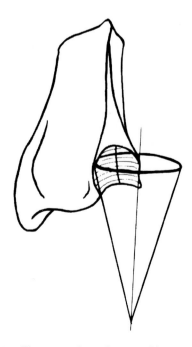

Figure 108-2. The sigmoid notch is roughly conical in shape, although there is substantial variability among individuals. (From Fernandez DL, Jupiter JB: *Fractures of the distal radius: a practical approach to management,* New York, 1995, Springer-Verlag.)

angular relationship and shortening of the radius with respect to the ulna are used both to guide initial treatment and to document residual deformity in studies of long-term results after fracture of the distal radius.

The ulnar inclination of the distal radial articular surface is measured from a radiograph in the coronal plane as the angle between a line connecting the tip of the radial styloid process and the ulnar corner of the articular surface of the distal radius and a line perpendicular to the longitudinal axis of the radius. This measurement is subject to substantial variation depending on the rotational positioning of the forearm when the radiograph is taken and the difficulty in determining the dorsal or palmar cortical rim of the end of the radius in repeated radiographs. The ulnar inclination may also be difficult to measure and interpret when the lunate articular facet is fractured and displaced. The average ulnar inclination in normal adult subjects has been reported to be between 22 and 23 degrees (Figure 108-3, A).[24]

The palmar inclination of the distal radial articular surface is measured from a radiograph in the sagittal plane as the angle between a line connecting the distal most points of the dorsal and volar cortical rims of the articular surface and a line perpendicular to the longitudinal axis of the radius. The palmar inclination can vary widely between 4 and 22 degrees in normal adults, but the average value lies between 10 and 12 degrees (Figure 108-3, B).[24]

There are two methods of measuring relative shortening of the distal radius with respect to the ulna. Measurement of the radial length is popular but is less useful because it measures the combined effect of loss of ulnar inclination and relative radial shortening, and it underestimates the amount of radial shortening in articular fractures involving the ulnar corner of the articular surface. The radial length is the distance in millimeters between a perpendicular line drawn along the longitudinal axis of the radius at the tip of the radial styloid and a second perpendicular line at the level of the distal articular surface of the ulnar head. The average value in normal subjects is between 11 and 12 millimeters (Figure 108-3, C).[26]

Measurement of the ulnar variance will more accurately reflect and isolate the relative shortening of the distal radius with respect to the ulna for most fracture patterns. The ulnar variance is the distance in millimeters between a line perpendicular to the longitudinal axis of the radius at the ulnar aspect of the distal radial articular surface and a second perpendicular line at the level of the distal articular surface of the ulnar head (Figure 108-3, D). The ulna becomes more prominent at the wrist as the radius shortens, resulting in positive ulnar variance. Hulten[30] noted that approximately 60% of normal adults have neutral ulnar variance, but it is important to keep in mind that normal ulnar variance can vary substantially between normal adults and even between extremities in a particular individual. Ulnar variance is affected by forearm rotation. Radiographs must be taken in the same manner to be consistent with the shoulder abducted 90 degrees, the elbow flexed 90 degrees, and the forearm in neutral rotation.

A measurement reflecting relative radial displacement of the distal fracture fragments, termed the *radial width* or *radial shift,* has been shown in some investigations to correlate with the functional result.[24] The radial shift is measured as the distance in millimeters between the longitudinal axis of the radius and a line parallel to the longitudinal axis passing through the lateral tip of the styloid process (Figure 108-3, E).

It is also important to evaluate the intercarpal and radiocarpal relationships because many fractures of the distal radius are the result of an impaction of the carpus against the distal radial articular surface, and the carpal bones or ligaments can also be injured.[57] The longitudinal axes of the third metacarpal, capitate, lunate, and radius on a true lateral radiograph should fall on a single line. It is important to ensure that the hand is placed in neutral position when the radiographs are taken because any amount of palmar or dorsal flexion will lead to corresponding angulation of the carpal bones, thereby clouding the interpretation. Dorsal or volar translation of the carpal axis with respect to the radial axis represents radiocarpal subluxation. Dorsal angulation of the

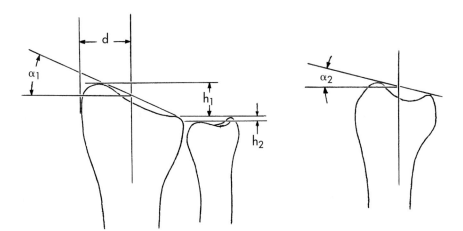

Figure 108-3. Several measurements made from standard radiographs can be used to characterize deformity of the distal radius. Among these are the ulnar inclination (α_1), the palmar tilt (α_2), the radial length (h_1), the ulnar variance (h_2), and the radial shift (d). See text for details.

lunate suggests disruption of the scapholunate interosseous ligament, whereas volar angulation suggests injury to the triquetrolunate interosseous ligament. If the angle between the longitudinal axis of the scaphoid and that of the lunate diverge by greater than 60 degrees, this also suggests injury to the scapholunate interosseous ligament. A gap between the scaphoid and lunate may be seen with this injury on the posteroanterior (PA) radiograph, and the normal clear space between the proximal and distal carpal rows may be narrowed.

The traditional teaching that the wrist adapts well to deformity has been displaced in recent years by an ever-increasing understanding of the association between anatomy and function.* Residual deformity after a distal radius fracture is unsightly, alters wrist motion to a less functional range, and affects hand function by interfering with the mechanical advantage of the extrinsic hand muscles. It may also lead to radiocarpal and distal radioulnar joint arthrosis, limitation of forearm rotation or pain as a result of a decreased contact area of the articular surfaces, incongruity of the distal radioulnar joint, ulnocarpal impingement, and carpal malalignment.

A decrease in articular contact area results in increased local pressures on the articular cartilage, which can lead to degeneration and arthrosis. Deformity of the distal radius can limit the articular contact area either through extraarticular malalignment, which decreases the congruity of opposing articular surfaces, or through intraarticular malalignment resulting in a step-off, with the more prominent areas in the articular surface taking a majority of the load. Arthrosis will develop in these situations despite the fact that the wrist is not a "weight-bearing joint" on the scale of the hip, knee, or ankle. Numerous studies have demonstrated that greater than 20 degrees of dorsal tilt of the articular surface[8,41,65] or 2 mm residual articular incongruity will lead to arthrosis.[36]

Incongruity of the distal radioulnar joint is one of the most common sources of disability after a distal radius fracture.[8,41,65] Incongruity can result from shortening, excessive dorsal tilt of the articular surface, and even loss of ulnar inclination or increased radial shift. The conical shape of the distal radioulnar joint makes it susceptible to shortening (as the ulnar head comes to articulate with a less congruous portion of the cone) and angulation, which causes the roughly cylindrical surfaces to rotate along distinct, nonparallel axes. Decreased rotational motion of the forearm and pain are notable immediately, and arthrosis of this joint will develop with time.

Instability at the distal radioulnar joint can also develop, in part related to the decreased congruity of the articular surfaces but also because of rupture or secondary elongation of the triangular fibrocartilage complex. If dorsal angulation of the distal radial articular surface exceeds 30 degrees, it is extremely likely that either the triangular fibrocartilage complex will be torn or the ulnar styloid will fracture at its base.[22]

Pain on the ulnar side of the wrist can also result from ulnocarpal abutment, which is a common sequel of the relative ulnar lengthening that occurs after a distal radius fracture.

---

*References 4, 8, 26, 39, 41, 65.

Excessive dorsal angulation of the distal radial articular surface also increases the amount of a load crossing the wrist, which is borne by the ulna.[52] A degenerative tear of the triangular fibrocartilage can develop, and there may even be cystic changes in the lunate.

Excessive dorsal tilt of the distal radial articular surface can result in a compensatory malalignment of the carpal bones.[62] A flexion deformity develops through the midcarpal articulation. The deformity is seen on a true lateral radiograph of the wrist, but disappears when the hand and wrist are extended to the same position as the distal radial deformity. This can become painful as the dorsal wrist capsule is repeatedly stretched with forceful flexion maneuvers. The carpal malalignment will often correct spontaneously if a distal radial osteotomy is undertaken early but may become resistant in late cases.

A dynamic midcarpal instability may also occur because the normal palmar displacement of the lunate with ulnar deviation is blocked by the dorsally displaced volar lip of the articular surface. In this situation, repetitive stretching may result in attenuation of the intercarpal ligaments.

Radiocarpal subluxation is often present when the dorsal angulation of the distal radius exceeds 35 degrees. In this case, the wrist is stable when the hand is extended and the carpus is reduced on the distal radius, but active volar flexion leads to dorsal subluxation and pain at the radiocarpal articulation.

CLASSIFICATION

The most common type of injury to the distal radius is a dorsally angulated, extraarticular fracture. Eponyms have long been used with the intention of distinguishing the less common fracture types from this so-called *Colles'* (or *Pouteau*) fracture. Unfortunately, the simplicity of eponymic descriptions increases their susceptibility to misuse and confusion. The eponym *Smith*, for example, is most appropriately applied to extraarticular bending fractures with palmar angulation of the distal fragment. It has been misapplied to anterior (volar) marginal shearing fractures, which have a more appropriate eponymic label of *Barton.*[63] Moreover, the term *Colles' fracture* has become almost synonymous with *distal radius fracture*, so that in many cases the only information it provides is misinformation when the fracture turns out to have articular involvement, radiocarpal subluxation, or associated injuries.

The large number of schemes developed for classifying distal radius fractures bears testament not only to the importance and complexity of these injuries, but also to our gradually increasing understanding of the myriad ways in which various fracture patterns can contribute to disability. Taken as a group, the early classifications demonstrate an understanding of the importance of such factors as the morphology of the fracture line, the direction and degree of displacement of the distal fragment, the extent of articular involvement, and involvement of the distal radioulnar joint. Unfortunately, a classification has yet to be developed that can account for all of these factors while accurately guiding prognosis and treatment in a simple, straightforward fashion.

Classifications that have enjoyed some popularity in recent times are those of Older et al[49] (Figure 108-4) and Frykman[25] (Figure 108-5). The Older et al classification separates dorsally displaced extraarticular fractures based on a number of factors known to be related to the functional outcome after distal radius fracture, including the degree of dorsal comminution, loss of articular surface palmar tilt, and shortening relative to the ulna. Frykman's classification, on the other hand, focuses on articular fractures, bringing attention to the fact that involvement of both the radiocarpal and distal radioulnar articulations must be considered, separating out those fractures with involvement of the distal ulna. These two examples illustrate the inability of most classifications to account on the one hand for the great variety of injury to the distal radius and on the other hand for all of the important elements of the injury. The weaknesses of the existing classifications may explain to a large degree the persistence of eponymic descriptions such as *Colles'* or *Smith's* fracture.

Recent developments include a valiant attempt at a comprehensive fracture classification, an increased understanding of articular fractures, and a separate classification of associated ulnar lesions. Müller et al[48] developed a detailed classification of fractures of the distal radius (Figure 108-6). The scheme, at first glance, appears overwhelmingly complex, but a closer look reveals that a wide variety of distal radius fractures has been organized in a relatively straightforward and accessible manner according to the principles of Müller et al[48] in *The Comprehensive Classification of Fractures of Long Bones.* Fractures are divided into types, groups, and subgroups according to pattern and increasing complexity. Type A distal radius fractures are extraarticular, type B partial articular, and type C complete articular fractures. Nearly every observable injury pattern is represented in varying degrees of comminution within the groups and subgroups.

It is now widely recognized that open reduction and internal fixation techniques can be used to treat complex articular fractures of the distal radius and ulna.[14,44-46] More frequent operative treatment has led to an improved understanding of the patterns of articular involvement, and these patterns have been codified into classification schemes. Melone[45] noted that radiocarpal articular fractures tended to separate into four basic parts: the radial shaft, the radial styloid, and dorsal and palmar medial fragments (Figure 108-7). He emphasized the stability of fragments in relation to the degree

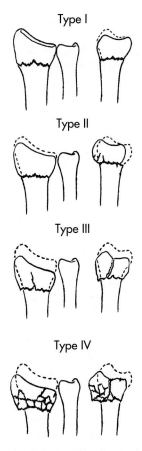

Type I

Type II

Type III

Type IV

Figure 108-4. Classification by Older et al of dorsal bending fractures of the distal radius based on magnitude of displacement, comminution, shortening, and articular involvement. (Redrawn from Fernandez DL, Jupiter JB: *Fractures of the distal radius: a practical approach to management,* New York, 1995, Springer-Verlag.)

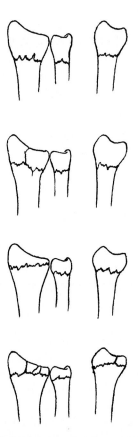

Figure 108-5. Frykman's classification was useful in drawing attention to involvement of both the radiocarpal and distal radioulnar articulations as well as the importance of the ulnar side of the wrist in these injuries. (Redrawn from Fernandez DL, Jupiter JB: *Fractures of the distal radius: a practical approach to management,* New York, 1995, Springer-Verlag.)

A1 Extraarticular fracture of the ulna, radius intact

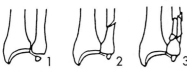

1 Styloid process
2 Metaphyseal simple
3 Metaphyseal multifragmentary

A2 Extraarticular fracture of the radius, simple and impacted

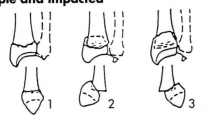

1 Without any tilt
2 With dorsal tilt (Pouteau-Colles)
3 With volar tilt (Goyrand-Smith)

A3 Extraarticular fracture of the radius, multifragmentary

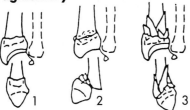

1 Impacted with axial shortening
2 With a wedge
3 Complex

A

B1 Partial articular fracture of the radius, sagittal

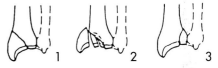

1 Lateral simple
2 Lateral multifragmentary
3 Medial

B2 Partial articular fracture of the radius, dorsal rim (Barton)

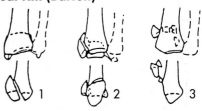

1 Simple
2 With lateral sagittal fracture
3 With dorsal dislocation of the carpus

B3 Partial articular fracture of the radius, volar rim (reverse Barton, Goyrand-Smith II)

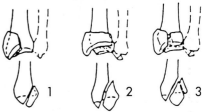

1 Simple, with a small fragment
2 Simple, with a large fragment
3 Multifragmentary

B

Figure 108-6. **A-C,** The Comprehensive Classification of Fractures organizes the wide variety of injury to the distal radius into a relatively straightforward and all-inclusive system. (From Fernandez DL, Jupiter JB: *Fractures of the distal radius: a practical approach to management,* New York, 1995, Springer-Verlag.)

Continued

of comminution. He also identified central articular fragments, which are impossible to reduce by closed means because they lack ligamentous attachments. The McMurty, Mayo, and Universal classifications were essentially variations on this theme.[14,44,46] These classifications identified the volar lunate articular fragments as particularly troublesome because the radiocarpal ligamentous attachments to these fragments tend to worsen alignment by causing dorsal rotation. Fractures without these separate volar fragments can often be treated by limited open manipulation and percutaneous fixation techniques, whereas the presence of a volar articular fragment often necessitates a volar operative exposure.

Involvement of the distal ulna, distal radioulnar joint, and triangular fibrocartilage has long been recognized as an integral part of injury to the distal radius. The ulnar element of the injury, however, has only occasionally been addressed in classification schemes, reflecting the fact that in most cases it is the distal radius fracture that will primarily be responsible for the final outcome. On the other hand, as Fernandez has emphasized, injury to the distal ulna can have a substantial influence on the final outcome if the function of the distal radioulnar joint is compromised. His classification of distal ulnar fractures emphasizes the necessity to evaluate the distal radioulnar joint for incongruity, instability, or malaligned articular fractures (Table 108-1).[22,27]

The distal radioulnar joint ligaments remain intact with type I lesions, and there is no articular incongruity. Avulsion fractures of the tip of the ulnar styloid and stable fractures of

C

C1 Complete articular fracture of the radius, articular simple, metaphyseal simple

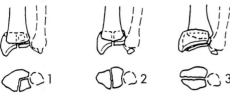

1 Posteromedial articular fragment
2 Sagittal articular fracture line
3 Frontal articular fracture line

C2 Complete articular fracture of the radius, articular simple, metaphyseal multifragmentary

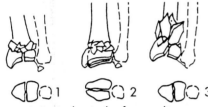

1 Sagittal articular fracture line
2 Frontal articular fracture line
3 Extending into the diaphysis

C3 Complete articular fracture of the radius, multifragmentary

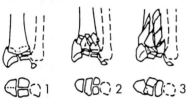

1 Metaphyseal simple
2 Metaphyseal multifragmentary
3 Extending into the diaphysis

Figure 108-6, cont'd. For legend see opposite page.

the ulnar neck are included within this group. Type II lesions are characterized by distal radioulnar instability as a result of either a massive tear of the triangular fibrocartilage complex or an avulsion fracture of the base of the ulnar styloid. Type III lesions are fractures involving the articular surface of either the ulnar head or the sigmoid notch of the radius. These lesions are potentially unstable.

These classification schemes are important and useful, but Fernandez developed a scheme that is simple, easy to remember, and easily applied (Table 108-2).[20] It provides a direct correlation with both the mechanism and epidemiology of the injury, as well as the treatment and prognosis. Moreover, it is easily tied into the more detailed Comprehensive Classification of Fractures by Müller et al.[48]

The central focus of the Fernandez classification is his separation of extraarticular bending fractures (type I), shearing articular fractures (type II), and compression articular fractures

(type III). Each of these types represents a distinct form of injury with a well-defined treatment algorithm. These three types represent the majority of distal radius fractures.

Two additional types are included to ensure that less common high-energy fracture patterns and their sequelae are recognized and treated appropriately. Radiocarpal fracture/dislocation (type IV) injuries have avulsion fractures of the ligamentous attachments, with dislocation of the scaphoid and lunate from their respective fossae in the articular surface of the distal radius. The type V classification is meant to identify those different cases in which there is marked articular or extraarticular comminution occasionally extending into the diaphysis, loss of bone, associated open wounds, injury to neurovascular or musculotendinous units, compartment syndrome, acute carpal tunnel syndrome, associated forearm or elbow injury, or associated ligamentous or bony carpal injury.

The value of the Fernandez classification is to provide a meaningful framework by which to organize the complex variety of skeletal injuries that occur at the distal radius and to apply it to the issues of indications, operations, and outcomes.

Extraarticular Bending Fractures

The dorsally displaced extraarticular fracture is the most frequently encountered fracture of the distal radius. Fractures with palmar displacement of the distal fragment are far less common. The mechanism of injury involves a fall onto an outstretched hand with the wrist extended, causing a bending force focused at the distal radial metaphysis. When the forearm is held in pronation and the body is rotating away from the planted hand, the metaphysis fails in tension volarly and in compression dorsally, resulting in dorsal displacement of the distal fragment, frequently with comminution of the dorsal cortex. The converse is true of palmar bending fractures, which occur when the forearm is supinated and the body is rotating toward the hand.

The stability of extraarticular bending fractures of the distal radius is defined in terms of the likelihood of success with nonoperative treatment.[22] Stable fractures are those that are able to resist displacement after manipulation into the anatomic position with only cast immobilization. The factors that predict instability can be identified on radiographs before a reduction attempt. These include the obliquity of the fracture line and degree of metaphyseal comminution for palmar bending fractures and marked displacement, metaphyseal comminution, and severe osteopenia for dorsal bending fractures.

The majority of palmarly displaced extraarticular fractures are inherently unstable because of either the obliquity of the fracture line or the degree of metaphyseal comminution or both. It is therefore useful, when faced with a palmar bending fracture, to consider the Fernandez classification into type A injuries with a transverse fracture line and minimal comminution, type B injuries with an oblique fracture line, and type C injuries with metaphyseal comminution (Figure 108-8).[17] Nonoperative treatment by manipulative reduction and long arm cast immobilization with the forearm in full supination and the wrist in slight extension should be considered only for

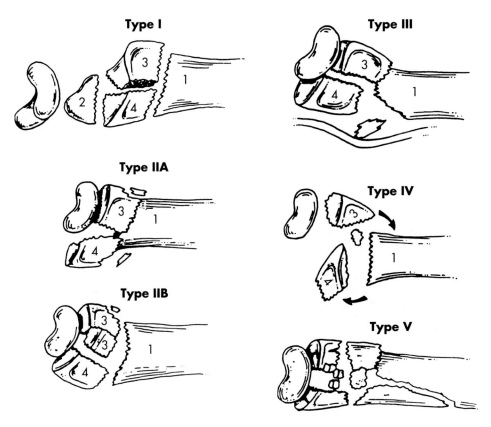

Figure 108-7. Melone captured the common patterns of articular disruption in his classifications, which emphasized the importance of a coronal split in the lunate fragment and central impaction (the so-called *die-punch fragment*). (From Melone CP: *Orthop Clin North Am* 15:217-236, 1984.)

patients with type A fractures. Types B and C fractures are best treated with volar plate fixation of the radius.

It is useful for treatment to subdivide dorsal bending fractures into minimally displaced, displaced but stable, and displaced unstable fractures. Nondisplaced or minimally displaced fractures are defined as those fractures that have less than 5 degrees of dorsal angulation of the radial articular surface and less than 2 mm of axial shortening as measured by ulnar variance.[22] These fractures are inherently stable and can be immobilized without reduction in a below elbow cast for 4 weeks, followed by a removable thermoplast splint for an additional 2 weeks. Radiographs are repeated within 7 to 10 days to monitor continued fracture alignment, and vigilance is maintained for the possibility of median nerve symptoms or spontaneous rupture of the extensor pollicis longus tendon. This latter complication is uncommon, but has been seen with minimally displaced fractures and is most common within 8 weeks of the injury. If tenderness, swelling, and/or crepitation are noted about Lister's tubercle, decompression of the third extensor compartment may avoid rupture of the extensor pollicis longus.

Displaced but stable fractures are those with between 5 and 20 degrees of dorsal angulation of the radial articular surface on the lateral radiograph and between 2 and 5 mm of shortening by ulnar variance on the PA radiograph.[22] These are the fractures for which a manipulative reduction and cast or splint immobilization are likely to be effective in restoring and

maintaining the anatomy and therefore the function of the distal radius. There is substantial variation in every aspect of the management of this subset of distal radial fractures, including the anesthetic technique, the method of manipulation, and the type, position, and duration of immobilization.

The most commonly used anesthetic is a hematoma block. The utility of this technique is widely recognized, but the quality of the anesthesia achieved can, on occasion, be suboptimal. There are a number of factors to consider that can improve the anesthesia obtained. First, the dorsal fracture line in a dorsal bending fracture can be difficult to find and enter. We prefer to inject 5 to 7 ml of 1% or 2% lidocaine without epinephrine into the more widely opened volar aspect of the fracture site. The anesthetic may enter the carpal canal with this method, altering median nerve function, and can create uncertainty about the nerve's status for approximately an hour and a half after injection. A separate injection of an additional 5 to 7 ml into the distal radioulnar joint and ulnar styloid may substantially enhance pain relief because these areas are also commonly involved in the injury.

The regional anesthesia provided by a Bier or brachial plexus block provides more predictable and complete anesthesia and a measure of muscle relaxation, but it is best performed by an anesthesiologist and has a slightly increased risk.

Closed reduction is performed by application of longitudinal traction while the distal fragment is pushed in a volar and ulnar direction and then locked into place by pronation of the

Table 108-1.

Classification of Distal Radioulnar Joint Lesions Associated With Fractures of the Distal Radius

	PATHOANATOMY OF THE LESION	DEGREE OF JOINT SURFACE INVOLVEMENT	PROGNOSIS	RECOMMENDED TREATMENT
TYPE I Stable (following reduction of the radius, the distal radioulnar joint is congruous and stable)	**A** Avulsion fracture tip of the ulnar styloid **B** Stable fracture of ulnar neck	None	Good	Fracture types **A** and **B:** Functional aftertreatment Encourage early pronation-supination exercises NOTE: Extraarticular *unstable* fractures of the ulna at the metaphyseal level or distal shaft require stable plate fixation
TYPE II Unstable (subluxation or dislocation of the ulnar head present)	**A** Substance tear of TFCC and/or palmar and dorsal capsular ligaments **B** Avulsion fracture of base of the ulnar styloid	None	Chronic instability Painful limitation of supination if left unreduced Possible late arthritic changes	Fracture type **A:** Closed treatment (reduce subluxation, sugar tong splint in 45 degrees of supination 4-6 weeks) Fracture types **A** and **B:** Operative treatment (repair TFCC or fix ulnar styloid with tension band wiring; immobilize wrist and elbow in supination (cast) or transfix ulna/radius with K wire and forearm cast)
TYPE III Potentially unstable (subluxation possible)	**A** Intraarticular fracture of the sigmoid notch **B** Intraarticular fracture of the ulnar head	Present	Dorsal subluxation possible together with dorsally displaced die punch or dorsoulnar fragment Risk of early degenerative changes and severe limitation of forearm rotation if left unreduced	Fracture type **A:** Anatomic reduction of palmar and dorsal sigmoid fragments; if residual subluxation tendency present, immobilize as in type-II injury Fracture type **B:** Functional aftertreatment to enhance remodeling of ulnar head If distal radioulnar joint remains painful, partial ulnar resection, Darrach, or Sauvé-Kapandji procedure may be performed at a later date

From Fernandez DL, Jupiter JB: *Fractures of the distal radius: a practical approach to management,* New York, 1995, Springer-Verlag.
TFCC, Triangular fibrocartilage complex.

Table 108-2.
Classification of Distal Radius Fractures According to Fernandez

FRACTURE TYPES (ADULTS) BASED ON THE MECHANISM OF INJURY	FRACTURE EQUIVALENT IN CHILDREN	STABILITY/ INSTABILITY*	DISPLACEMENT PATTERN	NUMBER OF FRAGMENTS	ASSOCIATED LESIONS†	RECOMMENDED TREATMENT
TYPE I Bending fracture of the metaphysis	Distal forearm fracture Salter II	Stable Unstable	Nondisplaced dorsally (Colles-Pouteau) Volar (Smith) Proximal Combined	Always two main fragments plus varying degree of metaphyseal comminution (instability)	Uncommon	Conservative (stable fractures) Percutaneous pinning (extrafocal or intrafocal) External fixation (occasionally bone graft)
TYPE II Shearing fracture of the joint surface	Salter IV	Unstable	Dorsal Radial Volar Proximal Combined	Two-part Three-part Comminuted	Less uncommon	Open reduction Screw/plate fixation
TYPE III Compression fracture of the joint surface	Salter III, IV, V	Stable Unstable	Nondisplaced dorsally Radial Volar Proximal Combined	Two-part Three-part Four-part Comminuted	Common	Conservative (closed, limited, arthroscopic assisted, or extensile open reduction) Percutaneous pins Combined external and internal fixation Bone graft

Type		Frequency	Stability	Displacement	Type of fracture		Treatment
TYPE IV Avulsion fractures, radiocarpal fracture/dislocation		Very rare	Unstable	Dorsal Radial Volar Proximal Combined	Two-part (radial styloid, ulnar styloid) Three-part (volar, dorsal margin) Comminuted	Frequent	Closed or open reduction Pin or screw fixation Tension wiring
TYPE V Combined fractures (I, II, III, IV); high-velocity injury		Very rare	Unstable	Dorsal Radial Volar Proximal Combined	Comminuted and/or bone loss (frequently intraarticular, open, seldom extraarticular)	Always present	Combined method

From Fernandez DL, Jupiter JB: *Fractures of the distal radius: a practical approach to management,* New York, 1995, Springer-Verlag.

*High risk of secondary displacement after initial adequate reduction.

†Carpal ligament, fractures, median and ulnar nerve, tendons, fracture ipsilateral upper extremity, compartment syndrome.

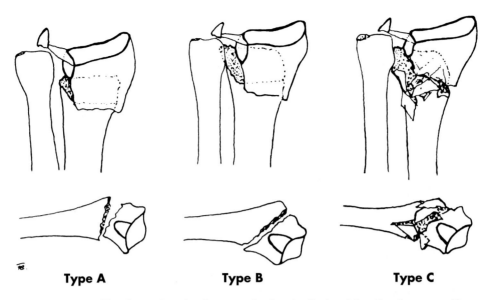

Figure 108-8. The Fernandez classification of palmarly displaced bending fractures. (From Fernandez DL, Jupiter JB: *Fractures of the distal radius: a practical approach to management,* New York, 1995, Springer-Verlag.)

hand and wrist. Finger trap traction may prove useful, particularly when the physician is lacking assistants, but it can tend to increase the dorsal angulation of the distal radial articular surface as the distal fragment pivots on the tightened intact dorsal periosteum and soft tissue structures. The simplest and most effective technique, as described by Jones,[31] puts dorsal pressure on the distal fragment with the thenar eminence of one hand while counter pressure is applied with the other hand against the proximal radius, with an assistant stabilizing the elbow. Relaxation of the intact dorsal soft tissue structures may be required in some cases by initially exaggerating the deformity to facilitate reduction.

A wide variety of immobilization techniques has been advocated in the literature, including splints, above or below elbow casts, and functional bracing with proponents of positioning in supination, pronation, and neutral rotation. The metacarpophalangeal (MCP) joints must remain free, and digital edema should be controlled in patients with casts. We advocate immobilization of the forearm and wrist in pronation, with the wrist in ulnar deviation and only slight flexion. Positioning the hand in extreme volar flexion–ulnar deviation (the so-called *Cotton-Loder position*) should be avoided because it increases the risk of acute carpal tunnel syndrome and also reduces the mechanical advantage of the extrinsic hand musculature, which contributes to digital stiffness. Careful three-point molding of the splint or cast will limit the risk of displacement, but if extreme positioning is required to maintain reduction, then operative fixation should be considered.

Our preference is to initially immobilize the fracture in a sugar tong splint with the hand and wrist pronated. This is changed to a below elbow cast after 3 weeks. Most displaced but stable fractures are immobilized for a total of 6 weeks.

Unstable fractures of the distal radius are defined as those that present with greater than 20 degrees of dorsal angulation, greater than 5 mm of shortening (by ulnar variance), have metaphyseal comminution extending volarly, or are associated with a large ulnar styloid or ulnar neck fracture.[22] These fractures are more common in elderly, osteopenic individuals and are more likely than not to displace after a manipulative reduction and cast immobilization. When a fracture that was initially considered stable displaces in a cast, it is reclassified as unstable unless there was a substantial deficiency in the technique of manipulation or immobilization indicating that a second attempt might be worthwhile. Operative fixation provides the most reliable treatment for unstable dorsal bending fractures of the distal radius.

Shearing Fractures of the Articular Surface

A shearing fracture of the distal radial articular surface is the result of a high-energy trauma. The radial styloid (scaphoid facet), lunate facet, dorsal or volar rim, or some combination of these may be involved.[22] The radial styloid shearing fracture is the most common of these uncommon injuries. The name *Chauffeur's fracture* was attached to this injury because backfire of the crank starter handle on early automobiles resulted in a forced dorsiflexion and radial deviation force, which caused a number of these fractures. Shearing fractures are commonly grouped under the eponym *Barton.* Volar shearing fractures are more common than dorsal shearing fractures that usually occur in association with radial styloid fractures.[22] Even when all of these fractures are considered together, this subclassification represents less than 3% of all fractures of the distal radius in most series.

Dorsal and volar shearing fractures of the articular surface require operative fixation not only to restore congruity of the articular surface but also to achieve stable reduction of the associated radiocarpal subluxation. The obliquity of the fracture line makes the fracture inherently unstable. Many radial styloid and lunate facet fractures can be reduced with closed or limited open manipulation and stabilized with percutaneously inserted Kirschner wires (K wires). Volar and dorsal marginal shearing fractures, however, are best treated by buttress plate fixation.[53,64]

These fractures are the result of a high-energy carpal impaction against the articular surface of the radius. One must therefore look carefully for associated carpal fractures or intercarpal ligamentous injuries. These patients should be treated by early open reduction and fixation, with vigilance for the development of complications such as carpal tunnel or forearm compartment syndromes.

Compression Fractures of the Articular Surface

A distal radial articular surface fracture most commonly results from an axial impaction of the carpal bones. Axial compression that occurs with radial or ulnar deviation can result in a shearing fracture of a single facet, whereas a more direct axial impaction results in fragmentation of the entire articular surface. The complexity of the fracture and the extent of metaphyseal comminution are determined by the strength of the bone and the magnitude of the injuring force. Concomitant injury to the carpus can occur.[57]

Recent investigations have corroborated the finding of Knirk and Jupiter[36] that residual articular malalignment will lead to painful arthrosis and restricted motion in an active adult. It may be possible to treat some stable fractures with minimal (less than 2 mm) separation between articular fragments in a cast, but most of these fractures are either widely displaced or associated with comminution in the metaphyseal bone supporting the articular fragments and are therefore unstable.[22] Operative fixation is therefore indicated. It may be possible with many simple articular fractures to obtain and stabilize an anatomic reduction under image intensification with closed or limited open manipulation and percutaneous wire fixation.[28] Open exposure with visualization of the articular surface is necessary for optimal treatment if there is fragmentation of the articular surface in the coronal plane or more extensive comminution is suspected.

Radiocarpal Fracture/Dislocation

Dislocation of the radiocarpal articulation is the result of a very-high-energy injury and is extremely uncommon. The injury is more appropriately considered a radiocarpal fracture/dislocation because the radiocarpal and ulnocarpal ligaments are avulsed from their origins on the distal ulna and radius. These patients often have severe soft tissue injury, other fractures to the ipsilateral limb, or have multisystem trauma. Fractures/dislocations with and without associated injury to the scapholunate or lunotriquetral interosseous ligaments should be distinguished by carefully evaluating the proximal carpal row on the radiographs because those with intact ligaments are likely to have a better prognosis.[22] Restoration of ligamentous stability is obtained

by operative fixation of the avulsed fragments of the distal radius and ulna.

High-Energy Combined Injuries

The category of high-energy combined injuries is intended to emphasize the fact that a complex fracture of the distal radius in a young adult is an extremely high-energy injury to the entire upper limb. The scope of these injuries often includes other injuries requiring expedient operative treatment, including neurovascular injury, open wounds, acute carpal tunnel syndrome and compartment syndrome, ipsilateral upper-extremity injury, and polytrauma. Treatment of these severely injured patients must be more comprehensive and can be far more challenging than treatment of the average elderly patient with an isolated fracture.

Ulnar Lesions

racture of the ulnar styloid or tearing of the triangular fibrocartilage complex are commonly associated with widely displaced fractures of the distal radius. These lesions have been well treated by the traditional distal radial fracture treatment regimens that involved 6 weeks of immobilization.[8] Nonunion of the ulnar styloid is common after displaced fractures of the distal radius, but it does not appear to detract from the functional result if the distal radioulnar joint is stable.

External and internal fixation techniques are now more routinely used, and prolonged immobilization of the distal radioulnar joint is less common. It may therefore be necessary to address the ulnar lesion at the time of operative intervention to ensure proper functioning of the distal radioulnar joint. The distal radioulnar joint should always be evaluated for articular congruity and stability after the distal radius fracture is reduced. Displaced articular fractures of the ulnar head require anatomic fixation.[22,27]

Persistent instability of the distal radioulnar joint despite restoration of distal radial alignment is adequately treated by 6 weeks of cast immobilization, with the forearm in 45 degrees of supination in most cases. Occasionally this does not restore stability, and temporary cross-pinning of the distal forearm with a 2-mm K wire is required. Consideration should be given to operative fixation when the ulnar styloid fragment, including its base, is widely displaced.[22,27]

The use of arthroscopy to visualize the articular surface has shown that injury to the triangular fibrocartilage is common. Many of these injuries can be repaired under arthroscopic guidance.[27,28]

MALUNION

Many patients with malunion present at a time remote from their injury with specific complaints referable to the malposition of the distal radius.[18,19,22] Patients with a malunited dorsal bending fracture may complain of pain localized to the radiocarpal, midcarpal, or distal radioulnar joints; limitation of forearm rotation caused by radioulnar incongruity; a weak grip; poor hand and wrist mechanics overall; instability of the distal radioulnar joint; or dissatisfaction with the appearance of the limb. Narrowing of the carpal canal and an extension posture of the distal radius can also contribute to the development of carpal tunnel syndrome. Patients with excessive palmar tilt of the distal radius may present with limitations in active wrist extension and supination. Many of these patients have already undergone extensive therapy, and operative treatment is the only remaining option. It is important to assess the radiocarpal and distal radioulnar articulations for evidence of arthrosis at this late stage because operative treatment may alter the operative approach.[19,22]

Traditional thinking has fostered the implementation of a thorough exercise program to maximize function and subsequently determine the need for a corrective osteotomy. We and others believe, however, that sufficient clinical and laboratory evidence has now been amassed to indicate that active patients with greater than 20 degrees of dorsal angulation of the distal radius articular surface, greater than 15 degrees of dorsal angulation of the lunate, greater than 2 mm step-off or gap in an articular surface, incongruity of the distal radioulnar joint, or radiocarpal subluxation are almost certain to develop problems.[33] Early corrective osteotomy of these malaligned fractures should be considered unless the patient is infirm or incapacitated. Our experience comparing early with late reconstruction of malaligned fractures of the distal radius would suggest that early correction is an easier and more predictable procedure, that return of motion is optimized by the limitation of soft tissue contracture, that the period of disability is markedly diminished, and that the overall costs are much less.[33] Many of the difficulties associated with the harvest of a structural iliac crest autograft are avoided with earlier correction because cancellous graft is usually sufficient.

INFORMED CONSENT

Percutaneous fixation methods can result in pin-tract sepsis and injury to sensory nerve blood vessels or tendons. Recurrence of the deformity is a potential concern, particularly if large bony defects were present and the pins are removed too soon, which can cause the fracture to settle somewhat. Open exposure of the distal radius also involves risks such as injury to neurovascular structures during exposure, infection, wound separation, and an unsightly scar. Placement of an implant on the bone risks a deep infection, implant failure, and/or irritation caused by the implant, requiring a second operation for its removal. The patient should be informed of all possible complications, including those associated with anesthetic, and must balance these with the potential for future disability with residual deformity, which are likely without surgery.

Patients should be forewarned that a number of factors important in determining the ultimate outcome are, to a large extent, beyond the control of the surgeon, such as articular cartilage injury and the possibility of developing complications such as sympathetic maintained pain.

OPERATIONS

ANESTHESIA

Either general or regional anesthesia can be used for operative procedures on the distal radius and ulna. Regional anesthesia may be safer in some medically ill patients; however, several factors make general anesthesia more appealing in most cases (e.g., correction of distal radius trauma in many cases requires the harvest of an autogenous bone graft from the iliac crest or prolonged use of a pneumatic tourniquet). General anesthesia also allows immediate postoperative evaluation of the neurologic status of the hand. If a regional anesthetic is used, it should be short acting to avoid delaying the diagnosis of an acute carpal tunnel or forearm compartment syndrome.

POSITIONING AND PREPARATION

The patient is positioned supine in most cases. A pneumatic tourniquet is applied to the most proximal aspect of the arm, but inflated only as necessary. The tourniquet is inflated routinely in most cases involving open reduction or elective osteotomy. One iliac crest is prepped for possible graft harvest.

BONE GRAFT

Anatomic reduction of fractures with extensive metaphyseal comminution or impacted articular fragments commonly results in the formation of bony defects.[37] These should be filled with autogenous cancellous bone graft to provide some structural support and enhance healing. In most cases, sufficient graft can be obtained with minimal morbidity through a small hole in the iliac crest, using an incision less than an inch in length. We have found trephine core biopsy needles to be particularly useful for the harvest of substantial amounts of graft through a small hole (Figure 108-9). Small

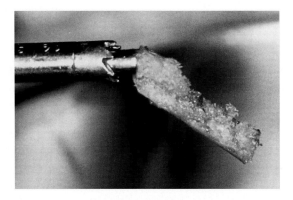

Figure 108-9. Trephine core biopsy needles provide a simple means by which to harvest small amounts of autogenous cancellous bone graft from the iliac crest through a small incision and hole in the iliac crest. This technique helps to diminish pain, deformity, and complications at the harvest site.

curettes can also be used. The periosteum is closed over the hole, leaving no defect or unstable fragment and little potential for hematoma or hernia formation.

Use of bone graft substitutes is becoming more popular as new products are developed. Ultimately some combination of an osteoconductive substance (e.g., collagen, coral hydroxyapatite, or freeze-dried allograft bone), an osteoinductive substance (e.g., demineralized bone or isolated growth factors such as bone morphogenic proteins), or perhaps an osteogenic substance (e.g., bone marrow aspirated from the iliac crest or cultured bone precursor cells) may prove to be equivalent or better than autogenous cancellous bone graft. Each of the many alternative substances presently have drawbacks that limit their appeal.[66]

A great deal of interest has been generated by the development of injectable bone graft substitutes that provide structural support and are remodeled, to some extent, into bone.[12] Injection of this type of substance into comminuted fractures with metaphyseal defects might eventually represent an alternative to operative fixation with K wires or external fixation (Figure 108-10).

OPERATIVE EXPOSURES

Dorsal Exposures

Exposure of the dorsal and radial surfaces of the distal radius, the distal radioulnar joint, and/or the distal ulna can be obtained through a number ofsssssss distinct intervals entering between extensor compartments. Dorsal exposure is advanta-

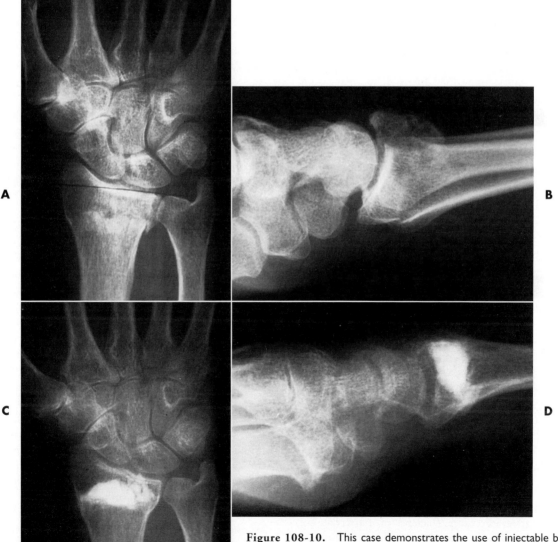

Figure 108-10. This case demonstrates the use of injectable bone graft substitutes. **A** and **B,** Radiographs demonstrate a dorsal bending fracture in an elderly female. A manipulative reduction was achieved in the operating room and Norian SRS (Norian, Cupertino, Calif.) was injected through a large-bore needle inserted into the fracture site through a small dorsal incision. **C** and **D,** Follow-up radiographs demonstrate healing with maintenance of alignment.

geous because the articular surfaces and intercarpal ligaments can be inspected through a dorsal wrist capsulotomy with little risk of destabilizing the carpus. Comminution requiring the application of bone graft or a buttress plate is most common on the dorsal aspect of the radius, and no major neurovascular structures are encountered. The primary disadvantage is that implants placed on the dorsal aspect of the distal radius can irritate the overlying extensor tendons.

A longitudinal incision that can be extended provides good access to the dorsum of the hand and wrist because of the mobility and elasticity of the dorsal skin. Cutaneous nerves should be identified and gently retracted to avoid a painful neuroma. Large veins should be preserved to limit edema formation after surgery. The skin incision is placed directly over the compartment of intended exposure.

The interval between the first and second extensor compartments provides exposure of the dorsoradial aspect of the radius. The approach is relatively straightforward, with the radial sensory nerve representing the only structure in immediate danger. Exposure through this interval is used most often for the treatment of radial styloid fractures. Accurate articular reduction of a comminuted fracture can be verified by incising the wrist capsule. This requires a more distal dissection, which places the radial artery and its dorsal carpal branch at risk as they course from palmar to dorsal through the anatomic snuffbox.

The interval providing the widest exposure, and that most appropriate for dorsal plate fixation, is that between the second

and fourth extensor compartments (Figure 108-11). The extensor retinaculum is incised immediately adjacent to the ulnar edge of the second dorsal compartment. The retinaculum is raised ulnarly until the third dorsal compartment is encountered and incised. If care is taken to preserve an ulnarly based retinacular flap, it may be placed under the radial wrist extensor tendons at the time of closure to help separate them from an underlying fixation device. The content of the third compartment, the extensor pollicis longus tendon, is mobilized proximally and distally and translocated radially within the subcutaneous tissues. No attempt is made to replace this tendon into its compartment at the time of closure. We have had favorable experience leaving the extensor pollicis longus in its translocated, subcutaneous position. Exposure of the dorsal surface of the distal radius is achieved through the third compartment. The integrity of the fourth dorsal compartment is preserved by elevating it subperiosteally from the distal radius in an attempt to limit adhesions and irritation. The second dorsal compartment is likewise mobilized. Incision of the dorsal wrist capsule is performed when inspection of the articular surface or the scapholunate interosseous ligament is indicated.

Exposure between the fourth and fifth extensor compartments is useful for direct manipulation of lunate facet fractures and inspection of the distal radioulnar joint. The interval between the fifth and sixth compartments is used for the repair of distal ulnar fractures, ulnar styloid fractures, and tears in the triangular fibrocartilage complex. Incisions on the dorsoulnar aspect of the wrist place the dorsal sensory branch of the ulnar nerve at risk.

Volar Exposures

The volar surface of the distal radius can be exposed from its radial or its ulnar aspect. A more ulnar exposure is obtained by entering the carpal tunnel and retracting the median nerve and flexor tendons radially. This interval is appealing for the treatment of high-energy injuries, in which median and ulnar nerve compression and forearm compartment syndrome are a substantial concern, because it results in extensive decompression. The more radial exposure between the flexor carpi radialis and the radial artery is more commonly used, but it can be difficult to gain access to the ulnar aspect of the distal radius through this exposure (Figure 108-12).

The skin incision for the ulnar volar exposure starts in the palm as the standard carpal tunnel incision. The transverse wrist creases are crossed obliquely, and a broad, radially based skin flap is fashioned to ensure coverage of the carpal canal in the event that excessive swelling prevents complete wound closure. The interval between the ulnar nerve and artery and the flexor tendons and median nerve is developed through the carpal tunnel by incising the transverse retinaculum. Adequate exposure is often obtained with only partial division of the pronator quadratus at its most distal aspect overlying the distal radioulnar joint (Figure 108-13).

For the radial volar exposure, the skin is incised between the tendon of the flexor carpi radialis and the radial artery, and this interval is developed. The flexor pollicis longus is identified in the proximal part of the wound and is retracted ulnarly, along

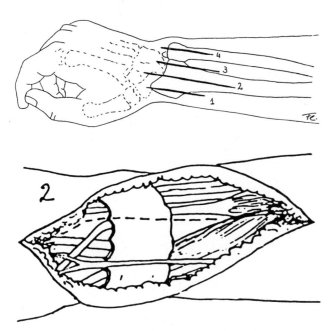

Figure 108-11. Exposure of the dorsal surface of the distal radius can be achieved through a number of distinct intervals between the dorsal extensor compartments. The most commonly utilized exposure is that between the second and fourth compartments, elevating the extensor pollicis longus out of the third compartment and leaving it dorsoradially in the subcutaneous tissues. (From Fernandez DL, Jupiter JB: *Fractures of the distal radius: a practical approach to management,* New York, 1995, Springer-Verlag.)

with its nerve supply, from the anterior interosseous nerve, as is the flexor carpi radialis tendon. The more distal pronator quadratus muscle is then divided along its most radial aspect, leaving a small cuff of tissue for reattachment at the time of closure.

Exposure of the Distal Ulna
The distal ulna can be approached either dorsally between the fifth (extensor digiti quinti) and sixth (extensor carpi ulnaris) extensor compartments (where access can be gained to the ulnar styloid and triangular fibrocartilage complex), or ulnarly between the extensor carpi ulnaris and flexor carpi ulnaris tendons.

Arthroscopy
The role of wrist arthroscopy in the treatment of distal radius fractures remains unclear. Use of arthroscopy in the treatment of high-energy injuries has been discouraged because of a concern that fluid extravasation might contribute to the formation of a compartment syndrome.[28] Moreover, image intensification represents a reliable means of verifying articular reduction of many simple fractures.[22]

Visualization of the radial articular surface through the arthroscope, however, may allow percutaneous fixation of some articular fractures that would otherwise require an operative exposure for capsulotomy. Arthroscopy also provides extensive visualization of soft tissue structures such as the scapholunate interosseous ligament and triangular fibrocartilage complex, both of which are commonly injured in high-energy fractures of the distal radius.[27,28]

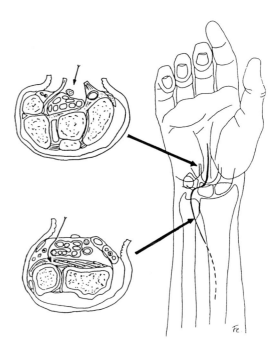

Figure 108-12. Volar exposure of the distal radius must be selected carefully. The ulnar exposure illustrated here represents the best choice for approaching fractures of the lunate facet because the ulnar border of the volar radial surface can be difficult to access from the more radial Henry approach (see Figure 108-13). High-energy injuries may benefit from this ulnar exposure because the carpal tunnel is released as part of the exposure. (From Fernandez DL, Jupiter JB: *Fractures of the distal radius: a practical approach to management,* New York, 1995, Springer-Verlag.)

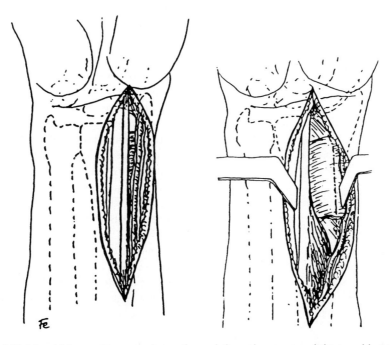

Figure 108-13. Volar exposure can be performed through a more radial interval between the flexor carpi radialis and the radial artery. (From Fernandez DL, Jupiter JB: *Fractures of the distal radius: a practical approach to management,* New York, 1995, Springer-Verlag.)

The technique utilized is identical to that for more elective procedures, with a few caveats. The landmarks for portal placement are often obscured by swelling and deformity, making it necessary to use small, open incisions and blunt dissection down to the capsule to ensure proper placement of the portals and to avoid injury to tendons or cutaneous nerves. The 3-4 portal should fall in line with the radial border of the long finger, and the 4-5 portal should fall along the midaxis of the ring finger. Needle insertion into the radiocarpal joint under image intensification can help verify proper portal position before incising the capsule. Visualization may be improved by delaying surgery until at least 3 days after the injury to optimize visualization by limiting active bleeding. The forearm should be wrapped in a compressive elastic bandage to limit fluid extravasation into the muscle compartments. Continuous distraction through an external fixator or small distractor represents an appealing alternative to finger trap traction in this setting.

FIXATION

External Fixation
External fixation is most often used to provide neutralization for percutaneous pins or internal fixation. Prolonged distraction through the fixator is poorly advised because this can cause tightness of the extrinsic hand muscles, leading to digital stiffness, and can also exacerbate carpal ligament injury.

External fixation has been used for over half a century. Steinmann pins or K wires were initially placed in the metacarpals and the forearm and then incorporated into a plaster cast in an attempt to immobilize comminuted intraarticular fractures of the distal radius in a distracted position. Modern designs, following that of Anderson[4] by connecting Schantz screws to a metal frame, have reduced the rate of complications, improved the results of treatment, and led to the development and wider use of external fixation. The popularity of external fixation for the treatment of distal radius fractures has led to an explosion in the number of different types of fixators available. Some devices allow limited wrist motion in the fixator. Dynamic fixators are more expensive and more difficult to apply correctly and to date have not improved the results in initial investigations.

We continue to use the simple pin-to-pin external fixator developed by the Arbeitsgemeinschaft für Osteosynthesefragen/Association for the Study of Internal Fixation (AO/ASIF) (Synthes, Paoli, Penn) and modeled after the original frame of Anderson.[4] The Schantz screws are inserted on the dorsoradial aspect of the second metacarpal in a plane midway between the sagittal and coronal planes of the palm to preserve thumb mobility. A corresponding plane is chosen for the pins in the radial shaft. These pins are placed at a point approximately 10 to 12 cm proximal to the radial styloid, avoiding the abductor pollicis longus and extensor pollicis longus muscles. Pin placement is planned under image intensifier control before incision of the skin. Insertion is planned so that the screws converge, creating a 45-to 60-degree angle between the two pins. This serves both to increase the

number of threads engaging the bone and enhance the stability of the construct. The planned pin orientation is drawn on the skin, and this determines the incision sites (Figure 108-14, B).

A small incision in the skin is made for each pin, and the soft tissues are dissected down to bone. The soft tissues are held apart and a protective drill sleeve is inserted directly onto the bone to ensure that neurovascular, muscular, and tendinous structures are not impaled. Some surgeons recommend larger incisions to facilitate direct visualization of all structures.[59] The holes for the metacarpal pins are predrilled with a 2-mm bit, and 2.5-mm Schantz screws are inserted. We predrill the radius with a 2.5-mm bit and insert 4-mm Schantz screws.

The wrist is immobilized in a neutral position and two carbon fiber rods can be used to connect the metacarpal to the radial pins. The first rod is placed as close to the skin as possible without risking pressure injury to increase the stability of the construct; the second rod is placed as far from the first rod as screw length will allow (about 2 cm).

When fixation is complete, residual skin tension around the pins should be released by extending the incisions as necessary. The pin sites are dressed with sterile gauze bolsters to limit motion at the skin-screw interface. The gauze is removed 3 to 6 days after the procedure, and pin care is initiated. This consists of cleansing the pins with hydrogen peroxide and releasing any areas of skin that become adherent to the pins. The patient may shower in the fixator.

Many of the problems associated with external fixation can be offset by early removal of the frame. Early frame removal is possible when it has been used to neutralize the wrist for percutaneous pin placement. The fixator can be removed as early as 4 to 6 weeks after the operation, whereas the percutaneous pins are removed when healing is assured, usually in 8 weeks.[22] Fractures with a large metaphyseal bony defect may require autogenous bone graft from the iliac crest. The fixator can often be removed as early as 4 weeks after grafting, and the limb is then placed into a splint.[22]

Kirschner-Wire Fixation
Many unstable fractures of the distal radius can be fixed with little operative morbidity using smooth K wires inserted percutaneously. Percutaneous pin fixation using 0.062-inch wires is suitable for dorsal bending fractures and many simple compression fractures of the articular surface. The use of an oscillating drill or dissection to bone through small incisions may be useful in limiting damage or irritation of sensory nerve branches. When fixation is complete, relaxing incisions are made as necessary to limit skin tension around the pins.

The pins are then either bent 90 degrees at the skin and left just outside the skin or cut off to lie just beneath the skin. In either case, if a below-elbow cast is applied a window should be cut over the pins to limit local irritation. The cast can generally be removed after 6 weeks, and the pins will remain in place for 8 weeks.

Screw Fixation
Screw fixation should be considered as an alternative to K wires when articular fragments are of sufficient size. Screws are stronger, gain better purchase by virtue of their threads, and

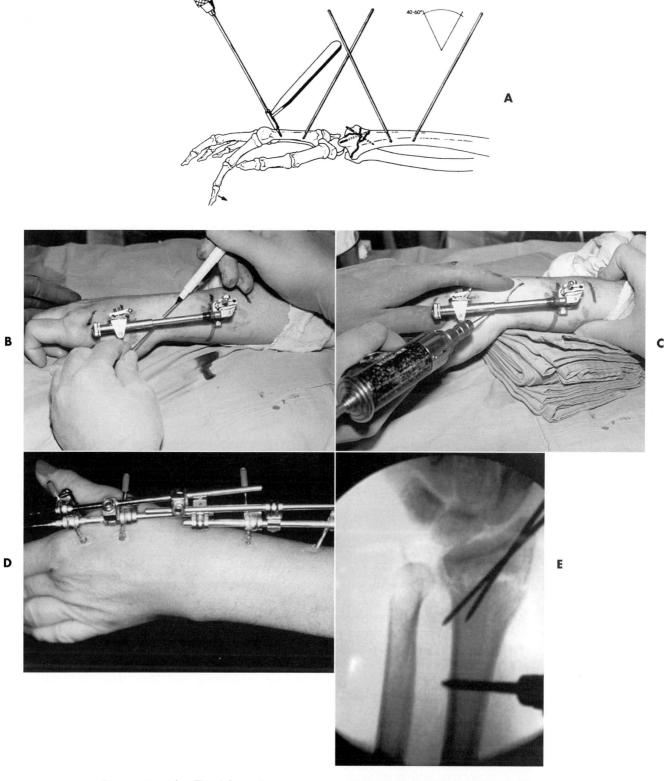

Figure 108-14. The AO small external fixator (Synthes, Paoli, Penn.) is well suited to the treatment of distal radial fractures. **A,** The Schantz pins should converge slightly both to increase purchase in the bone as well as to increase the overall stability of the construct. **B,** The intended site for a K wire is marked on the skin, using image intensification to facilitate accurate pin placement. **C,** The small distractor proves useful for obtaining and holding a manipulative reduction and can be applied to the two Schantz pins closest to the fracture. **D,** The fracture is reduced by manipulation, fixed wire, and a Kirchner wire, and the external fixator is applied. **E,** This radiograph from an image intensifier illustrates an exemplary final result.

can be used to apply interfragmentary compression where appropriate. Cannulated screws are more precise and effective because they allow insertion over an accurately placed provisional K wire.

Plate Fixation of the Dorsal Surface of the Distal Radius

Plate fixation is an appealing means of providing stable anatomic fixation for distal radius fractures. Use of plate fixation has been limited as a result of both the tendency of dorsally applied plates to irritate the overlying extensor tendons and the poor adaptation of current plate designs to the contour and fracture anatomy of the distal radius.

The oblique T-plate is representative of current standard distal radial plates. The plate is relatively thin, but the screw heads are prominent. The plate is broad and difficult to contour, contributing to its bulk. This plate nearly always causes synovitis of the extensor tendons and has to be removed. The screw insertion sites are few, and their distribution does not correspond with commonly encountered fracture patterns. Furthermore, only large fracture fragments can be fixed with the 3.5-mm screws because clinical guidelines suggest that fragments smaller than three times the size of the screw diameter are likely to fragment further with screw insertion.

Newer plate designs have focused on limiting irritation of the overlying extensor tendons by providing a lower profile plate with recessed screw heads. The so called π-plate, named for its resemblance to the Greek letter π, represents the result of the effort of the AO Hand Study Group (whose members include Ueli Buchler, Jurg Brennwald, Hill Hastings II, and Jesse Jupiter) to develop an implant for the dorsal surface of the distal radius that, in addition to being well tolerated, is also well suited to the treatment of acute articular fractures and for reconstruction of distal radius malunions.[55,56]

The resemblance to the Greek letter π derives from the combination of a distal juxtaarticular limb and two separate longitudinal limbs extending proximally. The distal limb is both precontoured to adhere to the curvature of the dorsal distal radius and tilted to match the radial inclination of the articular surface. The plates are built with 10 degrees of palmar tilt and are designed for left and right wrists (Figure 108-15).

A juxtaarticular band helps confine articular comminution while simultaneously providing numerous holes through which either 2.4-mm self-tapping screws or 1.8-mm buttress pins, which are proximally threaded and screw into the plate, can be utilized to stabilize articular comminution.

The fracture site is exposed dorsally between the second and fourth extensor compartments, and provisional reduction is accomplished with the aid of a distractor and K wires. A bending template is then used to verify plate length and contour. One or more holes can be trimmed from the plate as needed using the cutting pliers. Additional contouring of the distal limb is performed where necessary using the bending irons, which screw into adjacent screw holes and allow contouring of the intervening interconnecting band. The proximal plate limbs are contoured using the bending pliers.

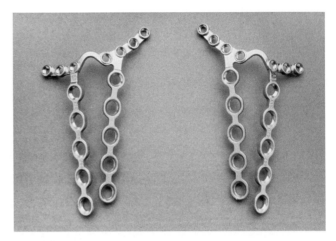

Figure 108-15. The π-plate is named for the resemblance to the Greek letter and results from the combination of two longitudinal limbs with a distal juxtaarticular limb. The plate is precontoured to reflect normal palmar tilt and ulnar inclination as well as the contour of the dorsal surface of the distal radius. Lister's tubercle is preserved and used as a landmark. Repair of the distal radial articular surface can be supported either with 2.4-mm self-tapping screws or buttress pins that thread into the distal limb of the plate, providing a fixed point of support analogous to that provided by a blade plate.

The plate is then applied to the distal radius, and the type, number, and location of the screws and buttress pins to be used are determined based on the individual fracture morphology. The 2.4-mm self-tapping screws are preferred in the distal juxtaarticular limb when the subchondral bone under the articular fragments is of sufficient size and quality to accept them without further fragmenting. The articular reconstruction is supported with 1.8-mm buttress pins in patients with severe comminution or poor bone quality. These 1.8-mm pins provide fixed anchor points that are not dependent on purchase between the screw thread and bone. The metaphyseal reconstruction is then stabilized by securing the proximal limbs of the plate with 2.7-mm self-tapping screws. The flexibility of the distal and proximal titanium limbs permits additional impaction of bony fragments as the screws are tightened into the bone and plate.

Irritation of radial wrist extensor tendons was encountered in the early trials of this plate. This was ascribed to the more radial extent of the π plate as compared with existing plates. The problem has been addressed by elevating an ulnarly based flap of extensor retinaculum that is created during the exposure and sutured over the plate in the floor of the second dorsal compartment at the time of wound closure.[55,56]

Plate Fixation of the Volar Surface of the Distal Radius

Plate and screw fixation of the volar surface of the distal radius is relatively straightforward. The plate is placed beneath the pronator quadratus and flexor pollicis longus muscles so that irritation of the overlying flexor tendons is uncommon. Volar plate fixation, on the other hand, has found limited application because most fractures of the distal radius require a dorsal buttress for cortical comminution or a dorsal capsulotomy to visualize an articular fracture. On the other hand, volar plate fixation is the most reliable method of stabilizing malrotated volar lunate facet fragments that often occur in complex articular injuries. Volar fixation is also necessary in the treatment of shearing fractures of the volar articular margin of the distal radial articular surface. Volar capsulotomy is discouraged because injury or attenuation of the volar radiocarpal ligaments may contribute to carpal instability.

OPERATIVE TREATMENT OF SPECIFIC RADIAL INJURIES

Bending Fractures

DORSAL BENDING FRACTURES. Percutaneous pin fixation represents the least invasive procedure that will reliably hold an unstable dorsal bending fracture of the distal radius after a closed reduction. A number of techniques have been described including the use of two pins placed through the radial styloid,[40] two pins with one inserted from the ulnar aspect of the distal radius and the other through the radial styloid,[9] intrafocal pinning within the fracture site,[34] ulnar to radial pinning with[54] or without[16] transfixation of the distal radioulnar joint, and one radial styloid pin with another across the radioulnar joint[47] (Figure 108-16).

We prefer the placement of pins through the radial styloid and occasionally insert a pin through the dorsoulnar aspect of the distal radius. A manipulative reduction is achieved and held while a smooth 0.062-inch (1.6-mm) K wire is inserted into the tip of the radial styloid using a power drill just dorsal to the first extensor compartment. The pin is advanced across the fracture site at an angle of 45 degrees and exits the dorsoulnar cortex of the radial shaft. A second wire is then inserted just distal to the first and inserted so that it diverges slightly from the first, crossing the fracture site at a slightly greater angle. An additional wire can be inserted, if necessary, into the dorsoulnar aspect of the distal radius between the fourth and fifth extensor compartments and directed to engage the volar-radial cortex of the proximal fragment. Wire placement and maintenance of reduction are verified at each step under image intensification.

Some surgeons use continuous longitudinal distraction through finger trap traction with 2.5 to 5 kg of weight to facilitate reduction. This technique has some drawbacks because it cannot provide the angular and rotational displacement required to obtain an anatomic reduction, and it limits the ability to position the arm during placement of the pins. A good alternative is available when an external fixator will be used as ancillary immobilization. A small distractor can be applied to the proximal metacarpal pin and one of the radial pins. Distraction across the pins will result in some ulnar deviation and volar flexion, facilitating an anatomic reduction. The distractor will not interfere with placement of the percutaneous pins, and the limb can be positioned as needed to facilitate their insertion. If the distractor is used, it is important

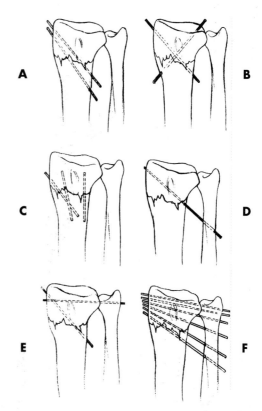

Figure 108-16. Several different techniques for percutaneous pinning of unstable dorsal bending fractures of the distal radius have been described. Illustrated here are two pins through the radial styloid **(A)**, one through the styloid and one through the dorsoulnar corner (Clancy) **(B)**, the intrafocal technique of Kapandji **(C)**, ulna-to-radius pinning without transfixation of the distal radioulnar joint **(D)**, one radial styloid pin and one crossing the distal radioulnar joint **(E)**, and ulna-to-radius pinning with transfixation of the distal radioulnar joint **(F)**. (From Fernandez DL, Jupiter JB: *Fractures of the distal radius: a practical approach to management,* New York, 1995, Springer-Verlag.)

to remember to apply definitive external fixation in a more neutral position to preserve hand function.

An alternative technique that is currently used by a number of surgeons was described by Kapandji.[34] This technique is known as *intrafocal pinning* and uses smooth K wires that are inserted into the fracture site to lever the fracture open, placing the distal radial fragment in proper alignment. This technique is most appropriate for younger patients with limited comminution. Maintenance of reduction may prove difficult in the presence of osteopenia.

One 0.062-inch smooth K wire is first introduced into the radial aspect of the fracture between the first and second extensor compartments and is followed by a second into the dorsal aspect between the third and fourth extensor compartments. Both pins are initially inserted parallel to the fracture site. Reduction is achieved by directing the pins distally, and fixation is achieved by driving them into the cortex of the proximal fragment. Additional pins can be used as necessary for either reduction or stabilization. Kapandji stated that cast or splint immobilization was optional,[34] but most advocates of the technique immobilize the fracture for 4 to 6 weeks after pin insertion. The pins are removed at the time of cast removal.

Definitive treatment with an external fixation device alone can be difficult. The principle on which external fixation is based is *ligamentotaxis*—the idea that traction across the wrist will pull the distal fracture fragments into an improved position through radiocarpal ligamentous attachments. Ligamentotaxis cannot, however, restore the palmar tilt of the distal radial articular surface. Tightening of the intact dorsal soft tissues causes pivoting of the distal fragment, leading to an increased dorsiflexion deformity (Figure 108-17).[1]

There are limitations of ligamentotaxis, and one commonly encounters patients in whom the external fixator has been manipulated into a position of volar flexion, ulnar deviation, and pronation with maximum distraction in an attempt to reduce the fracture. Some fixators are even designed so that manipulation can be performed by simple crank mechanisms after the fixator has been applied. This hand and wrist position is as harmful in an external fixator as it is in plaster. Digit stiffness is inevitable because the extrinsic hand muscles are placed at a mechanical disadvantage, and full digit flexion is impossible. Increased pressure within the carpal canal may contribute to median neuritis, sympathetic maintained pain, or even acute carpal tunnel syndrome. Marked distraction across the wrist may also aggravate intracarpal ligament injury. Prolonged distraction can lead to tightness of the extrinsic extensor tendons with MCP hyperextension and possible loss of radiocarpal and intercarpal mobility. The application of

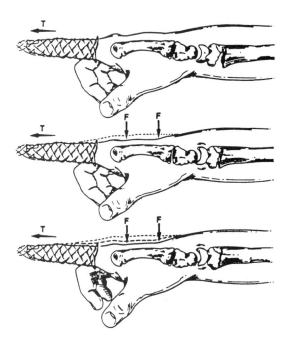

Figure 108-17. The ability of ligamentotaxis to facilitate reduction of dorsal bending fractures of the distal radius is limited. The combined effect of an intact dorsal soft tissue hinge, including periosteum, and the pull of the stout volar radiocarpal ligaments tends to increase the deformity. A palmar translation force *(F)* rather than direct axial traction *(T)* is required to achieve satisfactory reduction. (Courtesy Hand Biomechanics Lab.)

volar translation to the hand and carpus, rather than volar flexion as Agee had discussed,[1] represents a means of restoring palmar tilt while preserving normal hand mechanics and avoiding excessive distraction (see Figure 108-17).

PALMAR BENDING FRACTURES. Fixation of palmar bending fractures with obliquity or comminution is achieved with a volarly applied plate.[17] The radial volar (Henry) exposure is used in most cases. The size and shape of the plate to be used is determined by the size of the distal fragment and the degree of comminution. A stronger, thicker plate should be used when the plate is required to provide stabilization in bridging a metaphyseal defect. Early mobilization and functional use of the hand and wrist are allowed, provided stable fixation is achieved. Plate fixation is relatively well tolerated on the volar surface of the radius, and the plate only rarely has to be removed.

Shearing Fractures of the Articular Surface
FRACTURES OF THE RADIAL STYLOID. Shearing fractures of the radial styloid are stabilized with wires or, preferably, screws. The radial styloid fragment is reduced with longitudinal traction and ulnar deviation, and fixation is achieved with two smooth K wires. These wires must be directed proximal, ulnarward, and somewhat dorsally because the radial styloid lies anterior to the midaxis of the distal radius. Anatomic reduction is verified in multiple planes using image intensification. These fragments are often large enough to accept screws without further fragmentation. One can either exchange the wires for screws sequentially or place cannulated screws over the wires.

The accuracy of the articular reduction in a comminuted fracture cannot be determined using image intensification alone and must be verified through a dorsal capsulotomy. A dorsal radial incision between the first and second dorsal compartments is used, and the radial artery is protected as dissection proceeds distally within the snuffbox, or arthroscopy can be used to verify the articular reduction. Arthroscopy is also useful for inspecting the scapholunate interosseous ligament, which is commonly injured with this fracture pattern. If complete tear of the scapholunate interosseous ligament is detected, either radiographically with traction views, by arthroscopy, or during open capsulotomy, we recommend open repair of the ligament with sutures anchored in bone. Partial tears diagnosed during arthroscopy may be treated with percutaneous pin fixation.[27,28]

FRACTURES OF THE LUNATE FACET. Shearing fractures of the lunate facet off the distal radial articular surface can occasionally be reduced with traction and manipulation but often resist such maneuvers because of impaction. Limited exposure between the fourth and fifth extensor compartments will allow the insertion of a pointed awl.[21] The awl can be used to elevate the fragment into anatomic position under image intensification. The fragment is then stabilized with smooth K wires placed percutaneously through the radial styloid so that they lie just under the subchondral bone of the lunate facet to act as a buttress. Care must be taken to avoid penetrating the distal radioulnar joint with the wires. Neutralization of the fixation with ancillary external fixation is advised.

VOLAR MARGINAL SHEARING FRACTURES. Volar marginal shearing fractures require open reduction and fixation with a volar buttress plate.[22,53,64] A volar radial (Henry) exposure is used to reduce volar shearing fractures of the scaphoid facet. A volar ulnar exposure should be considered when the lunate facet is involved or the median nerve must be released. The fracture site is cleared of fracture hematoma using a dental pic and irrigation. Accurate articular reduction will correspond with an accurate metaphyseal reduction when there is no intraarticular comminution. Assessment of the articular reduction in comminuted fractures requires inspection of the joint through the fracture by elevating the volar fragment while leaving the volar capsule intact to avoid jeopardizing intercarpal stability.

Reduction is achieved by hyperextending the wrist over a rolled towel. Provisional fixation with 0.045-inch K wires facilitates the placement of a buttress plate. To avoid hindering plate placement, these wires can either be placed obliquely through the distal margin of the articular surface or driven out through the dorsal cortex and overlying soft tissues and skin.

Undercontouring of a 3.5-mm T-plate will result in compression of the fracture fragments to the intact radius as the screws are tightened. The screws are tightened sequentially from proximal to distal, bringing the plate into contact with the bone at its midportion and compressing the distal articular fragments (Figure 108-18, *C*). The buttress effect of the plate often provides adequate stabilization. It may be desirable to fix the fragments with screws entering either through the plate or independently when the volar rim fragment is comminuted. The new volar counterpart to the π-plate may prove useful in this endeavor by virtue of its juxtaarticular limb and small 2.4-mm screws. The reduction and fixation are evaluated under image intensification or biplanar radiographs. When metaphyseal comminution is present, autogenous bone graft should be placed into the defect that results from reduction of the fracture.

DORSAL MARGINAL SHEARING FRACTURES. Exposure of the dorsal surface of the distal radius through the second and fourth extensor compartments is achieved. A radial styloid fragment, if present, should first be reduced and stabilized with smooth K wires or threaded screws. The dorsal capsule can be incised to allow direct inspection, if verification of the articular reduction is necessary.

Fixation of the dorsal rim fracture has been limited in the past by the lack of a suitable implant. K wires and small T- or L-shaped plates have been used based on the size of the fracture fragments. The design of the π-plate, which includes a distal juxtaarticular limb through which either 1.8-mm buttress pins or 2.4-mm screws can be placed, may facilitate fixation in these cases. The radial extension of the juxtaarticular limb of the π-plate may also allow fixation of the radial styloid fragment with screws placed through the plate.

Compression Fractures of the Articular Surface
LIMITED OPEN REDUCTION. Many two-and three-part simple articular fractures are amenable to closed or limited open reduction and fixation with percutaneously inserted K wires.[21] The technique for three-part fractures is a combination of the techniques described for the management of isolated radial styloid and lunate facet fractures in the section on shearing fractures of the articular surface. The radial styloid fragment is reduced first and stabilized with two smooth 0.062-inch K wires. The lunate facet is then reduced through a limited open exposure between the fourth and fifth extensor compartments using a pointed awl and stabilized with two 0.062-inch K wires lying just under the subchondral bone (Figure 108-19). An external fixator is used to neutralize the wire fixation. The external fixator acts to bridge the metaphyseal defect when there is metaphyseal comminution (fracture type C2). This defect should be filled with autogenous bone graft.

OPEN REDUCTION AND FIXATION THROUGH A DORSAL EXPOSURE. More complex articular fractures (C3) require a dorsal exposure, both for visualization of the articular surface through an incision in the capsule and to facilitate accurate reduction and stable fixation of the fragments.[22] Operative exposure of some simple articular fractures (C1 and C2) may be required if a limited open technique is not successful. Open exposure of simple articular fractures may become more commonplace as newer plate designs are developed and perfected.

Fixation of complex articular fractures is commonly achieved using numerous smooth K wires to fix fragments to one another and to the radial shaft. A small distractor is useful to facilitate reduction and limit soft tissue dissection. This can be converted to external fixation at the end of the case, providing protection and neutralization of the pin fixation.

Previous plate designs were not well suited to the internal fixation of complex articular distal radius fractures, but the π-plate has been designed with this specific indication in mind. The juxtaarticular limb has seven holes through which up to seven screws or buttress pins can be inserted. The 2.4-mm screws can be used to fix individual fragments when they are large and the bone quality is good. Patients with extensive comminution or severe osteopenia can have 1.8-mm buttress pins threaded directly into the plate, providing fixed points to support repair of the articular surface. The two longitudinal limbs will bridge metaphyseal defects that should be copiously grafted with autogenous bone (Figure 108-20).

OPEN REDUCTION AND FIXATION THROUGH A VOLAR EXPOSURE. A dorsal exposure is generally preferred for the visualization, manipulation, and fixation of complex articular fractures because the dorsal capsule can be incised with relatively little risk to carpal kinematics. A fracture of the lunate facet in the coronal plane, however, will result in the volar lunate fragment rotating dorsally with ligamentotaxis. Reduction of this fragment requires an ulnar volar exposure in addition to the dorsal exposure. Fixation of this fragment is

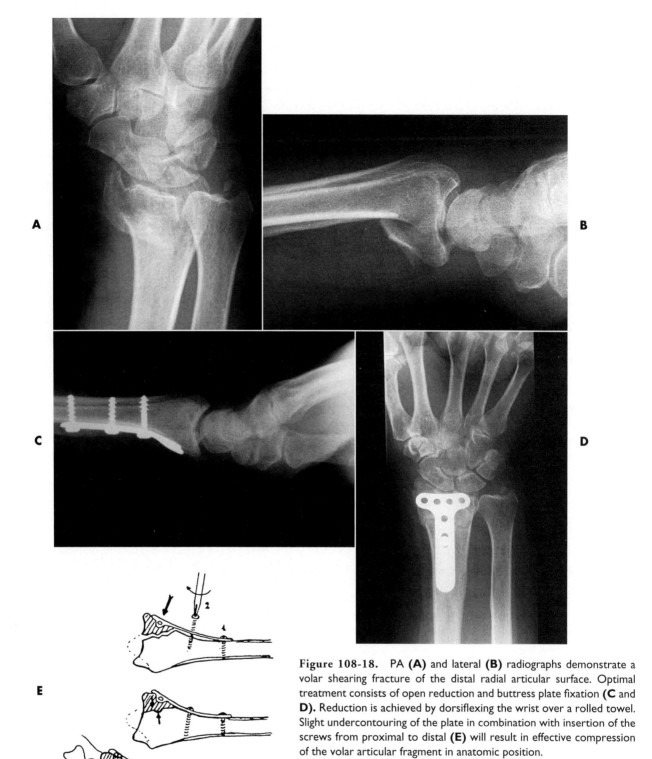

Figure 108-18. PA (**A**) and lateral (**B**) radiographs demonstrate a volar shearing fracture of the distal radial articular surface. Optimal treatment consists of open reduction and buttress plate fixation (**C** and **D**). Reduction is achieved by dorsiflexing the wrist over a rolled towel. Slight undercontouring of the plate in combination with insertion of the screws from proximal to distal (**E**) will result in effective compression of the volar articular fragment in anatomic position.

most predictably achieved using a small T- or L-shaped plate (see Figure 108-19).[21,22]

Radiocarpal Fracture/Dislocation

The carpus is relocated on the distal radius using longitudinal traction and rotation of the hand and wrist. An external fixator is then applied and used as a distractor to facilitate operative repositioning and repair of the radiocarpal ligaments and their avulsion fragments. The median and ulnar nerves are decompressed through an extensile ulnar volar incision, often incorporating a traumatic wound by opening the carpal tunnel and canal of Guyon. The radiocar-

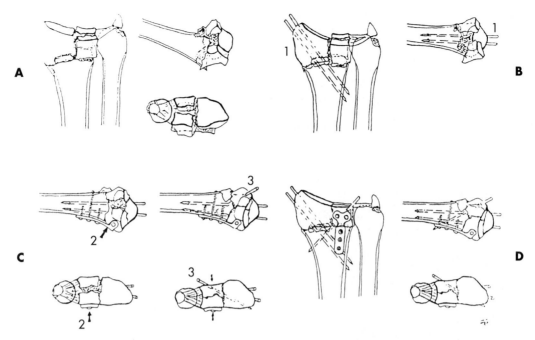

Figure 108-19. Illustration of the technique for reducing and fixing a four-part compression articular fracture of the distal radial articular surface **(A).** The radial styloid fragment is reduced first using traction, flexion, and ulnar deviation (often facilitated by the use of a small distractor) and pinned with two K wires **(B).** The next step requires open exposure of the lunate facet fragment and buttress plate fixation **(C).** Finally the dorsal lunate fragment is reduced and fixed with a K wire inserted into the dorsoulnar corner of the distal radius between the fourth and fifth extensor compartments **(D).** (From Fernandez DL, Jupiter JB: *Fractures of the distal radius: a practical approach to management,* New York, 1995, Springer-Verlag.)

pal articulation can be inspected and cleaned of any debris through the traumatic volar capsulotomy. The radial styloid, ulnar styloid, and volar articular rim fracture fragments are then reattached using either screws or paired K wires, based on the size of the fragments, and occasionally incorporating a tension band wire. Any fragments from the volar articular margin that remain attached to the capsule and that are too small to accept internal fixation are left in place to facilitate repositioning and hasten healing after the volar capsule is sutured back to the distal radius through drill holes or using suture anchors. Associated injury to the carpal interosseous ligaments may require concomitant dorsal exposure to allow repair of the ligaments. The external fixator should remain in place for 6 to 8 weeks to protect the repair. The forearm should be immobilized in midsupination with a sugar tong splint for 3 to 4 weeks if there is concern regarding injury to the soft tissue stabilizers of the distal radioulnar joint.

High-Energy Fractures

ASSOCIATED CARPAL INJURIES. We manage combined skeletal injury to the carpus and distal radius with stable operative fixation of both fractures to maintain normal carpal alignment and facilitate functional aftercare. Similarly, associated injury to the scapholunate interosseous ligament is managed with ligament repair using interosseous sutures through a dorsal exposure. Distraction can be used to facilitate

fixation of the distal radius fracture but should be released before addressing the carpal injury.

ASSOCIATED FOREARM AND ELBOW INJURIES. Injury to more proximal skeletal elements of the ipsilateral upper extremity should also be operatively managed. It is particularly important to recognize that the combination of distal and proximal forearm injury, the so-called *bipolar injuries,* may result in a radius without soft tissue attachments. Management of the floating radius is challenging.[32] The length and alignment of the radial head and distal radius, not to mention associated ulnar fractures, must be restored with sufficient stability to maintain the relationship of the radius to the ulna from the wrist to the elbow while the triangular fibrocartilage and interosseous, annular, and quadrate ligaments are healing. If the distal radioulnar joint remains unstable after internal fixation of all fractures, immobilization in supination should be tried. Persistent distal radioulnar subluxation or dislocation requires cross pinning of the distal radius and ulna at the distal radioulnar joint.

NEUROVASCULAR AND SOFT TISSUE INJURY. In the presence of severe soft tissue injury, it is necessary to achieve a stable soft tissue envelope before definitively addressing any bone loss. External fixation and limited fixation with K wires are used to maintain skeletal alignment while the

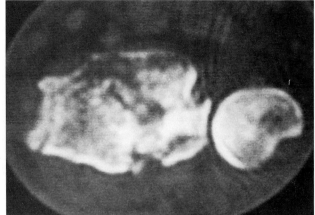

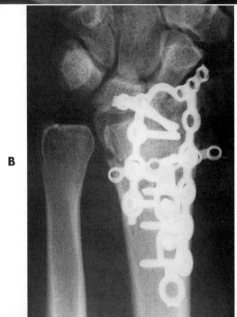

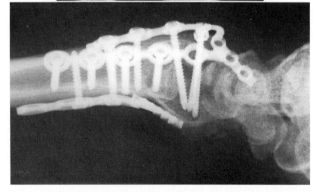

Figure 108-20. A, This computed tomography (CT) image demonstrates substantial disruption of the distal radial articular surface, including a coronal split in the lunate facet as well as articular surface impaction. **B** and **C,** PA and lateral radiographs illustrate the fixation technique applied. Exposure of the articular surface through a dorsal capsulotomy was required to ensure accurate reduction. A dorsal plate was applied to help support the articular reduction. A separate volar exposure and plate were required to address the volar lunate facet fragment. Autogenous bone graft was harvested from the iliac crest using trephines and applied to help support the articular reduction and to enhance healing.

health of the wound is ensured by serial soft tissue and skeletal debridement. Skin grafts and, occasionally, composite tissue flaps are used for wound coverage. Autogenous bone grafts can be inserted into the defect when the wound is stable, along with more extensive internal fixation where appropriate.

Severe injuries that devascularize the hand should first have definitive fixation of the distal radius fracture before revascularization. The stabilization will both facilitate and protect the vascular repair.

Acute carpal tunnel syndrome, forearm compartment syndrome, and compression of the ulnar nerve within the canal of Guyon can occur after a distal radius fracture. Constant vigilance of all patients with high-energy injuries is required by the surgeon because in many cases the condition takes over 24 hours to develop.[61] Decompression and fixation can be performed through either the ulnar volar exposure of the distal radius extended along the ulnar border of the forearm according to McDonnell's technique,[43] or with a radial volar (Henry) incision combined with a separate carpal tunnel incision.[22] Note that connection of the latter two incisions risks injury to the palmar cutaneous branch of the median nerve and should be avoided.

Malunion

Reconstructive osteotomy of the distal radius is guided by a preoperative plan based on tracings of radiographs of the involved and uninvolved wrists. Radiographs of the uninvolved wrist are used to guide the restoration of the level and alignment of the articular surface of the malunited distal radius.

NASCENT MALUNION. Reconstruction of a malaligned distal radius fracture should be undertaken within 12 weeks of injury because the fracture line can usually be identified and developed using a small osteotome.[33] Articular malunion can also be addressed. Fracture callus is resected using a small rongeur, and a distractor facilitates realignment. A distal Schantz screw can be placed directly into the distal fragment when it is of sufficient size and there is good bone quality.

Dorsal bending fractures and articular malunions with dorsal angulation of the metaphysis are exposed dorsally through the interval between the second and fourth compartments. Malunited palmar bending fractures or dorsal bending fractures that were overcorrected into excessive palmar inclination are addressed through a radial volar (Henry) approach. Once the fracture lines have been reestablished the articular fragments are secured in anatomic position either definitively or provisionally using screws and wires. The fracture is manipulated out to length through the metaphyseal fracture line, and the appropriate alignment of the articular surface is restored with the assistance of a distractor and a broad lamina spreader. Cancellous autograft is harvested from the iliac crest and placed in the metaphyseal bony defect. Stable fixation is achieved using a dorsally applied plate (Figure 108-21, *C-E*).[33]

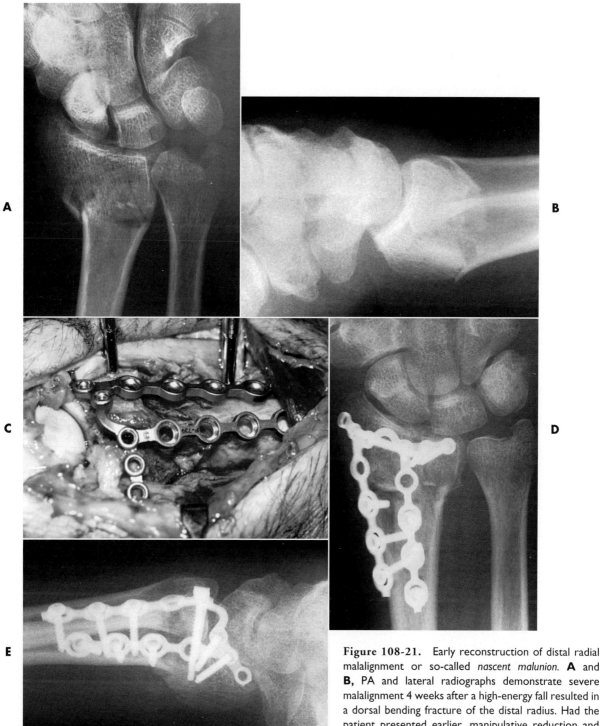

Figure 108-21. Early reconstruction of distal radial malalignment or so-called *nascent malunion.* **A** and **B,** PA and lateral radiographs demonstrate severe malalignment 4 weeks after a high-energy fall resulted in a dorsal bending fracture of the distal radius. Had the patient presented earlier, manipulative reduction and pinning would have been adequate treatment, but at this point early healing is established and an open exposure will be required to recreate the fracture site by resecting the callus. **C,** Reduction is facilitated and maintained using a small distractor, with one of the Schantz screws placed into the distal radial fragment. A dorsal plate is used for fixation. **D** and **E,** Radiographs demonstrating the early result.

MATURE MALUNION. Reconstruction of a wrist with a mature malunion requires careful preoperative planning.[18,19,22] Comparison with the contralateral uninvolved extremity provides the best template for realignment of the distal radius and facilitates accurate determination of the structural dimensions of the bone graft that will be required.

Malunited dorsal bending fractures are approached through a dorsal incision. The dorsal surface of the distal radius is exposed, and a fine K wire is placed into the radiocarpal joint to mark the orientation of the articular surface. A 2.5-mm K wire or Schantz screw is then inserted perpendicular to the radial diaphysis in the sagittal plane, proximal to the osteotomy site. A second wire is placed into the distal radius in the sagittal plane so that the angle subtended by the two wires represents the intended angle of correction according to the preoperative plan. The distal pin angulates 5 to 10 degrees more dorsal than the pin marking the orientation of the distal radial articular surface. A distal radial osteotomy is then performed at a site 2 to 2.5 cm proximal to the joint margin, parallel to the articular surface in the sagittal plane and perpendicular to the radial diaphysis in the transverse plane. The saw cut is not completed through the volar cortex. After the osteotomy is performed, distraction between these two pins (using a small distractor) restores the length and palmar tilt of the distal radius. A laminar spreader can be used to help open the osteotomy site dorsally and radially. The laminar spreader should have broad limbs to limit impaction of the metaphyseal bone with distraction. It is occasionally necessary to Z-lengthen the brachioradialis when a large amount of opening is required on the radial side. It may also be useful to insert a second set of stout K wires in the coronal plane, against which distraction can be applied to aid in restoring ulnar tilt.

Once the desired correction is obtained, the estimated dimensions of the bone graft, as determined through careful preoperative planning, are verified by direct measurement. An appropriate corticocancellous graft is then harvested from the iliac crest and contoured. The graft is then placed into the osteotomy gap, and the construct is stabilized with a K wire entering the dorsal articular margin of the distal fragment, skewering the graft and gaining solid purchase in the distal fragment. The distractor is then removed, and radiographs are obtained. A dorsal plate is applied if the correction is satisfactory (Figure 108-22), the provisional K wire is removed, and the wound is closed.

Malunions with excessive palmar angulation of the distal radial articular surface are approached through a volar (Henry) approach. Use of a flat, T-shaped plate will effect reduction of the rotational deformity while providing stable fixation of the lengthened and dorsiflexed distal fragment. One must be careful not to overcorrect beyond the 10-degree normal palmar tilt.

OPERATIVE TREATMENT OF ULNAR LESIONS

Fixation of the ulnar styloid fractured below its base is achieved through an exposure between the extensor digiti quinti and extensor carpi ulnaris tendons. A tension band wire can be passed through the proximal ulnar fragment and either around or through the ulnar styloid fragment, or two small K wires can be used to fix the fragment to the shaft. The forearm should be immobilized in neutral rotation for 6 weeks.[27,28]

Triangular fibrocartilage lesions discovered by arthroscopy can usually be treated through the arthroscope. Central tears are debrided; if the radial margin is avulsed with a bony fragment, the fragment is secured with a K wire. The forearm is otherwise immobilized for 6 weeks in neutral rotation. Ulnar peripheral tears can be repaired by making a small incision over the extensor carpi ulnaris tendon, which is retracted out of the way. An 18-gauge needle can then be inserted through the sheath of this tendon and into the articular disc. Sutures passed through the needle at spaced positions can then be tied in place. The forearm is immobilized for 4 weeks.[27]

FUNCTIONAL AFTERCARE

Active motion of the digits, use of the hand for daily activities, and control of edema are the essence of functional aftercare for fractures of the distal radius and ulna. Wrist immobilization in a cast or external fixator may be necessary for 4 to 8 weeks to protect percutaneous pins, but wrist mobilization may be possible within 2 weeks of injury when operative fixation with a plate has resulted in a stable construct. In many cases, however, the comminution is so extensive that even a plate will require protection for 4 to 6 weeks.

OUTCOMES

EVALUATION OF TREATMENT

Everyone agrees that a well-functioning, pain-free wrist is best for independent living and contributes substantially to the patient's overall health status, but many dispute the contention that deformity is incompatible with good function.[7] Fractures of the distal radius have been considered benign and simple to manage since Colles' original description of the injury, in which he optimistically proclaimed that good function was the rule despite residual deformity.[7] Support for the concept that good function is dependent on the anatomic restoration of fracture fragments has gathered slowly, only after the development of numerical scoring systems based on evaluation of subjective, clinical, and occasionally radiographic factors. The system developed by Garland and Werley[26] was the first such system, and most subsequent systems represent minor variations of this original.[60] Garland and Werley evaluated 60 fractures in their report, using a demerit point system to rate the results of treatment based on residual deformity, pain, limitation of function, loss of motion, and complications such as arthrosis, digital stiffness, or median neuropathy. They recorded 31.7% unsatisfactory (fair or poor) results using this system, which is actually relatively forgiving. An in-depth

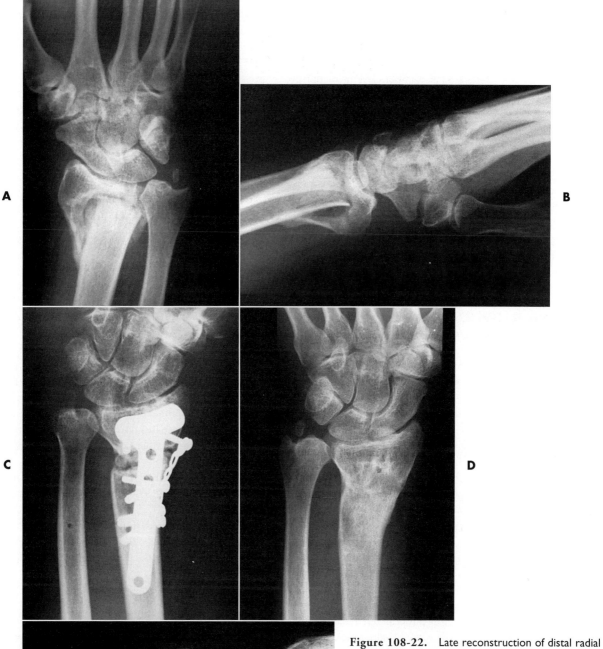

Figure 108-22. Late reconstruction of distal radial malalignment or so-called *mature malunion*. **A** and **B,** PA and lateral radiographs demonstrate severe shortening, loss of ulnar inclination, and some dorsal tilt of the distal radius. **C,** The anatomy was restored by osteotomy, Z-lengthening of the brachioradialis, and corticocancellous graft harvested from the patient's iliac crest. In addition to the oblique T-plate, a small plate was applied to the radial aspect of the radius to help buttress the restoration of ulnar inclination. **D** and **E,** Radiographs taken after removal of the hardware document restoration of distal radial anatomy.

analysis of risk factors led them to conclude that excessive dorsal tilt was most commonly associated with a poor result. They also emphasized that not all Colles' fractures are equivalent, and that fractures with displaced articular fragments are much more likely to lead to posttraumatic arthritis and an unsatisfactory result. They also emphasized the inability of cast or splint immobilization alone to maintain the closed reduction of a markedly displaced fracture and the tendency of such fractures to gradually return to their prereduction deformity over the course of treatment in plaster. In essence, they described all of the problems that current operative methods of treatment are intended to address.

The system developed by Green and O'Brian[29] for rating complex carpal injury has been applied, with minor modification, to distal radius fractures in recent times. This system is much more stringent in that a patient can regain just under 100% of motion and grip strength and if they have even mild occasional pain, they are rated a fair result. Systems that combine radiographic finding with subjective and objective clinical factors, such as those of Stewart et al[60] and the New York Orthopaedic Hospital wrist rating score[59] make it difficult to determine the association between anatomy and function because the numerical score is based on a combination of both. Despite the obvious weaknesses of the scoring system approach, these systems have been relatively successful at stratifying functional results in a meaningful way.

Presently there is limited application of patient-based appraisals or instruments for measuring improvements in the quality of life and general health status of patients in evaluating the outcomes of various treatments for distal radius fractures.[3,22,23] The importance of considering these issues, however, has been well recognized, and the patient's point of view has long been a focal point of the controversies regarding optimal treatment for distal radius fractures. Initial experience using outcome questionnaires to evaluate patients undergoing treatment of these fractures suggests that these measurement tools provide information regarding subjective symptoms and functional impairment that is not well reflected by traditional objective physical measurements.[3] In other words, a comparison of treatment based mainly on physical and radiographic examination does not capture the overall health impact of the injury and its treatment on the whole patient. Future investigations should try to capture these patient-based factors more completely by utilizing outcome questionnaires.

COST CONSIDERATIONS

There has been little in the way of cost-benefit analysis regarding the treatment of distal radius fractures. It was documented in a study of 2000 workers' compensation patients that distal radius fractures are commonly associated with disability.[5] What remains to be shown is that operative treatments reduce the number of patients permanently disabled or the degree of disability. Our comparison of early and late reconstruction of malaligned distal radius fractures suggested that early corrective osteotomy will reduce the

overall costs, primarily by limiting the time of disability.[33] Early surgical intervention should be considered for this and other reasons when the degree of malalignment suggests a high likelihood of permanent dysfunction.

The costs associated with various fixation devices and bone graft substitutes also need to be considered carefully. Use of the more costly and demanding dynamic external fixator, for example, may not have a significant advantage over standard static fixator designs to justify the added cost.[10] There is currently very little in the literature to guide such considerations.

COMPLICATIONS

One of the most important factors in determining outcomes is the occurrence of complications. Complications are common after both nonoperative and operative treatment of distal radius fractures. Cast treatment can be associated with digital stiffness as a result of excessive swelling or a cast or splint that restricts motion at the MCP joints. It may also contribute to compression of the median, radial, or ulnar nerves and Volkmann's ischemia. Sympathetic maintained pain is not uncommon and may be related to both the swelling and median nerve dysfunction in a cast. Lastly, a redisplacement requiring repeat reduction or leading to extraarticular or intraarticular malunion may occur in a cast or splint. Operative treatment is intended to limit these complications by providing stable and predictable fixation while facilitating early active motion and edema control.

The risks of operative fixation, as outlined above, are many and tend to balance the consideration to proceed with operative treatment. The most common complications, however, are related to irritation or injury to sensory nerves or extrinsic hand tendons and are, to a large degree, within the control of the surgeon.

REFERENCES

1. Agee JM: External fixation, *Orthop Clin North Am* 24:265-274, 1993.
2. Alffram PA, Bauer GCH: Epidemiology of fracture of the forearm: a biomechanical investigation of bone strength, *J Bone Joint Surg* 44A:105-114, 1962.
3. Amadio PC, Silverstein MD, Ilstrup DM, et al: Outcome after Colles' fracture: the relative responsiveness of three questionnaires and physical examination measures, *J Hand Surg [Am]* 21:781-787, 1996.
4. Anderson R, O'Neil G: Comminuted fractures of the distal end of the radius, *Surg Gyn Obst* 78:434-440, 1944.
5. Bacorn RW, Kurtzke JF: Colles' fracture: a study of two thousand cases from the New York State Workmen's Compensation Board, *J Bone Joint Surg* 38A:643-658, 1953.
6. Bengner U, Johnell O: Increasing incidence of forearm fractures: a comparison of epidemiologic patterns 25 years apart, *Acta Orthop Scand* 56:158-160, 1985.

7. Cassebaum WH: Colles' fractures: a study of end results, *JAMA* 143:963-965, 1950.

8. Castaing J: Les fractures récentes de l'extremité inférieure du radius chez l' adulte, *Rev Chir Orthop* 50:581-696, 1964.

9. Clancey G: Percutaneous Kirschner wire fixation of Colles' fracture, *J Bone Joint Surg* 66A:1008-1014, 1984.

10. Clyburn TA: Dynamic external fixation for comminuted intraarticular fractures of the distal end of the radius, *J Bone Joint Surg* 69A:248-254, 1987.

11. Colles A: On the fracture of the carpal extremity of the radius, *Edinburgh Med Surg J* 10:182-186, 1814.

12. Constantz BR, Ison IC, Fulmer MT, et al: Skeletal repair by in situ formation of the mineral phase of bone, *Science* 267:1796-1799, 1995.

13. Cook PJ, Exton-Smith AN: Fractured femurs, falls, and bone disorder, *J R Coll Physicians Lond* 16:45-49, 1982.

14. Cooney WP III, Agee JM, Hastings H II: Symposium: Management of intraarticular fractures of the distal radius, *Contemp Orthop* 21:71-104, 1990.

15. Crilly RG, Delaguerriere-Richardson LD, Roth JH: Postural instability and Colles' fracture, *Age Aging* 16:133-138, 1987.

16. Depalma AF: Comminuted fractures of the distal end of the radius treated by ulnar pinning, *J Bone Joint Surg* 34A:651-662, 1952.

17. Fernandez DL: Smith frakturen, *Z Unfallmed Berufskrankheiten* 3:110-114, 1980.

18. Fernandez DL: Correction of posttraumatic wrist deformity in adults by osteotomy, bone grafting, and internal fixation, *J Bone Joint Surg* 64A:1164-1178, 1982.

19. Fernandez DL: Radial osteotomy and Bowers arthroplasty for malunited fractures of the distal end of the radius, *J Bone Joint Surg* 70A:1538-1551, 1988.

20. Fernandez DL: *Fractures of the distal radius: operative treatment*, AAOS Instructional Course Lectures 42:73-88, 1993.

21. Fernandez DL, Geissler WB: Treatment of displaced articular fractures of the radius, *J Hand Surg [Am]* 16:375-384, 1991.

22. Fernandez DL, Jupiter JB: *Fractures of the distal radius: a practical approach to management,* New York, 1995, Springer-Verlag.

23. Fernandez JJ, Gruen GS, Herndon JH: *Outcome of distal radius fractures using the short-form 36 item health survey,* Paper 334 presented at the 64th Annual Meeting of the American Academy of Orthopaedic Surgeons, San Francisco, February 13-17, 1997.

24. Friberg S, Lundström B: Radiographic measurements of the radiocarpal joint in normal adults, *Acta Radiol Diag* 17:249-256, 1976.

25. Frykman GK: Fracture of the distal radius including sequelae— shoulder hand finger syndrome: disturbance in the distal radioulnar joint and impairment of nerve function: a clinical and experimental study, *Acta Orthop Scand Suppl* 108:1-155, 1967.

26. Gartland JJ, Werley CW: Evaluation of healed Colles' fractures, *J Bone Joint Surg* 33A:895-907, 1951.

27. Geissler WB, Fernandez DL, Lamey DM: Distal radioulnar joint injuries associated with fractures of the distal radius, *Clin Orthop* 327:135-146, 1996.

28. Geissler WB, Freeland AE: Arthroscopically assisted reduction of intraarticular distal radius fractures, *Clin Orthop* 327:125-134, 1996.

29. Green DP, O'Brien ET: Open reduction of carpal dislocation: indications and operative techniques, *J Hand Surg [Am]* 3:250-265, 1978.

30. Hulten O: Ueber anatomische variationen der handgelenkenknochen, *Acta Radiol* 9:155-168, 1928.

31. Jones R: *Injuries of the joints,* London, 1915, Henry Frowde and Hodder & Stoughton.

32. Jupiter JB, Kour AK, Richards RR, et al: The floating radius in bipolar fracture-dislocation of the forearm, *J Orthop Trauma* 8:99-106, 1994.

33. Jupiter JB, Ring D: A comparison of early and late reconstruction of malunited fractures of the distal end of the radius, *J Bone Joint Surg* 78A:739-748, 1996.

34. Kapandji A: L'ostéosythèse par double embrochage intrafocal: traitement functionnel des fractures non articulaires de l'extremité infériure du radius, *Ann Chir* 30:903-908, 1976.

35. Kapandji IA: *The physiology of the joints of the upper limb,* Edinburgh, 1982, Churchill-Livingstone.

36. Knirk JL, Jupiter JB: Intraarticular fractures of the distal end of the radius in young adults, *J Bone Joint Surg* 68A:647-659, 1986.

37. Leung KS, Shen WY, Leung PC: Ligamentotaxis and bone grafting for comminuted fractures of the distal end of the radius, *J Bone Joint Surg* 71B:838-842, 1989.

38. Lewis OJ, Hamshere RJ, Bucknill TM: The anatomy of the wrist joint, *J Anat* 106:539-552, 1955.

39. Lidström A: Fractures of the distal end of the radius: a clinical and statistical study of end results, *Acta Orthop Scand Suppl* 30(Suppl 41):1-118, 1959.

40. Mah E, Atkinson R: Percutaneous Kirschner wire stabilization following closed reduction of Colles' fractures, *J Hand Surg [Br]* 17:55-61, 1992.

41. Martini AK: Die sekundare arthrose des handgelenkes bei der in fehlstellung verheilten und nicht korrigierten distalen Radiusfracturen, *Aktuel Trauamtol* 16:143-148, 1986.

42. Mayfield JK, Johnson RP, Kilcoyne RF: The ligaments of the human wrist and their functional significance, *Anat Rec* 186:417-428, 1976.

43. McConnell AA: Approach to the median nerve in the forearm, *Dublin J Med Sci* 149:90-92, 1920.

44. McMurty RY, Jupiter JB: Fractures of the distal radius. In Browner BD, Jupiter JB, Levine AM, Trafton PG (editors): *Skeletal trauma,* Philadelphia, 1992, WB Saunders.

45. Melone CP: Articular fractures of the distal radius, *Orthop Clin North Am* 15(2)217-236, 1984.

46. Missakian ML, Cooney WP III, Amadio PC, Glidewell HL: Open reduction and internal fixation for distal radius fractures, *J Hand Surg [Am]* 745-755, 1992.

47. Mortier JP, Kuhlmann JN, Richet C, Baux S: Brochage horizontal cubito-radial dans les fractures de l'extremite inferieure du radius comportent un fragment posterointerne, *Rev Chir Orthop* 72:567-571, 1986.

48. Müller ME, Nazarian S, Koch P, Schatzker J: *The comprehensive classification of fractures of long bones,* New York, 1990, Springer-Verlag, pp 54-63.

49. Older TM, Stabler EV, Cassebaum WH: Colles' fracture: evaluation of selective therapy, *J Trauma* 5:469-476, 1965.

50. Owen RA, Melton LJ, Johnson KA, et al: Incidence of Colles' fracture in a North American community, *Am J Public Health* 72:605-607, 1982.

51. Palmer AK, Werner FW: The triangular fibrocartilage of the wrist: anatomy and function, *J Hand Surg [Am]* 6:153-162, 1981.

52. Palmer AK, Werner FW: Biomechanics of the distal radioulnar joint, *Clin Orthop* 187:26-35, 1984.

53. Pattee GA, Thompson GH: Anterior and posterior marginal fracture-dislocation of the distal radius, *Clin Orthop* 231:183-195, 1988.

54. Rayhack J: The history and evolution of percutaneous pinning of displaced distal radius fractures, *Orthop Clin North Am* 24:287-300, 1993.

55. Ring D, Jupiter JB: Dorsal fixation of distal radius fractures using the π-plate, *Atlas Hand Clin* 2:25-44, 1997.

56. Ring D, Jupiter JB, Brennwald J, et al: Prospective multicenter trial of a new plate for dorsal fixation of the distal radius, *J Hand Surg [Am]* 22:777-784, 1997.

57. Rosenthal DI, Schwartz M, Phillips WC, Jupiter JB: Fracture of the radius with instability of the wrist, *AJR* 141:113-116, 1983.

58. Ryu J, Cooney WP III, Askew LJ, et al: Functional ranges of motion of the wrist joint, *J Hand Surg [Am]* 16:409-419, 1991.

59. Seitz WH Jr, Putnam MD, Dick HM: Limited open surgical approach for external fixation of distal radius fractures, *J Hand Surg [Am]* 15:288-293, 1990.

60. Stewart HD, Innes AR, Burke PD: Factors influencing the outcome of Colles' fracture: an anatomical and functional study, *Injury* 16:289-295, 1985.

61. Stockley I, Harvey IA, Getty CJM: Acute volar compartment syndrome of the forearm secondary to fractures of the distal radius, *Injury* 19:101-104, 1986.

62. Talesnick J, Watson HK: Midcarpal instability caused by malunited fractures of the distal radius, *J Hand Surg [Am]* 9:350-357, 1984.

63. Thomas FB: Reduction of Smith's fracture, *J Bone Joint Surg* 39B:463-470, 1957.

64. Thompson GH, Grant TT: Barton's fractures—reverse Barton's fractures: confusing eponyms, *Clin Orthop* 122:210-221, 1977.

65. Villar RN, Marsh D, Rushton N: Three years after Colles' fracture: a prospective review, *J Bone Joint Surg* 69B:635-638, 1987.

66. Yaszemski MJ, Payne RG, Hayes WC, et al: Evolution of bone transplantation: molecular, cellular, and tissue strategies to engineer human bone, *Biomaterials* 17:175-185, 1996.

CHAPTER 109

Arthroscopy

Daniel J. Nagle

INTRODUCTION

Wrist arthroscopy is the natural extension of the minimally invasive endoscopic surgical techniques used throughout the body. Wrist arthroscopy can be divided into three main indications: diagnostic, staging, and surgical. Elements of any of these can be combined.

Diagnostic wrist arthroscopy is rapidly becoming the gold standard against which all other diagnostic techniques are compared. Arthrography was the predominant diagnostic technique in the past, but its role has progressively been usurped by arthroscopy. It is interesting to note how this gradual inversion of roles is mirrored in the evolution of arthrography and arthroscopy in the diagnosis of knee and shoulder pathology.

Many authors have evaluated the accuracy of arthrography compared to arthroscopy. Nagle and Benson[8] in their series of 84 wrist arthroscopies noted that arthrography completely demonstrated all lesions in the wrist in only 11% of cases.

Magnetic resonance imaging (MRI) holds great promise, but its use in the evaluation of wrist problems remains limited.[2] This is not to say that MRI does not have a role to play in the assessment of a painful wrist. It is quite useful, for example, in the evaluation of a patient suspected of having Kienböck's disease. However, in its current state, the resolution of community-based MRI machines is insufficient to permit accurate and complete assessment of the interosseous ligaments, articular surfaces, or triangular fibrocartilage. These structures are best evaluated arthroscopically.

Standard radiographs can provide much insight into the origin of a patient's wrist pain. Static and dynamic carpal instabilities can be diagnosed with appropriate radiologic techniques. Unfortunately, standard radiographs provide little insight into the more subtle changes that can occur in the articular cartilage or into the presence of a stretched or partially torn interosseous ligament.

All diagnostic imaging techniques used to evaluate the wrist interpose a greater or lesser degree of technical distortion between the physician and the reality he or she is trying to assess. Arthroscopy eliminates this distortion and permits the wrist surgeon to directly view the anatomy of interest.

INDICATIONS

Earlier, three types of wrist arthroscopy were listed. Let us first look at *diagnostic arthroscopy,* whose name defines its indication. Diagnostic arthroscopy is performed when the definitive diagnosis has not been established by less invasive techniques, such as standard radiographs and the clinical examination. The arthroscope permits a clear assessment of the articular surfaces of the distal radioulnar, radiocarpal, ulnocarpal, and mid-carpal joints; the scaphotrapeziotrapezoid (STT) and pisotriquetral joints; the interosseous ligaments; the triangular fibrocartilage; the extrinsic ligaments; and the synovium. Subtle dynamic carpal instabilities can be diagnosed by observing the intercarpal motion during dynamic stressing of the wrist. Even a "negative" wrist arthroscopy can be useful in that it can eliminate an intraarticular cause of symptoms and permit the clinician to investigate extraarticular etiologies.

The second broad indication for wrist arthroscopy is *staging arthroscopy.* This category of wrist arthroscopy is carried out in the face of known pathology in an effort to define the status of the articular surfaces. This information is critical in the formulation of a definitive treatment plan. For example, a frequent indication for staging arthroscopy is assessment of the articular surfaces of a patient with a scapholunate advanced collapse (SLAC) deformity. The condition of the lunate fossa has a great bearing on the definitive treatment. Degeneration of the articular surfaces in patients with an advanced SLAC wrist will be evident on standard radiographs, but this is not the case in less advanced cases. Staging arthroscopy permits accurate assessment of the lunate fossa. If the lunate fossa is involved in the degenerative process, a scaphoid resection and ulnar column fusion is unlikely to lead to resolution of the patient's pain and would therefore be contraindicated. Short of an arthrotomy, only an arthroscopy can provide this information.

Another indication for staging arthroscopy is in patients with Kienböck's disease. The articular surfaces of the radiocarpal and mid-carpal joints are assessed to determine what procedures are likely to successfully treat the disease. Clearly, if a radiograph indicates a disease process is benign but arthroscopic findings demonstrate diffuse advanced chondromalacia, extraarticular procedures are contraindicated.

Box 109-1.
Indications for Wrist Arthroscopy

DEBRIDEMENT
Synovium
Scar
Triangular fibrocartilage complex (TFCC) tears
Partial interosseous ligament tears
Capsule
Loose bodies
Abrasion chondroplasty
Ulnar shortening (Feldon)
Proximal row carpectomy
Carpectomy
Radial styloidectomy
Radial osteophytectomy
Ganglionectomy
Distal ulnar resection (Darrach, Bowers)

REPAIR
Peripheral TFCC tears
Scapholunate instability
Lunatotriquetral instability
Ulnocarpal ligament laxity
Distal radius fracture
Scaphoid fracture

The third indication for wrist arthroscopy is *surgery.* Surgical procedures performed through the arthroscope can be separated into two categories: debridement and repair (Box 109-1). In the future, capsular/ligamentous shrinkage and photostimulation of chondrogenesis may also be common indications for arthroscopy.

OPERATIONS

PATIENT PREPARATION

The preoperative discussion with the patient undergoing wrist arthroscopy will be influenced by the indication for the surgery. The morbidity associated with wrist arthroscopy is minimal. Infection, nerve damage, tenosynovitis, reflex sympathetic dystrophy (RSD), and stiffness can occur but are rare. In addition, specific surgical procedures accomplished through the scope carry their own morbidity.

The postoperative course is also influenced by the type of wrist surgery performed via arthroscopy. The patient will experience mild to moderate pain after arthroscopy performed for the purposes of diagnosis or staging. This pain will diminish rapidly over the first 3 to 7 days after surgery. Some swelling can be expected to persist for several weeks. A simple wrist splint is given to the patient on the first postoperative visit unless contraindicated based on the associated surgery, and gentle range-of-motion exercises are started. No heavy lifting is permitted for 6 weeks.

Alternative diagnostic procedures will most likely have been exhausted before proceeding with arthroscopy, although there is a trend to earlier use of the arthroscope for the diagnosis of wrist pathology. Alternate treatments for the surgical procedures carried out by arthroscopy would include arthrotomy combined with the definitive procedure.

TECHNIQUE

Successful wrist arthroscopy requires adequate distraction. Various manufacturers market wrist distraction devices. A shoulder distraction boom can also be used when combined with countertraction applied to the arm.

Tourniquet use is a function of surgeon preference. A synovectomy and other "ectomy" procedures, however, can be more easily accomplished under tourniquet control.

During arthroscopy of the wrist, the portals are carefully placed to avoid injuring any underlying neurovascular or tendinous structures. The portals are named according to the adjacent dorsal compartments. Figure 109-1 shows the dorsal anatomy of the wrist. The portals and their common uses are listed in Table 109-1.

The 1-2 portal is established between the first and second dorsal compartment tendons just distal to the radial styloid. This places the portal in the anatomic snuffbox. The radial artery and branches of the superficial branch of the radial nerve pass through this area and must be protected. Only careful blunt dissection should be used to establish this or any arthroscopic wrist portal.

The "work horse" portal is the 3-4 portal. This is established slightly distal to Lister's tubercle in the interval between the extensor pollicis longus (EPL) and the fourth dorsal compartment tendons. Care must be taken to enter this portal just at the dorsal rim of the distal radius. If this portal is placed too far distally, the arthroscope will strike the scaphoid and the distal placement will impede passing the scope to the ulnar side of the wrist.

The 4-5 portal is placed just distal to the triangular fibrocartilage complex (TFCC) between the tendons of the fourth and fifth dorsal compartments. It is the instrument portal used during ulnocarpal surgery such as TFCC debridement.

The 5-6 portal or 6R (radial) is established just distal to the TFCC between the tendons of the fifth and sixth dorsal compartments. It can be used in place of the 4-5 portal. The 6U (ulnar) portal is placed just palmar to the extensor carpi ulnaris (ECU) and just distal to the ulnar styloid. This portal, like the 6R and 4-5 portals, passes near the dorsal branch of the ulnar nerve. The 6P portal is often used as an outflow portal but it can be used for viewing and joint instrumentation.

There are two mid-carpal portals, one radial and one ulnar. The radial mid-carpal portal is established 1 cm distal to the 3-4 portal. This portal places the scope just ulnar to the extensor digitorum communis (EDC) tendon of the index finger. It also is used to evaluate the mid-carpal joint. The ulnar mid-carpal portal is occasionally easier to establish and is located approximately 1 cm distal to the 4-5 portal and just ulnar to the

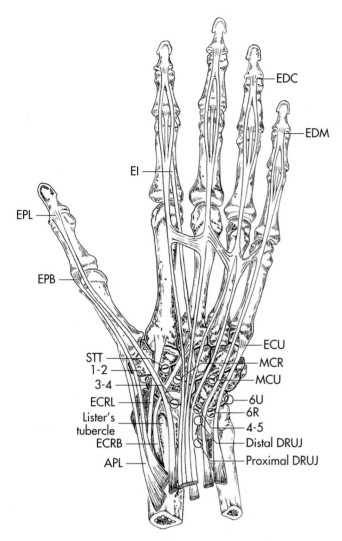

Table 109-1.
Arthroscopic Portal Use

PORTAL	USE
1-2	Radial styloidectomy Viewing for dorsal ganglionectomy
3-4	General viewing of radiocarpal joint Ulnocarpal surgery
4-5	General viewing of ulnocarpal joint Radiocarpal surgery
6R	Same as 4-5
6P	Outflow Ulnocarpal viewing Ulnocarpal surgery
Radial MC	General viewing of mid-carpal joint Viewing of ulnar mid-carpal surgery
Ulnar MC	Alternate general mid-carpal viewing Viewing of radial mid-carpal surgery (not STT)
STT	STT viewing and surgery
Distal DRUJ	Viewing DRUJ and proximal TFCC surface Ulnar head resection
Proximal DRUJ	Viewing DRUJ Distal ulnar resection

Figure 109-1. Wrist arthroscopy portals. This anatomic drawing depicts the true relationships of tendons and carpal bones as they rest in a slightly distracted wrist as one might see at arthroscopy. *APL,* abductor pollicis longus; *DRUJ,* distal radioulnar joint; *ECRB,* extensor carpi radialis brevis; *ECRL,* extensor carpi radialis longus; *ECU,* extensor carpi ulnaris; *EDC,* extensor digitorum communis; *EDM,* extensor digiti minimi; *EI,* extensor indicis; *EPB,* extensor pollicis brevis; *EPL,* extensor pollicis longus; *MCR,* midcarpal-radial portal; *MCU,* midcarpal-ulnar portal; *STT,* scaphotrapeziotrapezoid; *6R,* 6 radial; *6U,* 6 ulnar. (Redrawn from Poehling GG: *Arthroscopy of the wrist,* New York, 1994, Raven.)

EDC of the ring finger. This places the scope at the confluence of the capitate, hamate, lunate, and triquetrum.

There are two distal radioulnar joint (DRUJ) portals. One DRUJ portal enters the DRUJ just proximal to the TFCC and just proximal to the 4-5 portal. The more proximal DRUJ portal is established 1 cm proximal to the ulnar head and is oriented toward the proximal DRUJ capsule. The DRUJ portals are easier to make if the DRUJ is first distended with saline.

The 3-4 portal is the first to be established. Some surgeons prefer to inject lactated Ringer's solution into the radiocarpal joint through this 3-4 portal. This distends the capsule and displaces it away from the articular surface. However, care

should be taken to not injure the scaphoid with the needle. A small transverse incision is made through the skin at the 3-4 portal. Blunt dissection is then carried out using a Hartman hemostat. The Hartman has a tip that follows the palmar inclination of the radius. A "pop" is felt as the Hartman penetrates the capsule. The Hartman is then spread and the blunt trocar and cannula are introduced. The scope is introduced and infusion of lactated Ringer's solution is begun. The use of a fluid-control pump is optional. The surgeon then passes the arthroscope to the ulnar side of the wrist and the 6U portal is identified. A spinal needle is passed into the prestyloid recess under direct vision. This orients the surgeon in regard to the placement of the outflow portal. The position of the spinal needle is noted and then removed. A longitudinal nick is made in the skin to accommodate the relatively large bore of the outflow cannula assembly. This is then introduced under direct vision into the wrist. The outflow cannula is fixed in place using a Steri-Strip. Gravity drainage is sufficient.

The position of the 4-5 portal is determined by passing the spinal needle into the joint while the ulnocarpal joint is observed from the 3-4 portal. A transverse incision is made through the skin and the subcutaneous tissue is bluntly dissected using the Hartman hemostat, followed by the insertion of a probe once the capsule is penetrated.

Inspection of the joint is then performed. It is essential this be done in a systematic fashion in each case to avoid overlooking any pathology. The scaphoid, scapholunate interosseous ligament, and lunate are easily visualized. The lunatotriquetral ligament and triquetrum are not always quite as easily seen and should be viewed through the 4-5 portal later in the procedure.

Once the scope has reached the ulnar aspect of the wrist, it is angled proximally and palmarly and guided radially to view the ulnotriquetral, ulnolunate, long and short radiolunate, and radioscaphocapitate ligaments.

Finally, the scope is again swept from radial to ulnar while the surgeon inspects the articular surface of the radius and the triangular fibrocartilage. The scope is then passed into the 4-5 portal for final inspection of the ulnar aspect of the wrist, including the triquetrum, the lunate, and the lunatotriquetral ligament.

Once the radiocarpal and ulnocarpal joints have been examined, the scope is placed in the radial mid-carpal portal, which is not always easy. If the radial mid-carpal portal is difficult to create, the ulnar mid-carpal portal offers an easier access to the mid-carpal joint. The ulnar mid-carpal portal, however, does not always afford visualization of the scaphotrapeziotrapezoid joint. The ulnar aspect of the mid-carpal joint is evaluated first through the ulnar mid-carpal portal. The radial mid-carpal portal is then established under direct vision and the radial mid-carpal joint is examined. The scope, once in the radial mid-carpal portal, slides distally between the scaphoid and capitate until the scaphotrapeziotrapezoid joint is clearly visualized. It is then passed proximally and ulnarly to visualize the scaphocapitate, capitolunate, and triquetrohamate articulations. The ulnar limb of the deltoid ligament can be assessed with some probing and occasional clearance of the synovial layer; in some lax wrists, the triquetrohamate ligament can be viewed. The radioscaphocapitate ligament can also be viewed as it passes from the scaphoid to the capitate.

Dynamic carpal instability is best assessed through the radial mid-carpal portal. This is accomplished by manipulating the wrist, after releasing the traction, while keeping the scope in the radial mid-carpal portal. The wrist is flexed, extended, radially and ulnarly deviated and submitted to a shuck test. Abnormal motion at the level of the scapholunate articulation, particularly abnormal widening, is a sign of scapholunate instability. Often this condition is associated with chondromalacia of the mid-carpal scapholunate joint. Lunatotriquetral instability is evidenced by abnormal motion at the lunatotriquetral joint during the intraoperative shuck test.

The DRUJ can also be visualized arthroscopically. The joint is first distended with a lactated Ringer's solution. A proximal DRUJ portal is established approximately 1.5 cm proximal to the DRUJ and oriented to enter the dorsal and proximal DRUJ capsule. A distal DRUJ portal can also be established just proximal to the 4-5 portal, passing just proximal to the TFCC. The DRUJ portals are useful for assessing the articular surfaces of the DRUJ and the proximal surface of the triangular fibrocartilage, in addition to arthroscopic distal ulnar resection.

Box 109-2.
TFCC Tear Classification

CLASS 1: TRAUMATIC
A. Central perforation
B. Ulnar avulsion (with or without ulnar styloid fracture)
C. Distal avulsion (ulnocarpal ligament tear)
D. Radial avulsion (with or without sigmoid notch fracture)

CLASS 2: DEGENERATIVE (ULNOCARPAL ABUTMENT)
A. TFCC wear
B. TFCC wear + lunate/ulnar head chondromalacia
C. TFCC perforation + lunate/ulnar head chondromalacia
D. TFCC perforation + lunate/ulnar head chondromalacia + L-T ligament tear
E. TFCC perforation + lunate/ulnar head chondromalacia + L-T ligament tear + ulnocarpal arthritis

From Palmer AK: J Hand Surg [Am] 14:594-606, 1989.

The temptation to keep the scope in one portal must be resisted. The surgeon should be familiar with all portals and be ready to use them.

DEBRIDEMENT OF TRIANGULAR FIBROCARTILAGE TEARS

Debridement of TFCC tears, particularly in the patient with an ulnar negative variance, has proven to be quite successful.[9] The goal of TFCC debridement is to debride the tear back to stable edges. The technique has evolved to now include the use of the Holmium:Yag laser. Andrew Palmer has described a classification system of TFCC tears that is very useful (Box 109-2).

Without laser assistance, debridement technique involves the use of both the 3-4 and 4-5 portals. The initial debridement of the radial, palmar, and a portion of the dorsal tear is accomplished with a scope in the 3-4 portal and the instruments entering through the 4-5 portal. Various small-joint, angled punches, graspers, banana blades, and hook knives are available for use in this procedure.

The scope is introduced into the 4-5 portal once the radial aspect of the TFCC has been debrided and the instruments passed through the 3-4 portal. The instruments cross the radiocarpal joint to debride the ulnar aspect of the TFCC. Three points must be kept in mind. One is to not detach the TFCC from its insertion at the base of the ulnar styloid. The second is to remember to not injure the dorsal or palmar radioulnar ligaments because these ligaments are the primary stabilizers of the DRUJ. The final point is to avoid scuffing the radiocarpal joint articular surfaces while passing the cutting/

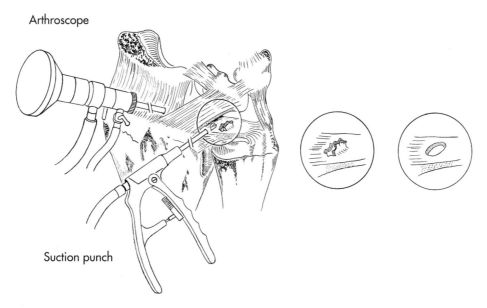

Figure 109-2. Debridement of a Palmer 1A central TFCC tear. The arthroscope and suction punch (and other instruments) are placed in either the 3-4 or 4-5 portals. The debridement of the radial aspect of the TFCC can be done with the instruments in the 4-5 portal, whereas the debridement of the ulnar edge requires the punch to enter the 3-4 portal and cross the radiocarpal joint.

grasping instruments into the ulnocarpal joint from the 3-4 portal (Figure 109-2).

The Holmium:Yag laser can also be used for TFCC debridement. The small size of the laser probe makes it ideally suited for small-joint arthroscopy. The scope is left in the 3-4 portal for TFCC debridement while the 70 degree, side-firing laser probe is introduced through the 4-5 portal. The entire debridement can be accomplished with a laser probe in the 4-5 portal, thus avoiding the danger of radiocarpal scuffing noted during mechanical debridement.

REPAIR OF THE TRIANGULAR FIBROCARTILAGE

Radial (Palmer 1D) and ulnar (Palmer 1B) detachments of the TFCC can be repaired arthroscopically. Two methods are routinely used for repair of an ulnar peripheral TFCC tear. One, described by Corso et al [3] and popularized by Whipple, [16] involves repair techniques similar to those developed for meniscorrhesis. The other, popularized by Poehling, uses a Tuohy needle. [1]

The Whipple technique places the scope in the 3-4 portal while the repair is accomplished through the 4-5 and/or 6R portal (Figure 109-3). A 2- to 3-cm incision is also made along the ECU just distal to the ulnar head to permit visualization of the ulnar capsule and tying of the repair sutures. Care is taken to avoid injuring the dorsal branch of the ulnar nerve or opening the sixth dorsal compartment proximal to the ulnar styloid. Subluxation of the ECU can occur if one is too liberal in releasing the ECU sheath. The torn edges of the TFCC are debrided and freshened using the full-radius cutters. The ECU is retracted with a Penrose drain, and the proposed reattach-

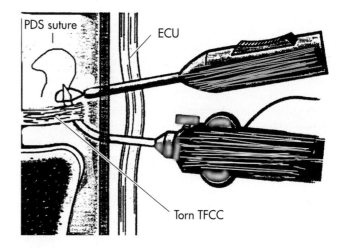

Figure 109-3. Repair of a Palmer 1B ulnar peripheral TFCC tear using the Whipple technique. The suture passer needle passes through the TFCC and feeds the 2-0 PDS suture through the retrieval loop. The suture ends are withdrawn and tied over the ulnar capsule. (Modified from Corso SJ, Savoie FH, Geissler WB, et al: *Arthroscopy* 13:78-84, 1997.)

ment points are defined by passing a 20-gauge spinal needle through the ulnar capsule under arthroscopic control. The "Inteq TFCC Repair Kit," or the "Instrument Maker" meniscal repair kit is used to pass a 2-0 polydioxanone (PDS) suture from outside-in through the TFCC repair needle following the path defined by the spinal needle. The needle passes through the ulnar capsule and through the free ulnar edge of the TFCC. A second needle containing a small wire

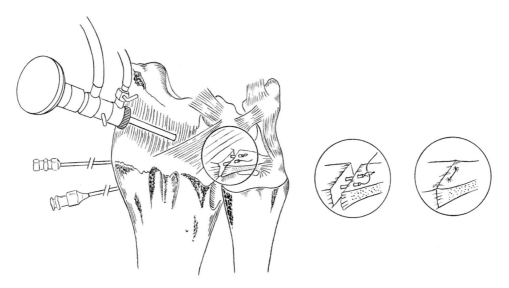

Figure 109-4. Repair of a Palmer 1B ulnar peripheral TFCC tear using the Tuohy needle. The arthroscope is placed in the 4-5 portal and the Tuohy needle enters the joint through the 1-2 portal. (Redrawn from Arujo W, Poehling GG, Kuzma GR: *Arthroscopy* 12:699-703, 1996.)

loop is passed either adjacent to the first needle to create a horizontal mattress stitch or just distal to the first needle to create a simple stitch. The suture is passed through the first needle and threaded through the wire loop of the second needle. The wire loop, along with the snared suture, is pulled through the ulnar capsule. The first needle is also removed, leaving the suture in place to be tied down over the ulnar capsule. This process is repeated two or three times as needed. An attempt should be made to avoid tying the knots within the ECU sheath, because this can lead to chronic tenosynovitis. The sheath should be repaired at the conclusion of this repair. It should be borne in mind there are two layers of the sheath—the deep sheath, which is the major stabilizer, and the superficial sheath, which is an extension of the dorsal retinaculum.

REPAIR USING THE TUOHY NEEDLE

Araujo and Poehling et al[1] described a relatively simple technique for the repair of peripheral (Palmer 1B) TFCC tears. This technique takes advantage of the blunt tip of the Tuohy needle, a needle used for epidural anesthesia. The scope is placed in the 4-5 portal. A 20-gauge Tuohy needle is passed through the 1-2 portal and engages the free edge of the TFCC. The needle continues through the region of the ulnar attachment of the TFCC, passing through the skin just palmar to the ECU. A 2-0 polydioxanone PDS suture is passed through the needle, leaving a tale extending out of the tip of the needle. The needle is pulled back into the joint, moved either dorsally or palmarly, and again passed through the free edge of the TFCC and out through the skin. The blunt

tip of the Tuohy needle pushes the suture through the TFCC and skin without cutting it. An incision is made in the skin at the exit site of the suture to permit tying the suture down on the ulnar capsule. Care must be taken to avoid injuring the dorsal branch of the ulnar nerve. The technique is repeated as many times as is necessary to affect a solid repair (Figure 109-4).

REPAIR OF RADIAL AVULSION OF THE TRIANGULAR FIBROCARTILAGE

Avulsion of the TFCC from the sigmoid notch of the radius can lead to DRUJ instability. The repair of these Palmer 1D lesions can be accomplished using a technique developed by Short and Sagerman.[12] This technique places the scope in the 3-4 portal and a motorized abrader is brought into the joint through the 6R portal. The abrader freshens the area of attachment of the TFCC to the radial sigmoid notch. A small incision is made over the interval between the first and second compartments. A 0.045 Kirschner wire (K wire) is passed through a 14-gauge hypodermic needle, which acts as a soft tissue protector, and is used to drill four tunnels from the dorsal aspect of the radius into the abraded surface of the sigmoid notch. Fluoroscopy is useful in these cases to guide placement of the K wires.

The arthroscope cannula is placed in the 6U portal, and long, meniscal repair needles armed with 2-0 PDS suture are passed through the cannula, through the radial edge of the TFCC, and into the tunnels drilled with the K wire. The sutures are tied over the dorsal aspect of the radius (Figure 109-5).

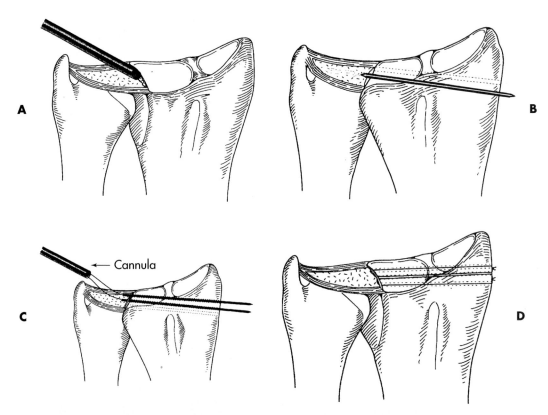

Figure 109-5. Repair of Palmer 1D radial peripheral TFCC tear. **A,** The distal edge of the sigmoid notch is prepared with a burr. **B,** Three tunnels are drilled from radial to ulnar, passing through the burred distal edge of the sigmoid notch. **C,** Meniscal repair needles armed with 2-0 polydioxanone suture are passed through the arthroscopic cannula in the 6U portal, passing through the tunnels created with the K wires and out through the radial side of the radius. **D,** The sutures, having been passed through the radial edge of the TFCC and distal edge of sigmoid notch, are secured over the lateral aspect of the distal radius. (From Sagerman SD, Short W: *Arthroscopy* 12(3):339-342, 1995.)

POSTOPERATIVE CARE

The postoperative care of patients undergoing debridement of TFCC tears includes the application of a bulky dressing and a volar splint. The patient is gradually weaned from this splint over a 6-week time frame. Our experience has been that premature return to activities can lead to an aggravation of postsurgical synovitis.

After repair of a peripheral TFCC tear, the arm must be placed in a cast in neutral rotation for 6 weeks. Therapy is begun after 6 weeks to regain wrist range of motion.

SOFT TISSUE "ECTOMY" SURGERY

Synovectomy can easily be accomplished using the arthroscope, either in combination with the laser or using full radius cutters and the suction punch. Partial tears of the interosseous ligaments can also be debrided. This simple procedure can be very beneficial. Chondral flap tears and chondromalacia can also be debrided.

REMOVAL OF LOOSE BODIES

Loose bodies are a relatively rare occurrence in my experience, but they can be treated arthroscopically. The appropriate portals are chosen and a grasping forceps is used to remove the loose fragments. A pituitary rongeur is occasionally needed to remove the loose body.

RADIAL STYLOIDECTOMY

Cases of radioscaphoid impingement can be successfully treated with a "mini" radial styloidectomy. This procedure carries with it certain risks not associated with the other procedures previously discussed. The contents of the first dorsal compartment can be compromised, as can the contents of the anatomic snuffbox. Care must also be taken to remove only that amount of styloid necessary to achieve the therapeutic end. An overzealous radial styloidectomy can lead to attenuation and/or rupture of the radioscapho-capitate and/or long radiolunate ligament. The loss of this ligamentous support can lead to ulnar translocation of the carpus.

A radial styloidectomy is accomplished using the arthroscope and fluoroscopy. The amount of radial styloid to be removed is determined, and the ulnar limit of the radial styloidectomy is marked with a K wire passed through the radial styloid into the radioscaphoid joint. Care is taken to not advance the K wire into the scaphoid. The wire's point should be barely visible in the joint. The styloidectomy can then be completed using a combination of portals, including the 1-2 and 3-4 portals with the scope introduced through the 4-5 portal. The styloidectomy is completed using the barrel abrader in combination with the laser. The arthroscopic monitoring of the procedure can be misleading, and serial fluoroscopic images are essential.

ARTHROSCOPICALLY ASSISTED ULNAR SHORTENING

The ulnar abutment syndrome, a combination of an ulnar plus variance and a TFCC tear, is the most common indication for arthroscopically assisted ulnar shortening (Figure 109-6, A).

Simple debridement of the TFCC in the face of an ulnar plus variance is inadequate treatment for patients with an ulnar abutment syndrome. The ulnar aspect of the wrist must be decompressed, and arthroscopically assisted ulnar shortening has proven to be very effective in this situation (Figure 109-6, B).[17] Arthroscopic ulnar shortening is accomplished by placing the scope in the 3-4 portal and introducing the instruments through the 4-5 portal. Occasionally the 6U portal can be used, as can the DRUJ portal. We have found the Holmium:Yag laser to be very useful for ulnar shortening. The laser is introduced through the 4-5 portal, and the cartilage and subchondral bone of the ulnar seat of the distal ulna are rapidly vaporized. The laser becomes less efficient once the trabeculations of the distal ulna are visible, and the 2.9-mm barrel abrader is brought in to finish the shortening. It is also important to avoid injury to the sigmoid notch. Frequent fluoroscopic monitoring of the amount of bone resected is mandatory. Care must be taken to fully supinate and pronate the wrist to adequately debride the ulnar head. A small ridge of bone will occasionally be left ulnarly; however, this usually does not impinge on the proximal carpal row. All instruments are removed at the end of the procedure, and the wrist is ulnarly deviated, axially loaded, and supinated and pronated to

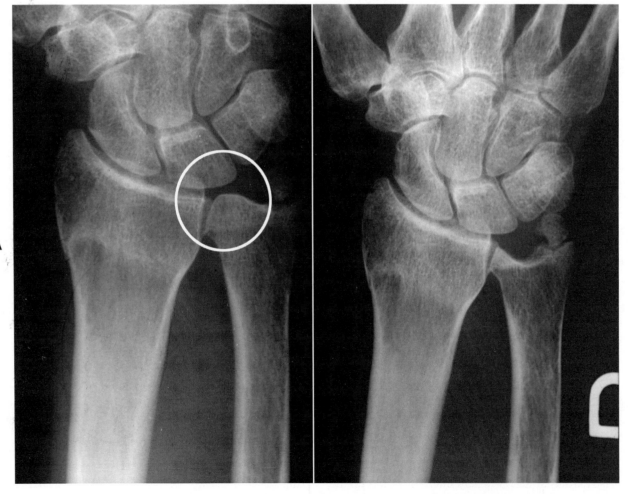

Figure 109-6. Arthroscopically assisted ulnar shortening. **A,** Preoperative radiograph of ulnar abutment syndrome. Note ulnar plus variance. **B,** Postoperative radiographs of ulnar abutment syndrome. Note arthroscopic ulnar shortening.

be sure no clicking or popping is noted. If any clicking or popping is noted and it appears to be emanating from the area of the surgery, further ulnar resection may be required. The goal of the surgery is to create an ulnar minus variance of 1 to 2 mm.

Any irregularities of the remaining distal ulna should be minimized. These do, however, have a tendency to flatten with the passage of time. Postoperative care of these patients includes the application of a volar splint followed by early range-of-motion exercises. Open ulnar shortening has been reported to be associated with a recovery period of up to 6 months,[4] whereas arthroscopic debridement requires a shorter recovery.

PROXIMAL ROW CARPECTOMY

Proximal row carpectomy can be achieved arthroscopically. It is, however, a tedious procedure and its advantage over open proximal row carpectomy remains to be demonstrated.

ABRASION CHONDROPLASTY

The use of abrasion chondroplasty in the knee has not been particularly beneficial. In selected cases, however, it can be useful in the wrist because of its non-weight–bearing status. It should be remembered that no series of carpal abrasion chondroplasty has been published. Abrasion chondroplasty is reserved for the treatment of grade IV chondromalacia. If the area of chondromalacia is in a portion of the carpus that when debrided leads to decompression of the involved joint, debridement of the subchondral bone and exposure of bleeding cancellous bone, combined with early range-of-motion exercises, can be curative. This is seen in patients with chondromalacia of the proximal pole of the hamate. If, on the other hand, it is impossible to "unload" the joint, as when the chondromalacia involves both articular surfaces of the radiolunate joint, a chondroplasty of both articular surfaces must be combined with early continuous passive motion to promote chondrognesis[13] and/or temporary interposition of silicone sheeting to inhibit intraarticular adhesions.

ARTHROSCOPICALLY ASSISTED TREATMENT OF CARPAL INSTABILITY

Scapholunate Instability

Whipple[16] has popularized arthroscopically assisted stabilization of the scapholunate joint. The indications for this procedure include recent reducible scapholunate instabilities with scapholunate diastasis of less than 5 mm. The goal of surgery is to create a "fibrous ankylosis" of the scapholunate joint by passing multiple K wires across that joint.

TECHNIQUE. The standard arthroscopic examination of the wrist is performed to rule out a SLAC deformity. An arthroscopically assisted reduction and internal fixation (ARIF) of the scapholunate instability is performed if the articular surfaces are intact. The scope is removed and 0.035 K-wire "joy sticks" are passed through 14-gauge hypodermic needles, one into the scaphoid and one into the lunate. These "joy sticks" allow manipulation of the scaphoid and lunate bones and facilitate the reduction of the scapholunate instability.

The scope is placed in the radial mid-carpal portal to visualize the scapholunate articulation. The scapholunate articulation is reduced using the joy sticks, and multiple (three to five) K wires are passed through the scapholunate articulation from radial to ulnar. This requires passing the K wires through the anatomic snuffbox. An incision is made in the snuffbox to protect the radial nerve and artery, which are identified and retracted. Fourteen-gauge hypodermic needles are then carefully passed through the snuffbox and positioned on the scaphoid to guide the placement of 0.045 K wires across the scapholunate articulation, protecting the soft tissues of the snuffbox. Some authors recommend passing the large-bore hypodermic needles percutaneously through the snuffbox, but it should be kept in mind that a 14-gauge hypodermic needle can lacerate the radial artery and nerve. The wires are placed under fluoroscopic and arthroscopic control. The adequacy of the reduction is verified through the scope, with the fluoroscopy unit, and with definitive standard radiographs. The joy sticks are removed and a long arm thumb spica splint is applied.

The patient's wrist is immobilized in the splint for 1 week. Any sutures are removed at 1 week, leaving Steri Strips in place. Another long arm thumb spica cast is applied and worn for 7 weeks. The long arm cast is replaced after 7 weeks by a short arm thumb spica cast, which is worn for 4 weeks. Some authors, however, immobilize the wrist for as little as 6 weeks. The wires are removed at the time of cast removal.

Occupational therapy is begun to restore wrist motion and upper-extremity strength. Whipple reports 83% good results in those patients with a scapholunate gap of less than 3 mm who underwent ARIF of the scapholunate instability within 3 months of the initial injury.

Lunatotriquetral Instability

Lunatotriquetral instability is a part of the spectrum of ulnar-sided wrist instability. Isolated lunatotriquetral instability, like scapholunate instability, lends itself to ARIF.[11] The technique used for scapholunate pinning can be transposed to the ulnar side of the wrist for lunatotriquetral pinning. The scope is introduced into the radial mid-carpal portal to control the reduction of the joint and to monitor placement of the K wires. Joy sticks are used to control the lunate and the triquetrum. An incision is made ulnar to the ECU and the dorsal branch of the ulnar nerve is identified and protected. Multiple K wires are passed under fluoroscopic/arthroscopic control through 14-gauge hypodermic needles/tissue protectors across the lunatotriquetral joint.

A long arm splint is applied postoperatively and converted to a long arm cast 1 week later. The cast is worn for 7 weeks, at which time it is replaced with a short arm cast. The pins are removed when the short arm cast is removed and occupational therapy is begun to restore wrist motion and upper-extremity strength.

Lunatotriquetral instability has also been treated by formal ulnar shortening. The ulnar shortening tightens the ulnocarpal ligaments, and stabilizes the lunatotriquetral joint. Savoie,[14] rather than shorten the ulna to tighten the ulnocarpal ligaments, has recently described the arthroscopic plication of the ulnocarpal ligaments for lunatotriquetral instability. This is a relatively new procedure, and the long-term results are still unknown.

Radio frequency and laser-assisted capsular shrinkage of the ulnocarpal ligaments have been proposed as alternative treatments of lunatotriquetral instability. These techniques have been used in the treatment of shoulder instability, but no clinical results of their use in the wrist have been published.

Ulnocarpal Instability (Capsular Shrinkage)

Capsular shrinkage using either laser or radio frequency (RF) energy has become commonplace in the shoulder. Its use in the wrist is in its infancy. One area that seems to lend itself well to capsular shrinkage is the treatment of subtle forms of ulnocarpal instability characterized by attenuation of the ulnolunate and ulnotriquetral ligaments. The controlled thermal energy transmitted to the tissues by either the laser or RF instruments disrupts the normal triple helix of capsular collagen. The helix unwinds and shortens. The denatured collagen is gradually (over 6 to 12 weeks) replaced by new collagen that is more tightly packed. The denaturation weakens the capsule, and it is for this reason that the shrunk capsule must be protected for several weeks. The tight configuration appears to be permanent and can lead to long-term "tightening" of the capsule.

Application of this technique to an attenuated ulnocarpal ligament complex offers a less-invasive approach to ulnocarpal instability as compared with ulnocarpal ligament plication or shortening ulnar osteotomy. Ulnocarpal capsular shrinkage is accomplished with the arthroscope in the 3-4 portal and the thermal device passed through the 4-5 portal. Just enough energy is applied to shrink the capsule without causing unwanted collateral damage. The energy setting for the Holmium:YAG laser for capsular shrinkage varies, but one should start with the lowest possible energy setting and gradually increase the power until the capsule is seen to shrink. The same approach can be applied to the use of RF devices.

No clinical series have been published reviewing the efficacy of ulnocarpal shrinkage. It is mentioned in this chapter because it is believed this technology will have an important impact on wrist arthroscopy in the years to come.

ARTHOSCOPIC GANGLIONECTOMY

Osterman[10] has reported excellent results in his series of arthroscopic dorsal wrist ganglionectomies. The ganglionectomy is accomplished with the arthroscope in the 6R portal. A 19-gauge spinal needle is used for the intraarticular localization of the ganglion. The full-radius cutter (or laser probe) is placed in the 3-4 portal and follows the scapholunate ligament dorsally and distally to the insertion of the capsule on the dorsal scapholunate ligament. A small "pearl" corresponding

to the origin of the ganglion is sometimes, but not always, seen at that level. A 1 cm × 1 cm segment of dorsal capsule is resected at the confluence of the dorsal capsule and scapholunate ligament, taking care not to injure the extensor tendons. After surgery, a bulky dressing reinforced with a volar wrist splint is worn for 1 week. Formal therapy is rarely needed. Heavy lifting is avoided for 6 weeks.

ARTHROSCOPICALLY ASSISTED REDUCTION AND INTERNAL FIXATION OF DISTAL RADIUS FRACTURES

Geissler[6,7] and others have published their technique of arthroscopically assisted distal radial fracture fixation. ARIF of distal radial fractures is best performed approximately 48 to 72 hours after the initial injury. Patients with distal radial fractures that reduce by preliminary closed manipulation but require "fine tuning" are the best candidates for ARIF. The arthroscope is used to verify how well the articular surface of the radius has been restored. The scope is placed in the 1-2, 3-4, and 4-5 portals as needed. Initial irrigation and debridement of the joint is critical to ensure adequate visibility. Care must be taken to avoid pumping irrigation fluid through the fracture fissures into the forearm and producing a compartment syndrome. A preliminary closed reduction is performed, and some form of external traction is applied either through finger traps or with an external fixator. Ligamentotaxis, multiple joy sticks, and intraarticular probes are used to manipulate the fracture fragments into position. They are then pinned in position under arthroscopic and fluoroscopic guidance. Small dorsal incisions over the distal radius are occasionally required to elevate impacted fragments and also allow the insertion of bone graft or bone substitute.

Postoperative care is dictated by the fracture pattern and rigidity of the internal/external fixation. Whether this technique offers any advantage over standard open reduction and internal fixation remains to be seen.

ARTHROSCOPICALLY ASSISTED REDUCTION AND INTERNAL FIXATION OF SCAPHOID FRACTURES

Whipple[15] has pioneered ARIF of scaphoid fractures. This technique is indicated in undisplaced and reducible scaphoid fractures. The technique requires the surgeon to be familiar with wrist arthroscopy and the Herbert-Whipple cannulated screw system.

In addition to the usual arthroscopy portals, one incision over the STT joint is needed for the placement of the Herbert-Whipple jig. The distal component of the jig is placed over the distal pole of the scaphoid after the STT joint has been opened and a palmar segment of trapezium is excised to permit placement of the jig. The distal hook of the jig is passed through a 1-2 portal. The radial mid-carpal portal is used to visualize the scaphoid fracture and verify its reduction. The 3-4 portal is used to guide the jig hook to the proximal scaphoid. The jig is tightened to hold and compress the scaphoid fracture and a guide pin is placed across the fracture. Its position is verified using fluoroscopy. A second pin is placed to control rotation. The screw hole is then drilled and the appropriate screw is placed. The STT capsule and skin are closed and a thumb spica splint is applied. Immobilization in Whipple's series was between 3 and 4 weeks and 19 of 20 fractures healed uneventfully.

OUTCOMES

Wrist arthroscopy is a relatively new technique and its indications and uses continue to expand. Formal outcome studies are lacking in this particular area of medicine. It is the general consensus that outcomes are good and patient satisfaction is high in those patients in whom the diagnosis is accurate, the pathology is well defined, and the surgical treatment is able to be conducted through the arthroscope. The best outcomes are found in the treatment of central or peripheral traumatic TFCC tears. Simple debridement of a central tear in a patient with an ulnar minus variance is likely to result in resolution of the patient's pain in over 80% of cases. The same is true for peripheral tears. The results of arthroscopic TFCC debridement for degenerative TFCC tears (palmar 2 lesions) are less predictable because of the associated degenerative changes noted in such wrists. The removal of an isolated loose body can also be expected to produce good results.

Synovectomy, radial styloidectomy, ganglionectomy, and debridement of partial interosseous ligament tears can be expected to provide the patient with a good functional outcome. More clinical studies are needed to refine the indications and outcomes of ARIF of distal radial fractures, scaphoid fractures, and abrasion chondroplasty. Fischer et al[5] and others have noted a very high incidence of associated ligamentous injuries with distal radial fractures. Whether all patients with distal radial fractures should undergo arthroscopic evaluation and treatment of these associated injuries remains to be seen. The arthroscopic treatment, like the open treatment of carpal instability, is still a challenge.

SUMMARY

Arthroscopy of the wrist continues to evolve. Just as arthroscopy has replaced arthrography and MRI in the knee it is also replacing these modalities in the wrist. Arthroscopy is the most accurate method of assessing most wrist pathology. This is not to say, however, that wrist arthroscopy can demonstrate all pathologic states. It will not demonstrate early phases of carpal avascular necrosis or subtle forms of mid-carpal instability. It is of no use in assessing extraarticular wrist pathology, except to the degree that it can eliminate an intraarticular source of a painful wrist.

REFERENCES

1. Araujo W, Poehling GG, Kuzma GR: New Tuohy needle technique for triangular fibrocartilage complex repair: preliminary studies, *Arthroscopy* 12(6):699-703, 1996.
2. Cerofolini E, Luchetti R, Pederzini L, et al: MR evaluation of triangular fibrocartilage complex tears in the wrist: comparison with arthrography and arthroscopy, *J Comput Assist Tomogr* 14:963-967, 1990.
3. Corso SJ, Savoie FH, Geissler WB, et al: Arthroscopic repair of peripheral avulsions of the triangular fibrocartilage complex of the wrist: a multicenter study, *Arthroscopy* 13:78-84, 1997.
4. Feldon P, Terrono AL, Belsky MR: Wafer distal ulna resection for triangular fibrocartilage tears and/or ulna impaction syndrome, *J Hand Surg [Am]* 17(4):731-737, 1992.
5. Fischer M, Denzler C, Sennwald G: Carpal ligament lesions associated with fresh distal radius fractures: arthroscopic study of 54 cases, *Swiss Surg* 2:269-272, 1996.
6. Geissler WB: Arthroscopically assisted reduction of intraarticular fractures of the distal radius, *Hand Clin* 11:19-29, 1995.
7. Geissler WB, Freeland AE: Arthroscopically assisted reduction of intraarticular distal radial fractures, *Clin Orthop* 327:125-134, 1996.
8. Nagle DJ, Benson LS: Wrist arthroscopy: indications and results, *Arthroscopy* 8:198-203, 1992.
9. Osterman AL: Arthroscopic debridement of the triangular fibrocartilage complex, *Arthroscopy* (6-2):12-24, 1990.
10. Osterman AL, Raphael J: Arthroscopic resection of dorsal ganglion of the wrist, *Hand Clin* 11:7-12, 1995.
11. Osterman AL, Seidman GD: The role of arthroscopy in the treatment of lunatotriquetral ligament injuries, *Hand Clin* 11:41-50, 1995.
12. Sagerman SD, Short W: Arthroscopic repair of the radial-sided triangular fibrocartilage complex tears, *Arthroscopy* (12-3):339-342, 1995.
13. Salter RB: History of rest and motion and the scientific basis for early continuous passive motion, *Hand Clin* 12(1):1-11, 1996.
14. Savoie FH 3rd: Personal communication.
15. Whipple TL: The role of arthroscopy in the treatment of scapholunate instability, *Hand Clin* 11:37-40, 1995.
16. Whipple TL: The role of arthroscopy in the treatment of intra-articular wrist fractures, *Hand Clin* 11:13-18, 1995.
17. Wnorowski DC, Palmer AK, Werner FW, Fortino MD: Anatomic and biomechanical analysis of the arthroscopic wafer procedure, *Arthroscopy* 8:204-212, 1992.

CHAPTER

Wrist Arthrodesis

110

Mark A. Deitch
Peter J. Stern

INTRODUCTION

Wrist arthrodesis is an established salvage procedure that is useful in a variety of clinical situations. This chapter reviews the indications for wrist arthrodesis, discusses the surgical techniques, and presents the results and complications of this procedure.

INDICATIONS

Wrist arthrodesis has been used since early in the twentieth century for a variety of disorders. Ely[10,11] used it for treatment of tuberculosis of the wrist joint, and Steindler[33] recommended it for patients with posttraumatic paralysis in the upper extremity. Liebolt[18] further expanded the indications, using wrist arthrodesis in patients with varied diagnoses, including posttraumatic deformities.

Currently, wrist arthrodesis is indicated for the management of a painful, deformed, or unstable wrist that interferes with function and is resistant to nonoperative treatment. Broad indications include noninflammatory arthropathy, inflammatory arthritis, and neurologic conditions.[40]

Many authors regard wrist arthrodesis as a "salvage" procedure that can be performed after failed motion-sparing procedures such as proximal row carpectomy, intercarpal arthrodesis, or total wrist arthroplasty.[7,9,20,40] With congenital deformities such as radial club hand, or in patients with a chronic scapholunate advanced collapse (SLAC) wrist, arthrodesis may be used as the initial surgical treatment. Procedures that preserve wrist motion in most cases should be considered before arthrodesis. Arthrodesis may be considered earlier in young, active patients with high load demands.

Posttraumatic osteoarthritis is the most common noninflammatory condition for which wrist arthrodesis is performed. The indications for surgery include malunited distal radius fractures, advanced Kienböck's disease, SLAC wrist, and neoplasms of the distal radius (such as a giant cell tumor), all of which require interpositional bone graft replacement.[20,38]

Rheumatoid arthritis is the most common inflammatory condition that leads to wrist-joint destruction. The inflammatory process damages the joint capsule and ligaments and destroys articular cartilage, leading to predictable patterns of deformity and instability.[35] Indications for wrist fusion include pain, instability secondary to wrist-joint destruction, ankylosis in marked flexion, and rupture of the wrist extensor tendons.[6]

Septic arthritis of the wrist, although an uncommon diagnosis, can lead to joint destruction. Guidelines have not been established for the length of antibiotic treatment required to eradicate an infection. A prolonged course of intravenous antibiotic therapy and a quiescent period of at least 6 months is generally advisable before any operative procedures are considered.[20]

Neurologic conditions for which wrist arthrodesis is indicated include posttraumatic paralysis, cerebral palsy, stroke, and polio. Arthrodesis may be indicated in patients with spastic conditions, such as cerebral palsy or stroke, or in patients who have severe flexion deformities as treatment for a dysfunctional posture or for hygienic purposes. Occasionally, wrist arthrodesis is performed in these patients to improve appearances.

Contraindications to wrist arthrodesis include an active infection, an open distal radius epiphysis, major sensory loss in the hand, quadriplegia with functioning wrist extensors, and conditions in which a procedure that preserves wrist motion is a better alternative.[9,20]

OPERATIONS

Many surgical techniques of wrist arthrodesis have been described.* Despite its long history, controversy exists with

---

*References 1, 5, 6, 14, 18, 24.

regard to the optimal surgical technique, wrist position, the use and source of bone graft, and the joints to be included in the fusion mass.

Abbott et al[1] used cancellous iliac crest bone graft and external immobilization to achieve fusion. More recently, Carroll and Dick,[5] described a "rabbit ears" corticocancellous iliac crest graft that was wedged in place between the bases of the second and third metacarpals and the distal radius. Today, this technique and similar others have become less popular because of the necessity for external immobilization, especially in patients with rheumatoid arthritis, and the risk of graft fracture.[8]

Currently, the two primary techniques of internal fixation are intramedullary rod fixation[6,22,24] and plate fixation.[14,23] Intramedullary rod fixation is indicated in patients with rheumatoid arthritis and osteopenic bone,[7,15,17] and plate fixation is preferred in those with noninflammatory arthritis.[13,16,37,40]

AO/ASIF PLATE FIXATION

Plate and screw fixation (Figure 110-1) is our method of choice for wrist arthrodesis in healthy, active patients with good bone stock.*

Plate Fixation Technique

A dorsal longitudinal approach is used for plate fixation, centered over Lister's tubercle (Figure 110-1, *A*). It extends from 4 cm proximal to Lister's tubercle to the level of the neck of the third metacarpal. Raising thick subcutaneous flaps off the extensor retinaculum decreases the chance of flap necrosis and injury to the superficial sensory nerves.

The extensor retinaculum is incised over the third compartment (Figure 110-1, *B*), and the extensor pollicis longus (EPL) tendon is retracted radially. Careful subperiosteal elevation of the fourth and fifth dorsal compartments exposes the distal radius and wrist-joint capsule (Figure 101-1, *C*).

The wrist capsule is then incised longitudinally. The distal radius and carpus are exposed in addition to the proximal 2 to 3 cm of the third metacarpal shaft. The joint surfaces are prepared by denuding articular cartilage and subchondral bone with osteotomes or rongeurs (Figure 110-1, *D*). The following joints are always included in the fusion mass: radiocarpal, capitolunate, capitohamate, scaphocapitate, and third metacarpal capitate. Fusion of the remaining intercarpal joints is optional.

We prefer the specially designed AO/ASIF wrist arthrodesis plate for fixation (Figure 110-2, *A* and *B*).[29] This plate is precontoured and has holes for 2.7-mm screw fixation in the metacarpal and carpal bones, and 3.5-mm screws for the distal radius. The plate is positioned over the third metacarpal to permit placement of three bicortical screws. The length of the plate should allow three or four screws to be placed in the distal radius and one or two lag screws in the carpal bones. Next, cancellous bone, usually obtained from the hip, is packed between the previously prepared articular surfaces.

*References 13, 14, 16, 23, 25, 37, 39.

The wound is closed in layers over a suction drain. The extensor retinaculum is transposed below the extensor pollicis longus tendon. A bulky dressing and a palmar splint are applied. Early finger motion is encouraged after surgery, and measures to control edema are employed. A splint is worn for approximately 4 weeks.

INTRAMEDULLARY ROD FIXATION

Patients with rheumatoid arthritis usually have poor bone stock and wound-healing capacity, which preclude the use of a plate. Clayton and Mannerfelt[6] and Malmsten[22] described the use of an intramedullary rod for wrist arthrodesis in this population. Millender and Nalebuff's[24] more recent description of this procedure is popular.

Intramedullary Rod Fixation Technique

A dorsal approach is also favored for intramedullary rod fixation. Often, there is tenosynovitis and pathology of the distal ulna that must be addressed. The extensor retinaculum is incised over the distal end of the ulna and reflected radially.[6,34] The extensor compartments are exposed, permitting tenosynovectomy and ulnar head resection when necessary.

The bony surfaces are prepared, and the third metacarpal head is exposed through a short longitudinal incision. The metacarpal head is dorsally penetrated using an awl to gain access to the medullary canal. Progressively larger Steinmann pins are inserted retrograde until there is snug contact between the medullary canal and pin. The pin is then driven through the carpus and down the shaft of the radius. Image intensification facilitates this process. If the pin and wrist position are acceptable, the pin is cut flush with the metacarpal head and countersunk into the third metacarpal (Figure 110-3, *A* and *B*). Alternatively, the pin can be placed between the second and third or third and fourth metacarpals. The use of the Steinmann pin places the wrist in neutral flexion/extension. The degree of radial/ulnar deviation depends on whether the pin exits in the second or third interspace.[6,24,34]

Bone graft is applied, usually from the ulnar head if it has been resected. The capsule is approximated, and the extensor retinaculum is transposed deep to the extensor tendons and repaired to stabilize the distal ulna.[6]

Postoperative management is similar to that for plate fixation. A short volar splint is worn for 4 weeks, and early digital motion is emphasized.

RADIOCAPITOHAMATE FUSION

Liebolt[18] recommended proximal row carpectomy for the correction of severe flexion deformities, such as in spastic cerebral palsy, followed by fusion of the radius to the distal carpal row. Louis[19] has more recently advocated this technique. Most of the proximal carpal row is removed, leaving only the distal 20% of the scaphoid to prevent proximal migration of the distal carpal row. The distal carpal row is then

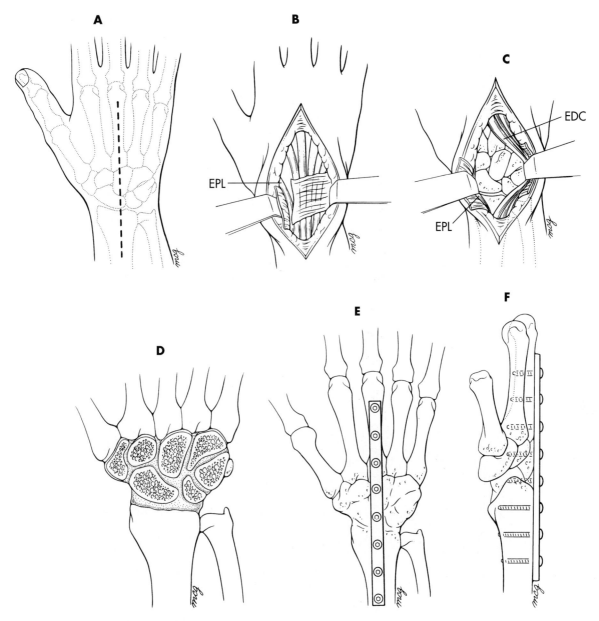

Figure 110-1. Surgical technique of wrist arthrodesis using plate fixation. **A,** A dorsal longitudinal skin incision is made in line with the third metacarpal. **B,** The extensor retinaculum is exposed and incised over the third dorsal compartment. **C,** The extensor pollicis longus tendon is retracted radially, and the fourth and fifth dorsal compartments are subperiosteally elevated. The wrist capsule is then incised to expose the distal radius, carpal bones, and the base of the third metacarpal. **D,** The joint surfaces to be fused are prepared by denuding articular cartilage and subchondral bone. **E** and **F,** The plate and screws are placed with three bicortical screws in the third metacarpal and three or four in the distal radius. Additional cancellous screws can be placed in the carpus.

fused to the distal radius. Kirschner wires (K wires) or staples are used for fixation.

SUPPLEMENTAL FIXATION

Supplemental fixation may be necessary if the methods described above fail to achieve a solid construct. Staples or K wires have been utilized, most often in patients with rheumatoid arthritis.[7,24] Staples, however, may loosen in osteopenic bone, and K wires may cause pin-track infections. We prefer a 22-gauge figure-of-eight tension band wire as described by Wood[38] (Figure 110-3, *B*). This technique stabilizes the bone graft and provides internal compression, especially when the arthrodesis is performed with an intramedullary rod.

Controversial Issues: Surgical Approaches

Most surgeons favor a dorsal approach, but Smith-Petersen[31] and MacKenzie[21] advocated an ulnar approach to minimize

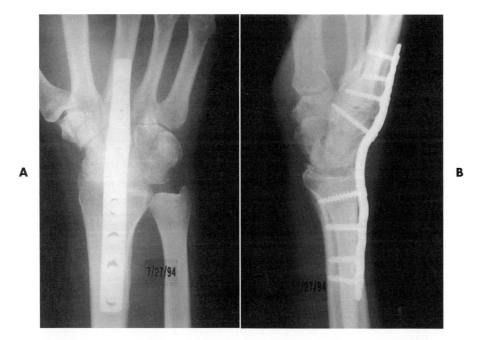

Figure 110-2. **A,** Anteroposterior (AP) wrist radiograph after arthrodesis with the AO/ASIF wrist arthrodesis plate. The plate is tapered distally to minimize its prominence over the third metacarpal. **B,** Lateral wrist radiograph after arthrodesis with an AO/ASIF plate. The plate has a low distal profile and is precontoured to provide slight extension of the wrist.

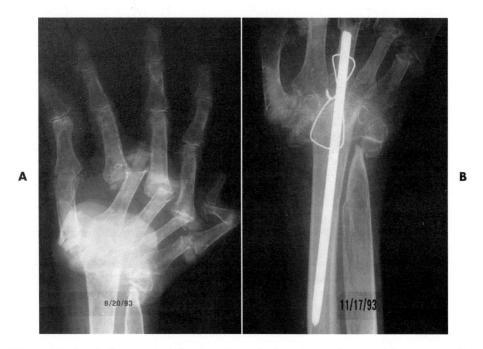

Figure 110-3. **A,** Preoperative AP wrist radiograph of a patient with severe deformity caused by rheumatoid arthritis. **B,** AP radiograph of the same wrist 3 months after wrist arthrodesis using intramedullary rod fixation. A figure-of-eight tension band wire was placed for supplemental rotational stability.

the chance of extensor tendon adhesions. The ulnar head is resected in this technique and used as bone graft.

Haddad and Riordan[12] recommended a radial approach between the first and second dorsal compartments. They placed a corticocancellous block from the iliac crest into a slot across the radius, intercarpal joints, and second and third carpometacarpal joints. This approach has the advantage of avoiding the distal radioulnar joint and the extensor tendons, thereby minimizing adhesion formation.

POSITION OF FUSION

Several authors have attempted to define the functional range of motion of the normal wrist joint to extrapolate the best position for wrist arthrodesis. Most activities of daily living are performed with 10 degrees of flexion, 30 to 40 degrees of extension, and a 25-to 40-degree arc of radial and ulnar deviation. Personal hygiene and activities requiring manual dexterity necessitate some wrist flexion.[4,26,30] Pryce[27] determined that ulnar deviation provides the optimum position for power grip and found no advantage of wrist extension over neutral. There was a decrease in grip strength with flexion of the wrist or more than 15 degrees of ulnar deviation.

There is no consensus, however, on the optimal position for wrist arthrodesis in clinical records. Larsson[16] noted increased grip strength in both rheumatoid and nonrheumatoid patients with wrist fusion in extension. Wright and McMurtry,[39] using AO plate fixation, failed to show any such improvement in either patient population.

Most authors support Clayton's assertion that the neutral position is most functional for hygiene and activities of daily living in patients with rheumatoid arthritis.* Clayton and Ferlic defined the neutral position for wrist arthrodesis as 0 degrees in the sagittal plane and 10 degrees of ulnar deviation in the frontal plane. They suggested that in this position, pronation and supination can best substitute for wrist flexion and extension. Millender and Nalebuff[24] found no functional difference in patients with rheumatoid arthritis whose wrists were fused in slight extension than those fused in neutral. Most authors position patients undergoing bilateral wrist arthrodeses with one wrist in neutral flexion/extension and the other wrist in slight flexion to aid in personal hygiene.[28,35]

Ten to 30 degrees of wrist extension is recommended in patients with high load demands, such as manual laborers. Plate fixation is commonly used in this patient population, and slight ulnar deviation is achieved by alignment of the radius with the third metacarpal.

Joints Included in Fusion Mass

It is generally agreed that the radiocarpal joint and the midcarpal joints around the capitate should be fused (Figure 110-4). Fusion of the remaining intercarpal joints is optional. The scapho-trapezial-trapezoid joint is usually avoided, unless it is involved in the degenerative process. The ulnar midcarpal joints are also usually left undisturbed. There is disagreement as to whether the second carpometacarpal (CMC) joint should be fused. Some authors advocate leaving these joints undisturbed, stating that this motion is important in power grip and may even increase after wrist fusion.[1,13] Bolano and Green[2] chose to fuse both the second and third CMC joints, out of concern that arthritis of the joints would develop after wrist fusion. Larsson[16] and Wright and McMurtry,[39] in contrast,

*References 6, 15, 22, 24, 34, 35.

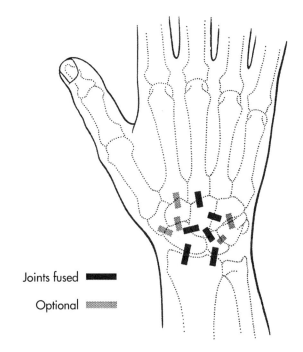

Figure 110-4. Diagram indicating joints to be included in the fusion mass when performing wrist arthrodesis (solid black bar). The shaded bars denote joints that may be arthrodesed if indicated (see text).

routinely remove the plate to leave the CMC joints unfused. O'Bierne et al[25] reported good results without fusing the CMC joints and without plate removal. Hastings et al[13] did not recommend plate removal but did recommend fusion of the third CMC joint. They were concerned that metal fatigue could lead to plate failure and pain. They did not recommend fusion of the second CMC joint unless degenerative changes were noted.

Bone Graft

Another point of controversy is the use of bone graft. The issue is whether a bone graft is necessary, what type of graft should be used, and from where should it be harvested. Most techniques use an iliac crest graft. Initially, structural corticocancellous grafts were harvested; however, with internal fixation, there was less need for structural grafts, and purely cancellous bone was utilized.[1,5] Hastings et al[13] found no difference in the time required for fusion with plate fixation in patients with autogenous corticocancellous graft compared with those with a purely cancellous autogenous graft.

Donor morbidity from the iliac crest graft has fostered a search for alternative sources of bone graft. Bone graft is usually taken from the resected ulnar head in patients with rheumatoid arthritis.[6,24] Weiss and Hastings[37] reported excellent results after wrist arthrodesis with plate fixation and cancellous bone graft from the distal radius. Several authors have used corticocancellous bone grafts taken from the distal radius.[6,32,38] Local bone graft harvest also permits the use of regional, rather than general, anesthesia.[38]

OUTCOMES

The diversity of diagnoses for which wrist arthrodesis is performed, and the varied techniques that have been used to achieve that goal, complicate any attempts to compare outcomes. No uniform method of objective or subjective evaluation has been established. Current objective parameters include radiographic evidence of fusion and strength measurements. Objective systems to evaluate function have been used but vary from study to study. Subjective evaluations of patient satisfaction are inconsistently reported, making comparisons difficult.

Excellent results have been reported using intramedullary rod fixation in patients with rheumatoid arthritis. Millender and Nalebuff[24] reported on 70 wrist fusions using an intramedullary Steinmann pin. Sixty-eight patients had successful fusion and relief of pain. Stability, strength, and dexterity were improved, but the method of assessment was not reported. Although some patients noted minor functional impairments, most adjusted to the lack of motion and felt the procedure was beneficial.[24] Kobus and Turner[15] reported 97% excellent or good results in 87 patients with wrist fusions performed using a Steinmann pin. Interestingly, the four dissatisfied patients had an arthroplasty on the contralateral wrist. Nine other patients with contralateral wrist arthroplasty were satisfied. Complications occurred in 23%, and half of these were caused by prominence of the Steinmann pin. Other complications included carpal tunnel syndrome and superficial wound slough.[15]

Patient assessments after wrist arthrodesis for posttraumatic arthritis also show excellent results. O'Bierne reported 100% union at an average of 10 weeks. Approximately 75% of these patients reported improvement in hand and wrist function.[25] Weiss and Hastings[37] reported a 100% fusion rate in 28 patients treated with plate fixation. Radiographic fusion was noted at an average of 10 weeks. Thirteen patients returned to full activity in their same job. The average period of disability was 10 weeks.

Hastings et al[13] retrospectively reviewed 89 patients after wrist fusion for posttraumatic osteoarthritis. They found statistically significant differences in the fusion and complication rates of wrists treated with plate fixation, compared with those fused by other methods. Approximately 98% of patients treated with plate fixation achieved fusion in 10 weeks, whereas with other methods an 82% fusion rate was noted, with union at an average of 12 weeks. Complications occurred less frequently in patients treated with plate fixation (51% compared with 79%), but the complications required operative treatment 59% of the time compared with 21% in the group treated with alternative techniques. The plate-fixation group returned to work at an average of 24 weeks after surgery, compared with 40 weeks for those without plate fixation. This difference, however, was not statistically significant.

Bolano and Green[2] compared 18 patients treated by radiocapitohamate arthrodesis with eight patients treated with compression plate fixation. The patients with plate fixation all fused, and there was one fibrous union in the group that received radiocapitohamate arthrodesis. Two patients in that group had painful CMC motion that required secondary surgery. There were no statistical outcome differences in the two groups.[2]

Plate fixation is generally not recommended in patients with rheumatoid arthritis because of poor screw purchase in osteopenic bone and diminished wound healing capacity. Bracey et al[3] reported a 17% nonunion rate in rheumatoid patients in which plate fixation was used. In another series, all three nonunions in a group of 46 arthrodeses occurred in patients with rheumatoid arthritis.[39] Larsson,[16] on the other hand, reported a 100% fusion rate using plate fixation in 17 patients with rheumatoid arthritis.

COMPLICATIONS

The complications of wrist fusion have been addressed specifically in two reports.[8,40] Clendenin and Green[8] reviewed the complications of 31 fusions using methods other than plate fixation. Major complications occurred in nine patients (29%) and included pseudarthrosis, graft fracture, deep wound infection, neuroma of the superficial radial nerve, and impingement of the Steinmann pin. The rate of pseudarthrosis was between 8% and 29%, depending on the surgical technique. Fourteen minor complications occurred in 13 patients (45%). The most common were skin necrosis and transient superficial radial nerve problems. Overall, wound problems occurred in 23% of patients and infection in 3%.[8]

Zachary and Stern[40] reported on the complications after 73 fusions in 71 patients using plate fixation. Eighty-two total complications in 50 patients were retrospectively identified, of which 63 resolved spontaneously. The complications were defined as short term, persisting for less than 3 months, and long-term, persisting more than 3 months. No pseudarthroses were encountered. The most common short-term complication was related to wound healing (25%), either at the wrist incision or the iliac graft donor site. The most common long-term complication was irritation caused by the plate. The next most common complication was distal radioulnar joint disorders secondary to arthrosis or ulnocarpal abutment. Secondary surgery was performed for plate removal, arthritis of the distal radioulnar joint, acute carpal tunnel syndrome, and extensor tendon adhesions. Unexplained wrist pain, fracture of the metacarpal or radius, scapho-trapezial-trapezoid arthritis, metacarpophalangeal (MCP) joint stiffness, and neurologic deficits were also encountered. The most common residual difficulty after arthrodesis was chronic pain, experienced by six patients.

Trumble et al[36] reported a series of three patients with ulnocarpal abutment after wrist arthrodesis with an AO plate and iliac crest bone graft. They treated all three cases with carpal resection to relieve pain that was occurring on forearm rotation. They recommended carpal resection rather than resection of the distal ulna because of concerns for instability of the distal ulna.

REFERENCES

1. Abbott LC, Saunders JBDM, Bost FC: Arthrodesis of the wrist with the use of grafts of cancellous bone, *J Bone Joint Surg* 24:883-898, 1942.

2. Bolano LE, Green DP: Wrist arthrodesis in post-traumatic arthritis: a comparison of two methods, *J Hand Surg [Am]* 18:786-791, 1993.

3. Bracey DJ, McMurtry RY, Walton D: Arthrodesis in the rheumatoid hand using the AO technique, *Orthop Rev* 9:65-69, 1980.

4. Brumfield RH, Champoux JA: A biomechanical study of normal functional wrist motion, *Clin Orthop* 187:23-25, 1984.

5. Carroll RE, Dick HM: Arthrodesis of the wrist for rheumatoid arthritis, *J Bone Joint Surg* 53A:1365-1369, 1971.

6. Clayton ML: Surgical treatment at the wrist in rheumatoid arthritis, *J Bone Joint Surg* 47A:741-750, 1965.

7. Clayton ML, Ferlic DC: Arthrodesis of the arthritic wrist, *Clin Orthop* 187:89-93, 1984.

8. Clendenin MB, Green DP: Arthrodesis of the wrist: complications and their management, *J Hand Surg [Am]* 6:253-257, 1981.

9. Dick HM: Wrist arthrodesis. In Green DP (editor): *Operative hand surgery,* ed 3, New York, 1993, Churchill Livingstone.

10. Ely LW: A study of joint tuberculosis, *Surg Gynecol Obstet* 10:561-572, 1910.

11. Ely LW: An operation for tuberculosis of the wrist, *JAMA* 75:1707-1709, 1920.

12. Haddad RJJ, Riordan DC: Arthrodesis of the wrist: a surgical technique, *J Bone Joint Surg* 49A:950-954, 1967.

13. Hastings H II, Weiss A-PC, Quenzer D, et al: Arthrodesis of the wrist for posttraumatic disorders, *J Bone Joint Surg* 78A:897-902, 1996.

14. Heim U, Pfeiffer KM: *Internal fixation of small fractures: technique recommended by the AO-ASIF Group,* ed 3, Berlin, 1988, Springer-Verlag, pp 145-178.

15. Kobus RJ, Turner RH: Wrist arthrodesis for treatment of rheumatoid arthritis, *J Hand Surg [Am]* 15:541-546, 1990.

16. Larsson SE: Compression arthrodesis of the wrist: a consecutive series of 23 cases, *Clin Orthop* 99:146-153, 1974.

17. Lee DH, Carroll RE: Wrist arthrodesis: a combined intramedullary pin and autogenous iliac crest bone graft technique, *J Hand Surg [Am]* 19:733-740, 1994.

18. Liebolt FL: Surgical fusion of the wrist joint, *Surg Gynecol Obstet* 66:1008-1023, 1938.

19. Louis DS, Hankin F, Bowers WH: Capitate radius fusion in the spastic upper extremity: an alternative to wrist arthrodesis, *J Hand Surg [Am]* 9:365-369, 1984.

20. Louis DS, Hankin FM: Arthrodesis of the wrist: past and present, *J Hand Surg [Am]* 11:787-789, 1986.

21. MacKenzie IG: Arthrodesis of the wrist in reconstructive surgery, *J Bone Joint Surg* 42B:60-64, 1960.

22. Mannerfelt L, Malmsten M: Arthrodesis of the wrist in rheumatoid arthritis: a technique without external fixation, *Scand J Plast Reconstr Surg* 5:124-130, 1971.

23. Meuli HC: Reconstructive surgery of the wrist joint, *Hand* 4:88-90, 1972.

24. Millender LH, Nalebuff EA: Arthrodesis of the rheumatoid wrist: an evaluation of sixty patients and a description of a different surgical technique, *J Bone Joint Surg* 55A:1026-1034, 1973.

25. O'Bierne J, Boyer MI, Axelrod TS: Wrist arthrodesis using a dynamic compression plate, *J Bone Joint Surg* 77B:700-704, 1995.

26. Palmer AK, Werner FK, Murphy D: Functional wrist motion: a biomechanical study, *J Hand Surg [Am]* 10:39-46, 1985.

27. Pryce JC: The wrist position between neutral and ulnar deviation that facilitates the maximum power grip strength, *J Biomech* 13:505-511, 1980.

28. Rayan GM, Brentlinger A, Purnell D, Garcia-Moral CA: Functional assessment of bilateral wrist arthrodeses, *J Hand Surg [Am]* 12:1020-1024, 1987.

29. Richards RR, Patterson SD, Hearn TC: A special plate for arthrodesis of the wrist: design considerations and biomechanical testing, *J Hand Surg [Am]* 18:476-483, 1993.

30. Ryu J, Cooney WP III, Askew LP, et al: Functional ranges of motion of the wrist joint, *J Hand Surg [Am]* 16:409-419, 1991.

31. Smith-Petersen MN: A new approach to the wrist joint, *J Bone Joint Surg* 22:122-124, 1940.

32. Sorial R, Tonkin MA, Gschwind C: Wrist arthrodesis using a sliding radial graft and plate fixation, *J Hand Surg* 19B:217-220, 1994.

33. Steindler A: Problems of the reconstruction of the hand, *Surg Gynecol Obstet* 27:317-325, 1918.

34. Straub LR, Ranawat CS: The wrist in rheumatoid arthritis: surgical treatment and results, *J Bone Joint Surg* 51A:1-20, 1969.

35. Taleisnik J: Rheumatoid arthritis of the wrist, *Hand Clin* 5:257-278, 1989.

36. Trumble TE, Easterling KJ, Smith RJ: Ulnocarpal abutment after wrist arthrodesis, *J Hand Surg [Am]* 13:11-15, 1988.

37. Weiss A-PC, Hastings H II: Wrist arthrodesis for traumatic conditions: a study of plate and local bone graft application, *J Hand Surg [Am]* 20:50-56, 1995.

38. Wood MB: Wrist arthrodesis using dorsal radial bone graft, *J Hand Surg [Am]* 12:208-212, 1987.

39. Wright CS, McMurtry RY: AO arthrodesis in the hand, *J Hand Surg [Am]* 8:932-935, 1983.

40. Zachary SV, Stern PJ: Complications following AO/ASIF wrist arthrodesis, *J Hand Surg [Am]* 20:339-344, 1995.

PART V

TENDONS

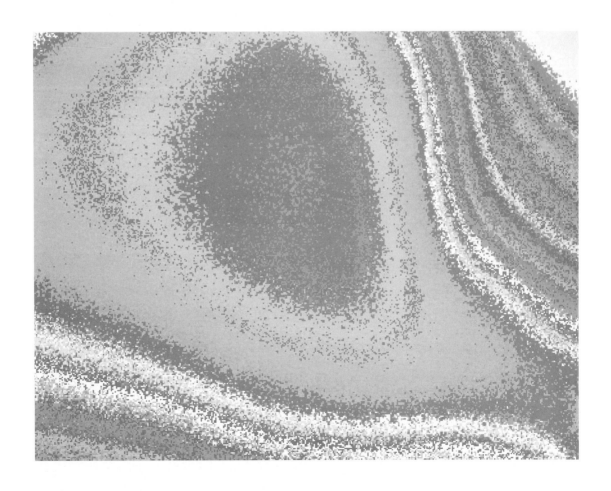

Flexor Tendons

111

W. P. Andrew Lee
Bing Siang Gan
Stephen U. Harris

INTRODUCTION

Flexor tendon injury is one of the most common hand injuries. It often occurs in young individuals in the prime of their lives, resulting in significant socioeconomic impact. The surgeon's goal for all patients with flexor tendon injuries is an expeditious return to full function.

Flexor tendon surgery historically has undergone continued evolution. In the second century, Galen strongly discouraged flexor tendon repair, stating that it would lead to convulsions. In the tenth century, Avicenna encouraged flexor tendon repairs, but his teachings were lost as a result of the prominence of the Galenian doctrine. Little progress was made until the mid-nineteenth century when Syme reported several successful cases of flexor tendon repair. The work of pioneer surgeons in the twentieth century such as Lexer, Mayer, Bunnell, Verdan, Mason, Allan, Kleinert, Manske, Pulvertaft, and Littler contributed significantly to the current practice and results.[31]

Despite modern advances, good results after flexor tendon repair are not uniformly obtained. Sterling Bunnell, in the early twentieth century, first promulgated the basic principles of flexor tendon repair that we still use today. He considered flexor tendon anatomy and physiology, advocated atraumatic surgical technique, described postoperative rehabilitation, and cautiously named the area within the digital flexor sheath "no man's land." Primary repairs in this area were found to perform so poorly that surgeons were advised not to repair the tendon injuries in this zone and to resort to secondary tendon grafting.

The techniques and indications of flexor tendon repair have evolved significantly in the last few decades. Primary repair of injured flexor tendons within the digital sheath is currently accepted as the preferred method of treatment. Laboratory and clinical investigations have been conducted to better understand the structure, function, and biomechanics of the flexor tendons, as well as their biological response to injury and repair.[67] Nevertheless, significant debate still exists regarding the specific methods of tendon repair and rehabilitation.

Much work remains to be done in the basic mechanisms of tendon healing and adhesion formation, adjunctive treatment for flexor tendon repair, and postoperative mobilization protocols.

ANATOMY

The flexor tendon system of the hand consists of intrinsic and extrinsic components. The extrinsic flexor tendons include the flexor digitorum profundus (FDP), flexor digitorum superficialis (FDS), and flexor pollicis longus (FPL). The distal interphalangeal (DIP) joints of index, middle, ring, and small fingers are flexed by their corresponding FDP tendons, whereas the proximal interphalangeal (PIP) joints are flexed by the FDS tendons. The interphalangeal joint of the thumb is flexed by the FPL tendon. The intrinsic flexor muscles include the lumbrical muscles, which flex the metacarpophalangeal (MCP) joints and extend the interphalangeal joints.

FLEXOR DIGITORUM PROFUNDUS

The FDP muscles arise from the proximal volar surface of the ulna and the ulnar half of the forearm interosseous membrane. Anatomic variations include an origin from the medial border of the proximal radius just distal to the radial tuberosity. The FDP muscle divides into an ulnar and radial bundle in the mid-forearm. The radial bundle travels to the index finger, and the ulnar bundle forms a common tendon to the middle, ring, and small fingers. The profundus tendon to each individual finger branches off proximal to the carpal tunnel and inserts on the volar proximal aspect of the respective distal phalanx. The FDP muscles to the index and middle fingers are typically innervated by the anterior interosseous nerve, which is a branch from the median nerve, whereas the FDP to the ring and small fingers are innervated by the ulnar nerve. The blood supply to the FDP muscle bellies arises from the ulnar anterior interosseous and the common interosseous arteries. The FDP tendons are vascularized at the wrist and mid-palm by branches of the superficial palmar arch. There is a segmental blood supply in the digits within each flexor tendon sheath arising from both digital arteries that reaches the tendon through the vincular system (Figure 111-1). (See section on tendon nutrition and healing, p. 1965.)

FLEXOR DIGITORUM SUPERFICIALIS

The FDS originates from two places. The ulnar head arises from the medial upper epicondyle of the humerus and the medial ligamentous complex of the elbow along with the other muscles that form the flexor pronator group. The radial head arises from a 6-to 8-cm area distal to the radial tuberosity. The superficialis muscle belly divides in the middle third of the forearm into four distinct bundles traveling to the four ulnar digits. The superficialis tendon to the small finger is subject to considerable variation and may be completely absent. Approximately 35% of all hands have some deficiency of the small-finger FDS, with a fifth of these hands having flexion power transmitted from the ring-finger FDS. The FDS tendons insert in the fingers along the volar aspect of the middle phalanx of the fingers. The superficialis muscles are innervated by the median nerve. The blood supply is provided by branches of the ulnar artery, as well as contributions from the radial artery. The FDS tendons are supplied at the wrist and palm through branches of the superficial palmar arch. As with the profundus tendons, the blood supply within the digital flexor tendon sheath is provided through the vincular system of the digital arteries.

FLEXOR POLLICIS LONGUS

The FPL originates in the mid-portion of the forearm from the volar radius, the interosseous membrane, and the coronoid process. It is the most radial tendon in the carpal canal. The FPL inserts on the volar proximal portion of the distal phalanx of the thumb. The FPL is innervated by the anterior interosseous nerve and its blood supply is through muscular perforators from the radial artery. The FPL is usually supplied by two distinct vincula within the tendon sheath of the thumb.

LUMBRICAL MUSCLES

The lumbrical muscles are unique because they arise from and insert into tendons. The lumbrical muscles to the index and middle fingers are unipennate, arising from the volar radial surface of the profundus tendons to the respective digit just distal to the carpal canal. The lumbrical muscles to the ring and small fingers are bipennate, arising from the profundus tendons of the corresponding digits and the radially adjacent profundus tendons. The muscles then pass through the lumbrical canal on the radial side of the digits volar to the deep transverse metacarpal ligament and insert into the radial aspect of the extensor mechanism dorsal hood. Their function is to facilitate interphalangeal (IP) joint extension irrespective of MCP joint position, and to initiate MCP flexion. The innervation to the lumbrical muscle corresponds to the nerve that innervates the associated profundus tendon. The lumbricals to the index and middle fingers are thus innervated by the median nerve, and those to the ring and small fingers are innervated by the ulnar nerve. The blood supply to the lumbricals arises from muscular branches of both the deep and superficial palmar arches.

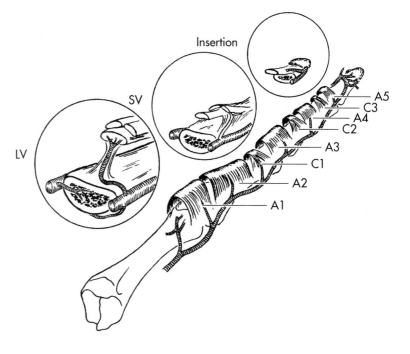

Figure 111-1. Flexor tendon perfusion within the tendon sheath is derived partly from the segmental branches of digital arteries via the vincular system.

ANATOMIC RELATIONSHIPS BETWEEN FLEXOR TENDONS

The FDS tendons in the distal forearm lie volar to the FDP tendons, with the FDS to the middle and ring fingers volar to the FDS to the index and small fingers. The FDP tendons to the digits lie in a single plane deep to FDS tendons. This configuration is maintained from the distal forearm through the carpal tunnel. The median nerve courses through the forearm in the deep fascia of the FDS muscles, superficial to the FDP muscles. Distal to the carpal tunnel the FDS tendons come to lie in a single plane volar to the FDP tendons. Each FDS tendon splits at the level of the distal palmar crease into two slips that diverge and wrap around the FDP tendon. The two slips of the FDS tendon then merge with one another dorsal to the FDP tendon and insert along the volar proximal aspect of the middle phalanx. The decussation of the FDS tendon immediately distal to where the FDP tendon pierces the two slips is called *Camper's chiasm.* The FDP tendon traverses beyond the DIP joint and inserts on the volar proximal aspect of the distal phalanx (Figure 111-2).

Fibroosseous Sheath/Vincular System

All digits have a synovium-lined flexor tendon sheath, which is reinforced by a fibrous pulley system. The synovial membrane of the flexor tendon sheath consists of two layers, a visceral layer around the structures within the sheath and a parietal layer covering the internal aspect of the pulley system. The flexor tendon sheath allows smooth tendon gliding and maintains an enclosed synovial sheath, facilitating tendon nutrition by synovial diffusion. Each flexor tendon also receives blood supply within the tendon sheath through the vincular system. In general, each tendon is supplied by a short vinculum (vinculum breve) and a long vinculum (vinculum longum) (Figure 111-3). The vinculum breve of the FDP (VBP) arises from the distal transverse digital artery from the radial and ulnar digital arteries at the level of the DIP joint and reaches the tendon through the mesotendon of the FDP. The vinculum breve of the FDS (VBS) arises from the central transverse digital artery at the level of the PIP joint, as does the vinculum longum of the FDP (VLP). The vinculum longum of the FDS (VLS) arises just distal to the MCP joint from the proximal transverse digital artery. The FPL in the thumb is also supplied by two vincula, one arising at the level of the IP joint and one arising at the level of the MCP joint.

PULLEY SYSTEM

The synovial flexor tendon sheath is reinforced by a system of fibrous pulleys, which increases the mechanical efficiency of the flexor tendons by preventing bow stringing of the tendons. There are five annular pulleys and three cruciform pulleys in the fingers (Figure 111-4).[14] In addition, it has been pointed out that the palmar aponeurosis serves a similar function as the digital pulleys and may be considered the most proximal part of the flexor pulley system.[55] The palmar aponeurosis pulley consists of transverse fibers that partially

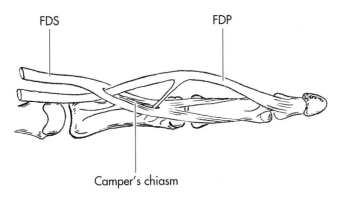

Figure 111-2. The relationship between FDP and FDS tendons along the volar aspect of the finger.

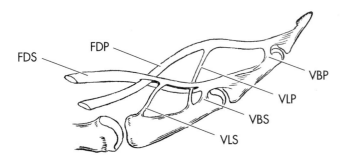

Figure 111-3. The FDP tendon is supplied by its vinculum breve (VBP) and vinculum longum (VLP). The FDS tendon is supplied by its vinculum breve (VBS) and vinculum longum (VLS).

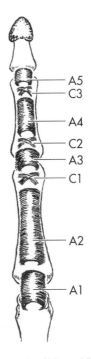

Figure 111-4. The annular (A1 to A5) and cruciform (C1 to C3) pulley systems of the flexor tendon sheath in the finger.

overlap the proximal end of the synovial flexor tendon sheath. It acts in conjunction with the two most proximal A1 and A2 annular pulleys. The A1 pulley is approximately 8 to 10 mm wide longitudinally and overlies the volar plate of the MCP joint. It becomes thickened in conjunction with flexor tenosynovitis and is the most common cause of trigger fingers. The A2 and A4 pulleys are located over the central aspects of the proximal and middle phalanges and are 18 to 20 and 10 to 12 mm wide, respectively. The A2 and A4 pulleys are generally considered the most important pulleys in that their disruption results in reduced mechanical efficiency during tendon excursion and consequently decreases flexion and grip strength. The smaller A3 and A5 annular pulleys are located over the volar plates of the PIP and DIP joints and are about 2 to 4 mm wide. The cruciform pulleys (C1, C2, and C3) are located proximal to the A3, A4, and A5 pulleys, respectively, and allow shortening of the pulley system in flexion.

The thumb pulley system is different because of its unique mobility and architecture of the thumb. There is one long oblique and two annular pulleys. The A1 and A2 pulleys are located over the volar plate of the MCP and IP joints, respectively, and the oblique pulley is located over the proximal phalanx. The oblique pulley is considered biomechanically the most important for thumb flexion.

FLEXOR TENDON ZONES

The level of flexor tendon injury carries a prognostic implication because of the different anatomic constraints to the flexor tendons over their course from the muscle belly in the forearm to their insertions in the phalanges. Verdan developed a uniform nomenclature that has now been accepted by most hand surgeons (Figure 111-5).[71] Zone I flexor tendon injuries occur in the area between the insertion of the FDS and FDP tendons. Zone II extends from the insertion of the FDS tendons to the level of the A1 pulleys. Zone III lies between the level of the A1 pulleys, and the distal limit of the carpal canal. Zone IV is the area of flexor tendons that lies within the carpal canal. Zone V is between the entrance to the carpal canal and the musculotendinous junction. There are also five zones in the thumb. Zone I lies distal to the IP joint, Zone II extends from the A1 pulley to the IP joint. Zone III is the area around the thenar eminence between the carpal tunnel and the A1 pulley. Zones IV and V correspond to Zones IV and V of the fingers. Zone II, where the tendons are enclosed within the fibroosseous sheath, has been termed *"no man's land"* because of the generally worse outcome associated with flexor tendon repairs in this area enclosed within the fibroosseous sheath.

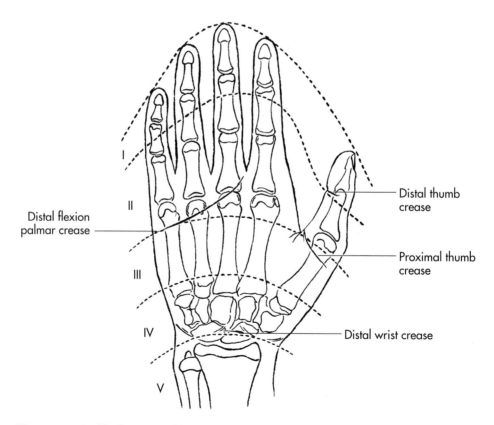

Figure 111-5. Verdan zones of flexor tendon injury are associated with prognostic implication.

INCISIONS

Incisions used to perform flexor tendon surgery should be extensile and aimed at providing sufficient exposure of the flexor tendons, the fibroosseous sheath, and adjacent neurovascular bundles. In addition, the incisions should not perpendicularly cross flexion creases to prevent later scar contracture. Placement of scars should also be minimized on important tactile areas of the hand, such as the ulnar side of the thumb and small finger or the radial side of the index, middle, and ring fingers.[9] The Bruner zigzag incision provides a superb exposure of the flexor tendons and all volar structures (Figure 111-6). Old scars from trauma or previous surgical procedures can often be incorporated in the incision, which can be readily extended into the palm. The neurovascular bundles do not need to be mobilized with the skin flaps and remain in their anatomic location. The mid-lateral incision, in contrast, preserves the tactile areas of the digits better than a Bruner incision (see Figure 111-6), and there is less likelihood of tendon exposure in cases of poor wound healing or infection. There is, however, an increased potential for injury to the dorsal nerve branches, particularly when the neurovascular bundles are mistakenly dissected with the volar flap. Combinations of a mid-lateral and volar zigzag approach have been advocated in an effort to combine their respective advantages.[23]

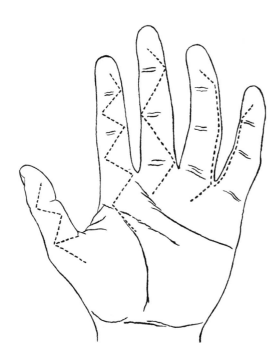

Figure 111-6. Surgical exposure to flexor tendons and other volar structures is best obtained through Bruner zigzag or mid-lateral incisions.

TENDON NUTRITION AND HEALING

Recent advances in the management of flexor tendon injuries have resulted from enhanced appreciation of tendon nutrition, healing, and biomechanics. Understanding the mechanism of flexor tendon healing has evolved over the last 2 decades. Flexor tendons within the digital sheath were regarded in the past as relatively inactive and poorly vascularized structures whose repair after injury required the ingrowth of cells and vessels from surrounding scar tissue. Experimental evidence has since demonstrated that the flexor tendon has a dual source of nutrition from both vascular and synovial diffusion. Furthermore, the tendons are capable of actively participating in the repair process through a process of *intrinsic healing*, independent of surrounding adhesions.[42]

The vascular anatomy of the flexor tendons has been well described. The tendons from the distal forearm to the digital sheath receive their blood supply through longitudinally oriented segmental vessels that run in the paratenon. The tendons receive vascular supply within the digital sheath through the vincular system, which leaves a relatively avascular area on the volar aspect of the tendons and a watershed area between the long and short vincular systems of both the FDS and the FDP tendons. Lundborg has shown that the diffusion of nutrients to the flexor tendons from synovial fluid within the digital sheath is more important than the vascular perfusion.[39,40]

The concept that tendon healing is dependent entirely on cells migrating into the repair area from outside the tendon is known as *extrinsic healing*. This idea was promulgated by Peacock[54] and Potenza.[56] This idea was challenged by in vivo and in vitro experiments that proved that tenocytes are capable of proliferating, producing collagen, and reconstructing their own gliding surface in the absence of adhesion ingrowth.[4] Further research has also shown that early tendon motion has a role in the modification of the repair response. Gelberman and Woo,[20] in a series of dog experiments, compared the strength and excursion characteristics of tendon repairs in dogs treated with immobilization, delayed motion, and early motion. Mobilized tendons showed progressively greater ultimate load compared with immobilized tendons. The strength of early mobilized tendons was also two to three times greater than the immobilized tendons at 3 weeks.[20] Histologic differences in the healing processes between immobilized and mobilized flexor tendons has also been demonstrated. These studies confirmed "Wolff's law" of connective tissue, which states that the strength of a healing tendon is proportional to the controlled stress applied to it.[43,44]

The dynamic phases of intrinsic tendon healing occur in three stages: inflammation, active repair, and remodeling.[8] The inflammatory phase is characterized by epitenon proliferation within 1 cm of the repair site. High levels of fibronectin are found within the repair site and are chemotactic for fibroblasts. Macrophages and other inflammatory cells accumulate in the repair site and function to debride nonviable tissues. During the phase of active repair, epitenon fibroblasts secrete type I collagen to unite the tendon ends. The repair site is biochemically weakest from 10 to 15 days after the repair, and thereafter begins to strengthen. The collagen in the repair site continues to strengthen during the remodeling phase. These processes are modulated by the stresses of controlled early motion.

No present-day tendon repair technique can predictably isolate the healing tendon ends from the ingrowth of adhesions from the surrounding tissues. Attempts at preventing the ingrowth of adhesions by wrapping the tenorrhaphy site or by the use of pharmacologic agents has not achieved widespread clinical use. Oral ibuprofen has been shown to significantly reduce adhesions at the tenorrhaphy site in a primate model.[32] In one prospective double-blind study, hyaluronate injected into the tendon sheath at the time of tendon repair had no statistically significant effect on subsequent total active motion.[22]

BIOMECHANICS OF DIGITAL FLEXION

A clear understanding of the biomechanical coordination of finger flexion is essential to the appropriate treatment and rehabilitation of patients with flexor tendon injuries. Electromyographic studies have shown that the FDP is the primary effector of finger flexion. The FDS and interosseous muscles also come into play with more forceful digital flexion.

The total effect or moment of a muscle at a joint is related to the force or tension times the leverage, defined as the *moment arm* or perpendicular distance between the axis of the joint and the tendon that crosses the joint. This explains why pulley resection, which causes bowstringing of the digital flexor tendons, results in decreased flexion efficiency. Increased tendon excursion is required to achieve the same degree of flexion. An increased moment arm also leads to diminished tendon excursion and joint flexion distally, a change in the balance of forces at that joint and the coordination of motion at other joints, decreased power of flexion, and an increased likelihood of flexion contracture and pulley rupture.[28]

It is important to appreciate the forces working across the IP and MCP joints to fully understand coordinated finger flexion. Landsmeer has shown that isolated extrinsic forces on the finger IP joints produces DIP-joint extension and PIP-joint flexion to achieve equilibrium while the PIP-MCP system collapses into a position of MCP-joint hyperextension and PIP-joint flexion. This is not seen in normal circumstances because of anatomic restraints and because of the presence of a third force that balances the biarticular systems of the DIP-PIP and PIP-MCP.[33] The FDP tendon is the only flexor of the DIP joint, but it can also flex the PIP joint. The DIP and PIP joints are linked by the oblique retinacular ligament (ORL), as well as differential loading of the extensor apparatus over the PIP joint. The ORL arises from the flexor sheath volar and proximal to the PIP joint and inserts into the dorsal aspect of

the DIP joint. When the FDP is activated, creating a flexion force at the DIP joint, the ORL is tightened. It will not allow DIP-joint flexion without PIP-joint flexion, thereby relaxing the ORL. Simultaneously, with PIP-joint flexion, the central slip and lateral bands of the extensor apparatus advance distally and relax the terminal extensor at the distal phalanx.

The third force in the PIP-MCP joint system is provided by the interosseous muscles. The interosseous muscles are silent in simple finger flexion. The extensor apparatus advances distally as the extrinsic finger flexors are activated and IP-joint flexion is initiated, thereby creating increased tension on the lateral bands at the level of the MCP joint. This affects simultaneous MCP-and PIP-joint flexion. Flexion of the MCP and PIP joints can be totally independent by the isolated pull of the intrinsic muscles with the extrinsic extensor tendon stabilizing the MCP joint in extension.[76]

ACUTE INJURIES OF THE FLEXOR TENDON

INDICATIONS

Mechanism of Flexor Tendon Injuries

The spectrum of hand injuries is varied, but the mechanisms by which flexor tendons can be injured can be classified as lacerations, avulsions, or ruptures. Flexor tendon lacerations can be partial or complete and are usually related to a known traumatic event. Flexor tendon avulsion is most commonly seen clinically at the distal phalangeal insertion of the profundus tendon. Ruptures may have several causes. A tendon would preferentially dehisce at the musculotendinous junction, through the muscle belly, or at its bony insertion,[52] but synovial inflammation is a common precipitating factor for tendon ruptures within their mid-substance in patients with collagen vascular disease. Avascular necrosis of the flexor tendons within the carpal tunnel has also been attributed to pressure from edematous synovial tissue in patients with rheumatoid arthritis.[15,16] Flexor tendon rupture in the rheumatoid patient most commonly results from attrition as the tendon moves across bone eroded by chronic synovitis.[17,70] Chronic attrition ruptures may also occur secondary to a Colles' fracture,[75] hamate fracture,[12] scaphoid nonunion,[41] and Kienböck's disease.[24,30,46] Finally, tendons may rupture as a result of intratendinous pathology in patients with gout or infection, or after a steroid injection.[25] The diagnosis and treatment of flexor tendon lacerations and avulsions will be described in this chapter, and those dealing with tendon rupture will be covered under the topic of rheumatoid arthritis.

Clinical Diagnosis of Flexor Tendon Injuries

The diagnosis of flexor tendon injury can usually be made by careful attention to the patient's history. The alert patient will complain of absent, weak, or painful flexion of the PIP and/or the DIP joints in the injured digit. It is important to ascertain the finger position at the time of penetrating injuries

(Figure 111-7). The level of tendon injury will be distal to the skin laceration if the finger was flexed at the time of injury. If the finger was in an extended position at the time of laceration, the level of tendon injury will correspond more closely to the skin laceration. The presence of digital-tip anesthesia or hypesthesia must be determined because the digital nerves may also be injured. Profundus tendon avulsion injuries most frequently result from a forced hyperextension of an actively flexed DIP joint. This often occurs in young athletes as the injured hand grasps the pants or jersey of the opposing player.

Keen observation is required during the physical examination for possible flexor tendon injury. First, the posture of the hand is noted. Interruption of both digital flexor tendons will lead to an obvious change in the normal flexion cascade of the uninjured hand. This observation may be essential to make the diagnosis in an uncooperative child or unresponsive adult. The absence of finger flexion in the injured digit at the PIP and/or DIP joints by the tenodesis effect during passive wrist extension also signifies complete tendon interruption.

Examination of the FDS tendon to each of the ulnar three fingers can be performed in the cooperative patient by holding the DIP joints of the fingers not being examined in extension. This maneuver isolates flexion of the FDS tendon in the digit being examined because the ulnar three FDP tendons have a common muscle belly (Figure 111-8). The integrity of the FDS tendon to the index finger is best tested by asking the patient to make an "OK" sign, thus holding the DIP joint in extension with the PIP joint in flexion.

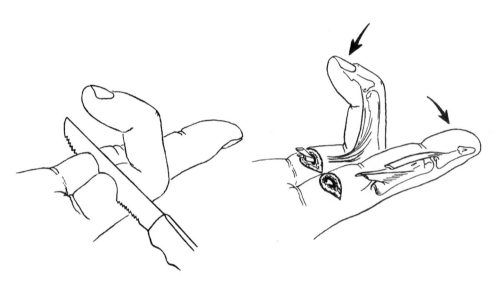

Figure 111-7. The finger position at the time of injury determines the level of flexor tendon laceration in relation to the skin penetration.

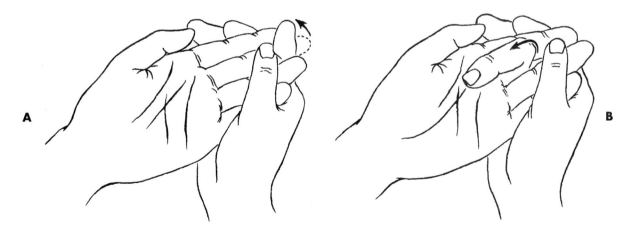

Figure 111-8. Examination of the FDP tendon is performed by isolated flexion at the DIP joint **(A).** Examination of the FDS tendon in the middle, ring, or small finger is performed by holding the other two digits in extension and asking the patient to flex the finger **(B).** The common muscle bellies of the ulnar three FDP tendons will prevent the digital FDP from contracting, thus isolating FDS movement.

The examination should test not only the patient's ability to actively flex the IP joints, but also the strength of flexion against resistance. An intact vinculum can flex the finger PIP joints and the thumb IP, even in the presence of complete FDP/FDS or FPL laceration. The strength of IP joint flexion in this case will be diminished. Patients with partial tendon lacerations will demonstrate weak flexion and pain with resisted flexion. In those patients who are reluctant to actively flex an injured digit, the examiner should place the digit in the flexed position and ask the patient to actively hold the finger in that position against resistance. Common anatomic variations of the FDS to the small finger and interconnections between the FDP to the index and FPL should also be remembered during the clinical examination.

Contraindication for Flexor Tendon Surgery

Primary repair of a lacerated or avulsed flexor tendon is the preferred treatment, but the overall general functional needs of the patient must be assessed. An isolated FDS laceration in an elderly or informed patient may not warrant the morbidity of a surgical repair. Similarly, a delay in seeking medical care, as sometimes occurs in athletes with FDP avulsion injuries that would require a two-stage reconstruction, may not be justified. Relative contraindications to immediate flexor tendon repair also include wound contamination and significant soft tissue loss. A delayed tendon repair after thorough debridement and stable coverage of the flexor system is favored.

Elements of the Informed Consent

The operative treatment is only a part of the total care required for patients with flexor tendon injuries. The informed consent for treatment obtained before surgery must include a discussion of the functional goals for surgery, the short-and long-term risks of surgical treatment, the expected functional deficits if no treatment is performed, the importance of rehabilitation to the restoration of flexor tendon function, and the expected time the patient will not be able to work or perform the activities of daily living.

The ideal functional goals include restoration of full digital motion and strength and return to previous levels of activity and employment. There is presently a lack of standardized methods in the literature to evaluate flexor tendon repairs. It may therefore be difficult to inform the patient of the expected rehabilitation time. The operative risks include infection, injury to adjacent neurovascular structures or components of the pulley system, and abnormal scarring along the volar aspect of the digit. Long-term complications of flexor tendon surgery include tendon adhesions or rupture, joint contracture, and, less commonly, triggering and tendon entrapment. Rehabilitation after surgery is required for 8 to 12 weeks, with the possibility of additional time required to treat adhesions or joint contracture. Resistance exercises are usually delayed for 6 to 8 weeks after a tenorrhaphy, and therefore return to regular work, sporting activities, or unrestricted activities of daily living may take up to 3 months. All of these considerations should be discussed with the patient before operative treatment is rendered.

OPERATIONS

Complete Flexor Tendon Lacerations

The principles of flexor tendon repair have been well described by Brooks and Seiler.[8] Repair should be performed by experienced hand surgeons in the operating suite within 7 days of injury. Tendons should be handled atraumatically and repaired with both core and epitendinous sutures. Meticulous hemostasis and careful wound closure should be performed after tenorrhaphy. Postoperative rehabilitation should include splinting in a position that protects the tendon repair and supervised therapy. These principles, combined with the basic science knowledge described in the previous section, can be applied to clinical practice to maximize hand function after flexor tendon injury.

Adequate surgical instrumentation, a pneumatic tourniquet, and loupe magnification are also essential to facilitate flexor tendon repair. General anesthesia, an axillary block, or intravenous regional anesthesia (Bier block) may be used in different situations depending on the patient and type of injury. We have found significant advantages in using an axillary block, including lower risk for patients with medical conditions, providing anesthesia of sufficient duration for more complicated injuries, and affording early postoperative analgesia.

TENDON PREPARATION. Planning the surgical exposure is the first step in treating flexor tendon injuries. An accurate history of the mechanism of injury helps in planning the incisions. The surgeon should consider the relation of the injured tendon at the time of injury to the corresponding vincular anatomy. The location and direction of the laceration should be considered when making proximal or distal incision extensions off the traumatic wound. Separate proximal incisions in the palm or distal forearm should also be anticipated and planned in selected cases. A volar zigzag Bruner incision or a mid-lateral approach may be utilized to gain the best exposure with the least tissue damage (see Figure 111-6). Frequently, a combination of these approaches is needed when incorporating a traumatic wound. The general principle in designing incisions is to avoid linear scars that cross flexion creases at right angles. These scars tend to contract and may limit finger motion after surgery. Care should be taken when extending an incision distally onto the digital pulp to avoid the tactile surface of the digit. Distal phalanx incisions should therefore be extended onto the ulnar side of the index, middle, and ring fingers, and the radial side of the thumb and small finger. Bruner incisions are preferred over mid-lateral incisions in FPL injuries.

The tendon ends should be retrieved through the flexor sheath in the least traumatic manner. The integrity of the annular pulley system, particularly the A2 and A4 pulleys, must be preserved. Lister has described creation of "retinacular windows" or funnel-shaped incisions in the cruciate pulleys proximal and distal to the A4 pulley.[36] Core sutures are placed in each tendon end through the closest retinacular window. The tendon ends are fed back into the tendon sheath with digital flexion and sutured together either proximal or distal to the A4 pulley. Another method for exposing the tendon ends through the flexor sheath was described by Callan and Morrison.[10] A transverse incision is made in the sheath 1 cm distal to the cut end of the distal tendon segment. Both tendon ends can be retrieved and repaired through this incision with full wrist and MCP-joint flexion. There are two advantages of this method when compared with Lister's technique. The Callan technique allows the suture lines in the tendon and tendon sheath to be at different levels, and a transverse sheath incision does not narrow the internal diameter of the tendon sheath.

Several methods have been described to retrieve the tendon ends into the retinacular windows, including milking the forearm with the wrist and MCP joints in full flexion, or wrapping the forearm with an esmarch bandage from proximal to distal. Blind retrieval with rigid hemostats should be done with caution to avoid injury to the sheath lining. No more than two attempts should be made. The use of flexible tendon retrievers and endoscopic visualization of the retracted tendon ends have also been described. When the tendon end cannot be retrieved with these techniques, a separate incision in the distal palm should be used to retrieve the proximal tendon ends under direct vision. The FDP tendon ends usually retract proximally only into the palm after a laceration at the digital level because they are held by the lumbricals, which originate in the palm. In contrast, the FPL tendon often retracts into the palm or distal forearm after injury at the thumb base, possibly because of its unique vincular anatomy. It is therefore prudent to make an incision proximal to the carpal tunnel to retrieve the FPL.

A pediatric feeding tube can be a useful adjunct in tendon retrieval when a separate proximal incision is required to identify the tendon stump (Figure 111-9). The tube is fed from distal to proximal and sutured to the end of the proximal tendon via a core suture, then pulled back through the sheath distally. Small-gauge needles (22 to 25 gauge) may be placed transversely through the tendons after retrieval to eliminate tension at the repair site and facilitate placement of the core suture. It is important that the relationship of the FDP tendon to the decussation of the FDS tendon be maintained. Another useful technique is to suture the feeding tube to the side of the proximal tendon segment at the distal palm. The proximal tendon end is advanced into the distal finger for repair as the tube is pulled distally. The tendon is pulled proximally after the repair has been completed and the tube is cut from the side of the tendon in the distal palm. Care must be taken in zone I injuries not to advance the FDP tendon more than 1 cm. This can lead to a flexion contracture of the DIP and PIP joints, as well as limited flexion of the adjacent fingers because of the quadriga effect.

SUTURE REPAIR. According to Strickland,[67] an ideal tendon repair should permit easy placement of sutures in the tendon, have secure suture knots with a smooth junction of tendon ends without gapping at the repair site, create minimal interference with tendon vascularity, and have sufficient strength throughout healing to permit early motion of the tendon. The difficulty in satisfying all these criteria by any

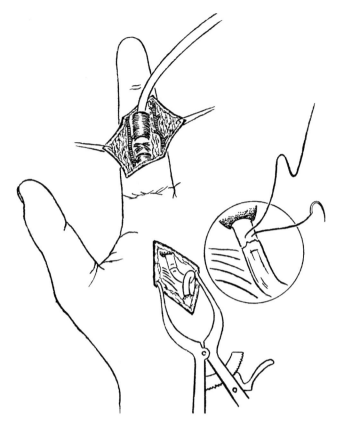

Figure 111-9. Retrieval of a retracted tendon stump is facilitated by passage of a pediatric feeding tube through the flexor tendon sheath into a proximal incision. The tendon end is sutured to the tube and pulled back through the sheath distally.

repair technique is probably reflected in the multitude of repairs described and currently utilized by practitioners.

Sutures used for tenorrhaphy may be classified into two types, the core suture and the peripheral epitendinous (or epitenon) suture. Clinical and laboratory studies support several conclusions regarding flexor tendon repair.[67] The strength of the tendon repair is proportional to the number of core suture strands that cross the tenorrhaphy site. The epitendinous suture significantly increases the overall repair strength and is important in resisting gap formation. Tendon-repair ruptures usually occur at the suture knots. Locking loops do little to increase the strength of the tendon repair and may actually lead to gapping with moderate loading.[47] There is no significant difference between monofilament polypropylene and braided polyester sutures with respect to strength, reactivity, handling, and elasticity, although many surgeons prefer 3-0 or 4-0 braided synthetic sutures.[69]

There are many variations in the technique of placing core sutures. The described techniques include the Bunnell, Tsuge, Tajima, Strickland, Kessler, modified Kessler, Savage, Becker, modified Becker (Massachusetts General Hospital or MGH repair), and Indianapolis repair (Figure 111-10). A recent survey of practicing hand surgeons found that 72% use the modified Kessler technique for flexor tendon repair.[50] Regardless of the particular technique used, core sutures should be placed in the volar half of the tendon to preserve the intrinsic

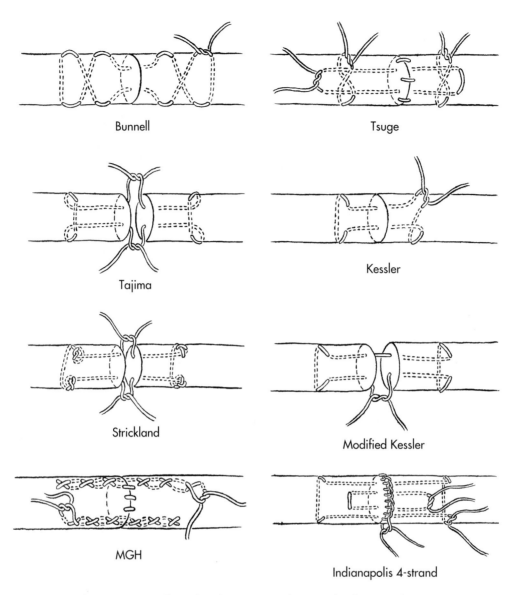

Bunnell

Tsuge

Tajima

Kessler

Strickland

Modified Kessler

MGH

Indianapolis 4-strand

Figure 111-10. Examples of core suture placement for flexor tendon repair.

vascularity, which enters the dorsal aspect of the tendon through the vincula.

The epitendinous suture, usually a running locked 5-0 or 6-0 Prolene, contributes significantly to the strength of flexor tendon repair. Other variations of the epitendinous suture include a Halsted running horizontal mattress or the cross-stitch technique described by Silfverskiöld and May.[60] It serves to compress the repair site when longitudinal stress is applied, similar to a Chinese finger trap. Diao et al[13] advocated placing the peripheral suture deeply, half the way to the center of the tendon, resulting in an 80% increase in repair strength compared with the more superficial technique.

Sanders[58] described an "epitendinous-first" technique of flexor tendon repair. The purported advantages of this technique include atraumatic handling of the tendon and minimal bulging of the tendon at the repair site. The core suture is also completely buried within the tendon, with the knot 1 cm away from the tendon juncture. Papandrea et al[53]

demonstrated in biomechanical testing that the epitendinous-first technique is 22% stronger than the modified Kessler technique.

Surgical repair of only the profundus tendon was recommended by earlier hand surgeons in patients with a zone II laceration of both the FDP and FDS tendons to decrease adhesions and improve the full range of digital motion. However, with the advent of modern repair techniques and protected-motion therapy programs, primary repair of both tendons is now generally recommended. The advantages of repairing both tendons include better tendon nutrition from restoration of vascularity from the vincular connection, potentially more independent digital motion with stronger and quicker PIP-joint flexion, a decreased tendency for PIP-joint hyperextension, and the preservation of a gliding synovial bed for the profundus tendon.

Repair of the flexor tendon sheath after the tendon repair was advocated by several authors. The tendon sheath serves as a barrier to the formation of extrinsic adhesions and helps mold the remodeling tendon after repair. It also enhances the reestablishment of synovial nutrition, and restores tendon sheath biomechanics.[67] Investigators have described primary tendon sheath repair and the use of synovial sheath grafts or the use of prosthetic material to reconstruct the tendon sheath. Despite these theoretical advantages, no studies to date have established the clinical benefits of tendon sheath repair.[37,57] We generally attempt to maintain sheath integrity by using carefully designed sheath incisions, atraumatic handling of tissue, preservation of the A2 and A4 pulleys, and sheath reapproximation after tendon repair. Despite these measures, however, gaps in tendon sheath often exist after tenorrhaphy, and their clinical significance is uncertain.

Hemostasis during and after surgery is essential to prevent a hematoma, which can lead to wound-healing complications, tendon adhesions, rupture, or infection. The arm tourniquet can be deflated before skin closure and then reinflated after hemostasis is secured. The wound is carefully approximated with simple or horizontal mattress sutures. A dorsal splint is usually applied to maintain the wrist in 30 degrees of flexion and the MCP joints in 50 to 70 degrees of flexion. Full extension of the PIP and DIP joints should be allowed in the splint. The surgeon should adjust the splint on a case-by-case basis, however, depending on the intraoperative findings and an assessment of the tenorrhaphy tension. Zone IV tendon injuries should be splinted with the wrist in near neutral position and the MCP joints flexed at 75 to 90 degrees to minimize bowstringing of the flexors in the carpal tunnel. The wrist is flexed at 50 degrees in FPL injuries, and the MCP and IP joints of the thumb are held in 15 to 20 degrees of flexion.

POSTOPERATIVE THERAPY. Hand-therapy rehabilitation after surgery is a critical part of the treatment for flexor tendon injuries. Rehabilitation strategies after flexor tendon repair are based on empirical observations. The tensile strength of immobilized tendon repair *decreases* 7 to 10 days after surgery.[48] Guarded motion and stress applied to a flexor-tendon repair, however, improves the ultimate tendon gliding. Controlled passive motion techniques have therefore become the most commonly used postoperative protocols. Dorsal blocking splints and controlled active motion protocols are also appropriate in selected patients. All rehabilitation after tendon repair can be divided into early, intermediate, and late phases.

Complete immobilization after tendon repair is indicated in patients under the age of 10, those with cognitive deficits, or those who have demonstrated an inability or unwillingness to comply with a controlled-motion protocol.[62] A splint is maintained at all times in these patients, with wrist and MCP joints in flexion during the early phase of healing, which lasts 3 to 4 weeks after repair. The splint is modified to bring the wrist into a neutral position during the intermediate stage, which begins at 3 to 4 weeks. Gentle, active, differential tendon gliding exercises are initiated out of the splint in cooperative patients at this time by active flexion and extension of the wrist, which (by tenodesis) causes digital extension and flexion. The splint is discontinued during the late phase,

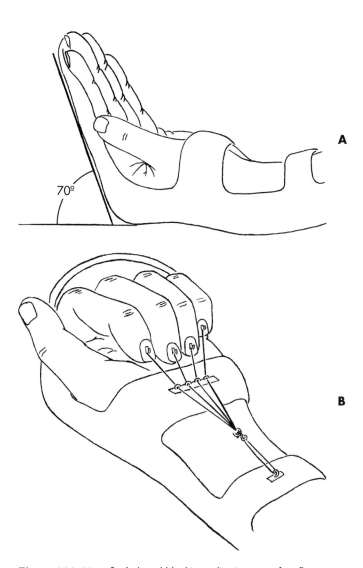

Figure 111-11. **A,** A dorsal blocking splint is worn after flexor tendon repair. **B,** In the Kleinert protocol, rubber bands are used to maintain digital flexion while allowing active extension.

beginning at 4 to 6 weeks. Active digital motion is then begun, focusing on blocking exercises that isolate either FDS or FDP motion. Exercises against resistance are initiated after 8 weeks. Additional modalities, such as neuromuscular electrical stimulation and ultrasound, may be instituted if necessary to decrease adhesions around the repaired tendon.

Early passive-motion protocols are the most commonly used methods to achieve flexor tendon gliding after repair. The Duran and Kleinert protocols both use a dorsal blocking splint to maintain flexion of the wrist and MCP joints after repair (Figure 111-11, *A*). Passive digital flexion is begun 2 to 3 days after repair, with the hand in a splint, which blocks full extension. The wrist and MCP joints are blocked in flexion, and the DIP and PIP joints are passively moved through a range of motion that produces excursion of the repaired tendon within the tendon sheaths. In the original Duran protocol, the splint was removed after 4½ weeks, and digital flexion was begun assisted by rubber bands attached to a wrist cuff. The modified Duran protocol avoids such extreme dynamic flexion to decrease the incidence of PIP-joint flexion contracture. Active flexion is initiated at 4½ weeks, resisted flexion is begun after 8 weeks.

The Kleinert protocol differs from that of Duran by using rubber bands to maintain digital flexion while allowing active extension in the early phase of rehabilitation (Figure 111-11, *B*). This method is based on the fact that the extrinsic flexor muscles are relaxed and electromyographically silent during active digital extension. Active extension moves the repaired flexor tendons without resistance from the relaxed flexor muscles. When the extensors are relaxed, the fingers are pulled back into flexion by the rubber bands without actual flexor muscle pull. Chow modified the Kleinert protocol by adding a "palmar pulley," which maintains the injured finger in full flexion to the distal palmar crease.[11] This strategy also achieves superior differential tendon gliding because it allows more MCP-joint extension and takes the repaired tendon passively through a greater excursion.

Early active motion is being used with increasing frequency after flexor tendon repair. This protocol requires an experienced therapist and surgeon, a reliable patient, and a strong tendon repair. Strickland has measured the strength of tendon repairs performed with two-, four-, and six-strand core sutures with and without epitendinous sutures (Figure 111-12).[67] The six-strand repair provides the greatest tensile strength, but a four-strand repair is considered safe from rupture during light, active motion in the early healing period. Strickland's data, however, did not account for the additional forces required to mobilize a repaired tendon in an edematous hand.

Another variation of the active motion protocol is the active place-and-hold technique, in which the patient passively places the injured digits in flexion and then maintains the flexed position by gentle muscle contraction. The place-and-hold technique often uses additional wrist tenodesis routines in which digital flexion is accompanied by wrist extension, followed by digital extension with active wrist flexion. There have been no controlled prospective trials involving early active mobilization despite a number of highly successful anecdotal reports.

Partial Flexor Tendon Lacerations

There is considerable debate in the literature regarding the management of partial tendon lacerations. Early studies suggested that partial flexor tendon lacerations should not be repaired. However, tendon entrapment, rupture, and triggering have been reported when partially lacerated tendons are not repaired. The benefits of avoiding sutures within the tendon must therefore be balanced against the potential complications of leaving partial tendon lacerations unrepaired.

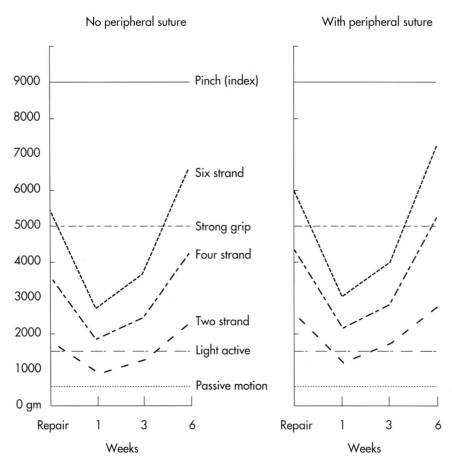

Figure 111-12. Strength of various flexor tendon repairs as a function of time in comparison with the forces necessary for postoperative mobilization.

A recent report by Bishop concluded that partial lacerations involving 60% or less of the flexor tendon substance are best treated by early mobilization without tenorrhaphy.[5]

Profundus Tendon Avulsions

Profundus tendon avulsion from its insertion on the base of the distal phalanx by forced hyperextension of the digit is the second most common type of flexor tendon injury after lacerations. Superficialis tendon avulsion has also been described, but it is an extremely rare injury. Most profundus-tendon avulsions occur in the ring finger, but any digit can be involved. There are several potential explanations for the frequent involvement of the ring finger. A common profundus muscle belly to the middle, ring, and small fingers may make the central ring finger more susceptible to a hyperextension injury.[21] Leddy theorizes that the inability of the ring finger to fully extend when the middle and small finger MCP joints are flexed is due to the juncturae tendinum between extensor tendons and makes the ring finger more vulnerable to forced hyperextension.[35] Finally, it has been shown anatomically that the profundus insertion into the ring finger is weaker than that in the middle finger.[45]

CLASSIFICATION OF PROFUNDUS TENDON AVULSIONS.
Several classification schemes have been described that correlate the anatomic findings with treatment and prognosis of these injuries. Leddy and Packer's[35] classification system is based on the level to which the avulsed profundus tendon retracts proximally and the status of the tendon vascular anatomy.

Type I injuries are those in which the profundus tendon has retracted proximally into the palm, with total disruption of the long and short vincula. The tendon is held in the palm by the lumbrical origin. The vascularity of the tendon is severely compromised because of the vincular rupture and the absence of synovial diffusion outside the tendon sheath. Surgery should be done within 7 to 10 days before development of a fixed muscle contracture or tendon resorption. Type I avulsion injuries are the least common pattern.

Type II injuries are those in which the profundus tendon has retracted to the level of the PIP joint after disruption of only the vinculum breve. The tendon's nutrition is preserved by the vinculum longum and its presence within the sheath, which allows it to be repaired up to 3 months after injury with a satisfactory result. A delay in treatment can, however, convert a Type II injury into a Type I injury if the vinculum longum subsequently ruptures from repeated contraction by the profundus musculotendinous unit.

Type III avulsion injuries are those that have an attached bone fragment that fractures off the volar base of the distal phalanx. The A4 pulley prevents proximal retraction of the bone and tendon, and both vincula are usually preserved. Radiographs demonstrate the large bony fragment and associated intraarticular fracture of the DIP joint. An additional type IIIa or type IV injury has been described, with further avulsion of the flexor tendon with a large osseous fragment.

TREATMENT OF PROFUNDUS TENDON AVULSIONS.
Early diagnosis and treatment facilitate repair of the avulsed profundus tendon. A distal digital incision is first made to ascertain the diagnosis and location of the avulsed tendon. A second distal palm incision will often be needed in type I injuries to identify the retracted tendon. The tendon should then be fed through the fibroosseous tunnel and reinserted into the base of the distal phalanx without injuring the tendon sheath or volar plate. A distally based periosteal flap is elevated with a small osteotome distal to the volar plate, and the tendon is sutured through drill holes in the distal phalanx using a pullout suture and button tied over the dorsal nail plate. More recently, small suture anchors have been developed that can be drilled into the distal phalanx to secure the avulsed tendon to the phalangeal base. Avulsion injuries are treated after surgery by maintaining flexion of the wrist and MCP joint of the injured digit in a dorsal blocking splint and beginning early passive motion. Active motion is instituted at 3 to 4 weeks after surgery.

The tendon in type II injuries can be identified using digital incisions for exposure. The profundus tendon is fed distally within the fibroosseous tunnel and reinserted into the distal phalanx as described for type I injuries. In type III and type IV injuries, attention is turned to open reduction and internal fixation of the bony fragment, as well as reinsertion of the FDP tendon in type IV injuries. Earlier active motion can be achieved with rigid internal fixation.

OUTCOMES

Evaluation Systems for Flexor Tendon Repair
There is presently no universally accepted system to evaluate the results of flexor tendon repair, making it difficult to compare the reported results from different clinical series. Boyes'[7] method measures the distance from the digital pulp to the distal palmar crease during maximal finger flexion. The Louisville system measures pulp-to-palm distance and any extension deficit at the DIP, PIP, and MCP joints.[38] Buck-Gramcko's system measures pulp-to-palm distance, the extension deficit, and composite digital joint flexion. The American Society for Surgery of the Hand devised a Total Active Motion (TAM) scale to assess digital motion after flexor tendon repair, in which any extension lag at the DIP, PIP, and MCP joints is subtracted from the total actual flexion of these joints. Strickland noted that MCP-joint flexion is dependent on intrinsic muscle function and is rarely affected by flexor tendon surgery; he recommended exclusion of MCP-joint movement from the assessment. His modified system measures flexion of the DIP and PIP joints, minus the respective extension loss, and is a more sensitive measurement of digital function after flexor tendon repair (Table 111-1).[64,66] So et al[61] prospectively compared five popular methods used to evaluate the results of flexor tendon repair and concluded that significant discrepancies exist among the different systems. Other parameters have been suggested as a way to assess hand function after flexor tendon repair, including finger flexion

Table 111-1.
Strickland's Evaluation System for Flexor Tendon Repair

DIP + PIP MOTION (°)	% OF NORMAL	RATING
132-175	75-100	Excellent
88-131	50-74	Good
44-87	25-49	Fair
<44	<25	Poor

(DIP + PIP) active flexion − (DIP + PIP) extension deficit ÷ 175° × 100 = % of normal (DIP + PIP) active motion

pressure, finger pinch pressure, key pinch strength, and grip strength.[18]

Chow used the Strickland modified TAM formula and reported superior results in military personnel after flexor-tendon repair using an early passive-flexion and active-extension protocol.[11] He studied 44 patients with zone II injuries who achieved 82% excellent results and 16% good results. Strickland reported the outcome of a controlled early active motion protocol after zone I and zone II flexor tendon repairs.[68] He measured 37 digits using the modified TAM system at the time of discharge from hand therapy and noted 9 digits (24%) had excellent results, 17 (46%) had good results, 9 (24%) had fair results, and 2 (6%) had poor motion. Long-term follow-up averaging 1.4 years after repair was performed on 19 digits with 11 (58%) rated as excellent, 5 (26%) good, 3 (16%) fair, and none poor. Extrapolation from any single study is difficult because of the variation in patients, surgical technique, and hand therapy, but these data nevertheless provide information on the outcome of flexor-tendon repairs in established hand-surgery centers.

Complications of Flexor Tendon Repair

Adhesion formation remains the most common complication after flexor tendon repair, despite the widespread use of early-motion protocols. Tenolysis should be considered when the patient's progressive gains in digital motion with hand therapy have plateaued, usually 3 to 6 months after repair. Another complication after repair is tendon rupture, which is often noted by the patient as a "popping" in the hand and is associated with acutely decreased active motion in the affected digit. A tendon ruptures most commonly between the seventh to the tenth postoperative day, when the tensile strength of the repair is the weakest. If the diagnosis is unclear, recent reports have demonstrated the use of magnetic resonance imaging (MRI) to diagnose a tendon rupture. Urgent reexploration and repair is generally the treatment of choice.

A flexion contracture of the digit can occur after a flexor tendon repair. Constant rubber-band traction that maintains the digit in a flexed position should be avoided. As previously noted, FDP advancement of more than 1 cm may also lead to a flexion contracture and weakened hand grasp because of the quadriga effect. Tendon triggering and entrapment have also been reported, especially when the flexor sheath has not been repaired. Finally, posttraumatic regional pain syndromes and cold intolerance have been reported in digits with flexor tendon injuries, even in those without concomitant nerve injuries.

LATE RECONSTRUCTION

Many surgeons in the early part of the twentieth century believed that primary flexor tendon repair was not indicated. Delayed tendon reconstruction using tendon grafts was therefore the standard of care. Primary flexor tendon repair now offers the best chance for functional return because of advances in our understanding of tendon healing, improved surgical technique, and modern postoperative mobilization protocols. Secondary flexor tendon reconstruction has therefore become less common and is now indicated only in situations when primary tendon repair is not possible because of special circumstances, such as a segmental tendon defect, loss of the pulley system, a compromised wound, a delay in diagnosis, or when there is excessive scarring or a rupture after primary repair. Such cases are almost always complicated by local adverse conditions, and secondary flexor reconstruction has thus become one of the most challenging procedures in hand surgery.

CONSIDERATIONS FOR FLEXOR TENDON RECONSTRUCTION

Failure of a primary tenorrhaphy caused by excessive scar formation or rupture of the repair results in lack of active motion. The resulting functional deficit, however, should be evaluated in the context of each individual patient and his or her required digital function. A lack of active DIP-joint motion in the index finger with good PIP function, for example, may best be treated by a joint-stabilizing procedure instead of flexor tendon reconstruction. The approach to each case should be individualized, and no single algorithm for tendon reconstruction can be universally applied to all patients. The important factors to consider include the severity, mechanism, and anatomic level of the injury; the presence of associated injury to nerve, bone, and soft tissue; the digit involved; and the hand dominance. Individual patient factors such as age, vocation, hobbies, and most importantly, the patient's motivation and ability to participate in hand therapy after surgery should also be considered. Patients who are unable to commit to the lengthy and demanding hand-therapy program after surgery should not be considered candidates for flexor tendon reconstruction.

The Boyes' grading scale of flexor tendon injury provides a guideline for determining the achievable outcome after flexor

Table 111-2.
Grading of Flexor Tendon Injury

Grade 1	Good (minimal scar, mobile joint, no trophic changes)
Grade 2	Skin scarring caused by injury or prior surgery; deep scarring caused by failed primary repair or infection
Grade 3	Joint scar or contracture with restricted range of motion
Grade 4	Nerve injury; damage to the digital nerves resulting in trophic damage in the finger
Grade 5	Multiple damage; involvement of multiple fingers with a combination of problems
Grade 6	Salvage

From Amadio PC, Wood MB, Cooney WP III, Bogard SD: J Hand Surg [Am] 13:559, 1988; and Boyes JH, Stark HH: J Bone Joint Surg 53A:1332, 1971.

tendon reconstruction (Table 111-2). A surgical history, including a prior unsuccessful treatment, implies a worse prognosis. The position of the digit to be reconstructed should also be considered. The ulnar ring and small digits require complete flexion to provide strong grasp, whereas full flexion of the IP joints of the radial fingers is less important because they are used for precision pinch. The thumb should provide a stable post for finger opposition. Full flexion at the IP and MCP joints of the thumb is therefore less important than providing a stable and sensate thumb of adequate length. A decision to recommend flexor tendon reconstruction should therefore only be made after the surgeon has a clear understanding of the patient's needs and determines the surgical goals are technically achievable.

PREREQUISITES FOR FLEXOR TENDON RECONSTRUCTION

Before tendon-reconstruction surgery can be undertaken, certain prerequisites must be met. These include adequate soft tissue coverage and digital vascularity, healed fractures, and passively supple joints. Active scars with persistent inflammation and hyperemia are a sign that tissue equilibrium has not been reached and that reconstruction is not yet indicated. Sensibility should optimally have returned, permitting useful function of the digit. The vascularity of the digit should be sufficient to avert postoperative healing problems or infection. The finger joints should be passively mobile from intensive hand therapy, because reconstruction of the flexor mechanism in a digit with stiff joints will not be successful. Adjunctive soft

tissue procedures should be performed if necessary before undertaking tendon reconstruction, including flap coverage, nerve grafting, joint capsulotomy or capsulectomy, and/or extensor tenolysis. Staged procedures with initial extensor tenolysis and dorsal capsulotomy followed by flexor tenolysis or reconstruction are frequently indicated.

CLINICAL ASSESSMENT

The status of the flexor mechanism should be carefully evaluated in the preoperative physical assessment, including the presence of contraction at the site of injury and the active and passive digital range of motion. However, attention should not be focused only on the flexor system. Other causes for diminished digital motion include fracture malunion, joint irregularities, periarticular scarring, extensor adhesions, and injury to the flexor motor unit. The status of the surrounding tissues, including the bones, joints, neurovascular bundles, and the intrinsic musculature, should all be evaluated. Radiographs may be necessary to identify bony nonunions, rotatory malalignment, or joint problems that are restricting digital motion.

RECONSTRUCTIVE MODALITIES

Reconstructive techniques to restore active digital flexion include tenolysis, tendon advancement, tendon transfer, and tendon grafts with or without creation of an artificial tendon sheath by prior silicone rod implantation. Alternatives to these procedures, such as amputation, joint fusion, tenodesis, and capsulodesis, should be discussed with the patient and should include a review of the relative advantages and disadvantages. A decision to reconstruct the flexor mechanism should only be made after the patient has a thorough understanding of the procedures involved, the morbidity of a tendon donor site, the length of postoperative rehabilitation, the potential for unplanned surgical procedures, and the chance of failure. It is not always possible to predict the etiology of the functional problem before surgery. A digit lacking active flexion after a primary tendon repair, for example, may have extensive adhesions around the repaired tendon, or there may be a complete rupture of tenorrhaphy. The former may be amenable to tenolysis, whereas the latter requires a staged tendon reconstruction. The patient must therefore be informed of the surgical options before surgery.

FLEXOR TENOLYSIS

INDICATIONS

Tenolysis is a controversial secondary procedure in the treatment of tendon injuries. Bunnell stated that "... a tendon released from cicatrix ... dropped back in its cicatricial bed will, of course, again adhere and in two weeks be as immobile as ever." Since then, however, the benefits of tenolysis have been clearly demonstrated, and the procedure is widely accepted to restore active motion by release of adhesions after a primary repair or graft.[65]

Tenolysis is considered one of the most technically difficult procedures and requires cooperation between the patient and surgeon. It is indicated when lack of active motion is attributed to excessive peritendinous scar formation and when the digital passive motion exceeds active motion. A full course of hand therapy aimed at breaking the adherent scars should always be instituted before performing a tenolysis. Surgery is indicated when continued therapy fails to increase the active digital motion and "plateaus" for at least 6 weeks. Scarring of a flexor tendon to the tendon sheath or an adjacent tendon limits motion distal to the zone of injury. Tenolysis is aimed at releasing the adhesions and should be combined with early motion protocols to avoid recurrent scar formation. The patient needs to be motivated and informed about the procedure, the possible complications, and the need for intensive rehabilitation.

Timing of Flexor Tenolysis

It is generally accepted that tissue "equilibrium" needs to be reached before performing tenolysis. Significant edema and active inflammation in the digit are therefore contraindications to performing the procedure. Full passive joint motion should always be achieved either by intensive hand therapy or by staged joint capsulotomy and extensor tendon tenolysis. The time interval between injury and tenolysis has been a subject of controversy. Most surgeons regard an interval of 3 months as a minimum before performing a tenolysis, although some studies have shown that range of motion continues to improve for up to 1 year after injury.[49] Many patients, however, often request surgical intervention after a plateau in progress has been reached in therapy. In our practice, tenolysis is usually recommended 4 to 6 months after injury as long as all prerequisites have been met.

OPERATIONS

Techniques of Flexor Tenolysis

Tenolysis is optimally performed with active participation of the patient during the surgical procedure, and therefore local anesthesia is generally used. The flexor sheath is exposed using a Bruner or midlateral incision, incorporating previous scars. All pulleys are preserved, and excision of any part of the flexor sheath should be discouraged. Transverse incisions made between the annular pulleys will avoid damage to the pulley system and prevent subsequent bow-stringing. All adherent scars are released using small periosteal elevators or special angled tenotomy blades, while avoiding damage to the pulley system and the tendon itself. The dissection should progress meticulously, and the digital range of motion should be continuously checked by pulling on the proximal tendon through a separate volar wrist incision. Once the target motion is achieved, no further release should be performed. It should

be remembered, however, that the range of motion obtained in the operating room will unlikely improve with postoperative therapy. On the contrary, the patient and therapists often struggle to maintain the active motion that had been achieved during surgery. The patient should be allowed to actively move the released tendon during surgery while observing the result. This serves to motivate the patient to comply with hand-therapy instructions after surgery by witnessing the progress achieved during surgery.

Adjunctive Procedures

Many adjunctive maneuvers have been described to improve the results of tenolysis by attempting to prevent scar recurrence. Local injection of steroids and placement of alloplastic sheath material, such as cellophane and silicone, to provide a gliding surface have generally not been found to be useful. A higher rate of tendon rupture and wound complications, such as infection and dehiscence, have been shown to occur after steroid injection. The routine use of these adjunctive measures in tenolysis is therefore not recommended.

Postoperative Care

It is crucial to start mobilization of the released tendon as soon as possible after surgery to prevent scar recurrence.[65] Adequate pain relief should be achieved by systemic analgesics or with local anesthesia through repeated injections or an indwelling catheter. Several authors have described the use of a continuous passive motion (CPM) device after surgery to mechanically put the digits through a full range of motion. Others have advocated motion protocols similar to those described for primary flexor tendon repair, such as the Duran program or Kleinert dynamic traction splinting. Active motion is more effective in achieving tendon excursion, and therefore active motion protocols have been increasingly recommended. The appropriate mobilization program after a tenolysis must be individualized and is determined by the strength and integrity of the tendon. If the tendon is found to be too weak to withstand active motion, then passive motion exercises should be instituted. The amount of active digital motion permitted after surgery should be enough to allow tendon movement without placing excessive tension to cause a secondary rupture. The surgeon should discuss the condition of the tenolysed tendons with the hand therapist after surgery and design an active and passive motion protocol to fit the situation.

OUTCOMES

Complications

The worst complication after tenolysis is tendon rupture. If, after the tenolysis, the tendon substance is noted to be significantly narrowed, a tendon graft should be considered to avoid rupture during postoperative therapy. Reconstruction of the pulley system is indicated if it is damaged during the tenolyses or when there is found to be preexisting injury. Concurrent pulley reconstruction and tenolysis, however, requires immobilization after surgery, which often leads to adhesion recurrence, and therefore staged reconstruction with a tendon rod may be a better alternative. Other complications after a tenolysis include reflex sympathetic dystrophy and devascularization of previously replanted digits. The degree of digital motion regained may be rapidly lost in the postoperative period despite appropriate rehabilitation therapy. Some surgeons have advocated early reexploration of these digits and have reported success using this aggressive approach.[63]

TENDON GRAFTING

INDICATIONS

Flexor tendon grafting is performed to salvage digital function when the injury has resulted in a tendon gap, or if primary tendon repair and/or subsequent tenolysis have failed. Tendon grafting can be carried out in one or two stages. One-stage tendon grafting is indicated after acute trauma when there is segmental flexor tendon loss in a clean, well-vascularized wound with an intact pulley system. This is infrequently the case. Immediate grafting may also be considered during tenolysis when the tendon is deemed inadequate to permit immediate postoperative motion, as long as the graft bed is relatively unscarred and the pulley system has maintained sufficient biomechanical strength and internal diameter.

Frequently, however, preexisting injury or the local wound condition precludes immediate tendon grafting, and staged tendon reconstruction is necessary. The goal of staged reconstruction is to create a supple pseudosynovial sheath by implanting a silicone rod.[27] Any necessary soft tissue coverage or pulley reconstruction should be performed at the time of rod placement. Formation of a pseudosynovial sheath takes approximately 8 weeks, after which the rod is replaced by a suitable tendon graft.

Indications for staged tendon reconstruction have been summarized to include the following:[26,59]

1. Segmental tendon loss in primary injuries when direct repair is not possible
2. A significantly scarred tendon bed in which primary tendon grafting has a low chance of gliding
3. Reconstruction of the profundus tendon with an intact sublimis and existing scars
4. As a salvage procedure to create a profundus or superficialis finger with a single tendon unit
5. After multiple digit replantation to simplify postoperative therapy and to avoid conflicting rehabilitation protocols for extensor and flexor mechanisms

Tendon grafting is a technically demanding operation, requiring meticulous attention to details. Sound surgical techniques with minimum handling of the tendon's gliding surface decrease scar formation and maximize the achievable range of motion. The status of graft bed, the type and size of the tendon graft, and the location of tendon repairs all have important implications for the final outcome. The ideal environment for a tendon graft is an undamaged or restored tendon sheath in a digit with supple joints and minimal soft tissue scarring.

OPERATIONS

Graft Bed Preparation

The graft bed preparation begins with a careful assessment of the local environment, such as the presence of scarred tendon remnants, damage to the pulley mechanism, and contraction of the fibroosseous tendon sheath. If the fibroosseous sheath has collapsed to an extent that it will not allow room for an appropriate tendon graft, then tendon sheath reconstruction should be considered. Surgical preparation should be aimed at minimizing reactive scar formation after the graft procedure and the preservation of critical structures such as the annular pulleys, volar plate, and phalangeal periosteum. A decision should also be made whether to graft from the digital tip to the palm or to the forearm.

Choice of Motor Unit

The choice of a motor unit to restore flexor tendon function is important. Myostatic contracture of the native motor unit often precludes its use because the required contraction amplitude has been lost. The status of the proximal myotendinous unit can be assessed by pulling on the end of its tendon. A minimum of 2 to 3 cm of excursion is generally necessary to motor a grafted FDP tendon. The FDS muscle has independent function and should be used over the FDP muscle as the motor unit when available. When the FDP muscle unit must be used, the tension on the graft must be carefully adjusted to prevent a flexor lag of the reconstructed digit (too loose) or the neighboring digits (too tight) caused by the quadriga effect of a single profundus muscle with four tendon slips.

Donor Tendon Selection

Selection of a donor tendon for grafting is dependent on the required length and diameter, ease of harvest, potential anatomical variations, and donor-site morbidity.[72] Recently, use of tendon grafts that include the synovial sheath, such as toe extensors, has been advocated over extrasynovial grafts, but clear differences in functional outcome have not been established.[1] Laboratory findings suggest that synovial tendon grafts lack epitenon fibroblast proliferation and exhibit a greater capacity for vascular ingrowth from the tenorrhaphy sites.[1,3,19] There was also less adhesion formation and deposition of more mature collagen. Despite these apparent advantages, harvest of synovial tendons has not become a standard practice probably because of a relative paucity of appropriate donor tendons. Many surgeons still favor thin extrasynovial tendons such as the plantaris or palmaris longus, which can be readily harvested with minimum donor-site morbidity.

The donor tendon should be carefully handled during harvest and placement because any damage can result in subsequent adhesion formation. The graft should be kept moist during surgery to avoid desiccation, and its paratenon should be preserved to provide a smooth gliding surface.

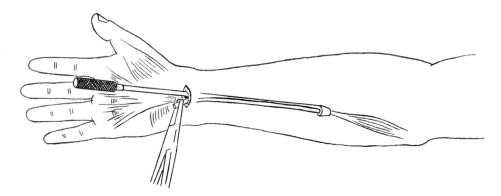

Figure 111-13. Harvest of the palmaris longus tendon graft through a volar wrist incision using a tendon stripper.

PALMARIS LONGUS. The palmaris longus tendon offers a graft of uniform size that is usually of sufficient length to graft from the digital tip into the palm. It can be harvested from the same operative field as the grafting procedure. The tendon is absent in about 15% of individuals, and its presence should be verified before surgery by having the patient simultaneously flex the wrist and oppose the thumb and small finger. Harvest can be performed through a short incision at the wrist crease using a Brand tendon stripper or through multiple small, transverse incisions on the forearm (Figure 111-13). Donor-site morbidity after harvest of a palmaris longus tendon is minimal.

PLANTARIS. The plantaris tendon is long and thin and provides an ideal donor when multiple tendon grafts are required. There is little donor-site morbidity associated with its harvest. The plantaris tendon is absent in 10% to 20% of patients; however, in contrast to the palmaris, no easy clinical test is available to confirm its presence. The most reliable method to determine the presence of a plantaris tendon is a computed tomography (CT) scan with transverse sections in the distal third of the lower extremity, but ultrasound may also be helpful. The plantaris is harvested through an ankle incision between the medial malleolus and the Achilles tendon. Use of the Brand tendon stripper facilitates its harvest and eliminates the need for a proximal incision.

EXTENSOR DIGITORUM COMMUNIS TO THE INDEX FINGER. The extensor digitorum communis tendon to the index finger is a relatively short tendon that can be harvested in the same operative field. Its sacrifice leaves the extensor indicis proprius as the sole MCP-joint extensor, and may result in a slight extension lag and/or weakness. The tendon can be harvested through a transverse incision proximal to the index MCP joint, and is identified as the more radial of the two index extensor tendons.

EXTENSOR DIGITORUM LONGUS. The extensor digitorum longus tendons to the second, third, and fourth toes can also be used as grafts. Harvest is performed from distal

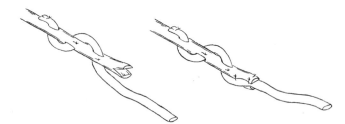

Figure 111-14. Pulvertaft weave for securing the tendon graft to the proximal tendon stump.

to proximal through a transverse incision at the level of the metatarsophalangeal (MTP) joints. The Brand tendon stripper is advanced toward the ankle, although a number of transverse incisions are often required on the dorsum of the foot to divide the junctures between adjacent tendons. These incisions may result in significant foot discomfort after surgery. The grafts may need to be harvested to a level proximal to the ankle to obtain sufficient length to reconstruct from the fingertip to the forearm, which may necessitate division of the extensor retinaculum.

EXTENSOR INDICIS PROPRIUS/EXTENSOR DIGITI QUINTI. The extensor indicis proprius and extensor digiti quinti tendons have the advantage of being in the same operative field and can be harvested without significant donor deficits. Specific, independent flexion of the digits appears not to be affected after harvest, but neither tendon is usually long enough to graft from the fingertip into the forearm.

Tendon Juncture and Tension Adjustment

There are a number of methods described to join the ends of a tendon graft, all with the common goal of obtaining a strong tenorrhaphy that will allow early digital mobilization and decreased adhesion formation. The authors favor performing the proximal juncture with a Pulvertaft weave, with two or more passes through the proximal motor tendons (Figure 111-14). An end-to-end proximal tenorrhaphy using a

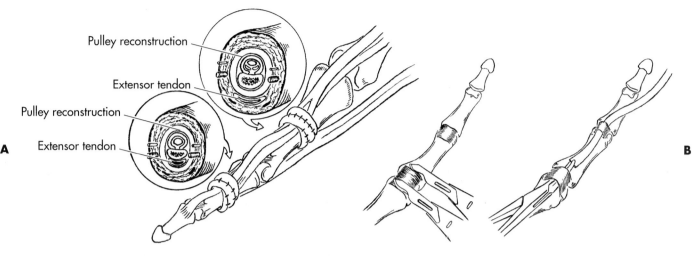

Pulley reconstruction

Extensor tendon

Pulley reconstruction

Extensor tendon

A

B

Figure 111-15. **A,** Pulley reconstruction using loops of autogenous tendon or fascia. Note A2 reconstruction is best performed by placing the loops dorsally beneath the extensor around the proximal phalanx, whereas A4 reconstruction is performed by placing the loops dorsal to the extensor. **B,** Pulley reconstruction using the "belt buckle" technique and the volar plates.

multiple-strand core suture augmented by an epitendinous suture can be employed but is weaker than a weave and is not recommended. Distally, the tendon graft may be secured to the distal phalanx in a number of ways. A pull-out suture technique without drilling holes in the bone may be used where the remaining distal profundus stump is raised from its periosteal insertion and the volar periosteum of the distal phalanx is removed. Care is taken to avoid damage to the volar plate of the DIP joint. The tendon graft is placed underneath the stump and a previously placed 3-0 Prolene core suture is passed around the distal phalanx as a pull-out suture, which is tied over a bolus protecting the nail. The distal FDP stump is then sutured over the tendon graft using nonabsorbable suture. Alternatively, a minisuture anchor drilled into the volar base of the distal phalanx may be used to secure the tendon graft. The suture anchor may be technically easier to perform, but care must be taken to avoid injuring the nail bed.

The proper tension of the tendon graft is essential to obtain optimal function. Normally, the distal tendon is inserted into bone, and the proximal weave into the motor unit is adjusted with the wrist in neutral to flex the finger into the cascade of the hand. We prefer to place the finger in a slightly more flexed position than what the normal cascade would dictate because some stretching of the reconstructed muscle tendon unit normally occurs after surgery. The reconstructed finger, for example, should be flexed equal to the adjacent ulnar digit. The wrist tenodesis effect may also be used to judge proper graft tension by placing the wrist through a range of motion. Wrist flexion should allow near normal digital extension, whereas full wrist extension should result in slightly more flexion than the normal cascade. If the tension appears incorrect, the proximal repair suture can be removed and the tension readjusted by sliding the weave one way or the other.

Pulley Reconstruction

A thorough evaluation of the pulley system must be undertaken during the first stage of a tendon reconstruction and any

deficiencies corrected when the silastic rod is used as a spacer. A well-healed pulley reconstruction surrounding a pseudosynovial sheath will facilitate early mobilization and gliding of the tendon graft. Pulley reconstruction during the second stage at the same time as tendon graft insertion increases the likelihood of pulley rupture and/or adhesion formation.

The A2 and A4 pulleys provide the most important biomechanical advantage for the flexor tendons and should be reconstructed if they are significantly damaged. The generated force along the tendon at the fingertip will be 30 times higher at the digital pulley. The material used for pulley reconstruction should therefore be strong, compact, and flexible to allow easy anchoring to the adjacent structures. The recommended width of a reconstructed pulley is approximately 5 mm. Autogenous tendon grafts of palmaris longus, plantaris, toe extensor, extensor indicis proprius, extensor retinaculum, or fascia lata are most commonly used, but synthetic materials have also been described by several authors. Various techniques using single, double, or triple loops circling the phalanx have been described, as well as "belt buckle" techniques using parts of the IP-joint volar plate (Figure 111-15). A common mistake is to underestimate the length of donor material required for pulley reconstruction. A double-loop reconstruction in an average digit, for example, may require approximately 10 cm of graft. Multiple pulley reconstructions, however, should not compromise available donor areas required for later tendon grafting.

Choice of Rod Size

In general, the largest size silicone rod possible should be placed underneath the remaining pulleys. A tight pseudosynovial sheath that forms around a small rod may lead to difficulties in mobilization after graft placement and the formation of adhesions or rupture at the tenorrhaphy sites. The tendon rod may be attached distally with a screw or sutured to the distal tendon remnant. The gliding of the implant after distal fixation should be tested by passively flexing and extending the finger. The implant should move freely without buckling between the pulleys. The appropriateness of the implant size may be confirmed during surgery by pulling and pushing on the rod proximally to note how easily it moves beneath the remaining pulleys.

Rehabilitation After Tendon Grafting

Tendon grafts were historically managed by prolonged immobilization to allow the proximal and distal graft junctures to heal.[74] More recently, the Kleinert controlled passive-motion protocol designed for patients who have had primary tendon repair has been applied for tendon graft rehabilitation with success.[29] We begin controlled passive motion in patients with tendon grafts immediately after surgery, with the initiation of active motion at 3 weeks and strengthening exercises at 6 weeks.

Superficialis Finger/Profundus Finger Reconstruction

In some patients with multiple flexor tendon injuries or extensive pulley-system damage, repair or reconstruction of both FDP and FDS tendons is not feasible. Creation of a superficialis *or* profundus finger with a single flexor may salvage partial digital function in these cases.[6] Staged reconstruction is performed with a silastic rod and subsequent tendon graft. The DIP joint needs to be fused or tenodesed in a superficialis finger.

OUTCOMES

Complications

The complexity of flexor tendon grafting predisposes the staged reconstruction to numerous potential complications. Infection may occur after silicone rod placement in a traumatized bed, necessitating rod removal. Synovitis secondary to the silicone rod can on occasions, however, mimic the symptoms and signs of an acute infection. An inappropriately tight pulley reconstruction during the first stage may lead to buckling of the rod and resultant implant failure. Pulleys that are not tight enough, on the other hand, may result in subsequent bowstringing of the tendon graft and a decreased range of motion. The tenorrhaphy or the graft itself may rupture during postoperative mobilization. If diagnosed early, immediate reexploration and repair may salvage the tendon graft. Other late complications include adhesion formation, decreased range of motion, and contracture. Excessive length of the tendon graft may result in a lumbrical plus deformity, with paradoxical extension at the IP joint when attempting digital flexion caused by transmission of the FDP contraction through the lumbricals to the extensor mechanism.

Long-Term Results

The assessment of flexor tendon reconstruction is hampered by the lack of a universal system to evaluate results. Outcomes data have not been reported uniformly from different centers. McClinton et al[51] studied 100 tendon grafts for the treatment of isolated profundus lacerations and concluded that two-stage

reconstruction is not required. The index finger in this study did poorly in regaining motion compared with the ulnar three digits. The patients in the study, however, were not classified according to the severity of injury. Amadio et al[2] demonstrated an improved outcome from staged tendon reconstruction when there was severe injury to the flexor system (Boyes stage 5 and 6). In his series, 54% of patients had a good or excellent result by the TAM method, expressed as a percentage of preoperative total passive motion (TPM). There was a complication rate of 15%, including 4% rupture, 4% amputation, and 1% reflex sympathetic dystrophy (RSD). Tenolysis was required after tendon grafting in 16% of patients. The results were gen erally poorer in zone I or II injuries, or in patients under 10 years of age. Similar findings were reported by LaSalle and Strickland,[34] who concluded that staged tendon reconstruction should be reserved for badly scarred digits. In their series, 47% of patients required subsequent tenolysis. The final outcome, according to the TAM percentage of TPM for only the IP joints, showed that 16% of the patients had a poor result, with the remainder equally divided between excellent, good, and fair results. In their review, Wehbe et al[73] found flexion contractures to be a significant complication in 41% of fingers after reconstruction. A successful outcome after flexor tendon reconstruction therefore demands the most meticulous patient selection, surgical techniques, and postoperative rehabilitation.

REFERENCES

1. Abrahamsson SO, Gelberman RH, Lohmander SL: Variations in cellular proliferation and matrix synthesis in intrasynovial and extrasynovial tendons: an in vitro study in dogs, *J Hand Surg [Am]* 19:259, 1994.

2. Amadio PC, Wood MB, Cooney WP III, Bogard SD: Staged flexor tendon reconstruction in the fingers and hand, *J Hand Surg [Am]* 13:559, 1988.

3. Ark JW, Gelberman RH, Abrahamsson, SO, et al: Cellular survival and proliferation in autogenous flexor tendon grafts, *J Hand Surg [Am]* 19:249, 1994.

4. Becker H: Intrinsic tendon cell proliferation in tissue culture, *J Hand Surg [Am]* 6:616, 1981.

5. Bishop A, Cooney W, Wood M: Treatment of partial tendon lacerations: the effect of tenorrhaphy and early protected motion, *J Trauma* 26:301, 1986.

6. Blackmore SM, Hunter JM, Kobus RJ: Superficialis finger reconstruction: a new look at a last-resort procedure, *Hand Clin* 7:461, 1991.

7. Boyes JH: Flexor tendon grafts in the fingers and thumb: an evaluation of end results, *J Bone Joint Surg* 32A:489, 1950.

8. Brooks F, Seiler J: Flexor tendon repair in zone II, *Atlas Hand Clin* 1:1, 1996.

9. Bruner JM: The Z-zag volar-digital incision for flexor tendon surgery, *Plast Reconstr Surg* 40:571, 1967.

10. Callan P, Morrison W: A new approach to flexor tendon repair, *J Hand Surg [Br]* 19:513, 1994.

11. Chow J, Thomes L, Dovelle S: A combined regimen of controlled motion following flexor tendon repair in "no man's land," *Plast Reconstr Surg* 79:447, 1987.

12. Crosby EB, Linscheid RL: Rupture of the flexor profundus tendon of the ring finger secondary to ancient fracture of the hook of the hamate, *J Bone Joint Surg* 56A:1076-1078, 1974.

13. Diao E, Hariharan J, Soejima O, Lotz J: Effect of peripheral suture depth on strength of tendon repairs, *J Hand Surg [Am]* 21:234, 1996.

14. Doyle JR: Anatomy of the finger flexor tendon sheath and pulley system, *J Hand Surg [Am]* 13:473, 1988.

15. Ehrlich G, Peterson L, Sokoloff L, Bunin J: Pathogenesis of rupture of extensor tendons at the wrist in rheumatoid arthritis, *Arthritis Rheum* 2:342, 1959.

16. Ertel A: Flexor tendon ruptures in rheumatoid arthritis, *Hand Clin* 5:177, 1989.

17. Ertel A, Millender L, Nalebuff E, et al: Flexor tendon ruptures in patients with rheumatoid arthritis, *J Hand Surg [Am]* 13:860, 1988.

18. Gault DT: Reduction of grip strength, finger flexion pressure, finger pinch pressure and key pinch following flexor tendon repair, *J Hand Surg [Br]* 12:182, 1987.

19. Gelberman RH, Seiler JG III, Rosenberg AE, et al: Intercalary flexor tendon grafts, *Scand J Plast Reconstr Hand Surg* 26:257, 1992.

20. Gelberman RH, Woo S: The physiological basis for application of controlled stress in the rehabilitation of flexor tendon injuries, *J Hand Ther* 2:66, 1989.

21. Gunter G: Traumatic avulsion of the insertion of flexor digitorum profundus, *Aust NZ J Surg* 30:1, 1960.

22. Hagberg L: Exogenous hyaluronate as an adjunct in the prevention of adhesions after flexor tendon surgery: a controlled clinical trial, *J Hand Surg [Am]* 17:132, 1992.

23. Hall RF Jr, Vliegenthart DH: A modified midlateral incision for volar approach to the digit, *J Hand Surg [Br]* 11:195, 1986.

24. Hallett J, Motta G: Tendon ruptures in the hand with particular reference to attrition ruptures in the carpal tunnel, *Hand* 14:283, 1982.

25. Hoffman S, et al: Unusual flexor tendon ruptures in the hand, *Arch Surg* 96:249, 1968.

26. Hunter JM: Staged flexor tendon reconstruction, *J Hand Surg [Am]* 8:789, 1983.

27. Hunter JM, Jaeger SH, Matsui T, Miyaji N: The pseudosynovial sheath: its characteristics in a primate model, *J Hand Surg [Am]* 8:461, 1983.

28. Idler R: Anatomy and biomechanics of the digital flexor tendons, *Hand Clin* 1:3, 1985.

29. Imbriglia JE, Hunter J, Rennie W: Secondary flexor tendon reconstruction, *Hand Clin* 5:395, 1989.

30. Inoue G: Attritional rupture of the extensor tendon due to long-standing Kienböck's disease, *Ann Chir Main Memb Super* 13:135, 1994.

31. Kleinert HD, Spokevicius S, Papas NH: History of flexor tendon repair, *J Hand Surg [Am]* 20:546, 1995.

32. Kulick M, Smith S, Hadler K: Oral ibuprofen: evaluation of its effect on peritendinous adhesions and breaking strength of a tenorrhaphy, *J Hand Surg [Am]* 11:110, 1986.

33. Landsmeer J: The coordination of finger-joint motion, *J Bone Joint Surg* 45A:1654, 1963.

34. LaSalle WB, Strickland JW: An evaluation of the two-stage flexor tendon reconstruction technique, *J Hand Surg [Am]* 8:263, 1983.

35. Leddy J, Packer J: Avulsion of the profundus tendon in athletes, *J Hand Surg [Am]* 2:66, 1977.

36. Lister G: Incision and closure of the flexor sheath during primary tendon repair, *Hand Clin* 1:85, 1985.

37. Lister G, Tonkin M: The results of primary flexor tendon repair with closure of the tendon sheath, *J Hand Surg [Am]* 11:767, 1986.

38. Lister G, et al: Primary flexor tendon repair followed by immediate controlled mobilization, *J Hand Surg [Am]* 2:441, 1977.

39. Lundborg G, Hansson H, Rank F, et al: Superficial repair of severed flexor tendons in synovial environment: an experimental, ultrastructural study on cellular mechanisms, *J Hand Surg [Am]* 5:451, 1980.

40. Lundborg G, Rank F: Experimental intrinsic healing of flexor tendons based upon synovial fluid nutrition, *J Hand Surg [Am]* 3:21, 1978.

41. Mahring M: Attrition flexor tendon rupture due to scaphoid non-union initiating an anterior interosseous nerve syndrome: a case report, *J Hand Surg [Br]* 10:62, 1985.

42. Manske P: The flexor tendon, *Orthopedics* 10:1733, 1987.

43. Manske P, Bridwell K, Lesker P: Nutrient pathways to flexor tendons of chickens using tritiated Prolene, *J Hand Surg [Am]* 3:352, 1978.

44. Manske P, Bridwell K, Whiteside L, Lesker P: Nutrition of flexor tendons in monkeys, *Clin Orthop* 136:294, 1978.

45. Manske P, Lesker P: Avulsion of the ring finger flexor digitorum profundus tendon: an experimental study, *Hand* 10:52, 1978.

46. Masada K, Kawabata H, Ono K: Pathologic rupture of flexor tendons due to long-standing Kienböck's disease, *J Hand Surg [Am]* 12:22, 1987.

47. Mashadi Z, Amis A: The effect of locking loops on the strength of tendon repair, *J Hand Surg [Br]* 16:35, 1991.

48. Mason M, Allen H: The rate of healing tendons: experimental study of tensile strength, *Ann Surg* 113:424, 1941.

49. May EJ, Silfverskiöld KL: Rate of recovery after flexor tendon repair in zone II: a prospective longitudinal study of 145 digits, *Scand J Plast Reconstr Surg* 27:89, 1993.

50. McCarthy D, Boardman N, Tramaglini D, et al: Clinical management of partially lacerated digital flexor tendons: a survey of hand surgeons, *J Hand Surg [Am]* 20:273, 1996.

51. McClinton MA, Curtis RM, Wilgis SEF: One hundred tendon grafts for isolated flexor digitorum profundus injuries, *J Hand Surg [Am]* 7:224, 1982.

52. McMaster P: Tendon and muscle ruptures: clinical and experimental studies on the causes and location of subcutaneous ruptures, *J Bone Joint Surg* 15:705, 1933.

53. Papandrea R, Seitz W, Shapiro P, Borden B: Biomechanical and clinical evaluation of the epitenon first technique of flexor tendon repair, *J Hand Surg [Am]* 20:261, 1995.

54. Peacock E: Biological principles in the healing of long tendons, *Surg Clin North Am* 45:461, 1965.

55. Phillips C, Mass D: Mechanical analysis of the palmar aponeurosis pulley in human cadavers, *J Hand Surg [Am]* 21:240, 1996.

56. Potenza A: Critical evaluation of flexor tendon healing and adhesion formation within artificial digital sheaths: an experimental study, *J Bone Joint Surg* 45A:1217, 1963.

57. Saldana M, et al: Flexor tendon repair and rehabilitation in zone II: open sheath technique versus closed sheath technique, *J Hand Surg [Am]* 12:1110, 1987.

58. Sanders W: Advantages of "epitenon first" suture placement technique in flexor tendon repair, *Clin Orthop* 280:198, 1992.

59. Schneider LH: Staged tendon reconstruction, *Hand Clin* 1:109, 1985.

60. Silfverskiöld K, May E: Flexor tendon repair in zone II with a new suture technique and an early mobilization program combining passive and active motion, *J Hand Surg [Am]* 19:53, 1994.

61. So Y, Chow S, Pun W, et al: Evaluation of results in flexor tendon repair: a critical analysis of five methods in ninety-five digits, *J Hand Surg [Am]* 15:258, 1990.

62. Stewart K, Van Strien G: Postoperative management of flexor tendon injuries. In Hunter JM, Mackin EJ, Callahan AD (editors): *Rehabilitation of the hand,* ed 4, St. Louis, 1995, Mosby.

63. Strickland JW: Flexor tenolysis, *Hand Clin* 1:121, 1985.

64. Strickland JW: Results of flexor tendon surgery in zone 2, *Hand Clin* 1:167, 1985.

65. Strickland JW: Flexor tendon injuries, *Orthop Rev* 16:137, 1987.

66. Strickland JW: Biologic rationale, clinical application, and results of early motion following flexor tendon repair, *J Hand Ther* 2:71, 1989.

67. Strickland JW: Flexor tendon injuries: foundations of treatment, *J Am Acad Orthop Surg* 3:44, 1995.

68. Strickland JW: The Indiana method of flexor tendon repair, *Atlas Hand Clin* 1:77, 1996.

69. Trail I, et al: An evaluation of suture materials used in tendon surgery, *J Hand Surg [Br]* 14:422, 1989.

70. Vaughan-Jackson O: Attrition ruptures of tendons on the rheumatoid hand, *J Bone Joint Surg* 40A:1431, 1958.

71. Verdan CE, Michen J: Le traitement des plaies des tendons flechisseurs des dogits, *Rev Chir Orthop* 47:285, 1961.

72. Wehbe MA: Tendon graft anatomy and harvesting, *Orthop Rev* 23:253, 1994.

73. Wehbe MA, Mawr B, Hunter JM, et al: Two-stage flexor-tendon reconstruction, *J Bone Joint Surg* 68A:752, 1986.

74. Wilson RL: Flexor tendon grafting, *Hand Clin* 1:97, 1985.

75. Younger C, DeFiore J: Rupture of flexor tendons to fingers after a Colles' fracture, *J Bone Joint Surg* 57A:562, 1975.

76. Zancolli E: *Structural and dynamic basis of hand surgery,* ed 2, Philadelphia, 1979, JB Lippincott.

CHAPTER 112

Extensor Tendons

William C. Pederson

INTRODUCTION

The care of injuries to the extensor tendons of the hand is often relegated to a position of less importance than that of the flexor tendons, yet improper management of these injuries can lead to problems no less debilitating to hand function than problems with the flexor system. A thorough understanding of the anatomy and function of the extensor system in both the finger and hand is necessary to properly manage these injuries. An appreciation of advances in postoperative management and the therapy of extensor-tendon injuries is also essential to optimize the outcome. This chapter will deal with the anatomy, management, and postoperative care of injuries to the extensor tendon system in the fingers and hand.

INDICATIONS

ANATOMY

The extensor system receives contributions from both the extrinsic muscles of the forearm and the intrinsic muscles of the hand. The long extensor muscles begin over the lateral epicondyle in their common origin—the "extensor wad." All of the extensor muscles of the hand and fingers are innervated by the radial nerve or its ultimate motor branch, the posterior interosseous nerve. These muscles terminate in tendons that cross the dorsal wrist in various extensor compartments underneath the extensor retinaculum. These compartments act as pulleys at the wrist to prevent bowstringing of the tendons with contraction of the proximal muscles. The tendons acting on the thumb—the abductor pollicis longus (APL), the extensor pollicis brevis (EPB), and extensor pollicis longus (EPL)—are the most radial of the extrinsic digital extensors and pass through the first and third dorsal compartments, respectively. The extensor indicis proprius (EIP) to the index passes through the fourth dorsal compartment with the common digital extensors, the extensor digitorum communis (EDC). The proper extensor to the little finger, the extensor digiti quinti (EDQ) passes alone through the fifth dorsal

compartment. The EIP and EDQ allow independent extension of the index and little fingers.

The extensor tendons proceed across the dorsum of the hand after passing through their various compartments. The common extensors of the fingers are interconnected over the distal third of the metacarpals by oblique slips of the juncturae tendinum, which promote extension of the fingers "en mass." At the level of the metacarpophalangeal (MCP) joints, the tendons are held in a central position over the joint by the sagittal bands, which connect palmarly to the volar plates and proximal phalanges. The EIP, which is on the ulnar side of the EDC to the index, fuses with the EDC at the level of the MCP joint and sagittal bands.

The intrinsic tendons become part of the extensor "apparatus" at the MCP joint. The intrinsic muscles contributing to digital extension are the *interossei* and *lumbricals,* and they are innervated primarily by the ulnar nerve, with contribution by the median nerve to the thumb intrinsic muscles and the radial lumbricals. The intrinsic tendons lie in a position volar to the axis of rotation of the MCP joint and thus at this level act as flexors of this joint. The extrinsic tendons continue through the dorsal apparatus at the MCP joint and terminate at the central slip with insertion on the dorsal base of the middle phalanx (Figure 112-1). The central slip is the primary extensor of the proximal interphalangeal (PIP) joint. The intrinsic tendons pass bilaterally along the mid-portion of the digit, with a lesser contribution to the central slip. The primary contribution of the intrinsic tendons is to the lateral bands, which continue from lateral to dorsal to become the conjoined tendon over the dorsum of the middle phalanx. This combined tendon then inserts on the proximal dorsal aspect of the distal phalanx and is the primary extensor of the distal interphalangeal (DIP) joint.

These various parts of the extensor apparatus in the finger are held in their proper place by various retinacular ligaments, which maintain the position and alignment of the system. All portions of the extensor system in the finger are interconnected, and therefore one can appreciate that damage to one part can affect the function of the whole system. Most surgery to repair extensor-tendon injuries or for reconstruction of problems of digital extension attempt to restore the delicate balance of this system. One of the best descriptions of the

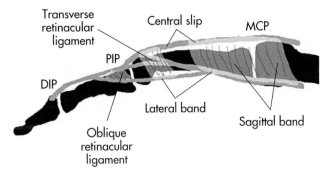

Figure 112-1. Diagram of extensor mechanism in the finger. *DIP,* Distal interphalangeal; *MCP,* metacarpophalangeal; *PIP,* proximal interphalangeal.

anatomy and actions of the extensor mechanism is given by Kaplan[22] in his classic work on functional anatomy, and this reference is suggested for further reading.

OPEN INJURIES

Open injuries to the extensor mechanism of the hand are common because the dorsal hand and wrist are frequently exposed to trauma.[2] This is particularly true of the "knuckles" of the hand, and injuries to the extensor tendons in this area can result from accidents in the workplace or home and from use of the hands in pugilistic activities. Lacerations at any of the joints of the fingers are common, and tooth injuries to the tendon and joint from fighting with the hands are common at the MCP joints.

The skin cover on the dorsum of the hand and fingers is relatively thin and it is not unusual to encounter tendon injury in combination with loss of the overlying soft tissue coverage in this area. Repair and reconstruction of these injuries must take this into account because skin coverage may take priority over tendon repair. This can mitigate against primary repair, and the surgeon must be acquainted with techniques of later tendon reconstruction. Although the extensor system is often assumed to be simpler than the flexor-tendon anatomy, this is in fact not the case. The interconnections of the extrinsic and intrinsic mechanisms for digital extension are finely balanced, and any disruption of this balance may lead to ineffectual extension and flexion of the fingers.[22]

CLOSED INJURIES

Closed injuries to the extensor mechanism are relatively less common than open injuries, but they do occur in certain circumstances. The most common closed injury to the extensor tendons, and one of the most common injuries overall, is the *mallet finger.* This is an injury to the extensor tendon at its distal insertion into the base of the distal phalanx of the finger. It can result from severe trauma, such as that which occurs in the forced flexion of the DIP joint while it is actively extended in a football player, or from seemingly insignificant trauma, such as the surgical resident rolling up his socks after a night on call. This injury is frequently seen initially by the patient's general physician, who may or may not be able to adequately treat it. It is not uncommon for the patient to be referred to the hand surgeon after several weeks of inadequate or inappropriate management. If left untreated, a simple mallet finger can lead to the so-called *Swan neck* deformity. The lateral bands on the finger in this lesion migrate dorsally as they tighten in an attempt to extend the DIP joint. In the severe lesion, the PIP joint becomes hyperextended as the volar plate stretches, with the DIP joint flexed.

Closed injuries are also seen in the more proximal extensor system, although somewhat less frequently than the mallet finger. Injuries at the PIP joint are fairly common and are usually the result of "jamming" the finger, or joint dislocation. Most patients presenting with a "jammed" PIP joint do not have significant central slip injuries, but this must be ruled out to avoid severe sequelae. Central slip tears, if left untreated, can result in a boutonniere deformity, and thus a seemingly trivial injury can lead to a marked decrease in digital function. A boutonniere deformity results from an injury to the central slip. The PIP joint becomes flexed, and the DIP joint eventually hyperextends. This happens from the pull of the lateral bands, which migrate volarly, and which now act to *flex* rather than *extend* the PIP joint. The DIP joint assumes a hyperextended position as the lateral bands tighten further.

The extensor system can also be injured at the MCP level, although this is less common than either of the above lesions. If the finger is forcibly adducted or abducted at the MCP joint, a tear in the extensor hood may result. This can lead to subluxation of the extensor tendon as it crosses the MCP-joint level. This injury, while not terribly disabling, may cause lack of full extension at this level and is usually painful to the patient. In my experience, this injury is usually seen by the hand surgeon late, and although splinting may heal an early injury, it seems to do little after a period of several weeks. Although making the appropriate diagnosis may be difficult, some authors feel that an exact diagnosis can be made by magnetic resonance imaging (MRI) of the injured joint.[12] Operative repair of the tear, with appropriate postoperative splinting, will usually alleviate symptoms. Severe bony injuries in the proximal wrist[28,35] and forearm[38] can lead to extensor-tendon rupture, but these injuries are decidedly unusual.

Other closed injuries to the extensor tendons are unusual in otherwise normal patients, but rupture of the EDC tendons from trauma has been reported.[36,37] Although this etiology is distinctly unusual, extensor-tendon ruptures are relatively common in patients with rheumatoid arthritis. Spontaneous rupture of the extensor tendons to the little and ring fingers occurs because of attenuation of the tendons over a protruding eroded ulna, a condition often referred to as the *Vaughan-Jackson* lesion,[40] after its first description. The loss of extension in these fingers in the rheumatoid patient can be confusing because loss of flexor/extensor balance or posterior interosseous nerve palsy can also lead to decreased extension in these patients.

OPERATIONS

ANATOMY

For the purposes of tendon repair of the extensor system, the hand and forearm have been divided into zones based on the anatomy and approach to repair of the injury (Figure 112-2). The odd-numbered zones in this system are located over joints, beginning with zone I over the DIP joint. Although the thumb is included in this general scheme, zones 2 and 3 are excluded in the thumb because it has only two phalanges. Injuries to the extensor system in the following discussion will be approached by zones, from proximal to distal.

REPAIR OF INJURY TO THE EXTENSOR SYSTEM

Zone IX

The most proximal zone covers the extensor muscles in the forearm. Injuries in this zone involving only the muscle bellies may be deemed insignificant by emergency room personnel and physicians. It is not uncommon for patients with lacerations through the muscle fascia to have management entirely in the emergency room with the usual "wash out and send out" technique. If the lacerations are deep or involve a significant portion of the muscle, it may be difficult to differentiate between a pure muscular injury and posterior interosseous nerve injury when the patient presents to the specialist's office. The patient who is left unsplinted for a while may present with an inability to fully extend the fingers and/or wrist from improperly treated injuries at this level. The diagnosis of the actual injury (muscle versus nerve) can be difficult, but a properly performed electromyogram (EMG) can usually rule out injury to the radial or posterior interosseous nerve.

When seen primarily by the hand surgeon, injuries through the fascia in zone IX should usually be treated in the operating room. One should be able to identify injury to the motor nerve with adequate exposure and lighting. Likewise, after thorough irrigation, the muscle fascia can be approximated to decrease separation of the ends. The tendon insertion into the muscle may on occasion be damaged and separated at this level, in which case the ends should be sought in the muscle and repaired. I prefer to splint the wrist and fingers in extension for 3 weeks after surgery, which should allow adequate time for the muscle to reapproximate. I then place the patient in a dynamic splint for another 2 to 3 weeks, which allows a gradual return of motion and avoids excessive stress on the healing muscle. Muscle-belly injuries, in contrast to injuries to the tendons alone, should not lead to a loss of motion if immobilized; however, in my experience, early motion may lead to dehiscence and stretching of the muscle.

Zone VIII

The musculotendinous junctions lie in this area. Tendon repair in this area is usually straightforward but can be difficult if the proximal tendon end retracts significantly within the structure of the muscle. Injuries in zone VIII are similar in this

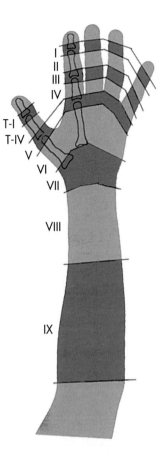

Figure 112-2. Diagram of extensor zones in the hand and forearm. Note that the thumb has only two zones.

regard to those in the more proximal zone IX. A muscle belly lacerated in this area should be brought back out to length and the tendon end reapproximated to the deep tendinous portion of the muscle or "woven" back into the substance of the muscle. If there has been damage to the proximal muscle and neither of the above options are practical, the tendon can be repaired in a side-to-side fashion. This is particularly applicable in the case of the EDC tendons because they normally work together. Significant scarring can occur in this area, and it is usually wise to begin protected digital motion early.

Zone VII

Zone VII injuries can be very problematic in my experience because this is the area in which the tendons run in their various synovial tunnels. Extensor-tendon repair in this zone is similar in many respects to repair of the flexor tendons within the digital pulley system of the fingers. Tendons repaired in this area have a tendency to scar together and to the extensor retinaculum, which can lead to poor results after repair.

Small wounds in this area can result in injury to several tendons because many of the tendons are grouped together. Good exposure before repair is therefore necessary. A portion of the retinaculum may need to be incised or excised to afford proper exposure to repair the injured tendons. The tendons in this zone are fairly round and are usually best repaired with a core suture of synthetic, nonabsorbable 4-0 suture. I prefer braided to monofilament suture because the knot from a monofilament is often palpable under the skin after healing has occurred. One should check for binding as the tendon passes through its respective compartment after repair. The thickened area of tendon at the site of the repair can bind or trigger as it goes through the compartment in the postoperative period, and the compartment should be released to prevent this if necessary. Leaving the retinaculum unrepaired, or excising a portion of it should not lead to bowstringing of the tendons.[23]

Traditionally, the wrist has been splinted after surgery in about 30 degrees of extension, with the MCP joints in slight flexion and finger IP joints splinted straight. This is continued for 10 days to 2 weeks, at which time careful protected motion is begun. The trend has been toward early protected dynamic splinting, which gives better overall results in terms of motion.[23] This type of motion and splinting should be initiated as soon as the condition of the wound permits, and is continued for 6 weeks after surgery.

Zone VI

The tendons in this zone are on the dorsum of the hand and tend to go from being round to rather flat as they proceed distally. The juncturae are present in this area as well, and these interconnections may make examination equivocal, even in the face of an injury. Injury to the extensor tendons in this zone is often combined with injury to underlying bony structures, which can lead to difficulties with scarring. Wounds with a combined loss of substance of the overlying skin and extensor tendons are common as well, and management of this type of injury is more difficult.

The repair of tendons on the dorsum of the hand is usually straightforward and is often performed in the emergency room. This should not be done unless the wound is very clean and there is no underlying fracture or soft tissue loss. Most patients with tendon injuries to the dorsal hand should have radiographs taken to rule out underlying metacarpal fractures, which may be missed in the emergency room. The patient's wound should be managed in the operating room when there are open fractures or complex soft tissue wounds. Repair of the tendons themselves is straightforward, and can usually be done with a core suture of synthetic, braided 4-0 suture. The more distal tendons have a tendency to be flatter, and repair can be accomplished with one or two figure-of-eight sutures placed in the tendon. The type of repair will depend on the cross section of the tendon at the injury site.

Closed rupture of the extensor tendons is relatively common in this zone in rheumatoid patients. This usually presents as the sudden loss of the ability to extend the involved finger and is usually painless. An isolated tendon rupture may not be too noticeable to the patient because of the presence of intact juncturae. The most commonly affected digit is the little finger, often followed rather rapidly by the ring and middle fingers (Figure 112-3). Direct repair of these ruptures is usually difficult, if not impossible, and I will usually repair a single rupture side-to-side to an adjacent tendon if this tendon is not also attenuated. Transfer of the EIP from the index finger can

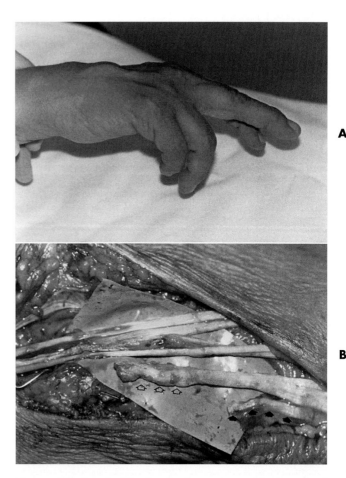

Figure 112-3. **A,** The hand of a patient with rheumatoid arthritis after spontaneous extensor-tendon rupture, with inability to extend little and ring fingers. **B,** The intraoperative findings, with rupture of the EDC to the small finger *(closed arrows)* and EDC to ring finger *(open arrows).*

be utilized in the case of multiple tendon ruptures. Further information on this problem is discussed in Chapter 128.

The wrist should be splinted in extension, with the MCP joints in slight flexion and PIP joints in full extension. This type of splinting has traditionally been applied for 4 weeks, but again, early motion is now advocated by many surgeons and therapists.

Zone V

Zone V covers the level of the MCP joint. The extensor tendon at this level is held in place over the joint by the extensor hood, and the intrinsic tendons are present at the lateral surfaces of the joint. Injury to the extensor tendon is common at this level because of scrapes or cuts of the knuckle in workers. It is also commonly injured in pugilists, with the "fight bite" being a common injury of the tendon and joint at the MCP level. This occurs when the closed fist strikes a tooth at the MCP joint level, leading to tendon injury and potential devastation to the joint if infection occurs. For this reason, most tendon injuries at this level require exploration, irrigation, and repair in the operating room. Most authors feel that small injuries to the hand at this level that have the appearance of puncture wounds should be considered tooth injuries and treated accordingly. All patients with injuries at this level should have radiographs taken to evaluate the metacarpal head for fractures or retained tooth elements.

If there is suspicion of a tooth-related injury, the wound must be explored, debrided, and irrigated in the operating room. The tendon is repaired and the wound left open. I prefer to place a small Penrose drain into the joint and usually remove it after 24 to 48 hours. Operative treatment should be followed by a course of intravenous antibiotics to cover the oral aerobic and anaerobic flora. I have seen patients late after injury (more than 24 hours) with destruction of both the extensor hood and bone from human tooth injuries at the MCP level. These patients are managed with operative debridement of the infected tissue and appropriate antibiotic coverage. This can be a devastating injury, however, and I have at least one patient who eventually required a ray resection of the finger because of injury and loss of substance in the MCP-joint area from a human bite injury that was treated late.

Simple open lacerations should also probably be managed in the operating room because the joint capsule has usually been violated by the trauma that injured the tendon. These lacerations require adequate debridement and irrigation to avoid joint infection. The skin wound and tendon injury can be at different levels, depending on the state of MCP joint flexion when injury occurred. The tendon will not retract when injured at this level, but if the finger was flexed, the level of tendon injury can be a centimeter or more proximal to the skin wound. The skin incision may therefore require extension to absolutely rule out injury to the tendon. Repair of a simple tendon laceration is straightforward and can be done as mentioned above with synthetic braided nonabsorbable 4-0 suture. I will usually perform a figure-of-eight repair at this level, with the knot placed on the deep surface of the tendon (Figure 112-4, *A* and *B*). Injuries to the extensor hood should be repaired as well because subluxation of the tendon can occur if this is not approximated.

Rehabilitation of these injuries has again traditionally been with immobilization in extension, but early passive motion has been advocated by many authors more recently. Merritt has developed a system of postoperative management utilizing a "relative motion extensor splint" (W. Merritt, personal communication). He has found that early active motion can be done if the repair is protected with a simple splint placed under the proximal portion of the proximal phalanx of the injured finger (Figure 112-5, *A*). This splint allows flexion and extension of all fingers, and he has demonstrated in clinical cases that this amount of splinting avoids any pull at the repair site (Figure 112-5, *B*). Merritt allows early return of motion and return to activity while wearing the splint. He has reported 96% total active motion in the injured digits after this therapy protocol (Figure 112-5, *C*). Merritt has also utilized this technique with good results for injuries in zones VI and VII.

A tear in the extensor hood or sagittal band at the MCP joint level as mentioned earlier in the section on closed injuries

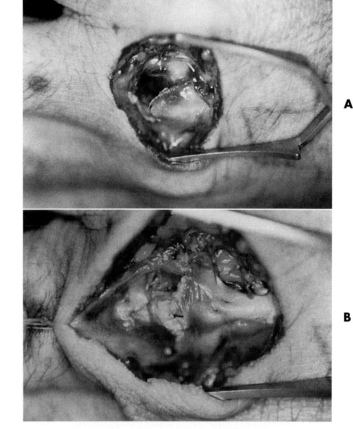

Figure 112-4. **A,** A saw injury to the extensor tendon in zone V. Note that a portion of metacarpal head was avulsed. **B,** The tendon after repair with a slight overlap of ends and the suture knots deep to dorsal surface.

is also a reasonably common injury.[21] These injuries are not usually seen initially by the hand specialist, and most commonly present several weeks after injury with obvious subluxation of the extensor tendon at the MCP joint with flexion. I have not had one of these injuries heal with splinting after 3 weeks and have had to operate to correct the tendon subluxation. Some authors suggest that closed injuries to the extensor hood with tendon subluxation can be effectively treated with splinting for up to 2 weeks but more chronic injuries will require surgical repair.[20] This would certainly agree with my experience, and I believe this is a reasonable approach.

I approach the joint through a longitudinal incision directly over the joint. There may be a great deal of scarring if the injury is quite old, but the defect in the extensor hood/sagittal band is usually obvious. The edges are freed up and the rent can usually be repaired directly with several interrupted, simple, 4-0 braided nonabsorbable sutures. If this repair is too tight or the extensor hood is attenuated, a loop made out of a portion of the extensor tendon is fashioned from the nondamaged side and sutured over to the intermetacarpal ligament on the side of injury.[20] I immobilize the hand for 5 to 7 days after surgery and then begin protected motion. Buddy

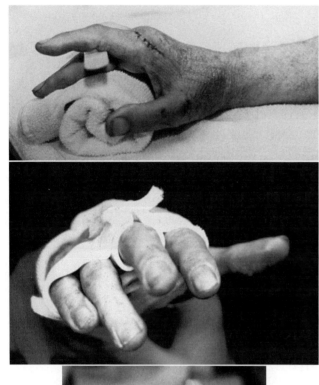

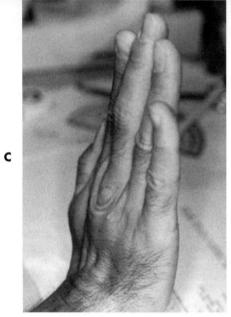

Figure 112-5. **A,** The patient immediately after surgery, with temporary "relative motion splint." **B,** The patient in fabricated Orthoplast splint that supports the repaired tendon at the middle-finger MCP joint but allows motion. **C,** The final result after therapy. (Courtesy Wyndell H. Merritt, MD, FACS.)

taping of the fingers is usually adequate to avoid undue tension on the repair. I have had good results from both of these techniques with no evidence of recurrent subluxation.

Zone IV

Injury to the extensor tendons in this zone primarily involves the central slip of the extensor mechanism. The lateral bands can also be injured as they come along the sides of the finger,

but this type of injury is relatively uncommon. Injuries to the tendon in this zone may be associated with fracture of the proximal phalanx; when present, this can lead to marked scarring of the tendon.

Simple tendon lacerations on the dorsal finger are easily repaired, and I prefer to do so with interrupted simple or figure-of-eight sutures of 4-0 or 5-0 braided, synthetic, nonabsorbable suture. Some injuries may be accompanied by loss or damage to the overlying skin, and this can be problematic. The soft tissue defect will usually have to be managed first, and the tendon loss addressed at a later time. These tendons are thin and easily shredded, and care should be taken in their repair. An attempt should be made to repair the periosteum after fracture stabilization if there is an associated underlying fracture because this can be helpful in decreasing adherence of the tendon to the fracture site. Injuries to the extensor tendon at this level are usually managed with 6 weeks of postoperative splinting followed by a program of progressive active and passive motion.

Zone III

Injuries to the extensor mechanism at this level can be either open or closed and result in the classic boutonniere deformity. Closed injuries to the central slip at this level can occur with forced flexion of the PIP joint while it is actively extended, which may cause an avulsion fracture of the proximal dorsal portion of the middle phalanx. Volar dislocations of the PIP joint can also lead to a tear in the central slip and development of a boutonniere deformity. Direct laceration of the central slip is also fairly common at this level, and this open injury can also lead to a boutonniere deformity. Acute closed injuries to the central slip can be difficult to diagnose because the lateral bands may be able to extend the finger at the PIP joint if they are intact. Some feel that the ability to extend the PIP joint against resistance is an excellent test of the status of the central slip because inability to perform this maneuver is indicative of a divided central slip.[9,13] Management of all injuries to the extensor tendon at this level are aimed at preventing development of a boutonniere deformity because treatment of this can be difficult once it is established.[16]

Open injuries to the central slip at this level merit exploration in the operating room because it may be difficult to rule out joint injury in the emergency room. The tendon is repaired with figure-of-eight sutures of braided, nonabsorbable, synthetic suture after exploration and irrigation of the joint. If a dorsal injury has resulted in an avulsion fracture of the middle phalanx, it should be repaired with Kirschner wires (K wires) or a fine interosseous wire. I will usually immobilize the joint with an oblique K wire for at least 4 weeks if there has been any concomitant bony injury or injury to the collateral ligaments of the PIP joint.

These injuries are usually managed after surgery by immobilization for 4 to 6 weeks. Some authors have proposed postoperative dynamic extension splinting after a short period of immobilization.[30,33] This technique is not widely practiced to date, but further study may prove it to be beneficial. In the usual protocol, the DIP joint is kept free to allow motion of this joint, which keeps the lateral bands in motion and decreases the chances of adherence. This motion also decreases contracture of the oblique retinacular ligaments. The finger is allowed to move after this period of immobilization, and often the patient may require a course of intensive therapy to regain motion. If a lag is noticed once active motion is begun, the finger is kept splinted in the extended position for another 2 to 3 weeks in between therapy sessions. Management of the late boutonniere deformity can present many challenges and is beyond the scope of this chapter. The reader is referred to more in-depth works covering the approach to this problem.[5,9,26]

Zones I and II

The last two zones will be considered together because injuries in these two zones cause essentially the same pathology and have the same management. An injury to the extensor tendons in one of these zones causes mallet finger—the inability to extend the DIP joint—and can be caused by closed or open injuries. The most common cause of mallet fingers in my practice is closed injuries, in which there is a sudden flexion force applied to the actively extended joint. If this is left untreated, it can lead to the development of hyperextension of the PIP joint, or swan-neck deformity, because of the position of the finger. This deformity is caused by the dorsal migration and tightening of the lateral bands, which leads to a hyperextension deformity of the PIP joint. Mallet fingers can be caused by seemingly trivial trauma, or may be the result of a significant force applied to the distal digit. All patients with mallet-finger injuries should have radiographs taken of the DIP joint, including a lateral view to evaluate for the presence of a fracture, although this may not change the ultimate management.

Most patients with a closed mallet-finger injury are often seen first by their primary care physician, who may place the injured finger in a splint. Sometimes patients won't seek medical attention for this injury for several weeks because it may be fairly asymptomatic in terms of pain. All patients with these injuries should have radiographic examinations, and the presence of an avulsion fracture from the dorsal proximal end of the distal phalanx does not necessarily mandate open treatment. Nearly all mallet fingers can be treated closed by some type of external splint (Figure 112-6). Reports on splinting techniques have utilized plaster, aluminum, plastic, and wire to keep the DIP joint in full extension.[4] I prefer to use a dorsally placed, foam-covered, aluminum splint in most patients. A portion of the foam overlying the joint must be trimmed to avoid problems with skin necrosis, which have lead some authors to eschew this technique. I use a Stack prefabricated splint placed on the volar side of the finger, held in place with either tape or Velcro straps in some patients. Any splint, however, that is too easy for the patient to take off can lead to poor tendon healing. I will generally treat the patient with continuous splinting for 6 weeks, after which I place the finger in a dynamic splint that allows some flexion. If the patient continues to have some extension lag at this point I will have him or her wear a static splint at night for an additional 2 to 4 weeks.

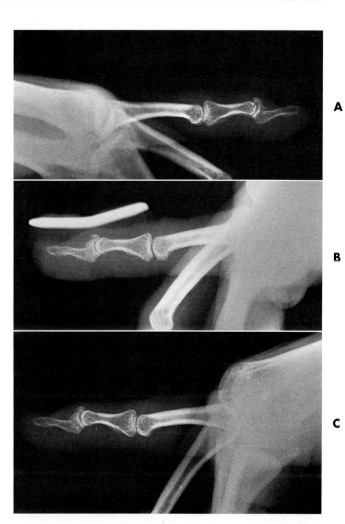

Figure 112-6. A, Radiograph of a closed mallet-finger injury with volar subluxation of the distal phalanx. This patient was referred for surgical consultation 3 weeks after injury. B, Radiograph of a finger with a dorsal aluminum splint in place. The patient wore the splint for 4 weeks. C, Radiograph after fracture healing. The patient had full extension with 45 degrees of flexion.

In my experience, the primary problem with conservative management of a mallet-finger injury is patient compliance. The splint must be worn continuously if it is to correct the injury, and it cannot be taken off without supporting the DIP joint by some other means. Many patients do not understand the necessity for this, despite being repeatedly told so. In this instance, a small nonremovable plaster splint may be the best option.[11] I will often treat patients who are intelligent and would have difficulty wearing an external splint with a buried 0.045-inch K wire across the DIP joint. The K wire can be placed in an outpatient procedure in the surgeon's office and left buried for 6 to 8 weeks. Infection is uncommon if the pin tract is properly cared for initially, although I have seen it occur with this technique. The pin is easily removed using digital block anesthesia in the office. A short, 2-to 4-week period of night splinting may be necessary after pin removal if an extensor lag develops. We have found that patients presenting up to 3 to 4 weeks after injury usually can be effectively treated

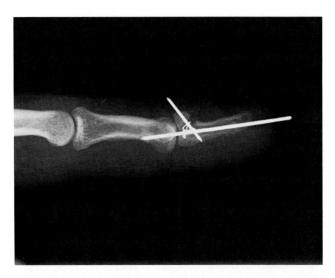

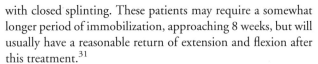

Figure 112-7. Radiograph of a finger with an injury similar to that in Figure 112-5, after correction of the subluxation by open reduction, wiring of the fracture, and K-wire pin fixation.

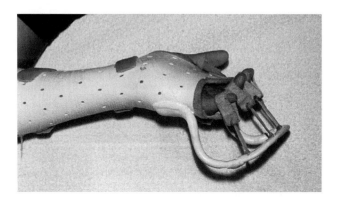

Figure 112-8. An example of a dynamic splint used for extensor-tendon injuries in zones VI through VIII.

with closed splinting. These patients may require a somewhat longer period of immobilization, approaching 8 weeks, but will usually have a reasonable return of extension and flexion after this treatment.[31]

The only patients with mallet-finger injuries on which I operate are those with open injuries and those with significant subluxation of the distal phalanx on the DIP joint in the case of fractures with a large intraarticular fragment (Figure 112-7). Open injuries are managed as mentioned above, with wash-out of the joint and tendon repair. The tendon is repaired with rather fine (4-0 or 5-0) braided, nonabsorbable suture, using simple or figure-of-eight technique. It is not unusual in open injuries to find that the tendon is raggedly torn and may be difficult, if not impossible, to properly repair. I routinely place a 0.045-inch K wire across the joint, with the joint held in slight hyperextension, in these instances. This will often allow approximation of the ends and tendon healing. I leave the pin in place for 4 to 6 weeks, and then place an external splint and begin protected motion. In cases with severe injury to the joint and loss of substance of the tendon, I will often opt for primary DIP-joint fusion rather than attempt to reconstruct the tendon at a later date. Secondary reconstruction will be necessary if the mallet finger is seen late and a swan-neck deformity is established. The reader is referred to other articles for a discussion of these procedures.[4,5,18]

REHABILITATION

The approach to rehabilitation of patients with extensor-tendon injuries has traditionally been one of a period of static splinting followed by mobilization. Although the benefit of controlled mobilization for gliding of repaired flexor tendons was appreciated in the 1970s,[24] it was not until the late 1980s and early 1990s that this approach was utilized for extensor tendons.[3] This approach was applied early to injuries proximal to zone V in the hand and forearm, with very good results in terms of motion. Chow et al[8] compared controlled mobilization to static immobilization and found excellent motion was obtained in 100% of patients in the first mobilized group. This compared favorably with the group who had immobilization, in whom only 40% obtained "excellent" motion, with 31% obtaining "good" motion, and 29% "fair" motion. The splint in this approach was applied so that the wrist was in 30 degrees of extension, with the MCP joint fully extended in a dynamic outrigger (Figure 112-8). Flexion at the MCP joint was limited to 30 degrees in the first postoperative week, 45 degrees in the second week, 60 degrees in the third week, and full flexion during the fourth and fifth weeks. There was no restriction of flexion of the IP joints. This approach has been evaluated by others for management of extensor tendon injuries on the dorsal hand, with equally gratifying results (Figure 112-9).[3,10,19,23,25]

Early motion has been advocated for injuries of the finger extensor tendons but to date has not met with universal acceptance. Most authors suggest an initial period of 2 to 4 weeks of immobilization followed by careful mobilization of the MCP and PIP joints.[15,30,33] Excellent to good results have been reported in 60% to 80% of patients using this approach.[30,33] Other authors note that the results of early mobilization in patients with zone III injuries are variable and generally worse than the results of this approach in the more proximal zones.[19] Most surgeons continue to manage finger injuries with a long period of immobilization, reserving early controlled mobilization for more proximal injuries.[10]

MANAGEMENT OF COMPOSITE DEFECTS

The dorsal hand is frequently involved in severe injuries in which skin cover is lost along with extensor tendons and/or

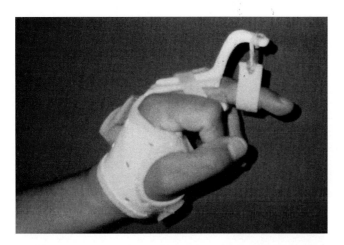

Figure 112-9. An example of a dynamic-type splint commonly used for injuries to the extensor tendons in zone V. Compare this with Merritt's splint in Figure 112-5.

bony structures. This type of injury can present many challenges to the reconstructive surgeon. The primary objectives are to obtain bony stability and provide soft tissue coverage to allow the bones to heal. A secondary objective is to provide tendons for finger extension. Sometimes these objectives can all be met with a single operation, whereas at other times the problem may require several stages to reconstruct the defect.

Traditionally, injuries involving multiple structures on the dorsal hand surface were managed in several stages: (1) bony fixation, (2) wound management or coverage, and (3) tendon and/or nerve reconstruction. The first two stages are generally accomplished in a single procedure; however, reconstruction of the tendons may take several stages.[7] Scheker et al[34] has reported good results by combining several stages to avoid a prolonged period of convalescence. Patients are managed in his approach with primary bone grafts to bony gaps, free-flap coverage utilizing cutaneous flaps, and immediate extensor-tendon reconstruction, which is accomplished by passing the grafts through individual tunnels made in the flap.[34] Only about 50% of his reported patients had "good" results, but there were few complications and none resulting in loss of the tendon or bone grafts. This approach is reasonable if one is comfortable with microsurgical flap transfer, and certainly should lead to fewer operative procedures and less time to accomplish the reconstruction.

The use of a flap, which may be taken including tendons, has been proposed by some for the dorsal hand. The primary flap of this type is the dorsalis pedis cutaneous flap,[9] which can be harvested with up to five tendons from the dorsal foot. The results using this flap in small series have been good, but the donor site on the foot is problematic.[1,6] I have treated injuries with a limited number of extensor tendons involved with the radial forearm flap. The palmaris longus tendon, if present, can be taken with this flap and utilized for reconstruction of one or two extensor tendons (Figure

112-10). The donor site from this flap is much less of a problem than that of the dorsalis pedis, and it provides very good cover even if the palmaris longus tendon is not present.

Secondary reconstruction is certainly a reasonable option if immediate reconstruction of the extensor tendons is not undertaken, and it is probably the approach used by most surgeons.[7] There are instances, however, in which a patient will have no extensor reconstruction for injuries on the dorsal hand and eventually get return of some extensor function. I have seen this phenomenon on several occasions, and it appears that the fingers extend from a scar band that connects the proximal tendons to the area of the extensor hoods. If reconstruction is necessary, however, it may be done as a two-stage or single-stage procedure, depending on the status of the soft tissues. I will often simply tunnel the tendon grafts through the fatty subcutaneous tissue of a flap with adequate soft tissue bulk and repair each end. When there is significant scarring of a flap or other procedures will be necessary later, I place silastic tendon rods before placing the tendon grafts. Both of these approaches seem to work, although tenolysis may be necessary after either a single-stage or two-stage reconstruction.

SECONDARY PROCEDURES

Function after extensor-tendon repair is generally good, but with dehiscence or adherence of the repair there can be significant loss of finger flexion and extension. The loss of flexion is often not appreciated, but if the extensor system becomes adherent to the bone, a loss of flexion is inevitable. Contractures left untreated can develop thickening and contracture of the joint capsules, particularly in the MCP joint. Release of the extensor tendon and joint release may be necessary to restore function.

Extensor-tendon tenolysis is usually best performed under "twilight" or neuroleptic anesthesia. This type of anesthesia allows for active motion by the patient during the operation to evaluate the adequacy of tendon and ligament release. I prefer a longitudinal incision placed directly over the center of the joint for release of the MCP and PIP joints. This type of incision allows complete exposure of the joint and usually won't dehisce during postoperative motion. Release of stiff fingers from extensor injury generally proceeds from tenolysis to capsular release to collateral ligament release.[39] Once the skin flaps are developed, the tendon is released. The extensor tendon is commonly adherent to the underlying bone, especially if a fracture of the metacarpal or phalanx was present. If release of the tendon fails to allow full extension and flexion of the digit, one must proceed to release of the dorsal and lateral joint capsule. Release of the MCP-joint capsule for patients with stiffness after injury offers some of the greatest gains with the least damage to other structures. One must proceed to release of the collateral ligaments if release of the joint capsule fails to provide full motion. The collateral ligaments are generally divided in stages from dorsal to volar. The finger

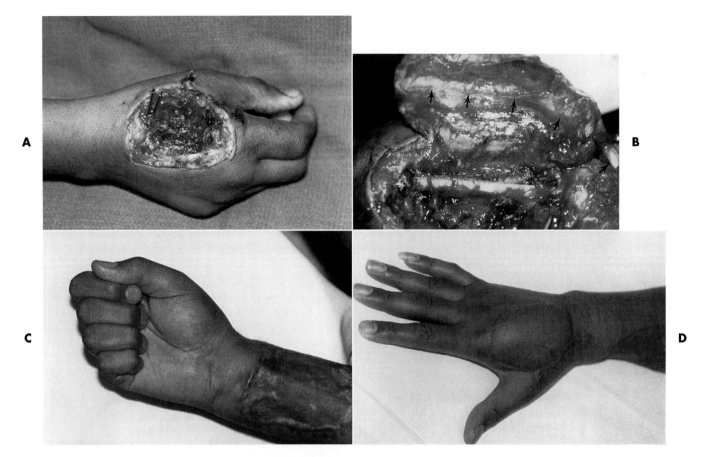

Figure 112-10. A, Patient who suffered a through-and-through shotgun wound to the hand, with loss of extensor tendons to the index finger. **B,** A radial forearm flap elevated with the palmaris longus tendon in the flap. The arrows point to the tendon within the fascia of the flap. **C,** The patient's postsurgical degree of flexion. **D,** The patient's postsurgical degree of extension.

is flexed and extended, and if the joint still will not move through its full range, further release is accomplished. The entire collateral ligament must be divided in some cases. This is generally safe, in terms of later joint stability, as long as the other structures, including the volar plate and lateral bands, are intact.

The patient is begun on a program of active and passive motion after release. If tenolysis was extensive, I will often protect the tendon with a dynamic extension splint that allows active flexion for a period of 3 to 6 weeks. A silastic sheet can be placed around the tendons in patients with extensive scarring to allow early motion and prevent scar formation. This technique suffers from the disadvantages of potential infection and the need to remove the sheet at a later date. Probably the best approach to this problem is to place a sheet of vascularized fascia, such as the temporoparietal fascia flap, around the tendons. This flap can be placed under, over, or around the tendons and has been shown to aid in return of motion by placing a nonscarred, smooth, gliding surface around the tendons.[32]

OUTCOMES

PRESENT DATA

The usual feeling is that the outcome from repair of extensor-tendon injuries is universally good. One report from the 1950s on 500 patients stated that the results after suture of the extensor tendons were always good.[17] This is unfortunately not always the case, but appreciation of this problem by objective studies has come only recently. Two recent studies have taken a close look at the outcomes from extensor-tendon repair, albeit from two slightly different perspectives.

In a 1990 report, Newport, Blair, and Steyers[29] looked at the results of extensor-tendon repair in 62 patients with 101 injured tendons. Most patients were treated after tendon repair with standard static splinting, with 60% sustaining some type of associated injury, including fractures, dislocations, and joint-capsule or flexor-tendon injuries. The mean follow-up in this group of patients was 5 years. The patients were evaluated using Miller's system, which is based on total extension lag and loss of flexion.[27] Evaluation of this group showed that distal injuries had good to excellent results in less than 50% of patients, whereas more proximal injuries had good to excellent results in 63% to 83% of cases. They also noted a marked loss of flexion in injured digits, with *more fingers having a loss of flexion after extensor-tendon repair than a loss of extension.* The average degree loss of flexion was greater than the average degree loss of extension in these fingers. Overall, 52% of fingers had a good to excellent result, but only 45% of fingers with associated injuries had good to excellent results. This compares with 64% of fingers in the good to excellent category for fingers that did not suffer associated injuries. The most important associated injury in terms of outcome was an underlying fracture, in which only 50% of fingers had a good to excellent result. The differences in these categories were found to be statistically significant. It should be noted that only four repairs failed (3%) and only one patient (1%) required a later tenolysis.

The effect on quality of life was evaluated, and 95% of patients who had extensor-tendon repair were satisfied with their functional result. Six patients (10%), however, had to change jobs because of their injuries. A total of seven patients (11%) had to change activities outside of their jobs, such as sports or hobbies, because of their injuries. It would appear from this study that extensor-tendon repairs are not universally successful, and that 10% of patients can expect this injury to adversely affect their lives in a significant manner.

The above study looked at the results of extensor-tendon repair by trained hand surgeons, whereas the following study evaluated the results after repair was performed by residents on staff in the emergency room. In a 1995 study in Nottingham, England, Evans et al[14] looked at the results of 46 extensor-tendon repairs in 42 patients. All repairs were performed in the emergency room under local anesthesia by emergency medicine residents. All patients were also treated with static splinting, and few received any postoperative therapy. The patients in this series were also assessed and graded according to Miller's system and, overall, 65% had a good or excellent result after extensor-tendon repair. Only 18% of patients with injury in the finger had a good or excellent result, whereas 80% of those patients with injury from the MCP joint proximally had good to excellent results. Four patients in their series had associated injuries, but only one of these patients (25%) had a good result. Twenty of 42 patients (47%) complained of some functional disability after extensor-tendon repair, and only two patients (4%) had to change jobs or hobbies. Evans et al suggests that because of their poor results, perhaps distal injuries should be treated by simple splinting to avoid the increased scarring from surgery. They also suggest that the use of dynamic postoperative splinting could improve the results in this group of patients.

These two reports obviously deal with a small number of patients and are incomplete, and further studies need to be done in the future. Obviously, extensor-tendon injuries are not as "benign" as is often taught, and care must be taken to ensure a reasonable outcome for the patient. Based on the available literature, the use of appropriate postoperative therapy with early motion should improve the results. This, of course, assumes that the future practice of medicine in a corporate profit–driven environment does not mitigate against the opportunity for patients to receive appropriate care.

REFERENCES

1. Balakrishnan C: Dorsalis pedis flap with vascularized extensor tendons for dorsal hand reconstruction [letter; comment], *Plast Reconstr Surg* 95:1335-1336, 1995.

2. Blair WF, Steyers CM: Extensor tendon injuries, *Orthop Clin North Am* 23:141-148, 1992.

3. Browne EZ Jr, Ribik CA: Early dynamic splinting for extensor tendon injuries, *J Hand Surg [Am]* 14:72-76, 1989.

4. Brzezienski MA, Schneider LH: Extensor tendon injuries at the distal interphalangeal joint, *Hand Clin* 11:373-386, 1995.

5. Burton RI: Extensor tendons: late reconstruction. In Green DP (editor): *Operative hand surgery,* New York, 1993, Churchill Livingstone.

6. Caroli A, Adani R, Castagnetti C, et al: Dorsalis pedis flap with vascularized extensor tendons for dorsal hand reconstruction [see comments], *Plast Reconstr Surg* 92:1326-1330, 1993.

7. Cautilli D, Schneider LH: Extensor tendon grafting on the dorsum of the hand in massive tendon loss, *Hand Clin* 11:423-429, 1995.

8. Chow JA, Dovelle S, Thomes LJ, et al: A comparison of results of extensor tendon repair followed by early controlled mobilisation versus static immobilisation, *J Hand Surg [Br]* 14:18-20, 1989.

9. Coons MS, Green SM: Boutonniere deformity, *Hand Clin* 11:387-402, 1995.

10. Crosby CA, Wehbe MA: Early motion after extensor tendon surgery, *Hand Clin* 12:57-64, 1996.

11. Doyle JR: Extensor tendons: acute injuries. In Green DP (editor): *Operative hand surgery,* New York, 1993, Churchill Livingstone.

12. Drape JL, Dubert T, Silbermann O, et al: Acute trauma of the extensor hood of the metacarpophalangeal joint: MR imaging evaluation, *Radiology* 192:469-476, 1994.

13. Elson RA: Rupture of the central slip of the extensor hood of the finger, *J Bone Joint Surg* 68B:86-88, 1986.

14. Evans JD, Wignakumar V, Davis TR, Dove A: Results of extensor tendon repair performed by junior accident and emergency staff, *Injury* 26:107-109, 1995.

15. Evans RB: Immediate active short arc motion following extensor tendon repair, *Hand Clin* 11:483-512, 1995.

16. Froehlich JA, Akelman E, Herndon JH: Extensor tendon injuries at the proximal interphalangeal joint, *Hand Clin* 4:25-37, 1988.

17. Hauge MF: The results of tendon suture of the hands: a review of 500 patients, *Acta Orthop Scand* 24:258-270, 1954.

18. Houpt P, Dijkstra R, Storm van Leeuwen JB: Fowler's tenotomy for mallet deformity [see comments], *J Hand Surg [Br]* 18:499-500, 1993.

19. Hung LK, Chan A, Chang J, et al: Early controlled active mobilization with dynamic splintage for treatment of extensor tendon injuries, *J Hand Surg [Am]* 15:251-257, 1990.

20. Inoue G, Tamura Y: Dislocation of the extensor tendons over the metacarpophalangeal joints, *J Hand Surg [Am]* 21:464-469, 1996.

21. Ishizuki M: Traumatic and spontaneous dislocation of extensor tendon of the long finger, *J Hand Surg [Am]* 15:967-972, 1990.

22. Kaplan EB: Mechanism of action of the fingers, the thumb, and the wrist. In Kaplan EB: *Functional and surgical anatomy of the hand,* Philadelphia, 1965, JB Lippincott.

23. Kerr CD, Burczak JR: Dynamic traction after extensor tendon repair in zones 6, 7, and 8: a retrospective study, *J Hand Surg [Br]* 14:21-22, 1989.

24. Lister GD, Kleinert HE, Kutz JE, Atasoy E: Primary flexor tendon repair followed by immediate controlled mobilization, *J Hand Surg* 2:441-451, 1977.

25. Marin-Braun F, Merle M, Sanz J, et al: Primary repair of extensor tendons with assisted post-operative mobilisation: a series of 48 cases, *Ann Chir Main* 8:7-21, 1989.

26. Massengill JB: The boutonniere deformity, *Hand Clin* 8:787-801, 1992.

27. Miller H: Repair of severed tendons of the hand and wrist, *Surg Gynecol Obstet* 75:693-698, 1942.

28. Minami A, Ogino T, Hamada M: Rupture of extensor tendons associated with a palmar perilunar dislocation, *J Hand Surg [Am]* 14:843-847, 1989.

29. Newport ML, Blair WF, Steyers CM Jr: Long-term results of extensor tendon repair, *J Hand Surg [Am]* 15:961-966, 1990.

30. O'Dwyer FG, Quinton DN: Early mobilisation of acute middle slip injuries [see comments], *J Hand Surg [Br]* 15:404-406, 1990.

31. Patel MR, Desai SS, Bassini-Lipton L: Conservative management of chronic mallet finger, *J Hand Surg* 11A:570-573, 1986.

32. Pederson WC: Free temporoparietal fascial flap and hand reconstruction. In Vastamaki M, Vilkki S, Raatikainen T, Viljakka T (editors): *Current trends in hand surgery,* Amsterdam, 1995, Elsevier.

33. Saldana MJ, Choban S, Westerbeck P, Schacherer TG: Results of acute zone III extensor tendon injuries treated with dynamic extension splinting, *J Hand Surg [Am]* 16:1145-1150, 1991.

34. Scheker LR, Langley SJ, Martin DL, Julliard KN: Primary extensor tendon reconstruction in dorsal hand defects requiring free flaps, *J Hand Surg [Br]* 18:568-575, 1993.

35. Schwartz MG, Green SM, Coville FA: Dorsal dislocation of the lunate with multiple extensor tendon ruptures, *J Hand Surg [Am]* 15:132-133, 1990.

36. Takami H, Takahashi S, Ando M, Suzuki K: Rupture of the extensor digitorum communis tendons caused by occupational overuse, *J Hand Surg [Br]* 16:70-71, 1991.

37. Takami H, Takahashi S, Inanami H: Post-traumatic rupture of the extensor digitorum communis tendon, *J Hand Surg [Br]* 16:327-328, 1991.

38. Uchida Y, Sugioka Y: Extensor tendon rupture associated with Smith's fracture: a case report, *Acta Orthop Scand* 61:374-375, 1990.

39. Uhl RL: Salvage of extensor tendon function with tenolysis and joint release, *Hand Clin* 11:461-470, 1995.

40. Vaughan-Jackson OJ: Rupture of extensor tendons by attrition at the inferior radioulnar joint: report of two cases, *J Bone Joint Surg* 30B:528-530, 1948.

CHAPTER

Tendon Transfers

113

Neil F. Jones

Eric T. Emerson

INTRODUCTION

Tendon transfers are reconstructive techniques that restore motion or balance to a hand with impaired function of the extrinsic or intrinsic muscle–tendon (MT) units of the forearm and hand. The origin or insertion of a functioning muscle in a tendon transfer is detached, mobilized, and then reattached to another tendon or bone to substitute for the action of a nonfunctioning tendon. The transferred donor tendon, unlike a tendon graft, remains attached to its parent muscle. A tendon transfer also differs from a free muscle transfer in that the neurovascular pedicle to the muscle of the transferred tendon remains intact.

INDICATIONS

There are three general indications for tendon transfers in the upper extremity: to restore function to a muscle paralyzed as a result of injuries of the peripheral nerves, the brachial plexus, or the spinal cord; to restore function after closed tendon ruptures or open injuries to the tendons or muscles; and to restore balance to a hand deformed from various neurological conditions. Tendon transfers are most commonly performed to restore function after peripheral nerve injuries, and they will be described according to each specific nerve palsy. The general principles for performing these procedures, however, apply to all transfers (Box 113-1).

GENERAL PRINCIPLES

Steindler[46] first suggested that tendon transfers cannot glide through edematous or scarred soft tissues nor can they flex or extend stiff metacarpophalangeal (MCP) and proximal interphalangeal (PIP) joints. He therefore advocated that tendon transfers be delayed until "tissue equilibrium" was restored.[46]

Fractures should be healed or rigidly fixed by internal fixation. Chronic scarred skin and subcutaneous tissues or skin grafts in the projected line of pull of a tendon transfer should first be resurfaced with a flap. If secondary tendon transfers are likely to be necessary, split-thickness skin grafting of hand or forearm soft tissue defects can be avoided by delayed primary coverage using pedicled flaps, such as the groin flap, reverse radial forearm flap, or free flaps, such as the lateral arm flap, contralateral radial forearm flap, or temporoparietal fascial flap. Occasionally silicone rods can be placed either beneath or through the subcutaneous fat of a transferred flap to create a smooth channel through which a tendon transfer may later be tunneled. The span of the thumb–index finger web space should be maintained by splinting, especially after median nerve injuries. A secondary adduction contracture should be released by a Z-plasty, skin grafting, or transposition flap before any opposition tendon transfer. A full passive range of motion of the MCP and PIP joints should be achieved by hand therapy and dynamic splinting before any tendon transfer. Preliminary capsulotomies of the MCP and PIP joints or tenolysis of adherent flexor or extensor tendons may occasionally be required to restore passive motion before performing a tendon transfer.

SELECTION OF THE DONOR MUSCLE–TENDON UNIT

The MT unit selected as a potential motor for transfer must be expendable. The ring-finger sublimis tendon, for example, may be used to correct clawing in patients with a low ulnar nerve palsy but it is not expendable in patients with a high ulnar nerve palsy who have no functioning profundus tendon to the ring finger. The availability of an MT unit to be used as a tendon transfer may also be influenced by the patient's occupation. The flexor carpi radialis (FCR) tendon, for example, may be a more appropriate transfer to provide finger extension in a working man rather than the more conventional flexor carpi ulnaris (FCU) because this muscle provides the important function of wrist flexion and ulnar deviation required for hammering. When multiple tendon transfers are

> **Box 113-1.**
> **Basic Principles of Tendon Transfer**
>
> - Soft tissue and bony healing
> - Full passive range of motion of involved joints
> - Adequate amplitude of donor muscle
> - Adequate excursion of donor muscle
> - Direct line of pull
> - Single function for each transferred tendon
> - Synergy of transfer

required, one wrist flexor, one wrist extensor, and one extrinsic flexor and extensor tendon to each digit should always be retained.

The surgeon must consider when selecting the appropriate donor muscle–tendon not only the strength of the muscle to be transferred but also the strength of the paralyzed muscle and that of the antagonist muscle. Brand[5,6] has shown that the maximum potential force of a muscle is directly proportional to its physiologic cross-sectional area. It has been calculated that a muscle can produce a force of 3.65 kg per cm^2 of its cross-sectional area. This potential force is maximal when the muscle is at its resting length, which is a position midway between the length when it is fully stretched passively and when it is fully contracted.

The potential amplitude or excursion of a donor MT unit must also be sufficient to restore the specific function lost. The finger flexors have an amplitude of 70 mm, the finger extensors 50 mm, and the wrist flexors and extensors 33 mm. The tenodesis effect of wrist flexion or extension may also increase the effective amplitude of a tendon transfer by 25 mm. The amplitude of a donor muscle may also be increased by extensive release of its surrounding fascia and is best exemplified by the brachioradialis muscle.

A tendon transfer should pass in a direct line from the origin of the donor muscle to its new insertion. Unless tendon transfers are being performed early when there is still a chance of reinnervation after nerve repair, the recipient tendons should be divided proximal to the site of the tendon repair to create a more direct line of pull rather than forming a Y-shaped end to side repair. Tendon transfers should only act across one joint and only perform a single function. A transfer may, however, be inserted into several recipient tendons as long as they perform the same function in adjacent digits. Finally, the donor muscle selected should preferably have a synergistic function to the muscle to be restored or the potential to be retrained by voluntary control.

The surgeon must determine the specific functions to be restored, select the appropriate donor MT units and decide on the timing of the tendon transfer. Every muscle in the forearm and hand should be tested to document which are functioning and to grade their individual strengths. The specific hand functions that need to be restored are then listed. The final step

is to match the available donor muscles with the functions that need to be restored based on the force, amplitude, and direction of the various muscles available. Arthrodesis of the wrist may need to be considered to release a wrist flexor or extensor tendon for transfer. Transfers that require postoperative immobilization with the wrist in flexion are usually performed at a first stage. Those transfers requiring postoperative immobilization with the wrist in extension are performed at a second stage.

TIMING OF TENDON TRANSFERS

The timing of tendon transfers may be classified as early, conventional, or late. A conventional tendon transfer is usually performed after reinnervation of paralyzed muscles fails to occur by 3 months after the expected time of reinnervation based on the rate of nerve regeneration of 1 mm per day. Brand,[6] Omer,[36] and Burkhalter[12] have advocated "early" tendon transfers in certain circumstances in which a tendon transfer is performed simultaneously with the nerve repair or before the expected time of reinnervation of the muscle. An "early" tendon transfer therefore acts as a temporary substitute for the paralyzed muscle until reinnervation occurs, acting as an "internal splint." If reinnervation is suboptimal, the "early" tendon transfer acts as a helper to augment the power of the muscle; if reinnervation fails to occur, it then acts as a permanent substitute.

SURGICAL TECHNIQUES

The success of any tendon transfer depends entirely on preventing scarring or adhesions around the path of the transferred tendon. Incisions should be carefully planned before elevation of the tourniquet so that the final tendon repairs lie transversely beneath skin flaps rather than lying immediately beneath the incisions. The donor muscle should be carefully mobilized to prevent damage to its neurovascular bundle, which usually enters in the proximal third of the forearm. The transferred tendon should glide in a tunnel through the subcutaneous tissues and not cross raw bone or pass through small fascial windows. Only the distal end of the tendon should be grasped during surgery, and care should be taken to prevent tendon desiccation. Tendon repairs are performed using a Pulvertaft weave technique. The donor and recipient tendons are sutured under normal tension, and after two nonabsorbable sutures have been inserted, the tension of the transfer is checked by observing digital flexion and extension of the digit during passive wrist flexion and extension. The hand is immobilized in the desired position after surgery for 3 to 4 weeks, at which time gentle active range-of-motion exercises are started, usually under the supervision of a therapist. The hand is protected for a further 3 weeks in a lightweight protective splint.

RADIAL NERVE PALSY

INDICATIONS

The functional deficit in a radial nerve palsy consists of the following:
- Inability to extend the wrist
- Inability to extend the fingers at the MCP joints
- Inability to extend and radially abduct the thumb

The most significant disability, however, is that patients are unable to stabilize their wrist, which results in impaired transmission of flexor power to their fingers and marked weakness of grip strength. Tendon transfers are therefore required to provide the following:
- Wrist extension
- Extension of the fingers at the MCP joints
- Extension and radial abduction of the thumb

Unlike the median and ulnar nerves, sensory loss after radial nerve injury is not functionally disabling unless the patient develops a painful neuroma.

The timing of tendon transfers to correct radial nerve palsy remains controversial. The two options are either to perform an "early" tendon transfer simultaneously with repair of the radial nerve (to act as a internal splint, which provides immediate restoration of power grip), or to delay any tendon transfers until there is lack of reinnervation of the most proximal muscles (the brachioradialis and extensor carpi radialis longus [ECRL]) within the time calculated for nerve regeneration. The latter is the more conventional option.

The more proximal the nerve injury, the less likely that functional muscle reinnervation will occur.[6,12] If the radial nerve is in continuity, most surgeons would agree that 3 months of observation are indicated to await spontaneous nerve recovery and return of muscle function. With respect to return of function after radial nerve repairs, Mayer and Mayfield[33] reported complete functional recovery after posterior interosseous neurorrhaphy (PIN) in 28 patients and partial recovery in 11 patients. Young et al[54] studied 51 patients with posterior interosseous nerve palsy, of which only 11 showed return of function by 3 months. Of the remaining 40 patients, 20 of the 23 who underwent neurolysis and 10 of the 12 who underwent nerve grafting eventually obtained excellent or good results. A conflicting study of radial nerve injuries demonstrated useful function in 65% of patients after nerve repair, but only 38% of patients who underwent fascicular grafting obtained useful motor function.[28] These studies demonstrate that injury and repair of the posterior interosseous nerve and radial nerves can provide significant return of function without the need for tendon transfers. The chances of successful reinnervation, however, are much less predictable in patients with extensive nerve gaps or associated soft tissue injuries, or in older individuals. Therefore it may be more appropriate for these patients to undergo the full set of tendon transfers early. It is important to maintain supple MCP joints capable of full extension and adequate thumb abduction with appropriate splinting and therapy in patients awaiting return of radial nerve function.

OPERATIONS

Zachary[55] emphasized the importance of retaining at least one wrist flexor—preferably the FCR—to facilitate wrist control. Other authors have suggested that the FCU is not an expendable tendon and therefore they prefer to use the FCR as the donor tendon to restore finger extension.[45] The advantage of using the FCR is that it preserves the important moment of flexion and ulnar deviation of the wrist, which is so important for power grip in a working person. This is especially true in the patient with a posterior interosseous nerve palsy in which ECRL function is preserved, but extensor carpi ulnaris (ECU) activity is lost. This leads to radial deviation of the wrist with attempted wrist extension. Use of the FCU transfer will further potentiate radial deviation of the wrist because only radially deviating wrist motors are preserved.

Several different tendon transfers have been reported to restore radial innervated muscle function.[3,16,51,55] Franke[21] provided one of the earliest descriptions of transferring the FCU to the extensor digiti communis (EDC) through the interosseous membrane. In 1899, Capellen described using the FCR to activate the extensor pollicis longus (EPL).[39] The pronator teres (PT) to the ECRL and extensor carpi radialis brevis (ECRB) transfer for wrist extension was first reported in 1906 by Sir Robert Jones. The use of the PT to provide wrist extension has become universally accepted, the only remaining controversy being whether to insert the PT into the ECRB alone or into both the ECRL and brevis. The three tendon transfers that have evolved for treatment of radial nerve palsy differ therefore only in the technique of restoring finger extension and thumb extension/abduction (Table 113-1).[3,16,51,55]

"Standard" Flexor Carpi Ulnaris Transfer

The FCU transfer is the authors' preferred technique for patients with a radial nerve palsy. The FCR transfer is preferred, however, in patients with a posterior interosseous nerve palsy. The FCU tendon is approached through an inverted J-shaped incision over the ulnar volar aspect of the distal forearm. It is transected at the wrist crease and released extensively from its fascial attachments up into the proximal third of the forearm, taking care not to damage the neurovascular pedicle and using a second incision in the proximal forearm, if necessary. The palmaris longus (PL) tendon is transected at the wrist crease through the same distal incision, and the muscle is mobilized into the middle third of the forearm. An S-shaped incision is then made beginning over the volar radial aspect of the middle third of the forearm, passing dorsally and ulnarly over the radial border of the forearm. The PT tendon is elevated from its insertion on the radius in continuity with a 2-to 3-cm strip of periosteum (Figure 113-1). The ECRB is transected at its musculotendinous junction if there is no chance of future reinnervation of the wrist extensors. The PT is then rerouted superficial to the brachioradialis and ECRL around the radial border of the forearm in a straight line, ready for insertion into the ECRB. A subcutaneous tunnel is made with a Kelly clamp from the dorsal incision around the ulnar border of the forearm into the proximal incision used to mobilize the FCU. The FCU tendon is passed through this subcutaneous tunnel to lie obliquely across the EDC tendons proximal to the extensor retinaculum. The EDC tendons can be transected at their musculotendinous junctions if no return of function is expected, so that a more direct line of pull can be achieved (Figure 113-2). Otherwise, an end-to-side repair is performed. The EPL tendon is divided at its musculotendinous junction, removed from the third dorsal extensor tendon compartment, and passed through a subcutaneous tunnel from the base of the thumb metacarpal to the volar wrist incision (Figure 113-3).

The proper tension in radial nerve tendon transfers should be tight enough to provide full extension of the wrist and digits without restricting full flexion of the digits. The distal ends of the four EDC tendons to the index, long, ring, and small fingers are woven through the FCU tendon proximal to the extensor retinaculum. The extensor digiti quinti (EDQ) is usually not included unless there is still an extensor lag when proximal traction is applied to the EDC tendon to the small finger. Starting with the index finger and finishing with the small finger, each individual EDC tendon is sutured with the wrist in neutral and the FCU under maximal tension to provide full extension at the MCP joint. Tension is then evaluated by checking that all four digits extend synchronously when the wrist is palmar flexed and, most importantly, ensuring that all four digits can be passively flexed into a fist when the wrist is extended. The PL and EPL are then interwoven over the radiovolar aspect of the wrist, with both

Table 113-1.
Tendon Transfers for Radial Nerve Palsy

STANDARD FCU TRANSFER	FCR TRANSFER	BOYES SUBLIMIS TRANSFER
PT → ECRB	PT → ECRB	PT → ECRB
FCU → EDC	FCR → EDC	FDS long → EDC long, ring, and small fingers
PL → EPL	PL → EPL	FDS ring → EIP and EPL
		FCR → APL and EPB

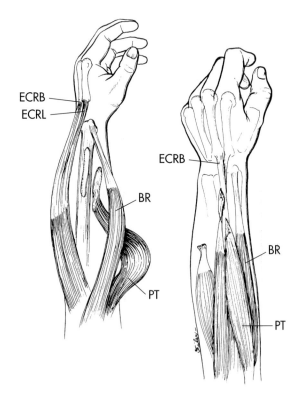

Figure 113-1. Transfer of pronator teres (PT) to extensor carpi radialis brevis (ECRB) to restore wrist extension.

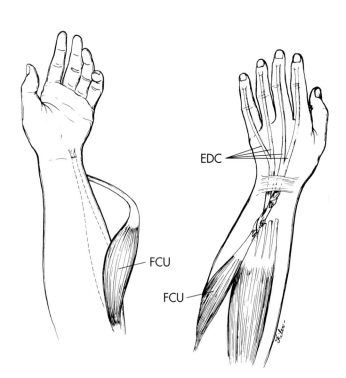

Figure 113-2. Transfer of flexor carpi ulnaris (FCU) to extensor digitorum communis (EDC) to provide finger extension.

tendons under resting tension with the wrist in neutral. The PT, under resting tension, is then woven through the ECRB, with the wrist in 45 degrees of extension (Figure 113-4). The wrist is immobilized in 45 degrees of extension in a volar splint, with the MCP joints positioned in slight flexion and the thumb in full extension and abduction.

Active flexion and extension of the fingers and thumb are begun at 3½ to 4 weeks; active exercises of the wrist begin at 5 weeks. Protective splinting is continued for 6 to 8 weeks after surgery.

Flexor Carpi Radialis Transfer

The skin incision extends from the radiovolar aspect of the mid-forearm and then courses dorsally over the third and fourth extensor-tendon compartments. The PT is transferred to the ECRB, and the PL is transferred to the EPL exactly as described in the standard FCU transfer. The FCR is divided at the wrist crease, mobilized approximately to the level of the mid-forearm, and rerouted around the radial border of the forearm. The four EDC tendons, and if necessary the EDQ, may be woven through the donor FCR tendon, but usually the extensor tendons need to be rerouted superficial to the extensor retinaculum to obtain a straighter line of pull (Figure 113-5). The small-finger EDC and EDQ may be sutured side to side to the ring-finger EDC, and the index-finger EDC may be sutured side to side to the long-finger EDC under appropriate tension to prevent a bulky tendon juncture. Only the two EDC tendons to the long and ring fingers are then weaved through the FCR tendon at a more proximal level. These tendon repairs are also performed with the wrist in neutral and the MCP joints in full extension, with the FCR tendon under maximal traction similar to FCU transfer.

Tenodesis of the abductor pollicis longus (APL) may occasionally be necessary to prevent a collapse flexion deformity at the carpometacarpal (CMC) joint of the thumb. The APL tendon, after transection in the distal forearm, is looped around the brachioradialis proximal to the radial styloid and sutured to itself, with the thumb metacarpal held in

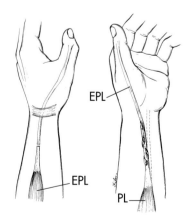

Figure 113-3. Transfer of palmaris longus (PL) to extensor pollicis longus (EPL) to provide thumb extension.

extension and the wrist in 30 degrees of extension. Postoperative management is similar to that for the FCU transfer.

Boyes Sublimis Transfer

Boyes[3] was the first to point out that neither the FCU nor the FCR has sufficient amplitude (30 mm) to produce full excursion of the digital extensor tendons (50 mm) without their amplitude being increased by the tenodesis effect of wrist flexion. He therefore advocated using the sublimis tendons to the long and ring fingers, which have an amplitude of 70 mm, to act as donor tendons to restore finger extension.[3,16] The advantages of the Boyes transfer are that it potentially allows simultaneous wrist and finger extension, it may allow independent thumb and index-finger extension, and it does not weaken wrist flexion. However, the long and ring fingers are deprived of sublimis function, and this may result in weak grip. Harvesting of the sublimis tendons may also lead to the subsequent development of either a "swan-neck" deformity or a flexion contracture at the PIP joint.

The sublimis tendons to the long and ring fingers are exposed between the A1 and A2 pulleys either through one transverse incision or two separate longitudinal incisions at the base of the fingers. The sublimis tendons are divided just proximal to their decussation and then withdrawn proximally through a longitudinal incision over the volar aspect of the middle third of the forearm. The PT tendon can be transected and rerouted through this same incision as described previously. Blunt dissection on either side of the flexor profundus muscles allows a window to be excised in the interosseous membrane just proximal to the pronator quadratus (Figure 113-6). This window should be made as large as possible, at least 4 cm long and as wide as the interosseous space, so that the muscle bellies of the two sublimis tendons can be passed through this window to minimize the development of adhesions. It is important to pass the sublimis tendons of the ring and long fingers to their respective side of the median nerve to prevent scissoring and compression of the nerve.

Thompson and Rasmussen[48] prefer to transfer the two sublimis tendons through subcutaneous tunnels around the radial and ulnar borders of the forearm (Figure 113-7). The extensor tendons are isolated together with the ECRB through a J-shaped incision passing transversely across the dorsum of the wrist and then extending proximally along the dorsum of the ulna. The PT was sutured to both the ECRL and the ECRB in Boyes' original description.[3] The PT, however, should only be woven end to end into the ECRB, with the wrist in 30 degrees of extension to prevent excessive radial deviation after radial nerve tendon transfers. The long-finger sublimis tendon is then passed to the radial side of the profundus muscles, and the ring-finger sublimis is passed to the ulnar side through the interosseous window into the dorsal incision. After transection of the EPL and extensor indicis proprius (EIP) tendons, they are woven end to end into the ring-finger sublimis tendon. Similarly, the transected EDC tendons to the index, long, ring, and small fingers are woven end to end into the long-finger sublimis tendon, although this arrangement can be reversed. The tendon repairs are per-

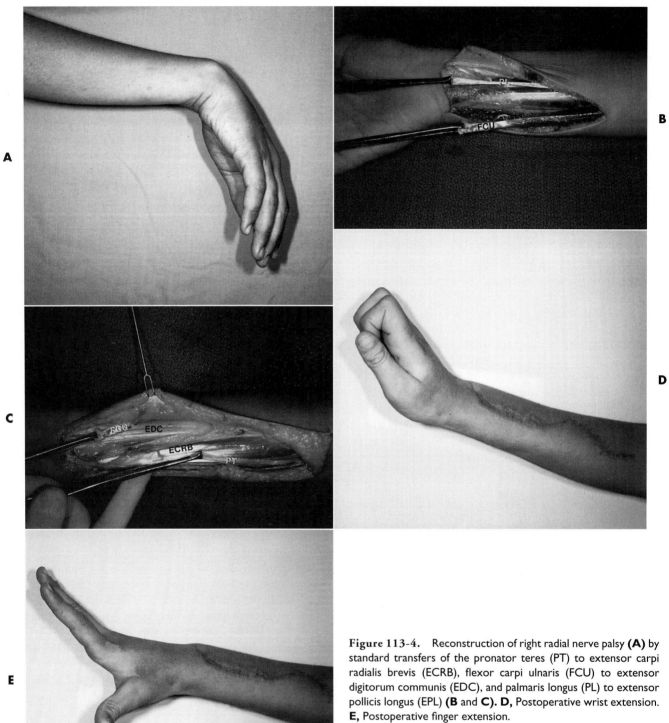

Figure 113-4. Reconstruction of right radial nerve palsy **(A)** by standard transfers of the pronator teres (PT) to extensor carpi radialis brevis (ECRB), flexor carpi ulnaris (FCU) to extensor digitorum communis (EDC), and palmaris longus (PL) to extensor pollicis longus (EPL) **(B** and **C). D,** Postoperative wrist extension. **E,** Postoperative finger extension.

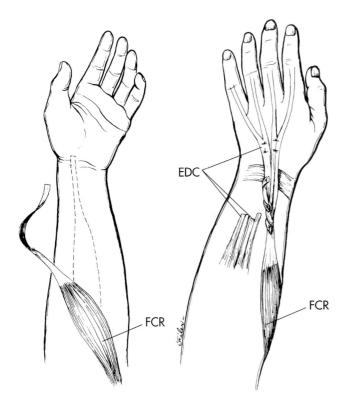

Figure 113-5. Flexor carpi radialis (FCR) to extensor digitorum communis (EDC) tranfer.

formed proximal to the extensor retinaculum, with resting tension in the donor sublimis tendons and full extension of the fingers at the MCP joints.

If necessary, the APL can be transected at its musculotendinous junction, passed through a subcutaneous tunnel from the base of the thumb into the volar forearm incision, and woven end to end with either the palmaris longus or FCR, which are transected at the wrist to provide abduction of the thumb and prevent a collapse deformity of the thumb metacarpal. The tourniquet should be deflated before the closure of the incisions because of the likelihood of bleeding from the anterior or posterior interosseous vessels.

OUTCOMES

The results of tendon transfers for radial nerve palsy are generally predictable if the basic principles are followed. Tsuge[51] reported his results in 69 patients over a 25-year period and described the evolution of his technique. He used the FCU transfer with insertion of the PT into both the ECRL and ECRB in the first 41 patients. He reported "fairly satisfactory" results, but felt that there were three problems with this transfer: development of radial wrist deviation, restricted wrist flexion, and marginal thumb abduction. Because of these concerns, the PT was subsequently transferred only to the ECRB, and the FCR was transferred through the interosseous membrane for

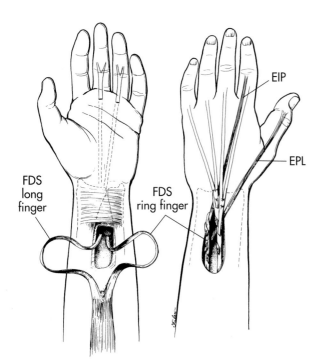

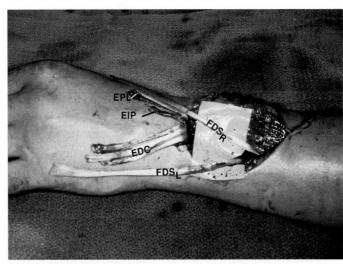

Figure 113-6. Transfer of the long-finger and ring-finger sublimis tendons (FDS$_L$, FDS$_R$) through a window in the interosseous membrane to restore function to the extensor digitorum communis (EDC) tendons and extensor indicis proprius (EIP) and extensor pollicis longus (EPL).

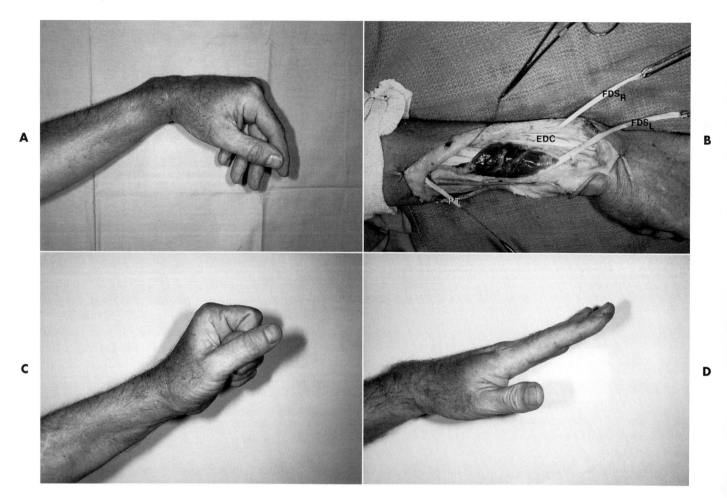

Figure 113-7. In this patient with left radial nerve palsy **(A)** the long-finger and ring-finger sublimis tendons were passed subcutaneously around the radial and ulnar border of the distal forearm **(B)** to restore wrist extension **(C)** and finger and thumb extension **(D)**.

finger extension, leaving the FCU intact. He reported good results in 24 of 27 cases treated with this method.

A study by Raskin and Wilgis[39] of the long-term functional results in six patients revealed adequate wrist mobility and power to perform daily activities with the FCU transfer. Patients in a work-simulation protocol were able to perform tasks without significant difficulty. Problems of inadequate ulnar deviation, grip strength, and wrist instability were not found. A subjective outcome report by Riordan[40] also confirmed satisfaction with the standard FCU transfer.

The Boyes sublimis transfer has also been reported to provide good results. The major advantage of this transfer is the potential ability to simultaneously extend the fingers and wrist. Chuinard et al[16] reported on 21 patients who had undergone this transfer, with excellent results in 10 patients, good results in 6, and only a fair result in 5 patients when assessed using the Zachary method.[55] Subjectively, 13 of these patients believed that they had obtained an excellent result, and 8 thought they had a good result. Complications requiring a second procedure were reported in five patients and included adhesions, pullout of the transfer, MCP joint and wrist extension contractures, and problems with obtaining the correct tension of the transfers.

A report by Fujiwara et al[22] in 1970 reviewing the results of 13 patients with radial nerve palsy and 5 patients with posterior interosseous nerve palsy found generally good results in those treated with the Boyes technique. No patients in any of these studies have developed postoperative median nerve compromise despite the potential for this complication with this transfer.

All three techniques described have been reported to yield good results. There are little quantitative data to substantiate most of the reported outcomes, and there are no comparative prospective trials evaluating the different techniques. The FCU transfer is the most straightforward procedure and provides reproducibly good results in patients with radial nerve palsy.

MEDIAN NERVE PALSY

INDICATIONS

The functional deficit after injury to the median nerve distal to the innervation of the extrinsic flexor muscles consists primarily of loss of thumb opposition and absent sensation over the thumb, index, and long fingers and radial half of the ring finger.

Opposition is a composite motion through three joints to position the thumb pad opposite the distal phalanx of the long finger. Abduction, pronation, and flexion occur at the CMC joint; abduction and flexion occur at the MCP joint; and either flexion or extension occurs at the interphalangeal (IP) joint. Approximately 40 degrees of thumb metacarpal abduction occurs at the CMC joint, and 20 degrees of proximal phalanx abduction occurs at the MCP joint. The thumb pronates approximately 90 degrees to achieve opposition to the long finger. Extension of the IP joint is required for pulp-to-pulp pinch, whereas slight flexion of the IP joint allows tip-to-tip pinch. Of the three intrinsic thenar muscles, the flexor pollicis brevis (FPB) muscle receives dual innervation from both the median and ulnar nerves. The FPB may therefore remain innervated by the ulnar nerve in approximately 70% of patients with a median nerve injury. These patients may not notice any significant functional loss, but careful testing will reveal a decreased range of abduction and pronation.

Patients with median nerve injuries should be instructed before any opposition tendon transfer to prevent the development of thumb adduction or supination contracture by a program of passive abduction exercises. A static splint may be used at night but usually interferes with the already compromised hand function if used during the day. Care should be taken to ensure that such splints abduct the thumb metacarpal rather than the proximal phalanx, otherwise the median nerve palsy will be compounded by attenuation of the ulnar collateral ligament of the MCP joint. If patients present with an established adduction or supination contracture of the thumb, release of the thumb–index finger web-space skin, fascia over the first dorsal interosseous muscle, or even the first dorsal interosseous and adductor muscles themselves may be required before performing an opposition tendon transfer.

Bunnell[10] first emphasized that the pull of an opposition tendon transfer should be in an oblique direction from the MCP joint of the thumb to the area of the pisiform and that the transfer should be inserted into the dorsoulnar base of the proximal phalanx to produce pronation. Generally, transfers that are directed along the radial aspect of the palm will produce a greater component of palmar abduction, whereas transfers that pass from the pisiform will produce both abduction and pronation. The more distal the transfer passes across the palm the greater the power of thumb flexion. Several methods of insertion for thumb opposition transfers have been advocated, including attachment to the dorsoulnar base of the proximal phalanx (Bunnell,[10] Royle-Thompson[42,49]); insertion into the abductor pollicis brevis (APB) tendon (Littler[30]); dual insertion into the APB tendon with continuation distally into the MCP joint capsule and EPL (Riordan[40]); insertion into the ABP, dorsal joint capsule, and adductor pollicis insertion (Edgerton and Brand[18]); and finally utilization of a distally based extensor pollicis brevis (EPB) tendon (Phalen and Miller[38]). A biomechanical study, however, has shown that opposition tendon transfers inserted

into the APB tendon alone will produce full abduction and pronation.[17] The more complex dual insertions therefore should probably be restricted for combined median and ulnar nerve palsies.

Several factors influence the likelihood of useful motor and sensory return after median nerve injury, including the patient's age, the level of injury, the length of the nerve defect, the quality of intervening graft, the repair technique, and length of time from injury to repair. The best results are realized in young patients with distal injuries requiring only primary repair. Associated injuries such as vascular damage, tendon injury, and concomitant ulnar nerve transection portend a worse prognosis. The chances of reinnervation of the thenar muscles after a group fascicular repair of a distal median nerve laceration should be reasonably optimistic. The conventional timing of an opposition tendon transfer may therefore only be required in those patients who fail to demonstrate signs of reinnervation within the usual calculated interval. Early tendon transfers should be considered in older patients or those with poor prognostic co-morbid factors.

Careful observation of thumb function after either a low or high median nerve injury will reveal whether an "early" opposition tendon transfer is necessary. The FPB remains innervated by the ulnar nerve in approximately 70% of median nerve injuries, and thumb function may not be significantly compromised. Consequently, an "early" opposition transfer should not be necessary. Some patients, however, will adapt to their loss of thumb opposition and abduction by substituting the APL to provide thumb abduction. This can only be achieved with the hand positioned in pronation and places the patient at an even greater disadvantage. Not only do these patients have absent sensation in the median nerve distribution, but with the forearm pronated they cannot even see the palmar surface of their hand to compensate for their loss of sensation. An "early" opposition tendon transfer should therefore be strongly considered if the surgeon or therapist observes the patient attempting to grasp objects by radial abduction of the thumb with the forearm pronated. If, however, the patient is able to pick up an object with the forearm in neutral or grasp an object with the forearm in supination, it is likely that the FPB remains innervated by the ulnar nerve and consequently the decision to perform an "early" opposition tendon transfer can be delayed.

OPERATIONS

Extensor Indicis Proprius Transfer

The EIP transfer by the Burkhalter method[13] is the authors' preferred technique except in elderly patients with thenar atrophy secondary to severe carpal tunnel syndrome. The EIP tendon is transected through a small transverse incision just proximal to the MCP joint of the index finger. The distal stump of the EIP tendon must be repaired to the EDC tendon of the index finger to prevent an extensor lag at the MCP joint. The EIP tendon is mobilized through two small transverse incisions: one proximal and one distal to the extensor retinaculum and the muscle belly mobilized through a longitudinal incision over the ulnar aspect of the dorsum of the distal forearm. A transverse incision is then made just proximal to the pisiform bone, and a subcutaneous tunnel is developed to connect this incision with the dorsal forearm incision. The EIP tendon is passed subcutaneously around the ulnar border of the distal forearm superficial to the ECU tendon into the pisiform incision. The APB tendon is identified through a small flap incision over the radial aspect of the MCP joint of the thumb, and a subcutaneous tunnel is developed across the palm, connecting this incision with the pisiform incision. The tendon transfer is passed obliquely across the palm and woven into the APB tendon under maximum tension, with the wrist in neutral position and the thumb in maximal palmar abduction (Figure 113-8). The tension of the transfer is then tested by the tenodesis effect of the wrist. Palmar flexion of the wrist should allow the thumb to be passively adducted. If dorsiflexion of the wrist produces excessive flexion or extension of the thumb at the MCP joint, this indicates that the transfer has been inserted either too far volarly or too far dorsally and should be adjusted accordingly. The thumb is immobilized in full abduction with the wrist in neutral position for 4 weeks, at which time active abduction and opposition movements are begun with protective splinting for a further 3 to 4 weeks. The only potential disadvantage of this tendon transfer is that the EIP tendon is only just long enough to reach the APB tendon.

Ring-Finger Flexor Digitorum Sublimis Transfer

In the ring-finger flexor sublimis transfer by Bunnell,[12] the ring-finger sublimis tendon is isolated through a small transverse incision just distal to the distal palmar crease and the tendon is transected between the A1 and A2 pulleys. A curved incision is made over the volar aspect of the distal forearm, and the ring-finger sublimis is delivered into this proximal incision. The FCU tendon is split longitudinally to create a distally based strip of the radial half of the tendon and this is then passed through a slit in the FCU tendon just proximal to the pisiform and sutured to itself to create a pulley (Figure 113-9). The distal end of the ring-finger sublimis tendon is passed through the pulley and through an oblique subcutaneous tunnel across the palm into a flap incision over the radial aspect of the MCP joint of the thumb. All the other incisions are then closed, and the tension on the tendon transfer is adjusted as previously described.

Simple looping of the ring-finger sublimis around the FCU tendon—rather than using a fixed pulley—rapidly becomes ineffective and the transfer becomes converted to a flexor of the MCP joint rather than a true opposition transfer. Less favored pulleys for the ring-finger sublimis transfer include passing the tendon through Guyon's canal or through a window in the transverse carpal ligament.

Compared with the EIP transfer, the ring-finger sublimis transfer is relatively stronger and has greater length. The ring-finger sublimis, however, is not available as a donor tendon in a patient with a high median nerve injury or in low median nerve injuries in which there have been associated injuries to the forearm flexor tendons. The ring-finger sublimis transfer should also not be selected in patients with a combined low median and high ulnar nerve palsy because the ring-finger sublimis is the only remaining flexor tendon in the ring finger. When treating a low median–low ulnar nerve palsy, the ring-finger sublimis may be required for correction of clawing. In addition, harvesting the sublimis tendon may result in either a flexion contracture or a "swan-neck" deformity of the PIP joint of the donor finger.

Palmaris Longus Transfer

The PL tendon transfer (Camitz[8,15,31]) is a simple transfer that will provide abduction of the thumb but little pronation or flexion and is particularly indicated in elderly patients with thenar atrophy caused by carpal tunnel syndrome. A strip of palmar fascia is dissected in continuity with the distal PL tendon through a standard carpal tunnel incision in the palm and extended proximally into the distal forearm. The strip of palmar fascia can be tubed with several tacking sutures. A subcutaneous tunnel is developed from the radial aspect of the distal forearm incision along the thenar eminence into a mid-axial incision on the radial aspect of the MCP joint of the thumb. The fascial extension of the PL tendon is passed through the subcutaneous tunnel and sutured to the APB tendon under maximal tension, with the wrist in neutral position (Figure 113-10).

Other Opposition Tendon Transfers

Huber[26] and Nicholaysen[35] described transfer of the abductor digiti minimi (ADM), which may occasionally be indicated in patients with a combined median and radial nerve palsy and also in children with congenital anomalies affecting the thumb. Because the muscle originates distal to the pisiform, this transfer provides excellent flexion and pronation of the thumb but little palmar abduction. The tendon insertion of ADM is transected from the ulnar lateral band through an ulnar mid-axial incision along the proximal phalanx of the small finger. The incision is then continued proximally along the radial aspect of the hypothenar eminence and the muscle is elevated in a distal-to-proximal direction, taking care to protect the neurovascular bundle that enters the muscle just beyond the pisiform. A wide subcutaneous tunnel is dissected between the APB tendon insertion at the MCP joint of the thumb and the hypothenar incision. Hemostasis is achieved after releasing the tourniquet, and the entire ADM muscle is rotated 180 degrees through the subcutaneous tunnel in the palm and sutured into the APB. This transfer has been compared to turning the page of a book.[26]

Phalen and Miller[38] advocate use of the EPB activated by the ECU. The EPB is divided at its musculotendinous junction in the distal forearm and retrieved through an incision at the MCP joint of the thumb. This distally based tendon is then passed through a subcutaneous tunnel obliquely across the palm to the area of the pisiform. The ECU tendon is transected at the base of the fifth metacarpal and routed subcutaneously around the ulnar border of the wrist to be interwoven with the EPB tendon.

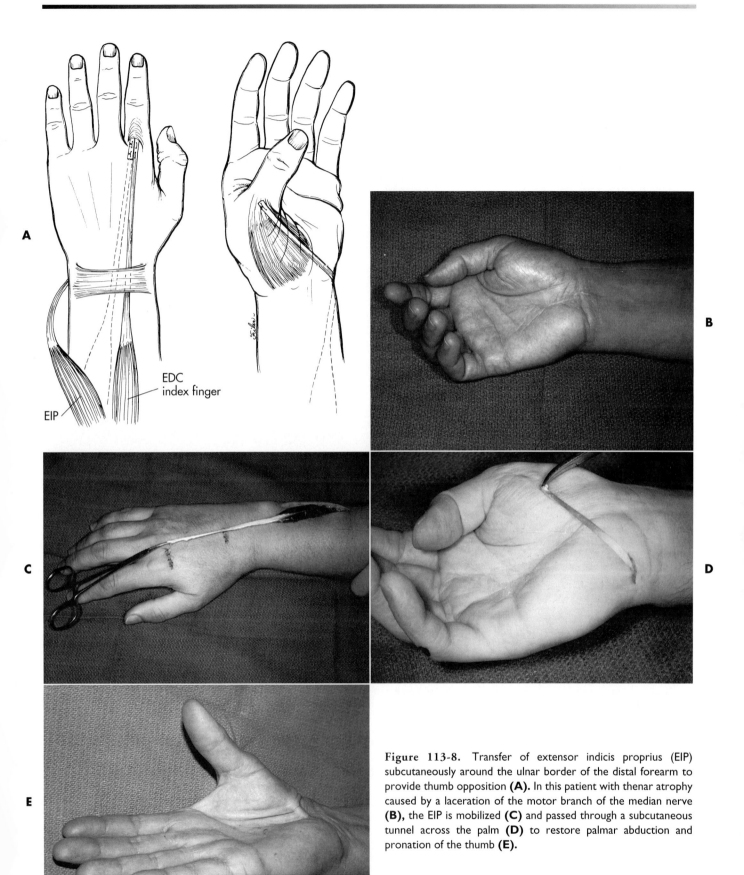

EDC
index finger

EIP

Figure 113-8. Transfer of extensor indicis proprius (EIP) subcutaneously around the ulnar border of the distal forearm to provide thumb opposition (A). In this patient with thenar atrophy caused by a laceration of the motor branch of the median nerve (B), the EIP is mobilized (C) and passed through a subcutaneous tunnel across the palm (D) to restore palmar abduction and pronation of the thumb (E).

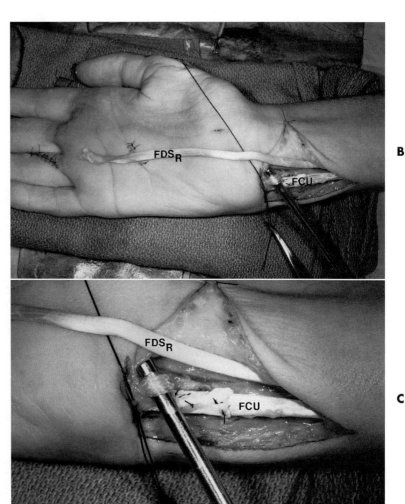

Figure 113-9. Transfer of the flexor digitorum sublimis from the ring finger to restore thumb opposition **(A)**. A distal-based strip of flexor carpi ulnaris (FCU) provides a pulley just proximal to the pisiform **(B** and **C)**, and the sublimis tendon is passed obliquely through a tunnel in the palm marked by the silk suture to insert into the tendon of the abductor pollicis brevis (APB).

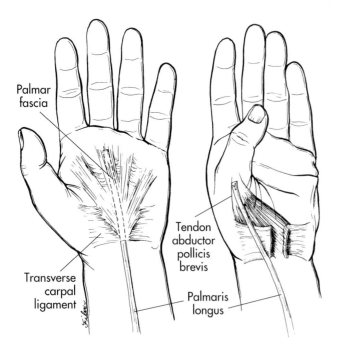

Figure 113-10. Camitz transfer. Transfer of palmaris longus extended by a strip of palmar fascia to provide palmar abduction of the thumb.

HIGH MEDIAN NERVE PALSY

INDICATIONS

The functional deficit after injury to the median nerve proximal to its innervation of the extrinsic flexor muscles results in an inability to flex the index finger at the PIP and DIP joints and the thumb at the IP joint, in addition to loss of thumb opposition. This is due to paralysis of all four flexor digitorum sublimis muscles, the flexor digitorum profundus (FDP) tendons to the index and long fingers, and the flexor pollicis longus (FPL) tendon. Patients are often still able to flex the long finger because of interconnections between the profundus tendons to the long, ring, and small fingers in the distal forearm. Therefore the two functions that need to be restored in patients with a high median nerve palsy are flexion of the IP joint of the thumb and flexion of the PIP and DIP joints of the index and long fingers, together with a conventional opposition tendon transfer.

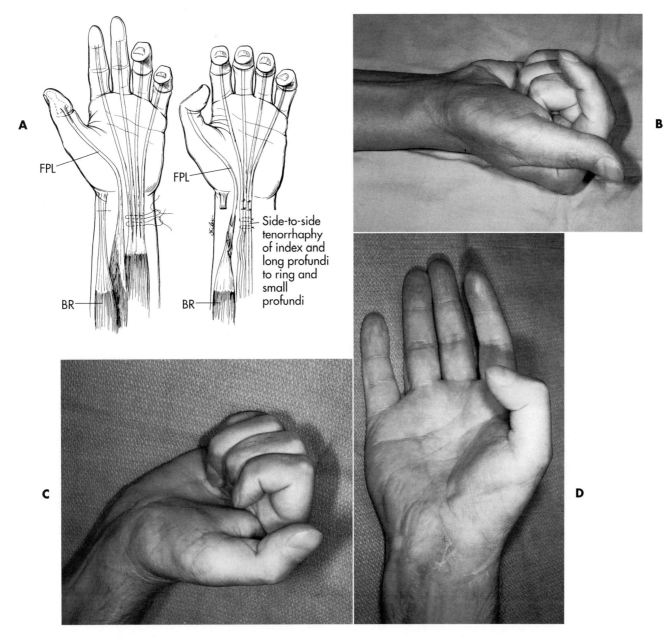

Figure 113-11. **A,** Brachioradialis (BR) to flexor pollicis longus (FPL) transfer and side-to-side tenorrhaphy of the profundus tendons to the index and long fingers to the ulnar innervated profundus tendons to the ring and small fingers for reconstruction of a high median nerve palsy. **B,** Loss of DIP-joint flexion of the index finger and IP-joint flexion of the thumb in a high median nerve palsy. **C** and **D,** Index finger DIP-joint and thumb IP-joint flexion restored by tenorrhaphy of the flexor digitorum profundus tendons in the distal forearm and brachioradialis to flexor pollicis longus transfer.

OPERATIONS

Flexion of the IP joint of the thumb is restored by transfer of the brachioradialis to the FPL (Figure 113-11). The brachioradialis is divided at its insertion on the distal radius and extensively mobilized from its investing fascia up into the proximal third of the forearm so that the freed muscle can develop approximately 30 mm of excursion. The FPL tendon can be divided at its musculotendinous junction and woven end to end into the brachioradialis tendon if reinnervation of the FPL longus muscle is not expected to occur after repair or grafting of the median nerve. If there is any possibility of reinnervation of the FPL, however, the brachioradialis tendon should be woven end to side into the FPL tendon, which remains in continuity.

The profundus tendons to the index and long fingers can be

2008 PART V TENDONS

sutured side to side to the ulnar innervated profundus tendons to the ring and small fingers through the same volar forearm incision (see Figure 113-11). If power flexion of the index and long fingers is required, then formal transfer of the ECRL tendon to the index-and long-finger profundus tendons can be performed. The ECRL is transected through a small transverse incision at the base of the index-finger metacarpal and passed subcutaneously around the radial border of the distal forearm into the volar incision. The profundus tendons to the index and long fingers are woven into the ECRL tendon so that with the wrist in 30 to 45 degrees of dorsiflexion, the tips of the index and long fingers almost touch the palm. Similarly, with the wrist in full palmar flexion, the fingers will assume an almost fully extended position. Adjusting tension on this transfer using the tenodesis effect of the wrist is absolutely critical because the donor ECRL tendon has only 30 mm of excursion, whereas the profundus tendons normally have 70 mm of excursion. If this transfer is sutured under too much tension, it will result in flexion contractures of these two fingers.

The timing of tendon transfers in a high median nerve palsy remains controversial.[12] There is usually a good chance for reinnervation of the extrinsic flexor muscles in a young patient if a good primary or delayed primary nerve repair can be performed. Consequently "early" brachioradialis to FPL or side-to-side repair of the index-and long-finger profundus tendons to the ring-and small-finger profundus tendons is not necessary. However, if the patient is seen late and requires secondary nerve grafting of the median nerve, then tendon transfers for restoration of thumb flexion and index-and long-finger flexion should be performed simultaneously with the nerve graft. The timing of "early" transfers for thumb opposition in both "low" and "high" median nerve palsies has previously been discussed.

OUTCOMES

There is no standard measure of thumb opposition in the literature. Some authors have developed functional scales to rate the outcome of opposition tendon transfers, and others have reported subjective patient satisfaction.[27,29] An anatomic and biomechanical study by Cooney et al[17] demonstrated that the long-finger FDS and the ECU best restored lost thenar strength, abduction, and rotation. The ECRL and the ring-finger FDS were found to be nearly as strong and replaced 60% and 40%, respectively, of required thenar muscle strength. The Camitz transfer provided good abduction, but weak flexion and pronation.

The results of the EIP opposition tendon transfer in patients with leprosy reported by Anderson et al[1] indicate that excellent or good results were seen in approximately 88% of patients. Similar results have been reported by other authors, but little data documenting thumb range of motion or rigorous functional outcome information exist.

The Bunnell sublimis transfer has few long-term results published with objective data. Brandsma et al[7] reported excellent results in 32% and good results in 51% of hands treated with the Bunnell procedure. A number of other patients in this study underwent FDS transfer for intrinsic replacement. Swan-neck deformities were seen in 15% of the 158 donor fingers, with DIP-joint flexion problems in 29%, and PIP-joint flexion contractures in 18%. Groves and Goldner[23] reported success in 75% of 16 patients with high median nerve or brachial plexus palsy undergoing sublimis opposition transfers.

Terrono et al[47] retrospectively reviewed their experience with the Camitz abductorplasty for severe median nerve compression at the wrist in 33 patients with a mean age of 65 years. Ninety-four percent (31 of 33) of patients felt that their thumb dexterity and speed were improved by the operation. Two patients were unhappy with the results. Braun[8] reported good results in 28 patients who underwent the Camitz transfer. Little objective mechanical data are available for this transfer.

Use of the ECU for restoration of thumb opposition is supported by experimental cadaver data. Phalen and Miller[38] reported good results with this transfer, but another study reported the development of significant radial deviation of the wrist in one third of cases.[53]

Most clinical trials report good results in all of the common opposition transfers (Table 113-2). Success is defined differently in each of these reports, and thus a cohesive evaluation and enlightened recommendation is difficult to make. Outcome data on tendon transfers for high median nerve palsy are even more scarce.

LOW ULNAR NERVE PALSY

INDICATIONS

Injury to the ulnar nerve distal to the innervation of the ring-and small-finger profundus tendons and FCU produces paralysis of all seven interossei, the ulnar two lumbricals, the three hypothenar muscles, and the adductor pollicis (AP). There is a resulting imbalance between the flexor and extensor forces at the MCP, PIP, and DIP joints of the fingers. Because the interossei are the main flexors of the MCP joints, extension of the proximal phalanges by the extrinsic extensor tendons is unopposed and is limited only by the weak volar plate. Extension by the extrinsic extensor tendons is concentrated at the MCP joints, and the interossei are unable to actively extend at the PIP and DIP joints. The increased tension in the flexor tendons is then unopposed at the PIP and DIP joints. This combination of forces produces the typical claw-hand deformity with hyperextension at the MCP joints and flexion at the PIP and DIP joints. Imbalance between the extrinsic extensor and flexor tendons also leads to reduced grip strength and asynchronous flexion of the fingers such that the MCP joints do not flex until after the IP joints have become completely flexed, resulting in curling of the tips of the fingers into the palm, with loss of ability to grasp large objects. The clawing and loss of integrated MCP and IP joint flexion are confined to the ring and small fingers, and to a lesser extent the long finger,

Table 113-2.
Opposition Transfers

OPPOSITION TECHNIQUE	ETIOLOGY	AUTHOR	YEAR	REPORTED SUCCESS
Huber	Trauma	Wissinger	1977	80%
	Neurologic disease			
	Congenital	Ogino	1986	100%
Camitz	Nerve compression	Terrono	1993	94%
	Mixed	Braun	1978	100%
EIP	Mixed	Anderson	1991	88%
	Trauma	Burkhalter	1973	88%
Bunnell	Leprosy	Brandsma	1992	83%
	Leprosy	Palande	1975	94%
	Trauma	Kirklin	1948	85%
	Trauma	Groves	1975	75%
	Polio	Goldner	1950	80%
	Mixed	Jensen	1978	78%
EDQ	Trauma	Schneider	1969	80%

in a low ulnar nerve palsy because the lumbrical muscles to the index and long fingers remain innervated by the median nerve. All four fingers are affected, however, with a combined median and ulnar nerve palsy. Fowler[20] has shown that the PIP joints can be extended by the extrinsic extensor tendons provided that the MCP joints are stabilized. Both the claw deformity and the asynchronous finger flexion may therefore be improved either by static techniques to prevent hyperextension of the MCP joints or by dynamic tendon transfers to produce either MCP-joint flexion alone or to provide both MCP-joint flexion and IP-joint extension.

The other significant impairment in patients with low ulnar nerve palsy is weak thumb–index-finger pinch, which may be only 30% of normal because of paralysis of the AP and the first dorsal interosseous muscles. There is dual innervation of the FPB muscle in 58% of patients with ulnar nerve injuries, which can to some extent provide MCP-joint flexion and key pinch to the index finger. Loss of key pinch is usually manifest by compensatory activation of the FPL, producing flexion at the IP joint (Froment's sign) and occasionally hyperextension at the MCP joint (Jeanne's sign). Tendon transfers will be required in such patients with weak pinch to restore adduction of the thumb and abduction of the index finger.

Patients may also develop an irritating ulnar deviation of the small finger in addition to the clawing at the MCP joint (Wartenberg sign), which is caused by the unopposed action of the extensor digiti minimi (EDM) tendon caused by paralysis of the third palmar interosseous muscle. A tendon transfer occasionally may be required to correct this ulnar deviation of the small finger.

The timing of tendon transfers for ulnar nerve palsy is dependent on two factors: the probability of motor recovery and the severity of the functional deficit. Primary microsurgical repair of the ulnar nerve at the wrist can be expected to yield acceptable function in about 75% of patients. Delayed nerve grafting has been reported to provide functional motor recovery in approximately 40% to 75% of cases, with a somewhat worse prognosis for sensory recovery. As in other peripheral nerve injuries, younger patients, those with shorter nerve defects, and those without other significant concomitant injuries have a better chance of obtaining useful results from ulnar nerve repair.

"Early" transfers should be considered for those patients with a debilitating claw deformity. Clawing can be treated conservatively using a lumbrical block splint during the waiting period after nerve repair, but some patients may benefit from either early static tenodeses or dynamic tendon transfers to prevent MCP-joint hyperextension and clawing. Trevett et al[50] studied the functional results after both high and low ulnar nerve repairs to better define the indications for tendon transfers. Patients continued to show improvement in intrinsic muscle power, grip strength, and sensation for at least 2 years after high ulnar nerve repairs and 3 years after low ulnar nerve repairs. A significant conclusion from this study was that early tendon transfers should only be performed in manual laborers who complain of poor grip or key pinch.

OPERATIONS

Clawing of the Fingers
STATIC TENODESES. Static procedures to prevent hyperextension of the proximal phalanges include capsulodesis and various tenodeses. Capsulodesis of the MCP joint as described

by Zancolli[56] is a very simple technique that involves proximal advancement of the volar plate and attachment into the metacarpal neck to hold the MCP joint in approximately 20 degrees of flexion. Parkes[37] described an effective tenodesis both to prevent hyperextension at the MCP joints and to provide extension of the IP joints. In this procedure, a tendon graft is attached to the transverse carpal ligament and passed volar to the deep transverse intermetacarpal ligaments to insert into the radial lateral band of each finger. Fowler has used tendon grafts from the radial lateral bands of each finger passed volar to the deep transverse intermetacarpal ligaments and then routed dorsally through the intermetacarpal spaces to be attached to the dorsal carpal ligament.[40] The Riordan tenodesis uses a similar dorsal route, but with two distally based strips of the ECRL and ECU tendons.[40]

TENDON TRANSFERS. The various dynamic tendon transfers that have been described to correct clawing differ primarily in whether they provide MCP-joint flexion alone or whether they also provide IP-joint extension. The surgeon can determine which general type of transfer is most appropriate by preoperative testing of PIP-and DIP-joint extension with the MCP joints passively flexed. If the extrinsic extensor tendons can produce full extension at the PIP and DIP joints with the MCP joints flexed, the transfer will only need to produce strong MCP-joint flexion. This can be achieved by insertion of the transfer either into the A1 pulley (Zancolli), the A2 pulley (Brooks-Jones[9]) or through a drill hole in the proximal phalanx (Burkhalter[14]). The central slip of the extensor mechanism may become attenuated, however, in patients with long-standing flexion deformities of the PIP joints. Consequently, if the patient cannot actively extend the PIP joints using the extrinsic extensor tendons when the MCP joints are passively flexed, the transfer will have to be inserted into the lateral bands so that potentially both MCP-joint flexion and PIP-joint extension can be restored.

If one of the sublimis tendons is used as a donor tendon to produce either MCP-joint flexion alone or both MCP-joint flexion and IP-joint extension, it does not produce any increase in power grip. Adding an extra MT unit to activate these transfers, such as a wrist flexor or extensor tendon, however, will potentially lead to increased grip strength.

Tendon Transfers to Provide Metacarpophalangeal-Joint Flexion Alone

The flexor digitorum sublimis tendons to the ring and small fingers are divided in the Zancolli "lasso" procedure distal to the A1 pulley through a distal palmar crease incision. Each tendon is withdrawn from the flexor sheath between the A1 and A2 pulleys, looped around the A1 pulley, and sutured to itself. The ring-and small-finger sublimis tendons cannot be used in patients with a high ulnar palsy. Consequently, the long-finger sublimis tendon is divided into two slips and each slip is passed under the A1 pulleys of the ring and small fingers and sutured to themselves (Figure 113-12).

All the sublimis tendons in patients with combined high median-ulnar nerve palsy are paralyzed and consequently an "indirect lasso" procedure is required. The sublimis tendons

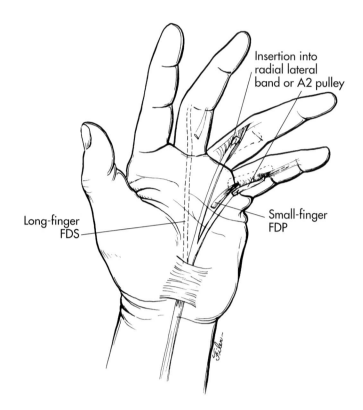

Figure 113-12. Correction of clawing of the ring and small fingers using the long-finger sublimis tendon. The modified Stiles-Bunnell transfer is shown in the ring finger with insertion into the radial lateral band to produce both MCP-joint flexion and IP-joint extension. In the small finger the slip of sublimis tendon is looped around the A2 pulley as in the "lasso" procedure to produce MCP-joint flexion only.

are passed around the A1 pulleys, and the proximal ends of the sublimis tendons are activated either by the ECRL or FCR. Brooks and Jones[9] have described a variant of this transfer in which the ECRL or FCR are elongated with plantaris or toe extensor tendon grafts through the carpal tunnel, with insertion more distally into the A2 pulley. Burkhalter and Strait[14] have also used the same donor tendons, the ring-finger sublimis and extensor carpi radialis longus, but with insertion through a transverse drill hole in the middle third of the proximal phalanx. In a low ulnar nerve palsy, the ring-finger sublimis is divided at the level of the PIP joint and withdrawn into the palm and divided into two slips. Each slip is then passed down the lumbrical canal and drawn into a transverse drill hole on the radial aspect of the middle third of the proximal phalanx of the ring and small fingers. In patients with a high ulnar nerve palsy or a combined high median–ulnar nerve palsy, the ECRL can be extended with either two or four tendon grafts. The grafts are then passed through the intermetacarpal spaces and down the lumbrical canals volar to the deep transverse intermetacarpal ligaments and again attached into a drill hole on the radial aspect of the middle third of the proximal phalanges of all four digits. These two transfers will produce MPC-joint flexion alone. Only those transfers powered by a wrist flexor, such as the FCR, or

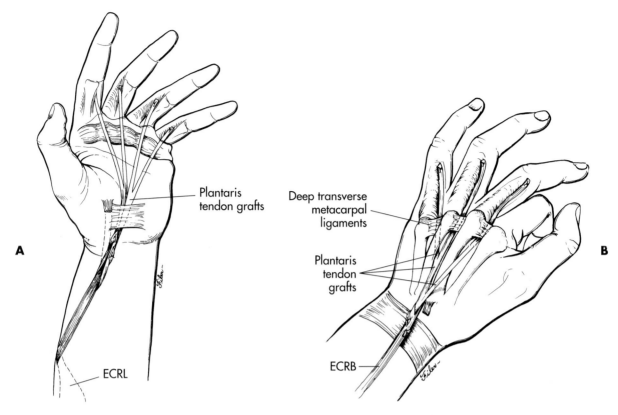

Figure 113-13. **A,** Brand transfer of extensor carpi radialis longus (ECRL) elongated with a four-tailed plantaris tendon graft to restore MCP-joint flexion and IP-joint extension. **B,** Dorsal route of the original Brand transfer using extensor carpi radialis brevis (ECRB) to correct clawing of the fingers.

extensor tendon, such as the ECRL, will lead to increased power grip.

Tendon Transfers to Provide Simultaneous Metacarpophalangeal-Joint Flexion and Interphalangeal-Joint Extension

MODIFIED STILES-BUNNELL TRANSFER. In the modified Stiles-Bunnell transfer,[11] patients with an isolated low or high ulnar nerve palsy need the long-finger sublimis tendon divided just proximal to the PIP joint through a radial mid-axial incision. The sublimis tendon is withdrawn through a transverse distal palmar crease incision and split longitudinally into two slips. The radial lateral bands of the ring and small fingers are approached through radial mid-axial incisions, and each slip of the long-finger sublimis tendon is passed down the lumbrical canals of the ring and small fingers. Each slip is sutured to the radial lateral band, with the wrist in neutral, the MCP joints in 45 degrees of flexion, and the IP joints fully extended (see Figure 113-12). Tension is tested using the tenodesis effect of the wrist, and the fingers should assume the "intrinsic-plus" position with dorsiflexion of the wrist. The hand is immobilized in a dorsal blocking splint for 3½ to 4 weeks, with the wrist in slight flexion and the MCP joints in 70 degrees of flexion. Occasionally the long-finger sublimis may need to be split into three slips should the long, ring, and small fingers need correction. Patients with a total intrinsic palsy need the sublimis tendons to the long and ring

fingers each divided into two slips and passed down the lumbrical canals to the radial lateral bands of the index, long, ring, and small fingers. Brand advocates insertion of the slip to the index finger into the ulnar lateral band to provide improved three-point pinch. This may, however, result in scissoring of the index and long fingers.

The disadvantages of the modified Stiles-Bunnell transfer are that the ring-finger sublimis is not expendable in a high ulnar nerve palsy or a combined high median–ulnar nerve palsy. Secondly, the transfer may result in progressive overcorrection of the claw deformity, eventually resulting in a "swan-neck" hyperextension deformity of the PIP joints. The modified Stiles-Bunnell transfer should therefore only be used in patients with mild PIP-joint flexion contractures or stable fingers that cannot be passively hyperextended at the PIP joints.

BRAND EXTENSOR CARPI RADIALIS LONGUS ZAND EXTENSOR CARPI RADIALIS BREVIS TRANSFERS. Brand,[4,5] from his extensive series of intrinsic transfers in leprosy patients, has convincingly documented increased grip strength after transfer of the ECRL lengthened with four plantaris tendon grafts passed through the lumbrical canals to the radial lateral bands of the long, ring, and small fingers and to the ulnar lateral band of the index finger (Figure 113-13, A). Two short transverse incisions are made over the second dorsal extensor tendon compartment and over the radial aspect of the mid-forearm to allow transection of the ECRL tendon, which is withdrawn into the mid-forearm. The tendon is then rerouted around the radial border of the forearm superficial to the brachioradialis into a transverse volar forearm incision approximately 2 to 3 inches proximal to the wrist crease. Each half of a folded plantaris tendon graft is then split longitudinally to make four slips, and its proximal end is sutured to the ECRL tendon projecting through the volar forearm incision. A tendon tunneling forceps is passed along the floor of the carpal tunnel through a 3-cm long incision just to the ulnar side of the thenar crease to exit through the ulnar side of the volar forearm incision. The four tendon grafts are then pulled distally through the carpal tunnel into the palmar incision. The proximal tendon juncture therefore now lies distal to the volar forearm incision but proximal to the transverse carpal ligament. Radial mid-axial incisions are made over the proximal phalanges of the long, ring, and small fingers. The tunneling forceps are passed through these incisions volar to the deep transverse intermetacarpal ligaments through the lumbrical canals and into the palmar incision, and the three tendon slips are pulled distally into each mid-axial incision. The tendon slip to the index finger may be tunneled through the first dorsal interosseous muscle to the radial lateral band or passed through the second intermetacarpal space to the ulnar lateral band as advocated by Brand.[44] This will produce supination of the index finger and may provide better three-point pinch. The hand is positioned on a lead frame with the wrist extended 40 degrees, the MCP joints flexed 70 degrees, and the IP joints fully extended. All slack in the four plantaris grafts is taken up and they are sutured to the lateral bands just proximal to the PIP joints. The hand is immobilized in this "intrinsic plus" position for 3 weeks.

Brand originally described this intrinsic transfer as a dorsal transfer using the ECRB to activate a four-tailed plantaris graft passed from dorsal to volar through the intermetacarpal spaces (Figure 113-13, B). The ECRB tendon is transected through a transverse incision overlying the bases of the metacarpals and withdrawn through a dorsal transverse incision at the level of the mid-forearm. The four-tailed plantaris graft is sutured to the ECRB tendon and then passed distally into the wrist incision superficial to the extensor retinaculum. Again, this places the proximal tendon juncture in unscarred tissues. The radial lateral band is identified through a mid-axial incision over the proximal phalanx of each finger, and the tendon tunneler is passed in a distal to proximal direction until it is opposite the metacarpal heads. The deep transverse intermetacarpal ligament can be felt by the nose of the tunneler, which is passed volar to the ligament. The fingers are then fully flexed and the tunneler is directed dorsally through the intermetacarpal spaces into the dorsal wrist incision. Each tendon graft can be pulled distally through the intermetacarpal spaces into the mid-axial incisions. The tunnel to the small finger is made by passing the tunneler volar to the deep transverse intermetacarpal ligament between the ring- and small-finger metacarpal heads and then passing it through the intermetacarpal space between the long- and ring-finger metacarpals. The graft to the index finger can either be tunneled

through the first dorsal interosseous muscle to the radial lateral band or, as Brand suggested, through the second intermetacarpal space to the ulnar lateral band of the index finger. The hand is then positioned with the wrist extended 45 degrees, the MCP joints flexed 90 degrees, and the IP joints extended. Slack is taken up in the four tendon grafts and they are sutured at the resting tension of the ECRB muscle. The hand is immobilized in this same position in a volar splint for 3 weeks. Relaxation of the ECRB and the tendon grafts during wrist extension is a relative disadvantage of this original dorsal route of the Brand transfer.

Riordan[40] has described a similar transfer using the FCR transferred dorsally around the radial border of the forearm and elongated with tendon grafts that are passed through the intermetacarpal spaces volar to the deep transverse intermetacarpal ligaments to the radial lateral bands. This transfer is mutually beneficial if there is an associated flexion contracture of the wrist. The dorsal route also forms the basis for the Fowler transfer in which the EIP and EDM tendons are each split longitudinally and passed through the intermetacarpal spaces to the radial lateral bands of the fingers.[19] The EIP tendon controls the index and long fingers; the EDM controls the ring and small fingers. Riordan, in a modification of this Fowler transfer, has described splitting only the EIP tendon into two slips and passing them through the third and fourth intermetacarpal spaces to insert into the radial lateral bands to correct clawing of the ring and small fingers.[19]

Tendon Transfers to Correct Ulnar Deviation of the Small Finger

A variant of the Fowler transfer has been advocated by Blacker et al[2] to correct the ulnar deviation of the small finger (Wartenberg's sign). The ulnar half of EDM is detached, passed volar to the deep transverse intermetacarpal ligament, and sutured into the insertion of the radial collateral ligament of the MCP joint on the base of the proximal phalanx, or if there is associated clawing of the small finger, it is looped under the A2 pulley and sutured back to itself (Brooks insertion).

Tendon Transfers to Provide Adduction of the Thumb

The most successful tendon transfers to restore adduction of the thumb have a transverse direction of pull across the palm deep to the flexor tendons, with insertion into the tendon of the AP. Littler[30] has advocated transfer of the ring-finger sublimis deep to the flexor tendons of the index and long fingers paralleling the transverse fibers of the AP into a drill hole just distal to the adductor insertion; with this approach, he has been able to document an increase in pinch strength to 71% of the opposite normal hand. Smith[43] described using the ECRB extended by a free tendon graft, passing through the second intermetacarpal space, and tunneling beneath the AP to its insertion. Other tendon transfers to provide adduction of the thumb have included either the brachioradialis (Omer) or the ECRL (Boyes) elongated with a tendon graft and passed through the third intermetacarpal space, and the EIP (Brand) passed through the second intermetacarpal space. Combined transfers to provide both thumb adduction and index-finger abduction have been described by splitting the EIP (Omer) or EDM (Zweig, Rosenthal, and Burns). Occasionally, arthrodesis of the IP joint or MCP joint of the thumb may be a simpler alternative to tendon transfers to provide strong key pinch.

RING-FINGER FLEXOR DIGITORUM SUBLIMIS. The ring-finger flexor digitorum sublimis tendon is transected between the A1 and A2 pulleys through a short oblique incision at the base of the ring finger.[30] The sublimis tendon is then passed transversely across the palm deep to the index-and long-finger flexor tendons to the ulnar aspect of the thumb MCP joint, if necessary using a short incision just to the ulnar side of the thenar crease. The transfer is either sutured to the AP tendon or passed into a drill hole through the proximal phalanx just distal to the adductor insertion and tied over a button. Tension is set with the wrist in neutral and the thumb adducted against the index finger, with the sublimis tendon at its resting length. This is then tested so that with palmar flexion of the wrist, the thumb can be passively abducted. Edgerton and Brand[18] have described a variation of this transfer in which the ring-finger sublimis is brought through a window in the palmar fascia and then passed subcutaneously to the adductor insertion. The ring-finger sublimis obviously cannot be used as an adductor transfer in patients with a high ulnar nerve palsy because this would deprive the ring finger of its only remaining flexor tendon.

EXTENSOR CARPI RADIALIS BREVIS. The ECRB is transected through a short transverse incision over the second dorsal extensor compartment just distal to the extensor retinaculum and withdrawn through a second transverse incision just proximal to the extensor retinaculum.[43] A small flap is then elevated over the ulnar aspect of the MCP joint of the thumb, and a palmaris or plantaris tendon graft is sutured to the AP tendon. A tendon passer is used to tunnel the tendon graft deep to the AP through a short transverse incision overlying the proximal third of the second intermetacarpal space and then directed dorsally through the second intermetacarpal space. The tendon graft is passed subcutaneously to the most proximal incision where it is woven into the ECRB tendon with the wrist in neutral and the thumb adducted (Figure 113-14). Tension is then checked by tenodesis of the wrist, where in palmar flexion the thumb should become strongly adducted and wrist dorsiflexion should allow easy passive abduction of the thumb. The thumb is immobilized for 3 weeks after surgery midway between full abduction and full adduction ,with the wrist in 20 to 30 degrees of dorsiflexion.

Tendon Transfers to Provide Index-Finger Abduction

Restoration of strong index-finger abduction is the second component required for powerful pinch. Bunnell[11] reported transfer of the EIP extended with a short tendon graft and inserted into the first dorsal interosseous tendon. Bruner divided the EPB tendon over the dorsum of the MCP joint of the thumb and tunneled it subcutaneously beneath the EPL

tendon into the first dorsal interosseous tendon. Neviaser et al[34] described elongation of an accessory APL tendon with a palmaris or plantaris tendon graft transferred to the insertion of the first dorsal interosseous (see Figure 113-14).

ACCESSORY ABDUCTOR POLLICIS LONGUS AND FREE TENDON GRAFT. A small skin flap is elevated over the radial aspect of the proximal phalanx of the index finger, and the palmaris longus or plantaris tendon graft is sutured to the first dorsal interosseous tendon just distal to the MCP joint. The proximal end of the tendon graft is then passed subcutaneously to a transverse incision over the first dorsal extensor compartment. The compartment is opened and one of the accessory APL tendons that does not insert on the base of the thumb metacarpal is transected. It is interwoven with the tendon graft, holding the wrist in a neutral position and the index finger radially abducted.

HIGH ULNAR NERVE PALSY

Many surgeons fail to realize the significant functional deficit experienced by a patient with high ulnar nerve palsy caused by paralysis of the FCU and profundus tendons to the ring and small fingers. The only remaining tendons on the ulnar side of the hand are the sublimis tendon to the ring finger and the usually diminutive sublimis tendon to the small finger. Paralysis of the profundus tendons to the ring and small fingers, however, will often be masked by interconnections between these two tendons and the long-finger profundus tendon in the distal forearm. Significant weakness of flexion of the ring and small fingers, which decreases power grip, can be restored by side-to-side tenorrhaphy of the ring-and small-finger profundus tendons to the long-finger profundus tendon. Independent flexion of the ring and small fingers can be restored with the sublimis tendon of the long finger used as the donor tendon to activate the profundus tendons to the ring and small fingers. Patients requiring strong ulnar deviation and flexion of the wrist may also need to be considered for transfer of the FCR tendon to the FCU.

OUTCOMES

There are a multitude of tendon transfers to restore synchronous finger flexion and pinch capability to the hand affected by an ulnar nerve palsy but very few reports are available to substantiate the relative effectiveness of each transfer. Hastings and Davidson[24] examined their results in 13 patients with high ulnar nerve palsy, 17 patients with low ulnar nerve palsy, and 4 other patients with combined injuries. Four techniques were used to correct a claw defect in 29 of the 34 patients: the Zancolli "lasso" and the Stiles-Bunnell, Brand, and Riordan transfers. Successful outcomes were seen in the majority of

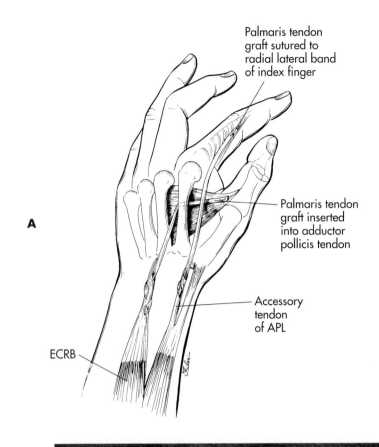

Palmaris tendon
graft sutured to
radial lateral band
of index finger

Palmaris tendon
graft inserted
into adductor
pollicis tendon

Accessory
tendon
of APL

ECRB

A

Figure 113-14. A and **B,** Restoration of power pinch by transfer of extensor carpi radialis brevis (ECRB) extended by a palmaris tendon graft into the adductor pollicis (AP) insertion, and transfer of an accessory tendon of the abductor pollicis longus (Ac APL) elongated with a palmaris tendon graft into the first dorsal interosseous (1st DI). Traction on the tendon grafts intraoperatively **(C)** demonstrates the strong adduction of the thumb and abduction of the index finger that can be achieved postoperatively **(D).**

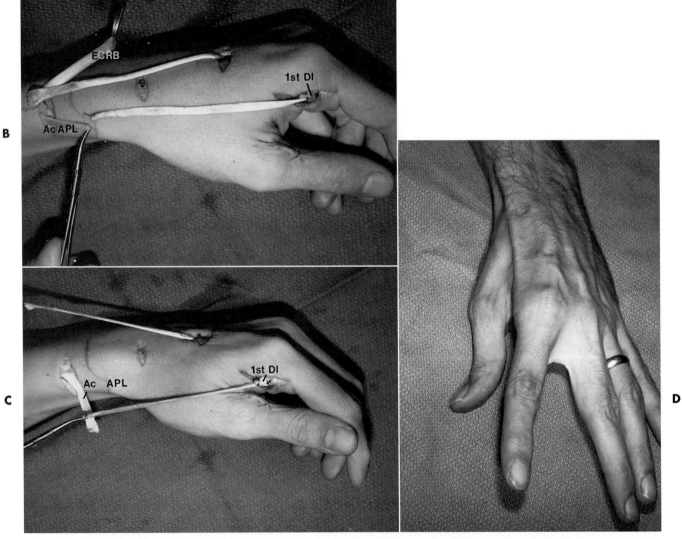

B

ECRB

Ac APL

1st DI

C

Ac APL

1st DI

D

cases (Zancolli 20/25, Stiles-Bunnell 15/22, Brand 11/11, Riordan 4/4). The majority of failures occurred in the small finger, and transfers utilizing the sublimis tendons were found to further weaken the hand. Only techniques using wrist flexors or extensors have been shown to increase grip strength. Another report examining the effectiveness of the FDS "lasso" procedure suggests similar results, with correction of clawing in 19 of 23 digits and no significant improvement in grip strength.[25] Brandsma et al[7] reported good (57%) or excellent (21%) results in the majority of patients undergoing sublimis transfers, but several complications did occur.

Thumb flexion is weakened by 75% and pinch decreased by over 80% in ulnar nerve palsy. Pinch strength has been shown to double after ECRB adductorplasty.[32] Hastings and Davidson[24] have also shown an approximate doubling of pinch strength in hands treated with the ECRB transfer, but it is interesting to note that only 18 of the 34 patients in this study felt that their pinch strength was compromised enough to warrant a tendon transfer. Robinson et al[41] studied the combined transfer of the ulnar slip of EDQ for thumb adduction and EIP for index-finger abduction in six patients and demonstrated an average improvement in pinch strength from 5% to a range of 40% to 50% of the normal side.

SUMMARY

Adequate quantitative outcome data are lacking for the plethora of tendon transfers but most surgeons and patients can attest to the significant benefits derived from them. Disability from peripheral nerve injuries has been well documented and is significant. Tendon transfers, if carefully selected and performed meticulously, will provide a gratifying functional improvement to the hand affected by radial, median, or ulnar nerve palsy. Comparative studies must be designed in the future to document the effectiveness of the many transfers and their ultimate impact on hand function and return to work.

REFERENCES

1. Anderson GA, Lee V, Sundararaj GD: Extensor indicis proprius opponensplasty, *J Hand Surg [Br]* 16:334, 1991.
2. Blacker GJ, Lister GD, Kleinert HE: The abducted little finger in low ulnar nerve palsy, *J Hand Surg [Am]* 1:190, 1976.
3. Boyes JH: Tendon transfers for radial palsy, *Bull Hosp Joint Dis* 21:97, 1960.
4. Brand PW: Tendon grafting illustrated by a new operation for intrinsic paralysis of the fingers, *J Bone Joint Surg* 43B:444, 1961.
5. Brand PW: *Clinical mechanics of the hand,* St. Louis, 1985, Mosby.
6. Brand PW, Beach RB, Thompson DE: Relative tension and potential excursion of muscles in the forearm and hand, *J Hand Surg [Am]* 6:209, 1981.
7. Brandsma JW, Ottenhoff-De Jonge MW: Flexor digitorum superficialis tendon transfer for intrinsic replacement: long-term results and the effect on donor fingers, *J Hand Surg [Br]* 17:625, 1992.
8. Braun RM: Palmaris longus tendon transfer for augmentation of the thenar musculature in low median nerve palsy, *J Hand Surg [Am]* 3:488, 1978.
9. Brooks AL, Jones DS: A new intrinsic tendon transfer for the paralytic hand, *J Bone Joint Surg* 57A:730, 1975.
10. Bunnell S: Opposition of the thumb, *J Bone Joint Surg* 20:269, 1938.
11. Bunnell S: Surgery of the intrinsic muscles of the hand other than those producing opposition of the thumb, *J Bone Joint Surg* 24:1, 1942.
12. Burkhalter WE: Early tendon transfer in upper extremity peripheral nerve injury, *Clin Orthop* 104:68, 1974.
13. Burkhalter WE, Christensen RC, Brown P: Extensor indicis proprius opponensplasty, *J Bone Joint Surg* 55A:725, 1973.
14. Burkhalter WE, Strait JL: Metacarpo-phalangeal flexor replacement for intrinsic muscle paralysis, *J Bone Joint Surg* 55A:1667, 1973.
15. Camitz H: Ueber die behandlung der opposition-slahmung, *Acta Chir Scand* 65:77, 1929.
16. Chuinard RG, Boyes JH, Stark HH, Ashworth CR: Tendon transfers for radial nerve palsy: use of superficialis tendons for digital extension, *J Hand Surg [Am]* 3:560, 1978.
17. Cooney WP, Linscheid RL, An KN: Opposition of the thumb: an anatomic and biomechanical study of tendon transfers, *J Hand Surg [Am]* 9:777, 1984.
18. Edgerton MT, Brand PW: Restoration of abduction and adduction to the unstable thumb in median and ulnar paralysis, *Plast Reconstr Surg* 36:150, 1965.
19. Enna CD, Riordan DC: The Fowler procedure for correction of the paralytic claw hand, *Plast Reconstr Surg* 52:352, 1973.
20. Fowler SB: Extensor apparatus of the digits, *J Bone Joint Surg* 31B:477, 1949.
21. Franke F: Sehnenüberpflanzug, *Arch Klin Chir* 52:87, 1896.
22. Fujiwara A, Ryo F, Kashiwagi D, Fujita H: Evaluation of the Boyes method in the treatment of radial nerve palsy, *Orthop Surg (Tokyo)* 21:954, 1970.
23. Groves RJ, Goldner JL: Restoration of strong opposition after median nerve or brachial plexus paralysis, *J Bone Joint Surg* 57A:112, 1975.
24. Hastings H, Davidson S: Tendon transfers for ulnar nerve palsy: evaluation of results and practical considerations, *Hand Clin* 4:167, 1988.
25. Hastings H, McCollam SM: Flexor digitorum sublimis lasso tendon transfer in isolated ulnar nerve palsy: a functional evaluation, *J Hand Surg [Am]* 19:275, 1994.
26. Huber E: Hilfsoperation bei medianus slahmung, *Dtsch Z Chir* 126:271, 1921.
27. Jensen EG: Restoration of opposition of the thumb, *Hand* 10:161, 1978.

28. Kallio PK, Vastamaki M, Solonen KA: The results of secondary microsurgical repair of the radial nerve in 33 patients, *J Hand Surg [Br]* 18:320, 1993.

29. Kirklin JW, Thomas CG: Opponen transplant: an analysis of the methods employed and results obtained in 75 cases, *Surg Gynec Obstet* 86:213, 1948.

30. Littler JW: Tendon transfers and arthrodeses in combined median and ulnar nerve paralysis, *J Bone Joint Surg* 31A:225, 1949.

31. Littler JW, Li CS: Primary restoration of thumb opposition with median nerve decompression, *Plast Reconstr Surg* 39:74, 1967.

32. Mannerfelt L: Studies on the hand in ulnar nerve paralysis: a clinical-experimental investigation in normal and anomolous innervation, *Acta Orthop Scand* 87(suppl):1, 1966.

33. Mayer JH, Mayfield FH: Surgery of the posterior interosseous branch of the radial nerve: analysis of 58 cases, *Surg Gyn Obstet* 84:979, 1947.

34. Neviaser RJ, Wilson JN, Gardner MM: Abductor pollicis longus transfer for replacement of the first dorsal interosseous, *J Hand Surg [Am]* 5:53, 1980.

35. Nicholaysen J: Transplantation des m. abductor dig v. die fenlader oppositions fehigkeit des daumens, *Drsch Z Chir* 168:133, 1922.

36. Omer JE: The technique and timing of tendon transfers, *Orthop Clin North Am* 4:243, 1974.

37. Parkes A: Paralytic claw fingers: a graft tenodesis operation, *Hand* 5:192, 1973.

38. Phalen GS, Miller RC: The transfer of wrist extensor muscles to restore or reinforce flexion power of the fingers and opposition of the thumb, *J Bone Joint Surg* 29:993, 1947.

39. Raskin KB, Wilgis EFS: Flexor carpi ulnaris transfer for radial nerve palsy: functional testing of long-term results, *J Hand Surg [Am]* 20:737, 1995.

40. Riordan DC: Tendon transplantations in median-nerve and ulnar-nerve paralysis, *J Bone Joint Surg* 35A:312, 1953.

41. Robinson D, Ashasi MK, Halperin N: Restoration of pinch in ulnar nerve palsy by transfer of split extensor digiti minimi and extensor indicis, *J Hand Surg [Br]* 17:622, 1992.

42. Royle ND: An operation for paralysis of the intrinsic muscles of the thumb, *JAMA* 111:612, 1938.

43. Smith RJ: Extensor carpi radialis brevis tendon transfer for thumb adduction: a study of power pinch, *J Hand Surg [Am]* 8:4, 1983.

44. Smith RJ: *Tendon transfers of the hand and forearm,* Boston, 1987, Little, Brown and Co.

45. Starr CL: Army experiences with tendon transference, *J Bone Joint Surg* 4:3, 1922.

46. Steindler A: Tendon transplantation in the upper extremity, *Am J Surg* 44:260, 534, 1939.

47. Terrono AL, Rose JH, Mulroy J, Millender LH: Camitz palmaris longus abductorplasty for severe thenar atrophy secondary to carpal tunnel syndrome, *J Hand Surg [Am]* 18:204, 1993.

48. Thompson M. Rasmussen KB: Tendon transfers for defective long extensors of the wrist and fingers, *Scand J Plast Reconstr Surg* 3:71, 1969.

49. Thompson TC: A modified operation for opponens paralysis, *J Bone Joint Surg* 24:632, 1942.

50. Trevett MC, Tucson C, de Jager LT, Juon JM: The functional results of ulnar nerve repair: defining the indications for tendon transfer, *J Hand Surg [Br]* 20:444, 1995.

51. Tsuge K: Tendon transfers for radial nerve palsy, *Aust N Z J Surg* 50:767, 1980.

52. Wissinger HA, Singsen EG: Abductor digiti quinti opponensplasty, *J Bone Joint Surg* 59A:895, 1977.

53. Wood VE, Adams J: Complications of opponensplasty with transfer of extensor carpi ulnaris to extensor pollicis brevis, *J Hand Surg [Am]* 9:699, 1984.

54. Young C, Hudson A, Richards R: Operative treatment of palsy of the posterior interosseous nerve in the forearm, *J Bone Joint Surg* 72A:1215, 1975.

55. Zachary RB: Tendon transplantation for radial paralysis, *Br J Surg* 23:350, 1946.

56. Zancolli EA: Claw hand caused by paralysis of the intrinsic muscles: a simple surgical procedure for its correction, *J Bone Joint Surg* 39A:1076, 1957.

PART VI

TENOSYNOVITIS AND INFECTIONS

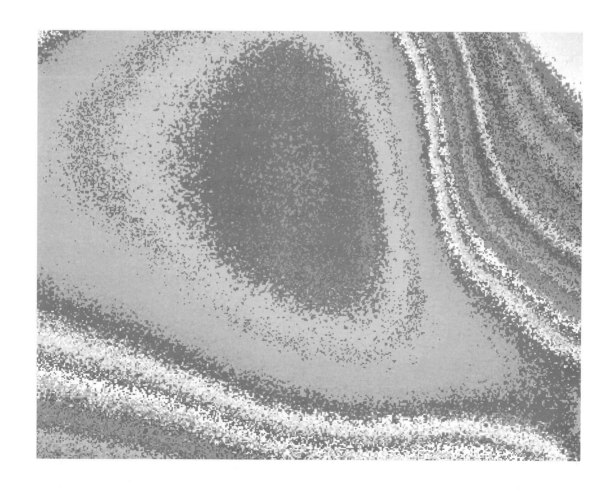

Tenosynovitis of the Hand and Forearm

114

Randy Sherman
Prasad G. Kilaru

INTRODUCTION

The hand contains an elegant series of ligamentous pulleys and fibroosseous canals that serve as restraining elements to facilitate change in tendon direction and maximize tendon pull. The dorsal and volar wrist surfaces are covered by thick retinacular ligaments, the dorsal carpal and the transverse carpal ligaments, respectively. The vertical septum from the dorsal carpal ligament separates the dorsal wrist area into six compartments. Each digit also contains a series of pulleys that contribute to the fibroosseous tunnel through which the flexor tendons travel. The tendons are covered by a filmy, areolar tenosynovium as they traverse these compartments. The tenosynovium acts to reduce friction and improves gliding of the tendons in the narrow spaces.[73] Any local or systemic condition that causes a change in the relative volume of the tenosynovium, the tendon, or the size of the fibroosseous canal can cause changes in the stress and friction forces. This mismatch and the subsequent inflammation may restrict tendon function and lead to pain and disability.

The tendons commonly affected with tenosynovitis are the abductor pollicis longus (APL) (de Quervain's disease), digital flexors (trigger finger), flexor pollicis longus (FPL) (trigger thumb), and flexor carpi radialis (FCR). Other tendons that are rarely involved include the flexor carpi ulnaris (FCU), tendon sheaths of the wrist extensors, extensor pollicis longus (EPL), and extensor digiti minimi (EDM).

Nonspecific, noninfectious tenosynovitis of the hand is seen after repeated and sustained hand stresses. The dominant hand is more frequently involved, and women are more frequently affected than men.[102] There is a higher incidence in patients with certain systemic diseases, such as diabetes mellitus, rheumatoid arthritis, and hypothyroidism.[47] It is believed that the pathophysiology for the various tenosynovial disorders is similar; because of this, common sense dictates that the therapeutic modalities used should also be similar. Rest, splinting, systemic nonsteroidal antiinflammatory agents, local steroid injections, and surgical release if conservative measures fail are the mainstay of treatment for most of these conditions.

FLEXOR STENOSING TENOSYNOVITIS (FINGER AND THUMB)

Stenosing tenovaginitis or tenosynovitis of the thumb or fingers is the most common form of flexor tendinitis in the hand.[39] The classic scenario is that of a middle-aged woman with gradual onset of pain in the distal palm that radiates to the proximal interphalangeal (PIP) joint. Patients tend to localize their symptoms to the PIP joint. Flexion and extension of the involved digit can be accompanied by a painful triggering or snapping. As this progresses, there can be a decrease in active flexion and eventually the finger can lock in a flexed position, requiring use of the other hand to straighten it.[38] Late, untreated cases can also present with PIP-joint contractures secondary to chronic flexion of the finger. Clinically, there may be a tender palpable nodule at the base of the MCP joint at the level of the A1 pulley.[70] The goal of treatment is the relief of symptoms and the restoration of full, painless range of finger motion.

Trigger finger may be described as primary or secondary. When no clear-cut etiology is noted the process is called *primary trigger finger.*[46] Typically, a middle-aged woman who notes gradual onset of distal palmar pain radiating to the PIP joint falls in this category. *Secondary trigger finger* is seen when associated disease processes are present, such as rheumatoid arthritis, diabetes, hypothyroidism, gout, or renal disease. Various other conditions involving the tendons or the sheath (e.g., neoplasms, schwannomas, mucopolysaccharidoses, and amyloidosis) also fall into this category.[20,45] Trigger finger and thumb are frequently associated with other forms of tenosynovitis, such as de Quervain's disease and carpal tunnel syndrome, because they probably share similar etiologies.[69]

A congenital form of trigger finger or thumb is seen in infants. This is much less common than the adult form and has a different etiology. This form of trigger finger or thumb usually involves a large tendon nodule that is caught at the A1 pulley, most often in the thumb. Spontaneous resolution occurs in about 30% of those trigger digits noted at birth and

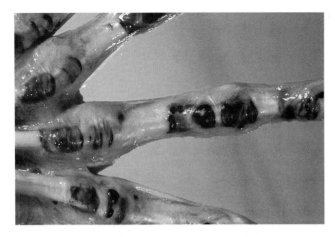

Figure 114-1. Contrast study demonstrating the digital annular and cruciate pulley system. Pulleys are stained blue. (From Johnson MK, Cohen MJ: *Hand atlas,* Springfield, Ill, 1975, Charles C. Thomas. Courtesy of Myles J. Cohen and Moulton K. Johnson.)

in only 12% of those noted between the ages of 6 months and 3 years.[27] If it does not resolve spontaneously, surgical release is required. Nonsteroidal antiinflammatory drugs or local steroid injections do not help in these situations because the process is not inflammatory in nature.[38]

ANATOMY

Doyle and Blythe[30,31] described the flexor tendon sheaths as being composed of a series of five annular and three cruciate pulleys, plus the palmar aponeurosis pulley. The A1, A3, and A5 pulleys overlie the MCP, PIP, and distal interphalangeal (DIP) joints, respectively, and the A2 and A4 pulleys overlie the proximal and middle phalanx, with cruciate pulleys present in between. The A1 pulley originates from the palmar capsule of the MCP joint and is the most proximal annular pulley. The palmar surface of the flexor digitorum superficialis (FDS) tendon makes direct contact with the inner surface of the A1 pulley through interposed visceral and parietal tenosynovium (Figure 114-1).[29] These two layers of tenosynovium create a closed bursal sheath that extends to the base of the fingers for the index, middle, and ring fingers and proximally into the wrist in the thumb and small finger. These bursal extensions are important in the spread of infection in suppurative tenosynovitis, which will be discussed later.[110]

The flexor tendon of the fingers and thumb enter the finger through a narrow fibroosseous tunnel formed by the groove in the palmar surface of the metacarpal neck and the first annular pulley.[20,64] Phalen[90] showed that the flexor sheath is narrowest at this level. The A1 pulley acts to prevent ulnar or radial drift of the flexor tendons and to fix the movement arm of the flexors so as to maintain a constant torque at the MCP joint. The A1 pulley is not indispensable, because transection of this ligament causes little functional deficit. Transection of the A2 pulley, however, causes a decrease in motion and loss of strength because of bowstringing of the flexor tendons off the proximal phalanx.[39]

PATHOLOGY AND ETIOLOGY

The first description of trigger finger was in 1850 by Notta[86] in Paris and subsequently in 1859 by Nelaton et al.[80] Notta described case series and cadaver dissections and postulated that the etiology of trigger finger was synovial engorgement or tendon nodularity. He even advocated surgical release of the A1 pulley as a form of treatment.

Several theories have been proposed regarding the pathophysiology of tenosynovitis. Finkelstein[41] proposed that with repeated use there is increased friction, which results in the development of sheath edema and leads to fibrosis in the sheath, causing it to take on a densely fibrous or even a fibrocartilaginous consistency. His work was initially on the retinacular changes seen in the first dorsal compartment in de Quervain's disease but has been extrapolated to flexor tendinitis. Thus fibrocartilaginous metaplasia of the A1 pulley, rather than tenosynovitis, is proposed as the initial cause of trigger finger.[99] This is backed by histological findings of sheath thickening in 66% of trigger releases in one series.[114]

The opposite view is that the tendon is the initial site of injury. Altered tendon nutrition[37] or vascularity[4] can cause flexor-tendon degeneration and fibrous proliferation. The thickening of the sheath with fibrocartilaginous metaplasia may be the secondary phenomenon. The FDS or FPL tendon histology under the A1 pulley in cases of trigger finger or thumb shows disruption of the parallel collagen bundles separated by vascular fibrous tissue.[39]

Given the two opposing views regarding the pathophysiology of trigger finger, the truth is probably somewhere in between, because both tissues are stressed in the disease process. Injury to the finger either as a direct contusion or a hyperextension may cause hemorrhage around the tendon, with secondary inflammation. This may in turn start a vicious cycle of tendon and sheath thickening. The tenosynovium is more vascular, so that the inflammatory response to injury is more likely to start in this tissue. Trigger finger pathology is therefore probably intratendinous and tenosynovial, with the contribution of sheath hypertrophy being secondary.[39]

PATIENT HISTORY

Patients who have trigger finger are more commonly older women who are otherwise healthy. Trigger fingers most commonly occur in the middle and ring fingers and are relatively rare in the index finger. Usually there is no history of direct or penetrating trauma, although there may be a history of repetitive use of the involved digit. One finger is usually involved in primary trigger finger, whereas in the secondary condition, multiple digits may be involved. The patient may also have other areas of tenosynovitis, such as de Quervain's disease or carpal tunnel syndrome.[20,69] A thorough history searching for metabolic or inflammatory conditions such as diabetes or rheumatoid arthritis should be obtained from all patients.

As stated earlier, the classic scenario is a gradual onset of pain in the distal palm that radiates to the PIP joint and is associated with intermittent snapping or triggering when the patient attempts active flexion or extension. Locking in flexion and pain at the PIP joint are the major complaints. Initially this may appear to be a "slow finger," which progresses to persistent locking that requires the use of other fingers or the opposite hand to release.[70] Further progression results in a finger that is fixed in flexion, or a patient that is reluctant to bend the finger secondary to the pain. Occasionally the finger may be locked in an extended position.

PHYSICAL EXAMINATION

A complete examination should be performed to rule out other associated conditions. Checks on the range of motion of the wrist, fingers, and palmar and dorsal tenosynovial areas and specific examinations to rule out de Quervain's disease and carpal tunnel syndrome should be performed. Joints should be checked for any inflammatory changes, extensor tendons examined for any injury, and the palms inspected for any masses, nodules, or Dupuytren's disease. Tenderness is almost always present in the area of the A1 pulley. A tender nodule at this level is usually palpable, especially with movement of the flexor tendons. Triggering can be elicited by repetitive flexion and extension of the involved finger. The finger may be locked in flexion in more advanced cases. In this situation, passive extension of the finger is most painful when pressure is exerted at the DIP joint compared with extension forces applied at the PIP joint. This is because extension at the DIP joint pulls both the flexor digitorum profundus (FDP) and the FDS tendons through the already tight A1 pulley area, whereas extension at the PIP joint only pulls the FDS tendon.[39] With time, patients learn to adapt to the discomfort by decreasing flexion at the DIP and the PIP joints, thereby decreasing the associated discomfort. This provides a clue to the duration of the symptoms.

DIFFERENTIAL DIAGNOSIS

Any condition that causes a feeling of stiffness in the fingers, decreased motion, flexion contracture, inflammation, locking, or snapping can be mistaken for trigger finger. These conditions can be broadly grouped into several categories:

1. *Remote tenosynovitis:* Although the A1 pulley is the most common site for triggering, the A2, A3, or A4 pulleys can be involved in this phenomenon.[96] If the A2 or A4 pulleys are involved, the pulleys should not be resected because a functional deficit would result. Instead, an internal wedge of tendon should be resected to restore gliding function.[104] Triggering can also occur at the wrist. Triggering can occur when flexor tendons catch at the transverse carpal ligament, either because of a tendon mass,[9,25,93] a partial laceration,[77] or an anomalous muscle belly.[19]

2. *Trauma:* Partial lacerations to the tendon sheath can cause triggering by either the healing tendon mass or a tendon flap getting caught in the flexor sheath.[3,58,77,103] This is more common in the open injury, although it may be seen in the closed setting as well.[112] Injuries to the extensor mechanism can also cause a snapping phenomenon.[39] Presence of fractures near the flexor sheath can impinge on the smooth gliding of the tendons and mimic flexor tendinitis.[56]

3. *Infection:* Granulomatous diseases such as tuberculosis, atypical mycobacterial infections, fungal infections, and parasitic infections can cause inflammation of the flexor sheath and mimic tendinitis.* This is also occasionally seen with suppurative tenosynovitis in the early stages of infection with organisms such as *Neisseria gonococci*.[87]

4. *Metabolic diseases:* Hyperglycemia in diabetes can lead to abnormal collagen[13] and palmar fascial thickening.[21] Hypercholesterolemia can result in tendon xanthomas from deposition of abnormal tissue.[51] Gouty tophus can be juxtaarticular and surround the flexor sheath.[78] The deposition of calcium pyrophosphate in pseudogout[66] or calcium oxalate in renal failure[97] can also impinge on the flexor sheath.

5. *Arthritis:* Rheumatoid arthritis should always be excluded when contemplating a diagnosis of trigger finger. In rheumatoid arthritis, multiple fingers are typically involved and there is the potential for tendon rupture. The surgical correction in this situation calls for preservation of the A1 pulley and excision of the diseased synovium. Other rare forms of arthritis, such as hemochromatosis,[32] chondrocalcinosis,[59] and Thiemann's disease,[98] may also involve the tenosynovium and result in a similar clinical picture.

6. *Neoplasia:* Masses within the flexor tendons or their sheaths can interfere with normal gliding function. Intratendinous fibromas,[49] giant cell tumors,[93] flexor-tendon xanthomas,[51] and lipomas[9] may all involve the flexor tendons. Additionally, tumors of the cartilage[108] or bone can impinge of the sheath and cause symptoms.

TREATMENT

Treatment for trigger finger ranges from conservative therapy to surgery. The usual course of treatment starts by using nonoperative modalities, reserving surgery for those patients in which nonoperative treatment has been unsuccessful. One exception is patients with a chronically affected finger that has an obvious flexion contracture and joint involvement. Conservative measures cannot be successful in these cases and only seem to prolong the pathologic state. Surgical correction is required.

Nonoperative Treatment

Conservative management of trigger fingers should be the initial mode of therapy in all patients except those with a neglected finger who present with a fixed PIP-joint flexion contracture. Splinting, avoidance of repetitive activity, rest, and oral antiinflammatory medication can improve the mild or early cases, with up to a 52% rate of symptom relief.[37,115]

---

*References 6, 17, 22, 34, 61, 95, 107.

The major nonsurgical adjunct treatment for trigger finger is the use of local steroid injections. A single injection within the sheath gives relief of triggering in an average of 49% of cases (range 25% to 73%).* Multiple injections increase the average number to 74% (range 41% to 88%).† Patients with diabetes or rheumatoid disease are less likely to respond to nonoperative treatment. The success rate of steroid injections decreases when secondary cases of trigger finger are included.[62] When more than one injection is required to relieve symptoms, the injections should be spaced at least 3 to 4 weeks apart.[102] Several authors caution not to exceed two or three injections because this can increase the incidence of possible complications associated with local steroid injections, especially tendon rupture.[14]

Several different combinations of steroid preparations have been described. Three milliliters of 1% plain lidocaine and 1 ml of Celestone (6 mg)[102] or 0.5 ml 1% plain lidocaine and 0.5 ml of Kenalog-40[39] can be used with equal success. The critical step is the accurate injection of medication into the synovial space of the tendon sheath and not into the tendon itself.[12] Three injection sites are commonly used to gain access to the flexor-tendon sheath. The region of the A1 pulley at the distal palmar crease,[89] the proximal finger flexion crease at the base of the finger,[79] or the mid-axial line over the proximal phalanx[11] have all been described. Various injection techniques have also been described. A ⅝-inch 25-gauge needle is passed through both tendons down to bone when injecting at the distal palmar crease or the proximal finger crease and is then gently withdrawn. The position of the needle within the tendon substance can be confirmed by passive motion of the finger while watching the movement of the needle. The needle is then slowly withdrawn, with simultaneous gentle pressure on the plunger. As the needle comes out of the tendon into the tendon sheath, there is a noticeable drop in resistance and injection can proceed without difficulty.[102] Visible and palpable filling of the tendon sheath should be noted as the fluid is being injected. The fingertip pulp may blanch temporarily secondary to the increased fluid in the sheath.[39] Complications are rare, especially if the number of injections is limited to two.

Operative Treatment

The gold standard for treatment of trigger finger is surgical release of the A1 pulley. This procedure can be performed under local anesthesia or intravenous regional anesthesia under tourniquet control. Either a longitudinal[106] or a transverse skin incision[46] at the distal palmar crease gives access to the proximal annular pulley. Anatomic studies show that the proximal edge of the A1 pulley corresponds to the distal palmar crease in the ring and small fingers, the proximal crease in the index finger, and halfway between the two creases in the middle finger.[46] The MCP flexion crease in the thumb corresponds to the pulley location (Figure 114-2).[71] A short transverse incision over these locations, followed by blunt

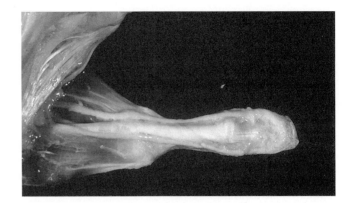

Figure 114-2. The thumb, dissected to demonstrate the FPL tendon passing through the A1, oblique, and A2 pulleys. (From Johnson MK, Cohen MJ: *Hand atlas,* Springfield, Ill, 1975, Charles C.Thomas. Courtesy of Myles J. Cohen and Moulton K. Johnson.)

longitudinal dissection, exposes the flexor sheaths. Loupe magnification and a bloodless field are essential to prevent injury to the adjacent neurovascular bundles. The neurovascular bundles are retracted with right-angled retractors, and the pulley is incised from proximal to distal with a #15 or a #11 blade. The pulley incision is stopped just proximal to the base of the finger flexion crease, which corresponds to the distal edge of the A1 pulley. Care is taken not to cut the A2 pulley, because this can cause tendon bowstringing and a loss of finger flexion. The patient then actively flexes and extends the digit to confirm that triggering has been relieved. The tourniquet is released, hemostasis is achieved, and the skin incision is closed with interrupted sutures. A small dressing that does not limit finger movement is applied, and the patient is instructed to start early hand movement. The two digital nerves of the thumb, especially the radial digital nerve, are at greater risk for injury because of their superficial location. Therefore while making an incision for trigger-thumb release, care must be taken not to carry the initial incision too deeply. Alternatively, a radially based V-shaped flap, like that made for a Brunner zigzag incision, can be used for access.[15]

Trigger fingers associated with rheumatoid arthritis should not be treated by release of the pulley. These patients should be treated with a more generous exposure, usually through a Brunner-type incision, and a more comprehensive flexor tenosynovectomy with preservation of as much of the pulley system as possible is indicated.[76]

PERCUTANEOUS TRIGGER-FINGER RELEASE. Trigger-finger release can be performed through a percutaneous approach by an experienced hand surgeon in appropriate patients. Scissors, arthromeniscotomes, or curved blades have been used through a small transverse incision,[46] or percutaneous release using a 19- or 21-gauge needle have been described.[33] The presence of a thickened annulus and digital locking is helpful because it can confirm release once the pulley is cut. This technique should not be used in patients with diabetes, rheumatoid arthritis, or excessive subcutaneous tissue.[46]

---

*References 5, 11, 18, 40, 55, 63, 85, 92.
†References 5, 11, 18, 40, 45, 48, 63, 85, 89, 92.

REDUCTION TENOPLASTY.   Occasionally there may be a bulbous enlargement of the flexor tendon distal to the A1 pulley. It is imperative that the A2 pulley be preserved, and therefore a reduction tenoplasty can be performed to narrow the involved tendon.[104] The flexor-tendon sheath is exposed through a mid-axial incision at the level of the PIP joint. The flexor sheath is incised at the cruciate ligament, and the bulbous tendon is exposed. A lateral incision is made on the tendon, the superficial fibers are retracted, and a central core of tendon material is excised to restore tendon contour sufficient to allow gliding under the annular pulleys.[46] The tenotomy is closed, and active range of digital motion is tested to ensure unrestrained digital motion. Active motion is instituted immediately after surgery.

COMPLICATIONS

The three well-documented complications of trigger-finger release are digital nerve injury,[15] bowstringing secondary to A2 pulley release,[53] and inadequate release. The radial digital nerve of the thumb is the most frequently injured nerve because of its superficial location. Complications are relatively uncommon and easy to avoid. Inadequate release can result in persistent symptoms. Testing of the release during surgery by having the patient actively flex and extend the digit can prevent this complication. Stiffness, especially in older patients, can occur if postoperative therapy is inadequate. Longitudinal tendon lacerations can occur with percutaneous release, which can create a tendon flap that catches distally and causes recurrent symptoms.[39]

DE QUERVAIN'S DISEASE

In 1895 De Quervain first described the entity of stenosing tenosynovitis of the first dorsal compartment involving the tendons of the extensor pollicis brevis (EPB) and the APL.[24] This condition was further elucidated by Finkelstein in 1930.[41] Patients with de Quervain's disease are usually middle-aged females with a history of repetitive stress or chronic sustained trauma to the area. The main complaint is radial-sided wrist pain, aggravated by wrist flexion and ulnar deviation.[46]

ANATOMY

The dorsal wrist contains six separate compartments under the extensor retinaculum. The first dorsal compartment is the one most radial, located over the radial styloid, and contains the APL and EPB tendons. These tendons pass through an unyielding osteoligamentous canal about 1 cm long that is formed by a groove in the radial styloid and the overlying

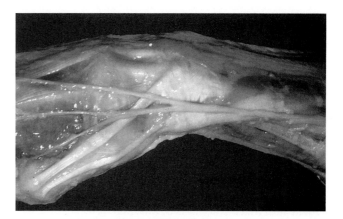

Figure 114-3.   Radial snuffbox demonstrating the retinaculum of the first dorsal compartment housing the APL and EPL tendons in relation to the radial styloid and superficial radial nerve. (From Johnson MK, Cohen MJ: *Hand atlas,* Springfield, Ill, 1975, Charles C. Thomas. Courtesy of Myles J. Cohen and Moulton K. Johnson.)

dorsal ligament. The classic anatomic description is a single compartment with one EPB and one APL tendon, but this is seen in less than 20% of the cases.[57,109] There are multiple variations in the first dorsal compartment tendon arrangement and failure to recognize this at surgery can result in recurrent symptoms caused by an inadequate compartment release.[7,8,72,100] The first compartment in 20% to 30% of the cases is subdivided into an ulnar compartment containing the EPB and a radial compartment containing one or more slips of the APL.[46] The APL is larger than the EPB and can have two or three slips with variable insertions into the base of the first metacarpal, trapezium, volar carpal ligament, opponens pollicis, or abductor pollicis brevis (APB). Any or all of these tendinous slips can be stenotic.[7]

The other important anatomic consideration is the location of the radial artery and nerve in relation to the first dorsal compartment. The radial artery passes diagonally across the anatomic snuffbox from the volar aspect of the wrist to the dorsum of the first web space, deep to the APL and EPB tendons. There is usually enough areolar tissue between the first compartment and the artery that it need not be exposed during surgery.[46] The radial sensory nerve, however, can be a problem. Two or three terminal branches of the radial sensory nerve lie immediately superficial to the first dorsal compartment and must be identified and preserved because they can form painful neuromas if they are cut (Figure 114-3).[1,94]

ETIOLOGY AND PATHOLOGY

The first dorsal compartment, like the flexor-tendon sheath and pulley system, is also a pulley system. It changes the direction of tendon pull and prevents displacement of the tendons. Any stimulus that causes hypertrophy of the tenosynovium can restrict the smooth gliding of the tendons. This in turn can cause inflammation of the tenosynovium underneath the ligament and start a cycle of edema, adhesions, and fibrosis, which leads to increased pain and decreased thumb mobility. As with trigger finger, the primary pathology of de Quervain's disease is probably in the tenosynovium, with the dorsal carpal ligament becoming secondarily thickened. This in turn causes a volume disturbance within the compartment, which produces the symptoms of the stenosing tenosynovitis.[74]

PATIENT HISTORY

The history is usually that of a middle-aged female with slow, progressive pain and occasionally swelling over the radial styloid area, which is aggravated by thumb movements. There is usually a history of chronic overuse of the hand and wrist, especially activity requiring repetitive thumb movements. Patients with severe cases can also show signs of numbness over the radial sensory nerve distribution, crepitus, and/or snapping sensation over the first dorsal compartment.[102]

PHYSICAL EXAMINATION

Pain, tenderness, and swelling over the first dorsal compartment, corresponding to the radial styloid area, are common. The pain can be exaggerated by simultaneous flexion of the thumb and ulnar deviation of the wrist. This maneuver forms the basis of the Finkelstein test,[41] which is pathognomonic for de Quervain's disease. The test is performed by asking the patient to flex his or her thumb into the palm, then ulnarly deviate the wrist, which will elicit pain in affected individuals over the radial styloid region. Another way to perform this test is to grasp the patient's thumb within the palm and ulnarly deviate the wrist to elicit the pain.[35] Alternately flexing and extending the wrist in the "Finklestein position"—with relief of pain on extension of the wrist and exacerbation with flexion—also confirms the diagnosis.[100] Overaggressive performance of the test can result in a false positive result because extreme ulnar deviation can cause pain even in the normal wrist. The extent to which ulnar deviation causes pain should always be compared with the contralateral, unaffected side whenever possible.[70]

Crepitus or a snapping sensation can be felt in later stages during movement of the tendons within the compartment; this is the so-called *wet leather sign*.[53] Entrapment of the radial nerve sensory branches in secondary adhesions and fibrosis can result in numbness and paresthesias along the nerve distribution.[94]

DIFFERENTIAL DIAGNOSIS

Other causes of radial-sided wrist pain must be considered and excluded whenever the diagnosis of de Quervain's disease is considered. Differential diagnoses include the following:

1. *Basal-joint arthritis:* Both de Quervain's disease and arthritis of the thumb carpometacarpal (CMC) joint are typically seen in middle-aged women who have pain in the base of the thumb. Infrequently, patients may have both conditions. Plain radiographs, including stress views and a Roberts view, show degenerative changes around the trapezium and can help diagnose basal-joint arthritis. Basilar arthritis is characterized by a positive "grind test," in which longitudinal compression and rotation of the thumb CMC joint produces a feeling of crepitus to the examiner's touch, and the patient experiences pain. The pain with basal-joint arthritis is also located more distally around the metacarpal base than with de Quervain's disease.[75,100,102]

2. *Intersection syndrome:* Intersection syndrome is typically characterized by pain approximately 4 cm proximal to the wrist joint and is associated with pain and swelling where the muscle bellies of the APL and EPB cross the two radial wrist extensors.[102] Crepitus may be noted with flexion or extension of the wrist. The basic pathology is a tenosynovitis of the second dorsal compartment and will be discussed in more detail later in the chapter.[50]

3. *Wartenberg's syndrome:* Wartenberg's syndrome is an entrapment neuropathy of the radial sensory nerve at the junction of the brachioradialis and extensor carpi radialis longus (ECRL). Both Wartenberg's syndrome and de Quervain's disease can cause pain in the dorsoradial wrist that is aggravated by ulnar deviation, and both can produce a positive Finkelstein's test. However, in Wartenberg's syndrome the area of maximal tenderness is located more proximally at the junction of the brachioradialis and the ECRL and is usually associated with a positive Tinel's sign.[23,101] Other conditions that can cause compression of the superficial radial nerve, such as, ganglia, tumors, or neuromas, should be considered.

4. *Miscellaneous conditions:* Carpal injuries (e.g., scapholunate dissociation or occult scaphoid fractures or nonunions), osteoporosis, periosteal reaction, and arthritic changes of the radial styloid can usually be detected by history and with plain radiographs. A careful history and physical examination and appropriate studies will usually be sufficient to establish the correct diagnosis.[100]

TREATMENT

Conservative, nonoperative treatment can be tried initially but the response rate is not as high as in patients with trigger finger. Some authors therefore advocate early surgical release to shorten the period of morbidity and prevent recurrence.[72,117]

Nonoperative Treatment

Conservative treatment consists of rest, splinting, oral nonsteroidal antiinflammatory agents, and the use of local steroid injections. A splint that immobilizes the wrist in neutral and the thumb base in extension while leaving the rest of the fingers free can give good symptomatic relief. The local steroid injection fluid is instilled into the first dorsal compartment. The compartment is entered proximally near the point of maximal tenderness, confirming the location of the needle tip in the compartment and being careful to avoid an intratendinous insertion. A bulging of the synovium distal to the first compartment is observed when a proper injection technique is utilized. A lag time of 1 to 2 weeks may be present, depending on the steroid preparation used, before relief of symptoms is noted. As with trigger finger, it is recommended that no more than two or three injections be given and that there be at least 3 to 4 weeks between injections.[39]

Several complications have been reported after steroid injection. The most dangerous is a hypersensitivity reaction that can develop after multiple injections. Suppression of the pituitary–adrenal axis can also occur with systemic slipover, especially when multiple sites are injected or if injections are not spaced far enough apart.[81] Multiple steroid injections have other complications as well. The risk of tendon rupture increases with the number of injections, especially after inadvertent intratendinous injection. Skin and subcutaneous fat atrophy, and skin depigmentation can also be seen.[65] Diabetic or immunocompromised patients are at increased risk of developing an infection around the injection site. Intraneural injection can give rise to painful neuritis or paresthesias.[88]

Patients may remain symptomatic after steroid injections. This is often secondary to a failure to infiltrate all of the subcompartments within the first dorsal compartment, which frequently subdivide into subcompartments containing the EPB and one or more slips of the APL. If any of these separate subcompartments is missed with the injection, the patient may have persistent symptoms. One may then consider a repeat injection to try to infiltrate all of the compartments or consider surgical release as the definitive treatment.[67,100]

Operative Treatment

The definitive treatment of de Quervain's disease is surgical release of the first dorsal compartment. This procedure can be performed under a local anesthesia or using intravenous regional anesthesia. A tourniquet is routinely used to facilitate a bloodless operative field. A 2-cm transverse incision is made about 0.5 cm proximal to the tip of the radial styloid, overlying the first dorsal compartment. This gives good exposure to the first compartment and usually produces a favorable scar.[46] Longitudinal incisions do provide a wider exposure but can cause problems with hypertrophic and painful scars.[100] One to three terminal branches of the radial sensory nerve must be identified as they cross the compartment and are then gently retracted. These branches are superficial and can be cut if the initial skin incision is too deep. The first dorsal compartment is identified using blunt longitudinal dissection. There are several methods for releasing the dorsal carpal ligament. One can simply incise the sheath[46,117] or excise the roof of the canal[68] for a more complete release. A third approach is to leave a radially based flap of retinaculum attached to the radius, open the dorsal ligament over the EPB, and release all intercompartmental septa.[12] This helps prevent subluxation of the EPB and APL tendons during wrist flexion.[1] A portion of the retinaculum may have to be excised to facilitate release in long-standing cases with peritendinous fibrosis and ligament hypertrophy. Every attempt should be made to ensure that the EPB and all slips of the APL are released. This can be done

intraoperatively by confirming the excursion of each tendon separately. A tenosynovectomy is performed if the synovium covering the tendons is thick and opaque, which is commonly the case in patients with rheumatoid arthritis. Once the decompression is completed, the tourniquet is released, hemostasis is achieved, and the skin incision is closed. The wrist is splinted in 30 degrees of extension for 2 to 3 weeks, and the thumb and fingers are left free for active range of motion.[46]

COMPLICATIONS

The most serious complication after release of the first dorsal compartment is injury to branches of the superficial radial nerve, resulting in painful neuroma formation.[1,8,72] Aggressive traction can also cause the formation of a neuroma in continuity. A bloodless field and loupe magnification, as well as caution while making the initial skin incision and during retraction of the skin edges all help to avoid this painful complication. Volar subluxation of the tendons may occur after extensive excision of the dorsal retinaculum. This can be avoided by limiting the dorsal excision and by placing the sheath incision more dorsally. When subluxation is present, it can cause a painful snapping of the thumb tendons over the radial styloid during wrist flexion and may necessitate reconstruction of the pulley system.[100]

Another common complication is recurrent symptoms secondary to an incomplete release. Subcompartmentalization of the first dorsal compartment, as mentioned earlier, is the rule rather then the exception. This must be kept in mind because a separate, inadequately released EPB compartment can result in persistent symptoms. The excursion of each tendon should be tested individually at surgery; if only APL function is noted, a further search for the EPB tendon should be undertaken. If the patient has persistent symptoms after a first dorsal compartment release, a useful clinical test is to hold the thumb metacarpal in maximal abduction and then flex the MCP joint. This position eliminates pull on the APL and one can specifically test for tenderness with movement of the EPB. If pain occurs with this movement, then most likely there is a separate unreleased EPB compartment.[72]

INTERSECTION SYNDROME

Intersection syndrome was first described in 1841 by Velpeau and is characterized by pain and swelling in the area of the muscle bellies of the APL and EPB where they cross the two radial wrist extensors.[28] In more severe cases, crepitus can be felt at this area, which is usually about 4 cm proximal to the wrist joint. The etiology was initially thought to be the result of friction between the muscle bellies of the APL and EPB with the radial wrist extensors.[10,28,116] In 1985 Grundberg and Reagan[50] showed the basic pathology to be a tenosynovitis of the second dorsal compartment. It is interesting to note that the pain and/or swelling is not seen over the second dorsal compartment, but more proximally. The tenosynovitis, however, is evident intraoperatively after incising the retinacular sheath.[102] This syndrome is frequently associated with repetitive wrist activity. As with other forms of stenosing tenosynovitis, work modification, splinting, nonsteroidal antiinflammatory agents, and local steroid injections into the second dorsal compartment produce good results with the majority of patients remaining permanently asymptomatic. Patients who experience persistent pain are treated surgically with a longitudinal incision over the radial wrist extensors and release of the second dorsal compartment. The wrist should be placed in a splint in slight extension for at least 10 days, after which movement is allowed as tolerated.[50] Most patients with intersection syndrome can be treated successfully provided an accurate diagnosis is made.

EXTENSOR POLLICIS LONGUS TENOSYNOVITIS

Tenosynovitis has been described involving all the dorsal compartments in one form or another. Tenosynovitis of the EPL tendon occurs rarely and is usually associated with rheumatoid arthritis, an old Colles' fracture, or, rarely, from overuse. It usually presents as pain and swelling just distal to Lister's tubercle, where the tendon changes direction. Once the diagnosis is made, early surgical release is advocated because this tendon is prone to rupture if left untreated, especially in patients with rheumatoid arthritis. A transverse skin incision (centered over Lister's tubercle) is made, and the EPL tendon is identified proximal to the tunnel, which is opened distally along its entire length. The tendon is then lifted out of the groove and transposed radially into a subcutaneous pocket. The tunnel is then closed to prevent later relocation of the tendon back into the groove.[46]

FLEXOR CARPI RADIALIS TENDINITIS

Tenosynovitis of the FCR tendon is a distinct clinical entity that is not widely appreciated. The patients usually complain of pain and tenderness over the FCR tendon just proximal to the scaphoid tubercle and trapezoid crest.[113] There is usually aggravation of pain with resisted flexion or radial deviation of the wrist. Occupations requiring sustained resistance against wrist flexion and certain sports (e.g., tennis or racquetball) can predispose to this condition.[2] Rest, nonsteroidal antiinflammatory agents, splinting, and corticosteroid injections at the point of maximal tenderness usually resolve the symptoms in most cases. Surgical release is done by opening the fibroosseous

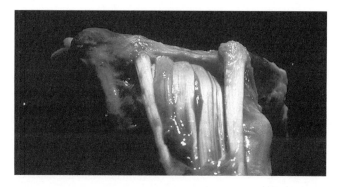

Figure 114-4. End-on view of the FCU (left) and the FCR (right) as they enter a fibroosseous canal at their insertion. (From Johnson MK, Cohen MJ: *Hand atlas,* Springfield, Ill, 1975, Charles C. Thomas. Courtesy of Myles J. Cohen and Moulton K. Johnson.)

FCR tunnel, which starts about 3 cm proximal to the wrist and ends at the insertion of the FCR. The roof of the tunnel can be incised through a transverse incision over the FCR at the wrist. Care should be taken not to injure the palmar cutaneous branch of the median nerve (Figure 114-4).[46]

OTHER FORMS OF EXTENSOR AND FLEXOR TENOSYNOVITIS

Other forms of tenosynovitis can involve the extensor carpi ulnaris (ECU),[26,52] extensor indicis proprius (EIP),[105] EDM,[54] and the FCU. Tendinitis of the FCU is similar to its counterpart on the radial side, with pain localized over the pisiform bone, especially during resisted ulnar wrist flexion.[102] All of these conditions respond to some degree to the regimen of rest, splinting, nonsteroidal antiinflammatory agents, and local steroid injections. Failure of nonoperative treatment can usually be managed by surgical release of the involved tendon.

SUPPURATIVE TENOSYNOVITIS

Infection of the tenosynovium is usually caused by penetrating injury, especially over the volar joint creases where the skin and flexor-tendon sheath are in close approximation.[83] It can also occur secondarily by extension of infection from felons, collar-button abscesses, or palmar-space infections, as well as from hematogenous seeding of a systemic infection (see Chapter 115). The flexor sheath in the index, middle, and ring fingers starts at the mid-palmar crease and ends just proximal to the DIP joint. The flexor sheaths of the small finger and thumb continue proximally into the forearm as the ulnar and radial bursa, respectively.

Flexor tenosynovitis is most commonly seen in the index, middle, or ring fingers.[83] Kanavel[60] described four cardinal signs of suppurative tenosynovitis that still remain important diagnostic aids: (1) the involved finger is held in a flexed position, (2) there is uniform swelling of the digit with (3) tenderness along the entire length of the involved tendon sheath, and (4) there is extreme pain on attempted extension of the digit. Not all four signs may be present initially. Pain on passive extension is the most reliable finding. An early infection without all four classic signs can be treated with elevation, splinting, and parenteral antibiotics. If the patient fails to improve after 24 hours of medical treatment, surgical decompression of the tendon sheath is warranted. Aspiration of the tendon sheath may give useful information if the diagnosis is in doubt, but there should be a low threshold for exploration if results are equivocal.[84]

Established pyogenic tenosynovitis is a surgical emergency and requires prompt drainage of the involved tendon sheath. Delays in treatment can result in tendon necrosis and even skin loss. Two basic approaches are available: open drainage and a closed tendon-sheath irrigation. If the tendon is necrotic, open drainage facilitates resection of the involved tendon. The entire tendon sheath is opened through mid-axial and palmar incisions, the involved tendon is debrided, and the wounds are left open to drain and heal secondarily. Delayed tendon reconstruction is carried out once the infection has subsided. Rehabilitation is prolonged and usually results in a permanently stiff finger.[36,42,43]

Closed tendon irrigation, introduced by Carter et al[16] in 1966 is most commonly used for established suppurative tenosynovitis without tendon necrosis. The technique involves a proximal palmar incision into the tendon sheath just proximal to the A1 pulley and a distal mid-axial or transverse incision at the distal edge of the A4 pulley. A 16- or 18-gauge irrigating catheter is placed distally, a small drain is placed proximally, and the wounds are closed.[84] Alternatively, an opening can be made in all the digital flexion creases to facilitate better irrigation and drainage. The hand is immobilized in a bulky dressing and elevated. The tendon sheath is then irrigated with an isotonic saline or antibiotic solution, either as a continuous drip or intermittent flush every 2 hours. Irrigation is continued for 48 to 72 hours, followed by gentle active and passive range of motion exercises after removal of the catheters and drains.[82,84,91] This technique facilitates quicker wound healing and earlier rehabilitation than the open drainage technique. This method cannot cure an already necrotic tendon, and considerable experience is required before deciding to use this closed method rather than opening and inspecting the sheath and tendon.

REFERENCES

1. Alegado RB, Meals RA: An unusual complication following surgical treatment of de Quervain's disease, *J Hand Surg* 4:185, 1979.
2. Allieu Y: The sportsman's hand. In Tubiana R: *The hand,* vol III, Philadelphia, 1988, WB Saunders.
3. Al-Qattan MM, Posnick JC, Lin KY: Triggering after partial tendon laceration, *J Hand Surg* 18B:241, 1993.
4. Amadio PC, Jaeger SH, Hunter JM: Nutritional aspects of tendon healing. In Hunter JM: *Rehabilitation of the hand,* ed 3, St. Louis, 1990, Mosby.
5. Anderson B, Kaye S: Treatment of flexor tenosynovitis of the hand ("trigger finger") with corticosteroids: a prospective study of response to local injection, *Arch Intern Med* 151:153, 1991.
6. Anderson GA, Chandi SM: Cysticercosis of the flexor digitorum profundus muscle producing flexion deformity of the fingers, *J Hand Surg* 18B:360, 1993.
7. Arons MS: De Quervain's release in working women: a report of failures, complications, and associated diagnosis, *J Hand Surg* 12A:540, 1987.
8. Belsole RJ: De Quervain's tenosynovitis: diagnostic and operative complications, *Orthopedics* 4:899, 1981.
9. Brand MG, Gelberman RH: Lipoma of the flexor digitorum superficialis causing triggering at the carpal canal and median nerve compression, *J Hand Surg* 13A:354, 1988.
10. Brooker AF Jr: Extensor carpi radialis tenosynovitis: an occupational affliction, *Orthop Rev* 6(5):99, 1977.
11. Buch-Jaeger N, Foucher G, Ehrler S, Sammut D: The results of conservative management of trigger finger: a series of 169 patients, *Ann Hand Surg* 11:189, 1992.
12. Burton RI, Littler JW: Soft tissue afflictions of the hand, *Curr Probl Surg* 12:16, 1975.
13. Cambell RR, Hawkins SJ, Maddison PJ, Reckless JPD: Limited joint mobility in diabetes mellitus, *Ann Rheum Dis* 44:93, 1985.
14. Carlson CS, Curtis RM: Steroid injection for flexor tenosynovitis, *J Hand Surg,* 9A:286, 1984.
15. Carozella J, Stern P, VonKuster LC: Transection of the radial digital nerve of the thumb during trigger release, *J Hand Surg* 14A:198, 1989.
16. Carter SJ, Burman SO, Mersheimer WL: Treatment of digital tenosynovitis by irrigation with peroxide and oxytetracycline, *Ann Surg* 163:645, 1966.
17. Chow SP, Stroebel AB, Lau JHK, Collins RJ: Mycobacterium marinum infection in the hand involving deep structures, *J Hand Surg* 8:568, 1983.
18. Clark DD, Ricker JH, MacCollum M: The efficacy of local steroid injection in the treatment of stenosing tenovaginitis, *Plast Reconstr Surg* 51:179, 1973.
19. Coenen L, Biltjes I: Pseudotumor of the palm due to anomalous flexor digitorum superficialis muscle belly, *J Hand Surg* 16A:1046, 1991.
20. Conklin JE, White WL: Stenosing tenosynovitis and its possible relation to the carpal tunnel syndrome, *Surg Clin North Am* 40:531-540, 1960.
21. Cronin ME: Metabolic bone and joint disease. In McCarty DJ, Koopman WJ: *Arthritis and allied conditions,* ed 12, Philadelphia, 1993, Lea and Febiger.
22. DeHaven KE, Wilde AH, O'Duffy JD: Sporotrichosis arthritis and tenosynovitis, *J Bone Joint Surg* 54A:874, 1972.
23. Dellon AL, MacKinnon SE: Radial sensory nerve entrapment in the forearm, *J Hand Surg* 11A:195, 1986.

2028 PART VI TENOSYNOVITIS AND INFECTIONS

24. De Quervain F: Ueber eine Form von chronischer tendovaginitis, *Correspondenz-Blatt F Schweizer Aerzte (Basel)*, 25:389, 1895.

25. Desai SS, Pearlman HS, Patel MR: Clicking at the wrist due to a friboma in an anomalous lumbrical muscle: a case report and review of the literature, *J Hand Surg* 11A:512, 1986.

26. Dickson DD, Luckey C: Tenosynovitis of the extensor carpi ulnaris tendon sheath, *J Bone Joint Surg* 30A:903, 1948.

27. Dinham JM, Meggitt BF: Trigger thumbs in children: a review of the natural history and indications for treatment in 105 patients, *J Bone Joint Surg* 56B:153-155, 1974.

28. Dobyns JH, Sim FH, Linscheid RL: Sports stress syndromes of the hand and wrist, *Am J Sports Med* 6:236, 1978.

29. Doyle JR: Anatomy of the finger flexor sheath and pulley system, *J Hand Surg* 13A:473, 1988.

30. Doyle JR, Blythe W: *The finger flexor tendon sheath and pulleys: anatomy and reconstruction,* AAOS symposium on tendon surgery in the hand, St. Louis, 1975, Mosby, p 81.

31. Doyle JR, Blythe WF: Anatomy of the flexor tendon sheath and pulleys of the thumb, *J Hand Surg* 2:149-151, 1977.

32. Duffy J: Arthritis and liver disease. In McCarthy DJ, Koopman WJ: *Arthritis and allied conditions,* ed 12, Philadelphia, 1993, Lea and Febiger.

33. Eastwood DM, Gupta MB, Johnson DP: Percutaneous release of the trigger finger: an office procedure, *J Hand Surg* 17A:114, 1992.

34. Ebelin M, Mariette X, Quillard J, et al: Tenosynovite d'aspect tuberculoide de la main, *Ann Chir Main* 10:151, 1991.

35. Elliott BG: Finkelstein's test: a descriptive error that can produce a false positive, *J Hand Surg* 17B:481, 1992.

36. Entin MA: Infections of the hand, *Surg Clin North Am* 44:981, 1964.

37. Evans RB, Hunter JM, Burkhalter WB: Conservative management of trigger finger: a new approach, *J Hand Ther* 13:59, 1988.

38. Fahey JJ, Bollinger JA: Trigger finger in adults and children, *J Bone Joint Surg,* 36A:1200, 1954.

39. Failla JM: Differential diagnosis of hand pain: tendinitis, ganglia and other syndromes. In Peimer CA: *Surgery of the hand and upper extremity,* New York, 1996, McGraw-Hill.

40. Fauno P, Anderson HS, Simonsen O: A long term follow-up of the effect of repeated corticosteroid injections for stenosing tenovaginitis, *J Hand Surg* 14B:242, 1989.

41. Finkelstein H: Stenosing tendovaginitis at the radial styloid process, *J Bone Joint Surg* 12:509-540, 1930.

42. Flynn JE: Modern considerations of major hand infections, *N Engl J Med* 252:605, 1955.

43. Flynn JE: The grave infections. In Flynn JE: *Hand surgery,* Baltimore, 1966, Williams & Wilkins.

44. Freiberg A, Mulholland RS, Levine R: Nonoperative treatment of trigger fingers and thumbs, *J Hand Surg* 14A:533-558, 1989.

45. Freiberg A, Mulholland RS, Levine R: Nonoperative treatment of trigger fingers and thumbs, *J Hand Surg* 14A:553, 1989.

46. Froimson A: Tenosynovitis and tennis elbow. In Green DP: *Operative hand surgery,* ed 3, New York, 1992, Churchill Livingstone.

47. Gould JS, Wissinger HA: Carpal tunnel syndrome in pregnancy, *South Med J* 71:144, 1978.

48. Gray RG, Keim IM, Gottlieb NL: Intratendon sheath corticosteroid treatment of rheumatoid arthritis-associated and idiopathic hand flexor tenosynovitis, *Arch Rheumatol* 21:92, 1978.

49. Grenga TE: Intratendinous fibroma of flexor tendon, *J Hand Surg* 15A:92, 1990.

50. Grundberg AB, Reagan DS: Pathologic anatomy of the forearm: intersection syndrome, *J Hand Surg* 11A:519, 1986.

51. Gunther SF, Gunther AG, Hoeg JM, Kruth HS: Multiple flexor tendon xanthomas and contractures in the hands of a child and familial hypercholesterolemia, *J Hand Surg* 11A:588, 1986.

52. Hajj AA, Wood MB: Stenosing tenosynovitis of the extensor carpi ulnaris, *J Hand Surg,* 11A:519, 1986.

53. Heithoff SJ, Millender LH, Helman J: Bowstringing as a complication of trigger finger release, *J Hand Surg* 13A:567, 1988.

54. Hooper G, McMaster MJ: Stenosing tenovaginitis affecting the tendon of the extensor digiti minimi at the wrist, *Hand* 11:299, 1979.

55. Howard LD, Pratt DR, Bunnell S: The use of compound F (hydrocortone) in operative and nonoperative conditions of the hand, *J Bone Joint Surg* 35A:994, 1953.

56. Inada Y, Tamai S, Kawanishi K, Fukui A: Fifth digit sesamoid fracture with tenosynovitis, *J Hand Surg* 17A:915, 1992.

57. Jackson WT, Veigas SF, Coon TM, et al: Anatomical variations in the first extensor compartment of the wrist: a clinical and anatomical study, *J Bone Joint Surg* 68A:923, 1986.

58. Janecki CJ: Triggering of the finger caused by flexor tendon laceration: report of two cases, *J Bone Joint Surg* 58A:1174, 1976.

59. Jensen PS: Hemochromatosis: a disease often silent but not invisible, *AJR* 126:343, 1976.

60. Kanavel AB: *Infections of the hand: a guide to the surgical treatment of acute and chronic suppurative processes in the fingers, hand, and forearm,* ed 7, Philadelphia, 1943, Lea & Febiger.

61. Kelly PJ, Weed LA, Lipscomb PR: Infections of the tendon sheaths, bursae, joints, and soft tissues by acid fast bacilli other than tubercle bacilli, *J Bone Joint Surg* 45A:327, 1963.

62. Kolind-Sorensen V: Treatment of trigger fingers, *Acta Orthop Scand* 41:428, 1970.

63. Kraemer BA, Young VL, Arfken C: Stenosing flexor tenosynovitis, *South Med J* 83:806, 1990.

64. Lapidus PW: Stenosing tenovaginitis, *Surg Clin North Am* 33:1317-1347, 1953.

65. Leadbetter WB: Corticosteroid injection therapy in sports injuries. In Leadbetter WB, Buckwalter JA, Gordon SL: *Sports-induced inflammation: clinical and basic science concepts,* Park Ridge, Ill, 1989, American Academy of Orthopedic Surgeons.

66. Leisen JC, Austad ED, Bluhm GB, Sigler JW: The tophus in calcium pyrophosphate deposition disease, *JAMA* 244:1711, 1980.

67. Leslie BM, Ericson WB, Morehead JR: Incidence of a septum within the first dorsal compartment of the wrist, *J Hand Surg* 15A:88, 1990.

68. Lipscomb PR: Stenosing tenosynovitis at the radial styloid process (de Quervain's disease), *Ann Surg* 134:110, 1951.

69. Liscomb PR: Tenosynovitis of the hand and the wrist: carpal tunnel syndrome, de Quervain's disease, trigger digit, *Clin Orthop* 13:164, 1959.

70. Lister G: *The hand: diagnosis and indications,* ed 3, New York, 1993, Churchill Livingstone, p 346.

71. Lorthier J: Surgical treatment of trigger-finger by a subcutaneous method, *J Bone Joint Surg* 40A:793-795, 1958.

72. Louis DS: Incomplete release of the first dorsal compartment: a diagnostic test, *J Hand Surg* 12A:87, 1987.

73. Lundborg G, Myrhage R: The vascularization and structure of the human digital tendon sheath as related to the flexor tendon function, *Scand J Plast Reconstr Surg* 11:195, 1977.

74. Meachim G, Roberts C: The histopathology of stenosing tenovaginitis, *J Pathol* 98:187, 1969.

75. Melone CP Jr, Beaves B, Isani A: The basal joint pain syndrome, *Clin Orthop* 220:58, 1987.

76. Millender LH, Nalebuff EA: Preventive surgery: tenosynovectomy and synovectomy, *Orthop Clin North Am* 6:765, 1975.

77. Minami A, Ogino T: Trigger wrist caused by a partial laceration of the flexor superficialis tendon of the ring finger, *J Hand Surg* 11B:457, 1986.

78. Moore JR, Weiland AJ: Gouty tenosynovitis in the hand, *J Hand Surg* 10A:291, 1985.

79. Murphy D, Failla JM, Koniuch MP: Steroid versus placebo injection for trigger finger, *J Hand Surg* 20A:628, 1995.

80. Nelaton A, Depres A, Jamain A: Tumeurs des doigts, *Elements Pathol Chir* 5:953, 1859.

81. Neustadt DH: Local corticosteroid injection therapy in soft tissue rheumatic conditions of the hand and wrist, *Arthritis Rheum* 34(7):923, 1991.

82. Neviaser RJ: Closed tendon sheath irrigation for pyogenic flexor tenosynovitis, *J Hand Surg* 3:462, 1978.

83. Neviaser RJ: Tenosynovitis, *Hand Clin* 5:525, 1989.

84. Neviaser RJ: Infections. In Green DP: *Operative hand surgery,* ed 3, New York, 1992, Churchill-Livingstone.

85. Newport ML, Lane LB, Stuchin SA: Treatment of trigger finger by steroid injection, *J Hand Surg* 15A:748,1990.

86. Notta A: Recherches sur une affectoin particuliere des gaines tendineuses de la main, characterisee par le developpment d'une nodosite sur le trajet des tendons flechisseurs des doigts et par l'empechement de leurs mouvements, *Arch Gen Med* 4(series 24):142, 1850.

87. Ogiela DM, Peimer CA: Acute gonococcal flexor tenosynovitis: case report and literature review, *J Hand Surg* 6A:470, 1981.

88. Otto N, Wehbe MA: Steroid injections for tenosynovitis in the hand, *Orthop Rev* 15(5):290, 1986.

89. Panayatopoulos E, Fortis AP, Armoni A, et al: Trigger digit: the needle or the knife? *J Hand Surg* 17B:239, 1992.

90. Phalen GS: Stenosing tenosynovitis: trigger fingers and trigger thumb, de Quervain's disease, acute calcification in the wrist and hand. In Flynn JE: *Hand surgery,* Baltimore, 1982, Williams & Wilkins.

91. Pollen AG: Acute infection of the tendon sheaths, *Hand* 6:21, 1974.

92. Quinell RC: Conservative management of trigger finger, *Practitioner* 224:187, 1980.

93. Rankin AE, Reid B: An unusual etiology of trigger finger: a case report, *J Hand Surg* 10A:904, 1985.

94. Rask MR: Superficial radial neuritis and de Quervain's disease: report of three cases, *Clin Orthop* 131:176, 1978.

95. Raturi U, Burkhalter W: Gnathostomiasis externa: a case report, *J Hand Surg* 11A:751, 1986.

96. Rayan GM: Distal stenosing tenosynovitis, *J Hand Surg* 15A:973, 1990.

97. Rosenthal A, Ryan LM, McCarthy DJ: Arthritis associated with calcium oxalate crystals in an anephric patient treated with peritoneal dialysis, *JAMA* 260:1280, 1988.

98. Rubenstein HM: Thiemann's disease: a brief reminder, *Arthritis Rheum* 18:357, 1988.

99. Sampson SP, Badalamente MA, Hurst LJ, Seidman J: Pathobiology of the human A1 pulley in trigger finger, *J Hand Surg* 16A:714, 1991.

100. Sampson SP, Wisch D, Badalamente MA: Complications of conservative and surgical treatment of De Quervain's disease and trigger finger, *Hand Clin* 10(1):73, 1994.

101. Saplys R, MacKinnon SE, Dellon AL: The relationship between nerve entrapment versus neuroma complications and the misdiagnosis of de Quervain's disease, *Cont Orth* 15:51, 1987.

102. Savage RC: Tenosynovial disorders of the hand and wrist. In McCarthy JG, May JW Jr, Littler JW: *Plastic surgery,* vol 7, Philadelphia, 1990, WB Saunders, 1990.

103. Schlenker JD, Lister GD, Kleinert HE: Three complications of untreated partial laceration of the flexor tendon: entrapment, rupture and triggering, *J Hand Surg* 6:392, 1981.

104. Seradge H, Kleinert HE: Reduction flexor tenoplasty: treatment of stenosing flexor tenosynovitis distal to the first pulley, *J Hand Surg* 6:543, 1981.

105. Spinner M, Olshansky K: Extensor indicis proprius syndrome: a clinical test, *Plast Reconstr Surg* 51:134, 1973.

106. Stefanich RJ, Peimer CA: Longitudinal incision for trigger release, *J Hand Surg* 14A:316-317, 1989.

107. Stern PJ, Gula DC: Mycobacterium chelonei tenosynovitis of the hand: a case report, *J Hand Surg* 11A:596, 1986.

108. Stockley I, Norris SH: Trigger finger secondary to soft tissue chondroma, *J Hand Surg* 15B:468, 1990.

109. Strandell G: Variations of the anatomy in stenosing tenosynovitis at the radial styloid process, *Acta Chir Scand* 113:234, 1957.

110. Strauch B, de Moura W: Digital flexor tendon sheath: an anatomic study, *J Hand Surg* 10A:785, 1985.

111. Strickland JW, Idler RS, Creighton JC: De Quervain's stenosing tenosynovitis, *Indiana Med* 83(5):340, 1990.

112. Takami H, Takahashi S, Ando M: Triggering of the finger secondary to partial flexor tendon tear after closed direct injury, *J Hand Surg* 18A:881, 1993.

113. Weeks P: A cause of wrist pain: non-specific tenosynovitis involving the flexor carpi radialis, *Plast Reconstr Surg* 62:263, 1978.

114. Weilby A: Trigger finger, *Acta Orthop Scand* 41:419, 1970.

115. Wolin I: The management of tenosynovitis, *Surg Clin North Am* 37:53, 1957.

116. Wood MB, Linscheid RL: Abductor pollicis longus bursitis, *Clin Orthop* 93:293, 1973.

117. Woods THE: De Quervain's disease: a plea for early operation—a report on 40 cases: *Br J Surg* 51:358, 1954.

CHAPTER 115

Infections

Stephen B. Schnall

He who wants to know man must look upon him as a whole and not a patched up piece of work. If he finds a part of the human body diseased, he must look for the causes which produce disease, and not merely treat the external effects.

Paracelsus, 16th Century

INDICATIONS

Hand and upper-extremity infections are a burden to the patient, the physician, and to society because of the potential for high treatment costs, the need for rehabilitation, and the likelihood of residual functional deficits. Hand infections are common problems that have multifactorial causes.

The principal of early antibiotic administration has been shown to decrease the overall infection rate in open hand fractures,[45,47] which may be as high as 11% in grossly contaminated wounds.[39] Delay in treatment is directly related to a slower resolution of the infection, particularly with infections of pulp spaces, tendon sheaths, and joints.[18] Despite the empiric selection of broad-spectrum antibiotics based on the patient's history,[59] high complication rates continue to occur.[11,56]

Histologically, infections that occur secondary to injuries sustained at home are most often caused by a single gram-positive organism.[33] *Staphylococcus aureus* or *Streptococcus* species are the single organisms that are most likely to cause hand infections.[25,26] However, bacteriologic flora cultured from hand infections between 1960 and 1980 have indicated an increasing number of gram-negative species and a decreasing number of gram-positive organisms.[60] Among their series of 69 patients, Spiegel and Szabo[57] reported that nearly 30% had mixed aerobic and anaerobic infections. Thus physicians treating patients with upper-extremity infections must know the history of each injury, and must have adequate knowledge of anatomy, bacteriology, and antibiotics appropriate to treat these infections.

A complete history and physical examination must be performed to identify any underlying physiologic condition (e.g., diabetes, rheumatic disease, or an immunocompromised status) that may predispose a patient to developing an infection or that may complicate treatment.[16,19,37,40] The final outcome may be dependent on gaining control of underlying metabolic problems. Conditions that may simulate infection include pyoderma gangrenosum, gout, brown recluse spider bites, metastatic lesions, and factitious injuries and must be considered in the evaluation of a patient with an "infection."[29]

Adequate tetanus prophylaxis is necessary in all cases and requires questioning the patient for a history of recent tetanus toxoid inoculation. If a patient was raised in a foreign country, the physician must ascertain whether an initial series of tetanus immunizations was given. If more than 5 years have passed since a patient's last booster immunization, 0.5 ml of tetanus toxoid should be administered. A hyperimmunoglobulin should be administered, along with an initial booster injection of tetanus toxoid, if no initial series of immunizations was given. The series of tetanus toxoid boosters subsequently should be completed.

Surgical drainage must be adequate and surgical debridement must be performed through incisions that allow exposure of all infected areas. Primary wound closure after debridement of upper-extremity infections was reported in the early 1950s by Scott and Jones.[54] The authors stressed that adequate excision, viable skin flaps, and no damage to major blood vessels were essential to performing primary closure. Primary wound closure is no longer advised after debridement, but may be attempted secondarily. Delayed wound closure and/or skin grafting is performed only after the wound shows good granulation tissue and no evidence of continued contamination based on negative wound cultures.[52] For most infections, however, wounds should be allowed to remain open and to heal by secondary intention unless vital structures become exposed and require skin grafting or flap coverage.

The correct choice of antibiotics is important in treating any patient with an upper-extremity infection. The physician is usually required to initiate treatment before definitive bacterial identification by culture and sensitivity occurs. Wound cultures should be taken before the initiation of antibiotic therapy. Cultures from patients with persistent infections who have already received antibiotics show a high

Table 115-1.
Penicillins

PENICILLINASE-RESISTANT	SECOND GENERATION	THIRD GENERATION	FOURTH GENERATION	NEW β-LACTAM
Methicillin	Ampicillin		Piperacillin	Imipenem
Oxacillin	Amoxicillin	Ticarcillin		Meropenem
Nafcillin				

Table 115-2.
Cephalosporins

FIRST GENERATION	SECOND GENERATION	THIRD GENERATION
	Cefuroxime	Cefotaxime
Cefazolin	Cefoxitin	Ceftriaxone
Cephalothin		Ceftazidime

Box 115-1.
β-Lactam and β-Lactamase Combinations

Amoxicillin-clavulanic acid
Ampicillin-sulbactam
Piperacillin-tazobactam

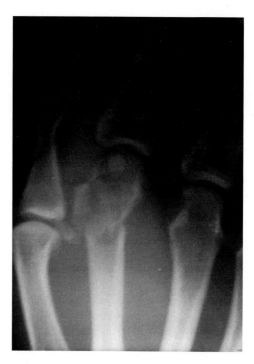

Figure 115-1. Unrecognized fracture of metacarpal head in patient treated for dog-bite wound.

percentage of mixed-flora infections, including anaerobic, mycobacterial, and fungal species.[60] A basic knowledge of antibiotics is therefore essential to treatment before the definitive results of an initial wound culture are received.

Antibiotics can be classified as cell-wall inhibitors, protein-synthesis inhibitors, or nucleic-acid inhibitors. Cell-wall inhibitors include the penicillins, cephalosporins, aztreonam, and vancomycin (Tables 115-1 and 115-2 and Box 115-1). The protein-synthesis inhibitors include aminoglycosides, tetracyclines, chloramphenicol, erythromycin, and clindamycin. Nucleic-acid inhibitors include the quinolones, such as ofloxacin, ciprofloxacin, norfloxacin, levofloxacin, and trovafloxacin; these inhibit DNA-gyrase, thus inhibiting DNA replication and repair.

The ultimate selection of antibiotics for the treatment of upper-extremity infections is determined by wound culture and sensitivity results. Table 115-3 lists the organisms that are covered by individual antibiotics, and Table 115-4 lists some empiric coverage suggestions that can be initiated before culture results are received.

Consultation with infectious-disease specialists may be helpful in difficult or resistant cases. Standard radiographs should be taken of any patient with an upper-extremity infection to determine the presence of foreign bodies, fractures (Figure 115-1), gas in the tissues, or bone changes consistent with osteomyelitis.

The initial hand and upper-extremity dressings and splints must appropriately position the digits and wrist to avoid potential persistent stiffness. Motion exercises, however, should be started as soon as possible to ensure maximum recovery of function. Coordination of care with appropriately trained hand therapists may be helpful.

OPERATIONS

An initially localized infection of the upper extremity can progress to involve multiple areas of the extremity. The

Table 115-3.
Antibiotics and Their Coverage

ANTIBIOTIC	COVERAGE
Penicillin G	Streptococci, enterococci, *Eikenella corrodens, Pasteurella multocida,* some anaerobes
Ampicillin	Same as for penicillin G but better for treatment of some enterococci
Oxacillin	Staphylococci (not methicillin or oxacillin resistant), streptococci
Piperacillin	Streptococci, Enterobacteriaceae, *Pseudomonas aeruginosa,* anaerobes
Ampicillin/sulbactam	Streptococci, *Staphylococcus aureus,* Enterobacteriaceae, anaerobe
First-generation cephalosporins	*S. aureus,* streptococci, some gram-negative species
Cefuroxime	Streptococci, *Haemophilus influenzae, S. aureus,* Enterobacteriaceae
Ceftazidime	Best cephalosporin for treatment of *P. aeruginosa;* poor choice for *S. aureus* and streptococcus anaerobes
Cefotaxime or Ceftriaxone	Streptococci, *H. influenza, S. aureus,* Enterobacteriaceae
Cefoxitin or imipenem	Anaerobes, Enterobacteriaceae, *Neisseria gonorrhoeae;* good general coverage except for treatment of some enterococci, including *Sterotrophomonas maltophilia*
Aztreonam	Gram-negative organisms only
Gentamicin	Aerobic and facultative anaerobic gram-negative bacilli
Tobramycin	Same as gentamicin; best aminoglycoside for treatment of *Pseudomonas*
Ciprofloxacin	Most gram-positive and gram-negative organisms except anaerobes
Ofloxacin	Same as ciprofloxacin
Levofloxacin	Same as ciprofloxacin, but covers more gram-positive organisms
Trovafloxacin	Same as levofloxacin, plus anaerobic coverage
Vancomycin	Gram-positive organisms, *S. aureus, S. epidermidis,* diphtheroids, streptococci, enterococci, clostridia
Clindamycin	*S. aureus,* streptococci, clostridia
Metronidazole	Anaerobic bacteria

Table 115-4.
Suggested Antibiotics by Infection Type

INFECTION	SUGGESTED EMPIRIC ANTIBIOTIC
Felon	Penicillins; clindamycin; cephalosporin
Tenosynovitis	Cephalosporins; ampicillin/sulbactam; vancomycin + quinoline; ceftriaxone
Intravenous drug abuse	Penicillins + aminoglycosides; ampicillin/sulbactam; vancomycin + aminoglycoside
Bite wounds	Penicillins + cephalosporins; ampicillin/sulbactam; clindamycin + quinolones
Pyarthrosis	Cephalosporins + aminoglycoside; penicillins; vancomycin; clindamycin
Osteomyelitis	Penicillins + quinolones; cephalosporins + aminoglycoside; vancomycin
Necrotizing fasciitis	Piperacillin + quinoline; imipenem

surgical treatment options for infections are best discussed by anatomic areas.

PULP-SPACE INFECTIONS (FELONS)

The pulp of the finger has numerous fibrous septa that connect the palmar skin to the underlying tuft of the distal phalanx. These septa reduce soft tissue shear and give structural support to the fingertip for the daily living activities of pinch and grasp. Most pulp infections occur after some type of penetrating injury, such as that caused by a rose thorn or wood splinter, although occasionally no such history is given. The patient usually experiences swelling and an intense fingertip pain in the pulp. The fingertip will be hot, red, and tender to the touch. Early in the course of the infection an area of "pointing" may be absent, but typically a specific area of tenderness or swelling can be identified (Figure 115-2). Progression of the infection can lead to osteomyelitis of the distal phalanx, or rarely to a purulent flexor tenosynovitis.[6]

Treatment by surgical drainage is accomplished by making an incision directly over the area of "pointing." Older texts describe a "fish-mouth" incision placed on the lateral aspect of the digit, just below the nail and not extending distally beyond the midline on the hyponychium.[6,10] However, this incision places the skin between the lateral incision and the pointing area at risk for necrosis and therefore should be avoided. All septal compartments must be decompressed and the distal phalanx should be probed to rule out soft bone that is indicative of osteomyelitis. The wound should be packed open to allow it to drain. The packing is removed after 24 to 48 hours to allow the fingertip to heal by secondary intention. If the bone is infected, debridement of the distal phalanx is necessary; in patients with extensive infection in the distal phalanx, a distal interphalangeal disarticulation with amputation at the joint may be necessary.

Staphylococcal organisms are the most common cause of felons and appropriate antibiotic coverage should be given.

PARONYCHIAL INFECTIONS

Paronychial infections are the most common infections of the upper extremity.[3] These infections can be isolated to the edge of the nail along the perionychium or can "run around" the proximal nail in the eponychial fold and involve both sides of the nail (Figure 115-3). Cellulitis can be treated early with warm soaks and oral antibiotics to cover the most likely organism, which typically is a Staphylococcus species. However, cultures from chronic cases may be positive for gram-negative bacteria and/or fungal elements such as *Candida albicans*.[3] The nail plate is formed in the proximal eponychial fold by germinal nail matrix and as it advances distally it is thickened by the sterile nail matrix. The skin along the radial and ulnar sides of the nail plate is the paronychia. Purulence under the nail plate must be drained by removing a portion of the nail either on one side along the paronychia or from the eponychial fold. Care is necessary to avoid injury to the underlying sterile and germinal matrix. Rarely, chronic cases are treated by marsupialization of the nail fold, which involves excising skin just proximal to the distal eponychium and allowing the wound to granulate.[3,31]

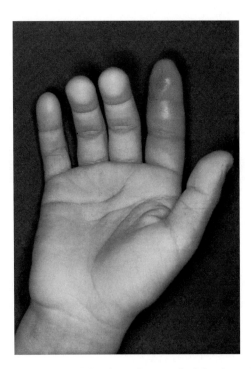

Figure 115-2. Felon (note "pointing" of the abscess).

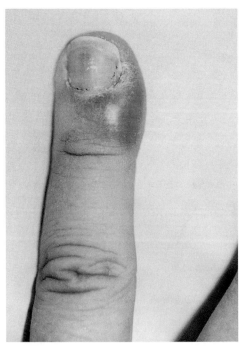

Figure 115-3. Chronic paronychia (note swelling and erythema extending to eponychium).

Most paronychial infections are acute problems that are easily treated by draining the infection. Patients with a chronic paronychia or one that appears difficult to control despite adequate drainage should alert the physician to the presence of underlying diseases (e.g., diabetes or scleroderma) that can cause a patient's peripheral circulation or immune system to be compromised.[19]

HERPETIC INFECTIONS OF THE DIGITS

The term *herpetic whitlow,* although commonly used, is probably an inaccurate description of superficial viral infections of the fingertip caused by the herpes simplex virus. These are not deep pulp-space bacterial infections, to which the Middle English term *whitlow* applies. Medical and dental personnel are at highest risk among the adult population for these infections,[5,26,35] which are also less commonly seen in the pediatric population.[61] Oral lesions in an infant or child may provide a helpful clue in determining this diagnosis. Clinically, these patients present with vesicles containing clear-to-turbid fluid. The turbid fluid can mimic pus but generally the fluid is more "watery" in consistency. Local erythema and tenderness also may be present, but to a lesser degree than in bacterial infections.[39] Patients with herpetic infections also may present with fever, lymphadenopathy, and lymphangitis.[61] The signs and symptoms generally occur over a 10- to 14-day period but shedding of the virus may continue for as long as 2 weeks after the initial presentation subsides. The diagnosis usually can be made clinically, but a Tzanck smear or a viral culture can be helpful. The treatment is

nonsurgical because an incision and drainage can lead to a secondary bacterial infection.[26,35] Acyclovir may be given intravenously in severe cases, or to immunocompromised patients; however, topical use of acyclovir is not indicated. Recently, the number of immunocompromised patients being hospitalized and tested for other medical conditions has increased. Medical personnel must recognize the increased risk for developing herpetic infections among this patient population to prevent cross contamination from hospital personnel to other patients.[19,58]

PALMAR-SPACE INFECTIONS

The palm of the hand has three spaces that are commonly susceptible to infections; these include the hypothenar, thenar, and mid-palmar spaces (Figure 115-4). Infections also can occur in the dorsal subaponeurotic and the interdigital web spaces; such infections may be confused with palmar-space abscesses. Parona's space in the distal forearm is also susceptible to infection.

The hypothenar space is an area beneath the hypothenar muscles and fascia. Incisions that are made to drain this space should avoid the ulnar border of the hand and are best made on the radial aspect of the hypothenar eminence. This prevents the formation of a tender scar on the ulnar side of the hand, where pressure is applied during daily use.[15,42]

The thenar space is bounded on the ulnar border by a fascial band from the third metacarpal to the palmar fascia, and radially by the fascia and musculature inserting on the proximal phalanx of the thumb. The space is bounded dorsally

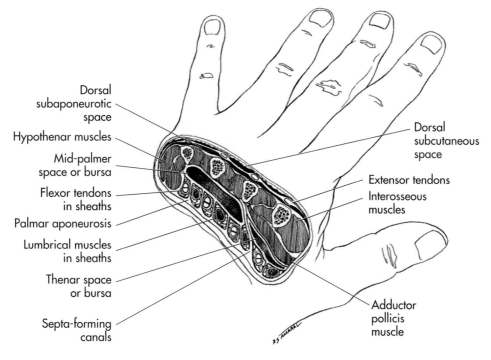

Figure 115-4. Palmar spaces.

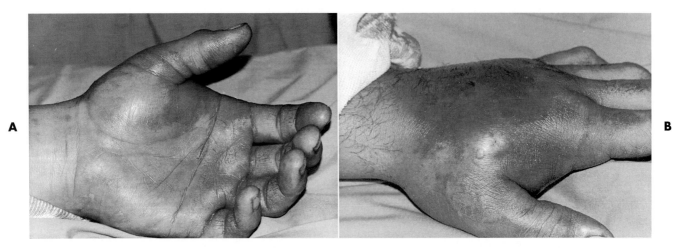

Figure 115-5. A, Thenar abscess. **B,** Thenar abscess with dorsal swelling.

by the adductor pollicis muscle and volarly by the flexor pollicis longus and flexor profundus to the index finger (Figure 115-5, *A* and *B*). Surgical drainage can be accomplished by a volar incision in line with the thenar crease, a dorsal straight line incision over the first dorsal web space, or both. Care must be taken to avoid injury to the recurrent branch of the median nerve when making the volar incision. Although continuous closed irrigation as described by Neviaser[15,41] can be used, I prefer open wound care after draining for all deep space infections.

The mid-palmar space is bounded on its radial side by the same fascia that forms the ulnar border of the thenar space. The ulnar border of the mid-palmar space is the hypothenar musculature. The mid-palmar space is deep to the extrinsic flexor tendons and is best drained through a palmar incision.

The diagnosis of a mid-palmar–space infection is sometimes difficult to make or delayed because the palmar space is deep to most of the soft tissue structures in the palm. Mid-palmar–space infections typically cause a loss of palmar concavity,[15] but also can cause swelling on the dorsum of the hand. The surgeon should maintain a high index of suspicion to avoid a delay in diagnosis based on negative aspirations from the dorsum of the hand.

WEB-SPACE (COLLAR BUTTON) ABSCESSES

The palmar fascia and its attachments to the skin at the level of the web spaces make it possible for infections to begin superficially in the palm, dissect through a small opening in the palmar fascia, and migrate dorsally.[7,34] These infections can present as a tender palmar-abscess pointing in the palm, or with relatively minimal swelling in the palm and great swelling in the dorsal web space (Figure 115-6). Treatment of web-space infections in either case requires the physician to drain any purulence through a volar and dorsal incision.[15,42]

The volar web-space incision should be oblique or zigzag to avoid contracture. Care must be taken during surgery because a web-space infection on the palmar surface is directly adjacent to the common digital nerves at their bifurcation.[8] A straight longitudinal incision is recommended on the dorsum of the hand.

The dorsal subaponeurotic space can develop purulent infections, although secondary swelling or cellulitis can make this diagnosis difficult. Aspirations can be performed but must be done aseptically to prevent secondary infections.

PURULENT FLEXOR TENOSYNOVITIS

The flexor-tendon sheaths are necessary to provide both tendon nutrition and a gliding surface through which the tendons can perform their excursion. The flexor-tendon sheaths for the index, long, and ring fingers begin approximately 1 cm proximal to the proximal border of the deep transverse metacarpal ligaments[30] and extend to the level of the distal interphalangeal joints. However, the sheaths of the little finger and thumb are essentially confluent with the ulnar and radial bursae, respectively, and therefore communicate proximally in the distal forearm (Figure 115-7). Infections can easily spread through the tendon sheaths of the thumb or little finger, whose bursal extensions into the distal forearm create the potential for migration of the infection at this level. Parona's space is a potential space between the pronator quadratus muscle and flexor profundus tendons in the distal forearm. A thumb or small finger flexor-tendon sheath infection can communicate at this level to create a "horseshoe abscess" or an infection extending into the distal forearm (Figure 115-8).

Penetrating trauma is the most common cause of purulent tendon sheath infections.[41,42] However, a hematogenous spread from another area also can occur, as has been reported with the development of gonococcal flexor tenosynovitis.[50]

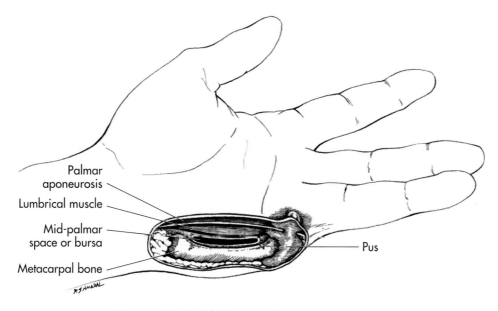

Figure 115-6. "Collar button" or web-space abscess.

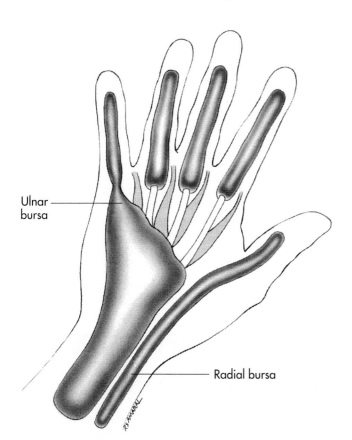

Figure 115-7. Bursae of hand.

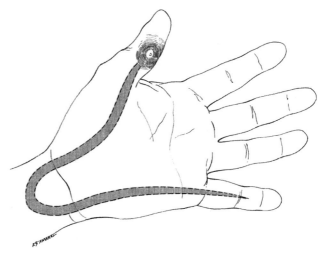

Figure 115-8. "Horseshoe abscess."

This emphasizes the need to obtain a complete history from patients with a hand infection. Tendon necrosis can occur secondary to pressure and loss of synovial nutrition within the tendon sheath.[15,53]

Four classic signs of infection, which were first described by Kanavel, have been used to make the clinical diagnosis of digital flexor tenosynovitis (Figure 115-9): (1) the digit is held in slight flexion, (2) fusiform swelling of the digit and (3) tenderness along the flexor sheath are present, and (4) the patient experiences excruciating pain with passive extension of the digit.[28] When used appropriately, these four signs can be quite helpful. The examiner must be able to differentiate a localized swelling, which may indicate cellulitis or a subcutaneous abscess, from true fusiform digital swelling. When attempting to elicit pain with passive extension, it is also useful to stabilize the finger and move only the distal interphalangeal joint. This helps to isolate flexor-tendon motion and to differentiate the pain of purulent tenosynovitis from more proximal joint pyarthrosis or local wound pain. The diagnosis of flexor tenosynovitis is a surgical emergency that, like an acute appendicitis, requires surgical intervention. Patients with diffuse cellulitis and no tendon sheath involvement may have a swollen, tender finger, which may be difficult to differentiate from a true flexor-tendon sheath infection. Hand cellulitis can be treated by immobilization, elevation, and parenteral antibiotics, but a true tenosynovitis necessitates adequate drainage of the tendon sheath.

Neviaser popularized the so-called *closed tendon sheath irrigation* method to accomplish drainage of the tendon sheath while allowing rapid wound healing and early motion.[41] An incision is made in the palm just proximal to the A1 pulley of the involved digit. A second small incision is made just proximal to the distal interphalangeal flexion crease and the tendon sheath is entered just distal to the A4 pulley. A 16- or 18-gauge angiocatheter is inserted approximately 1 to 2 inches into the proximal end of the tendon sheath, which is irrigated with sterile saline until the effluent is clear. The hand is immobilized in a bulky dressing and elevated. Tendon sheath irrigation is continued after surgery with 5 to 10 ml of saline every hour for 2 to 3 days. The catheter is subsequently removed and the patient begins active range-of-motion exercises. This method of treatment is very successful but requires patient cooperation and good ancillary care to ensure that the catheter remains in place and the irrigation is properly performed.

Alternative methods, which are modifications of the closed sheath irrigation technique, have been described by several authors.[15,27,53] Some advocate irrigation through an indwelling catheter for as many as 72 hours[27]; others remove the catheter during surgery after a thorough irrigation of the sheath produces clear effluent. All wounds are left open and the hand is dressed and splinted. Saline soaks are begun the next day, along with a supervised motion program, until wound healing of the incision sites occurs by secondary intention.[27,53]

It is important to emphasize that total exposure of the flexor tendon and/or excision of large portions of the sheath should not be performed because the resulting scar interferes with hand motion.

Parenteral antibiotics should be administered for at least 5 to 7 days, depending on the patient's progress.

MYCOBACTERIAL INFECTIONS

Tuberculosis

In 1984, reports indicated that the incidence of tuberculosis was declining in developed countries.[9] However, the number of new cases during the last 10 years has increased in the United States; these cases have been characterized by both pulmonary and musculoskeletal involvement.[63] A number of factors have influenced the increase in new cases, including an increasingly larger number of immunocompromised and elderly patients and increased international air travel. Currently an estimated 10 million people in the United States are infected with *Mycobacterium tuberculosis* and one fifth of newly diagnosed cases are associated with extrapulmonary disease.[39] Approximately 2% of patients have musculoskeletal involvement of the elbow, wrist, and hand.[63]

The clinical presentation of tuberculosis can be quite insidious because only one third of patients with bone involvement have a history of pulmonary disease.[6,63] A so-called *cold abscess* (i.e., swelling without erythema) or increased warmth may be the only visible sign. Radiographs show osteopenia, with a distinct lack of bone destruction. A slight periosteal reaction and joint narrowing may be the only subtle changes implicating tubercular involvement of the joints,[63] as seen in the radiograph of a patient who presented with minimal pain and swelling of the elbow (Figure 115-10). This patient's preoperative chest radiograph was in fact consistent with a diagnosis of tuberculosis (Figure 115-11). Skin tests may be helpful, although their false-negative rate is reported to be as high as 20%.[14,49]

Aspiration alone may not be diagnostic; biopsy specimens and cultures must be performed. All suspected hand infections should be cultured for aerobic, anaerobic, fungal,

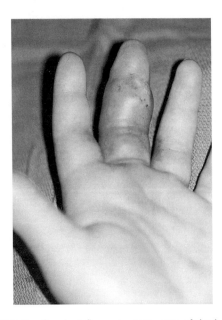

Figure 115-9. Purulent flexor tenosynovitis of the long finger.

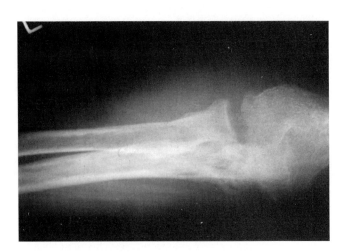

Figure 115-10. Tuberculosis of the elbow.

and mycobacterial organisms to determine the type of infecting organism. Biopsy specimens can be helpful if mycobacterial or fungal infections are suspected and may be the best method for obtaining a diagnosis. It is necessary to be specific in requesting the appropriate culture. *Mycobacterium tuberculosis* is grown on Lowenstein-Jensen medium at 37° C. Some atypical mycobacteria grow at cooler temperatures, such as 30° to 32° C.

Surgical treatment includes aggressive debridement of bone, joints, or tenosynovium. Primary wound closure is acceptable in treating mycobacterial infections, although inadequate debridement can lead to wound breakdown.[9] Appropriate pharmacologic agents are necessary, and cooperation with infectious-disease consultants is helpful.

Atypical Mycobacteria

The incidence of atypical mycobacterial infections has been increasing. A delay in diagnosis is common because of their indolent and progressive course.[32] A history consistent with occupational and/or recent exposure to locations known to harbor such organisms is helpful. *Mycobacterium marinum*, for example, is associated with aquatic exposure; *Mycobacterium terrae* is found in farm environments.[32] An increase in *Mycobacterium avium* complex has been seen in immunocompromised patients, particularly in those with acquired immune deficiency syndrome.[32]

Skin tests and acid-fast smears have proven unreliable despite an abundant reactive synovitis; as with tuberculous infections, a biopsy may be necessary to confirm the diagnosis. The clinician must request that cultures of *M. marinum* be performed at 30° to 32° C on Lowenstein-Jensen medium. Aggressive surgical debridement and appropriate pharmacologic agents should be initiated based on the clinical presentation and biopsy specimen histology because culture results may take as long as 3 to 6 weeks to obtain.[32] Antibiotic therapy is prescribed for a least 6 months. Minocycline is the primary drug of choice, but combination therapy may be necessary, empha-

sizing the need for a combined effort with infectious disease consultants.

INFECTIONS CAUSED BY PARENTERAL DRUG ABUSE

Addiction to injectable drugs causes major morbidity and mortality and is a significant economic cost to society.[51,55] A large county hospital reported that upper-extremity abscesses secondary to injection of illicit drugs were responsible for 28% of the infection-ward admissions. Associated secondary extremity infections have shown a high incidence of gram-positive organisms (Figure 115-12, *A-D*).[4,44,51,62,64] Gram-negative organisms, however, are also seen, particularly in patients over 40 years of age.[51] This may be related to physiologic changes caused by chronic drug use, such as the destruction of peripheral lymphatics.[43] Wide debridement and aggressive wound care are necessary to treat these infections. Broad-spectrum antibiotics should provide good aerobic, anaerobic, gram-negative, and gram-positive coverage. Illicit-drug users are at risk for acquiring human immunodeficiency virus and hepatitis. These patients must be identified and evaluated to rule out the presence of these conditions. Health care personnel must be vigilant to prevent inadvertent iatrogenic injury to themselves and others.

ANIMAL BITE WOUNDS

Approximately 1 to 2 million patients with animal bites are treated by physicians each year. Patients with dog, cat, or human bite wounds account for 1% of all emergency room visits.[1,21,65] It is estimated that one out of every two persons in the United States will be bitten by another person or an animal at some time during their lives.[21]

Dog and Cat Bites

Dog and cat bites occur seasonally and are more frequent in warmer weather. Dog bites comprise 80% of all animal bites in humans, and in nearly 70% of cases the dog is known to the victim.[21] Dogs exert significant pressure (as much as 450 pounds per square inch[1]) when they bite (Figure 115-13), but only 15% to 20% of dog bites become infected.[21] This is because dogs' teeth are relatively blunt and produce large, tearing lacerations (Figure 115-14). However, more than 50% of cat bites become infected,[21] perhaps because the sharp, needle-like teeth of cats essentially serve to "inject" bacteria into a wound (Figure 115-15). The bacteriology of dog and cat bites are similar and are characterized by a combination of aerobic and anaerobic bacteria.[1,22,65] *Pasteurella multocida* is a gram-negative bacteria that is both an aerobic and facultative anaerobic organism. It is present in many dog bites[2] and is found in 50% of infections caused by cat bites. *Pasteurella* is sensitive to penicillin, which is the drug of choice to prevent subsequent infection in animal bites.

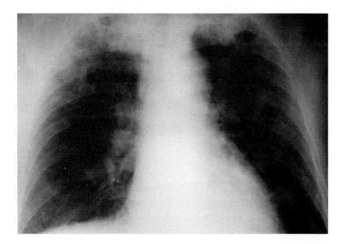

Figure 115-11. Radiograph showing pulmonary tuberculosis.

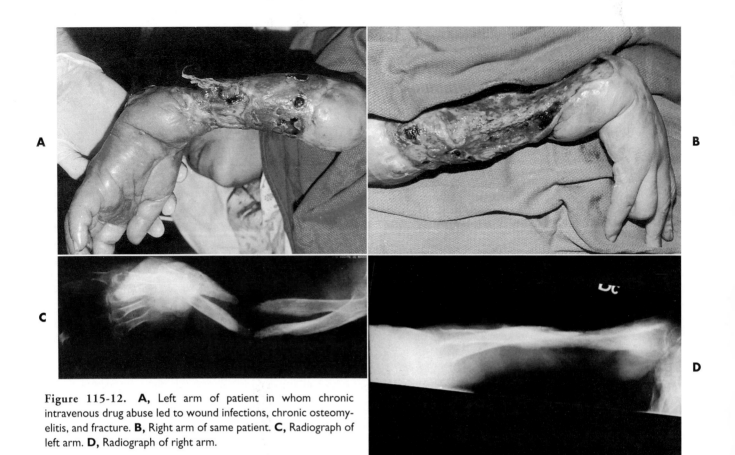

Figure 115-12. **A,** Left arm of patient in whom chronic intravenous drug abuse led to wound infections, chronic osteomyelitis, and fracture. **B,** Right arm of same patient. **C,** Radiograph of left arm. **D,** Radiograph of right arm.

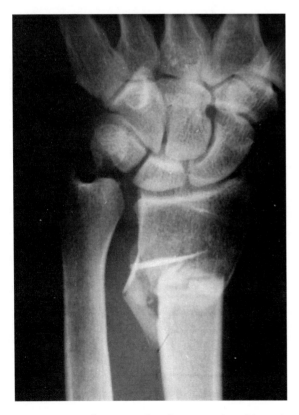

Figure 115-13. Fracture of radius in patient bitten by a large dog.

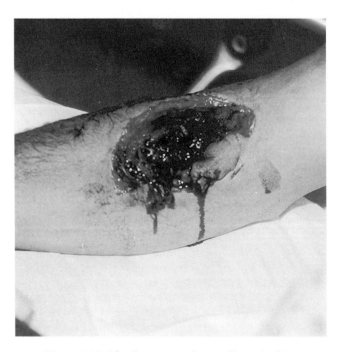

Figure 115-14. Large wound caused by a dog bite.

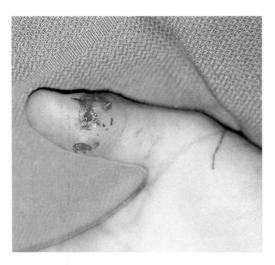

Figure 115-15. Wound caused by a cat bite.

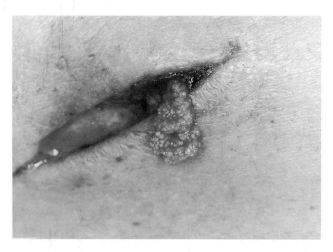

Figure 115-16. *Candida albicans* infection in patient with acquired immunodeficiency syndrome (AIDS).

HUMAN BITE WOUNDS

Human bite wounds resulting in infection can be categorized as self-inflicted, inadvertent, or true occlusional bite wounds. These wounds can be further subdivided into those involving traumatic amputation and those limited to skin penetration only, such as clenched-fist injuries.[38] Although the bacteriology of these wounds is similar, the nature of these injuries makes the underlying tissue injury different. True bite wounds are usually at the fingertip or phalangeal level; clenched fist injuries occur at the metacarpophalangeal level in nearly 85% of patients. Clenched-fist injuries are associated with a violated joint in 68% of cases, injured tendons in 20% of cases, and injured bone in 17% of cases.[46] These wounds should be surgically explored and irrigated with sterile saline. Human bites, like those caused by dogs and cats, have a mixture of aerobic and anaerobic organisms.[12,21,22,46,56] At least 42 different organisms have been isolated from normal human mouth flora,[56] but an organism that is likely to be encountered is *Eikenella corrodens*, a gram-negative facultative anaerobe.[20,21,48] Aerobic and anaerobic cultures and those performed in a 10% CO_2 atmosphere should be requested to achieve the most accurate identification of the infecting organisms.

Human bite wounds seen early, without bone or joint involvement and before the onset of established infection, may be treated on an outpatient basis with adequate wound lavage and broad-spectrum antibiotics, if the patient is compliant.[12,67] Noncompliant patients, and those with established infections[12] or bites that involve the bone or joint surface, should be treated with debridement and irrigation in the operating room, followed by hospitalization and intravenous antibiotics. Suggested antibiotics include combinations of cephalosporins and penicillins, or ampicillin/sulbactam (see Table 115-4). Patients with allergies to these drugs may be treated with clindamycin or vancomycin.

FUNGAL INFECTIONS

A high clinical suspicion is necessary to diagnose fungal infections of the upper extremity; thus the diagnosis frequently is delayed. Aside from cutaneous and nail infections, the most common fungal infection of the hand most likely is caused by *Sporothrix schenckii*. This is a saprophyte that is found in soil and plant materials; it exists in almost any climate. An isolated ulceration may develop initially at the site of injury. Subsequently the infection is characterized by lymphatic spread; the lymphatics become indurated and subcutaneous nodules develop along the path. These nodules may ulcerate with a violaceous appearance. Topical treatment with saturated solutions of potassium iodide (SSKI) has been recommended, although newer oral agents such as fluconazole may be effective in treating this and other fungal infections. Treatment should be continued for at least 6 weeks.

Other fungi, including coccidioidomycosis, histoplasmosis, mucormycosis, aspergillosis, and candidiasis can cause infections in humans (Figure 115-16). Therefore a careful patient history must be taken and must include information about travel, birth place, and possible immunocompromised status. Debridement is necessary, but the mainstay of treatment for these fungal infections of the upper extremity continues to be administration of appropriate pharmacologic agents such as amphotericin B.

NECROTIZING SOFT TISSUE INFECTIONS

Necrotizing soft tissue infections are characterized by rapidly progressing necrosis of skin, subcutaneous fat, and fascia, but not muscle. Several terms have been used to describe this entity since its first description in 1871 by Joseph Jones; these include Fournier's disease, Meleney's gangrene, and hemolytic streptococcal gangrene.

Clinically, this necrotic soft tissue infection is usually

characterized by a history of trauma, self-induced injury (e.g., intravenous drug abuse),[24] or previous surgery. The onset may mimic cellulitis but there is a rapid progression and significant morbidity and mortality; thus the physician must have a high index of suspicion to make the diagnosis. Edema occurs early in the course of the infection and extends beyond the associated erythema. Skin vesicles or bullae and subcutaneous gas may be present, but lymphangitis often is absent. Progression of the disease leads to skin anesthesia, ecchymosis,

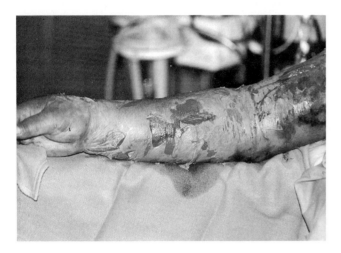

Figure 115-17. Necrotizing fasciitis.

induration, and necrosis, and associated symptoms include fever, hypotension, and eventually septic shock (Figure 115-17). The diagnosis may be missed because aspirations usually do not return frank pus. A gray necrotic fascia is noted at surgery, and Gram stain on frozen sections reveals thrombosis of small arteries and veins, fascial necrosis, and bacteria. The bacteria are usually combinations of non-group-A streptococci and staphylococcus species, gram-negative aerobes (e.g., *Proteus, Pseudomonas, Enterobacter, Escherichia coli,* and *Klebsiella*), and various anaerobes.

Treatment requires aggressive fluid resuscitation, electrolyte monitoring with blood replacement, and broad-spectrum antibiotics such as penicillin, aminoglycosides, clindamycin, ampicillin, piperacillin, and imipenem. The antibiotics must be altered based on results of wound cultures and sensitivity. The most important treatment for this disease is adequate surgical debridement of all necrotic and indurated tissue. The debridements must be extensive (Figure 115-18, *A, B,* and *C*), despite the fact that multiple debridements are often necessary.[24] The surgeon should not limit the initial debridement because of anticipated future debridement because these infections spread very rapidly, resulting in further necrosis. The overall mortality rates have been as high as 38%.

These patients are similar to those who have suffered a severe burn over a large body surface. Necrotizing infections are extremely difficult to treat. A team approach that involves

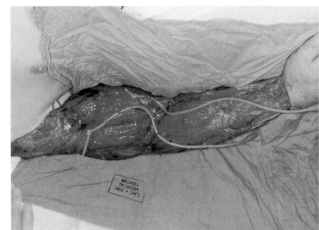

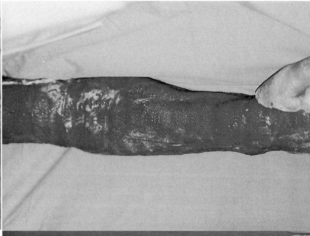

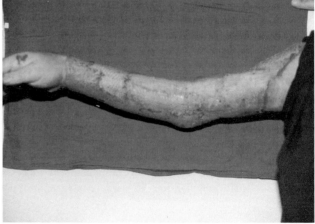

Figure 115-18. A, Debrided wound (red Robinson catheters used for intermittent irrigation of wounds between dressing changes). **B,** Debrided wound ready for skin grafts. **C,** Healed skin grafts.

surgeons, infectious-disease specialists, and therapists is necessary to provide the optimal surgical, antibiotic, nutritional, metabolic, and rehabilitation treatment for these very ill patients.

INFECTIONS OF JOINTS

Traumatic injuries are the most common cause of joint infection in the hand. *S. aureus* and streptococcus species are the most common causative organisms, except in joint infections resulting from bite wounds.[17] Septic joints create erythema, swelling, and pain with joint motion. The physician must be careful to determine that the joint motion is the source of pain and differentiate it from pain caused by a local abscess. The diagnosis is made when pain is produced by joint flexion, extension, or axial loading. If there is no history of a traumatic insult such as a laceration or puncture wound, the patient's immune status should be evaluated. The patient's sexual history also should be questioned because septic gonococcal arthritis can occur. Rheumatoid variants or crystalline deposition diseases such as gout also must be considered.[17]

Septic joint infections must be surgically opened and drained. Joint swelling in the fingers and destruction of the supporting structures can lead to a septic boutonniere deformity. Therefore surgical incisions and postoperative splinting should be planned to preserve the extensor mechanism and maintain its competence to prevent late deformity.[66] The joint should be copiously irrigated with normal saline during surgery. A small infusion catheter can be placed in the joint, which is left open and flushed with saline or antibiotic solution for 2 to 3 days after surgery.

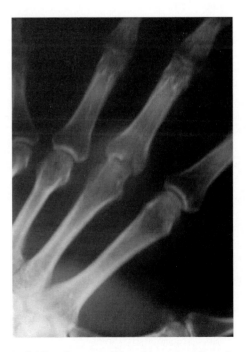

Figure 115-19. Osteomyelitis of metacarpal and proximal phalanx from infected clenched-fist injury.

Intravenous antibiotics should be continued for 2 to 4 weeks after the definitive surgical treatment; oral antibiotics sometimes are given for as many as 6 weeks after surgery.

OSTEOMYELITIS

Bone infection of the upper extremity is most often caused by penetrating trauma and/or predisposing conditions such as vascular connective tissue disease or diabetes,[17] or chronic intravenous drug abuse. The organisms may vary, depending on the underlying etiology of the osteomyelitis. Direct trauma that penetrates or fractures a bone may lead to *S. aureus* or streptococcal infection. Mutilating injuries have been associated with mixed gram-positive and gram-negative colonization,[13] and human bite wounds develop osteomyelitis from the skin and oral flora.[23] Bone infections that develop after open reduction and internal fixation procedures often are caused by *Staphylococcus epidermidis.*

Clinical signs of erythema and tenderness are usually present, but radiographs must be taken to determine whether there is bone involvement (Figure 115-19), which cannot be treated with antibiotics alone.

Surgical debridement is necessary primarily to remove necrotic bone so that antibiotic therapy can reach vascularized bone; no evidence suggests that even prolonged antibiotic therapy penetrates necrotic bone.[36] When an infection develops in a recently stabilized hand fracture in which transcutaneous pin fixation was used, the pins should be removed and alternative stabilization with an external fixation or splints should be used. Internal fixation with plates, screws, or buried pins that appear to rigidly immobilize the fracture may be left in place until the fracture heals, or such fixation may be replaced with another method of stabilization. An infected fracture that is unstable requires the removal of internal hardware and the use of alternative stabilization until the fracture heals. Widely infected bone must be excised, and reconstructive procedures involving flaps, large bone grafts, or the use of free fibular grafts may be necessary.

When to initiate antibiotic therapy is controversial and has been based primarily on empiric thought, depending on the clinical situation. It takes approximately 4 to 6 weeks before debrided bone is protected by revascularized tissue.[36] Therefore, intravenous antibiotics should be administered for at least 4 to 6 weeks, and subsequent oral antibiotic follow-up therapy should be given for a variable period of time, depending on the clinical setting.

OUTCOMES

The many etiologies of infections of the upper extremity make the determination of outcomes difficult. Certain factors, however, have been shown to improve results and decrease morbidity. Mann[38] reported that exploration and thorough debridement, coupled with hospitalization for at least 48 hours for the administration of intravenous antibiotics, resulted in a reduced incidence of amputations and/or finger stiffness. Kanavel[28] stated that early motion is of great benefit when treating hand infections that have been adequately drained. Several authors emphasize that early range of motion is a necessary adjunct to thorough irrigation and debridement when treating purulent flexor tenosynovitis of the hand.[27,41,53] Neviaser reported that 18 of 20 patients regained total active and passive range of motion after closed tendon sheath irrigation and debridement for the treatment of purulent flexor tenosynovitis of the hand.[41] Other authors have noted a relationship between the success of treatment and the severity of the infection, depending on how early treatment was begun. Patients treated early had less severe infections and better overall outcomes compared with those whose treatment was begun later, emphasizing the need for early diagnosis and aggressive treatment of these infections.[27,53]

The cost of treating infections varies, based on the severity of the infection and the presence of underlying systemic diseases. In 1986 Wallace[62] reported the treatment of drug-related abscesses during a 12-month period at a major metropolitan hospital and found that the average cost per patient was greater than $10,000—unless the patient developed a mycotic aneurysm, which increased the cost to more than $24,000. The length of hospital stay was affected by the patients' ability to care for their wounds on an outpatient basis. Schnall[52] found that many patients were unable to care for their wounds on an outpatient basis, but after delayed primary closure of some of these wounds, the hospital stay and associated costs were substantially reduced.

Avoiding delays in diagnosis, implementing early and aggressive surgical and antibiotic treatment, and beginning range-of-motion exercises as soon as possible after surgery are the best ways to optimize outcomes.

REFERENCES

1. Anderson CR: Animal bites, *Postgrad Med* 92(1):134-146, 1992.

2. Arons MS, Fernando L, Polayes IM: *Pasteurella multocida:* the major cause of hand infections following domestic animal bites, *J Hand Surg [Am]* 7(1):47-52, 1982.

3. Bednar MS, Lane LB: Eponychial marsupialization and nail removal for surgical treatment of chronic paronychia, *J Hand Surg [Am]* 16(2):314-317, 1991.

4. Biederman P, Hiatt JR: Management of soft-tissue infections of the upper extremity in parenteral drug abusers, *Am J Surg* 154:526-528, 1987.

5. Bleicher JN, Blinn DL, Massop D: Hand infections in dental personnel, *Plast Reconstr Surg* 80(3):420-422, 1987.

6. Bolton H, Fowler PJ, Manchester J: Natural history and treatment of pulp space infection and osteomyelitis of the terminal phalanx, *Orthop Clin North Am* 31B(4):499-504, 1949.

7. Bunnell S: *Surgery of the hand,* ed 2, Philadelphia, 1948, JB Lippincott.

8. Burkhalter WE: Deep space infections, *Hand Clin* 5:553-559, 1989.

9. Busch DC, Schneider LH: Tuberculosis of the hand and wrist, *J Hand Surg [Am]* 9(3):391-398, 1984.

10. Canales FL, Newmeyer WL III, Kilgore ES Jr: The treatment of felons and paronychias, *Hand Clin* 5(4):515-523, 1989.

11. Dellinger EP, Wertz MJ, Miller SD, et al: Hand infections bacteriology and treatment: a prospective study, *Arch Surg* 123:745-750, 1988.

12. Dreyfuss UY, Singer M: Human bites of the hand: a study of one hundred six patients, *J Hand Surg [Am]* 10(6)884-889, 1985.

13. Fitzgerald RH, Conney WP, Washington JA, et al: Bacterial colonization of mutilating hand injuries and its treatment, *J Hand Surg [Am]* 2(2):85-89, 1977.

14. Floyd WE III, Foulkes GD: Tuberculous, mycotic and granulomatous disease. In Peimer CA (editor): *Surgery of the hand and upper extremity,* New York, 1991, McGraw Hill.

15. Floyd WE III, Troum S, Frankle MA: Acute and chronic sepsis. In Peimer CA (editor): *Surgery of the hand and upper extremity,* New York, 1996, McGraw Hill.

16. Francel TJ, Marshall KA, Savage RC: Hand infections in the diabetic and the diabetic renal transplant recipient, *Ann Plast Surg* 24(4):304-309, 1990.

17. Freeland AE, Senter BS: Septic arthritis and osteomyelitis, *Hand Clin* 5:533-552, 1989.

18. Glass KD: Factors related to the resolution of treated hand infections, *J Hand Surg [Am]* 7(4):388-394, 1982.

19. Glickel SZ: Hand infections in patients with acquired immunodeficiency syndrome, *J Hand Surg [Am]* 13(5):770-775, 1988.

20. Goldstein EJC: Bite wounds and infection, *Clin Infect Dis* 14:633-640, 1992.

21. Goldstein EJC, Barones MF, Miller TA: *Eikenella corrodens* in hand infections, *J Hand Surg [Am]* 8(5):563-567, 1983.

22. Goldstein EJC, Citron DM: Comparative susceptibilities of 173 aerobic and anaerobic bite wound isolates to sparfloxacin, temafloxacin, clarithromycin, and older agents, *Antimicrob Agents Chemother* 37(5)1150-1153, 1993.

23. Gonzalez MH, Papierski P, Hall RF: Osteomyelitis of the hand after a human bite, *J Hand Surg [Am]* 18(3):520-522, 1993.

24. Gonzales MH, Thomas K, Weinzweig N, et al: Necrotizing fasciitis of the upper extremity, *J Hand Surg [Am]* 21(4):689-692, 1996.

25. Hausman MR, Lisser SP: Hand infections, *Orthop Clin North Am* 23(1):171-185, 1992.

26. Hurst LC, Gluck R, Sampson SP, et al: Herpetic whitlow with bacterial abscess, *J Hand Surg [Am]* 16(2):311-314, 1991.

27. Juliano PJ, Eglseder WA: Limited open-tendon sheath irrigation in the treatment of pyogenic flexor tenosynovitis, *Ortho Rev* 20(12):1065-1069, 1991.

28. Kanavel AB: *Infections of the hand,* ed 7, Philadelphia, 1939, Lea and Febiger, pp 453-469.

29. Kann SE, Jacquemin JB, Stern PJ: Simulators of hand infections, *J Bone Joint Surg* 78A(7):1114-1127, 1996.

30. Kaplan EB: *Functional and surgical anatomy of the hand,* Philadelphia, 1953, JB Lippincott.

31. Keyser JJ, Eaton RG: Surgical cure of chronic paronychia by eponychial marsupialization, *Plast Reconstr Surg* 58:66-70,1976.

32. Kozin SH, Bishop AT: Atypical Mycobacterium infections of the upper extremity, *J Hand Surg [Am]* 19(3):480-487, 1994.

33. Leddy JP: Infections of the upper extremity, *J Hand Surg [Am]* 11(2):294-297, 1986.

34. Linscheid RL, Dobyns JH: Common and uncommon infections of the hand, *Ortho Clin North Am* 6(4):1063-1104, 1975.

35. Louis DS, Silva J: Herpetic whitlow: herpetic infections of the digits, *J Hand Surg [Am]* 4(1):90-93, 1979.

36. Mader JT, Landon GC, Calhoun J: Antimicrobial treatment of osteomyelitis, *Clin Orthop* 295:87-95, 1993.

37. Mandel M: Immune competence and diabetes mellitus: pyogenic human hand infections, *J Hand Surg [Am]* 3(5):458-461, 1978.

38. Mann RJ, Hoffeld TA, Farmer CB: Human bites of the hand: twenty years of experience, *J Hand Surg [Am]* 2(2):979-1104, 1977.

39. Mann RJ, Peacock JM: Hand infections in patients with diabetes mellitus, *J Trauma* 17(5):376-380, 1977.

40. McLain RF, Steyers C, Stoddard M: Infections in open fractures of the hand, *J Hand Surg [Am]* 16(1):108-112, 1991.

41. Neviaser RJ: Closed tendon sheath irrigation for pyogenic flexor tenosynovitis, *J Hand Surg [Am]* 3(5):462-466, 1978.

42. Neviaser RJ, Butterfield WC, Wieche DR: The puffy hand of drug addiction, *J Bone Joint Surg* 54A(3):629-633, 1972.

43. Neviaser RJ, Green DP (editors): *Operative hand surgery,* ed 2, New York, 1988, Churchill Livingstone.

44. Orangio GR, Pitlick SD, Della-Latta P, et al: Soft tissue infections in parenteral drug abusers, *Ann Surg* 199:97-100, 1984.

45. Patzakis MJ, Harvey P, Ivler D: The role of antibiotics in the management of open fractures, *J Bone Joint Surg* 56A(3):532-541, 1974.

46. Patzakis MJ, Wilkins J, Bassett RL: Surgical findings in clenched-fist injuries, *Clin Orthop* 220:247-250, 1987.

47. Patzakis MJ, Wilkins J, Bassett RL: Factors influencing infection rate in open fracture wounds, *Clin Orthop Rel Res* 243:36-40, 1989.

48. Rayan GM, Putnam JL, Cahill SL, et al: *Eikenella corrodens* in human mouth flora, *J Hand Surg [Am]* 13(6):953-956, 1988.

49. Rooney JJ Jr, Crocco JA, Kramer S, Lyons NA: Further observations on tuberculin reactions in active tuberculosis, *Am J Med* 60:1517-1522, 1976.

50. Schaefer RA, Enzenauer RJ, Pruitt A, et al: Acute gonococcal flexor tenosynovitis in an adolescent male with pharyngitis, *Clin Orthop* 281:212-215, 1992.

51. Schnall SB, Holtom PD, Lilley JC: Abscesses secondary to parenteral abuse of drugs, *J Bone Joint Surg* 76A(10):1526-1530, 1994.

52. Schnall SB, Thommen V, Holtom P, Allari T: Delayed primary closure of infections, *Clin Orthop Rel Res* 335:286-291, 1997.

53. Schnall SB, Vu-Rose T, Holtom PD, et al. Tissue pressures in pyogenic flexor tenosynovitis of the finger, *J Bone Joint Surg Br* 78B(5):793-795, 1996.

54. Scott JC, Jones BV: Results of treatment of infections of the hand, *J Bone Joint Surg* 34B(4):581-587, 1952.

55. Senay EC: Drug abuse and public health: a global perspective, *Drug Safety* 6(Suppl 1):1-65, 1991.

56. Shields C, Patzakis MJ, Meyers MH, et al: Hand infections secondary to human bites, *J Trauma* 15(3):235-236, 1975.

57. Spiegel JD, Szabo RM: A protocol for the treatment of severe infections of the hand, *J Hand Surg [Am]* 13(2):254-259, 1988.

58. Stern H, Elek SD, Millar DM, et al: Herpetic whitlow: a form of cross infection in hospitals, *Lancet* 2:871-874, 1959.

59. Stern PJ, Staneck JL, McDonough JJ, et al: Established hand infections: a controlled, prospective study, *J Hand Surg [Am]* 8(5)Part 1:553-559, 1993.

60. Stromberg BV: Retreatment of previously treated hand infections, *J Trauma* 25(2):1163-1164, 1985.

61. Walker LG, Simmons BP, Lovallo JL: Pediatric herpetic hand infections, *J Hand Surg [Am]* 15(1):176-180, 1990.

62. Wallace JR, Lucas CE, Ledgerwood AM: Social, economic, and surgical anatomy of a drug-related abscess, *The Am Surg* 52:398-401, 1986.

63. Watts HG, Lifeso RM: Current concepts: review tuberculosis of bones and joints, *J Bone Joint Surg* 78A(2):288-299, 1996.

64. Webb D, Thadepalli H: Skin and soft tissue polymicrobial infections from intravenous abuse of drugs, *Western J Med* 130:200-204, 1979.

65. Wiggins ME, Akelman E, Weiss APC: The management of dog bites and dog bite infections to the hand, *Orthopedics* 17(7):617-623, 1994.

66. Wittels NP, Donley JM, Burkhalter WE: A functional treatment method for interphalangeal pyogenic arthritis, *J Hand Surg [Am]* 9(6):894-898, 1984.

67. Zubowicz VN, Gravier M: Management of early human bites of the hand: a prospective randomized study, *Plast Reconstr Surg* 88(1):111-114, 1991.

PART VII

CONTRACTURES

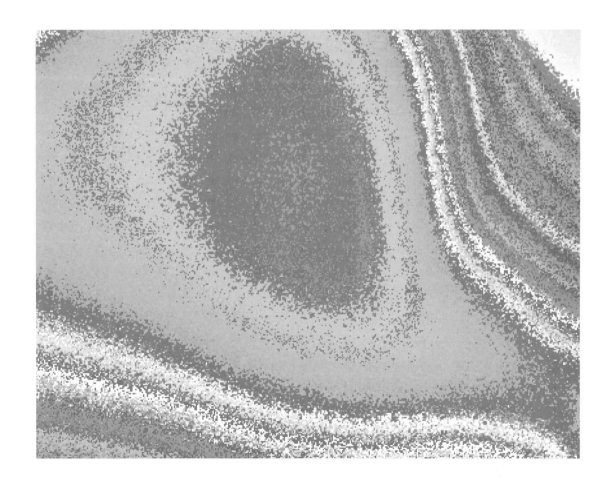

CHAPTER

Stiff Joints

116

Duffield Ashmead, IV
H. Kirk Watson

INTRODUCTION

Mobility is a prerequisite for normal hand function. Some measure of digital motion is essential for basic prehensile skills, and manipulative tasks demand even greater flexibility and dexterity. Loss of mobility, or "stiffness," is a frequent basis for hand surgical consultation and intervention. Evaluation and management of stiff joints are addressed in this chapter.

INDICATIONS

IDENTIFYING THE PROBLEM (PATIENT ASSESSMENT)

Digital mobility requires not only supple joints, including articular and capsular components, but also freely gliding flexor and extensor tendons, elastic extrinsic and intrinsic musculature, and a compliant soft tissue envelope. Compromise of any individual component may limit motion, and often multiple components are involved simultaneously. The principal challenge in patient assessment is to identify where the problem lies. Although the history may provide clues, a thorough physical examination is essential. We also have found the illustrated algorithm to be helpful (Figure 116-1).

Many patients who complain of joint stiffness in fact retain a full active range of motion but describe resistance or difficulty in demonstrating it. This "subjective stiffness" may be associated with mild soft tissue swelling, minimal intrinsic tightness, or early arthrosis. Frequently, however, it is without clear cause and is therefore poorly understood. Such subjective stiffness is almost never an indication for surgical intervention. Conversely, patients with demonstrable compromise of active or passive mobility typically have discrete, identifiable pathology that may be amenable to treatment.

If active mobility is compromised, it is essential to determine whether passive motion is limited. Full passive motion rules out significant joint pathology as well as static musculotendinous or soft tissue restrictions. When active mobility is limited but passive motion is full, primary neurologic conditions should be considered and must be distinguished from a loss of musculotendinous continuity, such as occurs with tendon lacerations or ruptures. The loss of a tenodesis effect indicates a loss of musculotendinous continuity. Tendon adhesions may restrict active motion while allowing passive motion. Isolated extensor adhesions, for example, may restrict active extension by limiting tendon pull through but do not compromise passive extension. However, if these same extensor adhesions compromise flexion, both active and passive modes will be equally impaired. Flexor tendons with adhesions in the flexor sheath may limit passive flexion by jamming within the constricted closed sheath.

Passive mobility of an individual joint often varies with the position of adjacent joints. This "seesaw effect" is the result of a restricting structure that bridges both joints. Extrinsic flexor tightness or a volar scar contracture may allow for passive proximal interphalangeal (PIP)–joint extension (provided that the distal interphalangeal (DIP) joint is flexed) and for passive DIP extension (provided that the PIP is flexed). Complementary restriction implies that the responsible structure lies entirely on the flexor (in this case) or extensor side of both joints. The Bunnell test of intrinsic muscle tightness is a demonstration of reciprocal restriction. The tight intrinsics lie volar to the metacarpophalangeal (MCP) joint and dorsal to the interphalangeal (IP) joints. As a result, full passive flexion of the IP joints is feasible in the context of MCP flexion, which takes tension off the intrinsics, whereas with MCP extension, residual intrinsic compliance does not allow for full passive IP flexion. Reciprocal and complementary restrictions focus on bridging structures that are external to the involved joints. Pathology intrinsic to a joint can be confidently excluded if any configuration of the adjacent structures allows full passive mobility of the joint in question.

If passive and active mobility are equally restricted, a joint problem almost certainly exists. Occasionally, combined flexor and extensor adhesions mimic this situation, either alone or in combination with joint restriction. In fact, combined pathology should not be surprising. Soft tissue contractures, tendon adhesions, and joint restrictions often develop concurrently in the aftermath of extensive trauma. An extrinsic restriction of

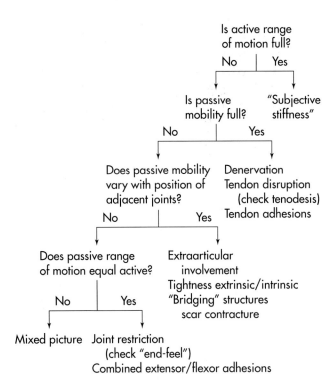

Figure 116-1. Algorithm for patient assessment.

joint motion by soft tissue constraints in a setting such as Dupuytren's contracture eventually leads to intrinsic joint pathology. These secondary joint restrictions continue to limit motion even if the soft tissue limitations are addressed.

A radiographic evaluation is essential when physical examination has implicated joint pathology, either alone or in combination with other pathology. Radiographic studies occasionally reveal an unsuspected explanation for the patient's stiffness. Ununited avulsions of either the volar plate or collateral ligaments are a frequent basis for chronic synovitis, pain, and restriction of terminal extension or flexion. These joints may be amenable to salvage. Any suggestion of significant joint incongruity or established arthrosis is a poor prognostic sign for the restoration of normal mobility.

PATTERNS OF PATHOLOGY

Joint stiffness follows predictable patterns that are easily understood in the context of normal anatomy. The MCP and IP joints are structurally quite different, particularly with regard to the volar plate and collateral ligaments (Figure 116-2). It is these structures that are most frequently implicated in restricted motion.

The MCP joint is not a simple hinge. The unique shape of the metacarpal head is such that, in extension, metacarpal-to-phalangeal contact is minimized, intraarticular fluid capacity is greatest, collateral ligaments are relatively lax, and abduction-adduction stability of the joint is minimal. Joint contact is greater during MCP flexion. Intraarticular volume

diminishes and a cam effect stretches the collateral ligaments to their full length. The volar plate is relatively elastic, changing in dimension from its full length in MCP extension to as much as 50% shorter in MCP flexion (unpublished research). Injury and swelling tend to favor MCP extension. Increased intraarticular fluid and capsular edema provide increased resistance to MCP flexion. Inadequate mobilization and the passage of time cause collateral ligament shortening and capsular fibrosis,[7] resulting in MCP joints that are stiff in extension. Flexion contractures of the MCP joints, when they occur, are almost exclusively caused by factors external to the joint, such as intrinsic tightness. The collateral ligaments are virtually incapable of restricting MCP extension. Volar plate shortening or surrounding fibrosis theoretically could result in a flexion contracture, but this does not occur with any frequency.

The PIP joint is bicondylar and has a negligible cam effect. The collateral ligaments are only slightly tighter during joint flexion than during extension. Joint contact and articular volume do not vary considerably. The IP volar plate is inelastic, maintaining comparable dimensions in flexion and extension. IP motion is permitted by proximal and distal translation of the plate as it hinges about its point of attachment at the base of the middle phalanx. The proximal tethers between the volar plate and the proximal phalanx are necessarily filmy and nonrestrictive. The IP joints occasionally become stiff in extension because shortening and fibrosis of the dorsal collateral ligaments restrict the available flexion arc. It is far more common, however, for IP joints to become stiff in flexion in response to restriction of the distal translation of the volar plate. The normally filmy proximal extensions of the volar plate become thickened and restrictive checkreins. Accompanying fibrosis of the pocket between the volar plate and the underlying proximal phalanx also may occur.

DIP-joint anatomy, including the structure and dynamics of the volar plate and collateral ligaments, is similar to that of the PIP joint. However, restriction of DIP extension is most commonly extrinsic to the joint, although checkreins and volar plate restriction are sometimes encountered. Similarly, restriction of DIP flexion is typically a function of extensor tendon adherence rather than collateral ligament tightness.

ALTERNATIVES

All patients who present with joint stiffness are entitled to a course of hand therapy. Active and passive range-of-motion exercises, as well as static and dynamic splinting routines, may afford significant benefit—particularly in cases of relatively recent onset. A spongy "endpoint" in response to passive stretching of the contracture suggests a measure of capsular elasticity, which may predict a beneficial response to conservative treatment. A solid endpoint suggests established fibrosis and may be a poor prognostic sign. In any case, surgery should be contemplated only when gains from nonoperative intervention have plateaued.

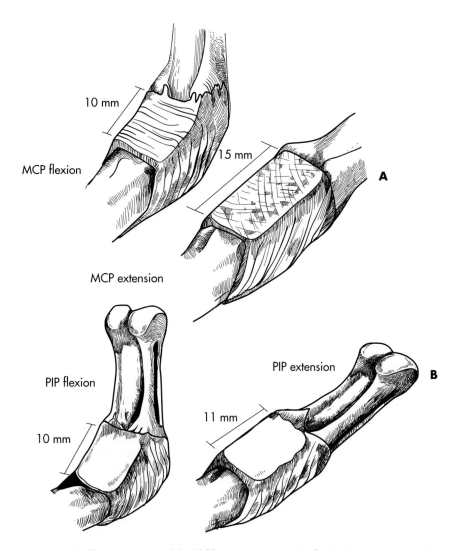

Figure 116-2. **A,** The volar plate of the MCP joint is composed of multiple criss-crossing fibers that have the ability to collapse from the fully extended to the fully flexed position. In flexion, the volar plate collapses to between one third and one half of its length in full extension. The volar plate pocket behind the MCP volar plate is smaller than at the IP joint, and there is no real tendency for the development of checkreins. (Sagittal microscopic views demonstrate these bundles of fibers as opposed to the more homogeneous collagenous arrangement in the IP volar plate.) **B,** The IP joint volar plate is similar to a unit in a suit of armor. It slides proximally and distally, protecting the joint. The volar plate is thick, allowing for extreme external loading over the joint. The volar plate pocket behind the proximal volar plate is large. The excursion of the volar plate between flexion and extension is great, and collapse of the volar plate itself between extension and flexion is minimal. Any limitation or fixation of the proximal volar plate, as with the development of checkreins, produces a significant restriction in extension of the IP joint. (From Watson HK, Turkeltaub SH: Stiff joints. In Green DP [editor]: *Operative hand surgery,* ed 2, New York, 1988, Churchill Livingstone.)

The surgical procedures described in this chapter are designed to improve joint mobility. This presupposes that increased mobility equates with increased function, which is not always true. Increased joint flexibility without voluntary control is of little functional benefit. Unless staged reconstruction is planned, it may be better for fingers without functional flexors and extensors to remain stiff. Similarly, increases in mobility at the expense of stability are counterproductive. Improved mobility in patients with advanced arthrosis may be associated with greater discomfort. Moreover, results of joint mobilization procedures may remain constrained by factors extrinsic to the joint. Extensive capsulotomy or capsulectomy affords little benefit if surrounding soft tissues are irretrievably fibrosed. Severe, long-standing PIP-joint contractures may prove particularly difficult to salvage because of neurovascular and skin envelope shortening. In each of the circumstances mentioned here, the patient may be better off pursuing a different type of treatment, such as joint-replacement arthroplasty, arthrodesis, or amputation. In some cases, the best option is to leave well enough alone.

INFORMED CONSENT

As with all surgical procedures, the term *informed consent* implies at least a basic understanding of the rationale for surgical intervention, the specific procedure planned, and the anticipated course of recovery. Realistic prospects for functional improvement, the inability to guarantee outcome, and the potential for complications must be disclosed. The patient must realize that circumstances surrounding joint-mobilization procedures vary tremendously from patient to patient, as do individual outcomes. Operative findings may dictate a change in operative plans or revised expectations for improvement. The patient may obtain a limited gain in motion or may experience greater disability after surgery. Wound-healing problems or infection may lead to a greater restriction of motion. Aggressive mobilization may result in compromise of joint stability, tendon continuity, or even neurovascular status. In rare instances, a finger may not survive surgery.

OPERATIONS

The joint capsule is responsible for the restriction of joint motion; thus it is not surprising that virtually all procedures designed to improve joint mobility are capsulotomies or capsulectomies. Improved understanding of pathologic anatomy has allowed some refinement in surgical technique, enabling the surgeon to leave all but restrictive structures minimally disturbed and to restore joint anatomy to as close to normal as possible.

PROXIMAL INTERPHALANGEAL FLEXION CONTRACTURES

Curtis[3] concluded that limitations of PIP extension were principally caused by volar plate restriction; consequently he described volar-plate resection techniques. More recently, emphasis has been placed on mobilization of the volar plate without excision, in the hope of preserving more normal joint anatomy. In our experience, even severe PIP-joint flexion contractures almost always can be released by checkrein resection alone, preserving the integrity of the volar plate and its distal attachments. Release of the volar collateral ligament fibers (accessory collaterals) and lysis of adhesions dorsal to the volar plate only rarely have proved necessary.[10]

Our technique[12,14] involves approaching the PIP joint from the volar side and elevating a Bruner triangular flap. This approach not only provides broad exposure, it also permits Y-to-V advancement of the flap for release of associated skin restrictions when necessary. The volar plate is approached through a flexor sheath window distal to the A2 pulley. The checkreins, which extend from the proximal edge of the volar plate to the margin of the flexor sheath, are identified. The

nutrient arteries to the vincular system are frequently identified where they branch from the digital arteries and pass beneath the checkreins. The attachments of the checkrein ligaments to the proximal edge of the volar plate are taken down, excising the checkrein while attempting to preserve the underlying nutrient vessel. After these checkrein ligaments have been resected, a gentle extension force on the PIP joint is typically sufficient to break up any residual fibrous restrictions. The joint space is left unviolated in this fashion. In the rare instance that full passive extension is not possible, gentle blunt dissection beneath the volar plate and/or sharp division of the volarmost fibers of the collateral ligaments is undertaken. However, these measures are infrequently necessary and are considered a last resort. A patient's inability to attain full passive extension after checkrein resection is more commonly a function of factors extrinsic to the joint, such as proximal flexor adhesions, volar displacement and shortening of lateral bands, or fibrosis of the oblique retinacular ligament. Measures to address these problems are outlined elsewhere.

After soft tissue closure, the PIP joint may be pinned or splinted in extension until the first dressing change 3 to 5 days after surgery. Active and passive mobilization should begin early, with the adjuvant use of dynamic splints during the day and Joint Jack or static splinting at night.

PROXIMAL INTERPHALANGEAL EXTENSION CONTRACTURES

PIP extension contractures are addressed by partial collateral ligament resection. The joint capsule may be approached through a solitary dorsal longitudinal incision or through paired dorsal lateral incisions. In either case, the transverse lamina of Landsmeer is divided, the lateral band is retracted dorsally, and the joint is approached from the side. A staged resection of the collateral ligament is carried out and enough of the ligament is removed to allow maximal passive PIP flexion. Relevant portions of the collateral ligament are not simply divided but are resected in an effort to minimize postoperative recurrence. Resection should be sufficient to enable passive ranging that is smooth and minimally resisted. A "jumping" phenomenon suggests residual collateral tightness and should be corrected by further release, beginning dorsally.

The extensor hood is assessed during the course of the exposure for adhesions over the proximal phalanx. These should be fully mobilized before the collateral ligaments are approached. Technical aspects of extensor tenolysis are addressed elsewhere. Given the remarkable frequency with which joint contractures are accompanied by tendon adhesions, it is frequently advisable to make a small flexor or extensor counter incision at the level of the wrist or distal forearm to ensure that the newly recovered passive joint mobility will be duplicated actively by the patient. An alternative is to perform PIP arthrolysis under digital block anesthesia, although this has not been our practice.

After soft tissue closure, the finger is immobilized in partial flexion pending early, aggressive mobilization during hand therapy 3 to 5 days after surgery. Active and passive range-of-motion exercises should be supplemented by dynamic splinting as warranted.

Occasionally PIP-joint mobility is restricted because of chronic synovitis rather than fibrosis. These cases typically are characterized by a loss of terminal extension and flexion. Preoperative radiographs occasionally identify nonunion of a small volar plate avulsion fragment, although a similar process may evolve without a discernible bone fragment. Exploration of the PIP joint, with resection of chronic inflammatory debris and the nonunion fragment (if present), has proven successful in our experience. The joint is approached from the volar side and the A3 pulley is taken down, providing broad exposure of the distal volar plate. The distal attachment to the middle phalanx is reflected on either the radial or ulnar side, preserving the attachment on the opposite side. Chronic inflammation is debrided using a fine soft tissue rongeur, and any loose fragments are removed. A shallow cancellous groove is created at the base of the middle phalanx. Provided that the volar plate remains tethered to the middle phalanx at either its radial or ulnar apex, the joint is not rendered hyperextensible and no formal reinsertion of the volar plate is undertaken. If surgery leaves the volar plate completely detached from the middle phalanx, a solitary suture is placed at the radial or ulnar apex, and the finger is protected briefly with an extension block splint. Postoperative hyperextension instability, as with acute avulsion injuries, is less problematic than residual flexion contractures.

METACARPOPHALANGEAL FLEXION CONTRACTURES

Flexion contractures of the MCP joint are encountered but are almost exclusively caused by factors extrinsic to the joint and its capsule. Palmar scarring, Dupuytren's contracture, or tight intrinsics can result in the restriction of MCP extension. The anatomy of the joint, however, is such that secondary contractures of the joint itself rarely occur. Release of the primary external constraint almost invariably facilitates the recovery of MCP-joint extension without the need for surgery directed at the joint itself. Thus it is not surprising that MCP flexion is a component of the "safe position" for long-term immobilization.

METACARPOPHALANGEAL EXTENSION CONTRACTURES

It is the nature of MCP joints to become stiff in extension. Not only do the mechanics of the joint favor a "neglected posture" of MCP extension, structures intrinsic to the joint perpetuate the problem. These structures include the dorsal capsule and principle collateral ligaments. When these structures thicken or shorten, active or passive flexion is adversely affected. Most procedures designed to mobilize stiff MCP joints consist of selective release of these structures.

Our preferred method[12] is a modification of the procedure described by Curtis.[4] The joint capsule is approached from the dorsal side, using a longitudinal incision for individual fingers or a single transverse incision when multiple fingers are addressed simultaneously. The superficial structures are retracted to either side and the extensor tendon is clearly exposed. The sagittal band fibers are retracted distally or, if necessary, may be divided on one side. The ulnar fibers typically are taken down because of the tendency for the extensor mechanism to prolapse ulnarly. This permits visualization of the underlying joint capsule and dorsal portions of the collateral ligaments on either side. Adhesions between the extensor tendon and underlying capsule are frequently identified, and these should be lysed. The normally diaphanous dorsal capsule typically is thickened and fibrosed; it is our practice to resect it. The principle step in mobilization of the joint is a graded release of the collateral ligaments. The dorsal fibers of the collateral ligament are taken down from their origin on the metacarpal head and resected in a fashion analogous to that described for PIP extension contractures. A graded resection permits increasingly supple flexion. Care must be taken to balance the radial and ulnar collateral ligament releases to allow the proximal phalanx to track within the normal axis of joint motion. A "jumping" phenomenon is a clear indication of residual tightness, which should be addressed by further resection.

We have rarely found it necessary to manipulate volar structures. A curved blunt instrument may be passed around the metacarpal head from a dorsal exposure, if necessary, to tease apart any adhesions dorsal to the volar plate. At the conclusion of the procedure, unresisted full, smooth, passive mobility of the MCP joint should be feasible. It may be necessary to check for proximal extensor tendon adhesions or other concurrent extrinsic restraints.

The operative dressing immobilizes the fingers in approximately 70 degrees of MCP flexion and is removed in 3 to 5 days for aggressive active and passive motion in hand therapy.

Variations in operative technique are principally related to exposure. A transverse skin incision allows the release of restricting skin and subcutaneous tissues and permits the possibility of skin grafting, if necessary. Unfortunately, when extensive soft tissue releases are necessary, the resulting wound bed typically consists of exposed tendons and joint structures. Such beds are not appropriate for grafts.

The extensor tendon may be divided longitudinally and subsequently repaired as an alternative to sagittal band division and repair. This technique preserves the sagittal bands, but care must be taken to avoid postoperative splitting of the extensor mechanism in the context of aggressive hand therapy.

OUTCOMES

Useful information on outcomes in the management of stiff joints is scarce. True outcomes instruments only recently have been developed in the field of hand surgery. A recent literature search restricted to small-joint mobilization yielded no information. The abundant literature on MCP and PIP mobilization predates this trend, and results typically are presented as range-of-motion data alone. As many of the authors themselves point out, the usefulness of this rather raw data is limited by several important factors.

Results vary tremendously depending on the primary etiology of the contracture. Contractures associated with neurologic conditions and injuries distant from the joint tend to respond because the joint and its surroundings remain relatively normal. Crush injuries and burns, in contrast, cause considerable damage to both the joint and other structures. Surgical release of a contracture in this context is invariably more demanding. Rehabilitation may be compromised by the need to protect skin grafts or other soft tissue reconstructions. The ultimate outcome reflects the recovery of not only the joint, but also its surrounding structures. The more complex the primary etiology and the more involved the surgical intervention, the less successful the joint release itself.

Results vary tremendously from patient to patient, even when patients are grouped by diagnosis. The severity within a diagnostic category may vary widely, and outcomes also depend on individual patient factors such as motivation and compliance. Standard deviation remains high within diagnostic groups, thus average outcomes are less meaningful. Individual projections based on group statistics may be particularly misleading.

Results also vary significantly over time. Virtually all authors point out that long-term results often show a loss of intraoperative gains. Early postoperative regression is the rule, and aggressive postoperative therapy is essential to reverse this trend. Moreover, raw range-of-motion data do not translate directly to functional status or overall patient satisfaction. Increased mobility is almost always of benefit, but for some patients joint-mobilization procedures are helpful despite a lack of net gain in the extension/flexion arc if the available motion is shifted to a more useful, absolute arc. For example, 30 degrees of PIP motion from 50 to 80 degrees is almost certainly preferable to 30 degrees of PIP motion from 0 to 30 degrees or from 80 to 110 degrees.

NONOPERATIVE MANAGEMENT

Weeks et al[15] reported on a large series of patients with stiff MCP and PIP joints who were treated nonoperatively with an aggressive course of active and passive range-of-motion exercises and dynamic splinting. Eighty-seven percent of the joints responded sufficiently and thus required no surgical intervention. Average active mobility almost doubled, and this translated to a significant reduction in the percentage of patients with permanent partial impairment; projected savings theoretically covered the cost of therapy tenfold. The dramatic improvement, as well as the fact that it was achieved with 2 weeks or less of therapy, reflects a patient population with modest pathology. It is clear, however, that conservative treatment is not simply an alternative to operative intervention but must be viewed as a prerequisite. Surgical intervention

should be contemplated only when gains from conservative measures have proved insufficient.

METACARPOPHALANGEAL JOINTS

Fowler[7] reported the results of MCP capsulotomy for extension contracture in more than 100 joints that had not responded to conservative treatment. He emphasized aggressive collateral ligament resection, and the importance of freeing the anterior capsule from the volar articular surface of the metacarpal head. Despite the complexity of his cases (a high percentage of which combined capsulotomy with other operations), he indicated that "results from capsulotomy are excellent and 80 to 90 degrees of motion may be confidently expected, if local tissues are good and the mechanics of the hand are satisfactory." In his published discussion of the paper, Sterling Bunnell corroborated the author's results, but reemphasized that the "dorsal skin and the surrounding parts must be in good condition." Although subsequent authors have reiterated the excellent results that can be obtained by MCP capsulectomy,[1,2,4] the data to substantiate these claims are sparse at best.

Results reported by Gould and Nicholson[8] were more modest. They reported on 100 MCP capsulectomies for extension contracture; gains in active motion averaged 21 degrees, for a total active flexion arc of 57 degrees, and total passive motion of 73 degrees. Passive mobility improved dramatically in patients recovering from stroke, but its functional benefit was questionable because these patients had no active control. The best results were obtained in young patients, independent of their diagnosis, with active flexion approaching 70 degrees.

The absolute measures of recovered flexion may be more modest than those achieved by Fowler and Bunnell, but the functional benefit afforded by MCP capsulectomy in these cases may be significant.

INTERPHALANGEAL JOINTS

In 1954, Curtis[3] reported on a series of 25 patients treated for IP-joint stiffness—principally extension contractures. Treatment consisted of aggressive collateral capsulectomy and/or volar plate division, usually in combination with intrinsic releases and/or flexor/extensor tenolyses. The results achieved in this report are somewhat difficult to interpret. The great value of the publication lies in its careful analysis of relevant anatomy.

Sprague[11] reported on 38 PIP-joint contractures treated surgically. Procedures ranged from capsulotomy with collateral ligament resection, for joints with extension contractures only, to far more involved releases of collateral ligaments, volar plate, extensor mechanism, and flexor sheath for joints with restriction of both flexion and extension. His results yielded several conclusions. The more extensive the surgery, the more disappointing the outcome. All cases followed over time showed significant postoperative regression. Even the simpler releases lost an average of 60% of operative gains, and in more complex cases the loss of surgical improvement increased to 80% or 90%. Sprague observed that fingers stiff in extension tended to fare better than those stiff in flexion. Harrison[9] encountered similar problems in a series of 30 PIP joints; fewer than 30% of those with flexion contractures improved their range by more than 40 degrees, and more than 70% of joints stiff in extension gained more than 40 degrees.

Gould and Nicholson[8] reported more modest results with 47 dorsal releases, yielding an average increase in active flexion of 14 degrees; in the same series, 65 volar releases yielded an average 13-degree improvement in extension. He emphasized that these results, as with his MCP results, reflected diverse etiologies and that neurologic patients had the best overall outcomes.

Diao and Eaton[6] reported the results of aggressive total collateral ligament resection for PIP-joint contractures, which yielded an impressive increase in mobility without apparent instability. The average arc of motion in these cases increased from 38 degrees to 78 degrees, with postoperative flexion in every case greater than 85 degrees. Modest residual extensor lag was present in most cases. The best results for the release of PIP extension contractures are those casually referenced by Curtis.[4,5] He indicates that the average flexion gain for 125 PIP-joint releases was 50 degrees.

Watson et al[13] focused specifically on flexion contractures, detailing the pathologic anatomy responsible for the loss of PIP extension. The checkrein release described avoids the need for volar plate resection and has yielded excellent intraoperative results. Long-term range-of-motion data have not yet been published.

Literature on surgical intervention for stiff joints supports the consensus that worthwhile functional gains may be achieved. Application of outcomes instruments in the coming years should provide a more objective and more useful interpretation of results. Physicians must move beyond striving for degrees of flexion and extension to assessing patient satisfaction and improving quality of life.

REFERENCES

1. Bodell LS, Gottlieb ME: Dorsal capsulectomy of the metacarpophalangeal joint. In Blair WF (editor): *Techniques in hand surgery*, Baltimore, 1996, Williams and Wilkins.

2. Buch VI: Clinical and functional assessment of the hand after metacarpophalangeal capsulotomy, *Plast Reconstr Surg* 53:452-457, 1974.

3. Curtis RM: Capsulectomy of the interphalangeal joints of the fingers, *J Bone Joint Surg* 36A(6):1219-1232, 1954.

4. Curtis RM: Stiff finger joints. In Grabb WC, Smith JW (editors): *Plastic surgery*, ed 3, Boston, 1979, Little, Brown, & Co.

5. Curtis RM: The interphalangeal joints. In Tubiana R (editor): *The hand*, vol II, Philadelphia, 1985, WB Saunders.

6. Diao E, Eaton RG: Total collateral ligament excision for contractures of the proximal interphalangeal joint, *J Hand Surg [Am]* 18:395-402, 1993.

7. Fowler SB: Mobilization of metacarpophalangeal joints, *J Bone Joint Surg* 29(1):193-202, 1947.

8. Gould JS, Nicholson BG: Capsulectomy of the metacarpophalangeal and proximal interphalangeal joints, *J Hand Surg [Am]* 4(5):482-486, 1979.

9. Harrison DH: The stiff proximal interphalangeal joint, *The Hand* 9(2):102-108, 1977.

10. Jabaley ME, Freeland AE: Capsulectomy of the proximal interphalangeal joint. In Blair WF (editor): *Techniques in hand surgery*, Baltimore, 1996, Williams and Wilkins.

11. Sprague BL: Proximal interphalangeal joint contractures and their treatment, *J Trauma* 16(4):259-265, 1976.

12. Watson HK, Dhillon H: Stiff joints. In Green DP (editor): *Operative hand surgery*, ed 3, New York, 1993, Churchill Livingstone.

13. Watson HK, Light TR, Johnson TR: Checkrein resection for flexion contracture of the middle joint, *J Hand Surg [Am]* 7(1):67-71, 1979.

14. Watson HK, Paul H: Pathologic anatomy, *Hand Clin*, 7(4):661-668, 1991.

15. Weeks PM, Wray RC, Kuxhaus M: Results of non-operative management of stiff joints in the hand, *Plast Reconstr Surg*, 61(1):58-63, 1978.

Dupuytren's Contracture

117

Lawrence N. Hurst

INTRODUCTION

Dupuytren's contracture is a fibroproliferative condition that primarily affects the palmar and digital fascia and can cause contractures of the metacarpophalangeal (MCP) and interphalangeal (IP) joints of the hand. As cited by Elliot,[10] Felix Plater of Basil first described fixed digital contractures in his book *Observations*, which was published in 1614. The disease was further discussed by the British surgeon John Hunter in 1777, and his student Henry Cline lectured on the disease and performed the first subcutaneous fasciotomy in Britain. In 1831, Dupuytren associated the disease with pathological changes in the palmar fascia and suggested surgical correction by open fasciotomy, thus initiating the surgical correction of Dupuytren's contracture.

INDICATIONS

INCIDENCE AND ETIOLOGY

The incidence of Dupuytren's contracture varies widely among races and is high among the descendants of the Celtic race, which originally inhabited northern Europe and the British Isles. In 1972 Mikkelsen[40] reported an incidence in Norway of 5.6%. He also found that the occurrence of Dupuytren's contracture was age and sex dependent; 9% of males and 3% of females were affected. The overall incidence was 7% among those younger than 40 years of age and more than 30% among those older than 65 years of age. McFarlane[33] reported a survey in which 82% of patients with Dupuytren's contracture were from Northern European families (Box 117-1). There was a higher incidence among males, with a male-to-female ratio of 82:16, which was consistent in all countries.[33] Bower[3] reported that the incidence of Dupuytren's contracture among individuals with human immunodeficiency virus (HIV) exceeds that of the general population.

Dupuytren's contracture is a genetic disease and is inherited by means of an autosomal-dominant gene with variable penetrance.[24] The expression of the gene is less complete in females, which accounts for the lower incidence and later onset among them.[29] The onset of Dupuytren's contracture usually occurs in the fifth decade in males, and the disease is gradually progressive. Trauma often is cited as a causative agent, but McFarlane[35] believes that evidence from epidemiological studies is insufficient to support this conclusion in most cases. However, a causal relationship may be considered in young patients who develop Dupuytren's contracture within 2 years of sustaining a single injury.

In 1996, Liss and Stock[25] reported that the incidence of Dupuytren's contracture among workers exposed to repetitive manual work was 5.5 times higher than the incidence among those in a similar control group. They also concluded that "there is good support for an association between vibration exposure and Dupuytren's contracture."

ASSOCIATED CONDITIONS

Dupuytren's contracture is associated with other malformations of fibrous tissue proliferation, including *knuckle pads* (Figure 117-1), *Peyronie's disease*, and *plantar fibromatosis* (Figure 117-2). Knuckle pads appear as nodular thickenings over the dorsum of the PIP joints. They can be tender but do not cause contractures and sometimes regress. The deposition of fibrous plaques on the dorsum of the penis in Peyronie's disease causes a painful penile contracture in response to erection. The plantar fascia proliferates in plantar fibromatosis in a fashion similar to that of the palmar fascia in Dupuytren's contracture. Flexion contractures rarely occur in the toes,[6] but nodules may appear in the plantar fascia. Hueston[17] described the clinical features of patients with particularly aggressive Dupuytren's contracture, which include a positive family history, the appearance of disease before 40 years of age, knuckle pads, plantar fibromatosis, and severe bilateral involvement. Such patients have a strong Dupuytren's diathesis and therefore should be identified because of a strong tendency for the disease to recur and progress.

Box 117-1.
Survey of 1227 Patients With Dupuytren's Disease Seen by 108 Surgeons in 12 Countries

FAMILY ORIGIN OF PATIENTS	
Northern European	82%
Southern European	2%
Black African	1%
Japanese and Chinese	1%
Polynesian	0%
American Indian	0.2%
Uncertain	12%
GENDER	
Male	82%
Female	16%
HAND DOMINANCE	
Right	94%
Left	5%
HAND INVOLVED	
Right	23%
Left	12%
Both	65%
AGE AT ONSET OF DISEASE	
49 years (males 49 years, females 54 years)	
AGE AT OPERATION	
58 years (males 58 years, females 62 years)	
FAMILY HISTORY OF DUPUYTREN'S DISEASE	27%
OCCUPATION	
Manual labor	45%
Nonmanual labor	41%
ASSOCIATED DISEASES	
None	62%
Diabetes	8%
Epilepsy	2%
Alcoholism	10%
Trauma	13%
OTHER AREAS INVOLVED	
Knuckle pads	22%
Feet	10%
Penis	2%

From McFarlane RM: Dupuytren's disease. In McCarthy JG (editor): *Plastic surgery*, Philadelphia, 1990, WB Saunders.

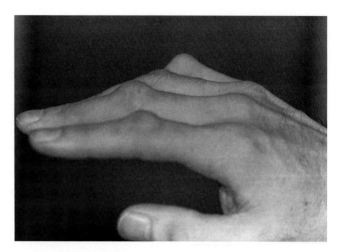

Figure 117-1. Patient's hand with knuckle pads.

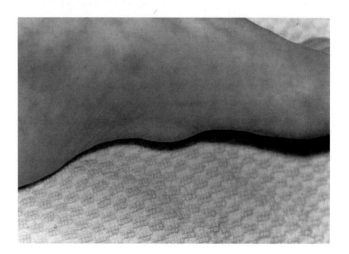

Figure 117-2. Patient with plantar fibromatosis.

epilepsy are affected equally; consequently, the increased incidence among this population is thought to be caused by the long-term effects of barbiturate therapy.[37]

Dupuytren's contracture is common among individuals with diabetes and the incidence increases with the age of the patient and the duration of the diabetes.[8,43] The distribution of the disease is more radial in the hand, with nodules typically appearing at the base of the middle and ring fingers. Involvement is mild and mainly in the palm, with few contractures of the fingers. Surgery may not be required. The connection between diabetes and Dupuytren's contracture is most likely related to diabetic microangiopathy, which causes disturbances in the structural macromolecules in the extracellular matrix and results in the inappropriate deposition of connective tissue.[8]

The association of Dupuytren's contracture with alcoholism, with or without cirrhosis, has been studied by many authors,[4,46,49] and reports show an increased incidence of Dupuytren's contracture among alcoholic patients. The

ASSOCIATED DISEASES

A greater incidence of Dupuytren's contracture occurs among individuals with epilepsy.[9] In these patients, the disease presents at an earlier age, has a normal distribution on the ulnar side of the hand, and is bilateral and aggressive. The incidence increases with the age of the patient and the duration of the epilepsy. Individuals with idiopathic and traumatic

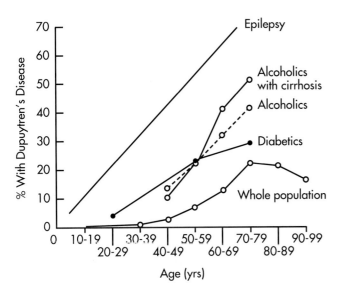

Figure 117-3. Graph showing the relationship between age and Dupuytren's disease, based on data from Mikkelsen's Norwegian study. Other superimposed graphs are based on data from multiple sources. Epilepsy drugs, alcoholism, and diabetes increase the incidence of this disease. (From Hurst LC: *Hand surgery update*, vol 1, Englewood, Colo, 1994, The American Society for Surgery.)

Table 117-1.
Factors That Affect Control of Symptoms of Dupuytren's Contracture

SUCCESSFULLY CONTROLLED	DIFFICULT TO CONTROL
No family history	Strong family history
Minimal involvement	Bilateral involvement
Late presentation	Early presentation
No intercurrent disease	Intercurrent disease (e.g., epilepsy, diabetes, alcoholism, infection with HIV)
No associated conditions	Associated conditions (e.g., knuckle pads, plantar fibromatosis, Peyronie's disease)
Patient is compliant with rehabilitation program	Patient is not compliant with rehabilitation program

distribution of the disease in such patients mainly involves a thickening in the palmar aponeurosis, without significant contractures. However, the disease can be very aggressive, leading to severe joint contractures in some cases. The association may be related to the amount of alcohol ingested and its effects upon the microcirculation. Dupuytren's contracture also has been strongly associated with both smoking and HIV infection (Figure 117-3).[41]

INFORMED CONSENT

It is clear that Dupuytren's contracture is caused by many factors, yet the progress of the disease can be predicted to some extent. Currently we cannot cure Dupuytren's contracture, but we can try to control the symptoms. Our success or failure in doing so depends on the patient, the presentation, and the associated conditions (Table 117-1). This topic is more fully discussed in the Outcomes section beginning on p. 2067.

NORMAL AND PATHOLOGICAL ANATOMY

A detailed knowledge of the normal (Figure 117-4) and pathological (Figures 117-5 and 117-6) anatomy of the palmar and digital fascia is mandatory for a safe surgical approach to the treatment of patients with Dupuytren's contracture. Stack[48] and Thomine[50] described the normal anatomy of the digital fascia, and Gosset[13] described the pathologic changes at the palmar digital junction. McFarlane[32] described the course and relationships of the diseased cords within the finger, the relationships of these cords to the normal digital fascia, and the

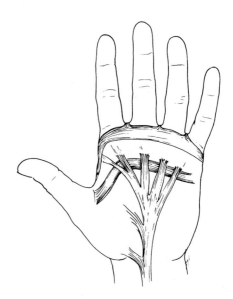

Figure 117-4. Components of the palmar fascia that are susceptible to disease. The pretendinous bands attach to the skin just distal to the distal palmar crease and also continue as spiral bands. The pretendinous band to the thumb and index finger is often deficient. The transverse fibers are at the level of the MCP joints of the fingers; only those in the first web space become diseased. The natatory ligament sweeps across the distal palm and terminates in the skin at the base of the thumb. (From Hall-Findlay EJ: The radial side of the hand. In McFarlane RM, McGrouther DA, Flint MH [editors]: *Dupuytren's disease: biology and treatment* (The Hand and Upper Limb Series), vol 5, Edinburgh, 1990, Churchill Livingstone.)

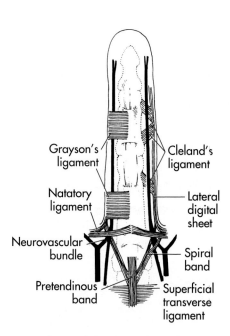

Figure 117-5. Parts of the digital fascia that are susceptible to disease. (From McFarlane RM: *Plastic Reconstr Surg* 54:31, 1974.)

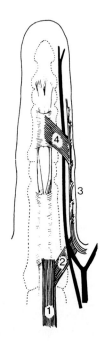

Figure 117-7. The normal parts of the fascia that produce the spiral cord. *1,* Pretendinous band; *2,* spiral band; *3,* lateral digital sheet; *4,* Grayson's ligament. (From McFarlane RM: *Plast Reconstr Surg* 54:31, 1974.)

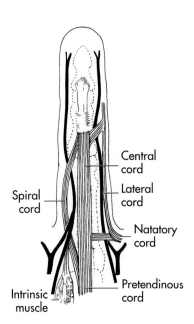

Figure 117-6. The diseased cords that cause contractures of the MCP and PIP joints. (From Chiu HF, McFarlane RM: *J Hand Surg* 3:1, 1978.)

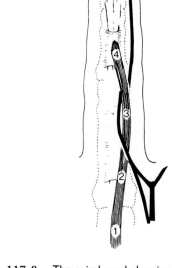

Figure 117-8. The spiral cord showing midaxial displacement of the neurovascular bundle and the four component parts of the spiral cord seen in Figure 117-7. (From McFarlane RM: *Plast Reconstr Surg* 54:31, 1974.)

involvement of the neurovascular bundles. His original diagrams are classics because of their simplicity and are reproduced here (Figures 117-7 and 117-8).

Narrative descriptions of anatomy are of little use to the operating surgeon, but clear mental images of the normal and

pathological anatomy are essential (Figure 117-9). Luck[27] suggested that normal fascia be called bands and that diseased tissue be called cords. Table 117-2 shows the normal bands that become diseased cords and in turn cause joint contractures. It should be emphasized that the pathologic anatomy in

Table 117-2.
Normal Fascial Bands and the Cords and Contractures They Form in Dupuytren's Contracture

NORMAL FASCIA	DISEASED CORDS	CONTRACTURE
Pretendinous band	Pretendinous cord	MCP-joint flexion
Pretendinous band, spiral band, lateral digital sheet, Grayson's ligament	Spiral cord	PIP-joint flexion
Lateral digital sheet	Lateral cord	PIP-joint flexion
None	Central cord	PIP-joint flexion
Natatory ligament	Natatory cord	PIP-joint flexion; MCP-joint adduction
Superficial transverse ligament, deep transverse ligament, Cleland's ligament, Landsmeer's ligament	Usually not involved	None

From Friedman RM: Dupuytren's disease. In Barton FE, Jr: *Selected readings in plastic surgery*, Dallas, 1995, Baylor University Medical Center.

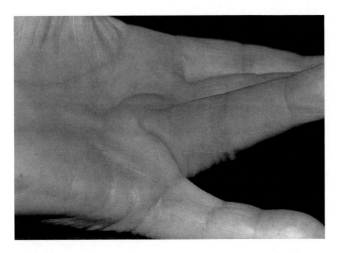

Figure 117-9. A typical pretendinous cord in early disease causing contractures of the right ring-finger MCP joint.

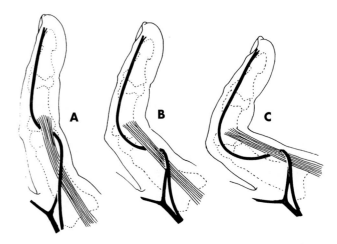

Figure 117-10. The neurovascular bundle is displaced (A) midaxially, (B) proximally, and (C) superficially with increasing contracture of the PIP joint. (From McFarlane RM: Dupuytren's contracture. In Green DP [editor]: *Operative hand surgery*, ed 2, New York, 1988, Churchill Livingstone.)

a severely contracted finger is more distorted than that shown in the Figures 117-4 through 117-8. However, the diagrams here serve to show the relationships between the cords and the neurovascular bundle. The spiral cord in a contracted finger can displace the neurovascular bundle to a more midaxial, superficial and proximal level (Figure 117-10). The spiral cord is the pathologic structure that combines the distal prolongation of the pretendinous cord through the spiral band, which courses dorsal to the neurovascular bundle at the MCP joint level. It subsequently joins the lateral digital sheet, which is lateral to the neurovascular bundle. Distally, this joins Grayson's ligament and attaches to the flexor tendon sheath volar to the neurovascular bundle. The spiral cord, therefore, includes the pretendinous cord, spiral band, lateral digital sheet, and Grayson's ligament. The spiral cord may also originate from the abductor digiti minimi and can cause severe

contractures of the PIP joint of the small finger. The natatory cord can narrow the interdigital web space and prevent separation of the fingers (Figure 117-11).

HISTOPATHOPHYSIOLOGY

Four major theories describe the pathogenesis of Dupuytren's contracture.

1. *Intrinsic theory.* McFarlane[32] reports that Dupuytren's contracture begins with activity in the perivascular fibroblast within the fibrous bundles of normal fascia. The pathologic cords form along the normal fascial bands, with

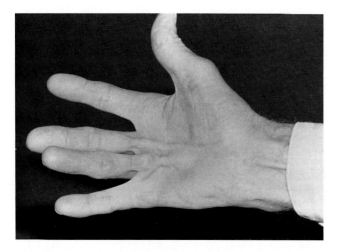

Figure 117-11. Advanced disease involving two pretendinous cords with a natatory cord from the ring finger to both the small and long fingers. Note the adducted long and ring fingers.

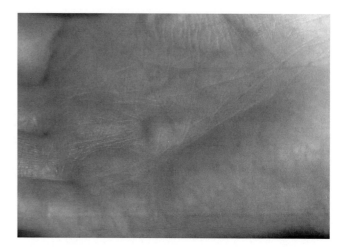

Figure 117-12. A patient with a painful early palmar nodule.

the exception of the central cord, which does not typically have a normal anatomical fascial precursor.

2. *Extrinsic theory.* Hueston[15] reports that the fibrous tissue proliferation starts de novo as nodules superficial to the normal palmar aponeurosis and progresses to cords overlying the aponeurosis.

3. *Synthesis theory.* Gosset[13] combines the intrinsic and extrinsic theories by suggesting that the nodules arise de novo and that the cords arise from the normal, preexisting palmar fascia.

4. *Murrell's hypothesis.* Murrell[19,43] believes that age and genetic and environmental factors contribute to microvessel narrowing with consequent localized ischemia and free radical generation. This can cause damage to the surrounding stroma and stimulate fibroblasts to proliferate.

Regardless of the source of the fibroblast, this cell structurally changes to become the myofibroblast described by Majno[28] and associated with Dupuytren's contracture in 1974.[12] The myofibroblast is present in actively contracting fascia. This process corresponds to Luck's[26] *proliferative phase,* which is followed by the *involutional phase,* in which a dense myofibroblastic network is aligned to the long axis of the collagen bundles. Collagen is actively produced in this subsequent phase, and contraction occurs while the ratio of type-III collagen to type-I collagen increases. In the third phase, known as the *residual phase,* the few myofibroblasts that persist are replaced by more dormant fibrocytes. Current research regarding Dupuytren's contracture is focused at this cellular level.

NONSURGICAL TREATMENT

Nonsurgical treatments, to date, have not been successful. Splints also cannot prevent or reverse contractures. Moreover, ultrasound, laser therapy, and radiation have been ineffective. Vitamin E, collagenolytic agents, and enzymatic fasciotomy

also have not been proven to be of long-term value unless combined with surgical treatment.[1,30,37] However, Ketchum[22] has produced beneficial results by the injection of steroids into early palmar nodules (Figure 117-12) to reduce symptoms. Skeletal traction also has been effective in reversing joint contractures in the preoperative patient.[18,39] Current research is focused at the cellular level to investigate macrophage growth factor, oxygen-free radicals, and the possible role of hypoxia and cytokines. Current studies suggest that transforming growth factor beta has a role in fibroblast proliferation, collagen deposition, and the neovascularization of the Dupuytren's nodule.[44] Perhaps with a clearer understanding of cellular biology we may improve control of the cellular activity. Currently, we are in the "stone age" with regard to the treatment of Dupuytren's contracture. Rather than carve out diseased tissue, genetic engineering should allow us to control the development of the disease. Until this is possible, surgery is our most effective treatment.

INDICATIONS FOR SURGERY

The development of a palmar nodule and cord in the early stages of Dupuytren's contracture are not necessarily indications for surgery. However, some manual workers, such as carpenters and mechanics, have difficulty because the developing nodules can be painful and can interfere with their occupations. If steroid injection of the nodule is ineffective in reducing symptoms, a limited excision of the painful nodule can allow the patient to continue working. The nodules become asymptomatic with time, but some patients require symptomatic relief.

Hueston's[15] "table-top test" determines when a patient has reached the stage of being unable to place the hand flat on a surface because of MCP-joint contracture. Early MCP-joint contractures may be followed, but an MCP-joint contracture of 30 degrees or more should be released.[34] Even severe MCP-joint contractures usually can be completely corrected. Contractures of the PIP joint are not as easily

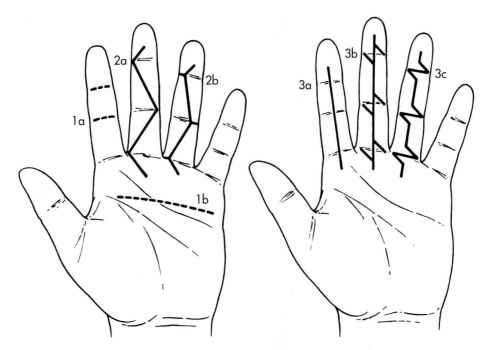

Figure 117-13. Some of the common incisions used to treat Dupuytren's contracture. *1a,* Incisions of both the fingers and palm are used in the "open technique"; *2a,* the most commonly used Bruner zigzag incision; *2b,* the Bruner incision can be closed by advancing the peaks as a Y-to-V closure to gain axial length; *3a,* the straight-line incision must be closed with Z-plasties *(3b)* to prevent a straight-line contracture and to gain axial length *(3c).*

corrected. A PIP-joint contracture of 30 degrees or more is an indication for surgery,[36] as is a severe adduction contracture, which can cause skin breakdown because of the patient's inability to separate the digits. Associated compression neuropathies or triggering digits can be released during the same procedure.

OPERATIONS

It is important to educate patients regarding the surgical treatment and rehabilitation of Dupuytren's contracture so that their expectations are realistic. The goal is to correct both the contractures in the fingers and the cords in the palm. Surgery cannot cure the disease itself. Correction of MCP-joint contractures is usually successful, but PIP-joint contractures are much more difficult to release, cannot always be fully corrected, and have a higher recurrence rate, particularly in the small finger.[36]

FASCIOTOMY

Multiple techniques have been developed since Henry Cline performed the first subcutaneous fasciotomy in England in 1808.[10] This procedure is still used for elderly or debilitated

patients, but in my opinion it has a very limited application. The recurrence rate is high,[7] and the patient is better served by a localized fasciectomy, which can be performed under distal regional block anesthesia with no more stress to the patient than that caused by subcutaneous fasciotomy.

FASCIECTOMY

Fasciectomy is the procedure most commonly performed for surgical treatment of Dupuytren's contracture. It may be limited, regional, or radical.

LIMITED FASCIECTOMY

The limited fasciectomy, as mentioned earlier, is reserved for the debilitated patient or the patient with strictly limited disease. It can be performed under local, median, or ulnar nerve block anesthesia at the wrist. Proximal infiltration of local anaesthetic in the upper arm, at the insertion of the deltoid muscle, blocks the lateral brachial cutaneous nerve of the arm. Medial infiltration at the same level blocks the posterior cutaneous nerve of the arm. No tourniquet discomfort occurs with this block. I prefer Marcaine (bupivacaine) without epinephrine for its extended duration of anesthesia.

Either a limited straight line or a Bruner[5] incision (Figure 117-13) is made over the cord and/or nodule, which is excised together with the surrounding palmar fascia. The tourniquet is released before closure, and meticulous hemostasis is achieved by bipolar coagulation. The skin is closed loosely, and a small Silastic drain may be used, depending on the surgeons' preference.

REGIONAL FASCIECTOMY

Regional fasciectomy is the most common fasciectomy performed for surgical treatment of Dupuytren's contracture. This procedure completely excises the diseased fascia in the palm and digits, but spares the normal-appearing fascia. This operation can be performed under block or general anesthesia, with tourniquet control and loop magnification. The most commonly used incision is the zigzag Bruner (Figure 117-14),[5] but the midaxial, straight-line, longitudinal incision may be used and closed with multiple Z-plasties. A disadvantage of this incision emerges if disease recurs in the finger: the flaps of the Z-plasty are tiny and require special attention during a second procedure in order to avoid ischemia of the flaps.

RADICAL FASCIECTOMY

The radical fasciectomy is reserved for patients with extensive disease, such as those with Dupuytren's diathesis as described by Hueston.[17] Both the diseased and the normal-appearing fascia are excised from the palm and affected fingers. This more extensive resection is accompanied by increased postoperative morbidity because of swelling and stiffness.

DERMATOFASCIECTOMY

Dermatofasciectomy was described by Hueston[16] for patients with aggressive diathesis and skin involvement; both the diseased fascia and the overlying skin are excised. The tissue

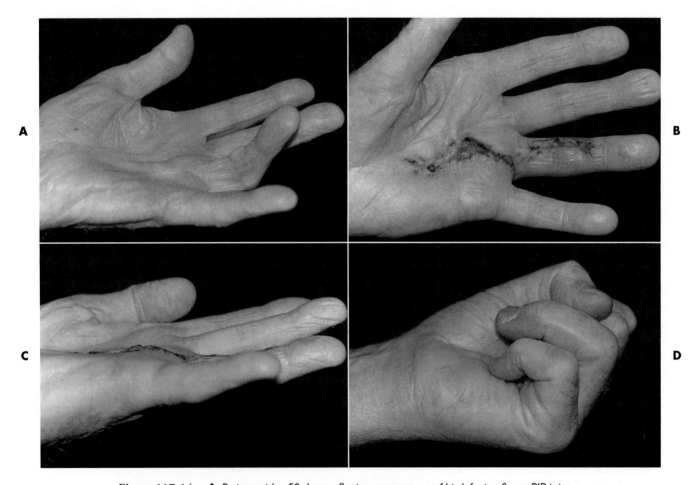

Figure 117-14. **A,** Patient with a 50-degree flexion contracture of his left ring-finger PIP joint, a 25-degree contracture of his MCP joint, and a pretendinous cord in the palm. **B,** Sutures removed 2 weeks after surgery, with healed skin flaps. **C,** Full extension of both MCP and PIP joints 2 weeks after surgery. **D,** Minimal loss of full flexion 2 weeks after surgery.

defect is replaced by a full-thickness skin graft; according to Hueston, this graft decreases the recurrence rate.[14]

OPEN-PALM TECHNIQUE

The open-palm technique described by McCash[31] involves transverse incisions in both the palm and the fingers that are not closed but left open to spontaneously reepithelialize, usually in 4 to 6 weeks. This technique avoids hematoma formation, is painless, and allows immediate mobilization of the fingers. However, daily dressings are required for an extended period.

SKELETAL TRACTION

As mentioned earlier, skeletal traction[39] has been successfully used to straighten contractures. Rapid recurrence takes place after the traction is removed, but the technique is useful for facilitating fasciectomy in severely contracted digits.

SECONDARY PROCEDURES

Surgical resection of the involved fascia cannot cure the disease but attempts to control its symptoms. Both recurrence and extension of the disease occur, and Gonzales[38] found that no patient followed longer than 10 years after the initial procedure was free of disease. Secondary disease presents a far more difficult problem than primary disease. Normal tissue planes are lost after the initial operation, and incisions are generally dictated by previous scars. Elevation of the skin flaps over newly formed diseased fascia necessitates an exacting technique. The neurovascular bundles are frequently very superficial in some areas. They require identification in virgin tissue first, and subsequent meticulous dissection into the diseased fascia. The patency of both the radial and ulnar vascular bundles should be checked because one or the other may have been previously damaged. Unfortunately, normal anatomy does not exist.

AMPUTATIONS

Amputations, as secondary procedures (particularly of the little finger), may result in many problems, including lack of extension, neuroma formation, and phantom limb symptoms. Jensen[21] et al advise alternatives to amputation. However, in specially selected patients who have both aggressive recurrent disease and severe contractures of the PIP joint of the little finger, I have found amputation to be very effective. I dissect the normal dorsal skin off the middle phalanx and perform a dermatofasciectomy, with excision of both the skin and diseased fascia over the volar aspect of the proximal phalanx. This technique com-

pletely frees up the MCP joint. The proximally-based dorsal skin is subsequently used to resurface the volar proximal phalanx. I have not had problems with recurrent flexion contractures, lack of extension, or recurrent disease in these fingers. Patient satisfaction with the procedure has been very high. Moreover, the full width of the palm is retained, which helps stabilize tools such as hammers during power grip.

PREFERRED MANAGEMENT PROGRAM

Initial Consultation

The management program that I prefer is to establish and document the medical status of the patient at the initial consultation, together with important data regarding intercurrent problems and medications. The patient must be advised to stop taking medications that affect coagulation at least 1 week before surgery. A full explanation of the etiology and natural history of Dupuytren's contracture should be given to the patient, together with an assessment of the extent of surgery, the rehabilitation program, and the anticipated outcome. A diagram of the extent of the disease and a measurement of the range of motion of the joints also should be documented. The patient should see a therapist for a full explanation of the postoperative rehabilitation and splinting programs. The patient will be much more compliant with the program when he or she understands what to expect.

Surgical Protocol

All patients are treated as outpatients with the rare exception of the extraordinarily debilitated patient. A regional or general anesthetic is used in addition to local, median, and ulnar nerve blocks with Marcaine (bupivacaine) to prolong postoperative analgesia.

All incisions are drawn; subsequently the arm is elevated and a tourniquet is inflated. Stripping the arm is unnecessary. I prefer to inflate the tourniquet for 90 minutes, with a maximum inflation time of 120 minutes). The tourniquet is inflated to 100 mm of mercury above systolic pressure. The dissection is aided by magnification loops with good quality lenses (approximately four power). The tourniquet is deflated before wound closure, and meticulous hemostasis is achieved with bipolar coagulation. The incisions are loosely closed, and a small Silastic drain is left in the proximal end of each incision. A well-padded dressing and splint are applied with the wrist in neutral and the digits extended but not under pressure. The hand is elevated postoperatively.

The patient is discharged after recovering from the anesthetic, asked to keep the hand at or above the level of the heart, and given a prescription for analgesics. When the patient returns to the clinic the next day, the drains are removed, and a light dressing is applied. The therapist fabricates a thermoplastic splint and immediately initiates a rehabilitation program.

Surgical Technique

I prefer a Bruner incision because the large flaps give excellent exposure and are much easier to dissect in recurrent disease. Alternatively, a midline incision may be used and closed with Z-plasties. The skin flaps are reflected to the radial and ulnar sides at the level of the diseased fascia. The flaps can be sutured to adjacent skin to keep them retracted and to give excellent exposure.

The pretendinous cord is incised proximally and carefully dissected with a scalpel to the level of the MCP joint. As the dissection continues distally, the flexion contracture of the MCP joint is released. It is unnecessary to remove the transverse fibers of the palmar aponeurosis because these are not involved in the disease process. The neurovascular bundles lie dorsal to the transverse fibers. It should not be necessary in primary disease to dissect the neurovascular bundles proximal to the level of the MCP joint.

The neurovascular bundles at this level become more superficial and are dissected. These bundles are subsequently followed distally, until the natatory cords are identified. When a spiral cord is present, the cord itself is usually straight, and the neurovascular bundles spiral around it. Great care must be taken to protect the neurovascular bundles because they are displaced midaxially and volarly. A neurosurgical nerve hook is helpful for retracting the bundle. I prefer to use sharp-pointed curved scissors for the dissection, and all resection must be carried out sharply.

Joint contracture is common at the level of the PIP joint and involves the central cord, the spiral cord, and the lateral cord. Full extension may not be achieved in long-standing cases of severe contracture. Excision of the volar checkrein ligaments as described by Watson[51] may be helpful. In long-standing contractures, another restricting structure at the PIP joint is the tendon sheath itself, which is shortened longitudinally. The sheath can be incised, but care must be taken to provide adequate skin cover for this area of exposed tendon.

Controversy exists regarding the benefit of capsulotomy of the PIP joint to gain more extension after fasciectomy alone. Weinzweig[52] reports "no statistically significant difference in the percentage of contracture correction in the capsulotomy group compared with the noncapsulotomy group at follow up." However, complications "tended to occur more commonly in the capsulotomy group."

Special attention should be paid to the little finger, which is frequently more severely affected than the other fingers.[38] Correction is not as successful in this finger and the recurrence of contracture is more frequent. McFarlane[37] favors skin closure by graft if the disease is extensive or if the PIP-joint contracture exceeds 45 degrees.

The disease is often extensive on the ulnar side of the small finger. Both the spiral cord and the lateral cord arise from the tendon insertion of the abductor digiti minimi into the proximal phalanx and contribute to the flexion contracture at the PIP joint. The neurovascular bundle is displaced and surrounded by extensively diseased cords, thereby making dissection difficult. The surgeon must use extreme care and

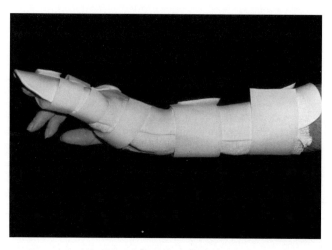

Figure 117-15. A dorsal-based forearm splint that allows application of a dynamic extension force.

accurate dissection using loop magnification, separating the neurovascular bundle and excising the diseased fascia. Less than complete extension of the PIP joint must be accepted in severe or long-standing cases. Attempts to gain full extension may result in compromise of the digital arteries, resulting in devascularization of the digit, which must be avoided.

Postoperative Management

Most patients undergo surgery as outpatients and return to the clinic the next day. The preoperative educational program is most beneficial at this time because the patient expects to conform to the protocol that was carefully explained at the initial consultation.

The dressings, splint, and drains are removed, and the hand is carefully checked for early problems such as undue swelling, hematoma formation, or wound complications. It is most unusual to encounter any of these potential difficulties at this stage. A light dressing is applied, and the patient's care is immediately referred to a hand therapist at the hand clinic.

The therapist already has a preoperative, well-documented baseline of the patient. Additional information from the surgical procedure, such as the amount of correction gained at surgery, the degree of any remaining contractures, the extent of the wound, and the reaction of the patient and the tissue to surgery is recorded. The splinting requirements of patients are assessed on an individual basis. Isolated palmar involvement without contracture does not require splinting, and a range-of-motion program with light hand use is initiated on the first postoperative day.

The hand of a patient with early disease may be easily positioned in extension with a volar-based hand splint. A forearm-based splint is used when there is more extensive involvement. The wrist position varies from zero to 20 degrees of extension, but is commonly in the neutral (zero-degree) position. This position improves the mechanical advantage of the splint to help counteract the shortened flexor tendons or tight volar structures. The forearm-based splint may be volar or dorsal. The dorsal splint (Figure 117-15) is used if maximum extension of the digits is not easily achieved. This

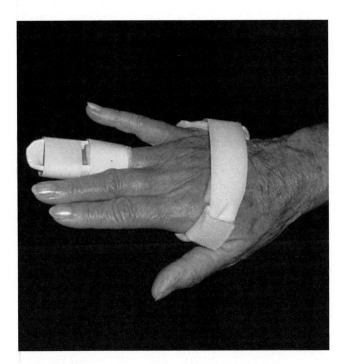

Figure 117-16. A hand-based extension splint.

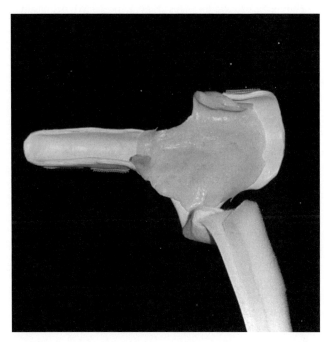

Figure 117-17. An elastomer insert to help control wound hypertrophy in a hand-based extension splint.

type of splint can add a "dynamic" component to the treatment because the individual digital straps can be progressively tightened to bring the digits closer to the splint base. A dorsal splint also avoids pressure on the healing skin flaps.

Therapy programs are tailored to each case. The patient is instructed to remove the splint for dressing changes with skin care as directed and to perform (four to six times per day) specific, gentle, active range-of-motion exercises, including composite flexion and extension. The patient's progress is carefully monitored, and the program usually can be upgraded at the end of the first week.

Sutures are removed 2 weeks after surgery and the patient's progress is reassessed. A dorsal splint may be remolded into a volar splint, which allows pressure to be exerted over the healing incision to assist in scar resolution. At the therapist's discretion, the program is upgraded to night splinting with intermittent day use to ensure that the patient achieves full flexion while maintaining active extension. Splinting is gradually decreased, but can be maintained at night for 3 to 6 months, depending on the patient's tendency to lose full range of motion. All patients are monitored closely by a therapist for at least 6 weeks, at which time the therapy program progresses to full hand use and strengthening.

Dynamic splinting is instituted if recurrent flexion contractures occur during the course of treatment. Edema is controlled by retrograde massage, elevation, icing, and self-adherent wrap (Coban) when necessary. Scar resolution is aided by friction massage after the sutures have been removed. Self-adherent wrap (Coban) with an interface of gel sheeting or silicone elastomer in combination with a volar splint have been very helpful in scar control (Figures 117-16 and 117-17). Ultrasound and laser treatments have been useful in patients

with very reactive tissues. However, continuous passive motion has not proven to be beneficial in the postoperative management of Dupuytren's contracture.[47]

The successful management of a patient with Dupuytren's contracture requires a team of highly trained, dedicated professionals; one physician cannot provide optimal management alone.*

OUTCOMES

COMPLICATIONS

Complications occur frequently. A large multicenter survey reported a complication rate of 19% (Box 117-2).[34] The incidence of hematoma can be decreased by ensuring that the patient discontinues aspirin, anticoagulants, nonsteroidal anti-inflammatory agents, vitamin E, vitamin B_{12}, and any other agent known to affect coagulation before surgery. These agents may be restarted on the first day after surgery.

Careful coagulation of bleeding vessels is completed using bipolar coagulation after tourniquet deflation and before wound closure. I leave a small Silastic drain in the proximal portion of each incision. The hand should be checked on the first postoperative day. If a hematoma is present, it must be thoroughly evacuated and copiously irrigated under sterile conditions; aspiration alone is usually not sufficient.

*This postoperative management section was written in conjunction with Ms. Carolyn Van Gool, Ms. Catherine Vandersluis, and the occupational therapists at London Health Sciences Centre, University Campus.

Flap necrosis can be caused by a neglected hematoma, devascularization of the flaps, or button holing of the flaps while reflecting the skin at the start of surgery. Dissection is made more difficult by palmar pits, severely contracted joints, or recurrent disease. Magnification loupes are invaluable in these situations because they allow the surgeon to remove all diseased tissue while preserving normal structures. The open-palm technique avoids hematoma formation and skin necrosis. Foucher[11] reports that postoperative complications associated with a modified open-palm technique were much lower than complications reported in comparable series of limited aponeurectomy. Infection is rare but can accompany a hematoma. When this occurs, the wound should be adequately drained and cultured. Appropriate systemic antibiotics, repeated local dressing changes, and elevation of the hand are also mandatory. Swelling from an infection is accompanied by joint stiffness; thus appropriate guarded therapy should be started early.

Nerve and vessel injuries can occur in the most expert hands, particularly during secondary procedures. Such injuries must be immediately recognized to avoid resection of nerve and vessel, which may compound the problem. A nerve injury should be repaired before closure by microsurgical technique. Even after uncomplicated fasciectomies, when the nerve is in continuity, sensation to the digit often is decreased. In a multicenter survey, decreased flexion was reported to occur at a rate of 6%, but McFarlane[36] believes that this complication is more common. Postoperative swelling must be approached aggressively, and if swelling occurs, the patient and therapist must work diligently on both flexion and extension of the IP joints during therapy.

Reflex sympathetic dystrophy has been reported in 4% of male patients and in 8% of female patients.[38] Dystrophy should be differentiated from the flare reaction that reflects soft tissue response to the trauma of surgery. Complaints of swelling, stiffness, and burning pain, sometimes occurring several weeks after surgery, should cause the surgeon to suspect reflex sympathetic dystrophy. Active therapy in conjunction with the use of nonsteroidal antiinflammatory agents, elevation, and sympathetic blocks are useful and help to alleviate these symptoms. I also have found it helpful to enlist the aid of our rehabilitation department in treating refractory cases.

CLINICAL OUTCOMES

Legge[23] reported that treatment outcomes for Dupuytren's contracture are influenced by many factors. The variables of significance in this series included the number of rays involved, the finger involved, the joint involved, and the preoperative degree of contracture ($p < 0.01$; Boxes 117-3 and 117-4).

"The age and sex of the patient, a family history of Dupuytren's disease, and the presence of involvement beyond the volar surface of the hand did not have any *predictable* effect on the results ($p < 0.01$)" in this series, which applied multiple regression analysis to these variables.

Rives[44] found a statistically significant difference in the mean improvement in PIP-joint extension in patients who complied with the postoperative dynamic extension splinting program, compared with patients who were noncompliant. This study suggests that "soft tissue responds to continuous dynamic extension stresses and can be remodelled over time."

The data in Table 117-3 confirm that the MCP joint usually can be significantly corrected. However, the interphalangeal joints are rarely completely corrected, particularly in the little finger. As indicated earlier, the little finger proximal interphalangeal (PIP) joint is frequently affected by more severe disease.[34]

Healy[2] reported the development of a "statistically valid outcome measure for assessing symptom and function scores and patient satisfaction after surgical correction of Dupuytren's disease" using the SF-36 questionnaire. Patient satisfaction strongly correlated with improved postoperative

---

Box 117-3.
Important Variables in Correction of PIP-Joint Contracture in the Little Finger

Preoperative contracture of MCP joint
Preoperative contracture of PIP joint
Number of rays involved
E (a constant)

From Legge JWH, McFarlane RM: Predictions and results of treatment of Dupuytren's disease, *J Hand Surg Am* 608:5, 1980.

Box 117-2.
Frequency of Complications After Surgery for Dupuytren's Disease

Hematoma, skin loss, or infection	3%
Nerve or arterial division	3%
Loss of flexion	6%
Reflex sympathetic dystrophy	5%
Overall	19%

From McFarlane RM: Dupuytren's disease. In McCarthy JG (editor): *Plastic surgery*, Philadelphia, 1990, WB Saunders.

Box 117-4.
Important Variables in Correction of PIP-Joint Contractures of the Index, Middle, and Ring Fingers

Preoperative contracture of PIP joint
Number of rays involved
E (a constant)

From Legge JWH, McFarlane RM: Predictions and results of treatment of Dupuytren's disease, *J Hand Surg Am* 608:5, 1980.

Table 117-3.
Correction of Flexion Contracture in Each Joint in Each Finger After 1202 Operations (6-18 Months After Surgery)

	LITTLE			RING			MIDDLE			INDEX			THUMB		
	N	PRE	POST	N	PRE	POST	N	PRE	POST	N	PRE	POST	N	PRE	POST
MCP joint	258	44.1±24.8*	3.2±11.1	251	36.3±20.0	2.5±8.4	126	28.1±16.3	2.3±7.5	27	23.3±15.2	4.6±9.3	16	19.6±11.6	8.8±17.2
Outcome[†]															
Perfect	84%	42.8±24.1	0	86%	34.3±18.9	0	87%	27.9±15.9	0	78%	21.1±12.2	0	69%	21.5±11.2	0
Improved	13%	54.9±25.3	14.3±11.2	12%	52.5±20.4	15.3±14.0	10%	31.1±20.8	14.8±8.1	11%	45.0±26.0	20.0±10.0	6%	35.0	30.0
Same/worse	3%	31.4±31.5	46.4±35.9	2%	22.0±16.8	29.0±21.3	3%	25.0±17.3	27.5±20.6	11%	16.7±5.8	21.7±2.9	25%	10.4±7.1	27.5±24.0
PIP joint	263	52.9±25.2	27.2±23.0	138	49.5±26.5	16.9±21.0	42	39.6±21.6	20.8±21.5						
Outcome															
Perfect	19%	46.5±23.8	0	45%	41.7±24.1	0	36%	30.3±14.3	0						
Improved	56%	63.2±21.3	28.8±17.4	42%	64.3±22.8	29.0±18.2	43%	50.4±20.7	26.4±13.4						
Same/worse	25%	34.9±22.7	44.9±23.3	13%	28.2±19.8	36.2±22.7	21%	33.7±25.6	44.2±22.1						
DIP joint	52	26.9±17.0	8.8±11.9	23	32.8±28.1	4.0±10.5	6	18.3±16.0	9.2±20.1						
Outcome															
Perfect	56%	20.9±15.2	0	82%	29.5±23.8	0	66%	12.5±5.0	0						
Improved	33%	38.6±15.4	16.6±7.7	9%	87.0±4.2	32.5±17.7	17%	10.0	5.0						
Same/worse	11%	23.0±13.7	29.7±8.9	9%	10.0±7.1	14.0±1.4	17%	50.0	50.0						

From McFarlane RM: Dupuytren's disease. In McCarthy JG (editor): *Plastic surgery*, Philadelphia, 1990, WB Saunders.
*Mean ± Standard deviation.
[†]Perfect: Flexion contracture was completely corrected.
Improved: Flexion contracture was less but not completely corrected.
Same/worse: There was no correction or the flexion contracture was worse.

function scores, improved postoperative symptom scores, and surgery on the dominant hand.

SUMMARY

Management of the patient with Dupuytren's contracture encompasses the whole spectrum of care of the surgical patient. Dupuytren's contracture is not life-threatening but also is not curable. Education is essential to ensure that the patient understands the natural history of the disease and the limitations of current treatment methods. Contractures of the MCP joint are in most cases completely corrected, but contractures of the IP joint often cannot be fully corrected and thus tend to recur more frequently. The disease has a strong genetic basis and is progressive.

Most patients are treated as outpatients, greatly reducing the cost to the health care system. However, surgical treatment and required postoperative rehabilitation significantly restricts the patient's personal and occupational activities for several months. This treatment protocol will change as we accumulate more information about the cellular biology of this disease and develop more sophisticated ways to exert control at a cellular level. Dupuytren's contracture has a strong genetic basis and the most productive avenue of research will likely involve genetic engineering. The future holds great promise!

REFERENCES

1. Berger A, Pelbruck A, Brenner P, et al: *Dupuytren's disease*, New York, 1994, Springer-Verlag.
2. Bodalamente MA, Healy W, Hurst LC, et al: An outcome study in Dupuytren's disease, *Am Soc Surg Hand* (51st meeting abstract) 24, 1996.
3. Bower M, Nelson M, Gazzard BG: Dupuytren's contracture in patients infected with HIV, *BMJ* 300:164, 1990.
4. Bradlow R, Mowat AG: Dupuytren's contracture and alcohol, *Ann Rheum Dis* 45:304-307, 1986.
5. Bruner JM: The zig-zag volar-digital incision for flexor tendon surgery, *Plast Reconstr Surg* 40:571, 1967.
6. Classen DJ, Hurst LN: Plantar fibromatosis: a case report of bilateral flexion contractures and review of the literature, *Ann Pl Surg* 28:475, 1992.
7. Coville J: Dupuytren's contracture: the role of fasciotomy, *Hand* 15:162, 1983.
8. Crisp AJ, Heathcote JG: Connective tissue abnormalities in diabetes mellitus, *J R Coll Physicians Lond* 18:132, 1984.
9. Critchley EMR, Vakil SD, Hayward HW, et al: Dupuytren's disease in epilepsy: result of prolonged administration of anticonvulsants, *J Neural Neurosurg Psychiatry* 39:498-504, 1976.
10. Elliot D: The early history of contracture of the palmar fascia, *J Hand Surg [Br]* 13:246, 1988.
11. Foucher G, Cornil C, Levoble E, et al: A modified open-palm technique for Dupuytren's disease: short and long term results in 54 patients, *International Ortho Abst* 19(5):285, 1995.
12. Gabbiani G, Majno G: Dupuytren's contracture: fibroblast contraction, *Am J Pathol* 66:131, 1972.
13. Gossett J: Dupuytren's disease and the anatomy of the palmodigital aponeurosis. In Hueston JT, Tubiano R (editors): *Dupuytren's disease,* London, 1985, Churchill Livingstone.
14. Hueston JT: The control of recurrent Dupuytren's contracture by skin replacement, *Br J Plast Surg* 11:152, 1969.
15. Hueston JT: Dupuytren's contracture: selection for surgery, *Br J Hosp Med* 13:361, 1974.
16. Hueston JT: Dermatofasciectomy for Dupuytren's disease, *Bull Hosp Joint Dis* 44:224, 1984.
17. Hueston JT: State of the art: the management of recurrent Dupuytren's disease, *Eur Med Bibliography* 1:7, 1991.
18. Hueston JT: Regression of Dupuytren's contracture, *J Hand Surg [Br]* 17:453, 1992.
19. Hueston JT, Murrell GA: Cell-controlling factors in Dupuytren's contracture, *Ann Chir Main* 9:135, 1990.
20. Hurst LC: *Hand surgery update,* vol 1, Englewood, Colo, 1994, The American Society for Surgery of the Hand.
21. Jensen CM, Hangegaard M, Rasmussen SW: Amputations in the treatment of Dupuytren's disease, *J Hand Surg [Br]* 18:781, 1993.
22. Ketchum LD: The use of the full thickness skin graft in Dupuytren's contracture, *Hand Clin* 7:731, 1991.
23. Legge JWH, McFarlane RM: Prediction of results of treatment of Dupuytren's disease, *J Hand Surg [Am]* 5:608, 1980.
24. Ling RSM: The genetic factors in Dupuytren's disease, *J Bone Joint Surg* 45B:709, 1963.
25. Liss GM, Stock SR: Can Dupuytren's contracture be work related? Review of the evidence, *Am J Indus Med* 29:521, 1996.
26. Luck JV: Dupuytren's contracture, *J Bone Joint Surg* 41A:635, 1959.
27. Luck JV: Dupuytren's contracture: a new concept of the pathogenesis correlated with surgical management, *J Bone Joint Surg* 41A:635, 1959.
28. Majno G, Gabbiani G, Hirschel BJ, et al: Contraction of granulation tissue in vitro, *Science* 173:548, 1971.
29. Matthews P: Familial Dupuytren's contracture with predominantly female expression, *Br J Plast Surg* 32:120, 1979.
30. McCarthy DM: The long term results of enzymatic fasciotomy, *J Hand Surg [Br]* 17:356, 1992.
31. McCash CR: The open-palm technique in Dupuytren's contracture, *Br J Plast Surg* 17:271, 1964.
32. McFarlane RM: Patterns of the diseased fascia in the fingers in Dupuytren's contracture, *Plast Reconstr Surg* 54:31-44, 1974.
33. McFarlane RM: Unpublished data from the Dupuytren's disease committee of the International Federation of Societies for Surgery of the Hand, 1985.
34. McFarlane RM: Dupuytren's disease. In McCarthy JG (editor): *Plastic surgery,* Philadelphia, 1990, WB Saunders.
35. McFarlane RM: Dupuytren's disease: relation to work and injury, *J Hand Surg [Am]* 16:775, 1991.

36. McFarlane RM: Dupuytren's contracture. In Green DP, (editor): *Operative hand surgery*, New York, 1993, Churchill Livingstone.

37. McFarlane RM: The current status of Dupuytren's disease, *J Hand Ther* 8:181, 1995.

38. McFarlane RM, Botz JS: The results of treatment. In McFarlane RM, McGrouther DA, Flint MH (editors): *Dupuytren's disease: biology and treatment* (hand and upper limb series), New York, 1990, Churchill Livingstone

39. Messina A, Messina J: The continuous elongation treatment by the TEC device for severe Dupuytren's contracture of the fingers, *Plast Reconstr Surg* 92:84, 1993.

40. Mikkelsen OR: The prevalence of Dupuytren's disease in Norway, *Acta Chir Scand* 138:695, 1972.

41. Murrell GA: An insight into Dupuytren's contracture, *Ann Roy Coll Surgeons England* 74:156, 1992.

42. Murrell GA, Francis MJ, Bromley L: Free radicals and Dupuytren's contracture, *Br Med J* 295:1373, 1987.

43. Noble J, Heathcote JG, Cohen H: Diabetes mellitus in the etiology of Dupuytren's disease, *J Bone Joint Surg* 66B;322, 1984.

44. Rabinovsky ED, Weinfeld AB, Barrows T, et al: The role of transforming growth factor (TGF-6) in Dupuytren's contracture, *Am Assoc Hand Surg* (27th meeting abs) 54, 1997.

45. Rives K, Gelberman R, Smith B, Carney K: Severe contractures of the proximal interphalangeal joint in Dupuytren's disease: results of a prospective trial of operative correction and dynamic extension splinting, *J Hand Surg [Am]* 17:1153, 1992.

46. Sabiston DW: Cataracts, Dupuytren's contracture, and alcohol addiction, *Am J Ophthalmol* 76:1005, 1973.

47. Sampson SP, Badalamente MA, Hurst LC, et al: The use of a passive motion machine in the post operative rehabilitation of Dupuytren's disease, *J Hand Surg [Am]* 17:333, 1992.

48. Stack HG: The palmar fascia and the development of deformities and displacements in Dupuytren's contracture, *Ann Roy Coll Surgeons England* 48:238, 1971.

49. Su CK, Patek AJ Jr: Dupuytren's contracture: its association with alcoholism and cirrhosis, *Arch Intern Med* 126:278, 1970.

50. Thomine JM: Le fascia digital development et anatomie. InTubiana R (editor): *La Maladie de Dupuytren*, ed 2, Paris, 1972, Expansion Scientific Francais.

51. Watson HK, Terry R, Light MD, et al: Checkrein resection for flexion contracture of the middle joint, *J Hand Surg [Am]* 4:67, 1979.

52. Weinzweig N, Culver JE, Fleegler EJ: Severe contractures of the proximal interphalangeal joint in Dupuytren's disease: combined fasciectomy with capsuloligamentous release versus fasciectomy alone, *J Plast Reconstr Surg* 97:521, 1996.

PART VIII

NERVE

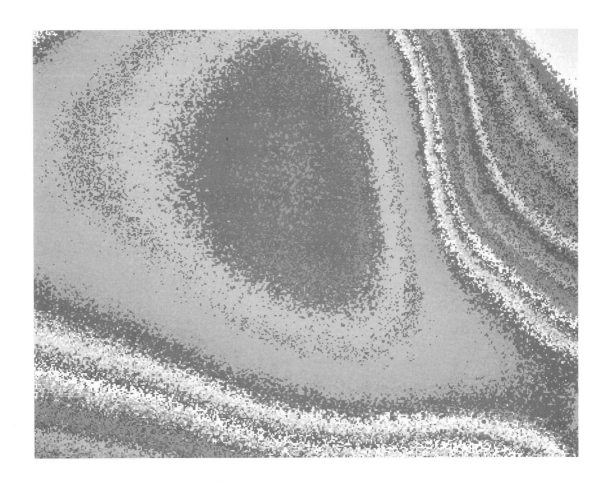

Brachial Plexus

118

Julia K. Terzis
Marios D. Vekris
Panayotis N. Soucacos

INTRODUCTION

Brachial plexus palsies are devastating injuries. They occur either during birth (because of a difficult delivery) or later in life. The majority are posttraumatic—usually caused by motor vehicle accidents and most often affecting young people during the most productive years of their lives.

Obstetric palsies, which have a better prognosis, have two primary characteristics. First, patients experience a functional compromise, which results from a paralyzed limb, and second, a limb-length discrepancy occurs, which develops over time from prolonged denervation of the growing skeleton.

The socioeconomic impact on patients with posttraumatic palsies is considerable. The patient faces either permanent disability (i.e., an inability to use the paralyzed extremity) or a prolonged recuperation. Many patients must be retrained in an occupation that requires less use of the extremity.

Precise and proper evaluation of the nerve lesion(s) is essential for primary management and to establish a reconstructive plan to provide the best function to the affected extremity. Intensive rehabilitation and psychological support are required to return these patients to society as quickly as possible.

The number of severe posttraumatic brachial plexus injuries that occur each year is increasing because of an increased survival rate after motor vehicle accidents, which currently are treated by advanced resuscitation techniques. Despite extensive experience and current sophisticated methods of treatment, debate continues regarding the best way to manage these devastating injuries.

Obstetric brachial plexus injuries typically are mild traction injuries of the upper brachial plexus and may show spontaneous recovery with conservative treatment. Posttraumatic brachial plexus lesions typically are severe and are characterized by a lack of functional return, except in cases of neurapraxia. Currently the method of choice for treating traumatic injuries and more extended and severe cases of obstetric brachial plexus palsy involves the use of aggressive early microsurgical reconstruction. Various modern techniques are used in combination, including neurotizations with ipsilateral and contralateral intraplexus and extraplexus nerve donors, free vascularized nerve grafts (e.g., vascularized ulnar nerve), and free vascularized and neurotized muscle flaps.

The goal of this multistage microsurgical management is the restoration of extremity function, even in patients with severe avulsion injuries involving distal targets such as the extrinsic and intrinsic muscles of the forearm and hand.

INDICATIONS

ESTABLISHMENT OF DIAGNOSIS

Meticulous evaluation of a brachial plexus injury is essential in reaching an accurate diagnosis of the lesion and in establishing a strategy for reconstruction. A comprehensive preoperative assessment includes a detailed history of the mechanism of injury, a thorough physical examination, and appropriate ancillary studies such as neuroradiologic studies, plain radiographs, occasional angiography, and electrophysiologic evaluations.

History

All possible information must be obtained from the patient and family and from any previous medical record related to the injury to determine the exact mechanism of injury to the plexus, such as traction, compression, or direct laceration (as occurs from a gunshot or knife injury).

Motor vehicle accidents are the most common cause of injury. The velocity of the collision is important because a high-velocity impact to the plexus can indicate possible root avulsion and/or severe and extended postganglionic damage. In contrast, application of a minor force may indicate the rupture of plexus elements.

The arm and head position in relation to the axis of the body at the time of injury may help identify the region of the plexus involved. Shoulder abduction of more than 90 degrees at the time of injury suggests a greater chance of a lower-plexus (C8 and T1) injury. The upper plexus (C5 and C6) is most likely involved when the arm has been pulled downward. Traction away from the body with the arm in 90 degrees abduction results in central plexus (C7) involvement.

The majority of brachial plexus lesions, with the exception of open injuries and lesions associated with concomitant vascular injuries, are not treated as emergencies but are managed in specialized centers. The reconstructive microsurgeon must be informed of associated injuries because they may alter the clinical picture and surgical planning.

Fractures and/or dislocations often indicate a coexistent distal lesion of brachial plexus components. Such lesions occur when nerves are severed either directly from bone fragments or from traction, or secondarily from scar tissue formation.

The following areas are of particular importance:

1. *Cervical spine:* Fractures of the transverse processes indicate preganglionic plexus injury.
2. *Clavicle:* A fracture indicates severe scarring of the retroclavicular plexus and may involve a compression lesion from bone fragments or iatrogenic injury from osteosynthesis material.
3. *Scapula:* Fracture of the suprascapular or spinoglenoid notch raises the suspicion of a lesion on the suprascapular nerve more distally.
4. *Shoulder dislocation:* The axillary nerve is frequently traumatized in a shoulder dislocation.
5. *Humerus:* The radial nerve may be torn or compressed with a midshaft humeral fracture or may be injured during osteosynthesis.
6. *Radius and ulna:* Fractures at the forearm may result in additional direct nerve trauma or can be the cause of a compartment syndrome, which can create secondary damage to nerves in the forearm.

Associated vascular injuries typically indicate a severe nerve injury. The majority of these vascular lesions involve the subclavian or axillary arteries. Transections of the subclavian artery typically are associated with major brachial plexus lesions. Emergency surgical intervention to repair the vascular supply to the limb invariably causes scarring, which makes subsequent microneural reconstruction extremely difficult. Moreover, alterations in the normal vascular anatomy of the region from placement of one or more interpositional vein grafts increase the potential for vascular injury during secondary nerve reconstruction.

Many patients have other types of associated trauma, which in some cases may be life threatening. Such trauma may include abdominal injury with intraperitoneal hemorrhage, or thoracic injury, such as chest contusion or pneumothorax. Patients who experience loss of consciousness must undergo a detailed neurologic examination to rule out intracranial hemorrhage; such patients can develop neurologic and/or psychologic deficits, which may prevent optimal rehabilitation because of the patient's inability to cooperate after surgery.

The presence or absence of pain, its initiation period, and its characteristics (including causal factors, frequency, intensity, duration, type, and responsiveness to treatment) are important considerations; they assist in determining a patient's diagnosis and prognosis and also play a role in surgical planning. Pain that appears at the time of injury or soon afterward and is persistent, severe, and localized in the hand typically indicates a C8 and/or a T1 root avulsion.

Physical Examination

INSPECTION. The upper extremity and scapulothoracic region should be inspected bilaterally and the extent of muscle atrophy and asymmetry should be determined. Wasting of the paraspinal muscles indicates a high cervical nerve avulsion injury. Loss of neck-to-shoulder symmetry or the presence of torticollis suggests trauma to the ipsilateral accessory nerve. Other observations may include subluxation of the shoulder and/or winging of the scapula, which characterize injury to C5, C6, and C7 nerve roots.

Wasting of the lower pectoral region and nipple area indicates a C8 and T1 involvement. The presence of Horner's syndrome (ptosis, miosis, and anhidrosis of the ipsilateral face) indicates injury to the white rami of the lower roots to the stellate ganglion and signifies a partial or complete avulsion of C8 and/or T1 roots.

Bone deformities and external scars may indicate multiple-level nerve lesions. Skin neurotrophic changes and discoloration, as well as joint contractures and abnormal postures, especially in the hand, should be recorded.

EXAMINATION. The muscles of the shoulder girdle and upper extremity are tested for strength and are compared with those of the opposite (normal) side. The evaluation begins proximally, and the strength of each muscle is tested precisely and graded by the manual muscle test of the British Medical Research Council Grading System. A scale of 0 to 5 is used, with 5 indicating normal strength, and the values are recorded on a brachial plexus chart. Passive range of motion of the joints in the cervical spine, shoulder, elbow, wrist, and hand also is measured. Maintenance of joint mobility is critical throughout the rehabilitation period; recovery is useless in the presence of joint contractures.

A full neurologic examination is carried out to detect any deficit in the ipsilateral lower limb or the contralateral upper limb, to rule out a Brown-Sequard lesion or severe medullary damage caused by root avulsions.

A thorough examination of the peripheral pulses, including an Allen's test, is essential to detect any differences in comparison with the normal extremity. The arterial pulses can be checked by Doppler in questionable cases.

A complete sensory evaluation is performed, which assesses touch, pain, static and moving two-point discrimination, joint position, and vibration submodalities (as tested with 30-and 256-cycle/sec tuning forks). The ninhydrin sweat test and thermography of the palms are carried out to measure sudomotor function and temperature changes. A positive ninhydrin test in an anesthetic territory indicates a lesion proximal to the rami communicantes of the autonomic nervous system and therefore an avulsion of the roots from the spinal cord.[7]

When these tests have been completed, the patient undergoes an examination for Tinel's sign. Each peripheral nerve is percussed (distally to proximally) along its anatomic pathway. The perception of a tingling sensation by the patient indicates the site of the most distal viable fibers of that nerve that have a central connection. The supraclavicular area, along the posterior border of the sternocleidomastoid muscle, is percussed last. The patient is asked to identify the area in the upper extremity in which he or she perceives a tingling sensation. The cutaneous distribution of each root is assessed by this technique. If there is perception in a skin region supplied by a specific root, that nerve root is considered to have continuity with the spinal cord. The examiner must be aware of dermatome overlap and variability in the sensory distribution of each spinal nerve.[14] The absence of a Tinel's sign in the supraclavicular region carries a grave prognosis because it signifies total plexus avulsion. Descent of Tinel's sign over time indicates the progression of regeneration and also can be used to determine the speed of regeneration.

Electrodiagnostic Studies

Electrodiagnostic evaluation involves electromyography, measurement of nerve conduction velocities and sensory potentials, and the percutaneous stimulation test (Lamina test).

Electromyography identifies fibrillations and positive sharp waves, which are indicators of denervation. These signals appear 2 to 4 weeks after a nerve injury, depending on the distance between the site of nerve injury and the examined muscle (the longer the distance, the later these signs develop). Electrodiagnostic studies are repeated at 6-week intervals when the cervical myelogram shows no evidence of root avulsion. If there is no evidence of recovery (even in the proximal musculature) after 3 months, surgical exploration and reconstruction are indicated.

A recording of polyphasic low-amplitude potentials or nascent reinnervation potentials constitutes a positive sign of reinnervation. Other positive signs of reinnervation in repeated electromyograms include a reduction in the number of fibrillations and positive sharp waves, and the increasing appearance (recruitment) of voluntarily activated motor units that form an "interference pattern." However, these electromyographic findings do not necessarily correspond to actual clinical muscle function and are not predictive of the exact level of functional recovery because a muscle may have near normal electrical activity without useful function. The interpretation of electrophysiologic data taken from patients with brachial plexus lesions should be carried out by a physician who has had experience with traumatic plexopathies.

Motor conduction velocity studies test the integrity of the peripheral motor neuron, indicate the severity of nerve involvement preoperatively, and measure the rate of recovery postoperatively. The number of motor units in innervated muscles can be estimated indirectly, by calculating the amplitude of the elicited compound-muscle action potential during motor conduction velocity studies.

The presence of a sensory nerve action potential (SNAP) and a normal sensory conduction velocity in the peripheral nerves innervating a clinically paralyzed and anesthetized extremity (after a brachial plexus injury) invariably implies root avulsion with preservation of the dorsal root ganglion. The clinically anesthetized arm with postganglionic lesions has an absence of SNAPs because of denervation of the sensory fibers distal to the lesion. However, this absence does not rule out the possibility of avulsion because a double-level lesion (rupture and avulsion) may be present.

The integrity of the sensory conduction from the peripheral nerves to the central nervous system can be assessed by the use of somatosensory evoked potentials.

In 1987 Liberson modified a technique of percutaneous lamina stimulation of the exiting spinal nerves that initially was adopted by MacLean.[48] This method allows the patient to identify the site or finger in which the stimulus is perceived. A positive response is strong evidence against avulsion injury in the stimulated spinal nerve.

Radiologic Examination

RADIOGRAPHS. Plain radiographs of the cervical spine, shoulder, clavicle, and other bones of the upper extremity are carried out as needed because, as previously mentioned, fractures may indicate secondary lesions to the involved nerves.

Inspiratory and expiratory chest radiographs and fluoroscopic studies are performed to determine whether the diaphragm is paralyzed, a condition that implies a high plexus lesion. In the presence of a thoracic injury, further investigation with chest and rib radiographs must be performed to rule out rib fractures. The intercostal nerves at sites along fractured ribs are not good donor nerves for neurotization.

NEURORADIOLOGY. Cervical myelograms have been used since the 1950s to provide an accurate impression of brachial plexus injury patterns. They can reveal pseudomeningoceles and deviation of the spinal nerve roots, indicating avulsion injuries. Despite reports of a high percentage of accuracy (84%), false-negative and/or false-positive results (9%) can occur during surgical exploration of the plexus. A cervical myelogram followed by axial computed tomography (CT) of the cervical spine has been used since 1983 in our center to evaluate the dorsal and ventral roots. This combination has considerably decreased false-negative or doubtful results (3.5% with CT myelography compared with 12% for standard myelography).[35]

A postmyelographic CT scan reveals slight intradural abnormalities, such as small diverticula or missing rootlets, which are not visible on a myelogram. It also can allow visualization of roots deviated by large meningoceles. However, a potential disadvantage of CT is poor imaging of the lower roots because of their oblique course and because of interference from the bulk of the shoulders. Despite its usefulness and low percentage of false-positive results (2.5%), a CT myelogram does not allow visualization of the distal extraforaminal part of the roots.[25]

MRI is a noninvasive method that can reveal the roots beyond the spinal foramina. Retroclavicular and infraclavicular lesions are best demonstrated with sections in an oblique coronal or sagittal plane. The percentage of false-negative results is similar to that of CT, but MRI provides a better image of distal lesions, especially in cases of brachial plexus tumors, with a reduced false-positive rate. However, the usefulness of MRI for distinguishing preganglionic from postganglionic lesions remains limited in our center, and the added expense of this test has not been justified.

A combination of the techniques described here can reveal the pathology of the entire plexus and provide a relatively accurate picture for various brachial plexus lesions.

Vascular Studies

Patients with a history of vascular injury and reconstruction or those scheduled for a free muscle transfer must have an angiogram of the upper extremity before surgery. If the angiogram indicates stenotic areas, or even a collateral network without major blood supply distally, flow studies must be used to determine the adequacy of the blood supply to the arm. Vascular reconstruction is indicated if there is not sufficient peripheral flow. Such reconstruction is performed by a vascular surgeon before microneural repair but during the same operative procedure.

TIMING AND INDICATIONS FOR RECONSTRUCTION

The timing for surgical exploration and reconstruction of the brachial plexus elements is determined by the evolution of the clinical picture. A debate continues regarding immediate or early exploration and reconstruction of the plexus in patients with open wounds caused by gunshots, blast injuries, or knife lacerations, or in patients who have brachial plexus trauma combined with vascular injury. However, it is generally agreed that during the immediate restoration of blood supply in cases of severe arm ischemia it is wise to carry out an exploration of the plexus to determine the extent and level of the nerve lesion(s).

Some authors[7] suggest an emergency repair of the nerve lesions when this is feasible. They support this thesis by pointing out two advantages of primary emergency nerve repair. First, an end-to-end repair or the use of short grafts is possible at this time, before retraction of the nerve stumps occurs. Second, difficulties arising from residual scar tissue during a secondary dissection, as well as the risk of injuring vascular grafts, are eliminated.

Compression lesions of the brachial plexus should be acutely decompressed, with evacuation of hematomas and excision or reduction of bone fragments.[24]

Alnot[2] prefers exploration of the traumatized plexus during vascular repair, and reconstruction at a secondary stage. Sedel[38] states that delayed primary repair (preferably after 4 to 6 weeks) is generally more successful; this time interval permits wallerian degeneration to occur, with formation of the proximal neuroma, which allows precise identification of the extent of the lesion. A delayed exploration permits more accurate decision making regarding the use of resection and

grafting or neurolysis alone. It also avoids exposing acute nerve repairs to possible local infection, especially when there are open contaminated wounds.

Controversies continue regarding the preferred method of treating closed traction injuries. Millesi[28] has suggested that observation is an option for any lesion that may have a chance for spontaneous recovery. However, unless the injury is a neurapraxia, the chances for spontaneous recovery are minimal. All other injuries should be explored and reconstructed. The optimal time for reconstruction has been discussed extensively in the literature.

Sedel[38] noted no significant difference in results obtained from repairs performed as many as 9 months after injury. However, these results are usually more favorable than those achieved after reconstruction is further delayed; there is minimal or no benefit in performing a nerve repair 2 years after denervation unless the nerve lesion is in continuity and there is electromyographic evidence of some target preservation.

Our preferred method of management is aggressive early reconstruction. The optimal time is 6 weeks to 3 months after injury. However, the timing of exploration frequently is dictated by the time the patient first visits our clinic.

PRIORITIES AND STAGES OF RECONSTRUCTION

The minimal goals of brachial plexus repair are to restore the paralyzed upper extremity to greater functional use and to avoid amputation. Stabilization of the shoulder restores the head of the humerus in the glenoid fossa and prevents subluxation. Our strategy for shoulder reconstruction consists of neurotization of the suprascapular nerve by means of intraplexus nerve donors, or more often directly from the distal spinal accessory nerve. Both options reverse the tendency for subluxation and provide 15 to 30 degrees abduction in the majority of cases. Restoration of external rotation of the shoulder is not as easily accomplished, despite the fact that both the supraspinatus and infraspinatus muscles are innervated by this nerve. If the axillary nerve can be repaired, the functional capability of the shoulder will be enhanced by the restoration of deltoid and teres minor muscle function.

Flexion is the first priority for elbow function restoration because it allows better arm-to-trunk prehension and the ability to bring the hand to the mouth. The musculocutaneous nerve can be restored by available intraplexus donors or by extraplexus donors, such as the intercostal nerves.

The restoration of sensation reduces trophic skin changes, prevents mutilating injuries, and corrects amblyopia of the hand. It also decreases pain in the paralyzed limb. In cases of avulsion, median nerve neurotization from sensory intercostal nerves or sensory branches of the cervical plexus provides some sensation to the hand. Return of sensation in the thumb and index finger is the primary goal. The same philosophy applies to providing some protective sensation to the dorsum of the hand, if adequate sensory donors are available for restoration of the radial nerve.

The options for reconstruction expand when there is an adequate number of nerve fibers to reinnervate the upper extremity and thus offer more function to the paralyzed limb.

The potential for hand reinnervation declines as the distance between the nerve repair sites and the target muscle and sensory receptor sites becomes greater. These repairs may have satisfactory results only when brachial plexus reconstruction is performed early. Finger flexion and extension are considered the first priorities in restoring hand function, followed by intrinsic substitution and thumb abduction and opposition.

FACTORS DETERMINING THE PROGNOSIS

The following factors determine the prognosis and influence the final outcome of a brachial plexus injury:

1. *Type of lesion* (e.g., avulsion or postganglionic injury)
2. *Total severity score.* The severity score assigned to each root is determined intraoperatively and can range from 0, for a root that is avulsed, to 5, for a root that is intact (0, avulsion; 1, rupture/avulsion; 2, rupture; 3, rupture/traction; 4, traction; 5, normal root). The sum of individual root severity scores determines the total severity score.
3. *Age* of the patient. Younger patients have better outcomes.
4. *Denervation time* (i.e., the time interval between the injury and the first stage of reconstruction). Early reconstruction gives a more favorable result.
5. *Degree of root involvement* (e.g., global, involving upper roots or lower roots)
6. *Reconstruction plan* in relation to the type of injury and the denervation time.
7. *Microsurgical technique.* Ideally a surgeon who is experienced in brachial plexus reconstruction combines meticulous atraumatic technique with adequate knowledge of the nature of these injuries.
8. *Patient's compliance* with the postoperative rehabilitation program.

OPERATIONS

EVOLUTION OF MANAGEMENT OF BRACHIAL PLEXUS INJURIES

But Hector, in his shining helm, while the other let his bow, hit him with the barren stone at the shoulder, where the clavicle divides the neck from the chest, a most opportune point, and broke the nerve. The arm fell numb to the wrist, he (Teucus) fell on his knees and lay still, the bow fallen from his hand.

Homer's *Iliad*

Upper-extremity palsies from brachial plexus injuries have been described since ancient times, but in 1827 Flaubert[34] published the first report of a traumatic brachial plexopathy after a shoulder dislocation. The 18th and 19th centuries were marked by clinical or anatomical observations and studies but not yet by surgical treatment of brachial plexus lesions.

New avenues were opened with the first report of surgical nerve coaptation by Nelaton in 1863, and with the experimental use of nerve grafts by Phillipeaux and Vulpian in 1870.

The dawn of the 20th century witnessed the first surgical repair of brachial plexus lesions by Thorburn in 1900. In 1903, Harris and Low proposed the intraplexus neurotization technique; soon other surgeons, such as Tuttle in 1913, began to use the method to reconstruct avulsion injuries.[34]

The surgical enthusiasm generated during the first decades of the 20th century later gave way to the pessimistic attitude of "wait and see"; this was in response to unrewarding results noted by Tracy and Brannon in 1958,[50] after the repair of traction injuries.

In 1934 Stevens[40] supported immediate repair of open brachial plexus lesions, but he was opposed to operating on traction injuries. In 1959, Bonney[6] reported poor results after surgical repair of brachial plexus injuries during wartime.

In 1965 Leffert and Seddon[24] stated that the overall results of operative treatment for plexus injuries sustained during World War II were so disappointing that a nonoperative approach was recommended for all lesions; exploration was recommended only to determine a lesion's prognosis.

Barnes[3] reviewed 63 closed injuries in 1949 and concluded that conservative management was best and that poor results were associated with the formation of endoneurial scar tissue.

Rehabilitative palliative procedures were introduced to enhance the functionality of the nearly paretic arm that often resulted from nerve surgery. Procedures that were initially established to correct the acquired deformities of poliomyelitis patients, such as muscle transposition or tendon transfers (e.g., Steindler flexorplasty in 1918, or various muscle transfers described by Marshall[27] et al in 1988) were eventually used to reconstruct the upper extremity after brachial plexus palsies.

Surgical management of the flail or anesthetic arm included several alternatives. One involved amputating the arm, fusing the shoulder, and fitting the patient with a prosthesis, as reported by Fletcher[15] in 1969. Another involved reconstruction with a tenodesis of the fingers, a posterior bone block at the elbow, and an arthrodesis of the shoulder. Another option involved the use of specialized splints, such as the flail arm splint described by Wynn Parry[51] in 1995.

Until 1950 the dilemma facing the surgeon involved differentiating a supraganglionic from an infraganglionic lesion. The former, as noted by Sunderland[41] in 1951, offered no chance of spontaneous recovery, but the latter did, depending on the severity of the lesion and whether it was in continuity. If continuity was lost, surgical reconstruction was necessary, either after bone shortening or using end-to-end nerve repairs under severe tension. Nerve grafting with cable grafts was used as a last resort before amputation.

The development of specialized tests during the late 1940s and 1950s allowed a more accurate diagnosis of the lesion; thus time was not wasted awaiting spontaneous recovery in lesions that needed surgical intervention. These tests included cervical myelography by Murphey in 1947, electromyography by Hodes in 1948, the recording of nerve action potentials by Dawson in 1949, and the histamine test by Bonney in 1954.[48]

In 1959 Bonney[6] advocated exploration after the acute inflammation stage to determine the site and extent of the lesion. Even with improved radiologic and electrodiagnostic techniques, surgeons currently must rely on the findings of surgical exploration to establish a final diagnosis and to determine a surgical plan and prognosis. In 1973 Lusskin et al[25] documented the use of intraoperative stimulation across the neuroma to determine the need for resection and nerve grafting.

In 1943 Seddon[36] established a classification system for nerve injuries based on the degree of the injury; this classification was expanded by Sunderland[41] in 1951. In 1963 Seddon[36] also used cable nerve grafts to bridge gaps in cases that involved a loss of continuity, and in 1961 Yeoman and Seddon[52] introduced neurotization by intercostal nerve transfer for reconstruction of the musculocutaneous nerve in cases of avulsion.

The operating microscope was introduced in 1964 by Kurze[23] for use in peripheral nerve surgery. In 1967 Millesi[30] and Narakas[32] reported the use of microsurgical techniques in peripheral nerve reconstruction.

The need to bridge long gaps in the reconstruction of severe and extended brachial plexus injuries led to the use of free vascularized nerve grafts. The first free vascularized nerve graft was performed by Taylor and Ham[42] in 1976.

Daniel and Terzis[12] described the superior ulnar collateral artery in 1975 during their search for future sites for neurovascular free flaps. In 1981 Terzis[45] transferred the entire ulnar nerve as a free microvascular nerve graft based on the superior ulnar collateral artery for the first time. Millesi[29] introduced the use of interfascicular interposition nerve grafting and in 1973 provided morphologic evidence of the harmful effects of tension at the coaptation site. Working independently in 1975, Terzis[47] provided electrophysiologic proof of the deleterious effect of tension at the repair site. She further showed that the results of an interpositional nerve graft were superior to those of an end-to-end repair under tension.

The 1980s brought several new approaches to brachial plexus reconstruction as more aggressive management was sought to restore some function to patients with supraclavicular lesions and multiple avulsions. Surgeons promoted intraplexus and extraplexus neurotizations in their efforts to restore some function to patients with a globally paralyzed limb.

Various donor nerves have been used for neurotizations. These include the intercostal nerves used by Yeomann[52] in 1961; the ipsilateral cervical plexus used by Brunelli in 1981[11]; the contralateral lateral pectoral nerve used by Gilbert[17] in 1992; the spinal accessory nerve used by Allieu[1] in 1988; the hypoglossal nerve and intraplexus donors used by Narakas[33]; the phrenic nerve and contralateral C7 root used by Gu[19,20]; and selective contralateral C7 root used by Terzis[43] in 1991.

In 1995 Carlstedt[9] demonstrated, in a large series of animal experiments, that severed roots could reconnect to the damaged spinal cord segment. These encouraging results led

him to use the same method in patients with lower root avulsions of the brachial plexus. He observed muscle reinnervation in response to this method, but the ensuing cocontraction handicapped the functional result. Further work is needed in this area to make this approach meaningful for clinical application.

Despite these advances, reanimation of the paralyzed hand remained an unattainable goal. The restoration of functional finger flexion and extension in devastating lesions was considered impossible. Reasons included the prolonged time necessary for nerve regeneration, which led to muscle atrophy and subsequent fibrosis, resulting in muscle strength that was inadequate to generate the force required to move the fingers. Subsequently, the microvascular transplantation of free neurotized muscle as described by Terzis[44,49] became the standard in the management of brachial plexus paralysis; it enabled surgeons to overcome distal target atrophy and restore finger flexion and extension.

Promising news regarding the use of growth factors to stimulate the nerve regeneration process is currently coming from the field of neuroscience, but their exact role in clinical practice remains to be seen.

BRACHIAL PLEXUS RECONSTRUCTION

Despite meticulous preoperative evaluation, with advanced special examinations, the final diagnosis of a brachial plexus lesion can be made only at the time of microsurgical exploration. However, the lesion's anatomical appearance during surgery can be misleading; intraoperative stimulation and recording can be employed in such cases. The final plan for surgical reconstruction is established during exploration.

The reconstructive plan is determined according to the level of injury, the anatomical findings, and the extent and type of the brachial plexus injury. The denervation time is also a predetermining factor in reconstruction of the paralyzed extremity. If the elapsed time between the accident and the first reconstruction is more than a year, the chances for reanimation of denervated muscles are less, and therefore secondary operations are mandatory to improve functional outcome in the paralyzed extremity.

Our preferred approach involves extensive exploration of the entire plexus to establish an accurate intraoperative diagnosis, and neurotizations from various intraplexus and extraplexus ipsilateral and contralateral donor nerves in combination with vascularized nerve grafts and secondary procedures such as free functional muscle transfers.

Brachial Plexus Exploration

The operative goal of brachial plexus exploration is to achieve adequate exposure of anatomic structures with minimal trauma. This entails preserving soft tissue (e.g., muscles such as the pectoralis minor and pectoralis major), blood vessels (e.g., the external jugular vein and transverse cervical vessels), and nerves (e.g., supraclavicular nerves). A meticulous atraumatic dissection increases the likelihood of retaining a good vascular bed for the nerve grafts. The exploration steps can be executed simultaneously by two microsurgical teams while a third team harvests nerve grafts from the lower extremities.

SURGICAL APPROACH. The incision follows the lateral border of the sternocleidomastoid muscle and curves postero-laterally to follow the superior border of the clavicle. Subsequently the incision is extended into the axilla, following the deltopectoral groove.

SUPRACLAVICULAR PLEXUS. The skin flaps are elevated in a plane beneath the platysma, and the supraclavicular sensory nerves and external jugular vein are exposed and preserved. The sternocleidomastoid muscle is retracted to medially expose the phrenic nerve and to identify the C4 mixed spinal nerve. The dissection proceeds in a caudal direction to expose the C5, C6, and C7 spinal nerves. The transverse cervical vessels and the omohyoid muscle are isolated as the C7 root is approached. The C8 and TI roots are identified on the first rib superior to the subclavian artery. The long thoracic, dorsal scapular, and suprascapular nerves are also identified.

INFRACLAVICULAR PLEXUS. The cephalic vein is circum-ferentially dissected and preserved in the deltopectoral groove. The pectoralis major and deltoid muscles are separated atraumatically and the pectoralis major is retracted to expose the pectoralis minor muscle, whose coracoid insertion is resected, if necessary. The lateral cord is encountered first and is traced distally to the median and musculocutaneous nerves. The posterior cord is found posterior to the lateral cord. The lateral pectoral nerve is dissected on the deep surface of the pectoralis major. When this area is scarred, the dissection commences in a normal area and proceeds from a distal to a proximal location.

The dissection continues to gain access to the space under the clavicle so that the supraclavicular and infraclavicular structures become connected. A clavicular osteotomy was performed in earlier times to gain better access to the retroclavicular plexus, and osteosynthesis of the clavicle was achieved at the end of surgery, using a compression plate. However, the clavicle has a great potential to develop delayed union or nonunion; thus clavicular osteotomy is rarely performed at our center.

Electrophysiologic stimulation studies are performed dur-ing the exploration as soon as each nerve is exposed, using a DC stimulator at 0.5 mAmp, 1.0 mAmp, and 2.0 mAmp. A chart of the muscular responses to various levels of stimulation is created. These data are used to develop a strategy for surgical reconstruction, particularly in cases involving lesions in continuity, in which the decision regarding the use of neurolysis or resection of the neuroma followed by nerve grafting must be made.

First, the brachial plexus is explored to identify the type and extent of injury. Subsequently the targets to be reconstructed are isolated and tagged with vessel loops of various colors. If extraplexus neurotizations are necessary, the identification and dissection of the various extraplexus ipsilateral motor donors

(e.g., the phrenic, cervical plexus motor nerves, and distal accessory nerve) can be accomplished through the same incision. Exposure of the hypoglossal and intercostal nerves requires different incisions.

The intercostal nerves are dissected through a curvilinear incision that starts proximally in the axilla, follows the midaxillary line, and curves forward after a short vertical course. The serratus anterior muscle is subsequently separated at the level of each intercostal space and the intercostal muscles are separated. Each intercostal nerve is retrieved from the lower margin of each rib. Stimulation of each intercostal nerve and its branches distinguishes motor from sensory branches. Each intercostal nerve subsequently is dissected free anteriorly to the midline of the trunk. Harvesting of T4 must be done with care, especially in women, so as to preserve the sensory branch that innervates the nipple.

The hypoglossal nerve is dissected through a small curvilinear incision 2 cm below the angle of the mandible. It is located deep to the posterior belly of the digastric muscle. A small, curved incision is used for exploration of the supraclav-icular plexus on the normal side to expose the contralateral C7 spinal nerve.

The harvesting of nerve grafts from the lower extremities is accomplished through small lazy-S incisions for the sural nerves, and the harvesting of saphenous nerves is performed with a proximal curvilinear incision at the medial side of the thigh and one or two smaller incisions at the medial aspect of the distal thigh and proximal calf. All explorations and dissections are performed under 4× loupe magnification, and all nerve repairs are executed under the operating microscope.

Biopsy specimens are routinely taken at the level of the spinal roots, proximal trunks, or cord stumps that will be used as intraplexus donors for repair or neurotization, to identify the presence of viable nerve fibers versus ganglion cells or scar tissue. Plexus elements that contain ganglion cells or scar tissue, with no evidence of myelinated nerve fibers, are not used as donors for nerve repairs. Biopsies are also taken from the distal end of a previously banked nerve to assess the maturity of regenerating fibers before its use as a motor donor for free muscle transplantation.

We routinely use modern histochemical techniques, as described in 1985 by Carson and Terzis,[10] to provide intraoperative evaluation of a candidate donor nerve and to discern the ratio of motor to sensory fibers.

Methods of Nerve Microreconstruction

The methods of nerve repair that are used for brachial plexus reconstruction include (1) microneurolysis, (2) direct nerve repair, (3) nerve grafting, and (4) neurotization.

The microcoaptations can be performed either end-to-end, which is the most common method of neurorrhaphy, or end-to-side. The end-to-side coaptation is used for obtaining nerve fibers from a healthy donor nerve without compromising the function of its distal targets (e.g., neurotization of a distal target from the phrenic nerve without jeopardizing the function of the diaphragm). Another type of "end-to-side" neurorrhaphy is used when the surgeon wants to increase the number of motor axons already functioning in a nerve.

MICRONEUROLYSIS. The degree of neurolysis is determined intraoperatively and is guided by the response of the peripheral nervous tissue to sequential decompression. The surgeon uses palpation and visualization to determine whether a simple epineuriotomy will suffice or whether he or she needs to proceed with interfascicular dissection. One must always respect the integrity of the perineural sheath during this procedure. Our instrument of choice for microneurolysis is the diamond knife.[46] During the neurolysis, methylene blue demonstrates the fascicles best and optimizes visualization under high magnification. Intraoperative palpation of the injured plexus provides the best feedback for determining the extent of neurolysis that must be performed. Fascicular bulging after decompression of the scarred interfascicular epineurium usually renders that nerve segment soft to palpation. The neurolysis is considered complete if all areas of fibrosis and compression are eliminated and the nerves feel soft in response to running the index finger and thumb over the decompressed region.

DIRECT NERVE REPAIR. Reconstruction by direct coaptation of the proximal and distal nerve stump is not usually feasible. Only in fresh, cleanly cut lesions is the nerve distensible enough that a primary repair without nerve grafts can take place without excessive tension at the area of coaptation.

NERVE GRAFTING. Nerve grafting is the most common technique for restoring continuity across a nerve defect in brachial plexus injuries. The most common type of nerve grafts involve fragments of nonvascularized cutaneous nerves. The sural, saphenous, medial antebrachial cutaneous, and superficial radial nerves are most commonly used. These thin cutaneous nerves are preferred because the donor site morbidity is minimal and because they have a better survival rate than thicker trunk nerve grafts because of their small diameter. If a nerve trunk is used for a free nerve graft, Millesi[29] recommends that the epifascicular epineurium be removed by microsurgical dissection and that the nerve be split into fascicular groups to provide grafts with a smaller diameter, which enhances the likelihood of their revascularization.

The other type of nerve graft that is currently used is the vascularized nerve graft. The most popular example involves the ulnar nerve, which is transferred as a pedicled or free vascularized graft in adults who have surgically documented C8 and TI avulsion injuries. In 1981 Terzis[45] first transferred the entire ulnar nerve based on the superior ulnar collateral artery as a free microvascular transfer. Other nerves used for vascularized nerve grafts include the sural, saphenous, superficial radial nerves.

The principles of nerve grafting for the management of obstetric brachial plexus lesions are different than those for the management of posttraumatic brachial plexus injuries in adults. Interpositional nerve grafts between the roots and the trunks or cords is preferred in children; in adults, bridging between the proximal donors with the distal nerves near the

muscle targets gives more rewarding results. Furthermore, reconstruction of C8, T1, or the ulnar nerve is of highest priority in patients with obstetric paralysis because restoration of hand function is an achievable goal. Thus the ulnar nerve is never used for nerve grafts in these cases, although it may be used in adults.

NEUROTIZATION. Neurotization allows reconstruction of a peripheral nerve when the proximal nerve stump is unavailable. The classic example of such a situation is root avulsion injury. Examples of donor nerves that are used for transfer include intraplexus donors (if available), ipsilateral intercostal nerves, terminal rami of the spinal accessory nerve, branches of the cervical plexus, partial phrenic and hypoglossal nerves, the contralateral pectoral nerve, and some sections of the contralateral C7. The transfer may be achieved by end-to-end repair or by interposition nerve grafts. The aim is to neurotize selected muscles to achieve stabilization and essential function in the shoulder, elbow, and hand.

The use of intercostal nerves continues to be a standard approach to the reconstruction of severe brachial plexus lesions, especially in patients with avulsion injuries. In 1982, Nagano et al[31] presented good results (82%) after direct neurotization of the musculocutaneous nerve, using intercostal nerves. They suggested that it is better to coapt the intercostals directly to the musculocutaneous nerve than to use interposition nerve grafts. We agree with this conclusion.

The accessory nerve also is considered a successful donor, especially for neurotization of the suprascapular nerve. It also can be used for neurotization of the axillary or musculocutaneous nerves.

In 1988 Allieu and Cenac[1] pointed out that the results obtained by neurotizations from unavulsed C5 and C6 roots are superior to those achieved with the use of extraplexus donors such as the accessory nerve, which should be considered a second-choice intervention.

In 1988 Kawai et al[22] reported satisfactory results in 64% of patients with avulsion injuries who had neurotizations that involved the use of intercostal or spinal accessory nerves for elbow flexion. Among these patients, the combined use of intraplexus and extraplexus donors provided a better outcome.

The anterior and/or posterior divisions of the contralateral C7 are powerful motor donors and are typically used in global avulsion injuries. They can give rewarding results in neurotizations involving vascularized ulnar nerve grafts, and also when they are used for neurotization of free muscle transfers through cross-chest banked nerve grafts.

Narakas and Hentz[33] viewed neurotizations as complementary methods to be used as part of a general plan for reconstruction. Plexoplexal transfers are far more reliable than those from extraplexal sources and are even superior to musculotendinous transfers for the restoration of shoulder abduction, elbow flexion, or wrist extension.

Strategy of Reconstruction

POSTGANGLIONIC INJURIES. Complete reconstruction of postganglionic injuries is more feasible compared with reconstruction of avulsion lesions. A rupture or traction injury typically is present and repair can be achieved by the interposition of vascularized or nonvascularized nerve grafts, or by neurolysis alone, if perineurial continuity can be guaranteed. Associated vascular injuries or fractures in this area predict a more difficult reconstruction with a less rewarding result. Injury of plexus elements at different levels must be investigated by extensive distal exploration. This is especially true for nerves that pass through narrow spaces or have an angulated course, such as the axillary or suprascapular nerves.

If the surgeon is faced with a neuroma in continuity but with clinical distal paralysis, the neuroma should be resected and grafted. If the neuroma serves targets that have an acceptable level of function, electrophysiological recordings are performed to determine the degree of nerve continuity across the neuroma; in such cases an extensive intraneural neurolysis is preferred, which preserves the bundles that show perineurial continuity and signal transmission. Resection and nerve grafting is performed for only those portions of the nerve that do not conduct or are involved in scar tissue. When the scar tissue is extensive and the function (distally) is minimal, the decision is made to proceed with neurotization of the distal nerve in proximity to its target instead of nerve repair at the scarred area of the lesion.

Direct muscle neurotization typically involves the use of interpositional nerve grafts with corresponding motor donors, if the nerves are avulsed from their muscle targets.

PREGANGLIONIC INJURIES

Avulsion of One or Two Roots. The chances of successfully reinnervating more structures in patients with avulsions involving only one or two roots are even greater. Typically the lower roots are avulsed and the other roots are involved to a variable degree. The further away a root is from the avulsion lesion, the less severe the injury. The prognosis is better if the lesion affects the upper plexus. Nerve repair is not beneficial in adult patients with avulsion of the lower roots because the intrinsic hand muscles atrophy very early. Neurotization can be performed with both intraplexus and extraplexus donors if C5 and/or C6 are avulsed. Thus if the ipsilateral C7 root has escaped injury, selective regions of the posterior division of the ipsilateral C7 are guided to posterior cord structures by direct coaptation, and selective segments from the anterior division are destined for anterior targets.

Avulsion of Three or Four Roots. The lower roots are most commonly avulsed (C7, C8, T1), but severe traction may also damage the C5 and C6 roots, which may be ruptured or may have a mixed injury involving rupture and avulsion. The chances for reconstruction are less than for injuries in the previous category because fewer intraplexus donors are available. However, in a pre-fixed plexus, repair of the injured plexus can be almost total if C5 and/or C6 can be used as proximal donors (except in reconstruction of the lower trunk, which has not been as successful in the adults).

Neurotization of the suprascapular nerve can be performed with the accessory nerve when only C5 is available to be grafted, whereas C5, if adequate, is coapted to loops of the

vascularized ulnar nerve and directed to the musculocutaneous and median nerves. Elements of the posterior cord, such as the axillary and radial nerves, can be neurotized from extraplexus donors. The goal is to obtain shoulder stability (with abduction and adduction of the arm), elbow flexion and extension, and improved sensibility in the forearm and hand.

The posterior cord also can be neurotized if both C5 and C6 are available for neurotization. Caution must be used to connect the anterior part of the donor roots to nerves destined for anterior targets (flexion) to maintain the correct cortical representation and to avoid co-contractions between antagonistic muscles. A vascularized ulnar nerve can be used in this type of lesion to simultaneously reconstruct two or three targets, using the "loop" technique introduced by Terzis[45] in 1981. The nerve fascicles are divided through epineurial and perineurial windows and connected to proximal spinal nerves and distal peripheral nerves, while the continuity of the epineurial blood supply is maintained.

Global Avulsions. Global avulsions are the most devastating lesions of the brachial plexus because they leave a totally flail and anesthetic limb, usually accompanied by severe, uncontrollable pain. It is important to convince patients who present with constant, intolerable pain and who beg for relief (even by means of an amputation) that an amputation is not going to solve their problem. Control of pain can be achieved by conservative methods, such as medication, and/or by electrical stimulation. Patients with refractory pain should be referred to specialized pain centers for treatment. The most popular treatment is the dorsal root entry zone (DREZ) procedure introduced by Nashold,[16] in which the neurosurgeon destroys the dorsal root entry zone in the spinal cord using coagulation. Preferably, this must be performed before nerve reconstruction.

The goals of primary repair are to provide shoulder stabilization and, if possible, a degree of shoulder abduction, elbow flexion and extension, wrist stabilization, and protective sensation to the upper extremity. An effort is made to reinnervate the latissimus dorsi for future transfer as a pedicled muscle flap. Placement of banked nerve grafts, for future free muscle transfers during secondary stages, also is an option. Because of the lack of proximal intraplexus donors, the surgeon must look for motor donors for neurotization using ipsilateral extraplexus nerves or those from the contralateral plexus. It is essential to identify whether there are associated lesions in other extraplexus nerves, which is not unusual in these severe injuries. The harvesting of an adequate number of nerve grafts from all available sources must be considered part of the surgical plan. The possibility of harvesting the ulnar nerve for a vascularized nerve graft also must be considered because the reconstruction of C8 and T1 is not an option in the adult.

Terzis' preferred strategy of reconstruction is as follows. The accessory nerve is used to directly neurotize the suprascapular nerve. The intercostal nerves are used to directly neurotize ipsilateral targets. The motor branches of the cervical plexus, the phrenic and hypoglossal nerves, and parts of the anterior and posterior division of the contralateral C7 are used with interposition nerve grafts to neurotize the musculocutaneous, median, axillary, radial, and thoracodorsal nerves; the branch to the triceps; and the long thoracic nerves. Sensory branches of the intercostals or supraclavicular sensory nerves are used to neurotize the median nerve to restore sensation. Moreover, nerve grafts are banked subcutaneously in the arm or elbow, for neurotization of future free muscle transfers after proximal coaptations. When the contralateral C7 is used as a donor for neurotization, a vascularized ulnar nerve, if available, is preferred as an interpositional nerve graft to bridge the gap.

Secondary procedures such as free muscle transfers and wrist arthrodesis typically are necessary to improve the function of the upper extremity.

SECONDARY RECONSTRUCTION

Secondary procedures are an integral part of brachial plexus reconstruction because only partial recovery of the brachial plexus can be achieved, especially in severe lesions such as avulsions and in palsies with prolonged denervation time. The goal for the shoulder region is abduction and external rotation, which can be achieved by local tendon transpositions or transfers, such as major rerouting of the latissimus dorsi and teres major for external rotation, or advancement of the trapezius to provide shoulder stabilization and abduction. External rotational osteotomy of the humerus also has been used to correct the internal rotation deformity that is usually present in brachial plexus patients.

In cases in which treatment was delayed, a free muscle transfer can be transplanted alone or as a double-muscle transfer for shoulder abduction and elbow flexion (e.g., transfer of the gracilis and the adductor longus on a common pedicle).[44] The reinnervation of these muscles is provided either by immediate neurotization, using local donors such as intercostals, or with previously placed "banked nerve grafts" that are connected to proximal ipsilateral or contralateral motor donors.

One option for elbow flexion is a pedicled ipsilateral latissimus dorsi transfer (if available), which was described by Zancolli in 1973.[27] Berger[5] uses this technique as his first choice to restore elbow flexion. The pectoralis minor alone or in combination with the pectoralis major also have been used.[44] A good rule for muscle transfer procedures is to use local muscles first, if they are available, rather than reinnervated free muscles.

Patients who have contractions of both the biceps and triceps can have elbow flexion restored by transferring the triceps. This relatively easy procedure gives strong elbow flexion. The disadvantages of this procedure, as noted by Brunelli,[8] involve an inability to extend the elbow above the shoulder to reach overhead objects or to stabilize an object on a table, and trouble engaging in other daily activities, such as running.

In 1918 Steindler[8] proposed proximal transposition of the forearm flexors from their origin on the medial epicondyle. This technique remained controversial, mainly because it creates the undesirable effect of pronation and simultaneous elbow and finger flexion. Brunelli[8] employed a modification of

the technique in 1995, which involved transfer on the anterior aspect of the humerus and separation of the transferred wrist flexors and pronator from the flexor digitorum superficialis; he recommends this procedure for treatment of C5 and C6 palsies.

Free vascularized and neurotized muscles currently are routinely used to strengthen elbow flexion and extension, or to provide finger flexion and extension when there is a lack of local motor units. The latter occurs when there is severe global injury to the plexus, especially in avulsions and in late cases in which the denervation time is more than 1 year. These procedures are usually performed in two stages, especially for hand reanimation. In the first stage, a nerve graft is coapted proximally to the available motor donor nerve and the distal end is placed where the new muscle will be transferred. Approximately 1 year later, a muscle is transferred by microvascular technique to the recipient site and the banked nerve is used to neurotize the muscle.

We have used the contralateral latissimus dorsi, or muscles from the lower extremity such as the gracilis, vastus lateralis, or rectus femoris, for biceps substitution. We have found that in heavy Caucasian adults the gracilis muscle is inadequate for strong elbow flexion restoration. However, the gracilis is the preferred muscle for finger flexion and extension.

Other surgeons, such as Berger,[5] propose one-muscle transfer for combined restoration of elbow flexion or extension with finger flexion or extension. Doi[13] proposed a procedure that involves the transfer of one free muscle for elbow and finger (two joints) reanimation. The transferred muscle passes under the flexor carpi radialis or brachioradialis and extensors at the level of the elbow joint, which act as a pulley for the free muscle transfer. The disadvantages of these free muscle transfers are that muscle strength is reduced because it is distributed over two joints, and difficulties occur in coordinating tasks that the new muscle has to perform simultaneously.

The wrist can be fused if it is unstable, especially in global avulsions or in late cases in which the restoration of wrist function is not feasible. This enhances hand function and may provide additional motor units in cases of residual wrist motion, which can be used to strengthen the overall function of the hand.

The thumb may be converted to a stable post by either arthrodesis or tenodesis, or partial restoration of its function may be obtained if local motor units are available for transfer (e.g., restoration of opposition with a ring flexor superficialis transfer) or with the use of a free muscle transfer. Intrinsic function is important for prehensile movements but is difficult to restore. An effort to replace intrinsic function can be achieved by various tendon transfers or tenodesis procedures and/or an additional free muscle transfer.

POSTOPERATIVE MANAGEMENT

The patient's upper extremity is placed in a prefabricated splint, which is custom made to immobilize the extremity based on the specific type of surgery that was performed. The patient is instructed to wear the splint for 6 to 8 weeks. The arm is maintained in a sling for an additional 4 weeks after the splint is removed. The patient subsequently starts a program of daily physical therapy that first includes gradually increasing passive range of motion followed by active range of motion, if there is any. Ultrasound treatment is used in the area of the incisions to avoid adhesions and scar tissue formation.

Daily application of slow-pulse electrical stimulation (20 minutes on/40 minutes off, five times per day, with a small portable unit) is recommended for every patient, even before surgery;* this treatment helps the muscles maintain their bulk and remain in good condition until reinnervation occurs.[48] The electrical stimulation also reduces pain, which is important for the patient's recovery.

Each patient must be supported psychologically through continuous communication with both doctor and physical therapist. Patients also should be encouraged to return to work with the help of special ergotherapy programs. In our experience, patients who follow the postoperative rehabilitation program and return to work have less pain and a better functional outcome.

OUTCOMES

During the last two decades surgeons have tried to improve the outcomes of brachial plexus reconstruction in posttraumatic palsies. The advent of microsurgery, a better understanding of the nature of these injuries, and cumulative experience gained over the years has yielded improved results. Despite the fact that general outlines in the management of brachial plexus lesions have been established, debates continue regarding the strategy of reconstruction and possible outcomes.

Our intent in this section is to present our series of patients and the possible functional outcomes that can be obtained with modern microsurgical schemes. Exemplary cases are displayed in Figures 118-1 through 118-3. Futhermore, we intend to discuss and compare our results with published outcomes from other centers.

Two hundred and fifty-one patients with posttraumatic brachial plexus lesions underwent surgery (performed by Terzis) in our center between 1978 and 1995. This is the largest series performed by a single surgeon in North America. The outcomes of brachial plexus reconstruction for 204 patients with adequate follow-up were evaluated by five reviewers who had not participated in any of the surgeries. The surgeon was not involved in the assessment process.

The ages of the 204 patients ranged from 15 to 62 years, with a mean of 25.9 ± 10.1 years. The most common cause of injury was high-velocity motor vehicle accidents. Seventy-three patients (36%) were injured in motorcycle accidents, and 46

(23%) were involved in car accidents as a driver or passenger. The speeds at which the accidents occurred ranged from 25 to 120 mph, with an average of 54.5 ± 30.0 mph.

One hundred and seventeen patients (57%) had concomitant fractures in the involved extremity, and 57 patients (28%) presented with an associated arterial injury involving the subclavian or axillary artery. The majority of patients had severe injury to the brachial plexus with a mean total severity score of approximately 5. One hundred and twelve patients (55%) had an avulsion lesion of one or more roots. Among these patients, 15 had a global avulsion of five roots, 30 of four roots, 30 of three roots, 24 of two roots, and 13 of one root. Forty-eight patients had a supraclavicular postganglionic injury, and in 43 patients (21%) trauma was located in the infraclavicular region.

The majority of patients (75%) underwent surgery less than 1 year after the accident and 45% had a denervation time of less than 6 months. A total of 577 nerve reconstructions were performed; of these, 140 were neurotizations without interposition nerve graft(s), and 437 nerves were reconstructed with grafts. One hundred and twenty repairs were performed by the interposition of vascularized nerve grafts (e.g., vascularized ulnar nerve). One hundred and twenty-one nerve grafts were banked to reinnervate future free muscle transfers. Microneurolysis was performed in 89 patients, in some cases alone but usually in combination with various restorations of nerve continuity (i.e., with nerve grafts and/or neurotizations).

The nerve reconstructions (either nerve repair or neurotization) and associated nerve donors are presented in Table 118-1.

Seventy-two patients underwent a secondary strengthening of various muscle targets after the first stage of brachial plexus reconstruction; 29 pedicled and 78 free vascularized muscle transfers were performed for this purpose. Additional secondary procedures, including shoulder arthroplasty and external rotation restoration with transposition of the insertions of the latissimus dorsi and teres major muscles, were performed in 15 patients. Wrist fusion was performed in 21 patients and tendon transfers to the hand were performed in 28 patients.

The results of postoperative muscle grading for all muscle targets were significantly higher than values obtained before surgery ($p < 0.05$), regardless of the type of injury (Table 118-2). Figures 118-4 to 118-9 show the mean muscle grading before and after reconstruction for the supraspinatus, deltoid, biceps, and triceps muscles, and for hand flexion and hand extension, by lesion type (A, avulsion; S, postganglionic supraclavicular; I, postganglionic infraclavicular.)

Statistical analysis of our results showed that postganglionic lesions have a better outcome ($p < 0.05$) than avulsion injuries. The results for postganglionic supraclavicular lesions were not significantly different from those obtained for infraclavicular lesions.

Factors such as age, denervation time, and severity score altered the results of reconstruction. For some muscle targets, a statistically significant difference in outcome was related to one or more of these factors. The greater the total severity in the reconstruction of the deltoid, the better the final outcome. A statistically significant inverse relationship ($p < 0.05$) between

---

*This regimen is described in detail in Liberson WT, Terzis JK: Contributions of clinical neurophysiology and rehabilitation medicine to the management of brachial plexus palsy. In Terzis JK: *Microreconstruction of nerve injuries,* Philadelphia, 1987, WB Saunders.

Text continued on p. 2092

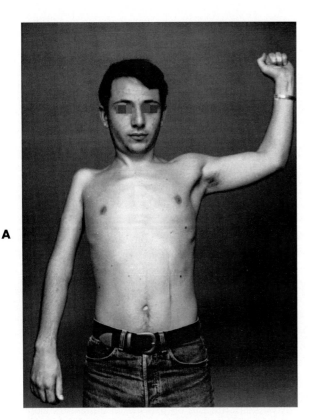

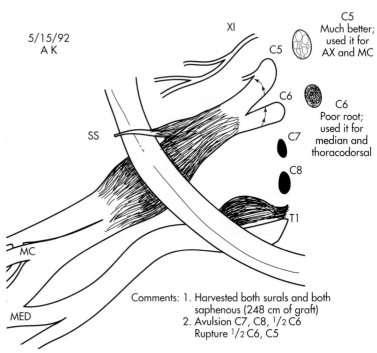

5/15/92
A K

XI

C5
Much better;
used it for
AX and MC

C5

SS

C6

C6
Poor root;
used it for
median and
thoracodorsal

C7

C8

T1

MC

MED

Comments: 1. Harvested both surals and both
saphenous (248 cm of graft)
2. Avulsion C7, C8, 1/2 C6
Rupture 1/2 C6, C5

Figure 118-1. **A,** 22-year-old male patient involved in a motorcycle accident on 9/28/91. The patient sustained a right brachial plexus injury associated with fracture of the right clavicle. **B,** Notes from surgery on 5/15/92: An exploration of the right brachial plexus revealed the following: C5 rupture, C6 rupture/avulsion, C7 and C8 avulsion, and T1 traction. **C,** Reconstruction of the brachial plexus included the following: microneurolysis; neurotization of the musculocutaneous and axillary nerves from the C5 by means of interposition nerve grafts; neurotization of the median, thoracodorsal branch to the triceps, and radial nerve from C6 by means of interposition nerve grafts; direct neurotization of the suprascapular nerve from the terminal branch of the accessory nerve. *Continued*

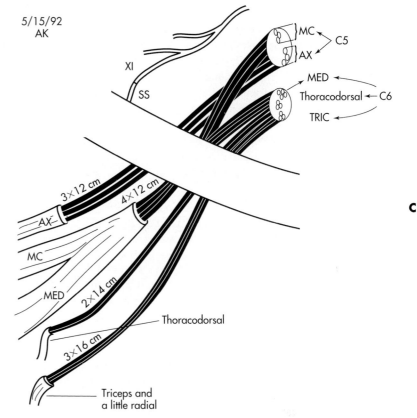

5/15/92
AK

XI

SS

MC
AX } C5

MED
Thoracodorsal ← C6
TRIC

3×12 cm

4×12 cm

AX

MC

MED

2×14 cm

Thoracodorsal

3×16 cm

Triceps and
a little radial

C

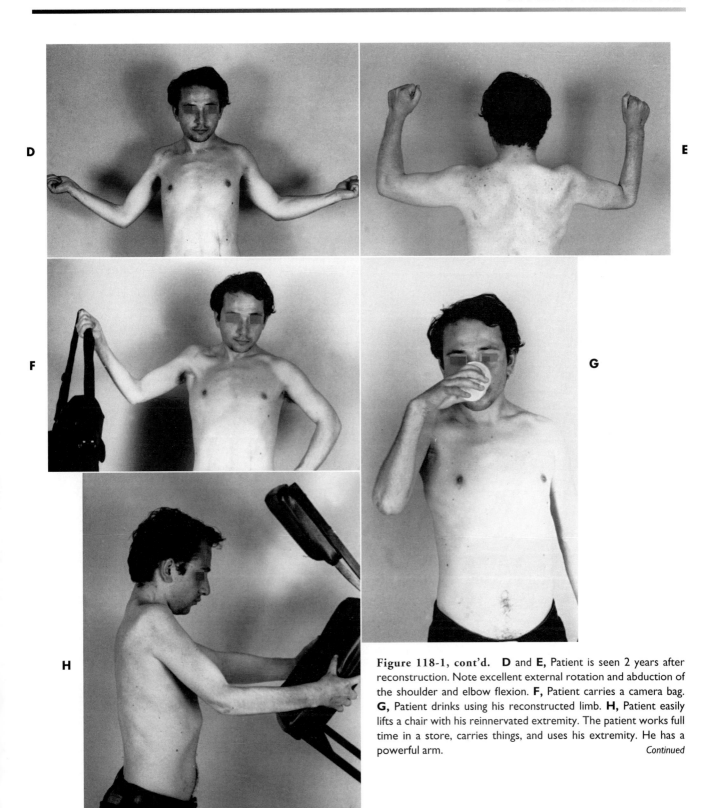

Figure 118-1, cont'd.   D and **E,** Patient is seen 2 years after reconstruction. Note excellent external rotation and abduction of the shoulder and elbow flexion. **F,** Patient carries a camera bag. **G,** Patient drinks using his reconstructed limb. **H,** Patient easily lifts a chair with his reinnervated extremity. The patient works full time in a store, carries things, and uses his extremity. He has a powerful arm.   *Continued*

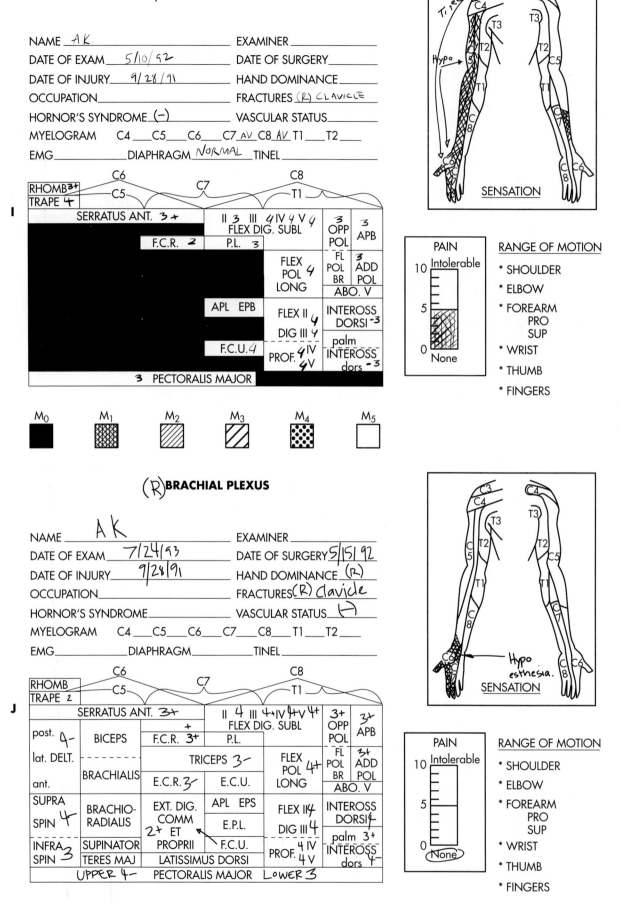

Figure 118-1, cont'd. I and J, Preoperative and postoperative plexus charts of the patient.

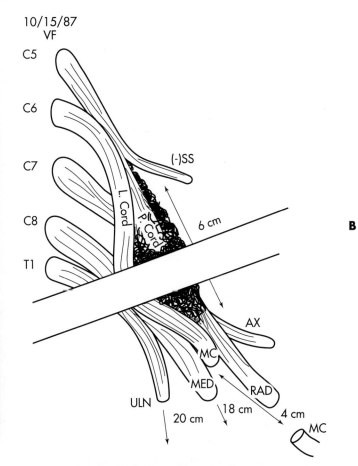

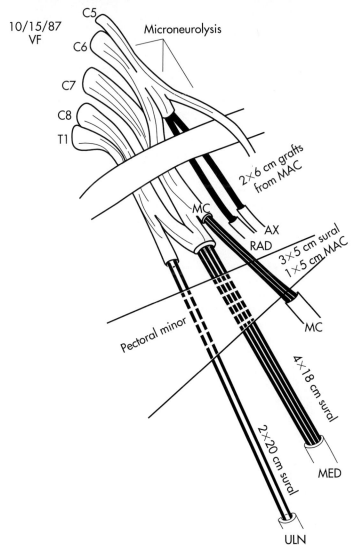

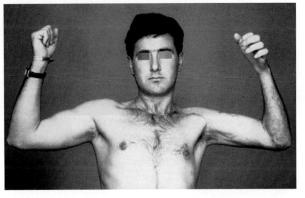

Figure 118-2. 24-year-old male patient who was involved in a motorcycle accident on 7/24/87. The patient sustained a left brachial plexus injury associated with fracture of the left humerus, which was treated by open reduction and internal fixation with plate and screws. **A,** Preoperatively, patient has a totally paretic left upper extremity. **B,** Notes from surgery on 10/15/87: An exploration of the left brachial plexus revealed a huge neuroma of the upper trunk and severe scarring. The lesion extended above and below the clavicle. **C,** The reconstruction included extensive microneurolysis and interposition nerve grafting from the lateral cord to the musculocutaneous nerve, and from the upper trunk to the axillary and radial nerves. The continuity of the median and ulnar nerves was reconstituted with interposition nerve grafts. **D,** 2 years after brachial plexus reconstruction (12/20/89). Note the degree of external rotation and abduction. He has a strong biceps and emerging finger flexion. On 12/21/89, a pedicled latissimus dorsi muscle was transferred to the triceps. The following tendon transfers were carried out in the hand: brachioradialis to extensor pollicis longus and flexor digitorum superficialis of the long finger for intrinsic substitution.

Continued

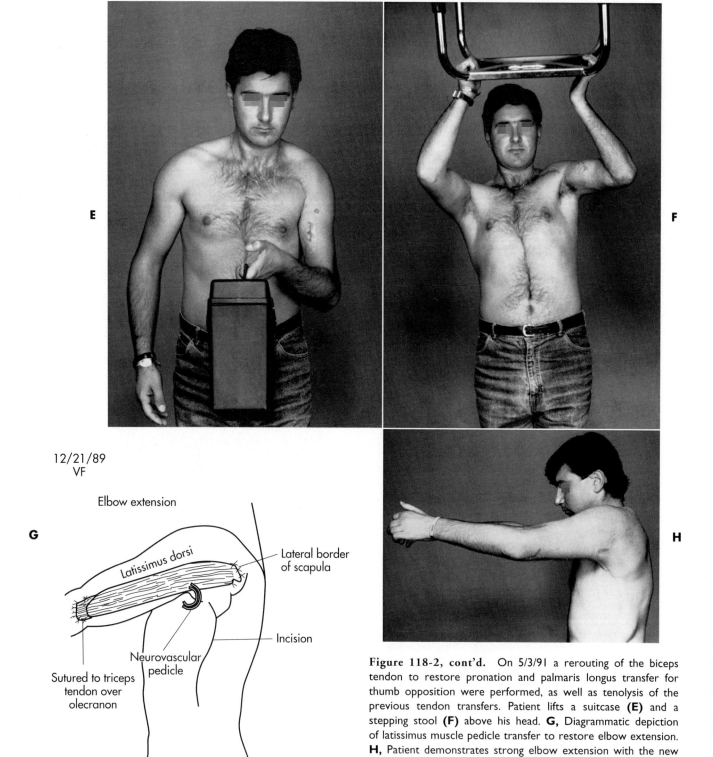

12/21/89
VF

Elbow extension

Latissimus dorsi

Lateral border
of scapula

Neurovascular
pedicle

Incision

Sutured to triceps
tendon over
olecranon

Figure 118-2, cont'd. On 5/3/91 a rerouting of the biceps tendon to restore pronation and palmaris longus transfer for thumb opposition were performed, as well as tenolysis of the previous tendon transfers. Patient lifts a suitcase **(E)** and a stepping stool **(F)** above his head. **G,** Diagrammatic depiction of latissimus muscle pedicle transfer to restore elbow extension. **H,** Patient demonstrates strong elbow extension with the new muscle.

Continued

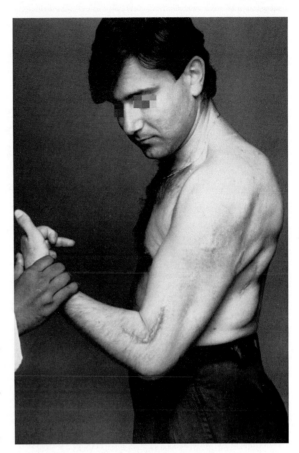

Figure 118-2, cont'd. I, Patient seen on 5/1/91, before his last stage of reconstruction. Three and a half years have passed since his initial brachial plexus reconstruction. Note powerful deltoid, biceps, and triceps (transferred latissimus). Patient is resisting elbow extension. The recovery of function to the left upper extremity is remarkable, and the patient can perform most daily activity tasks. **J** and **K,** Plexus charts of the patient's examination before and after surgery. *Continued*

I

BRACHIAL PLEXUS

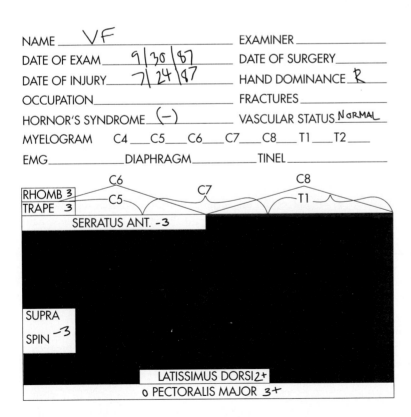

NAME _____ VF _____   EXAMINER _____

DATE OF EXAM ___ 9|30|87 ___   DATE OF SURGERY _____

DATE OF INJURY ___ 7|24|87 ___   HAND DOMINANCE __R__

OCCUPATION _____   FRACTURES _____

HORNOR'S SYNDROME ___(−)___   VASCULAR STATUS __NORMAL__

MYELOGRAM   C4 ___ C5 ___ C6 ___ C7 ___ C8 ___ T1 ___ T2 ___

EMG _____ DIAPHRAGM _____ TINEL _____

RHOMB 3
TRAPE 3
C5   C6   C7   C8   T1
SERRATUS ANT. -3
SUPRA SPIN -3
LATISSIMUS DORSI 2+
0 PECTORALIS MAJOR 3+

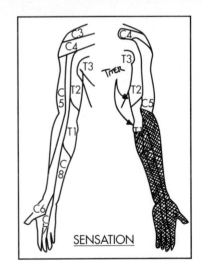

SENSATION

J

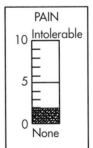

PAIN
10 Intolerable
5
0
None

RANGE OF MOTION

* SHOULDER
* ELBOW
* FOREARM
    PRO
    SUP
* WRIST
* THUMB
* FINGERS

 M_0 M_1  M_2 M_3 M_4 M_5

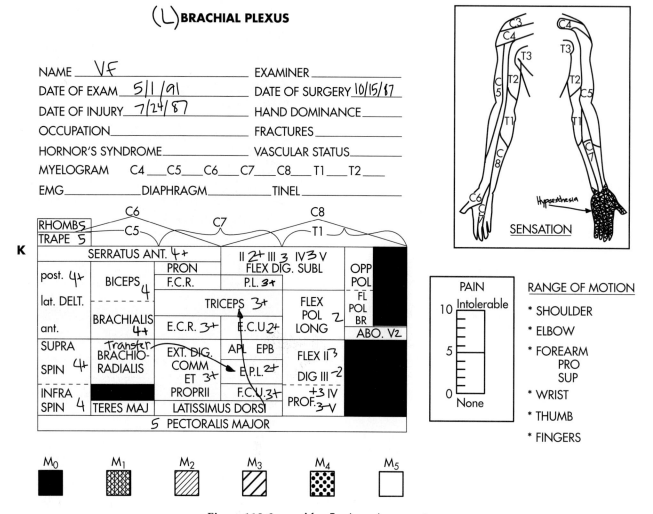

Figure 118-2, cont'd. For legend see previous page.

the age of the patient and the outcome was determined for the biceps and triceps (i.e., higher postoperative muscle strength was achieved in younger patients). Postoperative muscle grading was significantly higher ($p < 0.05$) for the biceps and triceps in patients who underwent reconstruction early, with a denervation time of less than 6 months.

Younger patients had significantly better outcomes ($p < 0.05$) in restoration of hand flexion and the results were significantly superior ($p < 0.05$) when early reconstruction (before 6 months of denervation) was employed. The lower the severity score, the less satisfactory the final outcome.

Protective sensation improved and pain decreased postoperatively before measureable improvement in muscle function in patients who underwent median nerve reconstruction. The mean pain score after reconstruction in avulsion injuries was 40% of the preoperative value. Protective sensation in the arm was present in 96% of patients postoperatively, in the forearm in 81% of patients, and in the hand in 65% of patients (Figure 118-10). This improvement in protective sensation came after neurotization of the median nerve with various sensory donors (e.g., sensory intercostal and supraclavicular nerves). Alnot[2] concurs that reinnervation provides a protective sensation, particularly in the area controlled by the median nerve.

Protective sensation allows the patient to recognize the position of an extremity in space and avoid injuries. Moreover, any return of afferent input, even protective sensation, dramatically blocks the nociceptive afferent pathways. Lack of pain permits the patient to focus on the rehabilitation of the extremity and to improve its dexterity and overall function.

Narakas[33] noted that among 208 patients who underwent surgery for brachial plexus avulsion injuries and who had severe deafferentation pain after extensive root avulsions, half were cured of their pain after neurotization. The positive effects of pain relief preceded the appearance of motor function by many months.

The postoperative muscle grade for each target was separated into four groups. An outcome was considered poor when the muscle grade was 0 to 2; it was considered fair when the grade was between 2+ and 3; good when the grade was between 3+ and 4-; and excellent when it was between 4 and 4+. The overall postoperative results for each muscle target are shown in Figure 118-11.

The most rewarding results were seen in patients who underwent suprascapular nerve reconstruction; approximately 70% had good or excellent results. Deltoid, biceps, and finger flexion restoration provided good or excellent muscle strength

Text continued on p. 2097

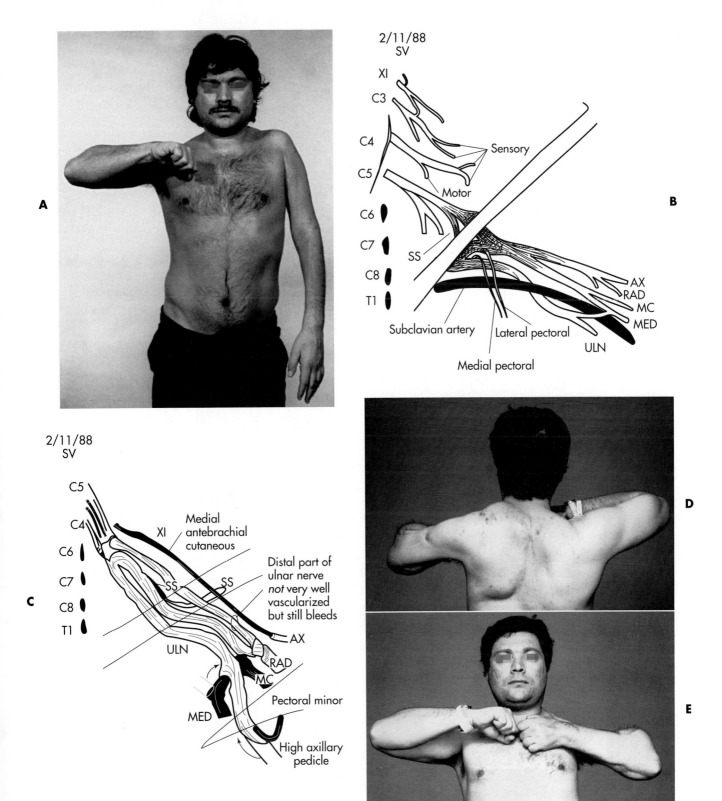

Figure 118-3. **A,** 32-year-old male patient who was involved in a high-velocity motorcycle accident on 9/6/87. The patient sustained a global left brachial plexus paralysis. He presented preoperatively with a flail, anaesthetic arm with severe, intolerable pain. A few weeks before brachial plexus reconstruction he underwent a DREZ procedure at the levels of C6 to T1. **B,** An exploration of the left brachial plexus revealed avulsion of all of the roots except C5. **C,** The reconstruction included the following procedures: neurotization of the axillary nerve from the accessory nerve by means of interposition nerve graft; direct neurotization of the suprascapular nerve from a motor branch of C4; and neurotization of the musculocutaneous, median, and radial nerves from C5 by means of a vascularized ulnar nerve graft. Banked nerve grafts also were placed and were neurotized with cervical motors. On 6/5/89, a wrist fusion and a free muscle transfer (gracilis) for finger extension were performed. On 12/10/90, a free latissimus dorsi was transferred for posterior deltoid and triceps strengthening. **D** and **E,** Patient demonstrates excellent shoulder abduction and elbow flexion 3 years after the initial reconstruction. *Continued*

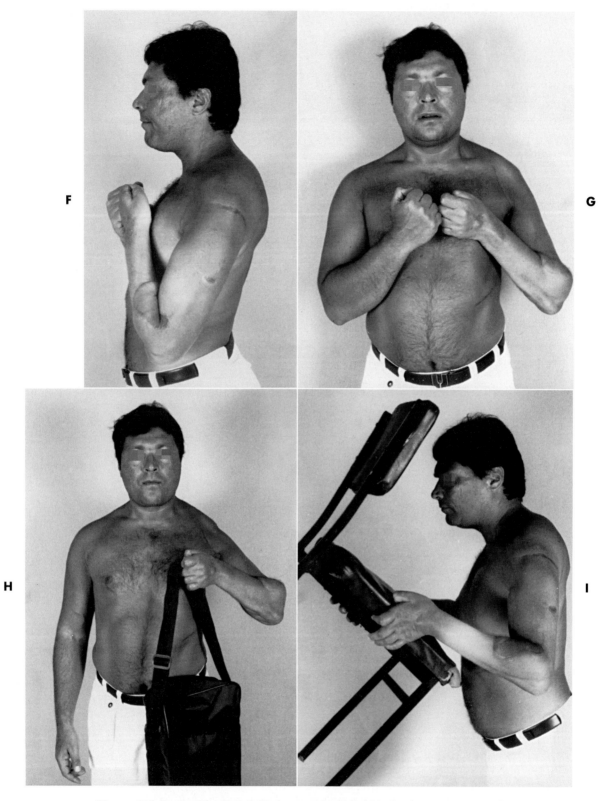

Figure 118-3, cont'd. **F** and **G,** 6 years after brachial plexus repair, patient demonstrates strong elbow flexion and finger flexion through median nerve neurotization. Patient easily lifts his shoulder bag **(H)** and a chair **(I)** with his reconstructed extremity. The patient is currently pain free, working as a security guard, and using his reconstructed extremity as an assisted arm.

Continued

(L) BRACHIAL PLEXUS

NAME _____ SV _____   EXAMINER _____
DATE OF EXAM _12/8/87_   DATE OF SURGERY _____
DATE OF INJURY _9/6/87_   HAND DOMINANCE _____
OCCUPATION _____   FRACTURES _Ø_
HORNOR'S SYNDROME _YES_   VASCULAR STATUS _Normal_
MYELOGRAM   C4 ___ C5 _N_ C6 _AV_ C7 _AV_ C8 _AV_ T1 _AV_ T2 _N_
EMG _____ DIAPHRAGM _____ TINEL _____

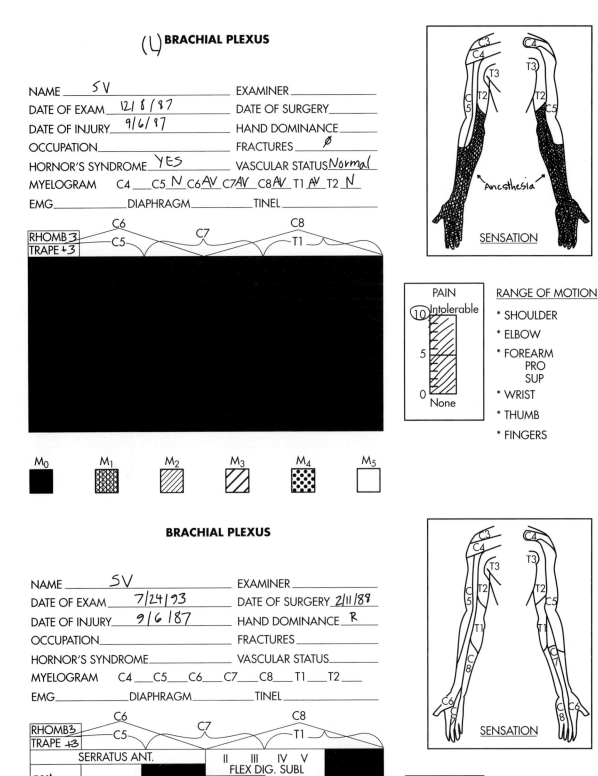

	C6	C7	C8	
RHOMB 3	C5		T1	
TRAPE +3				

RANGE OF MOTION
* SHOULDER
* ELBOW
* FOREARM   PRO   SUP
* WRIST
* THUMB
* FINGERS

PAIN — 10 Intolerable, 5, 0 None

M₀   M₁   M₂   M₃   M₄   M₅

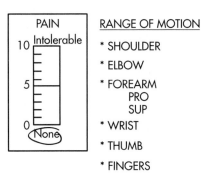

J

BRACHIAL PLEXUS

NAME _____ SV _____   EXAMINER _____
DATE OF EXAM _7/24/93_   DATE OF SURGERY _2/11/88_
DATE OF INJURY _9/6/87_   HAND DOMINANCE _R_
OCCUPATION _____   FRACTURES _____
HORNOR'S SYNDROME _____   VASCULAR STATUS _____
MYELOGRAM   C4 ___ C5 ___ C6 ___ C7 ___ C8 ___ T1 ___ T2 ___
EMG _____ DIAPHRAGM _____ TINEL _____

	C6	C7	C8	
RHOMB 3	C5		T1	
TRAPE +3				

SENSATION

SERRATUS ANT.		II III IV V FLEX DIG. SUBL	
post. 3	BICEPS -4		2
lat. DELT.		TRICEPS	FLEX POL +1 LONG
ant.	BRACHIALIS		
SUPRA SPIN +3	BRACHIO-RADIALIS	EXT. DIG. COMM -3 ET PROPRII	FLEX II DIG III 2+
INFRA SPIN	SUPINATOR		PROF. -3 IV V
	TERES MAJ	LATISSIMUS DORSI	
PECTORALIS MAJOR			

PAIN — 10 Intolerable, 5, 0 None

RANGE OF MOTION
* SHOULDER
* ELBOW
* FOREARM   PRO   SUP
* WRIST
* THUMB
* FINGERS

K

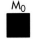 M₀    M₁   M₂   M₃   M₄   M₅

Figure 118-3, cont'd.   **J** and **K,** Plexus charts of clinical examination before and after surgery.

Table 118-1.
Nerve Reconstructions

DONOR NERVE TARGET	SUPRA SCAPULAR	AXILLARY	MUSCULOCUTANEOUS	TRICEPS	MEDIAN	RADIAL
Intraplexus	25	51	61	24	54	46
Cervical plexus	5	12	8	4	8	2
Accessory	50	9	5	5	—	—
Hypoglossal	—	—	2	—	2	—
Phrenic	—	1	5	4	—	—
Intercostals	—	7	21	21	2	4
Contralateral C7	1	4	7	3	9	5
Other*	1	16	18	9	22	14

*Other proximal donors include the proximal stumps of repaired nerves and distal parts of the plexus (cords).

Table 118-2.
Muscle Grading

MUSCLE	PREOPERATIVE MEAN MUSCLE GRADE	POSTOPERATIVE MEAN MUSCLE GRADE	p VALUE
Supraspinatus	−1	3	< 0.0001
Deltoid	0	−3	< 0.0001
Biceps	−1	3	< 0.0001
Triceps	0	−3	< 0.0001
Finger flexion	0	2+	< 0.0001
Finger extension	−1	−2	< 0.05

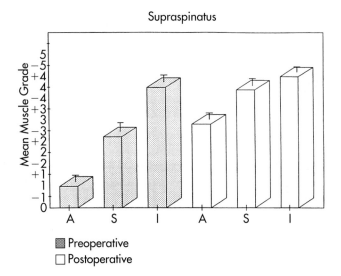

Figure 118-4. Mean muscle grading of the supraspinatus muscle before and after surgery, in relation to the type of injury. *A*, Avulsion; *S*, postganglionic supraclavicular; *I*, postganglionic infraclavicular.

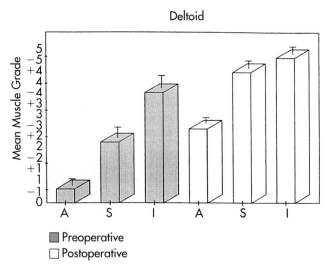

Figure 118-5. Mean muscle grading of the deltoid muscle before and after surgery, in relation to the type of injury. *A*, Avulsion; *S*, postganglionic supraclavicular; *I*, postganglionic infraclavicular.

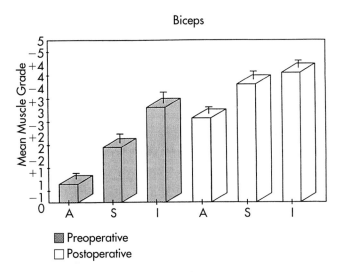

Figure 118-6. Mean muscle grading of the biceps muscle before and after surgery, in relation to the type of injury. *A,* Avulsion; *S,* postganglionic supraclavicular; *I,* postganglionic infraclavicular.

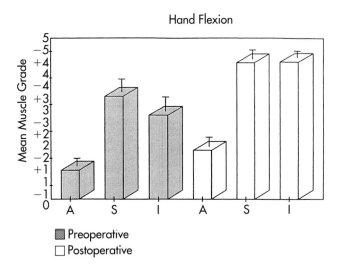

Figure 118-8. Mean muscle grading for hand flexion before and after surgery, in relation to the type of injury. *A,* Avulsion; *S,* postganglionic supraclavicular; *I,* postganglionic infraclavicular.

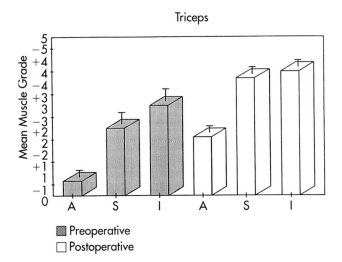

Figure 118-7. Mean muscle grading of the triceps muscle before and after surgery, in relation to the type of injury. *A,* Avulsion; *S,* postganglionic supraclavicular; *I,* postganglionic infraclavicular.

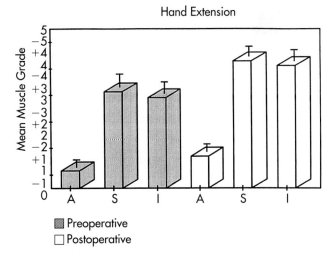

Figure 118-9. Mean muscle grading for hand extension before and after surgery, in relation to the type of injury. *A,* Avulsion; *S,* postganglionic supraclavicular; *I,* postganglionic infraclavicular.

in 35% to 45% of patients. We also found that among patients who underwent triceps restoration, approximately 60% had muscle strength grades between 2+ and 3, and 25% had a good or excellent outcome. The outcome was less satisfactory among patients who underwent restoration of finger extension: 15% of patients had fair results and 25% had good or excellent function.

The majority of our patients were satisfied with the results of microsurgery. Among those who have not completed their reconstruction, most want to proceed with further surgery to improve the function of their extremity.

We believe that a multistage approach, with aggressive early nerve reconstruction and the use of various modern techniques in combination with secondary procedures, such as free muscle

transfers, should be used for microsurgical management of all brachial plexus injuries. The only exceptions to this rule are lesions involving neurapraxia, which have a chance of spontaneous recovery.

Sedel[37] presented the results of brachial plexus reconstruction in 62 patients who had 29 avulsion injuries, 19 supraclavicular lesions, and 15 infraganglionic lesions. The reconstruction involved external neurolysis only in 10 cases; neurotization with intercostals, using interpositional grafts, was performed in eight cases (in three of these the spinal accessory with graft was used to reconstruct the lateral and posterior cord); a combination of intraplexus nerve grafting and neurotization with intercostals was performed in seven cases; and nerve grafting only was performed in the remaining cases. Sedel did not reconstruct the suprascapular nerve but did reconstruct the axillary indirectly by restoring the continuity at a more proximal trunk or cord level. His overall results were recorded as good or excellent in 13% of the patients at the shoulder, in 45% for elbow flexion, and in 22% for triceps

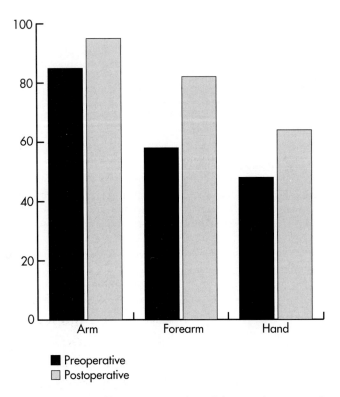

Figure 118-10. Protective sensation of the arm, forearm, and hand before and after surgery.

restoration. He obtained fair results for hand flexion in 16% of the patients with complete palsies. His results for infraclavicular lesions and supraclavicular lesions were better when at least two roots were available for neurotization. The outcome was considered disappointing when only one root was available.

In 1988 Millesi[29] compared results of surgery in patients who had complete brachial plexus lesions with loss of continuity. He found that between 1963 and 1973 he achieved shoulder stability in 18.6% of patients and strong elbow flexion in 62% of patients; between 1982 and 1984 his results improved to 76.2% and 83.7% of patients, respectively. He also used intercostals to neurotize the musculocutaneous nerve and obtained useful elbow flexion in 58.9% of patients. Millesi also neurotized the suprascapular and axillary nerves with the accessory nerve and achieved stability of the shoulder in 61% of patients who underwent this procedure. He states that a result is useful if strong elbow flexion returns and if the patient can stabilize the shoulder with some active motion. It is worth mentioning that he does not routinely reconstruct hand function.

In 1995 Alnot stated that overall results are better for repair of infraclavicular lesions and supraclavicular injuries involving the upper roots. Among his series of 810 patients who underwent surgery for traumatic brachial plexus injuries, 75% of injuries were supraclavicular, and 24% of these involved global avulsions. He obtained fair to good results (M3 to M4) after axillary and musculocutaneous repair, using nerve grafts in 90% of patients who had infraclavicular or retroclavicular lesions. Results were difficult to assess only in cases of retroclavicular plexus injuries associated with vascular injuries; these are traction injuries that can involve more than one level

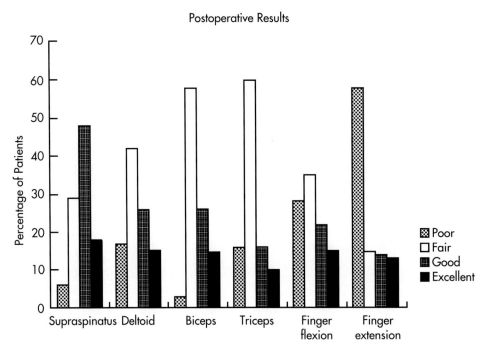

Figure 118-11. Overall postoperative results for each muscle target (*poor*, 0 to 2; *fair*, 2+ to 3; *good*, 3+ to 4-; *excellent*, 4 to 5).

of nerve trauma. The main problems concerned the median and ulnar nerves. Partial supraclavicular palsies of C5 and C6 were successfully repaired in 73% of patients; when C7 was also involved the percentage dropped to 49%. Alnot repaired the suprascapular nerve from the accessory nerve. He achieved elbow flexion of M3 to M4 in 75% of patients with global avulsion injuries by means of neurotization of the musculocutaneous nerve with the accessory and motor branches of the cervical plexus. He noted that shoulder and elbow function in patients with complete palsies and root avulsions was better if two roots were available. Hand function was also ignored in this series.

In 1988 Hentz and Narakas[21] analyzed data from 114 patients. They advocated early exploration in cases of complete palsies and suggested that outcomes are better in younger patients and in the presence of proximal healthy roots. Nerve grafts were performed in 61 patients; of these 16 underwent neurotization, and 23 patients underwent a combination of nerve grafts and neurotization. All muscle testing was performed by the authors. The average muscle recovery grade was −2 for biceps, 1+ for deltoid, and 1+ for supraspinatus muscles. Finger flexion was averaged −1. A total of 3100 muscles were analyzed in the 109 patients who were studied more closely and only 15% achieved results of grade 3 or better. Statistically significant improvement occurred in the average scores of patients with infraclavicular injuries. Statistically significant correlations also were present between the result and the patient's age, denervation time, and type of reconstruction.

In 1987 Gu et al[18] presented 20 years of experience with 108 patients who had avulsion injuries. They showed good results in 75% of musculocutaneous neurotizations using the phrenic nerve; in 50% of suprascapular and axillary neurotizations using motor branches of the cervical plexus; in 55% of radial neurotizations using the accessory nerve; and in 33% of median repairs with intercostals. Gu hypothesized that the poor results of the intercostal neurotizations were caused by fewer motor fibers in the donor nerves and the long distance between the site of nerve repair and the targets. The most satisfactory results after these nerve transfers were related to early surgery, following the principle of tension-free repair, in young patients without severe crushing trauma to the distal plexus elements.

Encouraging outcomes were also presented in 1995 by Songcharoen,[39] who reported on 350 patients treated by several methods. He performed primary nerve reconstruction, including 38 neurolyses, 23 nerve grafts, and 314 neurotizations (of which 250 used the accessory nerve), and/or secondary operations, including 16 free muscle transfers and 30 musculotendinous transfers. His outcomes were fair or good or excellent in 69% of patients who underwent neurolysis, and in 82% of patients who underwent nerve grafting. Better outcomes were obtained by neurotization from the accessory and phrenic nerves to the musculocutaneous, suprascapular, and axillary nerves (75%) and from the use of intraplexus donors (71%). Intercostal neurotizations to the musculocutaneous nerve were less satisfactory;

65% of patients who underwent this procedure had good or fair results.

In 1988 Narakas and Hentz[33] conveyed their experience with neurotization using the accessory nerve in 30 patients; they obtained good results in 35% of patients. Intercostals were used in 24 patients for musculocutaneous neurotization, with fair to excellent results in 60% of patients. For the remaining targets (median, radial, axillary, suprascapular, posterior cord) the results were fair to excellent in 38% of patients. Various intraplexus donors were used in 31 patients, with good results in 50% of these patients. The authors obtained good elbow flexion with these methods in more than 50% of patients; however, shoulder function was limited and no useful finger flexion was obtained.

In 1995 Berger[5] presented 12 years of experience treating 362 patients and stated that only the combination of primary nerve repair with secondary procedures can restore maximum function in the paralyzed extremity. He performed 104 neurolyses, 126 nerve grafting procedures, 87 neurotizations using the accessory nerve to axillary nerve and intercostal nerves to musculocutaneous and median nerves. He also performed 191 secondary operations in 96 patients in an attempt to reconstruct hand function using free muscle transfers. Because he did not provide results regarding the degree of muscle function restored to the hand, comparisons are not feasible.

The total severity score must be considered when comparing overall results from various large series. The mean total severity score for all patients in our series was approximately 5, which indicates that the majority of the injuries sustained were severe (i.e., most of the patients had multiple root avulsions). A severity score of 25 reflects a normal brachial plexus.

It is generally accepted that upper root palsies have a better overall outcome than lower root injuries or complete palsies. The reason for this is dual. First, hand function is preserved, and second, the muscle targets are closer to the plexus. The short distance between motor donor nerves and the target also explains the better outcome of injuries to the proximal muscles (e.g., supraspinatus, biceps, and deltoid).

The strategies for reconstruction differ in various series. Currently, the most prevalent method for treating complete severe brachial plexus palsies involves only reconstruction of the shoulder to provide stability and some motion and elbow flexion. This strategy ignores reconstruction of hand function.

No patient wants to undergo amputation of the paralyzed limb. Patients prefer even partial use of the limb. The surgeon must make every effort to maximize motor and sensory recovery by whatever means seem appropriate. Thus we consider it necessary to pursue the restoration of hand function.

One of the major concerns during neurotization or nerve grafting procedures must be the level of the distal coaptation. In 1995, Alnot[2] indicated that nerve grafting is more rewarding when the distal coaptation is near the muscle target. We agree with this assessment and advocate placement of the distal coaptations (for interpositional nerve grafts or neurotizations) near the muscle target to yield the best result. This method increases the number of nerve fibers that are directed to the muscle target because less dispersion of donor fibers occurs as the repaired nerve branch becomes more specific.

We also found that the results from our series were less rewarding in targets arising from posterior cord motors such as the deltoid, the triceps, and the finger extensors. Thus it seems that an inferior response to reconstruction occurs in certain muscle groups (e.g., shoulder abductors, external rotators, supinators, extensors). Similar observations were made by Narakas,[33] who mentions that this paradox can be partially explained by the embryologic origin of various muscles. There seems to be a built-in preference for restoration of the flexors, which are vital for the survival of the organism.

We prefer to use intraplexus rather than extraplexus motor donors for neurotizations, when the former are available. Intraplexus donors have a greater number of axons than extraplexus donors and therefore the chances for successful neurotization are greater. We use all possible ipsilateral intraplexus and extraplexus donors in severe complete palsies with avulsions, including the phrenic, hypoglossal, accessory, and cervical motor branches, the intercostals, and the contralateral motor donors, in an effort to reconstruct the largest number of critical targets either primarily or by banking nerve grafts for neurotization of future muscle transfers, especially for the hand. Some of the extraplexus donors have given constantly satisfactory results when used directly with certain targets (e.g., the accessory nerve for neurotization of the suprascapular nerve). Various Japanese surgeons, such as Nagano et al,[31] have noted the superiority of using the intercostal nerves for direct neurotizations of existing muscles or for free muscle transfers without an interpositional nerve graft.

SUMMARY

Nerve reconstruction can provide far more satisfactory function than the various secondary reconstructions with muscle transfers. Free muscle transfers and other secondary procedures are still necessary to improve the final outcome in global avulsion injuries, in cases in which a long period has elapsed between injury and repair, or in the reconstruction of distal targets such as the hand. All authors agree that the best overall outcomes are achieved in young patients who have proximal injuries of the brachial plexus that can be repaired by intraplexus donors and who are reconstructed early. The restoration of hand function is a difficult but feasible task and must be attempted. Preservation of the muscle targets and joints, especially the distal ones, must be a high priority, if functional restoration in the hand is to be pursued.

The socioeconomic issues involved in these injuries and their treatment must be considered in the evaluation of outcomes. These patients typically are young and active and in the most productive period of their lives; the accident, and the residual palsy, forces them to stop working. The reconstruction of these devastating injuries usually involves multiple stages. The postoperative course of rehabilitation includes immobilization in a custom made splint for 6 to 8 weeks, followed by intensive physical therapy.

The patient must cooperate with the prolonged time of recuperation and must realize that even the most successful surgeries offer a functional but not normal upper extremity. It is very important during this period to provide the patient with psychological support and encourage the patient to start working. It has been observed that patients who are not working have less rewarding outcomes and continue to have pain; this creates a vicious cycle that leads the patient to refuse further reconstruction, reducing the chances of improvement in the paralyzed extremity.

A comparison of the published literature shows that outcomes achieved in our center by aggressive early reconstruction are superior to those achieved elsewhere. This is an important observation, especially in view of the fact that the majority of the patients in our series had avulsion injury and furthermore the outcomes in our series were graded by a panel of five independent reviewers that did not include the senior surgeon. We are one of very few centers that has made hand reanimation a focal point in our overall reconstructive scheme.

We conclude that early, aggressive reconstruction with meticulous microsurgical techniques offers the best results, even in cases of severe brachial plexus injuries. Neurotizations with various intraplexus and extraplexus donors (both ipsilateral and contralateral), in combination with vascularized nerve grafts and secondary procedures such as free functioning muscle transfers, yield rewarding results, even in distal targets such as the hand, and avoids amputation, even in cases of global avulsion injury.

REFERENCES

1. Allieu Y, Cenac P: Neurotization via the spinal accessory nerve in complete paralysis due to multiple avulsion injuries of the brachial plexus, *Clin Orthop* 237:67-74, 1988.
2. Alnot J: Traumatic brachial plexus lesions in the adult: indications and results, *Hand Clin* 11(4): 623-631, 1995.
3. Barnes R: Traction injuries of the plexus in adults, *J Bone Joint Surg* 31B:10-16, 1949.
4. Berger A, Becker M: Brachial plexus surgery: our concept of the last twelve years, *Microsurgery* 15:760-767, 1994.
5. Berger A, Brenner P: Secondary surgery following brachial plexus injuries, *Microsurgery* 16:43-47, 1995.
6. Bonney G: Prognosis in traction lesions of the brachial plexus, *J Bone Joint Surg* 41B:4-35, 1959.
7. Brunelli GA, Brunelli GR: Preoperative assessment of the adult plexus patient, *Microsurgery* 16:17-21, 1995.
8. Brunelli GA, Vigasio A, Brunelli GR: Modified Steindler procedure for elbow flexion restoration, *J Hand Surg [Am]* 20:743-746, 1995.

9. Carlstedt TP: Spinal nerve root injuries in brachial plexus lesions: basic science and clinical application of new surgical strategies (a review), *Microsurgery* 16;13-16, 1995.

10. Carson KA, Terzis JK: Carbonic anhydrase histochemistry: a potential diagnostic method for peripheral nerve repair, *Clin Plast Surg* 12(2):227-232, 1985.

11. Chuang D: Neurotization procedures for brachial plexus injuries, *Hand Clin* 11(4):633-645, 1995.

12. Daniel RK, Terzis JK, Schwarz G: Neurovascular free flaps: a preliminary report, *Plast Reconstr Surg* 56(1):13-20, 1975.

13. Doi K, Sakai K, Fuchigami Y, Kawai S: Reconstruction of irreparable brachial plexus injuries with reinnervated free-muscle transfer, *J Neurosurg* 85:174-177, 1996.

14. Dykes RW, Terzis JK: Spinal nerve distributions in the upper limb: the organization of the dermatome and afferent myotome, *Philos Trans R Soc Lond B Biol Sci* 293(1070):509-554, 1981.

15. Flether I: Traction lesions of the brachial plexus, *Hand* 1:129, 1969.

16. Friedman AH, Nashold BS Jr, Bronec PR: Dorsal root entry zone lesions for the treatment of brachial plexus avulsion injuries: a follow-up study, *Neurosurgery* 22(2):369-373, 1988.

17. Gilbert A: *Neurotization by contralateral pectoral nerve.* Presented at the 10th Symposium on the brachial plexus, Lausanne, Switzerland, 1992.

18. Gu YD, Wu MM, Zheng YL, et al: Microsurgical treatment for root avulsion of the brachial plexus, *Chin Med J* 100(7):519-522, 1987.

19. Gu YD, Wu MM, Zheng YL, et al: Phrenic nerve transfer for brachial plexus motor neurotization, *Microsurgery* 10:287-289, 1989.

20. Gu YD, Zhang GM, Chen DS, et al: Cervical nerve root transfer from contralateral normal side for treatment of brachial plexus root avulsion, *Chin Med J* (Engl) 104:208, 1991.

21. Hentz V, Narakas A: The results of microneurosurgical reconstruction in complete brachial plexus palsy: assessing outcome and predicting results, *Orthop Clin North Am* 19(1):107-114, 1988.

22. Kawai H, Kawabata H, Masada K, et al: Nerve repairs for traumatic brachial plexus palsy with root avulsion, *Clin Orthop* 237:75-86, 1988.

23. Kurze T: Microtechniques in neurological surgery, *Clin Neurosurg* 11:128-137, 1964.

24. Leffert RD, Seddon H: Infraclavicular brachial plexus injuries, *J Bone Joint Surg* 49B:9-22, 1965.

25. Lusskin R, Campbell JB, Thompson WAL: Post-traumatic lesions of the brachial plexus: treatment by transclavicular exploration and neurolysis or autograft reconstruction, *J Bone Joint Surg* 55(A):1159, 1973.

26. Marshall RW, De Silva RDD: Computerized axial tomography in traction injuries of the brachial plexus, *J Bone Joint Surg* 68B:734, 1986.

27. Marshall RW, Williams DH, Birch R, Bonney G: Operations to restore elbow flexion after brachial plexus injuries, *J Bone Joint Surg* 70B:577-582, 1988.

28. Millesi H: Brachial plexus injuries: management and results, *Clin Plast Surg* 11:115, 1984.

29. Millesi H: Brachial plexus injuries: nerve grafting, *Clin Orthop* 237:36-42, 1988.

30. Millesi H, Ganglberger L, Berger A: Erfahrung mit der Microchirurgie peripherer nerven, *Chir Plast Reconstr* 3:47, 1967.

31. Nagano A, Tsuyama N, Ochiai N, et al: Direct nerve crossing with the intercostal nerve to treat avulsion injuries of the brachial plexus, *J Hand Surg [Am]* 14(6):980-985, 1989.

32. Narakas A: The surgical management of brachial plexus injuries. In Daniel RK, Terzis JK (editors): *Reconstructive microsurgery*, vol 1, Boston, 1977, Little-Brown.

33. Narakas A, Hentz V: Neurotization in brachial plexus injuries: indications and results, *Clin Orthop* 237:43-56, 1988.

34. Robotti E, Longhi P, Verna G, Bocchiotti G: Brachial plexus surgery: a historical perspective, *Hand Clin* 11(4):517-533, 1995.

35. Roger B, Travers V, Laval-Jeantet M: Imaging of posttraumatic brachial plexus injury, *Clin Orthop* 237:57-61, 1988.

36. Seddon HJ: Nerve grafting, *J Bone Joint Surg* 45:447, 1963.

37. Sedel L: The results of surgical repair of brachial plexus injuries, *J Bone Joint Surg* 64(B):54-66, 1982.

38. Sedel L: Repair of severe traction lesions of the brachial plexus, *Clin Orthop* 237:62-66, 1988.

39. Songcharoen P: Brachial plexus injury in Thailand: a report of 520 cases, *Microsurgery* 16:35-39, 1995.

40. Stevens JH: Brachial plexus paralysis. In Godman EA (editor): *The shoulder,* Brooklyn, NY, 1934, G. Mill.

41. Sunderland S: Classification of peripheral nerve injuries, *Brain* 74:491-516, 1951.

42. Taylor GI, Ham FJ: The free vascularized nerve graft: a further experimental and clinical application of microvascular techniques, *Plast Reconstr Surg* 57:413, 1976.

43. Terzis JK: *Contralateral C7: A powerful source of motor neurons for devastating brachial plexus paralysis.* Presented at the 7th annual meeting of European Association of Plastic Surgeons, Innsbruck, Austria, 1996.

44. Terzis JK: Personal communication, 1984.

45. Terzis JK, Breidenbach W: The anatomy of free vascularized nerve grafts. In Terzis JK (editor): *Microreconstruction of nerve injuries,* Philadelphia, 1987, WB Saunders.

46. Terzis JK, Faibisoff B, Williams HB: A diamond knife for microsurgical repair of peripheral nerves, *Plast Reconstr Surg* 54(1):102-103, 1974.

47. Terzis JK, Faibisoff B, Williams B: The nerve gap: suture under tension vs. graft, *Plast Reconstr Surg* 56(2):166-70, 1975.

48. Terzis JK, Maragh H: Strategies in the microsurgical management of brachial plexus injuries, *Clin Plast Surg* 16:605-616, 1989.

49. Terzis JK, Sweet RC, Dykes RW, Williams HB: Recovery of function in free muscle transplants using microneurovascular anastomoses, *J Hand Surg [Am]* 3(1):37-59, 1978.

50. Tracy JF, Brannon EW: Management of brachial plexus injuries (traction type), *J Bone Joint Surg* 40(A):1031, 1958.

51. Wynn Parry CB: Rehabilitation of patients following traction injuries of the brachial plexus, *Hand Clin* 11(4):517-533, 1995.

52. Yeoman PM, Seddon HJ: Brachial plexus injuries: treatment of the flail arm, *J Bone Joint Surg* 43B:493, 1961.

Nerve Repair and Nerve Grafting

119

Benjamin M. Maser
Nicholas Vedder

INTRODUCTION

Interruption of saltatory conduction along the axons of a peripheral nerve causes significant disability because of partial or complete loss of motor function and sensation. Nerve tissue does possess an intrinsic regenerative capability,[42] but functional recovery of untreated or very severely injured nerves is unpredictable and usually poor.[37] Accurate repair of a severed peripheral nerve is of paramount importance in restoring function. Repairs undertaken without meticulous attention to technique also lead to less than optimal results.

Techniques to repair transected peripheral nerves continue to evolve. The current approach focuses on early repair and the belief that "less is more" with regard to the repair technique. Despite our best efforts and the use of meticulous microsurgical technique, peripheral nerve function after a repair never returns to normal. The goal is to continue to find ways mechanically or biochemically to improve nerve regeneration.

INFORMED CONSENT

The following issues should be discussed with the patient after the diagnosis and decision to operate have been made:

1. *Planned incisions:* The surgeon should describe the incisions that will be necessary to expose the injured nerves and those that may be necessary to harvest a nerve graft.
2. *Potential findings:* The physician should describe, in lay terms, a normal nerve and general types of nerve injury that may be found, including a nerve that is contused, a nerve that has been partially lacerated but is still intact, and/or a nerve that has been completely transected (with possible segmental loss).
3. *Repair:* The physician should describe types of nerve repair that may involve suturing a partially lacerated nerve, repair of a completely transected nerve, and the use of interpositional nerve grafts if repair cannot be achieved without undue tension. The patient also should be informed that, depending on the extent of tissue damage and contamination, it may be necessary to debride and

tag the transected nerve ends for identification during subsequent repair.
4. *Nerve grafting:* The patient must understand that if nerve grafting is required, a neurologic deficit in the sensory or motor distribution of the donor nerve will occur. Our preferred donor nerve is the sural nerve; when this nerve is used the patient should be told that sensory deficit on the dorsolateral surface of the foot occurs in response to graft harvesting (Figure 119-1).
5. *Potential complications:* The potential complications of nerve repair merit careful discussion with the patient and include the standard complications of any operation (e.g., risks associated with anesthesia, bleeding, and wound infection). Complications that are unique to the repair of a peripheral nerve include neuroma formation at the site of repair, rupture of the nerve repair from excessive tension across the repair site, and inadequate nerve regeneration despite a technically acceptable repair.
6. *Recovery:* The patient must understand that splinting after surgery is necessary to allow the nerve to heal before motion of the extremity or digit is resumed. Return of function in a damaged nerve will not be immediate; complete motor and/or sensory return may take as long as 3 years. The level of nerve function that is ultimately achieved is unpredictable, but function never completely returns to normal.[16]

ANATOMY

A surgeon who hopes to carry out the best nerve repair technically possible must have a thorough knowledge of peripheral nerve anatomy.[32,53] The normal cross-sectional anatomy of a mixed peripheral nerve is shown in Figure 119-2. Groups of individual cell axons are separated from each other within the nerve and are surrounded by the collagenous endoneurium. Large motor and sensory axons are individually myelinated; smaller axons may be grouped together and wrapped by individual Schwann cells along the course of the axons. The greater the degree of myelination, the faster the conduction. Groups of axons are bundled together to make up individual nerve fascicles. Each fascicle is surrounded by the lamellar perineurium, which serves to control the intraneural ionic environment. Individual fascicles are arranged into fascicular groups. These groups are suspended in and surrounded by the inner epineurium, which also surrounds individual longitudinally arranged nutrient blood vessels. The periphery of the nerve is encased in the outer epineurium, which is a condensation of the collagenous internal epineurium. This layer is what gives the nerve strength.

Several types of nerve injury can occur. Degrees of nerve injury have been classified by both Sunderland and Seddon (Table 119-1).[45,50] Nerve injuries associated with closed fractures are usually neurapraxias; in these cases the nerve is intact but contused and temporarily dysfunctional, despite having intact axons. High-velocity missile injuries often produce an axonotmesis; in such injuries the nerve is intact externally but characterized by complete or partial discontinuity of axons internally. A nerve laceration that involves complete division of all nerve substance is termed a *neurotmesis*.[37]

The damage to the nerve observed during surgical exploration may take multiple forms. If, for example, the epineurium has not been disrupted in a crush injury, the nerve may appear edematous and contused or may appear normal. An avulsion injury can occur when longitudinal forces are applied to the nerve, causing a stretch injury. A severe stretch may leave the epineurium intact but may cause internal disruption of the axons, producing an axonotmesis; a nerve with this type of injury may be narrowed into a viable hour-glass deformity. Nerve lacerations can be partial or complete. The proximal and distal stumps retract after a complete transection because of the inherent elastic tension within the nerve. The degree of proximal and distal retraction and the extent of physical damage to the nerve determine the method and the timing of repair.

Primary end-to-end nerve repair without tension is most likely to restore function but may not be possible when there is segmental loss of nerve substance or when the proximal extent of nerve injury cannot be determined. Primary or delayed

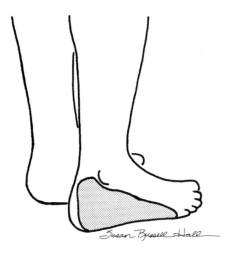

Figure 119-1. Expected region of anesthesia *(shaded area)* after harvesting of sural nerve graft.

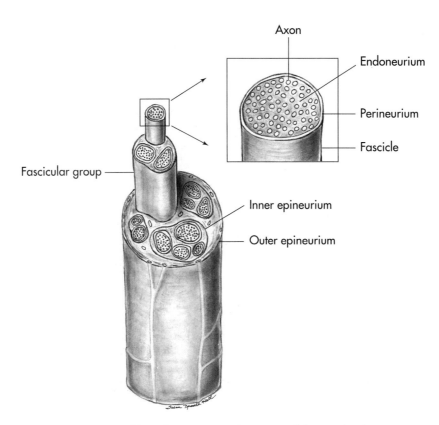

Figure 119-2. Normal cross-sectional anatomy of the peripheral nerve.

nerve grafting may be necessary in such cases to restore nerve continuity and function.

the number of axons that cross the repair sites and make end-organ contact.

INDICATIONS

PATHOPHYSIOLOGY OF INJURY

Axonal disruption leads to well-defined changes within the nerve cell, both proximal and distal to the zone of injury. These changes occur to prepare the nerve cell for regeneration. Axons within the proximal nerve stump first undergo degeneration, the extent of which depends on the mechanism and magnitude of the injury.[23] Each proximal axon subsequently begins to generate multiple axon sprouts, as soon as 5 hours after injury. These sprouts join to form a single axon, known as a *regenerating unit* or *growth cone.* The growth cones of each axon are guided and stimulated by biochemical neurotrophic factors, generated both locally and in the distal nerve stump, that influence the direction of axon growth. Regenerating axons grow toward the distal nerve stump, where they eventually make contact with it and continue into it. The nerve distal to the injury undergoes *wallerian degeneration,* a term derived from the initial description of this process by Joseph Waller.[6] Axoplasm and myelin in the distal stump are cleared away by macrophages and Schwann cells during this process. After the removal of neuronal debris is complete, the resulting connective tissue/Schwann-cell conduit becomes the new scaffolding for axons regenerating from the proximal stump.

The individual axon growth cones propagate distally along the bands of Bunger in the distal stump, which are composed of Schwann-cell columns resting on the basement membrane of the nerve. Propagation occurs at a rate of 1 to 2 mm/day.[47] Axons that establish end-organ contact survive; those that do not are cleared away.[1] The goal of nerve repair is to maximize

OPERATIONS

EVOLUTION

Nerve repair was performed as early as the thirteenth century. However, it was not until scientific confirmation of the regenerative capacity of nerves was pursued by Cruikshank[9] and Muller[35] in the late seventeenth century and by Ramon y Cajal[42] in the early twentieth century that suture repair of nerves became accepted practice.[5,17,42] Many of the major advances since that time grew out of wartime experience, including studies of nerve injury by Mitchell during the Civil War and by Tinel, Seddon, and Woodhall during World Wars I and II.[33,46,58,60] The latter surgeons also performed primary nerve repair and nerve grafting, setting the stage for the further development of these techniques. In the post-war period, Sunderland[50] defined the internal neuroanatomy of peripheral nerves, which provided the groundwork for the various anatomy-specific repairs used today. The evolution of microsurgical technique during the last 30 years also has significantly improved outcomes after peripheral nerve repair.

TIMING OF NERVE REPAIR

Nerve repair that is performed within the first 24 hours after injury is termed *primary repair.* The term *primary* here refers to timing, not to technique. Repairs that are carried out within 1 week of injury are referred to as *delayed primary repairs.* When repair is delayed more than 1 week after injury, it is termed *secondary repair.* A number of studies have examined the effect that timing of repair has on outcome.[4,46,49] Primary or delayed

Table 119-1.
Classification of Nerve Injury

SEDDON CLASSIFICATION	INJURY	SUNDERLAND CLASSIFICATION
Neurapraxia	Anatomic/axonal continuity	First degree
Axonotmesis	Axons transected; endoneurium intact	Second degree
Axonotmesis	Axonal transection; loss of endoneurial tube continuity; perineurium intact	Third degree
Axonotmesis	Epineurial continuity; additional disorganization of nerve architecture (e.g., neuroma in continuity)	Fourth degree
Neurotmesis	Loss of nerve trunk continuity	Fifth degree

Modified from Bowers HB, Carlson EC, Wenner SM, Doyle JR: *Hand Clin,* 5(3):445-453, 1989.

primary nerve repair usually gives the most favorable results, provided that appropriate conditions exist at the time of operation. The best conditions for primary repair involve a sharply transected nerve or one with a small crush component that can be clearly defined at the time of repair and excised back to normal nerve. There should be minimal wound contamination and a well-vascularized soft tissue bed surrounding the nerve repair. There should be no associated injuries in the extremity that might render it avascular or skeletally unstable, and there should be no associated life-threatening injuries to the patient. Secondary repair should be considered when these conditions cannot be met.

AVAILABLE NERVE-REPAIR TECHNIQUES

A number of techniques are available for the repair of injured peripheral nerves. Studies have yet to identify a single method that is clearly superior to all others. Regardless of the technique used, the repair and recovery of an injured peripheral nerve should generally involve adherence to certain principles proposed by Watchmaker and MacKinnon (Box 119-1).[57]

An end-to-end coaptation of the nerve ends is preferred when they can be connected under minimal or no tension. This procedure can be accomplished with or without the use of suture. Suture-free techniques may involve the use of fibrin glue, ring coupling, or CO_2 laser welding[57,59]; all of these are carried out at the level of the epineurium. Some of the advantages and disadvantages of these techniques are outlined in Table 119-2.[18,40,41,57,59] The vast majority of peripheral-nerve repair techniques currently are performed with a microsurgical suture technique. Suture repair techniques are based on the internal anatomy of the nerve, and include perineurial, group fascicular, and epineurial repairs. A perineurial repair joins the nerve ends at the level of the individual fascicles (Figure 119-3). A group fascicular repair joins anatomically separate fascicular groups by placing sutures through the internal interfascicular epineurium (Figure 119-4). An epineurial repair joins the nerve by placing sutures through the outer epineurium (Figure 119-5).

Box 119-1.
Principles of Nerve Repair

1. Quantitative preoperative and postoperative assessment of motor and sensory function
2. Microsurgical repair technique
3. Tension-free coaptation
4. Interpositional nerve grafting (to avoid end-to-end coaptation under tension)
5. Avoidance of postural maneuvers to decrease tension on repair
6. Primary repair when clinical and surgical conditions permit
7. Group fascicular repair when intraneural anatomy permits; epineurial repair when topography is indeterminate or mixed
8. Secondary repair if proximal or distal extent of nerve injury cannot be determined at time of injury
9. Sensory and motor reeducation to maximize results of repair

---

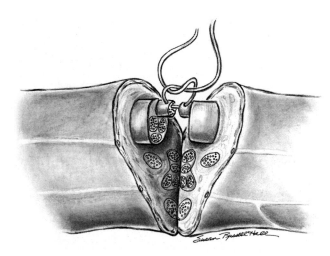

Figure 119-3. Technique of perineurial repair.

Table 119-2.
Nonsutured Repair Techniques

TECHNIQUE	ADVANTAGES	DISADVANTAGE(S)
Laser coaptation	Rapid	Results in decreased early tensile strength/high dehiscence rate; requires additional skills/training; expensive
Fibrin glue	Simple; minimizes trauma to nerve; leaves no foreign body (e.g., suture)	Risk of infection; results in poor early tensile strength
Ring couplers	Simple; rapid	Has no proven advantage over suture; leaves large amount of foreign body at repair site

Regardless of the method chosen, divided nerve ends should be anatomically aligned before repair. Proper fascicular alignment offers regenerating axons the best chance to repopulate their original positions in the nerve distal to the injury and consequently the best chance to reinnervate appropriate motor or sensory end-organs. The surgeon should examine both ends of the cut nerve and identify and/or draw the fascicular pattern observed in each end. This is best achieved by assessing the internal fascicular topography of the nerve in the proximal and distal stumps at the level of the injury, and by aligning the visible longitudinal surface vessels in the epineurium (Figure 119-6). When alignment based on

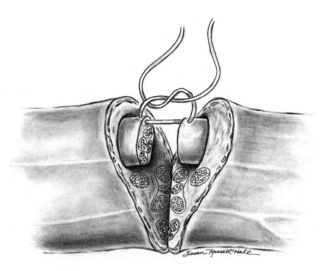

Figure 119-4. Technique of group fascicular repair.

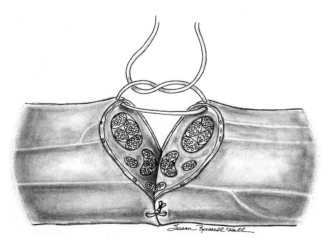

Figure 119-5. Technique of epineurial repair.

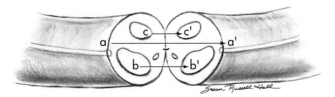

Figure 119-6. Technique using surface vascular anatomy and internal topography of the nerve for optimal alignment before nerve repair.

visual nerve anatomy is difficult, techniques employing electrical stimulation or immunohistochemical staining of the nerve can be used.[57] However, because these techniques can be cumbersome and time consuming, and because they may require the assistance of trained personnel, they are not commonly employed.

Nerve Grafting

Even minimal amounts of tension at the nerve repair site can adversely affect the functional outcome.[30] Thus nerve grafting should be performed when primary repair of severed nerve ends cannot be achieved in a tension-free fashion. Regardless of the repair technique used, the surgeon should attempt to restore anatomical alignment of the individual nerve fascicles. Measurement of the gap between the divided ends, which ranges from 1 to 5 cm,[58] has been used as the criteria for determining when grafting is required. The maximum distance between cut nerve ends that is acceptable for an end-to-end coaptation depends on the site of the lesion. Primary repair may not be possible without the use of a nerve graft in areas with short gaps (e.g., the digit), but end-to-end coaptation of a nerve with the same-sized gap may be easily achieved in the forearm. The surgeon must determine how much tension will be created by an end-to-end repair and, using judgment and experience, determine whether a nerve graft is warranted.

Nerve grafting techniques are similar to those of end-to-end repair. Any diseased or fibrotic nerve tissue in the proximal and distal stumps should be excised back to healthy nerve. Grafts should be of adequate length to minimize tension at the repair sites when the extremity is in a neutral position. The surgeon should strive to accurately match sensory and motor fascicles across the gap; this can be difficult in the proximal portion of the extremity, where fascicles contain mixed sensory and motor fibers. Distally, individual fascicles tend to be primarily either motor or sensory, thus allowing accurate alignment. Local "trophism" also assists regenerating axons in reaching their proper distal destinations.[42]

Nerve-to-graft coaptation can be carried out at the perineurial *(fascicular graft)*, group fascicular *(interfascicular graft)*, or epineurial *(trunk graft)* levels in a manner similar to that of an end-to-end nerve repair.[58] Cable grafts, created by "braiding" strands of a nerve graft into a single unit, are not commonly used. As with end-to-end repair, use of magnification and microsurgical technique is imperative.

Recent studies have examined the experimental and clinical use of allografts and the use of biologic and prosthetic conduits as bridging material for large nerve gaps.[24,25,54,57] Currently autografts remain the standard material for this purpose; they provide a successful scaffolding for the propagation of axonal regeneration into the distal nerve stump. Nerve tissue is usually transferred as a nonvascularized graft. Taylor and Ham[52] introduced the free vascularized nerve concept in the 1970s, and further study has demonstrated its usefulness in situations such as those involving a scarred or irradiated wound bed.[8]

The sural nerve is the most commonly used donor nerve. This pure sensory nerve can provide as much as 40 cm of graft length[23] and is found in the subcutaneous fatty tissue of the posterior leg. After harvest, the nerve can be split longitudi-

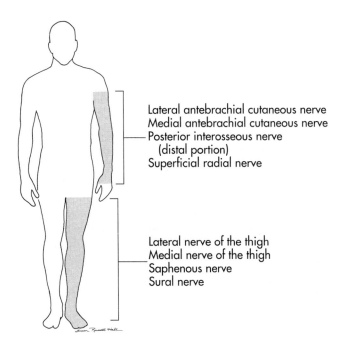

Figure 119-7. Potential donor nerves of the upper and lower extremities.

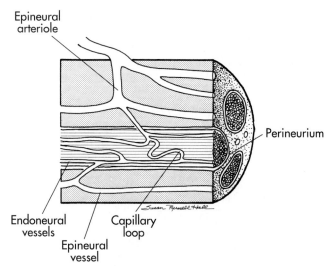

Figure 119-8. Cross-sectional vascular anatomy of the peripheral nerve.

nally into individual strands at the group fascicular level, each split increasing the length of available graft material and improving the total contact surface available for graft revascularization. Other sources of donor nerve are shown in Figure 119-7.

OUR PREFERRED METHOD

We believe that nerve injuries should be managed as early as possible. For open injuries, we prefer primary repair within 24 hours of injury whenever possible. Exceptions to this rule involve patients with associated life-threatening injuries, grossly contaminated wounds or wounds that lack adequate soft tissue to cover the repair, nerve tissue with questionable long-term viability (as can occur in crush injuries), or nerve gaps that require grafting. If primary repair is not possible, delayed primary or secondary repair is performed when such conditions are resolved.

We prefer early rather than late surgical exploration in closed injuries with associated nerve damage. When there is clinical or electromyographic absence of functional return, we generally explore the nerve within 2 months from the time of injury. Our hope is to find and treat any lesion that is impeding recovery.

Our approach to nerve repair begins by optimizing the conditions of the injured nerve and the surrounding wound. The wound should be debrided of all devitalized and contaminated tissue before the nerve is repaired. Adequate soft tissue also must be present to cover the repair. After the condition of the wound is acceptable, we sharply mobilize the proximal and distal nerve stumps with the aid of loupe magnification or the operating microscope. This can be performed safely over considerable distances without rendering the nerve ischemic because of the rich vascular plexus that exists within peripheral nerves.[44] The vascular supply to peripheral nerves consists of both extrinsic and intrinsic systems (Figure 119-8).[53] The extrinsic plexus is a series of segmentally arranged vessels that originate from neighboring arteries and veins. These segmental branches ramify in the epineurium and supply the intraneural plexuses through ascending and descending branches. The intrinsic system begins at the branch points of the extrinsic vessels and runs longitudinally in the interfascicular epineurium, where it forms an extensive plexus. Interconnections with the longitudinal perineurial plexus feed an endoneurial capillary "basket." The endoneurial and perineurial vessels can be safely separated from the segmental branches for 5 to 10 cm, facilitating extended proximal and distal nerve stump mobilization. However, the surgeon should attempt to identify the segmented vascular branches entering the epineurium along the course of the nerve from adjoining vessels and preserve these branches by means of a spreading dissection whenever possible.

The proximal and distal nerve stumps are subsequently sharply trimmed back to a point where they are healthy in appearance. We use a "razor and miter box" technique for this purpose to ensure clean transection of the nerve.[7] Nerves that are fibrotic tend to flatten; thus the nerve should be trimmed back until nerve tissue protrudes from the cut ends of the fascicles, which signifies that healthy nerve has been reached.

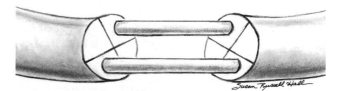

Figure 119-10. Technique for achieving proper spatial orientation of nerve grafts between the proximal and distal stumps.

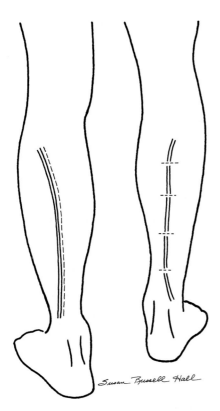

Figure 119-9. Incisions used to harvest the sural nerve graft *(dashed lines).*

This involves debridement of all devitalized nerve tissue for primary repair of acute open injuries. All fibrotic tissue associated with the nerve (including a neuroma, if present) is excised during secondary repairs by sharp transection back to healthy nerve, both proximally and distally.

End-to-end coaptation is subsequently performed if the mobilized nerve ends can be brought together under minimal or no tension and without significant postural joint positioning. Before the repair, we use the surface anatomy of the nerve and the fascicular pattern observed in each end of the nerve stump to achieve proper fascicular alignment, as previously described. We perform all nerve repairs with interrupted epineurial sutures of 8-0 or 9-0 monofilament nylon. Prospective studies have not yet demonstrated the superiority of one repair technique over another.[57,61] Therefore we generally do not employ perineurial or group fascicular repair techniques; instead we rely on epineurial repair, with attention to proper alignment of both internal fascicular and surface vascular anatomy.

We reserve nerve grafting for situations in which end-to-end coaptation of the nerve cannot be achieved in a tension-free fashion. We do not use the absolute nerve gap measurement criteria to determine when grafting is necessary. We prefer to use the sural nerve as our donor nerve when grafting is required; we harvest this nerve with the patient in the prone or lateral decubitus position, through a longitudinal incision on the posterolateral aspect of the leg (posterior to the medial malleolus) or through multiple small, transverse incisions along the course of the nerve (Figure 119-9). The sural nerve subsequently can be split at

the group fascicular level, as mentioned previously. Before placement of the graft, the proximal and distal nerve stumps are trimmed back to healthy nerve and all fibrotic tissue is removed. The nerve graft is sutured in place between the proximal and distal stump under magnification, using a group fascicular and/or epineurial repair technique. The nerve graft should be reversed so that the distal end of the graft is sutured to the proximal nerve stump and the proximal end of the graft is sutured to the distal nerve stump. Multiple small-caliber nerve grafts are used to bridge gaps in larger-diameter nerves because large-diameter grafts undergo central necrosis and degeneration before revascularization.[48] When multiple grafts are used, we strive to maintain the spatial orientation of graft placement between the proximal and distal stumps by sewing the proximal and distal ends of the nerve graft into the same quadrant that contains the proximal and distal stumps (Figure 119-10). This is accomplished to maximize the number of regenerating axons that reach their respective distal end-organ targets. It is essential to ensure that no tension exists across either graft suture line by using a graft of adequate length to bridge the existing nerve gap.

POSTOPERATIVE MANAGEMENT/ SECONDARY PROCEDURES

After surgery, splinting is performed where necessary to prevent joint motion from exerting tension on the nerve repair. Patients remain splinted for approximately 2 to 4 weeks after repair and often begin controlled active or passive motion exercises, which allow joint motion without placing tension on the nerve repair. Patients are followed closely so that the return of motor function or sensation can be monitored, depending on the type of nerve repaired. The progress of nerve regeneration can be followed by examining the patient and gently tapping along the course of the nerve to elicit a Tinel's sign; the Tinel's sign moves distally as the regenerating axons grow toward the end of the nerve. Other findings that indicate nerve regeneration include return of pseudomotor function in the form of sweating and the return of normal fingerprints. Some patients benefit from an intensive sensory reeducation protocol designed to maximize function after the repair of sensory nerves.[12]

Secondary procedures may be required for the treatment of neuromas, which can form at the repair site. Their management may require internal neurolysis, neuroma excision and recoaptation of the nerve, or bypass nerve grafting.

OUTCOMES

The functional results of nerve repair and grafting have been described in numerous reports. However, the vast array of nerve injuries, the difficulty in obtaining standardized and meaningful long-term follow-up, and the infinite number of levels along individual nerves at which these injuries can occur make the results difficult to quantify.

The overall predicted outcome of nerve repair has been correlated with several different factors.* Functional recovery is inversely related to age, to the amount of tension across the

_____

*References 2, 4, 11, 15, 22, 26, 29, 34, 55.

nerve repair, and to the time that elapses between injury and repair. A direct correlation exists between functional outcome and both the use of microsurgical technique and the patient's cognitive capacity. Moreover, the long-term recovery of sensation is greatly enhanced by sensory reeducation after surgery. Functional recovery after a clean nerve transection and repair is better than recovery after a crush-type injury. The level of the injury also affects recovery; generally, the more distal the injury, the better the long-term functional outcome. A proximal nerve transection and repair requires axons to regenerate and grow over huge distances (comparable to miles for an ivy plant). The axon cell body must generate enough intracellular neuron axoplasm to push the axon growth cone from the site of injury to the distal motor or sensory end-organs, which on a cellular scale are "miles" away. The farther the nerve must grow, the less likely it is to reach an end-organ.

The most commonly used grading systems for quantifying recovery after nerve repair include the British Medical Research Council (BMRC) scheme for motor recovery (Table 119-3), and several variations of the Highet classification for evaluating sensory recovery (Tables 119-4 and 119-5).[27,38]

MacKinnon and Dellon[23] have compiled an excellent and comprehensive collection of results following nerve repair and grafting. Modifications of the BMRC and Highet grading

Table 119-3.
British Medical Research Council Motor Function Classification

GRADE	OBSERVED FUNCTION
M_0	No contraction
M_1	Flicker or trace of contraction
M_2	Active movement, with gravity eliminated
M_3	Active movement against gravity
M_4	Active movement against gravity and resistance
M_5	Normal power

Table 119-4.
Highet Classification of Sensory Function

CLASSIFICATION	SENSORY FUNCTION
S_1	No sensation
S_2	Deep cutaneous pain in autonomic zone
S_3	Superficial pain and tactile sense in autonomic zone
S_4	Superficial pain and tactile sense in autonomic zone, with disappearance of over-response
S_5	Recovery of two-point discrimination in autonomic zone

Table 119-5.
Modified Highet Classification of Sensory Function (British Medical Research Council Scale)

CLASSIFICATION	SENSORY FUNCTION
S_0	Absence of sensation in anatomic zone
S_1	Recovery of deep cutaneous pain sensation in autonomous area of nerve
S_2	Return of some degree of superficial cutaneous pain and tactile sensation in autonomous area of nerve
S_3	Return of superficial cutaneous pain and tactile sensation throughout autonomous area, with disappearance of any previous over-response
S_{3+}	Some recovery of two-point discrimination in autonomous area of nerve
S_4	Complete recovery

systems were used in this review for standardization and to compare the results of different series.[18]

MEDIAN NERVE

The reported results of repair of low median-nerve transections were, until recently, relatively disappointing. However, great improvement in results has occurred during the past 20 years with good to excellent return of motor function and sensation after median-nerve repairs at the wrist level, and in more than a third of those in the forearm.[23] Birch and Raji[4] reported good to excellent results after primary repair of median-nerve injuries in the forearm in 19 of 26 patients. Hudson and de Jager[20] examined median nerve function after repair in patients with severe wrist injuries involving multiple structures; the return of motor function was at BMRC level 4 or 5 in 67% of patients who had undergone median nerve repair.[20] The outcome after repair of high median-nerve injuries in the proximal forearm or above the elbow generally has been less favorable than that for low median-nerve injuries. These findings are consistent with the general principle that the more proximal the injury, the poorer the functional result.[53]

Grafting of median-nerve injuries has yielded results that generally are fair to good, with most patients regaining at least M3 motor function and S3 sensory return.[23] Trumble et al[55] reviewed median nerve grafts at or distal to the elbow and found that both the length of the graft and the time that elapsed before nerve grafting correlated inversely with the percentage of muscle force recovered. Kalomiri et al[21] followed a series of 73 patients who underwent median nerve grafting and reported BMRC level 4 or 5 motor function and S_3 to S_4 sensory return in 55% of patients. In 1994 Daoutis et al[10] reported BMRC level 4 motor function and S_{3+} to S_4 sensory return in 24 of 47 patients. Patients in both series were followed for at least 2 years after undergoing median nerve grafting at various levels.

ULNAR NERVE

The results of ulnar nerve repair tend to be less favorable than those for repair of the median nerve.[23] This is especially true for the motor component of ulnar nerve function, which depends on accurate reinnervation of the numerous distally located intrinsic muscles of the hand. However, overall good results can be obtained after ulnar nerve repair.[4,14,36] The potential for sensory recovery is generally greater than for motor recovery, and, as with median nerve injuries, better outcomes have been reported after repair of distal (compared with proximal) injuries of the ulnar nerve.[23] Daoutis et al[10] reported on 41 patients who underwent ulnar nerve repair; 29 regained BMRC level 4 motor function, and 19 experienced S_3 to S_4 sensory return.

Ulnar nerve grafting also has produced good results. Millesi found that 49% of 39 patients who underwent ulnar nerve grafting regained BMRC level 4 or 5 motor function and that 20% achieved a sensory recovery of S_3 to S_4.[28,31] In 1994 Kalomiri et al[21] reported on a series of ulnar nerve grafts in 85 patients; 61% of patients achieved BMRC level 4 or 5 motor function and S_3 to S_4 sensory return.

RADIAL NERVE

Results after repair or grafting of the radial nerve historically have indicated motor return in the M4 range or better in 20% to 40% of patients.[23] More recent series have demonstrated higher success rates. Kalomiri et al[21] studied 35 patients who underwent grafting of the radial nerve and he reported BMRC level 4 or 5 motor function in 89% of patients.

DIGITAL NERVE

The results of digital nerve repair have varied historically. In 1988 a review of the literature by MacKinnon and Dellon[23] found that approximately 60% of patients eventually achieved S_{3+} or greater sensory return after nerve repair. Tadjalli et al[51] reviewed 150 patients who underwent digital nerve repair and found that recovery of sensation correlated with the severity of the hand injury. Such findings may help to explain the variability in outcomes. In 1991 Berger and Mailander[3] reported excellent results in 19% and good results in 27% of patients who underwent repair of digital nerves. Al-Ghazal et al[2] reviewed 75 digital nerve repairs in 71 patients; they reported excellent results in 17% and good results in 51.1% of patients. In 1995 Efstathopoulos et al[13] reviewed a series of 64 digital nerve repairs; they reported excellent results for 13% of the repairs and good results for 39%.

Two-point discrimination recovery after digital nerve grafting also has been variable. Historically, only 30% of patients recovered sensation of S_{3+} or better.[23] In 1988, however, MacKinnon and Dellon[23] reported on 33 patients who underwent digital nerve grafting, and 95% of these patients achieved S_{3+} sensory return postoperatively. Similar results have been reported for patients who received vascularized digital nerve grafts.[43] The results of nerve grafting in some cases, such those involving mild crush injuries, have been superior to the results of end-to-end coaptation of severed nerves.[56]

SUMMARY

Peripheral nerve injuries can manifest a wide variety of sensory and motor derangements, which may vary in severity. Successful management by direct nerve repair or grafting requires adherence to well-established surgical guidelines, including early intervention, use of microsurgical technique, careful realignment of the severed nerve stumps, and avoidance of tension across the repair (which may necessitate use of a nerve graft). Meticulous surgical technique and attention to detail are necessary regardless of whether the repair is epineurial, fascicular, or group fascicular. Precise, anatomical nerve repair maximizes the functional outcome in most cases.

REFERENCES

1. Aitken J: The effect of peripheral connexions on the maturation of regenerating nerve fibres, *J Anat* 83:32-43, 1949.

2. Al-Ghazal SK, McKiernan M, Khan K, et al: Results of clinical assessment after primary digital nerve repair, *J Hand Surg [Br]* 19:255-257, 1994.

3. Berger A, Mailander P: Advances in peripheral nerve repair in emergency surgery of the hand, *World J Surg* 15:493-500, 1991.

4. Birch R, Raji AR: Repair of median and ulnar nerves: primary suture is best, *J Bone Joint Surg* 73B:154-157, 1991.

5. Bowers WH, Carlson EC, Wenner SM, Doyle JR: Nerve suture and grafting, *Hand Clin* 5:445-453, 1989.

6. Boyes JH: *On the shoulders of giants,* Philadelphia, 1976, JB Lippincott.

7. Braum RM: Epineurial nerve suture, *Clin Orthop* 163:50-56, 1982.

8. Breidenbach WC, Terzis JK: Vascularized nerve grafts: an experimental and clinical review, *Ann Plast Surg* 18:137-146, 1987.

9. Cruikshank W: Experiments on the nerves, particularly on their reproductions and on the spinal marrow of living animals, *Philos Trans R Soc Lond* 85:177-189, 1795.

10. Daoutis NK, Gerostathopoulos NE, Efstathopoulos DG, et al: Microsurgical reconstruction of large nerve defects using autologous nerve grafts, *Microsurgery* 15:502-505, 1994.

11. Dellon AL: The moving two-point discrimination test: clinical evaluation of the quickly adapting fiber/receptor system, *J Hand Surg [Am]* 3:474-481, 1978.

12. Dellon AL, Jabaley ME: Reeducation of sensation in the hand following nerve suture, *Clin Orthop* 163:75-79, 1982.

13. Efstathopoulos D, Gerostathopoulos N, Misitzis D, et al: Clinical assessment of primary digital nerve repair, *Acta Orthop Scand Suppl* 264:45-47, 1995.

14. Gaul JS Jr: Intrinsic motor recovery: a long-term study of ulnar nerve repair, *J Hand Surg [Am]* 7:502-508, 1982.

15. Glickman LT, Mackinnon SE: Sensory recovery following digital replantation, *Microsurgery* 11:236-242, 1990.

16. Goldie BS, Coates CJ, Birch R: The long-term result of digital nerve repair in no-man's land, *J Hand Surg [Br]* 17:75-77, 1992.

17. Guy de Chauliac: *Guy de Chauliac (AD 1363) on wounds and fractures* (translated by WA Brennan), Chicago, 1923, Translator.

18. Highet WH, Sanders FK: The effects of stretching nerve after suture, *Br J Surg* 30:355, 1943.

19. Huang TC, Blanks RH, Berns MW, Crumley RL: Laser versus suture nerve anastomosis, *Otolaryngol Head Neck Surg* 107:14-20, 1992.

20. Hudson DA, de Jager LT: The spaghetti wrist: simultaneous laceration of the median and ulnar nerves with flexor tendons at the wrist, *J Hand Surg [Br]* 18:171-173, 1993.

21. Kalomiri DE, Soucacos PN, Beris AE: Nerve grafting in peripheral nerve microsurgery of the upper extremity, *Microsurgery* 15:506-511, 1994.

22. Lundborg G, Rosen B, Dahlin LB, et al: Functional sensation of the hand after nerve repair [letter], *Lancet* 342:1300, 1993.

23. MacKinnon SE, Dellon AL: *Surgery of the peripheral nerve,* New York, 1988, Thieme Medical Publishers.

24. MacKinnon SE, Dellon AL: Clinical nerve reconstruction with a bioabsorbable polyglycolic acid tube, *Plast Reconstr Surg* 85:419-424, 1990.

25. Mackinnon SE, Hudson AR: Clinical application of peripheral nerve transplantation, *Plast Reconstr Surg* 90:695-699, 1992.

26. McEwan LE: Median and ulnar nerve injuries, *Aust NZ J Surg* 32:89-104, 1962.

27. Medical Research Council: Memorandum no. 45. Her Majesty's Stationery Office, 1976, pp 1.

28. Millesi H: Interfascicular grafts for repair of peripheral nerves of the upper extremity, *Orthop Clin North Am* 8:387-404, 1977.

29. Millesi H: Interfascicular nerve grafting, *Orthop Clin North Am* 12:287-301, 1981.

30. Millesi H, Meissl G: Consequences of tension at the suture site. In Gorio A, Millesi H, Mingrino S (editors): *Post-traumatic peripheral nerve regeneration,* New York, 1981, Raven Press.

31. Millesi H, Meissl G, Berger A: Further experience with interfascicular grafting of the median, ulnar, and radial nerves, *J Bone Joint Surg* 58A:209-218, 1976.

32. Millesi H, Terzis JK: Nomenclature in peripheral nerve surgery. Committee report of the International Society of Reconstructive Microsurgery, *Clin Plast Surg* 11:3-8, 1984.

33. Mitchell S: *Injuries of nerves and their consequences,* Philadelphia, 1872, JB Lippincott.

34. Moberg E: Criticism in study of methods for examining sensibility in the hand, *Neurology* 12:8-19, 1962.

35. Muller J: *Elements of physiology,* London, 1842, Taylor and Walton.

36. Nicholson OR, Seddon H: Nerve repair in civil practice: results of treatment of median and ulnar nerve lesions, *BMJ* 2:1065-1071, 1957.

37. Omer GE Jr: Results of untreated peripheral nerve injuries, *Clin Orthop* 163:15-19, 1982.

38. Omer GE Jr: The evaluation of clinical results following peripheral nerve suture. In Omer GE Jr (editor): *Management of peripheral nerve problems,* Philadelphia, 1997, WB Saunders.

39. Palazzi S, Vila Torres J, Lorenzo JC: Fibrin glue is a sealant and not a nerve barrier, *J Reconstr Microsurg* 11:135-139, 1995.

40. Povlsen B: A new fibrin seal in primary repair of peripheral nerves, *J Hand Surg [Br]* 19:43-47, 1994.

41. Prevel CD, Eppley BL, McCarty M, et al: Mechanical anastomosis of nerves: a histological and functional comparison to conventional suturing, *Ann Plast Surg* 33:600-605, 1994.

42. Ramon y Cajal S: *Degeneration and regeneration of the nervous system,* London, 1928, Oxford University Press.

43. Rose EH, Kowalski TA, Norris MS: The reversed venous arterialized nerve graft in digital nerve reconstruction across scarred beds, *Plast Reconstr Surg* 83:593-604, 1989.

44. Rydevik B, Lundborg G, Nordborg C: Intraneural tissue reactions induced by internal neurolysis: an experimental study on the blood–nerve barrier, connective tissues, and nerve fibres of rabbit tibial nerve, *Scand J Plast Reconstr Surg* 10:3-8, 1976.

45. Seddon H: Three types of nerve injury, *Brain* 66:237, 1943.

46. Seddon H: *Surgical disorders of the peripheral nerves,* Baltimore, 1972, Williams & Wilkins.

47. Seddon H, Medawar P, Smith H: Rate of regeneration of peripheral nerves in man, *J Physiol (London)* 102:191-215, 1943.

48. Smith JW: Peripheral nerve surgery: retrospective and contemporary techniques, *Clin Plast Surg* 13:249-254, 1986.

49. Snyder CC: Epineurial repair, *Orthop Clin North Am* 12:267-276, 1981.

50. Sunderland S: *Nerves and nerve injuries,* Edinburgh, 1978, Churchill Livingstone.

51. Tadjalli HE, McIntyre FH, Dolynchuk KN, Murray KA: Digital nerve repair: relationship between severity of injury and sensibility recovery, *Ann Plast Surg* 35:36-40, 1995.

52. Taylor GI, Ham FJ: The free vascularized nerve graft: a further experimental and clinical application of microvascular techniques, *Plast Reconstr Surg* 57:413-426, 1976.

53. Terzis J, Smith K: *The Peripheral nerve: structure, function, and reconstruction,* New York, 1990, Raven Press.

54. Trumble TE: Peripheral nerve transplantation: the effects of predegenerated grafts and immunosuppression, *J Neural Transplant Plast* 3:39-49, 1992.

55. Trumble TE, Kahn U, Vanderhooft E, et al: A technique to quantitate motor recovery following nerve grafting, *J Hand Surg [Am]* 20:367-372, 1995.

56. Wang WZ, Crain GM, Baylis W, et al: Outcome of digital nerve injuries in adults, *J Hand Surg [Am]* 21:138-143, 1996.

57. Watchmaker GP, Mackinnon SE: Advances in peripheral nerve repair, *Clin Plas Surg* 24(1):63-73, 1997.

58. Wilgis E, Brushart T: Nerve repair and grafting. In Green D (editor): *Operative Hand Surgery,* New York, 1993, Churchill Livingstone.

59. Wong BJ, Crumley RL: Nerve wound healing: an overview, *Otolaryngol Clin North Am* 28:881-895, 1995.

60. Woodhall B: *Peripheral nerve regeneration: a follow-up study of 3,656 World War II injuries,* Washington DC, 1957, US Government Printing Office.

61. Young L, Wray RC, Weeks PM: A randomized prospective comparison of fascicular and epineural digital nerve repairs, *Plast Reconstr Surg* 68:89-93, 1981.

CHAPTER

Upper Extremity Compression Syndromes

120

Allen L. Van Beek
Marie-Claire Buckley

INTRODUCTION

The 1939 edition of Campbell's *Operative Orthopedics* does not contain a section on nerve compression syndromes.[7] A compression syndrome involving the ulnar nerve was recognized in 1908, and a compression syndrome affecting the median nerve was reported by Hunt in 1911,[25] but not until 1951 did reports by Phalen[45] lead to wider recognition and improved treatment of carpal tunnel syndrome and herald the recognition of other compression syndromes.[42,49,50] Different nerve irritation sites, etiologies, and secondary effects were described in the 1960s and 1970s. Improved electrodiagnostic studies confirmed focal sites of nerve injuries, and associations between some pain syndromes and compression syndromes were established.[10,22,25,33,57]

An epidemic of various "compression syndromes" began to emerge in the 1980s and 1990s and seemed to be associated with certain occupations and mechanisms of extremity use.* Expansion of the work force occurred during this period, and the majority of adult men and women were engaged in the production of goods and services outside the home. The development of an insurance system that compensated employees for time off work because of injuries sustained during work, combined with changes in the work place, produced an epidemic of "compression neuropathies." These maladies are well documented by objective electrodiagnostic evidence, but the exact etiology and, in some circumstances, the most appropriate treatment has been controversial.[56,59,46,52,42]

Worker's Compensation regulations designed to help injured employees have evolved into a complex political, litigious, and sometimes counterproductive system. Adverse opinion experts paid by third party insurance companies often deny the existence of focal work-related nerve injuries and patient advocate specialists advocate compensation for injured individuals when compensation is not justified. Moreover, huge sums of money are spent for legal representation by both sides of the controversy, further increasing cost without providing health care benefit.

Given this milieu of unresolved issues, how should the treating physician respond to a patient who complains of nerve injury? The surgeon must obtain a careful history documenting social, work, and medical issues; conduct a physical examination of the entire peripheral nervous system (PNS); understand the anatomical variations as reported by Tountas[54]; and obtain supportive electrodiagnostic data to accurately establish the diagnosis and its impact on the individual both at work and home. Physicians should avoid becoming routine adverse experts for insurance companies and should also be wary of being trapped as rope-a-dope specialist advocates for contriving patients.

Peripheral neuropathy does exist, has increased in frequency, and responds to treatment. However, controversies regarding its etiology and management continue. Some of the controversy is generated by the cost associated with compensating injured workers and by the efforts of health managers to decrease expenditures by shifting the cost to other entities.

The anatomy of the peripheral nerve is compartmentalized into an arborizing structure that uniquely connects to various end organs.* The nerve fibers provide a highly evolved, biologically based communication network. When this system is injured, the consequences can range from insignificant to devastating. This chapter discusses the diagnoses and treatment of only the most common compression syndromes affecting the upper extremity, including carpal tunnel syndrome, cubital tunnel syndrome, pronator–anterior interosseous nerve syndrome, and posterior interosseous nerve syndrome. Thoracic outlet syndrome, cervical disk syndromes, and combined compression syndromes are beyond the scope of this chapter, but readers are reminded of their importance in the differential diagnosis of nerve irritation maladies.

---

*References 1, 2, 14, 21, 32, 55.

*References 3, 4, 30, 43, 51, 52.

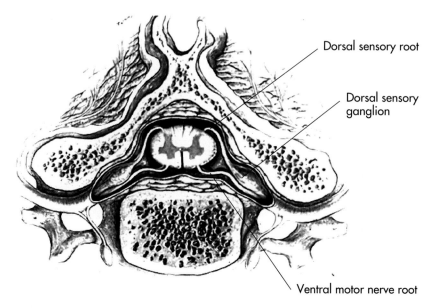

Figure 120-1. A peripheral nerve is formed when the dorsal sensory and ventral motor nerve roots from the spinal cord unite. The cell bodies of the afferent sensory nerve fibers are located outside the spinal cord in the dorsal sensory ganglion.

ANATOMY

The peripheral nerves originate where the dorsal and ventral nerve roots of the spinal cord coalesce. The controlling cell bodies and dendritic network of the ventral nerve root's efferent and motor fibers are located in the substance of the ventral spinal cord.[43] The dorsal root's afferent and sensory fibers originate in the dorsal spinal cord as a dendritic nerve complex, and the associated cell bodies are located outside the spinal cord in the dorsal root ganglion (Figure 120-1).

The unique location of the dorsal root ganglion (outside the spinal cord) provides one mechanism for the differential diagnosis of supraganglionic brachial plexus avulsion injuries. When supraganglionic injuries occur, the cell bodies are not disconnected from the nerve fiber leading to the periphery, and wallerian degeneration of the sensory fibers does not occur (Figure 120-2). However, the cell bodies are disconnected from the spinal cord, making sensory perception impossible. The intact afferent nerve fibers peripherally evoke nerve impulses along the nerve during electrical stimulation.

The efferent ventral root motor fibers do not have the same status. When their roots are avulsed, efferent motor fibers degenerate and fail to conduct nerve impulses, which leads to lost motor reflexes, spontaneous skeletal muscle electrical activity, muscle atrophy, and distinct patterns of muscle denervation.

The dorsal and ventral rootlets coalesce in the spinal canal to form the nerve root just distal to the dorsal root ganglion. The nerve root courses through the spinal foramen of the vertebral body and exits the protective skeletal confines of the central nervous system (CNS), forming the brachial plexus (Figure 120-3).

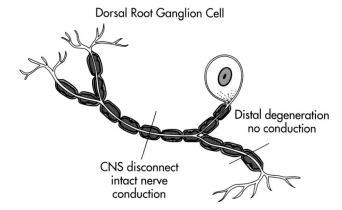

Figure 120-2. Dorsal sensory fibers have a bipolar fiber that permits nerve conduction even when the fiber has been disconnected from the spinal cord.

Each nerve element has unique characteristics and functions that are beyond the scope of this chapter. The structural components of the PNS are integral to the repair, documentation, and consequences of injury.

Nerve conduction studies are an essential adjunct to the diagnosis of peripheral nerve injuries[22,33,42,58,59] and the physician's understanding of these reports must go beyond the summary statement made by the electrodiagnostician. Nerves are capable of both retrograde and antegrade conduction from the point of nerve fiber stimulation. Important findings that may lead to the diagnosis of significant nerve pathology include decreased conduction velocity, fibrillation potentials, positive sharp waves, decreased recruitment, decreased M-wave amplitude, and loss of sensory perception or conduction.

A decrease in conduction velocity is best detected when it is measured across a short segment of the nerve.[57] Attempting to delineate a short segment of decreased conduction velocity

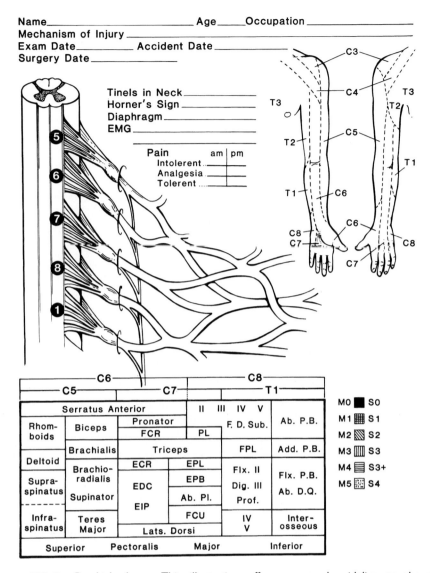

Figure 120-3. Brachial plexus. This illustration offers a general guideline to the anatomy, examination, and documentation of the peripheral nervous system status of the upper extremity.

when velocity is measured across a long segment of nerve is difficult if only a short portion of the nerve is diseased; in such cases the normal segment of conduction may mask or interfere with detection of the short segment of abnormal conduction. If injury to a nerve is so severe that degeneration of nerve fibers has occurred, spontaneous muscle activity will be evident. Muscle fibers that are separated from their nerve supply develop small bursts of spontaneous endplate activity referred to as *fibrillation potentials* or *positive sharp waves.* These findings are indicative of degenerated nerve fibers and are a clear sign of significant neuropathy. An increased motor or sensory latency means that the velocity of nerve conduction through the segment of nerve being analyzed has decreased. This occurs in response to demyelination of nerve fibers, intercalation of shorter internodal distances within segments of remyelinated nerve fiber, or conduction block caused by nerve ischemia. Likewise a decrease in motor unit potentials indicates that the number of muscle fibers innervated by an efferent nerve fiber

has decreased, resulting in a lower motor unit potential. This also is indicative of peripheral neuropathy.

Our diagnosis often is influenced by a comparison of ulnar nerve latency with median nerve latency, based on the assumption that the median nerve is entrapped but that the ulnar nerve is not. Because of differences in conduction characteristics and in the distances involved, ulnar nerve latency ordinarily differs from median nerve latency across the wrist by 0.2 to 0.4 msec. The physician should suspect median pathology if the latency difference is greater than 0.8 msec, even though the latency recorded is within normal limits. Because normal limits of conduction latency vary from lab to lab, many patients with abnormal nerves receive false-negative reports. This is ample justification for depending on our clinical diagnostic abilities, and using electrical studies only as an adjunct. However, this is sometimes impossible because of third-party interests, state mandated laws, a litigious environment, and distrust of the physician's motivation and diligence.

MECHANISM OF NERVE INJURY

The mechanism of nerve injury often can be determined by the patient's history, with the realization that injuries may occur at more than one level along the course of a nerve. Furthermore, an injury may occur because of an occult underlying disorder within the nerve, which may be caused by a disorder such as diabetes or multiple sclerosis. This chapter discusses injuries or irritation to peripheral nerves from compression or strain. It focuses on injuries to the nerves of the upper extremity, and readers are advised that similar problems are associated with nerves of the lower extremity.

The mechanism of injury delineated by a patient's history is important, but the clinician also must anticipate the type of injury that may have been produced. Two classifications of nerve injuries have been popularized and both consider the unique structure and function of various nerves (Table 120-1). Seddon's classification[46] is based on the clinical evaluation and clinical judgment of injury to a peripheral nerve. Sunderland's classification[51] is more specific and requires that the clinician understand what occurs histologically after a nerve injury. Clinically, the Seddon classification seems more applicable preoperatively, and the Sunderland classification seems more applicable after the status of the nerve has been explored or determined histologically.

Transection of a nerve by a sharp, blunt, crushing, or avulsive mechanism produces immediate and long-term consequences that can be devastating to the patient. Such injuries are readily detected. In contrast, metabolic, inflammatory, ischemic, partial stretch, compression, infectious, strain, and shear injuries may have an overwhelming impact on the patient but may be associated with clinical findings that are elusive or even normal. Shingles produced by herpes zoster virus, diabetic neurotrophic ulceration, and Parsonage-Turner syndrome are classic examples of diseases that have major clinical consequences without anatomical disruption of the nerve. The clinician must be aware of manifestations of PNS diseases that are not related to trauma, strain, or compression. Mechanical strain, compression, or stretch injuries superimposed on such diseases may further increase the difficulty in diagnosing the cause of pain.

We believe that mechanisms of peripheral nerve injury exist in addition to those caused by direct injury, vibration, compression, ischemia, and metabolic and traction injuries. These include strain-related injuries that occur because of repetitive glide friction, repetitive nerve impact, or repetitive fulcrum force directed against or across the nerve. When the median nerve is impacted between the two heads of the pronator teres, sometimes in combination with a tendinous hiatus formed by the sublimis muscles, a strain-related injury occurs. In some cases the median nerve undergoes repetitive fulcrum strain while crossing joint lines, such as those of the wrist carpus or elbow. Just as repetitive vibration activity can produce demyelination, it seems likely that a similar process of focal demyelination may occur across the various joint fulcrums of the body in response to frequent and persistent repetitive motion.

The nerve exhibits many clinical responses to injury. Loss of motor and sensory function are often the easiest to detect, although they may be difficult to understand or document. Careful electrodiagnostic studies can confirm losses associated with a nerve injury that produces wallerian degeneration.

Table 120-1.
Nerve Injury Classification*

	NERVE FIBER	SCHWANN CELL SHEATH	PERINEURIUM	EPINEURIUM	NERVE
SEDDON					
Neurapraxia	Intact	Intact	Intact	Intact	Intact
Axonotmesis	Disrupted	More or less disrupted	More or less disrupted	Intact	Intact
Neurotmesis	Disrupted	Disrupted	Disrupted	Disrupted	More or less disrupted
SUNDERLAND					
Degree					
First	Intact	Intact	Intact	Intact	Intact
Second	Disrupted	Intact	Intact	Intact	Intact
Third	Disrupted	Disrupted	Disrupted	Intact	Intact
Fourth	Disrupted	Disrupted	Disrupted	Disrupted	Together
Fifth	Disrupted	Disrupted	Disrupted	Disrupted	Separated

*Nerve injuries may comprise various combinations of these types of injuries.

Conduction block that occurs when the nerve fiber is intact and not undergoing wallerian degeneration also can be confirmed by electrodiagnostic studies in most cases. However, short segmental changes in the peripheral nerve may not be detected by electrodiagnostic studies because the short segment of injury may elude the detection of conduction changes, as previously mentioned. The problem is compounded when multiple areas of short segmental injury occur in series.

Definitive diagnosis in patients who manifest variable symptoms associated with the PNS is difficult without confirmatory studies. Pain is produced by the CNS in response to information from the PNS. The complexity of the CNS can lead to a myriad of presentations that the clinician must diagnose using limited resources when the insurance environment is suspicious. The clinical impression and diagnosis, even with the use of modern technology, remains the final word in the detection of neuropathology.

CLINICAL EXAMINATION

NECK AND SHOULDER

The impulse to examine only the area in which pathology is suspected (because of clinical symptoms) must be avoided. A focus on one area of pathology may result in a failure to detect multiple levels of pathology, which ultimately may lead to treatment failure. The physician must first determine whether the CNS is producing the patient's symptoms. Subsequently the physician determines whether cervical disk disease, thoracic outlet syndrome, scalenus syndrome, cervical rib compression, Parsonage-Turner syndrome, or brachial plexus traction injuries may be the cause of neural symptoms originating in this anatomic area. Clinical examination also involves a search for painful areas and for Tinel's sign in the neck and axilla. Adson's maneuver, the military posture test, hyperabduction, and range of motion strain are performed to detect pathology along the course of the nerve. Cervical radiography may be useful, but computed tomography (CT) typically is better for detecting anatomical variations that may be contributing to a neuropathy. Electrodiagnostic tests are helpful in advanced cases of neuropathy but the difficulties associated with short segment analysis in the cervicothoracic area may make detection of less severe nerve pathology difficult.

The elbow area and adjacent arm and forearm produce many focal neuropathies. Examination for focal areas of pain and Tinel's sign and the use of provocative positions and pressure are important in the detection of nerve abnormalities. Nerves that are sensitive to pressure or percussion typically are undergoing either changes in myelination or neural degeneration and regeneration. Direct digit pressure with the equivalent of 20 to 30 mmHg of force for 30 seconds over the radial, median, or ulnar nerve that results in distal changes in sensation or significant pain often is indicative of an irritable nerve. Sustained extreme range-of-motion maneuvers (e.g., elbow flexion, pronation, and supination) that reproduce neural symptoms or distal neural symptoms are indicative of irritable peripheral nerves. Muscle volumes should be compared with those of the contralateral extremity (by means of inspection, volume displacement, or circumference measurements) for evidence of atrophy, an indication of decreased or absent nerve function. Any atrophy should be documented and investigated.

Peripheral nerve abnormalities associated with the wrist have reached epidemic proportions; common examples of these abnormalities are discussed in this chapter. The wrist should be examined for Tinel's sign and to determine the presence of focal sites of pain, atrophy, unusual swelling or circulation disturbances, and sensation alterations. The specific anatomic pattern of sensory alteration also should be determined. Provocative compression and positioning are adjunctive forms of clinical examination that can detect focal areas of nerve irritation.

Examination of a nerve along its entire length often leads to the discovery of associated areas of nerve irritation in other nerves, or along the course of the same nerve. Initially, this may seem surprising; however, because compression is not the only mechanism of injury that produces nerve irritation and irritability, multiple sites of injury are common.

A careful history and examination typically leads to an accurate diagnosis. Electrodiagnostic tests may be used to confirm a diagnosis but never should be used to determine definitively whether a nerve is irritated or injured. An injury that is severe enough to produce detectable electrodiagnostic changes may have been ignored for too long and thus may not undergo complete recovery at the cellular level after decompression.

CARPAL TUNNEL SYNDROME

INDICATIONS

A prevailing symptom of carpal tunnel syndrome is numbness of the hand, which is manifested in the tips of the thumb and the index and middle fingers. Whether numbness extends into the base of the thumb and forearm must be determined. Cramps involving the muscles, dropping of objects, and swelling of the hand, especially during work, can be common complaints.[5,21,45,55] Proximal extension of pain up the arm caused by carpal tunnel syndrome was reported by Cherington.[10] Vascular disturbance[53] resulting in color change and/or cold intolerance is also a frequent symptom. In our experience tobacco use seems to increase the incidence of vascular changes associated with carpal tunnel syndrome.

Clinical examination may reveal a positive Phalen's sign,[44] a positive provocative compression sign over the median nerve, Tinel's sign, positive reverse Phalen's sign, evidence of thenar atrophy, or weak abduction of the thumb from the palm. Ulnar innervation of the thenar muscles can make the examination difficult in some patients. Monofilament tactile testing and vibratory testing are more reliable methods of testing sensation than two-point or light-touch testing.

Electrodiagnostic testing confirms the results of the clinical examination when the conduction time across the wrist is increased during either motor or sensory testing. Spontaneous muscle action potentials combined with increased latency across the wrist confirm the diagnosis of carpal tunnel neuropathy. Spontaneous muscle activity without an increase in latency across the wrist should increase the suspicion of a neuropathy at a more proximal site, such as the elbow or neck. This differential point is crucial in determining the site of a neuropathy. As mentioned earlier, a comparison of conduction latency (for median and ulnar nerves) across the wrist also may be used to confirm the results of a clinical examination. If more than a 0.8-msec difference in latency exists between the ulnar and median nerves, suspicion of neuropathy is warranted, even when the median latency is within normal limits for the lab. This is especially true when the clinical examination is strongly indicative of the diagnosis.

After the diagnosis of a focal neuropathy at the wrist is confirmed, the best method of treatment must be determined. The treatment of acute cases is different than that for chronic cases. Nonoperative treatment is unlikely to be successful in cases of long-standing carpal tunnel syndrome. Delaying surgical treatment of the chronically injured nerve while attempting various forms of nonoperative treatment may, in fact, lead to further damage and incomplete nerve recovery.

Nighttime splinting and, in some circumstances, splinting during working hours decreases the severity of symptoms in patients with neuropathy of recent onset. A static splint that comfortably fits the hand and wrist is recommended. It should block wrist motion, and keep the wrist in a neutral position while permitting flexion and extension of the digits. Systemic steroidal and nonsteroidal antiinflammatory medications may be used to decrease acute episodes of inflammation and swelling caused by acute episodes of nerve irritation; there is less justification for their use on a long-term basis. Many physicians advocate the injection of steroids around the nerve to decrease acute inflammation and to ameliorate symptoms. These steroids are placed adjacent to the median nerve, within the carpal tunnel. This practice is associated with a risk of direct injury to the nerve, either by the injected substance or by the hypodermic needle used for injection. Although steroid injection may be beneficial in some acute circumstances (when injected by a highly skilled physician), we do not use this form of treatment. After a nerve is inadvertently injected with a steroid preparation or punctured with a needle, the nerve injury becomes much more difficult to manage. The physician must determine whether the short-term benefit of injection justifies the risk of further injury.

Ergonomic adjustments in the workplace are another important factor in reducing the stress and strain that work requirements amplify. Adjustable chairs and wrist support devices may be necessary. Moreover, work schedules, work patterns, and even work activities may require modification if the physician believes they are contributing to the patient's problem. A visit to the work site or a video tape of the work site may be useful in complex circumstances, to ascertain whether a job is too intense and to determine how the workplace might be modified. Understanding the stress and emotions that each patient associates with the workplace is crucial. Fear, anger, frustration, and other emotions about work often are important factors that affect a patient's motivation to return to work.

When should conservative management be replaced by surgical management is a frequent question. Supportive care (with medications, splints, workplace intervention, and education) is applicable when a patient's symptoms have been present for less than 6 months and when nerve conduction studies (NCS) are normal. Patients whose symptoms have been present for more than 6 months and are refractory to supportive care must be considered surgical candidates. Surgical exploration and decompression is recommended when clinical findings are supportive and/or NCS are abnormal. Controversy frequently develops when a patient's symptoms and findings are positive but his or her NCS are normal. Third parties often use the lack of supportive NCS to confirm that surgery is not necessary. This point of view must not prevail when the clinical diagnosis is obvious. Similarly, not every patient with hand numbness requires nerve exploration. The final recommendations of the responsible treating physician must prevail if the patient is to have the best care.

Exploration of the median nerve at the wrist has changed in the past decade with the advent of endoscopic carpal tunnel release. The variable anatomy of the median nerve across the wrist area also has been more clearly delineated by Lanz.[30]

Important anatomical landmarks that must be assessed when planning or while performing median nerve exploration at the wrist include the palmaris longus, third metacarpal, wrist crease, thenar crease, ulnar artery and nerve, hook of the hamate, recurrent motor branch, digital flexor tendons, and lumbrical muscles (Figure 120-4). Open exploration of the nerve provides ample opportunity to evaluate all of these features (Figure 120-5) whereas endoscopic decompression does not.

OPERATIONS

Open Carpal Tunnel Release

Open exploration of the median nerve at the wrist often is performed with local anesthesia, Bier block, axillary block, or even general anesthesia; the appropriate choice of anesthesia

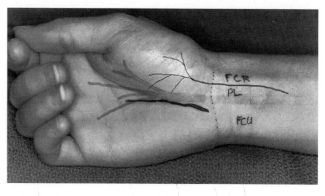

Figure 120-4. Unless the open carpal tunnel incision is carefully planned, palmar cutaneous neuromas *(thin black lines)* may cause sensitivity in the area of the incision. The incision shown here *(thick black lines)* is in a safe zone.

varies, depending on the circumstances of each case. Regardless of the choice of anesthesia, tourniquet control of bleeding is essential to prevent iatrogenic injury to structures located within the field of surgery.[29] The incision is designed to remain between the ulnar border of the third metacarpal and the radial border of the fourth metacarpal; such an incision avoids injury to the palmar cutaneous nerves of both the median and ulnar nerves.[9,52] It is impossible to avoid the small tertiary arborizations of these two nerves but extremely sensitive neuromas may occur if the nerve proper is injured during the skin incision. Cutaneous sensitivity in the mid to distal palm may be associated with dividing the smaller branches of these two nerves. Endoscopic release is the only way to avoid injuring these small branches, but this type of surgery has its own limitations. We prefer to avoid an incision that crosses the wrist flexion crease. If additional exposure is required to completely release the volar carpal ligaments proximal extension into the forearm fascia, I prefer to use a second transverse incision 1.5 cm proximal to the wrist crease. This incision permits more proximal release without the hazard of pinching or cutting the nerve while trying to reach the proximal extent of the volar carpal ligament.

The palmar fascia is identified and the hook of the hamate usually can be found after the palmar incision is completed. Opening the palmar fascia affords exposure of the superficial palmar arch and the common digital nerves, which should not be inadvertently injured. The ulnar side of the carpal tunnel is identified and the linear division of the transverse carpal ligaments is begun. The median nerve is directly under the transverse carpal ligament and must be protected during incision of the ligament. The nerve is readily visible after the ligament is transected. It should be inspected to evaluate the degree of compression, vascular inflammation, and epineurial thickening and to identify a median artery, more proximal nerve branching, or pseudoneuroma formation. Tendons are retracted out of the tunnel, which should be inspected for ganglions, thick synovium, abnormal anatomy, lumbrical muscle status, and

other potential abnormalities (Figure 120-6). The palmar fascia and palmar fat pad are approximated with absorbable suture and the skin is closed. Bupivacaine 0.5% containing adrenaline (10 ml) is injected adjacent to the skin incision and 10 ml is pushed through the closed incision into the surgical site using the syringe's needle connector. This injection provides surgical pain relief and partial median paralysis for 24 hours. Often a steroidal antiinflammatory drug is also irrigated into the surgical site. A removable splint is placed across the wrist for protection of the incision and for additional pain relief. Beginning the day after surgery, the patient removes the splint several times each day to actively exercise the wrist. Digit motion is permitted immediately after surgery. Lifting and extreme abduction of the thumb are avoided for 3 weeks after surgery to prevent incision disruption.

Recurrent carpal tunnel syndrome is possible and may create even more complex diagnostic and management issues, as reported by Cobb and Amadio.[13]

Endoscopic Carpal Tunnel Release

Endoscopic carpal tunnel release is used in selected cases of median nerve neuropathy at the level of the wrist.[12,20,36,37] It is estimated that only one third of the senior author's releases are performed endoscopically. This selection is influenced by the referral of a significant number of patients with recurrent or severe carpal tunnel syndromes, and also by the reluctance of some patients to assume the slightly increased risk of recurrence associated with endoscopic releases.

Before attempting endoscopic carpal tunnel releases, the surgeon must be familiar with the endoscopic appearance of the carpal tunnel and with the tools used for release; he or she must also be able to convert to an open release if necessary and must have supervised experience with the technique. The planning for a two-portal release is illustrated in Figure 120-7. Postoperative management is similar to that for open carpal tunnel release, with some acceleration of return to work

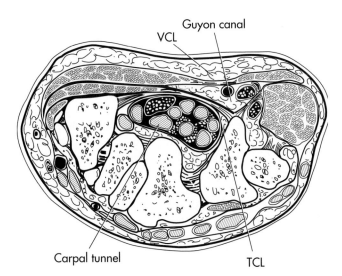

Figure 120-5. A cross-sectional comparison of the carpal tunnel and the Guyon canal. *TCL,* Transverse carpal ligament; *VCL,* volar carpal ligament.

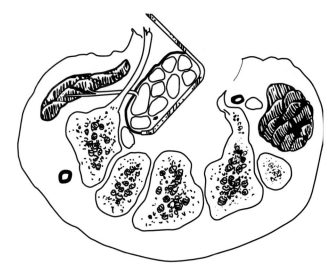

Figure 120-6. During open carpal tunnel release, the tendons are lifted out of the tunnel and the entire tunnel is inspected.

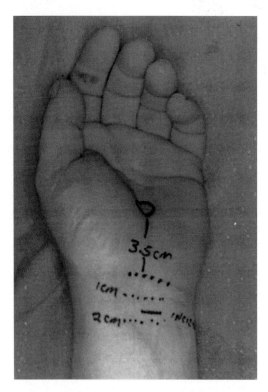

Figure 120-7. When an endoscopic release is planned, the ports should be located to avoid cutaneous nerve injury. The use of two ports and direct visualization of the cannula (distally) provides extra security against laceration of nerve and tendon structures.

because of less tenderness. The distal portal is used during endoscopic carpal tunnel release to directly inspect the canal to ensure that the common digital nerves are not engaged by the cannula. In addition to releasing both the transverse and volar carpal ligaments, Brown's recommendation that the surgeon release the proximal extension of the volar carpal ligament into the forearm fascia seems advisable.[6] The surgeon often can palpate the tightness proximal to the wrist where the volar carpal ligament transitions to the forearm fascia.

Return to work is possible 7 to 10 days after surgery if light or one-handed work is available. When restricted work is not available, patients may require 4 to 8 weeks of recovery before return to work can be expected. A change in occupation may be necessary if the patient's work contributed to the median neuropathy and is likely to cause a recurrence.

CUBITAL TUNNEL SYNDROME

Clearly we prefer to specify neuropathy by first identifying the nerve involved and subsequently determining the site. Although the site is crucial, the term *cubital tunnel syndrome* misleadingly implies that the problem occurs only at the elbow, when often the problem can occur at multiple sites along the ulnar nerve, as described by Miller.[35] Traditional

terms will not be replaced, but ulnar neuropathy should be described as cubital tunnel syndrome only when the examiner is completely satisfied that the cubital tunnel is the only site of nerve irritation or damage.

INDICATIONS

The cubital tunnel is the second most common location for surgical exploration and decompression of a peripheral nerve. Symptoms consist of pain and sensitivity behind the medial epicondyle and along the course of the ulnar nerve in that region.[1,17,32] Accompanying complaints of numbness of the ulnar two digits and dorsum of the hand are common. Muscle cramps, weakness, atrophy, and circulatory disturbances can accompany numbness and soreness and must be differentiated from thoracic outlet syndrome.[2,17,22]

During examination, the peripheral nerve is readily palpable behind the medial epicondyle. The examiner should determine whether Tinel's sign is present. Does the nerve sublux across the epicondyle during elbow flexion and is there any snapping of the triceps tendon associated with flexion? Do these responses occur during extreme elbow flexion or during direct digital compression of the nerve? Is numbness in the ulnar nerve distribution accentuated? The examiner should look for decreased pinch strength, difficulty in making the "wish sign" (crossing the middle finger over the index finger), presence of a Wartenberg sign (abduction of the small finger with no ability to adduct it to the ring finger), or intrinsic atrophy. Decreased strength in the profundus to the fifth finger or flexor carpi ulnaris are additional signs of ulnar neuropathy at or above the elbow.

Nerve conduction studies often are helpful in determining whether the problem with the ulnar nerve is located at the wrist, elbow, or thoracic outlet.[22,25] The conduction velocity across the elbow slows when the nerve is irritated at the elbow. The irritation at this level is significant if the conduction across the elbow is slowed by 20%. If signs of denervation are present in the flexor carpi ulnaris or profundus of the fifth finger, and latency is greater than 20% across the elbow, the diagnosis of neuropathy is confirmed at this level. Neuropathy at this level does not exclude neuropathy at other levels. It is not uncommon for a patient to return with symptoms and progressive atrophy after cubital tunnel release because of concomitant neuropathy under the pisohamate ligament of the wrist that was not previously detected.

Surgical decompression at the elbow is performed when clinical evidence and supportive diagnostic studies indicate the presence of significant neuropathy. The cubital tunnel has unique anatomy that mandates careful surgical technique; imprecise technique can lead to accentuated pain, even when the neuropathy has been improved.

OPERATIONS

Anatomical landmarks include the medial epicondyle, olecranon process, flexor carpi ulnaris fascia, and medial intermuscu-

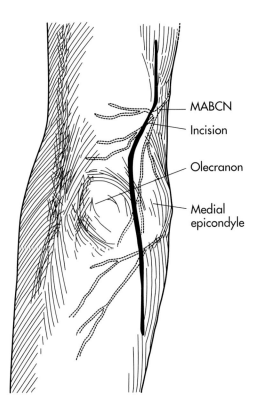

Figure 120-8. The incision must avoid the branches of the medial antebrachial cutaneous nerve *(MABCN)* and permit easy access to the ulnar nerve, medial intermuscular septum, and flexor carpi ulnaris aponeurosis. The articular sensory branch should be preserved while the ulnar nerve is transposed from its tunnel. The inferior ulnar collateral vessels should be transposed with the nerve.

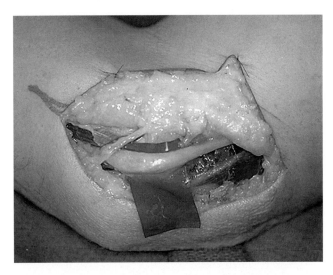

Figure 120-9. The cubital tunnel is opened across the elbow to expose the ulnar nerve. Branches of the medial antebrachial nerve have been dissected in the subcutaneous tissue and spared.

lar fascia.[4,18,31,32] The incision is located midway between the olecranon and the medial epicondyle. The incision extends proximally for approximately 8 cm and distally for approximately 6 cm (Figure 120-8). After the incision through the skin is completed, careful dissection and identification of the posterior branches of the medial antebrachial cutaneous nerve must be performed. This nerve is usually 2 to 3 mm in diameter and is ideally located in the proximal portion of the incision, often adjacent to the cephalic vein, and can then be traced distally. The posterior branch at this level is usually located posterior to the vein; the anterior branches remain anterior. The nerve and its branches should be traced through the surgical field and the branches should be retracted to prevent injury, as reported by Dellon.[18] When this process is completed, the ulnar nerve should be located and the cubital tunnel should be opened along its entire length; the flexor carpi ulnaris fascia also should be opened distally (Figure 120-9). The very small articular sensory branch and larger flexor carpi ulnaris motor branch should be identified because they must remain intact.

The nerve is subsequently lifted out of the tunnel, along with the accompanying vascular leash of the inferior ulnar collateral vessels. After this process is completed, the medial intermuscular septum located along the distal medial humerus and medial epicondyle will be readily apparent and must be excised. The decision regarding where to place the nerve is important. Success has been reported after simple decompres-

sion, medial epicondylectomy,[15] subcutaneous transposition,[57] and submuscular transposition.[31,32] We prefer submuscular transposition when the patient's work requires the use of hands and arms. This location is more likely to prevent direct impact against the nerve. The submuscular location is also preferred in cases of recurrent disease or when neuroma formation is present because it typically places the nerve in a deeper and less sensitive plane.

When surgery is completed and the tourniquet has been deflated, the skin edges are infiltrated with bupivacaine, which is also instilled into the surgical site after hemostasis and skin closure have been completed. A long-arm removable splint is applied, with the elbow in a 95- to 100-degree position for protection of the incision. Beginning on the day after surgery, the splint is removed by the patient three times each day and active range of motion is initiated. The splint is worn for 3 weeks to protect the incision from disruption and also to prevent pain from inadvertent trauma. Return to work in a restricted capacity usually may begin by 10 days after surgery and unrestricted return to work by 6 to 10 weeks after surgery. If a submuscular transposition was performed, a more conservative return-to-work policy is necessary to prevent the flexor muscle origins from separating from the epicondyle.

Permanent work restrictions, orthotic devices, or ergonomic changes may be necessary after ulnar nerve release at the elbow for patients with occupations that require extensive elbow use.

MEDIAN NEUROPATHY AT THE ELBOW

Pronator and anterior interosseous syndromes have become well-recognized examples of nerve irritation because of the work of Morton Spinner.[42,50] The symptoms of numbness, muscle cramping, and weakness mimic carpal tunnel syndrome.[28,40,58] Unfortunately, a patient who presents with textbook picture of perfect weakness of the muscles supplied by the anterior interosseous nerve[27] or numbness with weakness caused by median compression is uncommon.[24,26,50] It is more likely that weakness, cramping, numbness, and pain emanating from the region of the proximal forearm will herald this site of neuropathy. It is useful to know that the numbness associated with elbow level compression often extends more proximally in the hand and wrist, and that median nerve compression at the wrist is usually isolated to the fingertips.

INDICATIONS

Clinical examination demonstrates sensitivity over the nerve in response to direct palpation. Digital compression over the nerve or elbow flexion combined with pronation may provoke nerve irritation and illicit symptoms. Flexion of the thumb and index finger terminal phalanx should be isolated and compared with the strength of the opposite side and with results of other patient examinations. Volitional tremors, the amplification of symptoms or signs, or other questionable responses to the examination by patients will make the task of determining the exact etiology more daunting.

Routine electrodiagnostic studies seldom help the clinician detect this malady because the studies are designed to detect disorders at the wrist. Neuropathy of the median nerve across the elbow can be detected by asking the electromyographer to obtain latency studies across the elbow for the median nerve. Also important are electromyographic studies of the thenar muscles, flexor pollicis longus, and pronator quadratus. It is essential to review these studies because these areas are innervated by the anterior interosseous branches of the median nerve below the elbow. Data regarding the flexor carpi radialis and pronator teres also are important, but if their innervation occurs more proximally in the arm and implies compression by a ligament of Struthers, as described by Smith and later by Al-Qattan,[3,48] or perhaps compression in the neck.[2] If the latency across the elbow is prolonged and spontaneous muscle activity manifested by fibrillation potentials and positive sharp waves is present, pronator or anterior interosseous syndrome is clearly documented. Sometimes the wrist latency and elbow latency are normal but fibrillation potentials or positive sharp waves are present in the thenar muscles. Such findings most likely indicate compression at the elbow. Remember, neuropathy at the elbow can produce thenar muscle denervation as well as extrinsic muscle denervation. In our experience the elbow area can be a site of compression neuropathy and, more importantly, a synchronous site of neuropathy in at least 10% of patients presenting with significant median nerve symptoms.

OPERATIONS

The surgical anatomy and surgical planning for median neuropathy at the elbow are shown in Figure 120-10. Exploration of the median nerve as it crosses the antecubital fossa is begun by making a 6-cm incision just medial to the flexor muscle mass and just distal to the antecubital crease. This incision permits thorough exploration of the median nerve; it is seldom necessary to extend the incision across the flexion crease. The incision is extended through the subcutaneous fat until the lacertus fibrosus and forearm fascia are identified. The anterior branch of the medial antebrachial cutaneous nerve follows the cephalic vein and must be avoided. The lacertus fibrosus can be a site of median nerve compression and is often dense and thick; it immediately covers the brachial artery, brachial vein, and median nerve. Because of its potential to entrap the nerve, the lacertus (which is found clinging to the side of the flexor muscle mass and medial to the brachial artery) should be removed. The anterior interosseous nerve may have a short 1- to 2-cm trunk with arborization or may exist as several branches originating from the median nerve.

The superficial and deep heads of the pronator teres muscles are encountered by dissecting the anterior surface of the median nerve distal to the antecubital fossa. The biceps tendon is found lateral to the nerve and blood vessels. The median nerve passes under a tendinous hiatus formed by the deep head of the pronator, which originates over a length of 2 to 3 cm from the ulna and joins the superficial components, which orignate from the medial humerus. This tendinous arch leaves a narrow 2- to 3-mm indentation in the nerve, which presumably is caused by the tendinous component of the deep head impaling the nerve during rotation activities of the forearm. Approximately 2 to 3 cm distal to this hiatus is a second hiatus formed by tendinous bands within the origins of the sublimis muscles. This second hiatus (Figure 120-10) can be readily palpated after releasing the deep head of the pronator. However, the tendons or bands

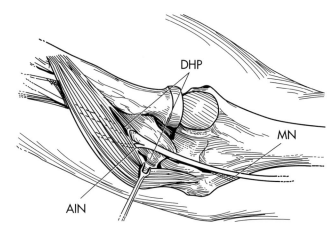

Figure 120-10. The deep head of the pronator teres (DHP) most commonly encompasses both the median nerve (MN) and the anterior interosseous nerve (AIN). The anterior interosseous nerve is rarely the only part of the nerve under only the fibrous portion of the deep head. The potential for sublimis band impingement cannot be detected until the deep head of the pronator is released. After the deep head is removed or released, the sublimis bands can be detected by palpation distal to the pronator arch.

responsible for the structure may not be directly visible because of the investing muscle covering the bands. These constrictions, if detected, are also released. The final step involves the use a lighted retractor to free and visualize the nerve proximal to the antecubital fossa. If a more proximal site of compression is likely, based on the clinical examination and electromyography, the incision can be extended proximally so that the ligament of Struthers or other reasons for neuropathy at a more proximal site can be found. In the past, the deep head of the pronator was sutured to the superficial head. In current practice the muscle and tendon are excised with caution to avoid the motor branches of the anterior interosseous nerve. This process completes the exploration and decompression of both the median and anterior interosseous nerves. The surgical site is closed after the tourniquet is deflated and hemostasis is established. To decrease postoperative pain, 15 ml of 0.5% bupivacaine containing 1/200,000 epinephrine and an appropriate injectable steroid are usually instilled into the surgical site after wound closure.

A long-arm removable thermoplastic splint is created preoperatively and is used for protection and pain relief after surgery. Active range-of-motion activity is started the day after surgery; the patient is instructed to remove the splint during daytime hours to exercise the elbow and forearm.

Recommendations regarding return to work parallel those following carpal tunnel release. Return to work typically occurs sooner than for patients who have undergone cubital tunnel release.

RADIAL NERVE COMPRESSION

INDICATIONS

Radial nerve entrapment is more difficult to diagnose because clinical symptoms are not as specific, lateral epicondylitis can complicate the diagnosis, and confirmatory electromyography is seldom positive. Antecedent trauma or tumors over the radial nerve often contribute to chronic entrapment of the radial nerve and can produce a classic picture.[6,8,16,39] However, radial neuropathy without prior injury or obvious etiology frequently occurs[49,16,60] and surgical procedures can cause unique circumstances, such as those reported by MacKinnon.[34]

The radial nerve can become entrapped in three areas.[49,57,42] These include the spiral groove through which the nerve courses from the medial to the lateral side of the arm behind the mid-humerus, the area extending from the radial head to the proximal half of the supinator muscle, and the area in which the nerve exits from under the brachioradialis tendon at the junction of the middle and distal thirds of the forearm. Irritation of the radial nerve at the elbow or in the spiral groove produces symptoms of pain that begin near the elbow and radiate proximally or distally. Posterior interosseous nerve irritation produces sensitivity to pressure approximately 5 cm distal to the lateral epicondyle. This symptom helps distinguish the diagnosis from lateral epicondylitis, which produces sensi-

tivity over the lateral epicondyle. The nerve can be detected by palpation between the mobile and immobile extrinsic extensor muscles. More proximal palpation of the nerve is complicated by the depth of the nerve under the muscle mass and also by the skeletal components of the elbow. The nerve also can be palpated approximately 8 cm above the elbow, in the intermuscular groove of the triceps and brachialis. Entrapment should be suspected at the spiral groove if examination is positive at this level.

The clinical examination and the patient's symptoms usually determine whether the radial nerve should be decompressed. Without evidence of neuropathy from the results of nerve conduction tests, the surgeon has a greater responsibility to ensure that the diagnosis is accurate. Symptoms, focal clinical findings, response to supportive treatment, and patient motivation become key factors in the decision regarding whether to operate.

OPERATIONS

Surgical exploration of the radial nerve and its posterior interosseous branch is most commonly performed because of suspicion that it is entrapped somewhere near the elbow.[60] Neuropathy in this area can be caused by the arcade of Froshe,[23] a tendinous arcade formed by the proximal edge of the supinator muscle. The radial nerve also can be entrapped by ganglions, synovium, or fibrosis around the area of the radial head. Entrapment suspected at the spiral groove requires exploration at the middle of the humerus and perhaps also at the elbow.

For exploration of the radial nerve at the elbow, we prefer to use a 6- to 8-cm incision starting 2 cm below the epicondyle and extending distally (Figure 120-11). The incision is located over the cleft between the brachioradialis and extensor carpi radialis longus muscles. The intermuscular plane leads to the

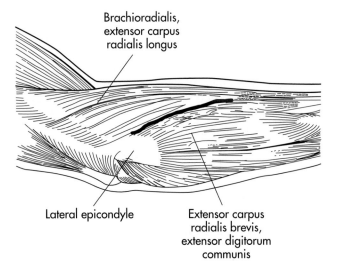

Figure 120-11. The incision *(heavy black line)* should be centered over an area 5 cm distal to the lateral epicondyle and can be extended proximally for management of problems involving the lateral epicondyle if necessary.

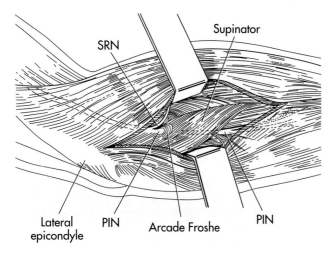

Figure 120-12. Location of the appropriate intermuscular plane is essential and facilitates location of the superficial radial nerve *(SRN)* and posterior interosseous nerve *(PIN)*. The entire fibrous edge of the supinator should be removed, avoiding injury to the motor branches that supply the supinator. The superficial branch of the radial nerve must be protected. To decompress the nerve, the arcade of Froshe and other tendinous bands should be removed.

proximal portion of the supinator and the fatty deposit that surrounds the radial nerve and the terminal branches of the profunda brachial artery and the radial collateral artery (Figure 120-12). The leading edge of the supinator is identified first, followed by identification of the posterior interosseous and superficial sensory branches of the radial nerve. The proximal tendinous edge of the supinator is subsequently excised, leaving only muscle fibers along the proximal 2 to 3 cm of the muscle. In some cases a pseudoneuroma is encountered, confirming the clinical diagnosis. The surgeon must be careful not to cut the motor branches to the supinator while excising the compressing bands or investing fascial bands of the muscle.

Compression syndromes often occur in constricted areas and in fulcrums of the extremities. The clinical diagnosis is the most reliable form of assessment; when other studies confirm the diagnosis, the decision regarding whether to operate is easy. The patient with multiple areas of nerve irritation presents a greater challenge when confirming diagnostic studies are not available. In such cases, the surgeon must rely on judgment, experience, and skill in evaluating pain symptoms.

OUTCOMES

CARPAL TUNNEL SYNDROME

The reported results of surgical decompression in patients with peripheral nerve compression syndromes are remarkably similar, despite the recent appearance of outcomes grading systems.

Perhaps a more standardized system of outcome measurement would have the sensitivity to detect differences between assessed groups. However, the level of injury, the mechanism of neuropathy, the degree of neuropathy, the age of the patient, and other variables make the study of results difficult.

Results after carpal tunnel release are often graded on a scale that includes three categories: excellent or good, poor, and no improvement. Studies of these results evaluate relief of symptoms, return of function, and often the return to work interval. Little data is presented in these studies regarding long-term results or recurrence.

Endoscopic carpal tunnel release seems to be associated with an earlier return to work compared with open surgical techniques, but the long-term functional outcome of this procedure is not yet well established. The final results with regard to the relief of symptoms appear to be the same with both endoscopic and open technique. When patients have no complicating medical problems and the time between diagnosis and treatment is not prolonged (years), recent studies indicate that approximately 80% of patients experience excellent or good results after carpal tunnel release; 10% to 15% experience fair results, and 5% to 10% experience poor results. The relief of pain is often immediate and is followed by a longer interval of improvement related to numbness, weakness, and muscle wasting. Most authors report that maximum recovery occurs 6 to 12 months after surgery. This parallels our experience. These results are long-lasting for a majority of patients, although recurrent problems can occur soon (6 to 12 months) after surgical release or as late as 5 to 10 years after surgical release. The rate of recurrence is estimated to be less than 1%.[11,19,59]

Common clinical predictors of outcomes are not noted in any clinical studies. However, factors that may influence the success of the surgical procedure include the patient's age, the severity and duration of symptoms, the degree of NCS abnormalities, and the presence of various systemic illnesses.

PRONATOR SYNDROME

Decompression of the median nerve in the proximal forearm produces results that are only slightly less successful than those associated with decompression at the wrist. This procedure is often complicated by the presence of multiple levels of synchronous neuropathy. Between 60% and 70% of patients experience improvement after median nerve decompression near the elbow. Postoperative results tend to shift from the excellent/complete category most often seen after decompression at the wrist to the good/partial relief category. Persistent symptoms of residual pain, paresthesias, or hypesthesia typically are reported after decompression near the elbow. An accurate diagnosis of pronator syndrome is difficult to make using NCS because these studies are more challenging to perform than some studies typically used to diagnose other neuropathies (e.g., CT scans). Some reports indicate that 10% to 20% of patients fail to improve after surgical decompression; we have not experienced this level of failure. Because fewer patients undergo surgery for this type of neuropathy, patient outcomes are more difficult to assess compared with those for patients who undergo carpal tunnel or cubital tunnel release. The poorer results may be related to a delay in diagnosis and treatment, which can result in more severe nerve injury such as Sunderland type II or greater injuries in the forearm that require nerve regeneration to occur over a greater distance.[41,24,58]

ULNAR NERVE COMPRESSIONS

For patients with cubital tunnel syndrome, more treatment options are available for decompression of the ulnar nerve than for compression of the median nerve; thus it is more difficult to analyze and compare the results of ulnar nerve release. Dellon[17] completed an exhaustive review of the literature on cubital tunnel syndrome and found that recovery of ulnar nerve function is dependent on the degree of compression before surgery. Excellent results were achieved in more than 90% of operative cases involving a minimal degree of compression. Results were excellent in 50% of cases involving moderate compression. The highest recurrence rate was associated with medial epicondylectomy. Anterior submuscular transposition of the ulnar nerve was associated with the lowest recurrence rate and an excellent outcome for 80% of patients. Less than 50% of patients achieved excellent sensory recovery; among these, only 25% of patients with motor loss experienced recovery. When detection and treatment were delayed for patients with severe compression, there was a 30% recurrence rate. More recent studies of single therapies indicate similar outcomes, with results lasting more than 1 to 4 years after decompression.[38,47]

REFERENCES

1. Adelaar RS, Foster WC, McDowell C: The treatment of the cubital tunnel syndrome, *J Hand Surg* 9A:90, 1984.
2. Adson AW: The classical surgical treatment for symptoms produced by cervical ribs and the scalenus anticus muscle, *Clin Orthop* 207:3, 1986.
3. Al-Qattan MM, Murray KA: The arcade of Struthers: an anatomical study, *J Hand Surg* 16B:311, 1991.
4. Apfelberg DB, Larson SJ: Dynamic anatomy of the ulnar nerve at the elbow, *Plast Reconstr Surg* 51:76, 1973.
5. Bell GE, Goldner JL: Compression neuropathy of the median nerve, *South Med J* 49:966, 1956.
6. Brown MG, Keyser B, Rothenberg ES: Endoscopic carpal tunnel release, *J Hand Surg* 17A:1009-1011, 1992.
7. Campbell WC: *Operative orthopedics,* St. Louis, 1939, Mosby.
8. Capener N: The vulnerability of the posterior interosseous nerve of the forearm, *J Bone Joint Surg* 48B:770, 1966.
9. Carroll RE, Green DP: The significance of the palmar cutaneous nerve at the wrist, *Clin Orthop* 88:24, 1972.
10. Cherington M: Proximal pain in carpal tunnel syndrome, *Arch Surg* 108:69, 1974.
11. Choi SJ, Ahn DS: Correlation of clinical history and electrodiagnostic abnormalities with outcome after surgery for carpal tunnel syndrome, *Plast Reconstr Surg* 102(7):2374-2380, 1998.
12. Chow JC: Endoscopic carpal tunnel release: two-portal technique, *Hand Clin* 10(4):637-646, 1994.
13. Cobb TK, Amadio PC: Reoperation for carpal tunnel syndrome, *Hand Clin* 12(2):313-323, 1996.
14. Cohen BE, Cukier J: Simultaneous posterior and anterior interosseous nerve syndromes, *J Hand Surg* 7:398, 1982.
15. Craven PR Jr, Green DP: Cubital tunnel syndrome: treatment by medical epicondylectomy, *J Bone Joint Surg* 62:986, 1980.
16. Cravens G, Kline DG: Posterior interosseous nerve palsies, *Neurosurgery* 27:397, 1990.
17. Dellon AL: Review of treatment results for ulnar nerve entrapment at the elbow, *J Hand Surg* 14A:688, 1989.
18. Dellon AL, Mackinnon SE: Injury to the medial antebrachial cutaneous nerve during cubital tunnel surgery, *J Hand Surg* 10B:33, 1985.
19. DeStefano F, Nordstrom DL, Vierkant RA: Long term symptom outcomes of carpal tunnel syndrome and its treatment, *J Hand Surg (Am)* 22(2):200-210, 1997.
20. Deune EG, Mackinnon SE: Endoscopic carpal tunnel release: the voice of polite dissent, *Clin Plast Surg* 23(3):487-505, 1996.
21. Ditmars DJ Jr, Houin HP: Carpal tunnel syndrome, *Hand Clin* 2:525, 1986.
22. Eisen A, Schomor D, Malmed C: The application of F-wave measurements in the differentiation of proximal and distal upper limb entrapments, *J Neurol* 27:662, 1977.
23. Frohse F, Frankel M: Die Muskeln des Menschlechen Armes. Bardelebenís Handbuch der Anatomie des Meuschildan, Jena Fisher, 1908.
24. Hartz CR, Lindscheid RL, Gramse RR, Daube JR: The pronator teres syndrome: compressive neuropathy of the median nerve, *J Bone Joint Surg* 63A:885, 1981.
25. Hunt JR: The thenar and hypothenar types of neural atrophy of the hand, *Am J Med Sci* 141:224-226, 1911.
26. Johnson RK, Spinner M, Shrewsbury MM: Median nerve entrapment syndromes in the proximal forearm, *J Hand Surg* 4:48, 1979.
27. Kiloh LG, Nevin S: Isolated neuritis of the anterior interosseous nerve, *BMJ* 1:850, 1952.
28. Knight CR, Kozub P: Anterior interosseous syndrome, *Ann Plast Surg* 3:72, 1979.
29. Kuschner SH, Brien WW, Johnson D, Gellman H: Complications associated with carpal tunnel release, *Orthop Rev* 20(4):346-352, 1991.
30. Lanz U: Anatomical variations of the median nerve in the carpal tunnel, *J Hand Surg* 2:44, 1977.
31. Learmonth JR: Technique for transplanting the ulnar nerve, *Surg Gynecol Obstet* 75:792, 1942.
32. Leffert RD: Anterior submuscular transposition of the ulnar nerve by the Learmonth technique, *J Hand Surg* 7:147, 1982.

33. Louis DS, Hankin FM: Symptomatic relief following carpal tunnel decompression with normal electroneuromyographic studies, *Orthopedics* 10:434, 1987.

34. Mackinnon SE, Dellon AL: The overlap pattern of the lateral antebrachial cutaneous nerve and the superficial branch of the radial nerve, *J Hand Surg* 10A:522, 1985.

35. Miller RG: The cubital tunnel syndrome: diagnosis and precise localization, *Ann Neurol* 6:56, 1979.

36. Nagle DJ: Endoscopic carpal tunnel release: in favor, *Clin Plast Surg* 23(3):477-486, 1996.

37. Nagle DJ, Fischer TJ, Harris GD, et al: A multicenter prospective review of 640 endoscopic carpal tunnel releases using the transbursal and extrabursal Chow techniques, *Arthroscopy* 12(2): 139-143, 1996.

38. Nathan PA, Keniston RC, Meadows KD: Outcome study of ulnar nerve compression at the elbow treated with simple decompression and an early programme of physical therapy, *J Hand Surg (Br)* 20(5):628-637, 1995.

39. Nielsen HO: Posterior interosseous nerve paralysis caused by fibrous band compression at the supinator muscle: a report of four cases, *Acta Orthop Scand* 47:304, 1976.

40. Nigst H, Dick W: Syndromes of compression of the median nerve in the proximal forearm (pronator teres syndrome; anterior interosseous nerve syndrome), *Arch Orthop Trauma Surg* 93:307, 1979.

41. Olehnik WK, Manske PR, Szerzinski J: Median nerve compression in the proximal forearm, *J Hand Surg* 19A:121-126, 1994.

42. Omer GE, Spinner M, Van Beek AL: *Management of peripheral nerve problems,* ed 2, Philadelphia, 1998, WB Saunders.

43. Pernkopf E: *Atlas of topographical and applied human anatomy,* ed 2, Philadelphia, 1980, WB Saunders.

44. Phalen GS: Spontaneous compression of the median nerve at the wrist, *JAMA* 145:1128, 1951.

45. Phalen GS: The carpal tunnel syndrome: seventeen years experience in diagnosis and treatment of 644 hands, *J Bone Joint Surg* 48A:211, 1966.

46. Seddon H: *Surgical disorders of the peripheral nerves,* Edinburgh, 1975, Churchill Livingstone.

47. Seradge H, Owen W: Cubital tunnel release with medial epicondylectomy factors influencing the outcome, *J Hand Surg* 23(3):483-491, 1988.

48. Smith RV, Fisher RG: Struthers ligament, a source of median nerve compression above the elbow, *J Neurosurg* 38:778, 1973.

49. Spinner M: The arcade of Frohse and its relationship to posterior interosseous nerve paralysis, *J Bone Joint Surg* 50B:809, 1968.

50. Spinner M: The anterior interosseous nerve syndrome, with special attention to its variations, *J Bone Joint Surg* 52A:84, 1970.

51. Sunderland SS: *Nerves and nerve injuries,* Edinburgh, 1978, Churchill Livingstone.

52. Taleisnik J: The palmar cutaneous branch of the median nerve and the approach to the carpal tunnel: an anatomic study, *J Bone Joint Surg* 55:1212, 1973.

53. Tosti A, Morelli R, DiAlessandro R, Bassi F: Carpal tunnel syndrome presenting with ischemic skin lesions, acroosteolysis, and nail changes (see comments), *J Am Acad Dermatol* 29 (2 Pt 2):287-290, 1993.

54. Tountas CP, Begman RA: *Anatomic variations of the upper extremity,* New York, 1993, Churchill Livingstone.

55. Tountas CP, MacDonald CJ, Mayerhoff JD, Bihrle DM: Carpal tunnel syndrome: a review of 507 patients, *Minn Med* 66:479, 1983.

56. Upton ARM, McComas AJ: The double crush in nerve entrapment syndromes, *Lancet* 2:359, 1973.

57. Van Beek AL: Management of nerve compression syndromes and painful neuromas. In McCarthy JG (editor): *Plastic surgery,* Philadelphia, 1990, WB Saunders.

58. Werner CO, Rosen I, Thorngren KG: Clinical and neurophysiologic characteristics of the pronator syndrome, *Clin Orthop* 197:231, 1985.

59. Wilbourn AJ, Gilliatt RW: Double-crush syndrome: a critical analysis, *Neurology* 49(1):21-29, 1997.

60. Young C, Hudson A, Richard R: Operative treatment of palsy of the posterior interosseous nerve of the forearm, *J Bone Joint Surg* 72:1215, 1990.

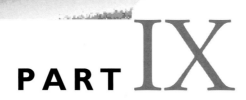

PART IX

MICROSURGERY

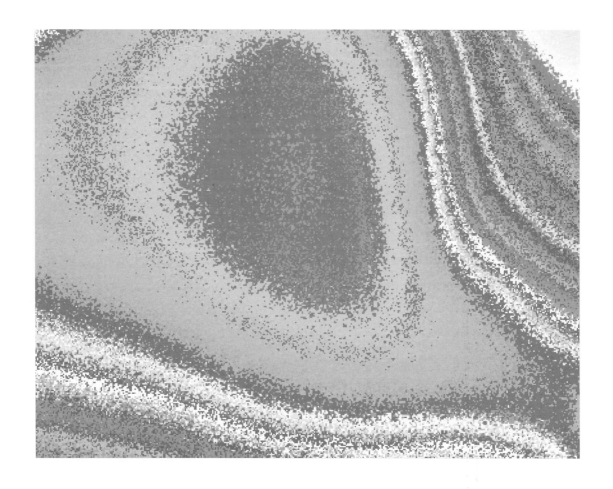

Replantation

121

Gregory M. Buncke
Harry J. Buncke
Gabriel M. Kind
Rudolf Buntic

INTRODUCTION

Replantation can be defined as the reattachment of an amputated part. Use of the operating room microscope is generally necessary to repair blood vessels and nerves, except in proximal amputations. Replantation of amputated parts, especially fingers, is one of the most difficult types of reconstructive hand surgery. The replantation effort can be very rewarding for both the injured patient and surgeon. Keys to a successful replantation include proper microsurgical techniques, a well-educated operating room and postoperative nursing staff, and good monitoring. Patience, personal conviction, and experience on the part of the surgeon are also essential. Many surgeons have been trained in microsurgical techniques; however, because of the many possible perioperative complications, the patient who requires replantation is often best treated in a replantation center. Successful replantation operations require a team effort, the expertise of several medical disciplines, and a center specializing in replantation and microsurgery. The replantation center should have operating rooms staffed with trained personnel who are available 24 hours a day for emergency replantation surgery. The following elements should be available to ensure success[6]:

1. An efficient network of ground and air transportation systems to transfer patients from referring hospitals to the replantation center.
2. An experienced microsurgical team working in 4-hour shifts.
3. A well-prepared emergency room staff to stabilize and quickly evaluate the patient through physical examination, radiographs, and laboratory tests.
4. Experienced anesthesiologists and operating room and microsurgical staff who are available 24 hours a day.
5. Proper microscopes, instruments, and sutures.
6. Trained nursing staff for postoperative care and monitoring.

7. Physical and occupational therapists trained in the rehabilitation of patients who have undergone replantation.
8. Psychologists and social workers to help the patient adjust to his or her injuries.

Efficient transportation is the key to minimizing unnecessary ischemic injury to the amputated part. Replantation surgeons should participate in educational seminars for emergency personnel from referring hospitals. Educational posters concerning replantation transportation protocols are extremely helpful for the staff at emergency rooms of referring hospitals.[8]

After the patient with an amputation has been stabilized, the amputated part should be placed in dry or nearly dry gauze. The gauze and amputated part should be placed in a zip-lock bag, which should be placed on ice. Care should be taken not to freeze the amputated part; the goal is to keep the part cold to avoid the negative effects of warm ischemia. Digits that have remained cold have been replanted as many as 48 hours after amputation. Parts with muscle that have remained cold have been replanted as many as 12 hours after injury.

Arrangements should be made to transport the patient to the replantation center as quickly as possible. Often air transport is not required because the patient can arrive faster by ground. Inappropriately delaying transfer to obtain unnecessary studies (such as an electrocardiogram or arteriogram) at the referring hospital can increase the total ischemia time. The amputation stump should be covered with a saline-moistened sponge, loosely wrapped, and perhaps splinted for pain relief. Under no circumstances should a digital block be performed because this procedure may interfere with the blood flow across the microvascular repair.

After the patient arrives at the replantation center, the surgeon should examine the radiographs, amputated part, and stump, if possible. The surgeon must know the patient's age and general medical condition and the functional requirements for the patient's vocation and avocations. Subsequently a discussion should take place among the operating surgeon, the patient, and the patient's family. The surgeon should describe the typical scenario of a replantation operation and associated rehabilitation time as a treatment option versus completing the amputation. The patient should know that replantation surgery typically requires 3 to 6 hours per replanted digit; he or she also should be aware of the possible need for a blood transfusion, which is commonly required for patients who take heparin. Patients who undergo hand replantation receive an average of five units of blood during hospitalization. Patients who undergo proximal upper-and lower-extremity replantation require an average of 15 units of blood perioperatively.[17] The patient should be aware of the risks associated with receiving a blood transfusion. A recent report describes the risks of acquiring a transfusion-transmitted viral infection as follows:[41]

Human immunodeficiency virus (HIV) 1:493,000
Human T-cell leukemia/lymphoma
   virus (HTLV)   1:641,000
Cytomegalovirus (CMV)   1:103,000
Hepatitis B virus (HBV)   1:63,000

The surgeon also should discuss the length of stay in the hospital and compare the possible need for secondary surgery among patients who undergo a replantation with that for patients who undergo completion of an amputation.

If the surgeon is confident that the patient has understood the discussion and the patient wishes to proceed with replantation the patient should be taken as quickly as possible to the operating room for attempted replantation.

HISTORY

Experimental replantation surgery was first performed in the early 1900s. Carrell and Guthrie[12] performed homograft transplantation of canine limbs that lasted as long as 22 days. It was not until the early 1960s that Malt and McKhann[31] performed the first clinical case of replantation. Small-vessel anastomosis was becoming a clinical reality because of experimental work by Buncke and Schulz.[9] Clinical reports of the microvascular repair of small vessels followed. Kleinert et al[26] reported the first vascular repair in fingers in 1963; subsequently Komatsu and Tamai[27] reported thumb replantation after a total amputation. The scope of replantation surgery expanded greatly with the refinement and standardization of microsurgical instruments, needles, and sutures, and with the establishment of microsurgical replantation centers.

INDICATIONS

Patient motivation and intelligence are among the major factors that influence functional outcome after replantation.[6] In an extraordinarily motivated and intelligent patient, even a single-digit, crushing amputation through zone 2 of an index finger in a nondominant hand can result in excellent long-term functional results (Figure 121-1). Unfortunately, factors such

as worker's compensation or litigation may have a negative influence on the patient's interest in having the best functional return possible.

Absolute contraindications to replantation of a replantable part include associated life-threatening injuries and severe underlying medical problems that preclude undergoing a long anesthetic procedure. The replantation surgeon should discuss these issues with the referring physician before transporting the patient so needless transport of a patient in critical condition can be avoided. Cigarette smoking after replantation surgery has been proven to have a deleterious effect on blood flow for as long as 3 months after surgery; however, no correlation exists between preoperative smoking and the survival of replanted parts.[13] I have had several patients who had such a strong addiction to nicotine that they were unwilling to stop cigarette smoking in the perioperative period and subsequently elected not to undergo replantation. All other replantation cases should be dealt with on a case-by-case basis.

Single-digit replantation is a controversial issue. An amputation distal to the sublimis tendon insertion is a favorable level for replantation, even if the distal interphalangeal (DIP) joint requires arthrodesis (Figure 121-2). Neuroma formation in finger amputation stumps is a common problem and can be avoided by replanting the finger. The need for secondary operations is rare in zone-1 distal replants. Replantation of amputated parts distal to the DIP joint frequently can be very demanding technically. Patients should be aware that the surgeon may be able to repair only an artery and may not be able to repair a vein. In such cases, heparinization, the use of leech therapy, and blood loss is anticipated. Because of poor functional return and disuse of the replanted finger, single-digit amputation at the level of zone 2 most likely is not an indication for replantation in the patient who does not need that digit for work or avocation.

In general, single-digit replantation is indicated in patients with amputations distal to the sublimis insertion. If the amputation is in zone 2, flexor and extensor tendons can adhere to healing bone and may require secondary tenolysis to improve motion; frequently the results in such cases, even after tenolysis, are not good. However, replantation of a single digit may be indicated in cases involving an intelligent, motivated patient who may require 10 fingers for his or her occupation; in cases in which cosmetic considerations are important; or in cases involving children.[4]

In contrast, the thumb is by far the most important digit in the hand, and replantation of an amputated thumb should be performed whenever possible. In some cases the thumb may be "banked" and replanted at a later date to permit other reconstruction before replantation.[51] Some authors believe that a thumb avulsion injury with bilateral digital nerve avulsion off the median nerve may be a contraindication to thumb replantation.[39] However, in such cases the surgeon can use the long, distal ends of the digital nerves to the thumb and perform microsurgical neurorrhaphy to branches of the dorsal sensory nerve in the first web space. Sensory return, especially in the young patient, is adequate to give protective sensation; in many patients this procedure provides useful sensation.[6]

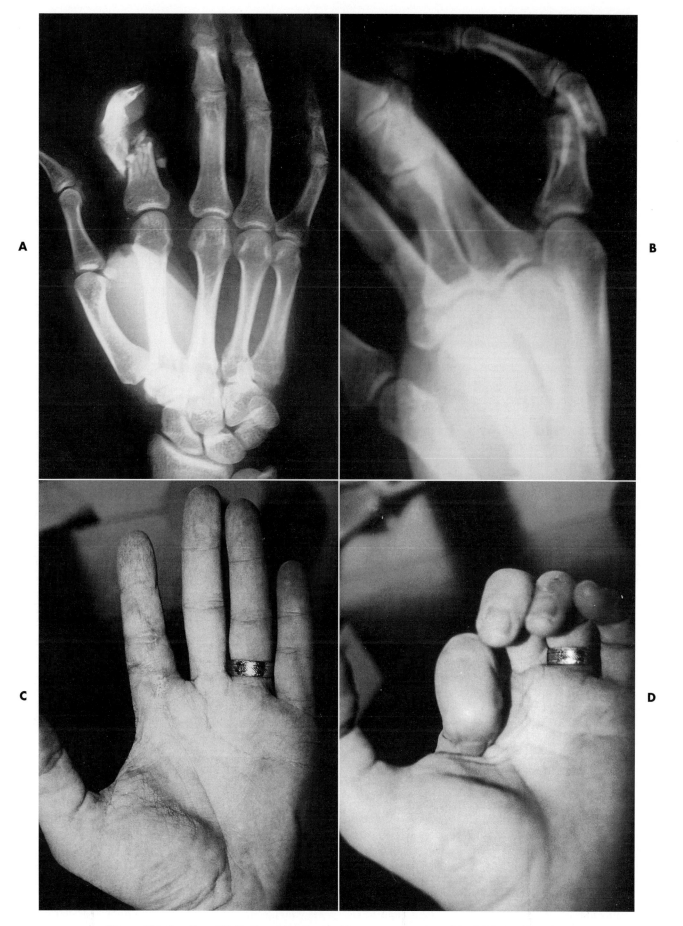

Figure 121-1. **A** and **B,** Radiographs of a crushing near-amputation of the left index finger in a 43-year-old, right-hand-dominant ophthalmologist, with laceration of the flexor tendon, extensor tendons, digital nerves, and digital arteries, and a comminuted fracture of the proximal phalanx. A phalangeal nonunion was repaired 2 months later with a plate, and simultaneous extensor tenolysis was performed. Flexor tenolysis was performed in a third operation 4 months later. Extension **(C)** and flexion **(D)** 3 months after flexor tenolysis.

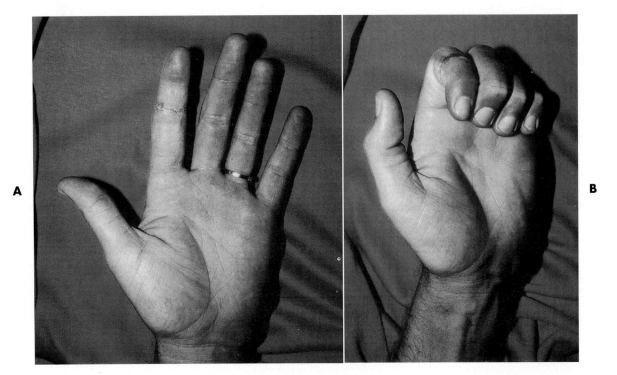

Figure 121-2. Extension **(A)** and flexion **(B)** of a single-digit replant distal to the superficialis insertion. No secondary surgery was necessary.

After saw-type injuries, ring avulsion injuries are perhaps the most common type of injury seen at our microsurgical service. These occur when a patient's ring (typically on the nondominant ring finger) catches a nail or ladder and temporarily suspends the patient's entire body weight on the ring, which strips the finger's soft tissue distally. Rather than a clean injury to the artery and veins of the amputated or nearly amputated digit, there is an area of segmental injury to arteries, nerves, and veins. Vein grafts are frequently needed to repair the segmental arterial loss. The vein usually can be mobilized proximally to perform direct repair. The nerve often can be repaired end-to-end, although the nerve may be damaged for several centimeters. Because these injuries frequently do not involve damage to the flexor or extensor tendon system proximally, or bony fracture in the zone-2 region, motion after a ring avulsion injury can be quite good. The traction injury to the nerve may result in less sensory return than occurs in patients after a sharp amputation injury (Figure 121-3).

Our general philosophy is to examine all patients with ring avulsion injuries in the operating room and to attempt repair of all structures, if possible. Although return of sensation in the digit may not be good, metacarpophalangeal (MCP) and proximal interphalangeal (PIP) joint motion is frequently excellent. Most patients with ring avulsion injuries prefer a successfully replanted digit (even with decreased sensation) to a ray amputation.

Replantation in patients with multiple-digit injuries is nearly always attempted unless the patient does not desire the operation or there are medical contraindications (Figure 121-4). We generally begin by replanting the most ulnar digit and work radially because this sequence is logistically easiest to perform and the ulnar digits are more important for grip span and strength. The replantation surgeon should try to replant the appropriate finger in the appropriate position; however, ulnar digits should take precedence over radial digits. If, for example, the patient has an amputation of the index and middle fingers, and the middle finger is not replantable, the surgeon should consider replanting the index finger in the middle finger position to prevent a gap in the normal architecture of the hand. The surgeon may consider ray amputation of the index finger at the time of the initial surgery or at a later date. The same holds true for multiple-digit amputations, including amputation of the thumb. If the thumb is not replantable, a digit should be replanted in the thumb position.

Replantation in cases of multiple-digit amputations through the palm should be attempted in almost all circumstances. Secondary tendon transfers may be necessary to balance the hand's intrinsic function because of the destruction of intrinsic muscles. Replantation may not be advisable when there is significant skeletal loss or MCP-joint destruction.

In most cases, replantation of amputations through the carpus or distal forearm should be attempted because this level of amputation has an excellent chance for good return of function. Structures at this level tend to be large and easier to repair. Because there is no intrinsic muscle damage, these muscles ultimately become reinnervated and frequently func-

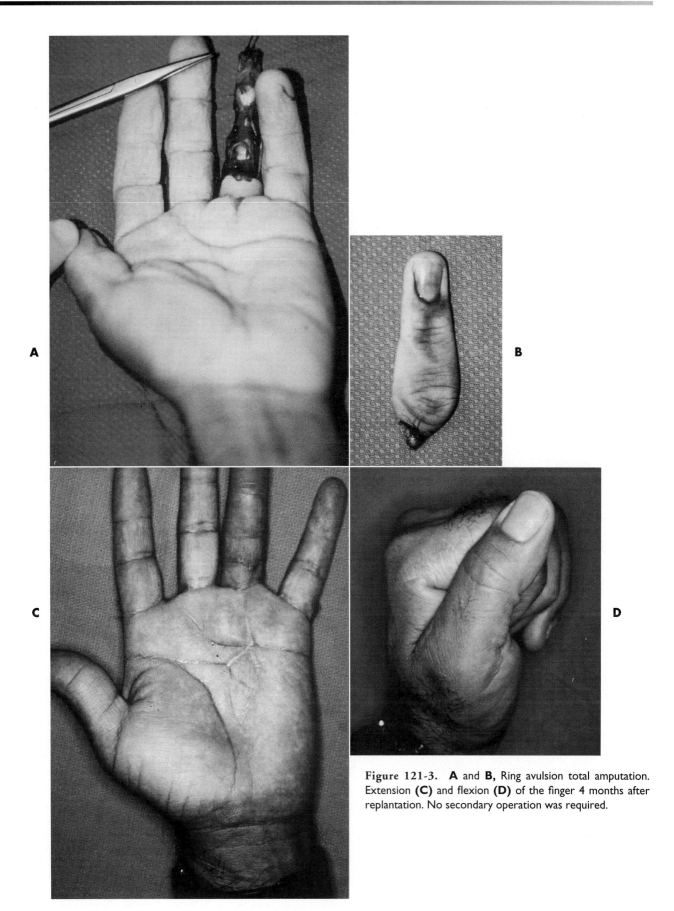

Figure 121-3. A and **B,** Ring avulsion total amputation. Extension **(C)** and flexion **(D)** of the finger 4 months after replantation. No secondary operation was required.

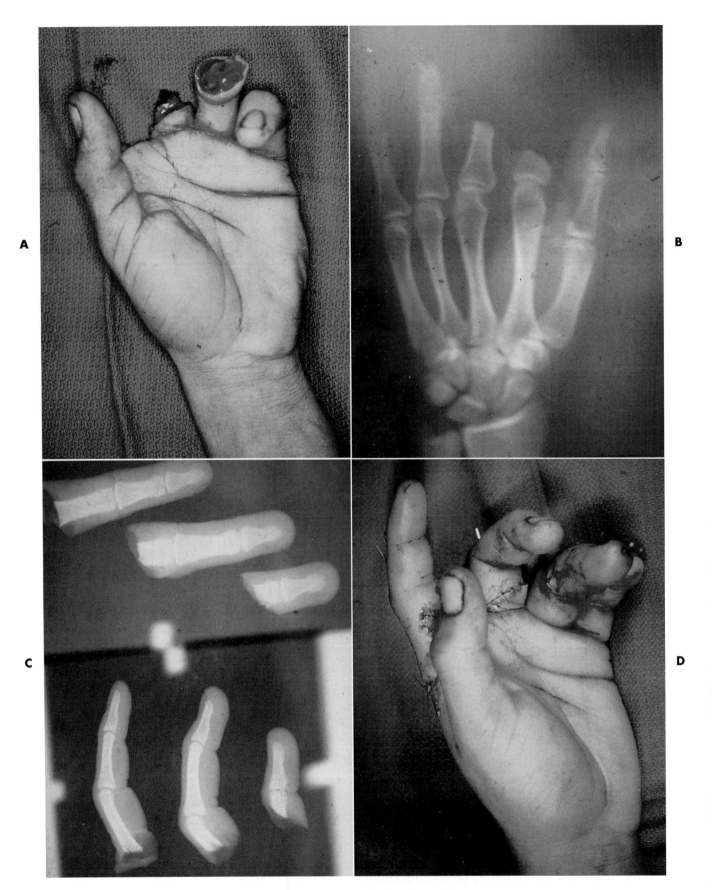

Figure 121-4. **A-C,** Multiple-digit amputations sparing the PIP and MCP joints. **D,** The immediate postoperative result.

Continued

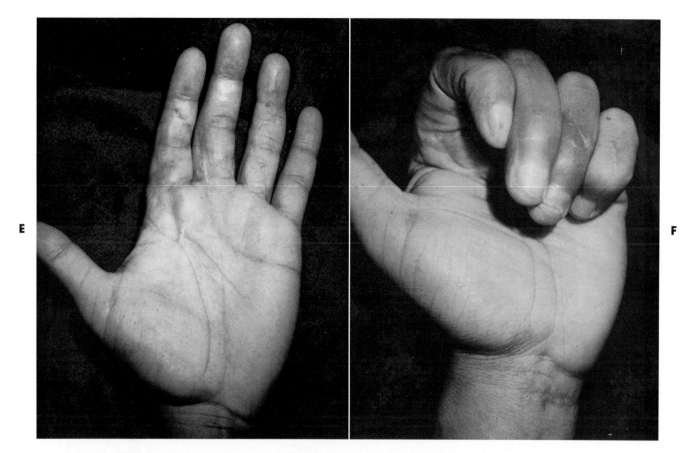

Figure 121-4, cont'd. **E** and **F,** The result after a secondary dorsal capsulotomy, extensor tenolysis, and flexor tenolysis.

tion after rehabilitation (Figure 121-5). Knobby T-shaped shunts[33] should be used to set up arterial inflow as the first step in the sequence of replantation. This shortens the warm ischemia time and limits muscle necrosis in the hand. The shunt can be removed after osseous fixation and arterial repair are performed (Figure 121-6).

More proximal forearm injuries unfortunately have poorer functional outcome than distal forearm injuries. Replantation should be performed when no more than 4 to 6 cm of radius and ulna must be removed. Amputations proximal to the elbow are frequently avulsive and crushing in nature; thus functional restoration of finger motion in such cases is unlikely except in the very young. However, replantation at this level may be indicated in the adult patient to establish elbow joint control and possibly to power a below-elbow prosthesis.[50]

The ischemia time should be measured from the time of the amputation until arterial inflow can be reestablished. Replantation usually is not recommended if the warm ischemia time is greater than 6 hours for an amputation proximal to the wrist or greater than 12 hours per digit, although survival of a replanted part has been documented after 42 hours of warm ischemia.[3] Moreover, replantation is not performed when the cold ischemia time for proximal amputations is greater than 12 hours. However, digits can be reliably replanted after 24 to 30 hours of cold ischemia.[6]

In cases of complex, multiple-digit, multiple-level injuries, better function often can be achieved by salvaging parts of amputated extremities, which can be used as microvascular transplants to reconstruct remaining stumps or open wounds of the hand.[1,22,24] The guiding principle is to use the parts that are available to restore as much extremity function as possible. An experienced surgeon should make such decisions on an individual basis. The surgeon should accomplish as much as is feasible during the initial operation because it may provide the only chance to restore a functional extremity. The surgeon's ability to assess the immediate situation and develop a long-range plan for reconstruction from the beginning significantly influences the patient's care and final outcome.

OPERATIONS

Replantation surgery can be tedious and time consuming; however, the time spent on aggressive debridement and precise microsurgical technique typically pays off in terms of the patient's long-term functional outcome. We generally plan on 3 to 4 hours of surgery per amputated digit.

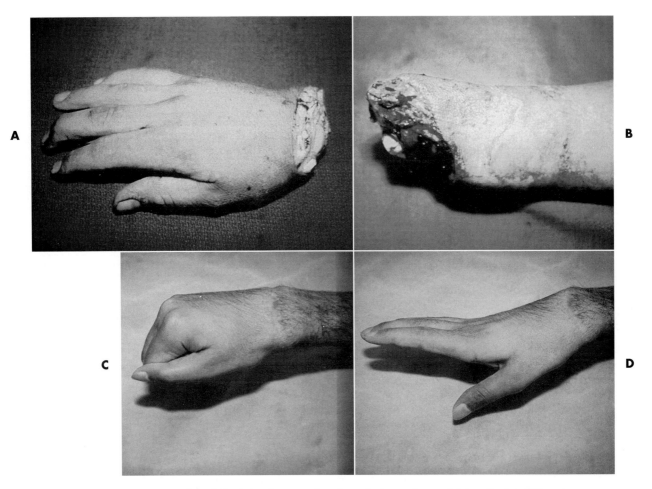

Figure 121-5. **A** and **B,** A hand amputation through the radiocarpal joint. Flexion **(C)** and extension **(D)** are shown after flexor tenolysis.

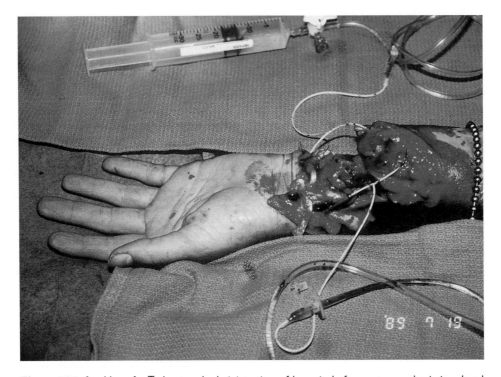

Figure 121-6. Use of a T shunt and administration of heparin before osteosynthesis in a hand replant.

Hand and forearm amputations often take 8 to 12 hours. Because of these time demands, we frequently try to relieve the primary surgeon so that no surgeon is required to operate more than 4 to 6 hours at a time. We believe that general anesthesia is appropriate because of the length of these operations. Other surgeons have recommended axillary blocks and sedation; however, we have found that patients frequently are uncomfortable after several hours on the operating table. Recently, we have administered brachial plexus blocks, even in patients undergoing general anesthesia, to help relieve vasospasm and improve pain control in the immediate postoperative period.

OPERATIVE SEQUENCE

After the decision to replant has been made, the parts should be taken to the operating room immediately for tagging. The surgeon should make two mid-lateral incisions in the mid-axial line and, using loupe magnification or the microscope, find the vital structures for replantation (Figure 121-7). Both neurovascular bundles should be tagged with 6-0 silk or a purple marking pen. The flexor and extensor tendons should be identified and trimmed. One or two dorsal veins should be identified and also tagged. These maneuvers can be performed without an assistant if the skin flaps are tacked back with 4-0 nylon. The edges of bone are trimmed to obtain the best bony contact. Two Kirschner (K) wires subsequently can be placed longitudinally or crossed through the cut end of the amputated digit, depending on the level of the amputation. The surgeon should avoid crossing joint lines with these K wires, if possible. Next, the finger is placed in a sterile container, which is placed on ice in the operating room.

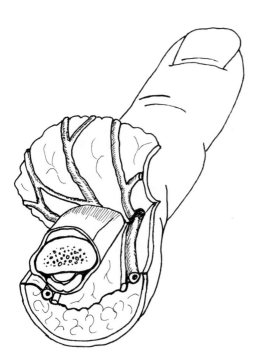

Figure 121-7. Lateral incisions for exposure of volar and dorsal structures of the amputated part.

At the same time, the patient is brought to the operating room, transferred to a well-padded operating room table, and given general anesthesia. An interscalene brachial plexus block frequently is also performed to promote vasodilation and reduce perioperative pain. A Foley catheter is inserted. Pneumatic tourniquets are placed on the proximal part of the injured extremity and on a donor leg for nerve, vein, or skin graft harvest.

The injured extremity is prepared and draped, and the amputation stump is copiously irrigated with warm normal saline. Careful debridement of the amputation stump under tourniquet control is performed. Gross contamination is sharply debrided and devitalized tissue is removed. Six-0 silk or a marking pen is used to tag the arteries, nerves, and dorsal veins. Ragged bone ends are trimmed to obtain the best bony contact with the amputated part. Flexor and extensor tendons are also trimmed to permit a clean tenorrhaphy.

Temporary knobby plastic shunts are used in proximal extremity amputations to allow rapid reperfusion of the extremity, which in turn allows a less hurried examination and identification of structures. Bony fixation subsequently can be performed without extending the ischemic time. The shunt is placed in the artery to reperfuse the extremity. Bleeding should be permitted from the venous system and cut muscle edges to flush the toxic by-products of muscle ischemia from the amputated part. The patient is generally allowed to bleed approximately one unit of blood.

Almost all major amputations require fasciotomy to prevent potential or impending compartment syndromes that develop with the significant muscle edema that occurs after revascularization. In cases of arm replantation, dorsal and volar forearm fasciotomies, carpal and Guyon tunnel releases, and intrinsic compartment decompression should be performed during replantation surgery.[32,38]

Subsequently osteosynthesis is performed. Bone shortening is frequently performed to permit primary tension-free anastomosis of vessels and nerves without compromising length and function. Primary soft tissue coverage is also facilitated by bone shortening. We generally use two longitudinal or crossed K wires for bony fixation of digital amputations. Plates or interosseous wires[28] are sometimes used in amputations through the phalangeal shaft because it is frequently difficult to stabilize this level of amputation without rigid fixation.[5]

Arterial repairs are performed next to quickly reestablish circulation and perfusion and to assess the viability of the amputated part. Venous and arterial anastomoses are performed with similar microsurgical techniques. This part of the operation should be performed with utmost precision to prevent thrombosis at the sites of anastomoses. Surgeons should sit comfortably with wrists and hands well supported to avoid fatigue and to improve control of the microsurgical instruments. The tourniquet should be released before arterial or venous repairs are begun and there should be good flow from the proximal artery or distal vein. The artery should be examined under the microscope for damage. Normal vessel color is opalescent, or pearly gray. Stretched or traumatized vessels are frequently speckled because of multiple ruptures of the vasovasorum, which produces a "measles" or "paprika" sign. The vessel ends should be inspected and cleared of any blood or platelet clots. A damaged artery also undergoes separation or loss of the endothelial layer. A normal vessel should have no separation between the endothelium, muscularis, and adventitia. Vessels should be trimmed both distally and proximally until normal vessel is found. If a tension-free vessel repair cannot be performed after trimming, a vein graft should be harvested from the wrist region and placed in reversed fashion to bridge the gap.[2]

The vessel ends are mechanically dilated with jeweler's forceps and heparinized saline is gently injected, with a blunt catheter, both distally and proximally beyond the level of the vascular clamps. Every attempt should be made to repair the ipsilateral artery; however, this repair may not be possible in some cases involving traction injuries. Arterial anastomosis in these cases also can be established by a cross-over vessel technique (e.g., the radial digital artery to the ulnar digital artery), although this technique makes secondary tenolysis precarious. The surgeon also can transpose the digital artery from an adjacent uninjured digit for proximal inflow.

Microvascular anastomosis subsequently is performed, for which we generally use the back-wall technique.[21] Two or three sutures are placed in the back wall and sutures are progressively placed toward the front wall, allowing direct visualization of the entire repair. If there is a size discrepancy between the two vessel ends, then , two or three back-wall sutures are placed, a front-wall stitch is placed, and sutures are placed on either side of these two stitches, thus bisecting the area that remains to be repaired. The microclamps are removed after the vessel is repaired and the vessel is bathed in papaverine. The replanted part should become pink within several seconds of clamp release. Frequently signs of perfusion occur almost immediately after removal of the clamps. If the part does not perfuse after papaverine and warm irrigation, the vascular repair must undergo a filling test to determine whether blood passes through the anastomosis. If the filling test indicates a lack of flow, the surgeon should remove the sutures to examine the inside of the vascular anastomosis or should cut out the anastomosis entirely and perform a reanastomosis of the vessel. If the filling test indicates good flow across the anastomosis, vascular spasm distal to the anastomosis most likely exists. In such cases, the vessels should be dissected distally and all side branches should be tied off or cauterized with bipolar cautery because unsatisfied side branches may cause segmental spasm in the artery. If perfusion still cannot be established in the part, the part must be perfused intraarterially with more heparin, or in some cases with approximately 50,000 to 100,000 units of streptokinase or urokinase. If perfusion is not reestablished after these maneuvers, the part may not be replantable, in which case the part should be removed and an amputation should be completed.

Microdigital neurorrhaphies are performed after reperfusion of the part has been established. Most nerves can be repaired without tension after adequate bone shortening. The nerve ends are examined under the microscope for *les yeux d'escargot* sign, or fascicles protruding from the ends of the cut nerve that verify uninjured repairable nerve. The ends of the nerves generally require some trimming before anastomosis. The digital nerves are subsequently repaired, using 9-0 or 10-0 microsuture and placing only as many epineural stitches as necessary to coapt the ends without tension.

Primary neurorrhaphy is often impossible in cases of severe crush injuries because of a loss of nerve substance, which creates a gap between the nerve ends. Primary nerve grafting should be performed only in an ideal situation, which rarely exists in a true replantation case. Nerve grafting should not be performed unless the wound is clean and can be closed primarily. Traumatic replantation sites may become secondarily infected or undergo partial skin loss, and replantation may fail completely after vessel thrombosis, all of which place primary nerve grafts at considerable risk. Therefore secondary nerve grafting typically is performed a few months after replantation, when the success or failure of the replantation has been determined and minor complications have been corrected.

The flexor tendons should be repaired using a modified Kessler stitch with 3-0 nonabsorbable suture and an epitendinous stitch with 5-0 nylon. A primary tendon transfer from a nonreplantable digit stump can be used in some cases if the proximal flexor tendon is not available in the replanted digit. Stiffness caused by flexor tendon adhesions is a significant problem after replantation; thus rehabilitation of the flexor tendons should be started as soon as possible, despite the risk of tendon rupture.

At this time a few stitches are placed in the skin to close the volar laceration. The hand is subsequently turned over and the extensor tendons are repaired using either 4-0 Vicryl or 4-0 Supramid sutures in a figure-eight tendinous stitch.

The microscope is brought back into the field and dorsal veins are repaired by a method similar to that used for repair of the artery. We generally repair one vein per digit; however, if outflow through that vein is poor, a second vein is repaired. A digit may survive even without venous repairs by means of leeching and heparinization. The skin on the dorsum of the finger is loosely approximated and skin grafts often are placed on the mid-lateral incisions, or the incisions are left open and allowed to heal by secondary intention to prevent tight skin closure.

Nonadhering gauze is placed over the wounds, avoiding constriction. To prevent compression by the dressing when the digit swells after surgery, circumferential dressings should not be placed around the digits. Care also should be taken not to place gauze between the digits (as in standard postoperative hand dressing). Unfortunately, the dressing can become caked with blood postoperatively and consequently may cause vascular compromise.

A dorsal protective splint is placed and held in position with a bias-cut stockinette. The patient's extremity is subsequently placed on two or three pillows, with the hand and replanted digits positioned above the level of the chest.

Replantation of the hand or distal forearm is begun with a palmar incision similar to that used for carpal tunnel release, which helps expose the flexor tendons and the median and ulnar nerves for proper identification and tagging before the initiation of surgical repair. Maintaining the delicate balance between flexor and extensor tendons is the surgical goal when replanting a hand. Bone shortening of as much as 3 to 5 cm is acceptable in subtotal amputations with bone loss. However, further shortening causes tendon imbalance that seriously compromises finger motion and hand function. Both the extensor and flexor tendons can be shortened and balanced appropriately in patients with total amputations and in such cases the bone can be shortened more than 5 cm. Occasionally further bone shortening is not an option; in such cases an emergency free tissue transfer for soft tissue coverage of repaired structures may be indicated either at the time of replantation or within the first week after surgery.[29]

POSTOPERATIVE CARE

The most important goals in the postoperative management of patients after replantation are to maintain adequate hydration and fluid balance, to perfuse the replanted part, to prevent peripheral vasoconstriction, and to closely monitor the blood flow into and out of the replanted part. The patient must be returned to the operating room immediately if there are uncorrectable signs of vascular compromise. Most patients are kept in the intensive care unit for the first 48 hours after surgery to facilitate these goals. Properly trained nursing and support staff are essential to appropriately manage these patients.

Adequate hydration is critical to optimizing the systemic and capillary blood pressures within the replanted part. Hematocrit levels should be kept in the high 20s to maintain perfusion and prevent peripheral vasoconstriction. All patients are given low-molecular-weight dextran (25 ml/hour) in the operating room at the time of the first anastomosis, and administration of dextran is continued for 5 days after surgery. Systemic heparinization is used only if intraoperative or postoperative thrombosis occurs, or for artery-only replants. Patients are given chlorpromazine (10 mg three times a day) to help prevent vasoconstriction[7] and to provide mild sedation. Patients also are given aspirin (325 mg) on a daily basis because of its antiplatelet activity.

Monitoring can be performed in a variety of ways. Examining the color and capillary refill of the replanted part continues to be the standard for many microsurgical groups. We routinely use the quantitative fluorescein washout technique[20] for monitoring our replants. This technique entails taking a reading at time zero with a quantitative fluorometer and injecting 1 ml of fluorescein intravenously. At 10 minutes a second reading is taken from the digit and also from a control area; there should be a rise in both readings if there is good arterial inflow. A third reading is taken at 60 minutes after injection; the numbers should go down at this time, indicating good venous outflow. These data, together with clinical evaluation, have been very effective in the diagnosis of early thrombosis (Figure 121-8). Other types of monitoring devices have included temperature probes, laser dopplers, and transcutaneous oxygen monitors. Evaluating color, turgor, and capillary refill are effective when

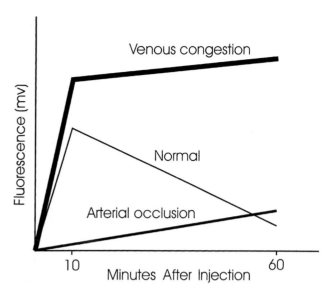

Figure 121-8. Normal, arterial occlusion, and venous occlusion rates using the fluorescein washout technique.

performed by experienced surgeons but are less reliable when performed by physicians less experienced in replantation surgery.

TREATMENT OF A FAILING DIGITAL REPLANT

When a replanted digit appears pale and deflated, and demonstrates very slow capillary refill and poor rise during quantitative fluorometry, the surgeon should assume that there is inadequate inflow into the digit. In such cases the dressing should be removed while the patient is kept calm and warm. The finger should be gently massaged, especially at the site of arterial anastomosis. A bupivacaine block can be administered in the appropriate nerve at the wrist. Papaverine can be gently injected through the skin incision site and over the site of anastomosis to reverse any vasospasm. The patient should be returned to the operating room for evaluation if these efforts do not increase perfusion to the digit. If thrombosis exists at the repair site, this area should be resected and repaired with or without a vein graft to avoid tension at the repair. The patient should be given a loading dose of 5000 units of heparin; subsequently the patient should receive heparin at a continuous IV rate to double the partial thromboplastin time (PTT).

A digit that appears plump and bluish in color, exhibits fast capillary refill, and exhibits a slow fall at the 60-minute fluorometry reading most likely has poor outflow. In such cases, the dressing should be removed to avoid any external constriction and some skin sutures can be removed if external skin tension appears to be a problem. If there is no improvement in the color of the digit within the first 48 hours after surgery, the patient should be returned to the operating room to undergo another venous anastomosis or a separate venous repair. A significant amount of wound maceration occurs after 48 hours, making another microvascular repair nearly impossible; in such cases

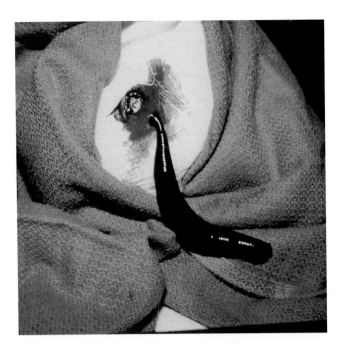

Figure 121-9. Leech therapy.

patients are treated with medicinal leeches and heparin (Figure 121-9).

Leeches are quite effective in treating venous outflow problems in failing replants. After the leech is placed on the digit it bites through the skin; it sucks a small amount of blood and ultimately falls off the patient within 10 to 15 minutes of eating. The leech is subsequently discarded. Bleeding from the site of the leech bite occurs for as many as 3 to 4 hours after the leech has fallen off the finger. Leech saliva contains a substance called *hirudin,* which acts as a very effective regional anticoagulant. Leeches are generally applied on an as-needed basis, but can be used as often as every 3 to 4 hours.

A wound infection secondary to a leech bite can pose significant problems. *Aeromonas hydrophila,* a species of bacteria that naturally occurs in leech saliva and in the leech gut, can infect a finger and is not sensitive to first-generation cephalosporins. Thus when leeches are used, we usually administer a third-generation cephalosporin; otherwise, the patient remains on first-generation cephalosporins throughout the perioperative period.[10]

The early introduction of hand therapy is extremely important to the patient's functional and psychological well being. The hand therapy unit at Davies Medical Center is a large room where therapists may treat several patients in a setting of informal group therapy. Patients at different levels of rehabilitation can discuss their problems openly with hand therapists and other patients. Patients with mutilating hand injuries often become withdrawn and depressed without the environment surrounding hand therapy.

Hand therapy[36] is generally begun on the day that anticoagulation is discontinued. A dorsal protective splint is fabricated and early protected motion (EPM) is begun. The patient visits the hand therapist daily, on an outpatient basis, for dressing changes and progressive range-of-motion exercises

(EPM 2). Hand therapy continues until the patient's progress plateaus, usually at 2 to 3 months after surgery. At that time a decision is made concerning the need for secondary surgery.

OUTCOMES

The replantation of amputated parts currently is a clinical reality. Survival rates from a variety of centers vary from 70% to 95%. Several groups have analyzed functional outcome and patient satisfaction as well as their survival rates. This section reviews these studies and describes the functional outcome of several types of replantation at varying levels.

Establishing a general scoring system for the evaluation of functional return after hand and digital replantation has been difficult. In 1982 Tamai,[44] the first surgeon to successfully replant a thumb, presented a scoring system. His system established an overall score for a replanted part, giving a numerical score for motion, sensation, subjective symptoms, appearance, and patient satisfaction (Figure 121-10). Of 181 patients with successful upper extremity replantations in his series, 72% were placed in the excellent-to-good range in terms of overall functional results.

Chen and Yu[14] also established criteria for functional return. Their four variables included (1) the patient's ability to work, (2) the range of motion of the joint, (3) the recovery of sensation, and (4) the recovery of muscle power. They evaluated 243 successfully replanted upper extremities 3 years after replantation; 38% had grade-I recovery, 37% had grade-II recovery, 28% had grade-III recovery, and 3% had grade-IV recovery (Table 121-1).

FUNCTIONAL OUTCOME DATA FOR DIGITAL REPLANTATION

Several authors have evaluated sensory recovery after digital replantation. Glickman and McKinnon[18] reviewed several series of digital replantation procedures performed between 1977 and 1989. They studied 367 fingers and 87 thumbs that were successfully replanted. The mean value for static two-point discrimination was 9.3 mm in cleanly amputated thumbs compared with 12.1 mm in crushed/avulsed thumb replants. The mean value for static two-point discrimination was 8 mm in cleanly amputated fingers compared with 15 mm in crushed/avulsed finger replants. The overall mean value for static two-point discrimination was 11 mm for all thumb replants and 12 mm for all finger replants. Sixty-one percent of replanted thumbs and 54% of replanted fingers gained useful static two-point discrimination (i.e., less than 15 mm, or greater than or equal to S3+).[42] The factors that influenced return of digital sensation included the patient's age, the level and mechanism of injury, and postoperative sensory reeducation. Recovery of sensation in the replanted digits was believed to be comparable

I. Motion—40
(1) Range of motion—20
    Thumb. Opposition: Possible—(10); Difficult—(5); Impossible—(0)
        MCP joint: Flexion/extension = / ; IP joint; Flexion/extension = /
        Total ROM: More than 50% of normal—(10); Less than 50% of normal—(5); Stiff thumb—(0)
    Finger.

	MCP joint	PIP joint	DIP joint	Sum of flexion	Lack of extension	Total ROM
II Flexion/extension	/	/	/			
III Flexion/extension	/	/	/			
IV Flexion/extension	/	/	/			
V Flexion/extension	/	/	/			

        Total ROM: More than 151°—(20); 111°-150°—(15); 71°-110°—(10); Less than 70°—(5); Stiff digit—(0)
(2) Activities of daily living
    1. Pushing
    2. Tapping
    3. Hanging or drawing
    4. Grasping a soft material
    5. Grasping a hard material
    6. Power grasping
    7. Picking up coin
    8. Picking up needle
    9. Wringing towel
    10. Dipping up water
    11. Washing face
    12. Knotting
    13. Buttoning
    14. Writing
    15. Scissoring
    16. Hammering
    17. Using screwdriver
    18. Using clothespin
    19. Fumbling in pocket
    20. Showing "scissors," "paper," and "stone"
        Easy—(1); Difficult—(0.5); Impossible—(0)

II. Sensation (using British Medical Research Council criteria)—20
    S_0 S_1 S_2 S_3 S_{3+} S_4
    (0)   (4)   (8)   (12)   (16)   (20)
III. Subjective symptoms—20
    Such as pain (rest pain or motion pain), cold intolerance, numbness, paresthesia, tightness, etc.
        Severe—(−3); Moderate—(−2); Mild—(−1)
IV. Cosmesis—10
    Such as atrophy, scar, color change, deformities (angulation, rotation, mallet, swan neck, buttonhole, intrinsic plus or minus, etc.), etc.
        Severe—(−3); Moderate—(−2); Mild—(−1)
V. Patient satisfaction—20
    Highly satisfied—(20); Fairly satisfied—(15); Satisfied—(10); Poorly satisfied—(5); Not satisfied—(0)
    Job status: Same—(0); Changed—(−5); Cannot work—(−10)

Figure 121-10. The Tamai functional scoring system.

Table 121-1.
The Chen Functional Scoring System

GRADE	FUNCTION
I	Able to resume original work; range of motion (ROM) exceeds 60% of normal; complete or nearly complete recovery of sensation; muscle power of grades 4 and 5
II	Able to resume some suitable work; ROM exceeds 40% of normal; nearly complete recovery of sensation; muscle power of grades 3 and 4
III	Able to carry on daily life; ROM exceeds 30% of normal; partial recovery of sensation; muscle power of grade 3
IV	Almost no function of survived limb

to recovery after simple nerve repair. These data were substantiated by Chiu et al,[15] who performed a multivariate statistical analysis to study the influence of four preoperative variables (age, mechanism of injury, level of injury, and type of amputation) and one postoperative variable (rehabilitation) on the functional recovery of replanted fingers. As expected, the younger the patient, the cleaner the injury, the more distal the amputation, and the sharper the amputation, the better the sensory return. The patients who underwent rehabilitation also had better functional recovery, with better scores in motion, sensation, and patient satisfaction.

Tark et al[45] reviewed 261 replantations and revascularizations and determined that digital sensation was significantly better in patients with sharp amputations. They also concluded that accelerated return of sensory function correlated with repair of two digital arteries and two veins rather than repair of one. They noted that cold intolerance, although present in all of their patients, was more troublesome among patients in whom only a single artery was repaired during digital replantation.

The range of motion for digital replants was most closely correlated to the level of injury. Amputations distal to the sublimis tendon insertion had better total active motion than replantations proximal to the sublimis insertion. Chiu and Lee[16] evaluated 82 consecutive cases, concentrating on the influence of joint injury on the functional recovery of a successfully replanted or revascularized finger. Total active motion of the finger minus the contribution of the metacarpophalangeal joint was 15 degrees for patients with PIP-joint injury. DIP-joint injury had a relatively minor effect on total active finger motion. Total active motion minus the contribution of the metacarpophalangeal joint for patients with middle phalanx amputations was 85.5 degrees, and for patients with proximal phalanx amputations was 80 degrees. The authors recommended joint preservation during replantation surgery whenever possible, especially for the PIP and the MCP joints. Other authors have substantiated these data.[45,52]

Our microsurgical service performed silastic arthroplasty on 77 patients for PIP-joint replacement. Two arthroplasties were placed immediately and had approximately 10 degrees of active motion; the others were placed during a second operation and averaged 44 degrees of motion.

The need for secondary operations among patients in our service also was evaluated.[11] The overall frequency of secondary operations was 60%. The overall frequency of secondary amputations for thumb replants and digital replants distal to the sublimis insertion was 11%. Secondary surgery was very common (93%) among patients with replants proximal to the sublimis insertion. The majority of these patients required extensor and/or flexor tendon tenolysis and release of joint contractures (67%). Open reduction and internal fixation of nonunions was necessary in 22% of patients.

Jupiter et al[23] evaluated the results of flexor tenolysis and demonstrated that total active motion increased from an average of 72 degrees before the procedure to an average of 130 degrees after tenolysis. Potential active motion increased

from a mean of 43% before the procedure to 70% after tenolysis. Tenolysis of thumb replants had less favorable results; however, only four tenolyses of thumb replants were performed.

Single-digit replantation has been an extraordinarily controversial issue. Most authors currently believe that replantation of amputations distal to the sublimis insertion is indicated.[25,43,46] However, replantation of a single finger proximal to the sublimis insertion is not indicated except in extraordinary circumstances. Urbaniak[47,48] supported this opinion with data showing that the average range of motion after replantation was 82 degrees for amputations distal to the insertion of the sublimis tendon and only 35 degrees for amputations proximal to the sublimis insertion.

Several authors have reviewed patient satisfaction after replantation. Replanted digits often demonstrated marginally satisfactory function by objective criteria, but were subjectively rated as more satisfactory by patients. Patients were happier to have replanted digit(s), despite their stiffness and reduced sensation, than to be without finger(s), perhaps partly for cosmetic reasons. However, Lukash et al[30] reviewed the socioeconomic impact of 47 digital replants in 21 patients. The mean cost per patient for each replanted part was $16,953. This figure included the surgical fee, operating room charges, hospital charges, and the cost of hand therapy. The authors stated that the majority of patients were dissatisfied with the emotional cost of replantation and the number of subsequent operations. By comparison, finger prostheses, which cost approximately $3000 per finger, last only 2 to 3 years if worn frequently. This can amount to a large sum of money over a patient's lifetime, yet patient satisfaction with finger prostheses is often quite high.[35,37]

FUNCTIONAL OUTCOME DATA FOR THUMB REPLANTATION

Most microsurgeons believe that the thumb should be replanted if at all possible. Several authors have supported this view. However, Goldner[19] reviewed 111 patients who sustained isolated, complete thumb amputations; 69 had successful replants and 42 had revision amputations. All underwent routine postoperative evaluations. Additional testing focused on 25 patients who underwent replantation and 18 patients who underwent revision amputation. Among these patients, there was no statistical difference in grip strength, lateral pinch strength, or ability to perform activities of daily living. Cold intolerance was more common among patients in the replant group. However, results of the questionnaire and interview section of the study revealed that patients who had proximal amputations of the thumb clearly had more difficulty performing activities of daily living. The authors concluded that replantation should be considered for all traumatically amputated thumbs. However, their study could not demonstrate uniform superiority of replantation over amputation for isolated thumb amputations distal to the proximal third of the proximal phalanx.

FUNCTIONAL OUTCOME DATA FOR HAND REPLANTATION

Fortunately, hand amputations are significantly less common than digital amputations; accordingly, however, less data regarding hand amputations are available for analysis. Most authors[40] agree that patients have better function with a hand replantation than with a prosthesis. Although the majority of patients who undergo replantation have disappointing long-term recovery of hand sensation, most patients are highly satisfied with their results.

Vanstraelen et al[49] reported the results for eight patients whose hands were amputated at the wrist or distal forearm. Six patients were available for review 1.5 to 7.5 years after injury. Only one patient had usable return of function. Only one of the six patients evaluated had an excellent result according to the Tamai score. Two had a good result and two had a fair result.

Lister[29] noted the following statistics after hand replantation. Protective sensation was restored in only 36% of patients. Range of motion of the replanted part averaged only 50% of normal. Eighty percent of patients required at least two additional procedures. The average amount of time off work was 7 months. The total cost of replantation exceeded that of revision of amputation by a factor of 5 to 10 times that of a wrist amputation and 10 to 15 times that of a digital amputation.

FUNCTIONAL OUTCOME DATA FOR PROXIMAL UPPER EXTREMITY REPLANTATION

Above-elbow and other proximal upper limb amputations, although technically easier to perform, result in outcomes that are significantly less satisfactory than those of more distal injuries. The majority of injuries to the proximal forearm and upper arm are avulsive in nature. Wood and Cooney[50] evaluated seven patients with complete transhumeral limb amputations. Five of the seven patients had useful elbow control, two patients had useful distal function of the wrist and hand, and all but one patient required multiple secondary operations. The authors suggested that limb replantation at the transhumeral level was of value for the recovery of elbow function. Recovery of useful hand function may be achieved in only a few patients (Figure 121-11).

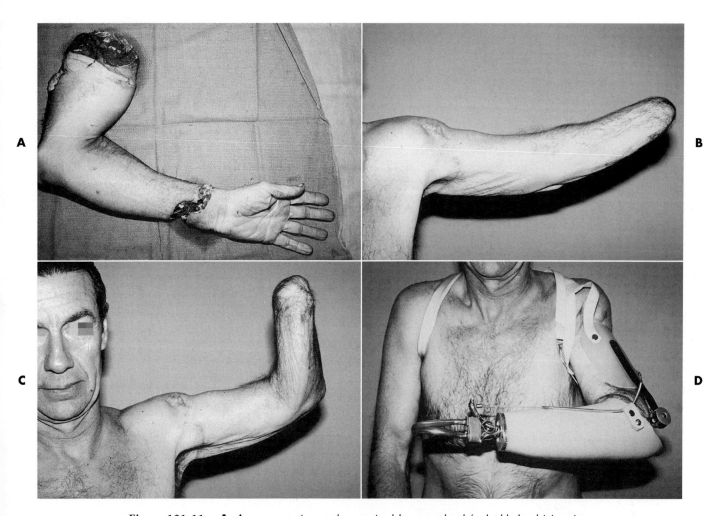

Figure 121-11. **A,** Arm amputation at the proximal humerus level (a double-level injury in a 55-year-old man with diabetes) in which we elected not to replant the hand. **B** and **C,** Return of biceps function. **D,** Adequate elbow control allows use of a below-elbow prosthesis.

Peacock and Tsai[34] reported the functional results for a 12-year-old girl who underwent traumatic, bilateral proximal humeral amputations at 7 years of age. Successful replantation of the nondominant arm was performed with subsequent nerve grafts and tendon transfers to improve function. The contralateral side was fitted early with a battery-powered prosthesis. Five years after replantation, this patient preferred the replanted side for activities of daily living, such as combing her hair. Sensory return, although poor compared with that of her normal hand, allowed the patient when blindfolded to identify objects placed in the hand. The authors believe that the replanted arm offered better function than a prosthesis for most activities.

SUMMARY

Urbaniak[47] succinctly summarized standard expectations after replantation surgery. He believed that most microsurgeons should have at least an 80% viability rate for replantations in patients with complete amputations. Regarding long-term recovery, Urbaniak determined the following:

1. Nerve recovery should be comparable to that following repair of an isolated severed peripheral nerve.
2. Approximately 50% of normal active range of motion should be restored but restoration of motion varies, depending on the level of injury.
3. Cold intolerance is problematic but typically resolves within 2 years of injury.
4. Cosmetic acceptability after replantation is generally better than that associated with amputation revision or prosthesis.
5. Replantation of the thumb, replantation of the hand at the wrist or distal forearm level, and replantation of fingers distal to the insertion of the superficialis tendon result in the best outcomes.

ACKNOWLEDGMENTS

A special thanks to Peter Siko, MD; Gedge Rosson, MD; and Matina Coulouris for their assistance.

REFERENCES

1. Alpert BS, Buncke HJ: Mutilating multi-digit injuries: use of free microvascular flaps for a non-replantable part, *J Hand Surg* 3:196, 1978.
2. Alpert BS, Buncke HJ, Brownstein M: Replacement of damaged arteries and veins with vein grafts when replanting crushed amputated fingers, *Plast Reconstr Surg* 61:17, 1978.
3. Baek SM, Kim SS: Successful digital replantation after forty-two hours of warm ischemia, *J Reconstr Microsurg* 8:455, 1992.
4. Baker GL, Kleinert JM: Digital replantation in infants and young children: determinants of survival, *Plast Reconstr Surg* 94:139, 1994.
5. Black DM, Mann RJ, Castine RM, et al: The stability of internal fixation on the proximal phalanx, *J Hand Surg,* 11A:672, 1986.
6. Buncke HJ: Replantation surgery. In Buncke HJ (editor): *Microsurgery: transplantation-replantation, an atlas text*, Philadelphia, 1991, Lea and Febiger.
7. Buncke HJ, Blackfield HM: The vasoplegic effects of chlorpromazine, *Plast Reconstr Surg* 31:353-361, 1963.
8. Buncke HJ, O'Hara M: Transportation protocol. In Buncke HJ (editor): *Microsurgery: transplantation-replantation, an atlas text*, Philadelphia, 1991, Lea and Febiger.
9. Buncke HJ, Schulz WP: Experimental digital amputation and replantation, *Plast Reconstr Surg* 36:62, 1965.
10. Buncke HJ, Valauri FA, Lineaweaver WC: Use of medicinal leeches in microsurgery. In Buncke HJ (editor): *Microsurgery: transplantation-replantation, an atlas text*, Philadelphia, 1991, Lea and Febiger.
11. Buncke HJ, Whitney TM: Secondary reconstruction after replantation. In Buncke HJ (editor): *Microsurgery: transplantation-replantation, an atlas text*, Philadelphia, 1991, Lea and Febiger.
12. Carrell A, Guthrie CC: Results of replantation of a thigh, *Science* 23:393, 1906.
13. Chang LD, Buncke GM, Slezak S, et al: Cigarette smoking in plastic surgery and microsurgery, *J Reconstr Microsurg* 12(7):467-474, 1996.
14. Chen ZW, Yu HL: Current procedures in China on replantation of severed limbs and digits, *Clin Orthop* 215:15, 1987.
15. Chiu HY, Chieh SJ, Hsu HY: Multi-variant analysis of factors influencing the functional recovery after finger replantation or revascularization, *Microsurgery* 16(10):713-717, 1995.
16. Chiu HY, Lee JW: Influence of joint injury on motor and functional recovery of finger replantation, *Microsurgery* 15:848-852, 1994.
17. Furnas HJ, Lineaweaver WC, Buncke HJ: Blood loss associated with anti-coagulation in patients with replanted digits, *J Hand Surg* 17A:226, 1992.
18. Glickman LT, Mackinnon SE: Sensory recovery following digital replantation, *Microsurgery* 11:236-242, 1990.
19. Goldner RD: 111 thumb amputations: replantation vs, revision, *Microsurgery* 11:243-250,1990.
20. Graham BH, Gordon L, Alpert BS, et al: Serial quantitative skin surface fluorescence: a new method of postoperative monitoring for vascular perfusion of revascularized digits, *J Hand Surg* 10A:226, 1985.
21. Harris G, Finseth F, Buncke HJ: Posterior wall first technique in microvascular surgery, *Br J Plast Surg* 34:47, 1981.
22. Hing D, Buncke HJ, Alpert BS: To replant or to transplant. In Mutaza H (editor): *Advances in plastic and reconstructive surgery*, Chicago, 1987, Year Book Medical Publishers.
23. Jupiter JB, Pess GM, Bour CJ, et al: Results of flexor tendon tenolysis after replantation of the hand, *J Hand Surg* 14A:335-344, 1989.

24. Keiter JE: Immediate pollicization of the amputated index finger, *J Hand Surg* 5:584, 1980.

25. Kim WK, Lim JH, Han SK: Fingertip replantations: clinical evaluations of 135 digits, *Plast Reconstr Surg,* 98:470, 1996.

26. Kleinert HE, Kasdan ML, Romero JL: Small blood vessel anastomosis for salvage of severely injured upper extremity, *J Bone Joint Surg* 45A:788, 1963.

27. Komatsu S, Tamai S: Successful replantation of a completely cut off thumb: case report, *Plast Reconstr Surg,* 42:374, 1968.

28. Lister G: Interosseous wiring of the digital skeleton, *J Hand Surg,* 3:427, 1978.

29. Lister G, Scheker L: Emergency free flaps to the upper extremity, *J Hand Surg(A)* 13A:22, 1988.

30. Lukash FN, Greenberg GM, Gallico GG, et al: A socioeconomic analysis of digital replantation resulting from home use of power tools, *J Hand Surg* 17A:1042-1044, 1992.

31. Malt RA, McKhann C: Replantation of severed arms, *JAMA,* 189:716, 1964.

32. Matsen FA III: Compartment syndrome: a united concept, *Clin Orthop* 113:8, 1975.

33. Nunley JA, Koman LA, Urbaniak JR: Arterial shunting as an adjunct to major limb revascularization, *Ann Surg* 193:271, 1981.

34. Peacock K, Tsai TM: Comparison of functional results of replantation vs. prosthesis in patients with bilateral arm amputation, *Clin Orthop* 214:153, 1987.

35. Pereira BP, Kour A-K, Leow E-L, et al: Benefits of use of digital prosthesis, *J Hand Surg* 21A:222-228, 1996.

36. Petrilli J: Hand therapy. In Buncke HJ (editor): *Microsurgery: transplantation-replantation, an atlas text,* Philadelphia, 1991, Lea and Febiger.

37. Pillet J: Aesthetic hand prostheses, *J Hand Surg* 8:78-81, 1983.

38. Rowland SA: Fasciotomy. In Green DP (editor): *Operative hand surgery,* ed 3, New York, 1993, Churchill Livingstone.

39. Russell RC, Bergman B, Graham B: Amputations: revascularization and replantation. In Cohen (editor): *Mastery of plastic surgery,* Boston, 1994, Little Brown.

40. Russell RC, O'Brien BMc, Morrison WA, et al: The late functional results of upper limb revascularization and replantation, *J Hand Surg [Am]* 9A:623,1984.

41. Schreiber GB, Busch MP, Kleinman SJ, et al: The risk of transfusion-transmitted viral infections, *New Engl J Med* 334(26):1685-1689, 1996.

42. Seddon H: *Surgical disorders of peripheral nerves,* ed 2, Edinburgh and London, 1975, Churchill Livingstone, pp 303.

43. Tamai S: Digital replantation, *Clin Plast Surg,* 5:195, 1978.

44. Tamai S: Twenty years' experience of limb replantation: review of 293 upper limb replants, *J Hand Surg,* 7(6):549, 1982.

45. Tark KC, Kim YW, Lee YH, et al: Replantation and revascularization of hands: clinical analysis and functional results of 261 cases, *J Hand Surg [Am]* 14(1):17-27, 1989.

46. Tsai TM, McCabe SJ, Maki Y, et al: A technique for replantation of the finger tip, *Microsurgery* 10:1 1989.

47. Urbaniak JR: Replantation in operative hand surgery. In: Green DP (editor): *Operative hand surgery,* ed 3, New York, 1993, Churchill Livingstone.

48. Urbaniak JR, Roth JH, Nunley JA: The results of replantation after amputation of a single finger, *J Bone Joint Surg* 67A(4):611, 1985.

49. Vanstraelen P, Papini RPG, Sykes PJ, et al: The functional results of hand replantation: the Chepstow experience, *J Hand Surg(B)* 18B:556-564,1993.

50. Wood NB, Cooney WP: Above-elbow replantation: functional results, *J Hand Surg [Am]* 11(5):682-687, 1986.

51. Yousif JN, Dzwierzynski WW, Anderson RC, et al: Complications and salvage of an ectopically replanted thumb, *Plast Reconstr Surg* 97:637-40, 1996.

52. Zumiotti A, Ferreira NC: Replantation of digits: factors influencing survival and functional results, *Microsurgery* 15:18-21, 1994.

CHAPTER 122

Free Flaps

William M. Swartz

INDICATIONS

Free flaps have become a widely accepted modality for treating a variety of reconstructive problems in the upper extremity. Historically, most open wounds of the hand and forearm have been treated with local flaps or pedicle flaps from the groin or chest. These techniques were used mostly for closing open wounds and achieving primary wound healing, with functional restoration of movement or sensory rehabilitation performed as a secondary procedure. A multiple-staged approach has been the accepted method of treatment in complex wounds involving fractures or injury to tendons. Soft tissue coverage is provided first, followed by staged bone reconstruction, and then by tendon grafting. These procedures would often take many months to accomplish, with the end result being a long period of disability with increased edema and joint stiffness. The widespread use of microsurgery has resulted in an increased use of free tissue transfers to solve these complex reconstructive problems, often bypassing the multiple-staged procedures required in previous times.

The principal advantages of using microsurgical techniques over conventional pedicle flaps for soft tissue coverage include the following:

1. The opportunity to use donor sites that are distant from the injured upper extremity, preserving both function and appearance of the forearm
2. The ability to mobilize the hand and wrist, preventing the joint stiffness and dependent edema that are common when using a pedicle groin flap or thoracoabdominal flap
3. The opportunity to provide multiple tissues, such as skin, tendon, and bone, to solve a complex wound problem, often with a single operative procedure
4. The tissue transferred to the hand by microsurgical technique brings with it its own blood supply, which often augments the blood supply to the wounded area and improves the overall circulation to the hand

The principal indications for a free flap reconstruction include soft tissue coverage of the hand and forearm for wounds caused by trauma or tumor extirpation, restoration of the critical sensory functions of the thumb and other digits, treatment of compound wounds requiring skeletal or tendon restoration as well as soft tissue reconstruction, and finally, replacement of whole digits lost through trauma, tumor resection, or congenital absence. Functional muscle restoration for digital flexion or extension is covered in Chapter 123. Free joint transfers are addressed in Chapter 124, and thumb reconstruction by microsurgical techniques is covered in Chapter 125.

Preparation of a patient for microsurgical reconstruction entails a frank discussion of the risks, complications, and alternatives. The risks of microsurgery today have been largely overcome with advancements in surgical technique, monitoring of microvascular free tissue transfers, and critical patient selection. Nevertheless, thrombosis of an artery or vein necessitates early detection and a return to the operating room to prevent loss of the entire free tissue transfer. Patients are informed that a thrombotic event occurs in 4% to 10% of cases, and total loss of the free tissue transfer occurs on an average of 2% to 6% of the time. Early identification of a vessel thrombosis and a timely return of the patient to the operating room results in successfully salvaging approximately 75% of these thromboses. The risk of smoking as it pertains to thrombosis has been evaluated and shown to increase the risk of thrombosis in digital replantation.[9] There does not, however, appear to be an increased risk for patients undergoing elective free tissue transfers.[15,25] Nevertheless, it is my practice to request that the patient cease smoking 2 weeks before surgery, if possible. Preoperative assessment of the upper extremity before performing a microsurgical procedure should be done to identify suitable recipient arteries and veins. Both the radial and ulnar arteries and the superficial and deep venous systems are available in young, healthy individuals. Preoperative vascular assessment with angiography is recommended in traumatic situations or in patients with advanced vascular disease. If a pulse cannot be palpated, in general the vessel is not suitable for a microsurgical anastomosis.

Alternative methods of therapy must be considered for soft tissue coverage of the upper extremity. These include the use of soft tissue flaps from the forearm based on distal vascular pedicles. The forearm flap based either on the ulnar or radial artery has enjoyed widespread popularity for covering the dorsum of the hand or palmar defects. Likewise, the posterior interosseous flap based on the distal branch of the posterior interosseous artery and located in the dorsal aspect of the forearm similarly reaches the dorsum of the hand for soft tissue coverage. These flaps are reliable, but they cause significant donor-site scarring, often requiring skin grafts for donor-site closure. The distally based radial and ulnar forearm flaps deprive the upper extremity of one of two major blood supplies; the integrity of the palmar arch must be assessed before sacrificing either the radial or ulnar artery for this flap. The scarring from these flaps is significant. Patients should be advised about the options because they might otherwise choose a distant flap with less visible donor-site deformities. Finally, the option of the conventional pedicle groin flap must be considered. In my opinion, the groin is an ideal donor site for upper-extremity reconstructive tissues. It can be utilized as a free flap or as a pedicle flap. Although the groin pedicle flap is a highly reliable and useful method for reconstruction, the drawback of having the hand attached to the groin for 3 weeks is less desirable to most patients than having this surgery performed as a free tissue transfer.

OPERATIONS

SOFT TISSUE COVERAGE FOR THE DORSUM OF THE HAND

Microsurgical options for soft tissue coverage of the hand include fasciocutaneous flaps, fascia flaps with skin graft, and for more extensive defects, musculocutaneous flaps. The patient's size and the degree of obesity must be considered in choosing a flap site that should ideally provide a thin flap that fits the contour of the hand. This problem is significant when there is soft tissue loss over the fingers or in the thumb–index finger web space. A wide variety of skin flaps have been identified, but my preference is to use a free groin flap, if possible, or a fasciocutaneous flap, such as the lateral arm flap. The donor site with each of these techniques can generally be closed without a skin graft, and the donor scar is more acceptable than that produced by the radial forearm free flap, particularly in young individuals. Another preferred flap is the temporoparietal fascia flap covered with a split-thickness skin graft. This flap is most useful for women in which the donor sites previously described have significant aesthetic consequences. Each of these flaps and their use will be discussed in detail.

The Free Groin Flap

The groin flap has been used for many years as a pedicle flap and has enjoyed widespread success and popularity. The vascular anatomy of this flap was well-known to early microsurgeons, and the groin flap was the first elective free tissue transfer performed in 1972 by Daniel and Taylor.[4] The vascular anatomy of this flap has been described by Ohmori and Harii,[23] who documented the contributions of the lateral femoral circumflex artery and superficial inferior epigastric arteries. Preoperative assessment of the circulation can be performed with a Doppler flow probe to identify the lateral femoral circumflex artery lateral to the anterior superior iliac spine. Venous drainage is typically through the superficial inferior epigastric vein, which communicates with the lateral circumflex iliac system (Figure 122-1). The flap is thin in slender individuals, and moderately thick in heavy individuals. Secondary defatting of the groin flap can be performed, should it be necessary, once collateral circulation has been established. The principal advantages of the groin flap as a free tissue transfer are that the donor site is well hidden in conventional underwear, and the procedure is well tolerated. Flaps up to 15 cm in width can be harvested with primary donor-site closure. The flap is hairless and is often the correct thickness for upper-extremity reconstruction. I prefer using the groin flap for coverage of the dorsum of the hand and the thumb–index finger web space. It is often a preliminary procedure to providing thumb reconstruction with a toe-to-thumb transfer for patients with avulsion injuries of the thumb. The drawbacks to the groin flap, however, include the short pedicle length and moderate complexity to the vascular pedicle. The short pedicle length in the hand, however, is not a problem because the radial artery is generally well positioned for wounds about the dorsum of the hand and thumb–index finger web space. The use of the groin flap for soft tissue coverage is demonstrated in the following example.

A 52-year-old woman sustained a severe thumb–index finger web-space contracture after ischemic necrosis caused by a prolonged, drug-induced coma. Release of the thumb–index finger web space created a large soft tissue defect that was

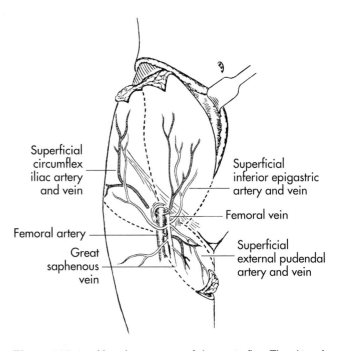

Figure 122-1. Vascular anatomy of the groin flap. The skin of the groin may be transferred on cutaneous vessels supplied by the superficial circumflex iliac artery and vein and superficial inferior epigastric artery and vein, which derive from the femoral artery and vein distal to the inguinal ligament.

covered with a free groin flap. The groin flap was defatted on two successive occasions once circulatory stability had been achieved (Figure 122-2, *A-D*).

Donor-site morbidity from the groin flap is low. The scar that results is well hidden in conventional underwear or bathing suits and typically does not interfere with ambulation or other activities.

The Lateral Arm Flap

A fasciocutaneous flap from the lateral aspect of the upper arm was described by Katsaros and others[13,14] for use in upper-extremity reconstruction after trauma. This flap is reasonably thin in most individuals, particularly in the distal-most portion over the lateral elbow. The vascular supply is a branch of the posterior collateral artery of the arm that, when dissected into the triceps muscle, provides a pedicle 6 to 8 cm in length.[8] Flaps up to 6 cm in width can be harvested and still permit primary donor-site closure. The length of the flap extends from the deltoid groove distally to the lateral aspect of the elbow. The lateral cutaneous nerve of the upper arm courses through the flap and innervates the distal portion. This flap is therefore

suitable as a sensory free flap. A significant drawback to the use of this flap is the donor-site scar, which is well tolerated in some individuals, but is unsightly when it extends to the elbow. Use of the lateral arm flap would not be my first choice for a young woman or a child.[7] Nevertheless, it does provide skin and subcutaneous tissue of the proper thickness for dorsal hand reconstruction. The donor site is much better tolerated in older patients. The vascular anatomy of the lateral arm flap has been well described. The posterior collateral artery and its vena commitans run within the mesentery of the intermuscular septum between the triceps and biceps muscles. The flap is designed so that its central axis lies along a line from the mid-portion of the deltoid groove to the lateral epicondyle (Figure 122-3). The flap is elevated from distal to proximal with inclusion of the investing fascia of the biceps and triceps muscles. The vessels are visualized beneath the fascia as it is elevated. The vascular pedicle is readily identified as the flap is dissected proximally and then dissected beneath the triceps muscle to gain additional length.[22] It is important to note that the radial nerve courses along this intermuscular septum with the lateral cutaneous nerve of the upper arm and the lateral

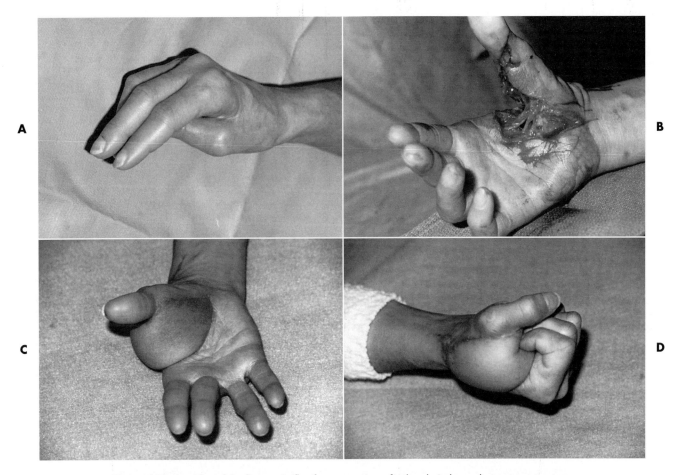

Figure 122-2. Use of the free groin flap for correction of a thumb–index web-space contracture. **A,** A 52-year-old woman sustained an ischemic injury to her right hand after a drug-induced coma. **B,** Release of the thumb–index web-space contracture created a large soft tissue defect. **C** and **D,** This tissue was provided with a free groin flap with vascular anastomosis performed to the radial artery and vena commitans. Secondary defatting was performed approximately 6 months later after collateral circulation had been established.

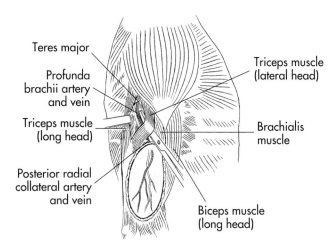

Figure 122-3. Anatomy of the lateral arm flap. The flap is centered over the mid-lateral line of the upper arm. The vascular supply is derived from the posterior radial collateral artery and vein. The radial nerve courses along the intermuscular septum along with the lateral cutaneous nerve of the upper arm. The lateral cutaneous nerve of the arm may be included in the flap dissection to provide an innervated flap.

cutaneous nerve of the forearm, which, if sacrificed, will render the proximal portion of the upper forearm anaesthetic. The lateral cutaneous nerve of the arm is included in the flap if a sensory flap is desired and dissected proximally as a nerve pedicle. The diameter of the artery is typically 1.5 to 2 mm, and the vein is typically 2 to 3 mm in diameter. Closure of the donor site is accomplished with skin and subcutaneous closure only. Donor-site complications include a widened scar and numbness in the forearm as noted above.[9,10]

The lateral arm flap is particularly useful in treating soft tissue loss in the same upper extremity. Two teams can operate simultaneously on both the donor and recipient sites with the arm abducted and extended, shortening the total operating time. The following cases illustrate the versatility of this flap for upper-extremity reconstruction.

A 20-year-old patient sustained a total degloving injury to his right upper extremity. He was initially treated by placing the degloved hand into an abdominal flap. The initial procedure included use of the abdominal flap as a free tissue transfer to provide coverage for the dorsum of the hand as well as the circumferential coverage of the digits. A sensory lateral arm flap was used in a second-stage procedure to restore soft tissue to the palm. The lateral cutaneous nerve of the arm was sutured to a branch of the median nerve, and the blood vessels were sutured end to side to the radial artery. There was protective sensibility in this flap 5 years after surgery, which was perceived as sensation in the middle and ring fingers. A great toe-to-hand transfer was performed for thumb reconstruction in a third procedure. This patient has useful sensation in both the thumb and the palm (Figure 122-4, *A-E*).

A 57-year-old man presented with a severe soft tissue injury to the forearm, with exposure to the flexor tendons. A lateral arm flap measuring 23 cm × 7 cm was harvested from the ipsilateral upper arm, and the flap blood vessels were sutured end to side to the radial artery. This flap provided stable soft tissue coverage compatible with the soft tissue requirements and an acceptable donor-site deformity in this older patient (Figure 122-5, *A-D*).

The lateral arm flap is typically a fasciocutaneous flap that provides skin and subcutaneous tissues with a rich vascular supply. The fascia component is necessary only to protect the blood vessels from separation during the dissection. A wide variety of these fasciocutaneous flaps have been described, including the deltoid flap[5,26] and the medial arm flap,[1,21] both from the upper extremity. These two flaps are useful for hand reconstruction, but they suffer from variability in their blood supply, particularly the medial arm flap. The donor site for a larger deltoid flap requires a skin graft for closure, rendering it cosmetically unacceptable in most patients. Other fasciocutaneous flaps from the lower extremity may be considered. Donor-site deformity, visible scars, and vascular anatomy that may be compromised in elderly patients are often relative contraindications for these flaps. In general, fasciocutaneous flaps are preferred to musculocutaneous flaps, which are usually too thick for aesthetic upper-extremity reconstruction.

The Temporoparietal Fascia Flap

The final alternative for upper-extremity soft tissue coverage is a fascia-only flap derived from the tissues beneath the scalp.[10,17,27] The temporoparietal fascia is composed of two layers, one superficial and the other deep, which overlie the temporalis muscle and extend from the temporal to the occipital scalp. The dimensions of this fascia are approximately 8 cm × 10 cm. The deep fascia that covers the temporalis muscle directly may be developed as a separate flap from the superficial fascia, thus expanding the surface area that it can cover. The principal indication for use of this tissue is to cover the dorsal hand surface, where protection of tendons is required, or for palmar resurfacing, in which case thin tissue is desired. The flap must be covered with a split-thickness skin graft. Additional possible applications include isolation of the median nerve from surrounding tissues in severe cases of median neuritis after repeat carpal tunnel surgeries.

The blood supply to the temporoparietal fascia is derived from the superficial temporal artery and its accompanying vein. These vessels are located in front of the ear and are readily palpated. The flap is dissected through a T-shaped incision in the temporoparietal scalp, and the hair-bearing scalp is elevated from the fascia under loupe magnification. The temporoparietal fascia itself is substantial and encompasses a rich vascular plexus. This fascia is readily dissected from the galia and deep temporal fascia, with a loose areolar plane between the two. The dissection is begun from superior to inferior, approaching the vascular pedicle in front of the ear. A deep branch of the superficial temporal artery at the level of the zygoma separates to supply the deep temporal fascia from the temporalis muscle (Figure 122-6, *A* and *B*). This architecture can be used to a surgeon's advantage by dissecting the deep temporal fascia as a

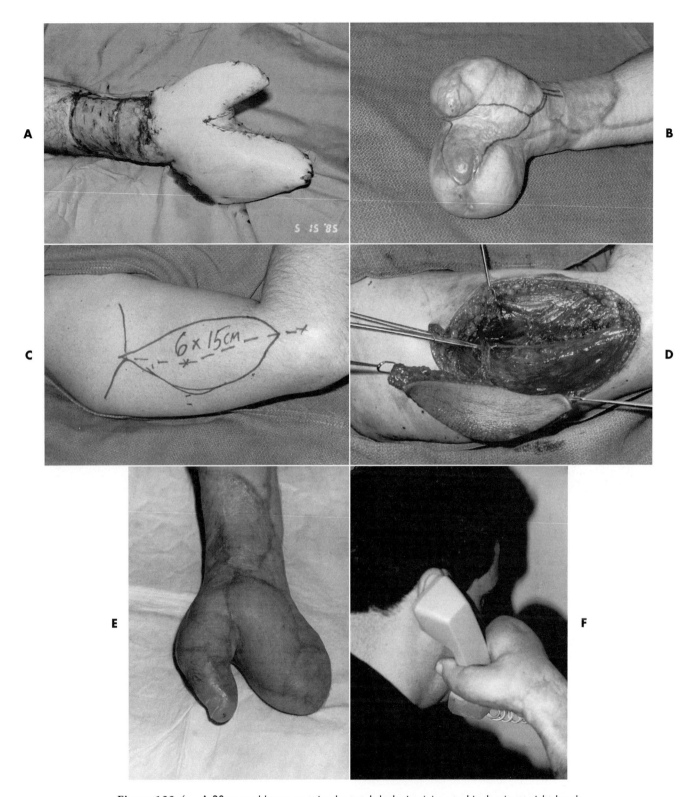

Figure 122-4. A 20-year-old man sustained a total degloving injury to his dominant right hand, requiring staged reconstruction for sensate soft tissue restoration. **A,** Initial treatment included placement of the hand in an abdominal flap, followed by secondary division of the flap **(B). C,** A sensory restoration of the palm was planned using an innervated lateral arm flap. The flap was centered along the intermuscular septum of the upper arm and measured 6 cm × 15 cm. **D,** The flap was elevated on the posterior radial collateral artery and vein. **E** and **F,** Postoperative views of the hand after an innervated lateral arm and great toe wraparound flap transfer were performed, providing prehensile grasp with sensation in both the palm and thumb.

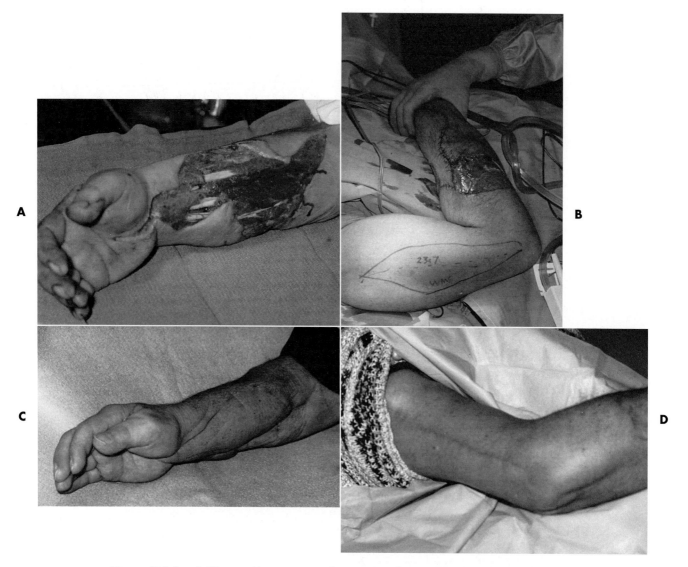

Figure 122-5. A 57-year-old man sustained a severe soft tissue avulsion injury of the volar and dorsal aspects of his forearm, with exposure of flexor tendons and median nerve. **A,** Preoperative view of volar forearm before flap coverage. **B,** A lateral arm flap was planned, measuring 20 cm × 7 cm. **C** and **D,** Postoperative views showing excellent soft tissue coverage and acceptable donor-site scars.

Figure 122-6. The blood supply to the superficial temporal fascia is derived from branches of the superficial temporal artery and vein. These vessels course anterior to the tragus of the ear, superficial to the zygomatic arch. The superficial temporal and deep temporal fascia are separated by a loose areola plane. A deep vessel at the level of the zygomatic arch supplies the temporalis muscle and fascia as a separate layer. *TPF,* Temporoparietal fascia.

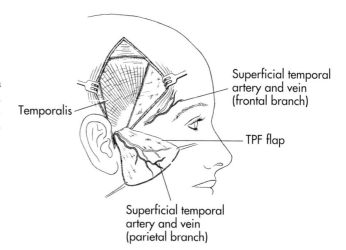

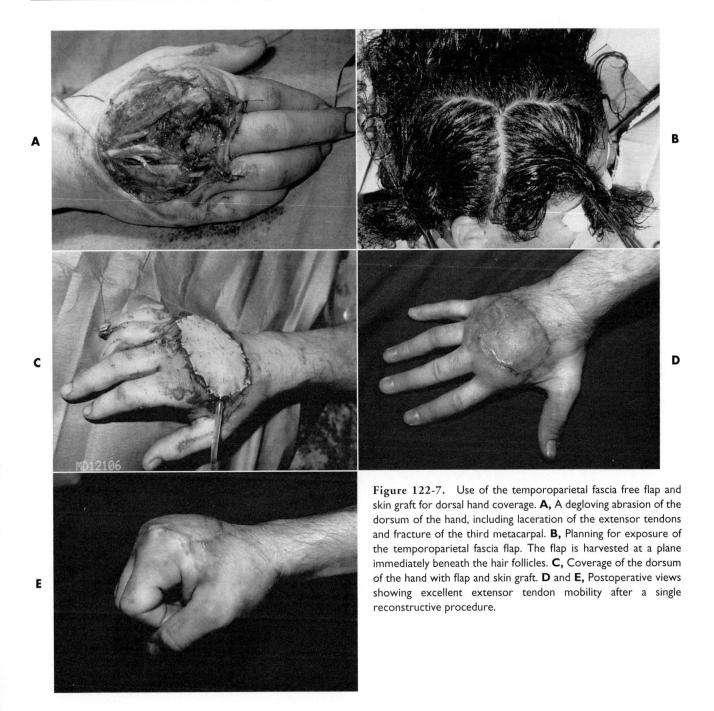

Figure 122-7. Use of the temporoparietal fascia free flap and skin graft for dorsal hand coverage. **A,** A degloving abrasion of the dorsum of the hand, including laceration of the extensor tendons and fracture of the third metacarpal. **B,** Planning for exposure of the temporoparietal fascia flap. The flap is harvested at a plane immediately beneath the hair follicles. **C,** Coverage of the dorsum of the hand with flap and skin graft. **D** and **E,** Postoperative views showing excellent extensor tendon mobility after a single reconstructive procedure.

separate component, increasing the effective size of the flap. Dissection of the vascular pedicle is somewhat tedious, because the vein is often fragile, but this flap is still highly reliable. The donor site is closed directly over a suction drain. Potential donor-site complications include injury to the frontal branch of the facial nerve and alopecia. These complications are avoidable if care is taken to avoid injuring the hair follicles during the subcutaneous scalp dissection. The main advantage of this flap is its inconspicuous donor site. This flap is particularly useful in women in which external scars are of concern. The quality of tissue provided is ideal for the thin dorsum of the hand and palm, in which bulk is a detriment to hand function. The vascular pedicle readily reaches the radial or ulnar arteries for most dorsal hand defects. Finally, the thin temporal fascial tissues are the best choice that I can identify

for reconstruction of finger skin.[2] The following cases illustrate the versatility of this flap.

A soft tissue injury to the dorsum of the hand occurred in a young woman who was thrown from an automobile. The injury included a fracture of the third metacarpal and abrasion lacerations of the extensor tendons to the ring, long, and index fingers. A temporoparietal fascia flap was utilized to cover the soft tissue defect. The fracture was pinned, and the extensor tendons were repaired with a short segmental tendon graft. The temporoparietal fascia flap was then used as two leaves, the first isolating the extensor tendons from the underlying bone fracture and the second placed over the tendons and then covered with a skin graft. Follow-up photographs at 3 months show full flexion and extension, with no further surgical procedures required (Figure 122-7, *A-E*).

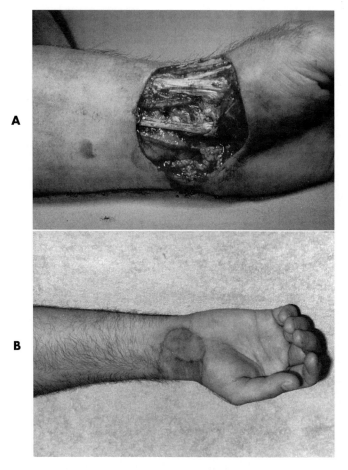

A

B

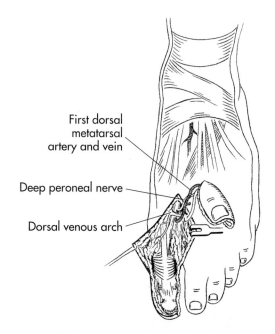

First dorsal
metatarsal
artery and vein

Deep peroneal nerve

Dorsal venous arch

Figure 122-9.   The median aspect of the great toe has a blood supply that is derived by branches of the first dorsal metatarsal artery as well as the plantar artery and vein. Either circulatory system may be utilized. The nerve supply to this area, however, is derived from the plantar digital nerves. Extension of the first dorsal metatarsal artery to the dorsalis pedis artery will provide a long vascular pedicle, allowing vascular anastomosis to be performed in the wrist.

Figure 122-8.   Use of the temporoparietal fascia flap for soft tissue coverage of the volar wrist. **A,** After excision of a malignant fibrous histiocytoma, the flexor carpi radialis and first dorsal compartment tendons were exposed. **B,** Result 3 months after coverage with a temporoparietal free flap and skin graft.

A second case shows the soft tissue defect in a young man after resection of a malignant fibrous histiocytoma of the flexor carpi radialis (FCR) tendon. A temporoparietal fascia free flap was transferred, with a split-thickness skin graft providing thin soft tissue coverage (Figure 122-8, *A* and *B*). There was no additional donor-site morbidity to the forearm. Other methods of soft tissue coverage can be used, but in this case the aesthetic considerations were significant. Alternative treatments, including a rotation of forearm tissues or mobilization of a forearm flap, would have created significant additional scarring.

RESTORATION OF DIGITAL SENSIBILITY

Soft tissue loss of the digital pulp results in the loss of stability in pinch and grip, as well as the loss of sensation. This loss of sensibility in the thumb, index, and long fingers diminishes the usefulness of these fingers for critical prehension. Methods of reconstruction to date have included the cross-finger flap, thenar flaps, or other local flaps to restore pulp contour; however, restoration of sensibility has been difficult. The ideal donor tissues are those with specialized nerve endings found only in glabrous skin.[11] Attempts at restoration of sensibility

began with the island pedicle flap of Littler,[18] in which a digital nerve from an adjacent finger is incorporated in a vascular island pedicle and then is transferred to the injured finger or thumb. This procedure is complicated by the fact that sensation remains cortically oriented to the donor finger. Additionally, the quality of sensation is diminished when compared with the original donor two-point discrimination. An alternative to this technique is the innervated cross-finger flap described by Cohen.[3] An adjacent digit is used to transfer the dorsal skin between the proximal interphalangeal (PIP) and distal interphalangeal (DIP) joints based on a dorsal digital nerve. This procedure requires a 2-week period of attachment of the donor to the recipient finger, and in older patients the procedure can be complicated by joint stiffness of the PIP joint. Nevertheless, the quality of sensation is adequate. It does require that a digital nerve be present adjacent to the soft tissue defect.

An alternative to these methods of treatment has been the transfer of soft tissues from the toes of the foot—notably the web space of the big toe and/or the second toe pulp.[29] Additionally, the nail bed can be transferred as part of this reconstruction in the form of a wrap-around toe flap. These procedures are discussed in greater detail in Chapter 125 on thumb reconstruction.

The medial aspect of the great toe may be transferred based on an extension of the first dorsal metatarsal blood supply and the plantar digital nerve.[28] The dorsalis pedis artery may be included to extend the length of the vascular pedicle, depending on the recipient-site requirements (Figure 122-9).

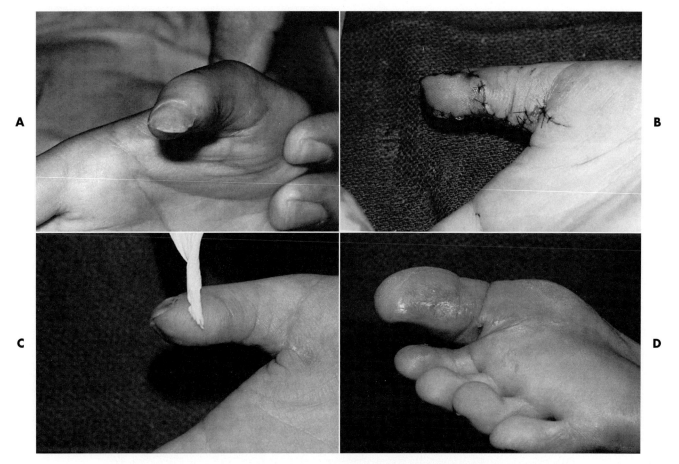

Figure 122-10. Use of the medial great toe pulp for restoration of thumb pulp with sensibility. **A,** A 19-year-old nursing student sustained an injury to the pulp of her thumb in a crushing accident. A tender neuroma was present at the level of the IP joint. **B,** A medial toe pulp was transferred to the thumb based on the first dorsal metatarsal artery. A plantar digital nerve was sutured to the radial digital nerve at the site of laceration. **C,** Follow-up at 6 months after surgery shows early restoration of sensibility in a well-healed thumb pulp flap. **D,** The toe donor site was closed with a full-thickness skin graft with no significant morbidity.

If vascular anastomoses are to be done in the finger, then the first dorsal metatarsal artery only is required. The quality of sensation in the toe flap improves from its recipient site once it is transferred to the hand. Critical two-point discrimination of 4 to 6 mm can be obtained. This can be increased to 2 to 4 mm with sensory reeducation. The plantar digital artery and veins are used in cases in which the first dorsal metatarsal artery is absent.

Preoperative assessment with digital Doppler and/or angiograms is required to determine the contribution of the first dorsal metatarsal artery to the vascular anatomy of the plantar surface of the great toe. Advantages of this method for digital pulp restoration include the improved quality of sensory rehabilitation compared with the previously discussed alternatives. Donor-site scarring is also significantly less because adjacent digits are not compromised. The following case illustrates the use of the great toe pulp for restoration of thumb pulp tissue loss.

A 19-year-old nursing student sustained an injury to the pulp of her thumb when her hand was closed in a car door. The wound was allowed to heal by secondary intention and she

was left with a painful digital neuroma and an unstable scar over the atrophic distal thumb. Reconstruction was accomplished with a great toe pulp flap. The plantar digital nerve to the toe was anastomosed to the proper digital nerve of the thumb, and the first dorsal metatarsal artery was sutured to the proper digital artery of the thumb at its base. Two years after surgery, the two-point discrimination was 4 mm (Figure 122-10, *A-C*).

A second example was a 35-year-old male who sustained a severe traumatic injury to his right, dominant hand. This injury included amputation of the ring, long, and index fingers and the tip of the thumb. The soft tissues of the thumb were degloved circumferentially. He was initially treated with a pedicle groin flap and then with elective sensory reconstruction accomplished with a first and second toe web-space innervated free flap. The medial aspect of the great toe was dissected along with the plantar digital nerve. The vascular supply was the first dorsal metatarsal artery and vein extended with the dorsalis pedis vascular system. Vascular anastomoses were performed in the forearm and a direct coaptation of the digital nerve to the thumb branch of the median nerve was achieved. Two years

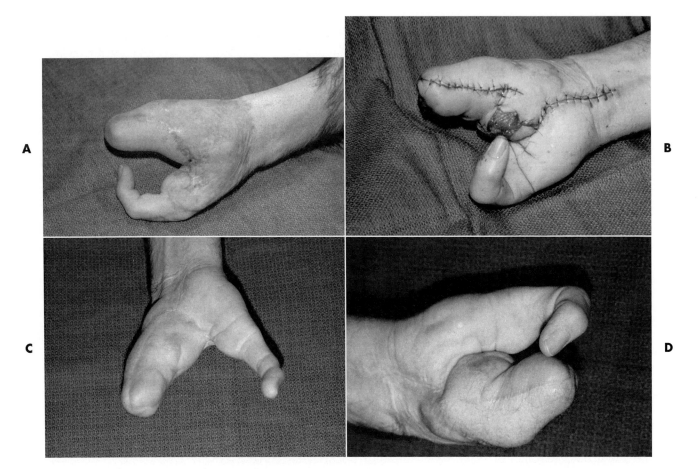

Figure 122-11. Use of the first and second toe web space for restoration of digital sensibility to a severely traumatized hand. **A,** A 35-year-old male sustained a traumatic injury to his hand, with loss of the ring, long, and index fingers, as well as the tip of the thumb. Initial wound coverage was achieved with a groin flap. **B,** Transfer of a thumb–index web-space flap for opposition sensibility was performed. The plantar digital nerves were anastomosed to branches of the median nerve, and the dorsalis pedis artery and vein were anastomosed to the radial artery and vein. **C** and **D,** Excellent opposition between the little finger and the thumb remnant was obtained, with protective sensibility in the thumb pad after 2 years.

later, the patient had excellent protective sensibility in the thumb-pad reconstruction, providing him with sensation in an area of critical opposition (Figure 122-11, *A-C*).

SKELETAL RESTORATION WITH VASCULARIZED BONE FLAPS

Major trauma to the upper-extremity skeleton resulting in segmental bone loss of the humerus, radius, and/or ulna, or resection of these bones after tumor removal creates a difficult reconstructive problem for restoration of skeletal integrity. Conventional bone grafting techniques are useful for segmental defects of up to 6 cm in length. However, larger defects treated with conventional bone grafting can lead to delayed healing and a high incidence of nonunion. The principal reason for this is that these bone grafts must heal by bone conduction and creeping substitution, a process that takes many months in longer defects. The use of vascularized bone

grafts in these circumstances has significantly improved the healing process and at the same time provides early structural stability. Each end of a vascularized bone graft placed into a segmental defect heals by primary bone union, a process similar to fracture healing.[20] Methods of external fixation can be employed for a shorter period, typically 6 to 12 weeks, with the observation that rapid bone healing occurs followed by bone hypertrophy. Useful bone flaps for upper-extremity reconstruction include the fibula, iliac crest, and occasionally the scapula.

The Fibula Vascularized Bone Flap

The free vascularized fibula flap was initially described by Taylor et al[31] in 1975 for lower-extremity reconstruction with great success. The fibula is even more versatile in the upper extremity for restoring segmental loss in the humerus, radius, and ulna. The fibula itself is almost identical in diameter to the ulna and is only a little smaller than the radius. There is normally a slight bow to the radius and ulna, but the straight

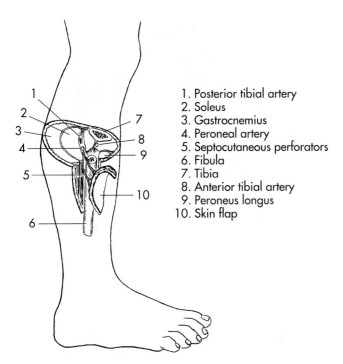

1. Posterior tibial artery
2. Soleus
3. Gastrocnemius
4. Peroneal artery
5. Septocutaneous perforators
6. Fibula
7. Tibia
8. Anterior tibial artery
9. Peroneus longus
10. Skin flap

Figure 122-12. Anatomy of the fibular osteocutaneous free flap. The peroneal artery and veins supply the distal two thirds of the fibula through periosteal vessels and a medullary branch. The proximal third of the tibia, including the growth plate, is supplied by the anterior tibial artery and vein. The fibular osteocutaneous flap based on the peroneal artery is elevated to include the skin of the lateral aspect of the leg. Septocutaneous perforating vessels supply the overlying skin up to 6 cm in width.

course of the fibula does not require an osteotomy in most circumstances. Up to 25 cm of length can be obtained in the fibula, making it an ideal replacement for the humerus in cases of bone-tumor resection. Fixation of the fibula is obtained with a variety of conventional techniques, including external fixation devices, rush rod pin fixation, or internal fixation with plates and screws. The thick cortical bone readily accepts this orthopedic hardware, providing stable osteosynthesis and early return of joint mobility. Skin of the lateral lower leg may be included in cases in which soft tissues are also required.[33]

The blood supply to the fibula is derived from the peroneal artery and its vena comitans. This vessel provides a medullary artery that enters at the junction of the proximal third and distal two thirds and also supplies periosteal vessels along the distal two thirds of the fibula. The proximal third of the fibula, including the growth plate, is supplied by branches of the anterior tibial artery.[30] This configuration is important to consider when transferring the growth plate of the fibula for distal radial reconstruction, particularly in children (Figure 122-12).[19] The fibula, as in other long bones, will survive on either the medullary or periosteal blood supply. The fibula may be harvested with skin from the lateral aspect of the leg based on perforating branches through the lateral intermuscular septum. A skin island 15 cm to 20 cm in length and as wide as 6 cm may be harvested and still allow primary donor-site closure.[6]

DISSECTION TECHNIQUE. The fibula may be harvested with or without a tourniquet, depending on the surgeon's preference. A mid-lateral incision along the lateral intermuscular septum is preferred if only the bone is to be harvested. If a skin island is required, then a skin paddle—with a maximum width of 6 cm—may be centered over the perforating vessels, which should have been identified before surgery using transcutaneous Doppler. The perforators are usually present in the junction of the distal and proximal two thirds. The skin island is elevated along with the fascia of the lateral compartment until the perforating vessels are seen emerging through the intermuscular septum. Occasionally, these muscles will course through the soleus as well. The common peroneal nerve is identified and protected as it courses around the neck of the fibula and then follows the anterior tibial vessels in the anterior compartment. The origins of the peroneus longus and brevis muscles are divided from their attachments to the fibula, and a thin cuff of muscle is included. The extensor hallucis muscle is also separated from the fibula. Once the lateral half of the fibula circumference has been dissected, an osteotomy is performed distally. The distal 10 cm of the fibula should be left intact to prevent instability of the ankle. Next, the intermuscular septum is divided, and the distal peroneal artery and vein are located. This vessel may be ligated and divided. The fibula will gain additional freedom once this intermuscular septum is divided, permitting direct visualization of the vascular pedicle. The medial and posterior attachments of the flexor hallucis longus, the tibialis posterior, and the soleus muscles are divided as the dissection proceeds from distal to proximal. The deep peroneal nerve must be preserved in this dissection. A proximal osteotomy is then performed, permitting free mobility of the fibula. The vascular pedicle can then be dissected all the way to its junction with the common tibial vessels. Once the peroneal artery and its vena comitans have been isolated, the bone is allowed to perfuse for several minutes before ligating and dividing these vessels.

The donor site is closed directly with sutures in the investing fascia layer, and a Jackson-Pratt or other type of suction drain is placed in the muscle cavity. Muscle is loosely approximated and the skin is closed. A plaster splint and compression dressing are applied, and the patient is permitted to use crutches while walking on the second day after surgery, with full weight-bearing at the end of 1 week.

The two most serious problems associated with fibula harvest are possible injury to the peroneal nerve, which results in a foot drop, and ankle instability if the fibula is harvested too close to the lateral malleolus.[6] There often is temporary weakness of the extensor muscles of the leg and foot after this dissection; however, recovery is rapid. Should ankle instability occur, distal fibula fixation to the tibia may be achieved with lag screw fixation. Additional complications are possible if the skin closure after skin island resection is too tight. It is recommended that a skin graft be used rather than have the patient experience delayed wound healing.

Clinical examples of the use of the fibula for upper-extremity reconstruction follow. The first patient is a 20-year-

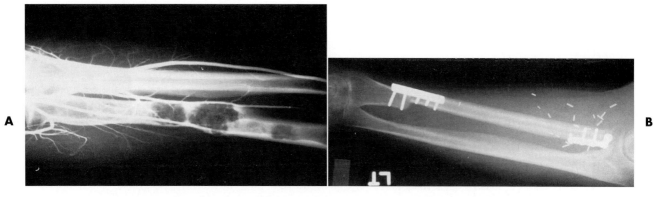

Figure 122-13. Use of a free fibula for reconstruction of the radius. **A,** A patient with osteogenic sarcoma has undergone preoperative angiography to determine the vascular anatomy before free tissue transfer. **B,** Use of the fibular osseous free flap for reconstruction of the radius. The proximal and distal bone fixation was provided with many plates. Bone union is identified at 6 weeks.

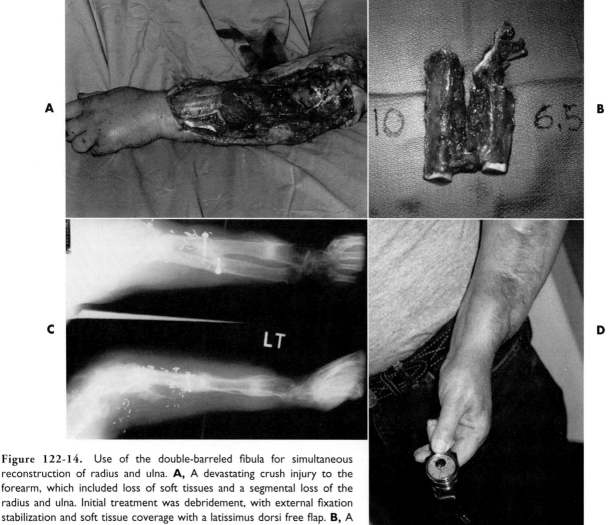

Figure 122-14. Use of the double-barreled fibula for simultaneous reconstruction of radius and ulna. **A,** A devastating crush injury to the forearm, which included loss of soft tissues and a segmental loss of the radius and ulna. Initial treatment was debridement, with external fixation stabilization and soft tissue coverage with a latissimus dorsi free flap. **B,** A double-barreled fibula flap with two bone segments based on the peroneal artery and vein. **C,** Bone healing with bone segments placed in both the proximal radius and ulna. **D,** Postoperative result showing excellent forearm stability. Pronation and supination were restricted because of unresolved elbow-joint problems.

old woman with osteogenic sarcoma of the proximal radius. A compartmental resection was performed, and immediate reconstruction was accomplished with a free fibula transfer. The bone fixation was provided with small plates. Early postoperative healing was observed at 6 weeks, and full, unprotected use of the arm was possible at 12 weeks (Figure 122-13, A and B).

The second patient required the use of two segments of fibula on a single vascular pedicle for replacement of both the proximal radius and ulna after a devastating crush injury to the forearm. External fixation was used initially for stability, and soft tissue cover was achieved with a latissimus dorsi free flap. A double-barreled fibula free flap[12] was used as a second-stage procedure to provide vascularized bone for both the radius and ulna. Primary bone union and soft tissue healing were achieved. The patient developed an ankylosis of the elbow, which restricted pronation and supination of the forearm and hand (Figure 122-14, A-D).

The Iliac Crest Vascularized Bone Graft

The iliac crest has enjoyed wide use as a source for conventional bone grafts. A vascularized iliac bone graft may be used for reconstruction of short segmental defects in the long bones of the forearm, or it may be used as a wider graft in fusions of the wrist in unusual circumstances. The skin overlying the iliac crest may be carried with this flap; however, it is often somewhat bulky, especially in heavier individuals. Nevertheless, it can provide both skin and bone for complex, three-dimensional upper-extremity reconstructions.

The blood supply to the ilium is derived principally from the deep circumflex iliac artery and vein.[32] These vessels originate proximal to the inguinal ligament from the iliac artery and vein, and course along the inner border of the ilium (Figure 122-15). They send branches to the overlying skin distal to the anterior superior iliac spine. The first branch of this system supplies the internal oblique and transversus abdominis musculature. A muscle flap can be isolated on this vessel as a separate pedicle from the bone flap.[24] Accompanying the deep circumflex iliac artery and vein is the lateral femoral cutaneous nerve, which exits the groin just proximal to the anterior superior iliac spine to supply sensation to the lateral thigh. Vena comitans accompany the artery and usually merge with the inferior epigastric artery and vein at its origin. The ilium itself is a bicortical bone with a thickened apex and a curvilinear shape extending from the anterior superior iliac spine to the posterior iliac spine. This distance measures approximately 14 cm in adult males. The ilium is not particularly useful for reconstruction of long defects because of its curvature, unless an osteotomy is performed. The inner cortex and cancellous bone alone may be harvested, leaving the outer cortex intact for selected reconstructive problems.

DISSECTION TECHNIQUE. When a skin island is not required, an incision is made from the pubic tubercle continuing along the inguinal ligament over the iliac crest. The external oblique fascia is divided in the direction of its fibers

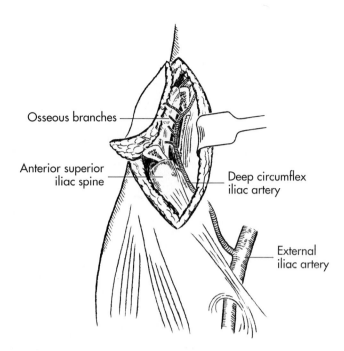

Figure 122-15. Anatomy of the iliac crest osteocutaneous free flap. The deep circumflex iliac artery and vein courses on the inner surface of the ilium distal to the anterior superior iliac spine. Perforating vessels supply the overlying skin and fascia.

and the internal oblique muscle is encountered in the more lateral portion. This is incised as far laterally as necessary to accommodate the length of bone required. Just inside the iliac crest the conjoined fibers of the internal oblique muscle and transversus abdominis muscles are incised, leaving approximately 1 cm between the incision and the iliac crest. The dissection is then carried above the inguinal ligament, where perivascular fat is encountered. Immediately adjacent to the ilium, the deep circumflex artery and vein can be palpated. These vessels are then dissected distally under loupe magnification, with care taken to identify and preserve the lateral femoral cutaneous nerve. The bone may be isolated at this point using a combination of oscillating saws or osteotomes and preserving the deep inferior epigastric arterial system on its medial border. The anterior superior iliac spine is preserved to avoid a cosmetic deformity of the hip. The vascularized bone flap is removed, and the donor site is closed in layers by anchoring the transversus abdominis and internal oblique muscles to the remaining iliac crest with permanent sutures placed through drill holes. This closure encompasses the tensor fascia lata laterally. The external oblique fascia is then closed as a separate layer.

Potential complications of this flap include development of an abdominal-wall hernia if the fascial closure is not secured to the iliac crest. Additional problems may include division of the T12 or ileoinguinal nerves that may cause some loss of sensation in the lateral thigh. A painful neuroma may result if these nerves are closed in the incision.

CLINICAL EXAMPLE. A 27-year-old male sustained a punch-press injury to the wrist that involved a traumatic

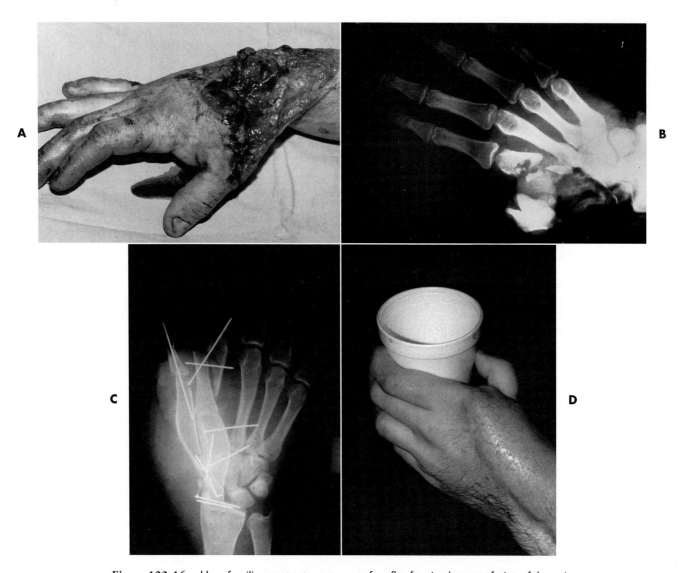

Figure 122-16. Use of an iliac crest osteocutaneous free flap for simultaneous fusion of the wrist and soft tissue coverage. **A** and **B,** A devastating punch-press injury to the right wrist resulting in loss of dorsal radial soft tissues and the metacarpal bones of the index finger and thumb, as well as the trapezium, trapezoid, navicular, and lunate bones. **C,** Bone restoration was accomplished with a vascularized iliac crest flap. The wrist was primarily fused to the index-finger metacarpal and a separate, nonvascularized bone graft was used for the thumb metacarpal. **D,** After secondary defatting, primary bone union of the wrist and index metacarpal was achieved. The thumb metacarpal underwent resorption, resulting in a shortening of the thumb.

injury to the distal radius with loss of the navicular, lunate, and a portion of the capitate. The injury also caused loss of the thumb and index metacarpal. An osteocutaneous groin flap was planned, with primary fusion of the radius to the adjacent carpal bones and a remnant of the first and second metacarpals. Primary wound healing was achieved, however secondary surgeries were required to debulk the thick skin paddle on the dorsum of the wrist (Figure 122-16, *A-D*).

Additional vascularized bone donor sites include the scapula and the radius. These donor sites are useful in selected circumstances usually involving the loss of a metacarpal bone.

Additional information concerning these procedures can be obtained in the cited references.

In summary, use of vascularized bone grafts for upper-extremity long bone and wrist reconstruction is an unusual, but very useful, tool for restoring skeletal integrity. These bone flaps offer the possibility of primary bone union when conventional bone grafts have failed. They provide skeletal integrity and obviate the necessity for prolonged external skeletal support. They are primarily indicated for situations in which a scarred wound bed will not support conventional bone grafts or when both bone and soft tissues are required in a complex reconstruction.

OUTCOMES

The clinical success of microvascular free tissue transfers has increased to between 94% and 96% in a recently reported study by Khouri et al[15] taken from cases performed in a 20-center cross section of microsurgical reconstructions done from 1994 through 1996. Success rates in upper-extremity free flaps approaches 98% and appear to be greater than similar procedures performed in the lower extremity. Soft tissue coverage in the upper extremity is effectively provided by these procedures; however, the usefulness of this procedure in helping patients to return to work and to activities of daily living has not been measured in any reported series to date. The time for recovery, however, is substantially reduced when compared with conventional pedicle flap techniques, with fewer surgical procedures required to obtain the final result.

In a recently reported series on reconstruction of soft tissue defects of the digits utilizing flaps from the first web space of the foot, the clinical outcome for successful reconstruction was 100%. Sensibility in free tissue transfers was recorded to improve from a 2-point discrimination in the toe of 11.3 mm to 16.4 mm to a postoperative 2-point discrimination in the hand at 7.2 mm to 10 mm. The authors ascribe this improved 2-point discrimination to the increased cortical representation of the recipient nerve on the brain and to the increased stimulation of the flap during continuous use in the hand as compared with the foot.[34]

Free tissue transfers for bone reconstruction have been noted to provide primary bone union at a more rapid rate than the conventional bone grafting techniques for segmental bone defects. Alternative methods of reconstruction have not been uniformly successful in large, segmental bone defects. Malizos et al[20] reported primary bone union by 6 months in 84.6% of patients (12 out of 14) after elective reconstruction of tumor defects compared with 76.5% of reconstruction in trauma patients. Bone union in the upper extremity was observed in a considerably shorter time frame than in the lower extremity, averaging approximately 3 months. Kumta et al[16] reported the use of free vascularized bone grafts in treatment of juxtaarticular bone tumors in 26 patients with upper-extremity tumors. All but one achieved bone union, with a pain-free, functional wrist achieved in 17 of 18 patients.[16] The advantages of these vascularized bone grafting techniques compared with conventional bone grafting have permitted more rapid bone union and mobilization of the affected joints in the patients described.

SUMMARY

The outcomes from reconstruction of upper-extremity defects using microvascular techniques in a selected series of patients have demonstrated an improved restoration of digital sensibil-ity in the case of sensory free tissue transfers and a more rapid bone union and restoration of joint mobility when these flaps have been used in the area of the distal radius and wrist. Microsurgical techniques are more demanding than conventional techniques to replace soft tissues and bone, but these more sophisticated reconstructions provide solutions to problems that would previously have ended in amputation.

REFERENCES

1. Budo J, Finucan T, Clarke J: The inner arm fasciocutaneous flap, *Plast and Reconstr Surg* 73:629, 1984.

2. Choudary RP: Use of temporoparietal fascia free flap in digital reconstruction, *Ann Plast Surg* 23:543-546, 1989.

3. Cohen BE, Cronin ED: An innervated cross finger flap for fingertip reconstruction, *Plast Reconstr Surg* 72:688, 1983.

4. Daniel RK, Taylor GI: Distant transfer of an island flap by microsurgical anastomoses, *Plast Reconstr Surg* 52:111, 1973.

5. Franklin JD: The deltoid flap: anatomy and clinical application. In Buncke HJ, Furnes DW (editors): *Symposium on clinical frontiers in reconstructive microsurgery, vol 24,* St. Louis, 1984, Mosby.

6. Ganel A, Jaffe B: Ankle instability of the donor site following removal of the vascularized fibular bone graft, *Ann Plast Surg* 24:7-9, 1990.

7. Graham B, Adkins P, Scheker LR: Complications and morbidity of free donor and recipient sites in 123 lateral arm flaps, *J Hand Surg [Br]* 17:189, 1992.

8. Harpf C, Papp C, Ninkovic M, et al: The lateral arm flap: a review of 72 cases and technical refinements, *J Reconstr Surg* 14:39-48, 1998.

9. Harres G, Finseth F, Buncke H: The hazards of cigarette smoking following digital replantation, *J Microsurg* 2:403-404, 1980.

10. Hing DN, Buncke HJ, Alpert B: Use of the temporoparietal fascia flap in the upper extremity, *Plast Reconstr Surg* 81:534-544, 1988.

11. Johnsson RD, Volbo AB: Tactile sensibility in the human hand: relative and absolute densities of four types of mechanoreceptive units in glabrous skin, *J Physiol* 286:283, 1979.

12. Jones NF, Swartz WM, Mears DC, et al: The "double barrel" free vascularized fibular bone graft, *Plast Reconstr Surg* 81:378-385, 1988.

13. Katsaros J, Schusterman M, Bepper M, et al: The lateral arm flap: anatomy and clinical applications, *Ann Plast Surg* 12:489-499, 1984.

14. Katsaros J, Tau E: The use of the lateral arm flap in upper limb surgery, *J Hand Surg [Am]* 16:598-604, 1991.

15. Khouri R: *Practice patterns and outcome data in a prospective survey of 495 microvascular free flaps.* Presented at the 11th annual meeting of the American Society for Reconstructive Microsurgery, Tucson, January 16, 1996.

16. Kumta SM, Leung PC, Yip K, et al: Vascularized bone grafts in the treatment of juxta-articular giant cell tumors of the bone, *J Reconstr Microsurg* April 14:3:185-190, 1998.

17. Lipton J, Rogers C, Durban-Smith G, Swartz W: Clinical applications of free temporoparietal flaps in hand reconstruction, *J Hand Surg [Am]* 11:475-483, 1986.

18. Littler JW: Neurovascular pedicle transfer of tissue in reconstructive surgery of the hand, *J Bone Joint Surg* 38A:917, 1956.

19. Mack GR, Lichtman DM, MacDonald RI: Fibular autografts for distal defects of the radius, *J Hand Surg [Am]* 4:576-583, 1979.

20. Malizos KN, Nunley JA, Goldner RD, et al: Free vascularized fibula in traumatic long bone defects and in limb salvage following tumor resection: comparative study, *Microsurg* 14: 368-374, 1993.

21. Matloub H, Ye Z, Yousif NJ, Sanger JR: The medial arm flap, *Ann Plast Surg* 29:517-522, 1992.

22. Moffett TR, Madison SA, Derr JW, Acland RD: An extended approach for the vascular pedicle of the lateral arm free flap, *Plast Reconstr Surg* 89:259-267, 1992.

23. Ohmori K, Harii K: Free groin flaps: their vascular basis, *Br J Plast Surg* 28:238-246, 1975.

24. Ramasastry SS, Tucher JP, Swartz WM, et al: The internal oblique muscle flap: an anatomic and clinical study, *Plast Reconstr Surg* 73:721-730, 1984.

25. Reus WF, Colen LB, Straker DJ: Tobacco smoking and complications in elective microsurgery, *Plast Reconstr Surg* 89:490-493, 1992.

26. Russell RC, Guy RJ, Zook EG, et al: Extremity reconstruction using the free deltoid flap, *Plast Reconstr Surg* 76:586, 1985.

27. Smith RA: The free fascial scalp flap, *Plast Reconstr Surg* 66:204-209, 1980.

28. Strauch B, Tsur H: Restoration of sensation in the hand by a free neurovascular flap from the first web space of the foot, *Plast Reconstr Surg* 62:361, 1978.

29. Swartz WM: Restoration of sensibility in mutilating hand injuries, *Clin Plast Surg* 16:515-529, 1989.

30. Taylor GI, Miller GDH, Flan FJ: The free vascularized bone graft: a clinical extension of microvascular techniques, *Plast Reconstr Surg* 55:533, 1975.

31. Taylor GI, Townsend P, Corlett R: Superiority of the deep circumflex iliac vessels as the supply for free groin flaps, *Plast Reconstr Surg* 64:595-604, 1979.

32. Taylor GI, Wilson KR, Rees MD, et al: The anterior tibial vessels and their role in epiphyseal and diaphyseal transfer of the fibula: experimental study and clinical applications, *Br J Plast Surg* 41:451-469, 1988.

33. Wei FC, Chou HC, Chuang CC, et al: Fibular osteoseptocutaneous flap: anatomic and clinical application, *Plast Reconstr Surg* 78:191-199, 1986.

34. Woo SH, Choi BC, Oh SJ, et al: Classification of the first web space free flap of the foot and its applications in reconstruction of the hand, *Plast Reconstr Surg* 103:2:508-517, 1999.

Free Muscle Flaps

Ronald M. Zuker

INDICATIONS

Free muscle transplantation can be used not only to provide soft tissue coverage but also to restore function. The use of the gracilis muscle as a functioning unit and the role of functional muscle transplantation in the upper extremity will be discussed.

Functional muscle transplantation is indicated for the reconstruction of a major segmental skeletal muscle loss that has resulted in a significant functional deficit. The loss of a functioning muscle unit can be caused by trauma or surgical excision and is commonly seen as a late sequela of Volkmann's ischemic contracture. There is essentially complete loss of muscle, which is generally static and will remain so indefinitely. Patients who are candidates for a functional muscle reconstruction must maintain passive joint mobility, otherwise stiffness will ensue and limit the options available for reconstruction. In cases in which some muscle function remains but is insufficient for effective hand use, it is possible to advance the involved muscle origins and improve range of motion. Muscle advancement techniques are only effective in volar forearm muscles that are minimally involved by the contracture process but can be very worthwhile in selected cases. Advanced cases in which the musculature is missing from trauma or surgical excision can also be reconstructed with a variety of tendon transfers, depending on the circumstances. Transfers are much easier to perform than free muscle transplantation, but they are often less effective and by definition must reduce function of the donor component. Muscle transplantation is therefore our procedure of choice.

The gracilis muscle is harvested from the thigh and transplanted to the upper extremity. It is appropriately positioned under optimum tension so that with contraction it will perform the function required. The muscle is revascularized through microvascular anastomoses, and proper reinnervation is critical. A regional motor nerve that is appropriate for the activity that is to be reconstructed is used to reinnervate the free muscle flap. The nerve that reinnervates the muscle must be a motor nerve and it should normally have performed the function that is to be restored. Thus the patient will not be required to relearn use

of the muscle transplant, and return of function should proceed in a straightforward manner.

The possible complications of free muscle transplantation can be either acute or chronic. Thrombosis of the vascular pedicle may require emergent reoperation and, if not corrected, will result in death of the transplant and a total failure of the procedure. Lack of muscle function after an appropriate time for reinnervation may be a result of poor innervation from a compromised recipient nerve. It is critical to be certain of the adequate functional status of this nerve before using it to reinnervate the gracilis muscle. Distal tendon adhesions may also limit excursion of the new musculotendinous unit after reinnervation has taken place. This can be improved dramatically by tenolysis, which should be considered in all cases in which normal or close to normal range of movement is not achieved.

The anatomy of the involved area may be severely distorted by the causative trauma, resultant contractures, or surgical interventions. Electrophysiologic testing can be helpful to define the remaining function of the residual muscle units or the integrity of the major peripheral nerves. Angiography can be used to demonstrate the condition of the extremity vasculature and its use should be routine before surgical intervention.

The overriding goal throughout the planning process must be to improve the functional capabilities of the patient. This will mean a truly significant increase in range of motion, with adequate power to make this complex reconstruction and the rehabilitative effort the patient must expend worthwhile.

OPERATIONS

The history of free muscle transplantation began in the laboratory. Tamai et al[8] in 1970 reported successful muscle transplantation by microvascular technique in the dog model. Three years later, clinical experience began in Shanghai when a portion of the pectoralis major muscle was transplanted to the forearm. Harii et al[1] in 1973 also carried out the first clinically successful functioning muscle transplantation for reanimation of facial paralysis. Subsequent to these initial clinical descriptions, Terzis et al[9] in 1978 provided a functional assessment of muscle transplantation in laboratory animals. A number of clinical reports followed, specifically by Ikuta et al,[2] Schenk,[7] O'Brien and Morrison,[5] and Manktelow and McKee.[2] Excellent long-term follow-up has been favorably reported by Manktelow[3,4] and Zuker[10] and has established the operation as the procedure of choice for specific muscle deficits in the upper extremity. Regional muscle slides or advancements can be helpful for minor contractures, but only free muscle transplantation can make a significant improvement in patients with major contractures or actual muscle loss. Tendon transfers are also not as effective in reestablishing functional movement, particularly for volar forearm deficiencies.

PATIENT PREPARATION

Certain prerequisites must be met in all patients before performing a functional muscle transplantation. There must first be an available and appropriate motor nerve to reinnervate the muscle, otherwise the procedure is not possible. There must be a good passive range of motion in the joints of the extremity that will be motored by the transplant. There should be good skeletal stability of the extremity, with all fractures healed, that will allow the muscle to be effective. The hand or end-organ should have good sensibility and preferably some degree of intrinsic muscle function. A stable wrist is required for finger and thumb flexion and/or extension reconstruction. There must be an appropriate bed and soft tissue cover for muscle and tendons to glide effectively. This may require a staged reconstruction to provide appropriate soft tissue coverage before performing a free muscle transfer. Lastly, consideration must be given to the personality and motivation of the patient. The rehabilitation program that will be necessary after a muscle transplantation procedure is arduous and prolonged, and patient compliance is required and indeed essential if optimum results are to be achieved.

PATIENT EVALUATION

The extremities should be evaluated in detail, with a particular emphasis on the specific anatomic reconstruction that will be required at the recipient site. These include the recipient artery and vein, the motor nerve that will power the transplant, the tendon bed and soft tissue cover, the stability of the proximal bone or joints, and the range of motion of the distal joints. Angiography is often necessary to clarify the vascular supply to the limb and also to specifically locate the arteries to be used for revascularization of the transplant. It is not uncommon in Volkmann's ischemic contracture, for example, to see gaps in the brachial artery that require reconstruction before undertaking a functional muscle transplant. Angiography can also help in planning how to position the muscle and in selection of a healthy recipient artery.

During patient evaluation, one can often gain valuable in-

formation about the status of an appropriate motor nerve. The clinical examination in patients with partial nerve loss will help provide evidence of an available motor nerve. However, if there is uncertainty about the motor nerve, assessment of the vascular pedicle with which it is associated is often helpful. If the nerve is in a deep, protected position or the adjacent vascular system seems intact on angiography, then it is highly likely that the nerve will also be protected and thus available for use. A common clinical situation is to reconstruct finger and thumb flexion after Volkmann's ischemic contracture. The preferred motor nerve is the anterior interosseous nerve, which lies in a protected position deep to the flexor digitorum superficialis (FDS), where it is only rarely injured. Angiography can be extremely helpful by demonstrating a healthy, uninjured, adjacent anterior interosseous artery. It can then be safely assumed that the anterior interosseous nerve will be uninvolved and available for use.

Another laboratory test that can sometimes be of value is electromyography of the pronator quadratus muscle. One can assume that the anterior interosseous nerve is available for use if this muscle is functioning. The skin cover should also be carefully evaluated. It is crucial to have good quality, appropriate skin and soft tissue cover in the region of the tendon reconstruction to facilitate tendon gliding. The muscle belly itself could potentially be skin grafted, but there must be an adequate bed and skin cover for the tendinous portion.

STAGE-SETTING PROCEDURES

Various other procedures may be necessary in certain situations to either facilitate the transfer itself or to optimize the function of the transfer. For example, vascular grafts may be required to reconstitute the arterial supply to the limb after a Volkmann's ischemic contracture that resulted from a supracondylar fracture in which the brachial archery is damaged. Segmental nerve defects may need to be bridged by grafting to provide sensibility to the hand and intrinsic muscle function. The tendon bed and skin cover may need to be reconstructed before the transfer with either a pedicle flap, a free skin flap, or by regional tissue expansion. Stability proximal to the transfer and appropriate joint mobility to the joints that the transfer will mobilize should be present before the actual transfer.

MUSCLE SELECTION

The selection of a muscle to be used as a functioning muscle transplant involves many factors, including transplant characteristics, dynamic requirements, and functional loss, that have been discussed in detail by Manktelow and McKee in 1978.[3]

Transplant characteristics refer to the vascular and neural supply of the muscle. The vessels must be of sufficient caliber to perform reliable microvascular anastomoses. The vascular pattern within the muscle is also very important. The classification system developed by Mathes and Nahai[5] in 1981 outlines the various types of vascular supply to muscle. One vascular pedicle is present in muscles with a type 1 pattern, such as the tensor fascia lata. One dominant pedicle and several minor pedicles are present in type 2 muscles, such as the gracilis. Type 3 muscles, such as the gluteus maximus, have two dominant vascular pedicles. Muscles with segmental vascular pedicles, such as the sartorius, are designated as type 4 muscles. Finally, type 5 muscles, such as the latissimus dorsi, have a dominant vascular pedicle plus several secondary segmental pedicles. Mathes and Nahai noted that free tissue transfer would be possible in type 1, 2, and 5 muscles.

The motor nerve anatomy must also be considered for appropriate function. It should be of adequate size and of sufficient length to facilitate the microneural repair. For free muscle transplantation to the extremity, it is preferable when only one single and pure motor nerve innervates the muscle.[3]

The dynamic factors outlined by Manktelow and McKee should be considered in choosing a muscle for transfer, including potential muscle strength and its range of movement. The potential strength of the muscle after transfer can be estimated directly from the cross-sectional area of the muscle fibers. The greater the cross-sectional area, the greater the potential for strength. A muscle transplant, to be effective, must produce the required range of motion, which is a factor of the resting muscle-fiber length. It is clear in the assessment of human muscles that the internal fiber anatomy may be different in different muscles. Bipennate muscles for example, generally have shorter fiber lengths than strap muscles. The strap muscles therefore have a longer excursion than bipennate muscles. It is also logical to anticipate some loss in the range of muscle excursion after transfer. Therefore it is best to select strap muscles that will have a remaining range of excursion sufficient to motor the involved part.

The third consideration in muscle selection is the functional loss at the donor site. This may be of crucial importance in patients with other conditions, such as hemiplegia, paraplegia, or limb amputations. Consideration should be given to the location of the donor-site scar in some individuals.

The preferred donor muscle for upper-limb reconstruction is the gracilis. It is relatively simple to harvest because it lies close to the surface and is easily accessible. It has a reliable neurovascular pattern and fulfills the neurovascular characteristics for a transplantable muscle. Its range of movement as a strap muscle is optimal. A 30-cm long gracilis muscle will contract more than 50% of its muscle-fiber length. This will fulfill the dynamic requirements for any limb reconstructive procedure. There is no functional loss when the muscle is removed from an otherwise normal leg, and there is very low donor-site morbidity. The donor scar on the medial thigh is usually well accepted, although care should be taken to keep it as posterior as possible to make it less visible from the anterior view.

SURGICAL TECHNIQUE

A two-teamed approach is used during muscle transplantation, with one team preparing the recipient site and the second harvesting the muscle. To minimize ischemic time, the muscle is removed from the thigh and transplanted to the upper extremity only after the recipient site is fully prepared.

The recipient site is dissected under tourniquet control whenever possible. Skin flaps are designed to ensure healthy soft tissue cover over the tendinous portion of the reconstruction. This aids in tendon gliding during muscle contraction. Preparation of the recipient site is often time consuming, tedious, and extremely difficult because of previous trauma and fibrosis. It is always best to begin the dissection, if possible, in an area of unscarred tissue, identifying the required structures in normal tissue and working into the area of scarring. The vascular and neural components are assessed in detail by direct examination during surgery to determine the best location for the vascular and nerve coaptation. The recipient vessels are identified and clearly dissected over a sufficient distance to reach as many normal vessels as is possible within a given surgical field. It is preferable in most extremity cases to do an end-to-side repair of the artery, and an end-to-end repair of the vein. The motor nerve that will be used to reinnervate the muscle is then identified. There are often small segments of remaining arm muscle that are still innervated by the motor nerve. This provides excellent reassurance that the nerve selected for muscle flap reinnervation is indeed a motor nerve and appropriate to reinnervate the muscle. The nerve is carefully prepared and marked to anticipate a tension-free neurorrhaphy.

The bed is then prepared to receive the muscle flap. This involves dissection of the origin and insertion sites, as well as the intervening new muscle bed, which is often heavily scarred. Often, some scar tissue must be excised to provide a healthy bed for the muscle flap. It is also often necessary to clearly dissect the major nerves of the extremity that are encased in the scar to confirm their continuity, improve their function if impaired, and place them in a position where they can receive additional vascularity from the muscle. It is not uncommon to have partial or complete defects in the major nerves in the extremity that require either secondary repair or grafting at the time of muscle flap transposition. This should all be done before the muscle is removed from the recipient site to minimize the ischemia time.

The origin is prepared so that a broad area of muscle attachment is available. This is generally 4 to 5 cm in width and should provide anchorage to healthy periosteum. The muscle can also be attached to bone using a Mitek anchor. The distal tendinous elements of the proposed insertion must be cleared of any adhesions. The forearm tendinous units should be placed in balance so that the fingers and thumb act in unison. The most common situation is reconstruction of the forearm flexors. The distal tendons of the flexor digitorum profundus (FDP) and flexor pollicis longus (FPL) are woven into distal muscle flap to provide independent motion of the fingers and thumb, if possible. The FDP flexor tendons are dissected free and then sutured together so that when traction is applied they flex in unison and cascade normally into the palm. They are sutured together in the desired position with an interweaving type of suture. The thumb can be placed into this weave with the tension adjusted to make sure its flexion is initiated only after the fingers begin to move. The correct tension prevents the thumb from flexing into or beneath the fingers but allows it to flex after the fingers have flexed into the palm. The distal muscle flap can also be split longitudinally into two separate muscle segments that are independently innervated by one of the major nerve fascials in the motor nerve. This natural division can be identified before moving the muscle from its donor site by individually stimulating separate fascicular groups and noting the contraction that occurs longitudinally along the muscle. The finger profundus tendons are sutured into the larger muscle mass, whereas the FPL tendon to the thumb is woven into the smaller distal muscle segment. Care should be taken to ensure there is good vascularized flap cover over the distal tendon repair. The arm tourniquet is released after site preparation but before muscle flap transfer to assess the vascularity of the bed and particularly to assess the arterial inflow at the proposed site of flap revascularization. Everything must be prepared at the recipient site before making the muscle flap ischemic.

The gracilis muscle is dissected and prepared for harvest by a second team while the recipient site is being prepared. The entire muscle must be removed and therefore a medial thigh incision is planned to expose the full length of the muscle. It is important not to extend the incision proximally beyond the groin crease because this may be a source of irritation from clothing in the future. The incision is therefore planned to begin about 2 cm distal to the groin crease and courses distally in a longitudinal fashion to the junction of the middle and distal thirds of the thigh. It is placed just posterior to the adductor insertion, which can be easily palpated when the hip is abducted. The gracilis muscle lies just posterior to the adductor muscle. An incision made about 2 cm posterior to the adductor origin will therefore afford excellent exposure to the gracilis muscle and its neurovascular pedicle. The incision is carried through the subcutaneous fat and the fascia overlying the gracilis down to the muscle itself. One can often get a very good idea of the location of the main neurovascular pedicle by the position of a large musculocutaneous perforator that arises from the mid-portion of the muscle. It lies at the exact level of the entry of the main pedicle into the muscle. The anterior border of the muscle is then dissected free and the pedicle is identified. Care must be taken not to injure any branches of the motor nerve that may branch away from the main body of the nerve into the muscle itself. Very commonly, fine "short-cut" branches can be identified and should be preserved. The vascular elements are then dissected to their origin, with ligation of branches coursing superiorly to the adductor musculature. Usually there is a single central artery with paired vena comitantes. A pedicle length of 6 cm is easily obtained in adults. The nerve runs proximally at a 45-degree angle between the vascular pedicle and the muscle toward the obturator foramen. A sufficient length of nerve is easily obtained because the nerve to the gracilis is easily separated from the obturator nerve proximally. The muscle is dissected circumferentially and the accessory pedicles are carefully ligated. The dissection should proceed proximally to include the fascial origin of the muscle, which will enhance anchoring it in the forearm.

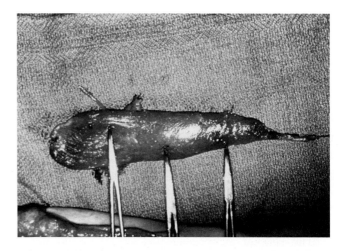

Figure 123-1. Diagram of muscle fully elevated and ready for transplantation.

The dissection extends distally to the tendon of the gracilis. A second incision is made in the medial distal thigh directly over the tendon, which is sometimes difficult to identify. The tendon is divided and the muscle is now fully prepared for removal and transplantation (Figure 123-1).

It is important to suture the muscle under appropriate tension when it is moved to the recipient site. The muscle is marked before it is divided and removed by abducting the hip and extending the knee to place it under maximum physiologic stretch. Marking sutures are then placed at 5-cm intervals along the entire length of the muscle. The natural resting tension can be recreated at the recipient site by stretching the muscle to restore the 5-cm increments.

Once the muscle and the recipient site have been fully prepared, the muscle is divided distally and then proximally, taking care to remove it with its fascial elements. The nerve is divided next, followed by the vessels. Careful inspection of the donor site is then carried out for any remaining bleeders, and the wound is closed by one team. A drain is not necessary unless there has been considerable interoperative blood loss at the time of the dissection. The wound is closed in layers and an occlusive dressing is applied.

The muscle is then moved to the upper extremity. Its actual location is planned so that the time required for reinnervation will be minimized. To do this, the donor nerve should be connected to the gracilis nerve as close to the muscle as possible. The muscle is placed into position and anchored proximally with nonabsorbable mattress sutures. Secure fixation of the origin is imperative. The muscle is then placed in position and the vascular repairs are performed. The operating microscope is moved into position and the vena comitantes are first anastomosed end to end to suitable recipient veins. The artery is anastomosed end to side to the recipient artery. Technically perfect vascular repairs are imperative because anastomotic revisions are time consuming and may lead to excessive muscle ischemia and/or necrosis. One should see excellent perfusion to all areas of the muscle after the vascular clamps are released. The motor nerve is then repaired. A technically perfect nerve repair in a tension-free, well-vascularized environment is imperative.

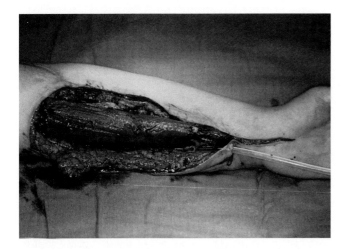

Figure 123-2. Diagram of muscle transplanted to the forearm with microneural and microvascular anastomoses.

It is crucial to have the recipient nerve identified as a motor nerve before muscle transfer. Preferably, it should also have been innervating muscles with a function similar to what the transferred muscle is expected to perform.

The distal tendon repair is performed after the vascular and nerve repairs have been completed. The muscle should again be stretched to its normal resting tension as determined by the previously placed, 5-cm apart marking sutures so that when it begins its activity, it is under physiologic stretch. Next, the recipient tendons are positioned to reflect the initiating position of the desired activity (Figure 123-2). If the muscle is used to reconstruct finger flexion, for example, then the maximum stretch position would be with the wrist and fingers fully extended. The tension on individual finger tendons should be adjusted to restore the normal cascade of digits into the palm from the radial to the ulnar side of the hand. The location of the tendon repairs is then marked, and the tendons are woven into the muscle tendon. The tension of the repairs can be checked by moving the wrist through a full range of motion and observing the position of the fingers, which should passively flex and extend with wrist extension and flexion. A full range of mobility will then be possible without overstretching the muscle. It will also place the maximum power of the muscle in the initiating position where it is most needed.

The skin flaps are closed after the insertion is secured. Care is taken to have appropriate skin-flap coverage over the distal tendon repairs. Skin closure should not be tight, particularly over the area of vascular repair. The belly of the muscle itself can be grafted, if necessary, at this initial stage to avoid excessive pressure from a tight skin closure. The skin graft can then be removed at a later date to create a better forearm contour.

The incisions are dressed with sterile gauze, and a protective splint is made in the operating room to decrease tension at both the origin and insertion. Patients who undergo finger-flexor reconstruction, for example, would have the elbow partly flexed, the wrist maintained in neutral, the metacar-pophalangeal (MCP) joints in flexion and the interphalangeal (IP) joints in extension. This would place the muscle at rest and not compromise later joint function.

POSTOPERATIVE MANAGEMENT

It is important during the postoperative period to provide adequate circulating fluid volume and pain management. Patient-controlled analgesia (PCA) is usually extremely effective in these situations. The extremity is splinted in a relaxed position for approximately 3 weeks. Passive stretching of both the origin and the tendon repair area is then initiated. The two sites are initially stretched alternately; after approximately 3 more weeks they can be stretched simultaneously. Full passive extension can usually be achieved by 7 to 10 weeks after surgery.

It is extremely important to initiate an active exercise program when the muscle begins to reinnervate. The time frame for innervation will depend on the distance between the nerve repair and the muscle belly itself. Reinnervation usually begins in 3 to 4 months. Active exercises to increase muscle excursion and strength are begun when the first signs of contraction are seen. This program is gradually increased to resistance exercises and may continue for 1 to 1½ years until the range of motion and strength have plateaued. The motivation and exercise tolerance of the patient will be extremely important during this process and will have a definite effect on the outcome.

SECONDARY PROCEDURES

Occasionally, despite good hand therapy, there will be inadequate muscle excursion with a limited range of motion. A tenolysis may be very helpful in such cases. This will allow whatever functional contraction the muscle has regained to be fully transferred to the fingers.

OUTCOMES

The results of this procedure are quite predictable if patients are carefully selected (Figure 123-3). Precise operative technique is crucial, and an involved, committed rehabilitation program is essential. The goal is to achieve a useful range of motion and grip strength that will improve the patient's functional capabilities (Figure 123-4). It should be noted, however, that at times the tendinous insertion may become adherent before activation of the muscle and may limit the actual range of motion achieved. Once strengthening exercises have plateaued, it may be worthwhile to perform tenolysis. This is necessary in approximately 33% of patients. It is extremely effective, but should only be done after the muscle is completely reinnervated and no further gains in active range of motion are achieved.

Postoperative range of motion may not reach 100% but should subsequently improve the patient's functional capa-

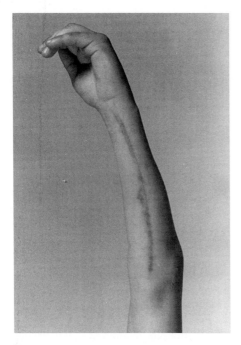

Figure 123-3. The preoperative functional capabilities of a child with Volkmann's ischemic contracture.

bilities. One can anticipate achieving a range of motion at least 50% of normal, although this can approach 100% in certain situations. Again, tenolysis may be helpful in improving the range of motion. The increase in strength after muscle transplantation compares favorably to other situations of muscle reinnervation. One can anticipate achieving 25% to 50% of normal strength in a transplanted muscle for forearm reconstruction. The functional capabilities of the patient with this amount of recovery should be substantially improved, although it is unrealistic to expect normal function. Muscle transplantation in the upper limb can be extremely important from an economic point of view in providing the patient with the added functional capability to return to a gainful employment. It can transform a limb that was essentially a helper only, with little or no grasp function, to one that is a major asset to the individual.

The aesthetic issues relate to the extent of the initial injury. The contour of the limb can be improved by muscle transplantation if the overlying skin cover is adequate. A relatively poor contour will result if there is inadequate skin cover and split-thickness skin grafting has been performed on the surface of the muscle. It may be necessary to revise the soft tissue at a later date by performing scar revision, graft excision, or even more complex interventions such as using tissue expansion of adjacent healthy skin. A smooth, relatively anatomic contour is the desired goal in this procedure and should be attainable.

A clear and realistic awareness of what is possible preoperatively will be very important to the final satisfaction of both the patient and the surgeon.

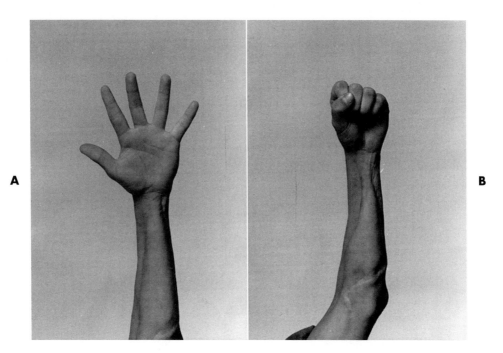

Figure 123-4. The postoperative functional capabilities after a free gracilis muscle transplantation. **A,** Full active extension. **B,** Flexion.

REFERENCES

1. Harii K, Ohmori K, Torii S: Free gracilis muscle transplantation with microneurovascular anastomoses for the treatment of facial paralysis, *Plast Reconstr Surg* 58:407-411, 1976.
2. Ikuta Y, Kubo T, Tsuge K: Free muscle transplantation by microsurgical technique to treat severe Volkmann's contracture, *Plast Reconstr Surg* 58:407, 1976.
3. Manktelow RT, McKee NH: Free muscle transplantation to provide active finger flexion, *J Hand Surg [Am]* 3:416-426, 1978.
4. Manktelow RT, Zuker RM, McKee NH: Functioning free muscle transplantation, *J Hand Surg [Am]* 9:132, 1984.
5. Mathes SJ, Nahai F: Classification of the vascular anatomy of muscles: experimental and clinical correlation, *Plast Reconstr Surg* 67:177, 1981.
6. O'Brien BMc, Morrison W: *Reconstructive microsurgery,* New York, 1987, Churchill Livingstone, pp 272-274.
7. Schenk RR: Rectus femoris muscle and compositeskin transplantation by microvascular anastomosis for avulsion of forearm muscles: a case report, *J Hand Surg [Am]* 3(1):60, 1978.
8. Tamai S, Komatsu S, Sakamoto H, et al: Free muscle transplants in dogs with microsurgical neurovascular anastomoses, *Plast Reconstr Surg* 46:219-225, 1970.
9. Terzis JK, Sweet RC, Pyker RW, et al: Recovery of function in free muscle transplants using microvascular anastomosis, *J Hand Surg [Am]* 3:37-59, 1978.
10. Zuker RM, Manktelow RT: Functional and aesthetic muscle transplants. In *Advances in plastic and reconstructive surgery,* vol 9, St. Louis, 1993, Mosby.

Free Joint Transfers

Todd Williams
Kimball Maurice Crofts

INTRODUCTION

The hand represents one of the most complex biomechanical systems in the human body. It functions with a meshed interplay of brute force and exquisite finesse. A powerful grasp is complemented and controlled by a delicate touch. Consummate hand function comes to fruition in the grand symphony of its individual components, opposing forces, balanced motions, and keen perceptions. The human hand gives man an amazing repertoire that can be used to physically promote his interests and solve his problems. An individual may become severely incapacitated and even dysfunctional in his or her element when this wonderful ability is lost or altered. Loss of just one component of hand function can in fact lead to incapacitation of virtually the entire hand and loss of that individual's livelihood.

The finger and thumb joints are the fulcrums of hand function. They must move smoothly through a normal range of motion (ROM) but be able to resist the lateral force vectors generated during pinch and grasp functions. There are many potential deficits that can impair the hand, one of which is loss of joint function. A joint may be absent, fused, stiff, or painful for a variety of reasons, including trauma, neoplasm, disease, or a congenital anomaly. A stiff or painful joint results in diminished digital and total hand function. The hand surgeon faced with this problem must choose the best option for the individual patient after considering many factors, including the patient's age, the importance of the digit or joint's contribution to overall hand function, and the patient's anticipated future hand use.

HISTORY

In 1902 Tietze first reported use of a proximal phalanx from the big toe as a nonvascularized bone graft to reconstruct a bone defect in the hand.[6] In 1913, Goebbel discussed the use of a nonvascularized toe-joint transfer for reconstruction of a finger.[15] Several small and a few larger studies have subsequently examined the use of toe joints to reconstruct defective finger joints. A portion of this work has examined the fate of the epiphyseal growth centers and cartilage surfaces in both vascularized and nonvascularized transfers. A few studies have reported growth in nonvascularized transfers,[13,28-30,42] and other studies have reported no growth in nonvascularized transfers.[30,31] Single case reports have also shown success with some degree of growth.[25,26,28,51,54] Two studies that examined growth in nonvascularized transfers seemed to indicate retaining the periosteum was beneficial, and the best success also seemed to be in patients around 6 months of age.[27,55] Entin et al[12] reported relatively normal architecture in nonvascularized joints up to about 15 weeks after transfer. This was followed over time, however, by joint degeneration, including loss of joint space with destruction of the cartilage, invasion of the joint space by fibrous tissue, and fragmentation of adjacent bone with widening of the bone ends. These findings have been confirmed in other studies.[13,33] Despite the apparent success in isolated cases, growth and long-term viability are not reliable in nonvascularized transfers.

Several studies, however, confirm epiphyseal growth and long-term bone and cartilage survival in vascularized joint transfers.* Retention of articular cartilage architecture is an important factor in long-term painless joint function. Some authors have tried articular cartilage grafts, without predictable success.[2,7,8] Articular cartilage is dependent on synovial fluid for its survival, which in turn requires an intact blood supply to the joint. This blood supply must be reestablished within 14 days after surgery to prevent replacement of the joint space with fibrocartilage.[13] In a primate study by Tsai et al[49] there was significantly more morphologic damage and necrosis in subchondral bone and loss of cartilage in nonvascularized transfers when compared with vascularized transfers.

The first vascularized transfer of a metacarpophalangeal (MCP) joint to an adjacent proximal interphalangeal (PIP) joint was performed by Buncke in 1967 as an island flap.[1] Foucher[21] reported the first free vascularized toe-joint transfer in 1976 and now has one of the largest series in the literature to date.[19,22] In 1992 Tsai and Wang compiled all the cases reported in the world literature to that date.[50] In these case

---

*References 11, 35, 40, 43, 48, 57.

reports, the vast majority of joint transfers were done using the second toe as the donor site, harvesting either the metatarsophalangeal (MTP) or PIP joints. In some traumatic situations in which an unsalvageable finger is present in conjunction with a destroyed joint in a viable finger, some authors have used a joint from the unsalvageable finger to reconstruct a damaged joint in an otherwise viable digit.[18,20,24,46] Others have used the transferred joint as a flow-through graft in a segmental loss of an amputated finger.[37] In addition, two joints have been transferred on a single pedicle.[47]

INDICATIONS

Despite the theoretical advantages of free joint transfer, other options are more preferable in many situations. The main two alternatives to a free vascularized joint transfer are either arthrodesis or arthroplasty. Arthrodesis is an excellent choice for patients with distal interphalangeal (DIP)–joint pain or disease in almost all situations. Fusion of this joint in 15 to 30 degrees of flexion provides good pain relief with minimal or no functional deficit. Fusion of the PIP joint is also a good option in an elderly patient, or in patients who do not require much digital dexterity. The PIP joint should be fused in 40 to 55 degrees of flexion, increasing from the radial to the ulnar side digits. Fusion of the MCP joints also decreases the functional mobility of the finger but is still an option in some patients who are not candidates for other types of reconstruction. Fusion of the MCP joint of the thumb causes less functional loss if the carpometacarpal (CMC) joint is supple and functional, and the result is more functional in elderly patients. Children on the other hand may have growth abnormalities after an arthrodesis if the epiphysis is destroyed during the traumatic event or during the surgery. Kowalski and Mansk,[38] however, showed that fusion could still be performed with minimal disturbance of the growth plates.

Arthroplasty using a silicone implant, a technique popularized by Swanson,[44,45] has become the standard treatment for MCP-joint replacement, primarily in patients with rheumatoid arthritis. This procedure provides relatively supple joints, with an average ROM of 45 degrees and good pain relief. The implants may also be used in the PIP joint in selected cases. The largest limitation of this procedure is decreased lateral stability when compared with a natural joint, and the potential injury to the epiphyseal growth plates in children. Patients who have rheumatoid arthritis have relatively weak hands that generate minimal forces on their reconstructed digits when compared with younger, healthier patients who have otherwise normal hands. Silicone implants do not tolerate the stresses placed on joints by young, active hands and eventually disintegrate; in addition, patients may develop silicone synovitis.[14,56] Silicone implants are best suited for use in older patients in whom the level of hand activity during the remaining years of their lives would not be expected to wear out the implants.

The patients best suited for free joint transfers are children and young, active adults with normal, functioning flexor and extensor tendons. Masear and Meyer[39] and Tsai and Wang[50] have outlined the indications for free joint transfer, including painful posttraumatic arthritis, posttraumatic joint instability, and posttraumatic deformity in patients under 40 years of age who cannot be treated by joint arthroplasty because of youth and/or high activity level, or when maintenance of motion is essential. Free joint transfers are also useful when soft tissue and skin are required in the reconstruction. The toe extensor mechanism and a skin island can be harvested with the donor joint for use as a composite tissue transfer.

Despite these advantages, toe transfer is not without risks and morbidity. Foucher[17] noted that the procedure is long (lasting several hours) and must be performed under general anesthesia, with an average hospitalization of 5.3 days. As with any microsurgical procedure, there is always a chance of failure. Donor-site morbidity is also a factor that must be discussed with the patient.

ANATOMY

The blood supply to the toes is from both the dorsal arch through the dorsalis pedis artery and from the plantar arch through the posterior tibial artery (Figure 124-1). In the majority of cases, the dorsal system provides the dominant blood supply to the second toe through the first dorsal metatarsal artery (FDMA).[53] The dorsalis pedis artery generally branches near the base of the metatarsal to create the FDMA. The FDMA provides a communicating branch to the plantar system in the mid-metatarsal region between the first and second metatarsals and then continues to eventually divide into the digital arteries to the lateral side of the first toe and the medial side of the second toe.[23] Before this terminal division, a small articular vessel branches laterally to supply the MTP joint of the second toe.[5,9,52] Branches from the proper digital artery supply the PIP joint. The FDMA can be sacrificed near its origin from the dorsalis pedis artery, or to gain as much pedicle length as possible the dissection may include a length of the distal dorsalis pedis artery. Foucher also describes identifying the plantar digital vessels and incorporating these as vascular pedicles if the dorsal arteries are of insufficient size for microvascular anastomosis.[16,22] The lateral digital artery to the great toe is sacrificed with the flap, and therefore a skin paddle on the lateral aspect of the great toe can be raised on its own digital vascular pedicle with the remainder of the flap (Figure 124-2).[10] This gives more freedom for the location of the skin paddle than can be achieved when the skin is taken on the dorsal aspect of the second toe.

The extensor mechanisms of the toe and finger vary significantly. The finger has a complex three-dimensional mechanism that relies on both intrinsic and extrinsic muscles to flex the MCP joint while simultaneously extending the IP joints. This delicate balance can be greatly affected by only

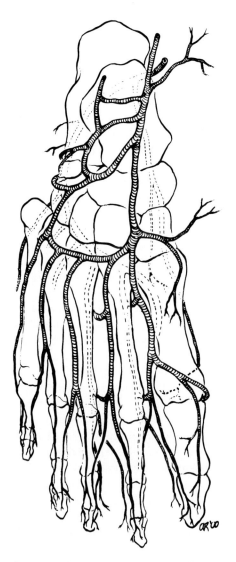

Figure 124-1. The blood supply to the toes from the dorsum arch through the dorsalis pedis artery and from the plantar arch through the posterior tibial artery.

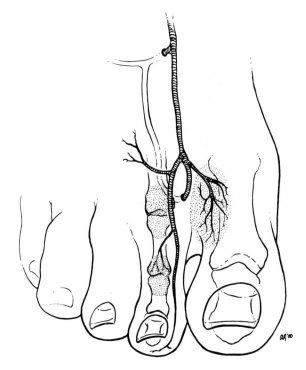

Figure 124-2. A skin paddle can be designed and elevated on the lateral aspect of the great toe.

minimal change in length of any of its components. A central slip that is too lax causes an extensor lag that may eventually lead to a boutonniere deformity. A central slip that is too tight may cause hyperextension and lead to a swan-neck deformity. Because the central slip inserts very proximally on the middle phalanx, it must either be sacrificed with the joint or saved by way of a step-cut osteotomy.[35] Tsai and Wang[50] recommend saving the native extensor mechanism in this fashion when it is intact and functioning. The flexor digitorum superficialis (FDS) inserts over a longer distance on the middle phalanx and can be left intact with less difficulty. The extensor mechanism of the toes includes the extensor digitorum brevis, which inserts into the proximal phalanx and has no real counterpart in the hand. Additionally, the extensor mechanism of the toes is simply not designed for fine control in the same fashion as that of the hand.

The ROM of the toe joints is also very different from that of the finger joints in both direction and magnitude. Normal ROM of the finger joints is 90 degrees flexion and 0 degrees extension at the MCP joint, 120 degrees flexion and 0 degrees extension at the PIP joint, and 80 degrees flexion and 0 degrees extension at the DIP joint. Despite the greater degree of flexion at the PIP joint, the MCP joint provides more motion to the total flexion arc. Useful joint function, however, does not need to meet these normal values. In a study by Hume et al,[32] during 11 daily activities the useful range of motion of the MCP, PIP, and DIP joints was only 61, 60, and 39 degrees, respectively. Normal ROM of the toe MTP joints is 20 to 25 degrees of flexion and 60 to 80 degrees of hyperextension. Normal ROM of the toe PIP joint is 70 degrees of flexion and 0 degrees of extension. Because of this, the MTP joint can be rotated 180 degrees around its long axis to increase flexion of the finger. The other option to overcome natural hyperextension of the MTP joint is to create an angled osteotomy on the recipient metacarpal. This allows the transferred joint to remain in hyperextension on radiographs during digital extension with the digit at 0 degrees and permits the transferred joint to move through its entire range of flexion.

The location of epiphyseal growth plates is important in children. The growth centers for the middle and proximal phalanges of the toes are at their proximal end. The growth plate of the metatarsal is at its distal end. This allows transfer of a growth plate on each side of the joint when the MTP joint is transferred, matching that of the hand. As noted by O'Brien et al,[41] transferring both growth centers when reconstructing an MCP joint in a child allows the digit to maintain growth of both the metacarpal and proximal phalanx, keeping pace with the other digits. Two growth plates are not required in adults or in reconstruction of the PIP joint in children and therefore the toe PIP joint may be a better donor site because of its size, ROM, stability, and decreased donor-site morbidity.

OPERATIONS

TRANSFER TECHNIQUES

Many different techniques have been described for both elective and emergent joint transfer. Tsai and Lim[47] and Chen et al[3] have described transfer of two joints on a single pedicle. Koshima et al[37] have also used the transfer as a flow-through flap to revascularize the distal portion of an amputated finger. Other variations have included a DIP-to-PIP joint transfer on the same finger and transfer of joints between fingers. The thumb CMC joint has also been reconstructed with a joint transfer, but this is more commonly performed as part of a complete thumb reconstruction.

Angiography may be useful to help identify the dominant arterial system or vascular foot anomalies, but its use is not absolutely necessary. A one- or two-team approach may be used. Foucher[17] believes the use of a single team helps prevent size mismatch of arteries, bones, veins, nerves, and tendons. The donor site in this case is usually dissected first under tourniquet control, which can be let down to allow the flap to perfuse while the recipient site is prepared. Others prefer a two-team approach to decrease operative time.[50]

The dissection of either the PIP or MTP joints is nearly identical, with the notable exception of the location of the osteotomies. Harvest of the PIP joint of the second toe is started with creation of a skin paddle over the PIP joint and middle phalanx. Both digital arteries of the toe can be identified through this incision. The FDMA can be visualized through a more proximal extension of this incision onto the dorsum of the first web space. If the distal toe is to be preserved, the medial digital artery is divided at the level of the DIP joint and dissected proximally to the edge of the skin paddle while preserving the branches to the PIP joint.

The lateral digital artery is carefully dissected from the PIP joint, dividing the branches to the joint and leaving the main vessel intact to supply the distal toe. The dorsal longitudinal incision continues proximally, and the proximal FDMA and dorsalis pedis with their vena comitantes are identified. If additional length is required, the dissection can also include the more proximal dorsalis pedis artery. The vena comitantes are dissected to include the greater saphenous vein, providing enough length to reach the cephalic vein on the dorsum of the hand. The extensor tendons are divided over the proximal metatarsal. Osteotomies in the middle and proximal phalanges may be made at any time and may be useful early to aid in the dissection. This may also aid in identification of the plantar vessels and the communication between the dorsal and plantar arteries. To include the communicating branch between the dorsal and plantar systems, both plantar and dorsal systems are dissected from the PIP joint proximally until the communicating branch is identified. The plantar system can then be transected just proximal to its communication with the dorsal

system. If the plantar system appears to be the dominant system, it can generally be dissected through the dorsal approach up to the plantar arch where it is divided. Dissection of the plantar system more proximal than the head of the metacarpals causes significantly more trauma to the foot. Innervation of the joint is generally not required,[1,12,36] but innervation of the skin paddle can be maintained by dissecting the dorsal digital branch of the deep fibular nerve, which runs with the FDMA and dorsalis pedis arteries as described by O'Brien et al.[41]

One problem with taking a skin paddle over the extensor surface of the toe is that the extensor mechanism of the finger must be sacrificed and reconstructed with that from the toe. Ellis et al[10] have described creation of a skin paddle over the dorsal aspect of the great toe based on a small cutaneous branch from the FDMA. This allows greater freedom in placement of the skin paddle and allows use of the finger extensor mechanism if it is intact.

The leg tourniquet is released after adequate dissection of all components and the foot is allowed to perfuse while the finger is prepared. A dorsal longitudinal incision is created on the back of the hand, and the cephalic vein and dorsal branch of the radial artery are identified and prepared for microvascular anastomosis. The PIP joint is exposed through an incision between the central slip and lateral band if it is going to be preserved or if the extensor mechanism over the joint is resected. If the extensor mechanism is to be maintained, a step-cut osteotomy is made in the dorsal cortex of the middle phalanx, leaving the central slip insertion intact.[35] If the MCP joint is being reconstructed, it is generally exposed through a longitudinal incision in the central slip. Care is taken to prevent injury to the flexor mechanism of the finger during resection of the joint. The donor joint is then transferred to the hand and any adjustment to bone length is performed at this time. Foucher[17] feels it is better for the bone flap to be too short than too long. Joint fixation is achieved with Kirschner (K) wires, and the arterial microvascular anastomosis is performed generally in an end-to-side fashion to the dorsal radial artery. At least two veins should be anastomosed and can be done in an end-to-end fashion. If the extensor mechanism is to be reconstructed, the extensor digitorum longus from the toe is sutured to the extrinsic finger extensor and the extensor digitorum brevis is sutured to the intrinsic finger extensors.

Dissection of the MTP joint is nearly identical to that of the PIP joint, with the exception of the level of osteotomies. One difference, however, is placement of the flap. Because of the mechanics of the MTP joint, it is either rotated 180 degrees around its long axis, placing the volar plate in a dorsal location in the finger, or an angled osteotomy is performed on the metacarpal to compensate for the normal hyperextension present at the MTP joint. Rotation of the joint around its long axis creates its own problems. Most notable of these is that the skin paddle is now located on the volar aspect of the recipient finger. The stability of a normal joint provided by the volar plate is also now lost to the dorsal aspect of the finger.

Despite these limitations, a good result can be achieved. Figures 124-3 through 124-8 are those of an 18-year-old

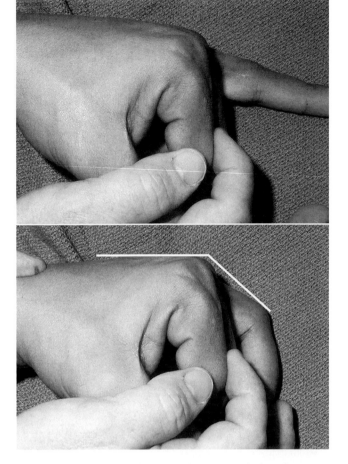

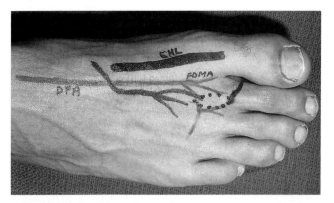

Figure 124-5. Preoperative markings for dissection of the MTP joint.

Figure 124-3. Passive flexion and extension before free joint transfer.

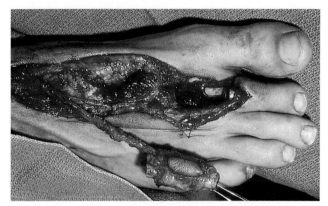

Figure 124-6. Elevation of the flap.

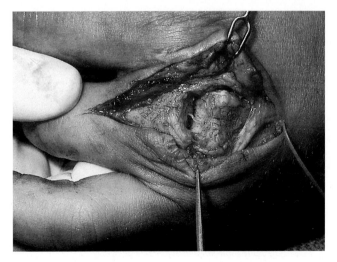

Figure 124-4. Intraoperative joint destruction.

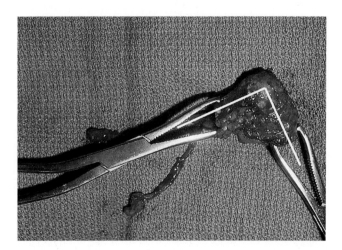

Figure 124-7. Intraoperative passive flexion of the rotated toe joint.

laborer who underwent free toe MTP joint transfer to the ring finger MCP joint. This patient had an initial injury that resulted in fusion of the left ring finger MCP joint. Initial attempts at tendon arthroplasty followed by joint capsulotomy resulted in improved ROM, but with significant pain. A second toe, vascularized, MCP joint transfer, rotated 180 degrees around the long axis, was performed followed

by an extensor tenolysis. Final ROM of the MCP joint was 80 degrees, with 95 degrees of flexion and a 15-degree extensor lag.

After surgery, the hand is initially splinted for 4 weeks, followed by gentle active motion if the extensor mechanism was intact, or a dynamic assisted extension splint is used if the extensor mechanism was reconstructed.

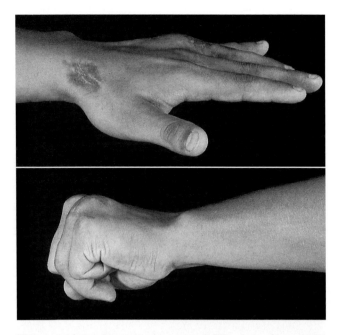

Figure 124-8. Postoperative active ROM of the finger MCP joint.

OUTCOMES

A number of authors have examined the results of free joint transfers to the hand. Most have seen improvement to a varying degree, whereas others have not. Foucher has reported his single surgeon experience of 28 vascularized joint transfers in 25 patients in 1990.[24] Average follow-up was 156 months, and average ROM was 35 degrees at the MCP joint and 23 degrees at the PIP joint. Tsai compiled all reported joint transfers in the literature up to 1991, including a review of his own experience of 32 transfers.[50] This review included 89 joints that were transferred in 79 patients. The donor site was usually the MTP or PIP joints, and recipient sites were 44 PIP joints, 33 MCP joints, six thumb interphalangeal (IP) joints, two thumb MCP joints, and one CMC thumb joint. The average ROM was 32 degrees, with 63% of transfers obtaining a range of motion greater than 30 degrees and 28% having a range of motion less than 10 degrees. The joint space of 42 cases in this combined series was evaluated by radiographs, and only one joint was found to have degeneration. In 1992 Imamura et al[34] reviewed their series of 11 free joint transfers for trauma and infection. The average postoperative range of motion was 31 degrees compared with 16 degrees preoperatively. Radiographs showed destruction of four joints thought to be related to vascular failure in two and infection in two. Finally, Chen[4] reviewed his experience of 29 free joint transfers in 1998. The average follow-up was 32 months, and the mean ROM was 34 degrees for the MTP-to-MCP transfer, 32 degrees for PIP-to-MCP transfer, and 24 degrees for PIP-to-PIP transfer.

The major complication of free joint transfer is extensor tendon adhesions. Tenolysis was required in 48% of patients

reported in Tsai's series.[10] As with any other microvascular transfer, arterial or venous thrombosis with subsequent flap failure is expected to be in the range of 5% to 10%.[39] Other reported complications include infection, loss of the skin island flap, and potential lack of growth in children. Donor-site morbidity may also be a consideration, with the most commonly reported problem being nonunion or delayed union in the toe. This problem may be circumvented by performing a complete ray amputation of the second toe. Leaving the second metatarsal in place combined with toe amputation or ray amputation if the angle between the first and second metatarsal is greater than 20 degrees, can lead to a hallux valgus deformity.

SUMMARY

Vascularized joint transfers in specific situations can result in significantly improved hand function despite the fact that a "normal" range of motion will not be achieved. The overall complication rate approaches 50%, but the majority of these cases may be salvageable with additional procedures, including tenolysis or scar revision. Less than 150 vascularized joint procedures have been reported in the world literature, making this a rarely indicated procedure, with the majority of these cases having been performed by three surgeons. It therefore seems wise to familiarize oneself with the experience of these three authors before considering performing this procedure. The potential gain in hand function and donor-site morbidity must be discussed with the patient so expectations are not too high. Currently, vascularized joint transfer is the procedure of choice for young, active patients who require long-term mobility in their finger joints and for children who will require growth of the digit.

REFERENCES

1. Buncke HI, Daniller AI, Schulz WP, Chase RA: The fate of autogenous whole joints transplanted by microvascular anastomoses, *Plast Reconstr Surg* 39:333-341, 1967.
2. Campbell CJ, Ishida H, Takahoashi I-I, Kelly F: The transplantation of articular cartilage: an experimental study in dogs, *J Bone Joint Surg* 45A:1579-1592, 1963.
3. Chen IC, Tsai TM, Firrell JC: Single pedicle vascularized double joint transfer: anatomic study of two models, *Microsurgery* 18(5):312-319, 1998.
4. Chen SH, Wei FC, Chen HC, et al: Vascularized toe joint transfer to the hand, *Plast Reconstr Surg* 98(7):1275-1284, 1996.
5. Chen YG, Cook PA, McClinton MA, et al: Microarterial anatomy of the lesser toe proximal interphalangeal joints, *J Hand Surg [Am]* 23(2):256-260, 1998.

6. Colson P, Hovot R: Chirurgie reparatrice du pouce: greffe articulaire, *Lyon Chir* 42:721-724, 1947.

7. DePalma AF, Sawyer B, Hoffmann JD: Fate of osteochondral grafts, *Clin Orthop* 22:217-220, 1962.

8. DePalma AF, Tsaltas TT, Mauler GG: Viability of osteochondral grafts as determined by uptake of S (35), *J Bone Joint Surg* 45A:1565-1578, 1963.

9. Edwards EA: Anatomy of the small arteries of the foot and toes, *Acta Anat* 41:81-96, 1960.

10. Ellis PR, Hanna D, Tsai TM: Vascularized single toe joint transfer to the hand, *J Hand Surg [Am]* 16:160-168, 1991.

11. Ellis PR, Tsai TM, Kutz JE: Joint transplantation with microvascular anastomosis. In Meyer VE, Black MJM (editors): *Microsurgical procedures,* New York, 1991, Churchill Livingstone.

12. Entin MA, Alger JR, Baird RM: Experimental and clinical transplantation of autogenous whole joints, *J Bone Joint Surg* 44A:1518-1536, 1962.

13. Erdelyi R: Experimental autotransplantation of small joints, *Plast Reconstr Surg* 31:129-139, 1963.

14. Ferlic DC, Clayton ML, Holloway M: Complications of silicone implant surgery in the metacarpophalangeal joint, *J Bone Joint Surg* 57A:991-994, 1975.

15. Foucher G: Vascularized joint transfer. In Green DP (editor): *Operative hand surgery,* ed 2, New York, 1988, Churchill Livingstone.

16. Foucher G: Computerized study of the functional results of a second toe transfer in finger mutilation, *Chirurgie* 115:572-576, 1989.

17. Foucher G: Vascularized joint transfers. In Green DP (editor): *Operative hand surgery,* ed 4, New York, 1998, Churchill Livingstone.

18. Foucher G, Citron N, Merle M, Dury M: Free compound transfer of the distal interphalangeal joint: a case report, *J Reconstr Microsurg* 3:297-300, 1987.

19. Foucher G, Hoang P, Citron N, et al: Joint reconstruction following trauma: comparison of microsurgical transfer and conventional methods: a report of 61 cases, *J Hand Surg [Br]* 11:388-393, 1986.

20. Foucher G, Lenoble E, Sammut D: Transfer of a composite island homodigital distal interphalangeal joint to replace the proximal interphalangeal joint, *Ann Hand Surg* 9:369-375, 1990.

21. Foucher G, Merle M: *Transfer articulaire au niveau d'un doigt en microchirurgie,* G.A.M., lettre d'information du GAM, No. 7, 1976.

22. Foucher G, Moss ALH: Microvascular second toe to finger transfer: a statistical analysis of 55 transfers, *Br J Plast Surg* 44:87-90, 1991.

23. Foucher G, Norris RW: The dorsal approach in harvesting the second toe, *J Reconstr Microsurg* 4:185-187, 1988.

24. Foucher G, Sammut D, Citron N: Free vascularized toe-joint transfer in hand reconstruction: a series of 25 patients, *J Reconstr Microsurg* 6:201-207, 1990.

25. Freeman BS: Reconstruction of thumb by toe transfer, *Plast Reconstr Surg* 17:393-398, 1956.

26. Freeman BS: Growth studies of transplanted epiphysis, *Plast Reconstr Surg* 23:584-588, 1959.

27. Goldberg NH, Watson HK: Composite toe (phalanx and epiphysis) transfers in the reconstruction of the aphalangic hand, *J Hand Surg [Am]* 7:454-459, 1982.

28. Graham WC, Riordan DC: Reconstruction of a metacarpophalangeal joint with a metatarsal transplant, *J Bone Joint Surg* 30A:848-853, 1948.

29. Haas SL: Experimental transplantation of the epiphysis with observations on the longitudinal growth of bone, *JAMA* 65:1965, 1915.

30. Haas SL: The transplantation of the articular end of bone including the epiphyseal cartilage line, *Surg Gynecol Obstet* 23:301-332, 1916.

31. Haas SL: Further observation on the transplantation of the epiphyseal cartilage plate, *Surg Gynecol Obstet* 52:958-963, 1931.

32. Hume MC, Gellman H, McKellop H, Bruinfield RH Jr: Functional range of motion of the joints of the hand, *J Hand Surg [Am]* 15:240-243, 1990.

33. Hurwitz P: Experimental transplantation of small joints by microvascular anastomosis, *Plast Reconstr Surg* 64:221-231, 1979.

34. Imamura K, Nagatani Y, Hirano E: Vascularized toe-to-finger joint transplantation: 11 patients followed for 4 years, *Acta Orthop Scand* 63(4):457-461, 1992.

35. Ishida O, Tsai TM: Free vascularized whole joint transfer in children, *Microsurgery* 12:196-206, 1991.

36. Kettelkamp DB: Experimental autologous joint transplantation, *Clin Orthop* 87:138-145, 1972.

37. Koshima I, Inagawa K, Sahara K, et al: Flow-through vascularized toe-joint transfer for reconstruction of segmental loss of an amputated finger, *J Reconstr Microsurg* 14(7):453-458, 1998.

38. Kowalski MF, Mansk PR: Arthrodesis of digital joints in children, *J Hand Surg [Am]* 13:874-879, 1988.

39. Masear V, Meyer R: An overview of free vascularized joint transfers, *Alabama J Med Sci* 25:164-167, 1988.

40. Mathes SJ, Buchannan R, Weeks PM: Microvascular joint transplantation with epiphyseal growth, *J Hand Surg [Am]* 5:586-589, 1980.

41. O'Brien BM, Gould JS, Morrison WA, et al: Free vascularized small joint transfer to the hand, *J Hand Surg [Am]* 9:634-641, 1984.

42. Ring PA: Transplantation of epiphyseal cartilage: an experimental study, *J Bone Joint Surg* 37B:642-647, 1955.

43. Singer DI, O'Brien BM, McLeod AM, et al: Long-term follow-up of free vascularized joint transfers to the hand in children, *J Hand Surg [Am]* 13:776-783, 1988.

44. Swanson AB: Arthroplasty in traumatic arthritis of the joints of the hand, *Orthop Clin North Am* 1:285-298, 1970.

45. Swanson AB, Maupin BK, Gajjar NV, Swanson GD: Flexible implant arthroplasty in the proximal interphalangeal joint of the hand. *J Hand Surg [Am]* 10(6 Pt 1):796-805, 1985.

46. Tsai TM, Jupiter JB, Kutz JE, et al: Vascularized autogenous whole joint transfer in the hand: a clinical study, *J Hand Surg [Am]* 7:335-342, 1982.

47. Tsai TM, Lim BH: Free vascularized transfer of the metatarsophalangeal and proximal interphalangeal joints of the second toe for reconstruction of the metacarpophalangeal joints of the thumb and index finger using a single vascular pedicle, *Plast Reconstr Surg* 98(6):1080-1086, 1996.

48. Tsai TM, Ludwig L, Tonkin M: Vascularized fibular epiphyseal transfer, *Clin Orthop* 210:228-234, 1986.

49. Tsai TM, Ogden L, Jaeger SH, et al: Experimental vascularized total joint autografts: a primate study, *J Hand Surg [Am]* 7:140-146, 1982.

50. Tsai TM, Wang WZ: Vascularized joint transfers: indications and results, *Hand Clin* 8:525-536, 1992.

51. Vercauteren ME, Van Vynckt C: Free total toe phalanx transplant to a finger: a case report, *J Hand Surg [Am]* 8:336-339, 1983.

52. Watanabe M, Katsumi M, Yoshizu T, Tajima T: Experimental study of autogenous toe-joint transplantation: anatomic study of vascular pattern of toe joints as a base of vascularised autogenous joint transplantation, *Ofthop Surg* 29:1317-1320, 1978.

53. Wei F, Silverman RT, Hsu W: Retrograde dissection of the vascular pedicle in toe harvest, *Plast Reconstr Surg* 96(5):1211-1214, 1995.

54. Whitesides ES: Normal growth in a transplanted epiphysis: case report with 13 year follow-up, *J Bone Joint Surg* 59A:546-547, 1977.

55. Wilson JN: Epiphyseal transplantation: a clinical study, *J Bone Joint Surg* 48A:245-256, 1966.

56. Worsing RA, Engber WD, Lange TA: Reactive synovitis from particulate Silastic, *J Bone Joint Surg* 64A:581-585, 1982.

57. Wray C, Mathes SM, Young VL, et al: Free vascularized whole-joint transplants with ununited epiphyses, *Plast Reconstr Surg* 67:519-525, 1981.

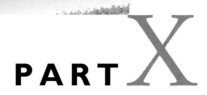

PART X

THE THUMB

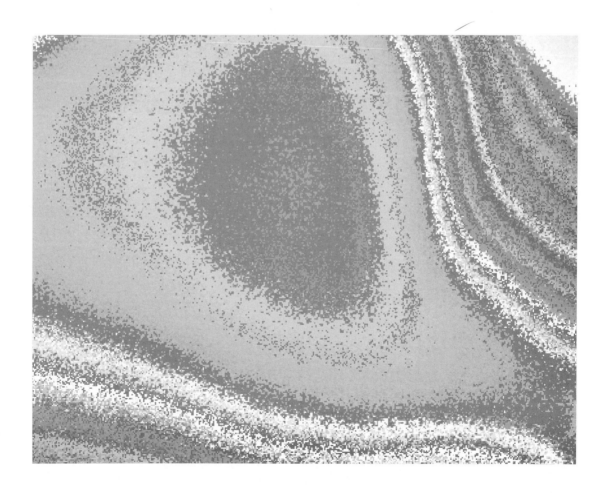

Thumb Reconstruction

Harry J. Buncke
Gregory M. Buncke
Gabriel M. Kind
Rudolf Buntic
Peter P. Siko

INDICATIONS

DEFINING THE PROBLEM

Loss of the thumb deprives the hand of 40% to 60% of its total function. Its importance increases with each additional finger lost. Restoration of key pinch to a hand with no digits accounts for 100% of function in such a hand (Figure 125-1). The thumb is the prime digit, and its reconstruction is considered mandatory by some persons in present-day society. However, there are patients who resist efforts to restore function out of fear of failure or complications, or because they are unwilling to accept the loss of another vital body part. These patients have difficulty understanding that they are not just losing a toe during the reconstruction procedure but are gaining a thumb. Many patients do not understand that the anatomic defect is being transferred from the hand to the foot, where it is better tolerated. Other patients may hope to gain economically by preserving the disability. Still others have unrealistic expectations regarding the potential restoration of function with a prosthesis.

The level of amputation and the side of the injury (dominant versus nondominant hand) are important considerations. Amputation through the distal joint on the dominant side is not as critical as the same injury on the nondominant side. Many tools and instruments can be manipulated with a short thumb. However, length is critical on the nondominant side, which must grasp and stabilize objects for the tool-handling, dominant side. Flexion of the distal joint of the thumb provides a "vice grip" ability to the nondominant thumb. The nondominant hand can hold large objects or heavy timber with this type of grasp, such as 2 × 6 or 4 × 4–inch boards or awkward-sized sheets of plywood. Strength of grasp is therefore more critical on the nondominant side than on the dominant side. Dexterity also is greatly enhanced with useful flexion of the distal joint (Figure 125-2).

Sensation is also more important on the nondominant side because the "eyes" of the hand—the sensory pulp pads of the index finger and thumb—must be able to identify and position objects such as nails, nuts, bolts, and wires for the tool-operating dominant side, sometimes in places where visual coordination is impossible.

The age of the patient is also an important consideration. Congenital absence of the thumb is often part of a complex hand anomaly in which many fingers may be involved. Reconstruction is more difficult when there is agenesis of the part because the nerves, blood vessels, and tendons may be absent for a variable distance proximally. Reconstruction is almost always possible, however, with conditions such as congenital amputations and amniotic bands, particularly when nubbins are present, because the critical structures are usually present down to the level of the anatomic amputation. Reconstruction using a toe transfer is often impossible with complete loss of the first ray. Pollicization of an index finger is then the operation of choice.

Toe transplants to repair congenital amputation of the thumb can be considered at age 2½ to 3 years if the child is of normal size. Arteriograms are not usually done in young children, and the vascular architecture of the blood supply to the foot is unknown. One can evaluate the arterial supply to the first metatarsal area with fairly good, predictable success, however, by using an ultrasonic Doppler probe.

The second toe can often be used in congenital reconstructions rather than the great toe because the transplanted digit tends to hypertrophy and develop to a greater extent than the corresponding digit on the opposite foot. The second toe is anatomically less thumblike than the great toe, but its use is often preferred in children, women, and persons who frequently wear thong-type slippers or shoes. The second toe is expendable from a functional and physiological standpoint. Loss of the great toe results in a weight-bearing shift to the lateral four metatarsal heads, and this is usually well tolerated. All of these choices involve some sacrifice, but follow-up evaluations and gait analysis have shown that loss of the great toe does not produce a severe functional defect.[21] Patients

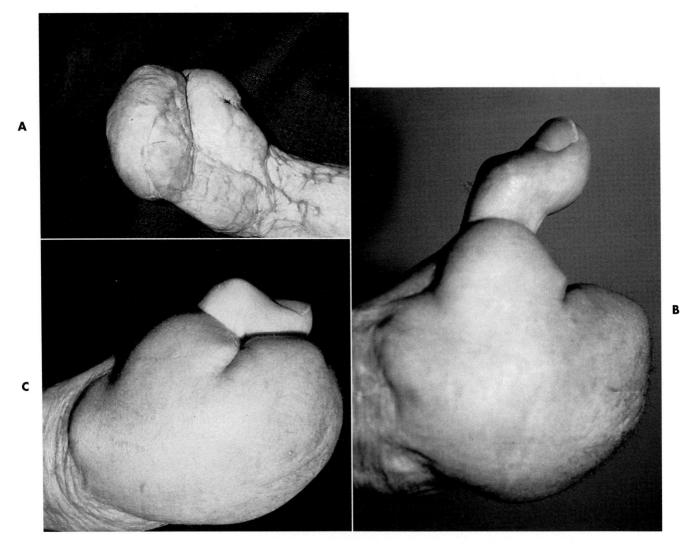

Figure 125-1. **A,** A pre-med student lost all of his fingers from his dominant right hand and his left hand and forearm in an automobile accident and fire. A great-toe transplant **(B)** and a first web space–plasty **(C)** restored key pinch and permitted the patient to complete medical school and specialty training in psychiatric counseling for patients who have suffered severe trauma. (From Buncke HJ: *Microsurgery transplantation-replantation: an atlas text,* Philadelphia, 1991, Lea & Febiger.)

can participate in almost every type of sport and activity (Figure 125-3).

Children adapt rapidly to the loss of a digit and change hand dominance quite easily. This adaptation is much more difficult for older patients. Once the thumb is reconstructed on the dominant hand, dominance returns almost immediately to the original side. The dominant hand may also be involved in congenital amputations. This becomes apparent when the child starts using the hand after the ability to pinch has been created with a toe transplant (Figure 125-4).

The great toe is wider than the normal thumb, but not longer. The width of the nail bed is within 1 to 3 mm of the size of the thumb. In addition, the transplanted great toe atrophies from 30% to 40% after it is placed on the hand, a phenomenon caused by temporary intraoperative denervation. The great toe on the foot in its dependent position is edematous and flat-

tened. It shrinks when transplanted to the elevated hand (Figure 125-5). Several operations have been devised to decrease the size of the toe at the time of transplantation or later. One such procedure, known as the *wraparound,* places the skin envelope of the great toe around a bone graft placed in the thumb position.[18] The critical flexion and extension of the distal joint is sacrificed in this procedure. and the functional result seldom equals that of a complete great-toe transplant.

INFORMED CONSENT

Most patients who have lost a thumb from an injury, tumor, or other cause are quite amenable to reconstruction. It is important to carefully discuss the details of the operation with the patient and inform him or her of the possibility of

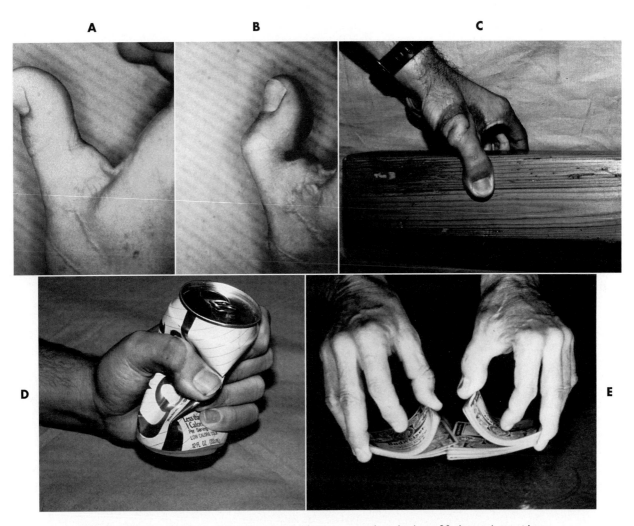

Figure 125-2.   Flexion of the distal joint of a toe transplant (at least 30 degrees) provides a vice grip, powerful grasp, and dexterity. **A** and **B,** Sixty degrees of active flexion. **C,** Vice-grip grasp. **D,** Strength. **E,** Dexterity. (From Buncke HJ: *Microsurgery transplantation-replantation: an atlas text,* Philadelphia, 1991, Lea & Febiger.)

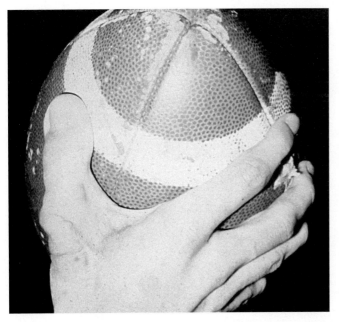

Figure 125-3.   Hand of a young man who lost his thumb in a water-skiing accident. Unfortunately, the thumb could not be retrieved from the bottom of the lake. After a great-toe transplant, he went on to become captain of his high school football and basketball teams and later created his own jazz band called "Rule of Thumb." Loss of the great toe does not significantly compromise foot function or gait. (From Buncke HJ: *Microsurgery transplantation-replantation: an atlas text,* Philadelphia, 1991, Lea & Febiger.)

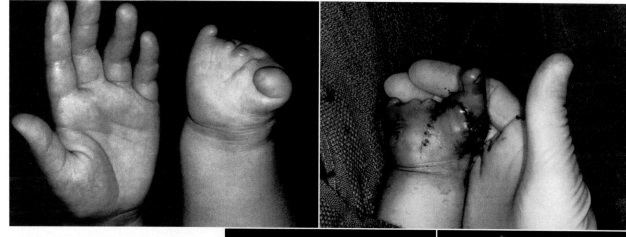

Figure 125-4. A, Hand of a child with congenital amputations of all of the digits of the right hand. The "nubbins" are mobile, which confirms the presence of normal proximal structures. **B,** The second toe from the right foot was transplanted to the thumb position. **C,** Six months later, the second toe from the left foot was transplanted to the ulnar border of the hand, producing the capability for pulp-to-pulp pinch. **D,** The child gradually began using her reconstructed right hand preferentially, proving that she was genetically right-handed, not left-handed. (From Buncke HJ: *Microsurgery transplantation-replantation: an atlas text,* Philadelphia, 1991, Lea & Febiger.)

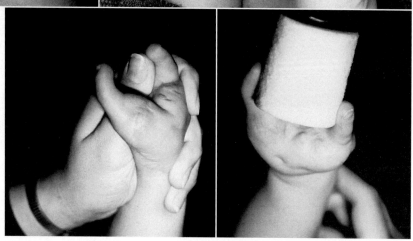

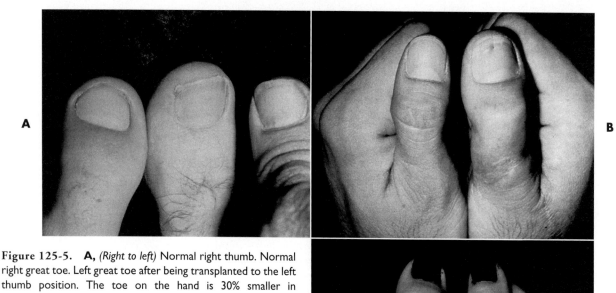

Figure 125-5. A, *(Right to left)* Normal right thumb. Normal right great toe. Left great toe after being transplanted to the left thumb position. The toe on the hand is 30% smaller in cross-sectional area than the other toe on the foot. **B,** The discrepancy in toe size is seldom appreciated unless both digits are displayed together. **C,** The size difference is even less apparent in this great-toe transplant to a woman (the first ever). (From Buncke HJ: *Microsurgery transplantation-replantation: an atlas text,* Philadelphia, 1991, Lea & Febiger.)

transplant loss. The success rate, however, is 98% or higher with current techniques. If the transplant fails, part of the bone can sometimes be salvaged with a tubed pedicle flap and a neurovascular island transfer, so all is not lost (Figure 125-6).

Patients with a traumatic thumb amputation when replantation is not possible or fails can be offered an immediate toe transplant (Figure 125-7). Many patients will have difficulty accepting immediate reconstruction, whereas others will welcome the opportunity of regaining a thumb, saving them many months of disability. Occasionally, vital parts of the thumb must be covered temporarily with a tubed pedicle flap. The patient then has time to consider further reconstruction with or

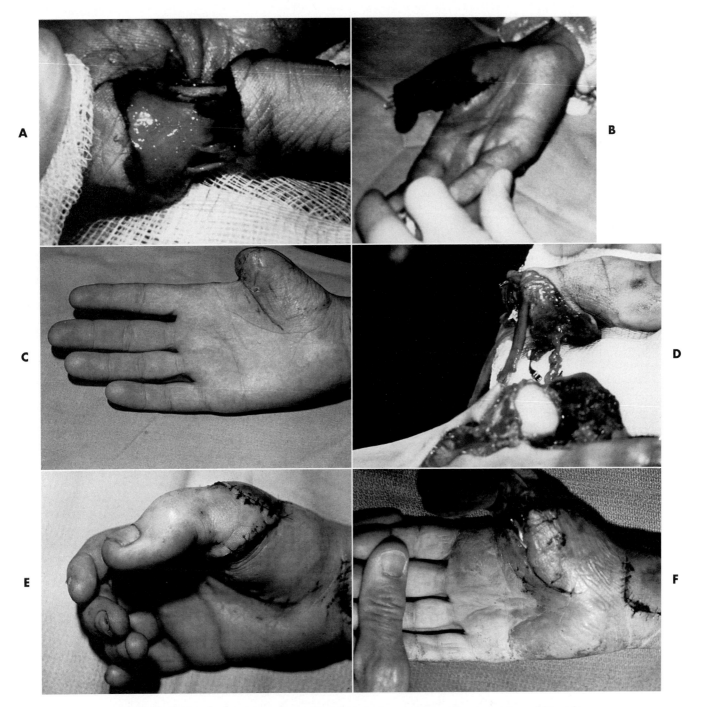

Figure 125-6. **A,** A construction worker sustained a partial avulsive amputation of his right thumb. **B,** An attempt at replantation and revascularization failed and the patient was referred to our center for a great-toe transplant. **C,** Preoperative view of the hand showing the amputated thumb. **D,** The right great toe is ready for transplantation. **E,** Problems developed postoperatively because of vascular spasm, possibly caused by nicotine because the patient smoked surreptitiously. **F,** Despite repeated attempts to reestablish circulation, the transplant failed. *Continued*

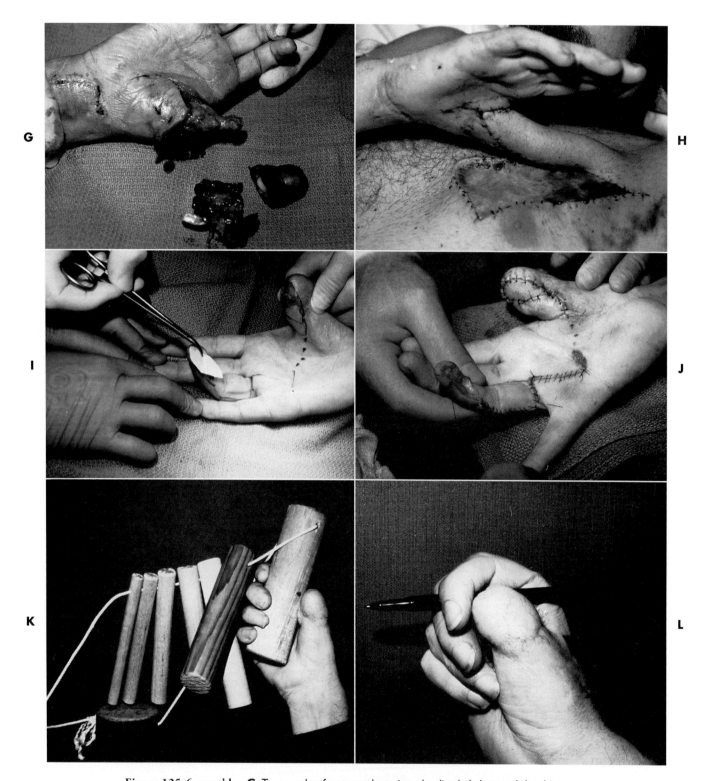

Figure 125-6, cont'd. **G,** Two weeks after transplantation, the distal phalanx and the skin cover of the toe were removed, preserving the proximal phalanx of the toe, which showed some evidence of neovascularization. **H,** The proximal phalanx was then encased in a tubed pedicle cross-chest flap rather than a groin flap, which often results in marked swelling of the hand because of the dependent position. **I,** After detaching the tubed pedicle flap, a sensory neurovascular island flap was transferred from the ulnar half of the ring finger. **J,** The neurovascular island flap was placed on the tactile surface of the new thumb. **K,** Useful sensate grasp was restored. **L,** The patient has functioned well with his new thumb, which is part original thumb, part toe transplant, part chest skin, and part ring finger.

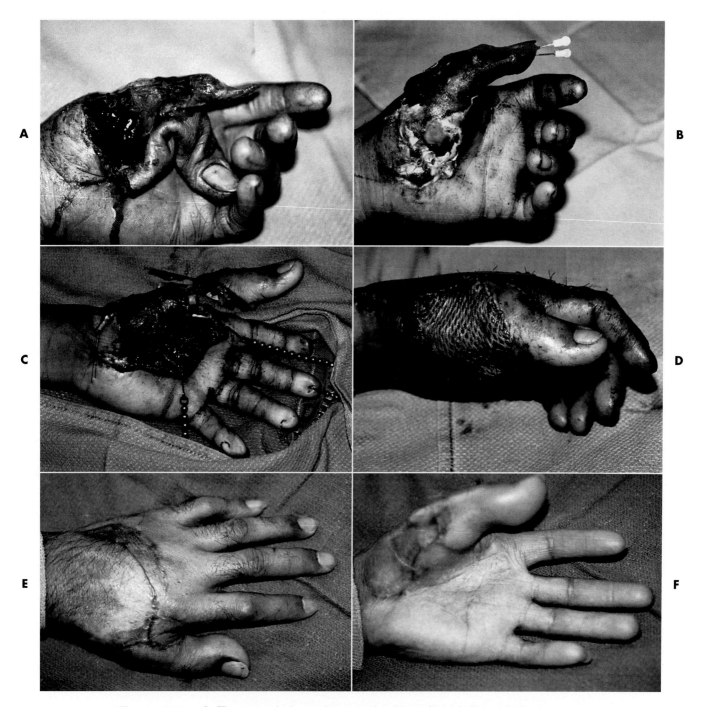

Figure 125-7. **A,** This patient had a crushing partial avulsion of his left thumb. **B,** An attempt at revascularization failed. **C,** The patient was counseled about the advantages of an immediate reconstruction with a great-toe transplant and he agreed to the procedure. **D,** The transplant was completed 10 days after the initial injury. Skin grafts were needed to cover the base of the debrided thumb. **E** and **F,** Postoperative views. The patient was discharged from the hospital 3 weeks after the initial injury and was able to return to work in 6 months rather than a year or 2. (From Buncke HJ: *Microsurgery transplantation-replantation: an atlas text,* Philadelphia, 1991, Lea & Febiger.)

without a toe transplant. In two cases, we replaced a tubed pedicle flap covering the proximal portion of the thumb and proceeded with a toe transplant rather than continuing with a tubed pedicle, bone graft, and neurovascular island flap reconstruction (Figure 125-8). In our practice, great-toe transplants were done immediately in 34 (28%) of 122 cases within 2 weeks of the injury.

The informed consent discussion must include counseling the patient on the need for blood transfusions. Patients can donate one or two units of their own blood before surgery on

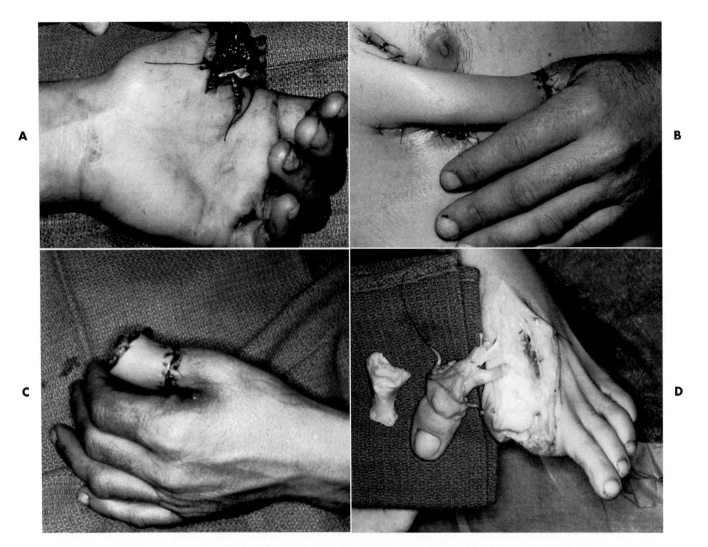

Figure 125-8. **A,** This patient sustained a rope avulsion of his left thumb, losing the distal phalanx and the soft tissue over the proximal phalanx. **B,** The avulsed thumb was not replantable; the exposed proximal phalanx and tendon structures were covered with a cross-chest tubed pedicle flap for temporary protection. The patient was counseled about the eventual reconstruction of his thumb with a great-toe transplant at a later date. **C,** The patient decided to proceed with the toe transplant immediately rather than wait for the tubed pedicle flap to be detached. **D,** Seven days after the injury, the left great toe was harvested and filleted, and the proximal phalanx was discarded after preserving the soft tissue skin cover that would be needed to surround the denuded proximal phalanx of the thumb. (From Buncke HJ: *Microsurgery transplantation-replantation: an atlas text,* Philadelphia, 1991, Lea & Febiger.) *Continued*

an elective basis or have several units of donor-designated blood available. With present blood-banking techniques and sophisticated tests, the risk of acquiring human immunodeficiency virus (HIV) from a blood transfusion is 1 in 493,000. Other diseases and their transmission rates during transfusion include the following: human T-cell leukemia/lymphoma virus (HTLV): 1 in 641,000; cytomegalovirus (CMV): 1 in 103,000; and hepatitis B virus (HBV): 1 in 63,000. New screening techniques should reduce these risks even further.[23]

We have found it very useful for patients contemplating thumb reconstruction by toe transplantation to talk to other patients who have been similarly injured and to review the literature on the subject. The surgeon must take time and help patients make the decision on their own and without pressure. When the patient is a child, other family members must be brought into this discussion and all of their questions must be answered in detail. In spite of the possibility of restoring 80% to 90% of function, there are patients who adamantly refuse this type of surgery for a variety of reasons, both cultural and psychological. Others may take weeks or months to make up their minds. Patients may schedule surgery, cancel, and then reschedule. This behavior should alert the surgeon that the patient may not be a candidate for such complex surgery. A good "rule of thumb" is to reschedule with caution the patient who cancels once, and never reschedule the patient who cancels twice.

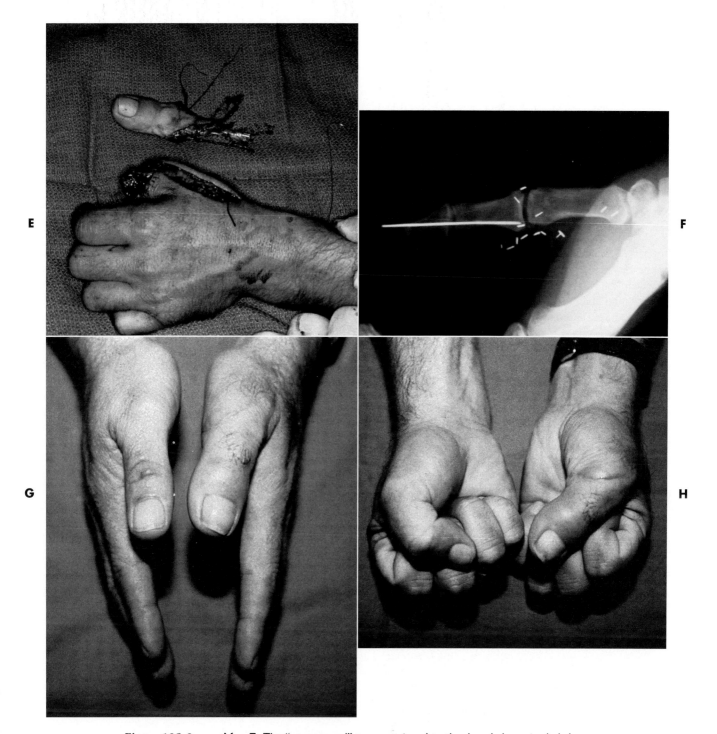

Figure 125-8, cont'd. **E,** The "wraparound" toe was pinned to the denuded proximal phalanx of the thumb, creating a compound distal joint, half toe and half thumb. **F,** Radiograph shows the compound joint pinned with Kirschner (K) wires. **G,** The transplanted toe has acceptable appearance and length. **H,** Strength and dexterity have been restored to the patient's hand.

OPERATIONS

Thumb reconstruction by toe transplantation was first described by Nicoladoni[19] in the late 1800s. He used a technique of sewing the hand to the foot for 4 to 6 weeks, using a delayed tubed pedicle type of transfer. This was later modified by Davis,[10] who realized that the superficial metatarsal artery and dorsalis pedis systems could be incorporated within a tubed pedicle flap and elevated so that the positioning employed by Nicoladoni would be less uncomfortable. Pollicization procedures and neurovascular island flaps perfected by Littler and others laid the groundwork for toe-to-hand transfers by microvascular techniques. Experimental toe-to-hand transfers were first accomplished in monkeys in the early 1960s and later in humans in the late 1960s and early

1970s.[4,5,9] Today, thumb reconstruction by toe transplantation is widely accepted and practiced throughout the world.

AVAILABLE TECHNIQUES

Reconstruction of the thumb at any level can be considered, to include a pulp transfer, a distal phalanx transfer, a partial toe transfer, or an entire toe transplant. When microsurgical skills and techniques are not available, a prosthetic post can be strapped to the thumb position to provide crude pinch and grasp. A tubed pedicle flap wrapped about a bone peg will provide a permanent, minimally sensate post. Campbell Reid[8] and others modified this approach by adding a Littler-like neurovascular island flap transfer from the ulnar side of the ring finger to the open end of the tubed pedicle flap at the time of detachment.[16]

Pollicization of an index finger, particularly if injured, provides the next level of nonmicrosurgical functional reconstruction.[15] However, such a four-finger hand has a spiderlike appearance and feel, particularly when it is on the right hand—the hand customarily used for hand-shaking.

Other digits have been pollicized, including the ring finger, the little finger, and even digits from the opposite hand. Kelleher and Sullivan[13] have shown that when the little finger is transposed to the thumb position the finger hypertrophies with time and function and becomes more thumblike (Figure 125-9). In a unique case, the thumb has been replaced using a modified Nicoladoni technique to transfer the thumb from the opposite hand from a paralyzed and functionless donor upper extremity. In another case, the entire hand has been transferred from a paralyzed limb to a seriously traumatized normal limb.[22]

The advent of microsurgical techniques may permit thumb reconstruction to be accomplished with a great-toe transplant, partial great-toe transplant, or second-toe transplant. We

believe that the great toe is the best choice, except when the entire first metatarsal is missing. In this situation, the second toe with the second metatarsal can be used to replace the first ray. The surgeon must first transfer or transplant additional tissue to the thumb area, however, to cover the second metatarsal shaft and reconstruct the first web space. This can be accomplished in one operation with a double microvascular transplant of the second toe and metatarsal head, plus a lateral arm flap or muscle flap to cover the second metatarsal shaft, thenar area, and first web space. Unfortunately, the final result is a small digit that does not look like a thumb.[11] The great toe—with the dorsal half of the first metatarsal, or even the entire first metatarsal—can be used in similar fashion without compromising foot function.

Homotransplantation of the thumb is now technically possible, but is still not a feasible alternative because the skin provokes the strongest immune response. Present-day immunosuppressive strategies for homotransplants are acceptable only when they are life-saving for the recipient. Other tissues, such as bone and nerves, are less antigenic, and their immune response can be suppressed even further by freezing. Thumbs have been reconstructed in China using frozen cadaver bone, joint, and tendon complexes covered with the skin envelope of the recipient's great toe. Loss of articular cartilage and bone resorption are unfortunately common in long-term follow-up.

PERTINENT ANATOMY

Understanding the arterial supply from the dorsalis pedis and plantar systems to the first metatarsal space is critical. The dorsalis pedis artery may continue as a dominant superficial first metatarsal artery out to the web space, providing the major arterial supply to the great or second toe. In our experience with over 300 toe transplants, this anatomic configuration is present in 40% of patients. The second most common condition is when the plantar first metatarsal artery is dominant, either from the plantar system arising from the posterior tibial artery or from the dorsal system through a large perforator extending from the dorsalis pedis artery in the proximal portion of the first metatarsal space. In the third most common condition, the first dorsal system begins superficially, then goes into the muscle and becomes deep, or intramuscular, throughout the entire first metatarsal space.

Arteriograms of the injured hand and donor foot are performed on the day before surgery, except in young children. A dominant dorsal metatarsal artery remains on the anteroposterior (AP) views in the mid-metatarsal space, from the proximal perforator to the distal perforator. If the plantar artery is dominant, it passes immediately medially under the shaft of the first metatarsal down to the metatarsal head, where it joins the distal perforator after passing medial or lateral to the sesamoid (Figure 125-10).

The ideal vascular system for transplantation is a dominant dorsal system. A long vascular pedicle can be mobilized up over the dorsum of the foot, including the dorsalis pedis artery, which can be dissected even into the ankle and up the leg. We have transferred the dorsalis pedis flap and the extensor brevis

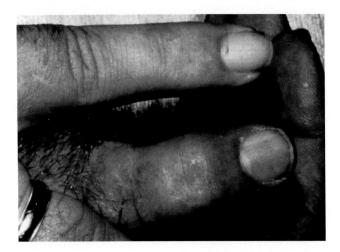

Figure 125-9. This patient had the little finger of her right hand pollicized to the thumb position. The digit has hypertrophied over the years because of the heavy duty in its new thumb position and is appreciably bigger in circumference than the left little finger. (Courtesy John Kelleher, MD, Toledo, Ohio.)

muscles on long pedicles to reconstruct defects around the ankle and the lower half of the leg.[12] The great toe on long arterial pedicles of this type can be developed to reach healthy vessels in the mid and proximal forearm when the upper extremity is severely traumatized and no acceptable vessels are present in the distal hand. Long venous pedicles are seldom a problem because the major draining veins from the great toe or second toe can be traced far proximally on the saphenous system (Figure 125-11).

If the arterial supply to the first metatarsal space is plantar dominant or intramuscular, it is wiser and saves time to start dissection distally in the web space and dissect the plantar system as far back as the transverse metatarsal ligament. An interpositional vein graft can then be used to lengthen the pedicle as needed.

An ultrasonic Doppler probe can be used to trace the dorsalis pedis artery in the first metatarsal space if arteriograms are not available or if the patient is a child. If it is a dominant artery,

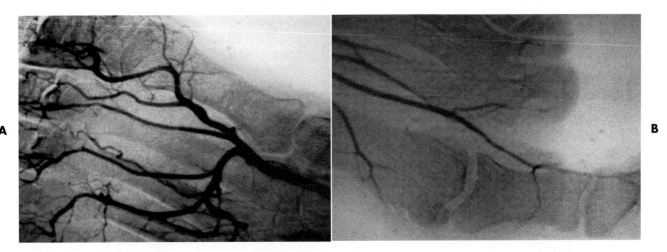

Figure 125-10. The first metatarsal artery may be dorsal dominant or volar dominant. **A,** Arteriogram of a plantar metatarsal system. The dorsalis pedis artery dips through the base of the first metatarsal space, communicating with the deep first metatarsal artery, which travels under the shaft of the first metatarsal. The Doppler signal of the dorsalis pedis is lost at the base of the first web space. **B,** Arteriogram of a dominant dorsal first metatarsal artery. The dorsalis pedis continues in a subcutaneous plane in the middle of the space between the first and second metatarsal shafts. The Doppler signal can be followed throughout the length of the metatarsal shafts to the web space, where it bifurcates and supplies the digital vessels to the lateral side of the great toe and the medial side of the second toe. (From Buncke HJ: *Microsurgery transplantation-replantation: an atlas text,* Philadelphia, 1991, Lea & Febiger.)

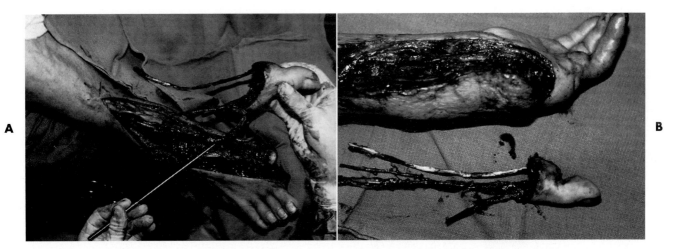

Figure 125-11. This patient sustained a crushing, avulsive injury to his right hand and forearm, with loss of his index finger, thumb, and soft tissues over the distal radial half of his forearm. **A,** Fortunately, the patient had a dominant dorsal metatarsal artery, which permitted the great toe to be mobilized on a long vascular pedicle above the ankle. The flexor hallucis was also detached above the ankle for similar length. **B,** The toe is next to the arm, showing a vascular pedicle of over 20 cm in length.

the signal can be heard all the way down the middle of the first metatarsal space to the web space and then into the second or great toe. The surgeon can presume that the system is plantar and plan accordingly if the signal disappears at the base of the first metatarsal space.

PREOPERATIVE PLANNING

The length and orientation of the transplant and flaps must be planned once the vascular anatomy of the first metatarsal space has been determined. Clay models of the transplant are very helpful in planning the orientation of skin flaps from the toe and the recipient area on the hand and also help the patient and family visualize the result (Figure 125-12). Compound joints of half toe and half thumb can be constructed if the articular surface is present on the end of the proximal phalanx of the thumb or the metatarsal.[27] A solid, bony junction can be created between the proximal phalanx and the transplanted toe by hollowing out the base of the great-toe proximal phalanx when the metacarpal joint is present, even with a flake or spicule of proximal phalanx. The thumb proximal phalanx can then be pinned in place, plated in place, or, if there is a relatively long spicule of proximal phalanx, secured with a four-cortical screw. The proximal dart of dorsal skin on the toe and the shorter dart of the plantar skin should be constructed so that the foot wound can be closed without tension. Many surgeons tend to take skin from the toe to cover the vascular anastomoses on the hand. Tight wound closure on the foot results in delayed healing, prolonged recovery, and painful scarring. The surgeon should take less tissue with the toe and plan for skin grafts on the hand. Skin grafts are better tolerated on the hand than they are on the foot and will be successful over interpositional vascular grafts and anastomoses.[17] Additional protective cover can also be provided for the vascular pedicle during the dissection on the foot by carrying tissue as a flange around the vessels beyond the skin island of the toe. This creates a vascularized fascial flap around the vascular pedicle.

Photographs of the hand that document its preoperative function should be taken before surgery, having the patient use instruments such as scissors, hammers, screwdrivers, and pieces of timber (e.g., 2 × 4, 4 × 4, and 2 × 6–inch boards) to demonstrate the lack of grip or pinch. A room set aside for preoperative photographs should have one wall painted black so that it can be used for backgrounds, plus sheets of similarly colored cloth to be placed on tables and chairs so that the hand and foot can be photographed without shadows. The principal surgeon should write out a scenario of the photographs he or she wishes to have taken during surgery and designate one member of the team as the responsible photographer. Intraoperative photographs should be taken from the same position and orientation, usually over the shoulder of the operating surgeon.

Operating-room equipment should be checked in advance for proper alignment of the tips and cutting edges of the scissors, and to ensure clamps are functional. This procedure is usually routine in a well-organized replantation and transplan-

tation microsurgical center. Nonetheless, the surgeon should anticipate the need for special instruments and problems unique to the particular case. The operating microscope should also be checked before each procedure to be sure that lenses are clean. Objective lenses are not easily visualized, and a large mirror placed under the objective lenses helps to visualize blood spots and dirt. Acceptable microsutures and needles are available commercially from several companies. The surgeon should use a needle–suture combination proportional to the size of the vessel. Vessels 1 mm or less in diameter require 10-0 sutures, vessels of 0.5 mm or less require 11-0 sutures. For 2-mm vessels, 9-0 sutures are quite acceptable. Vessels 3 mm or larger require 8-0 sutures. External cuffing devices, particularly on the venous side, save time as long as they are not in the subcutaneous tissue where the devices can be palpated.[20]

The size of the needle should be as close to the size of the following suture thread as possible. An electroplating technique was developed in the early 1960s that produced a suture needle of 50 microns plated on a nylon thread of 30 microns.[6] The points on these needles were created by first holding the end of the metalized nylon at a 60-degree angle against an extremely fine grinding disk. The needle was then rotated 90 degrees and again placed against the disk, creating an extremely "sharp" point. Today's needles are attached to the suture material mechanically by drilling a hole in the end of the needle with a laser beam. The suture is then glued into the hole. Previously, swedging techniques were used to flatten the special steel, which was then wrapped around the suture with a microcrimping device. In the late 1960s the S&T Company of Germany was first to make microneedles of acceptable suture-and-needle-diameter.[1] Once this was accomplished and microsutures became available worldwide, the field of microsurgical replantation and transplantation developed rapidly. A variety of vascular clamps are available commercially. Most importantly, they should not have a blade pressure of more than 30 to 40 g/sq mm; otherwise, endothelial injury results.[25] We prefer the curved, serrated, seraphin type of vascular clamp, which is quite large but works nicely on these small vessels because it can hold vessels away from the wound surface, relieving tension.

INTRAOPERATIVE DRUGS

Heparin in saline, 100 units/ml, is used to irrigate the operative field, wash out vessel ends, and irrigate the vascular pedicles without washing the entire transplant. Systemic, low-molecular-weight dextran is started at the beginning of microvascular repairs. Near the completion of the vascular repairs, papaverine in saline at 60 units/ml is sprayed on the operative field and anastomoses. A fine, snowy precipitate will be noted. If severe vascular spasm is encountered, papaverine in saline at 6 units/ml is used intraarterially. If further problems with clotting develop, intraarterial streptokinase and urokinase should be available. The smallest-sized Fogarty balloon catheters should also be on hand. Special forms are used to record preoperative, intraoperative, and postoperative data (Figure 125-13).

Text continued on p. 2204

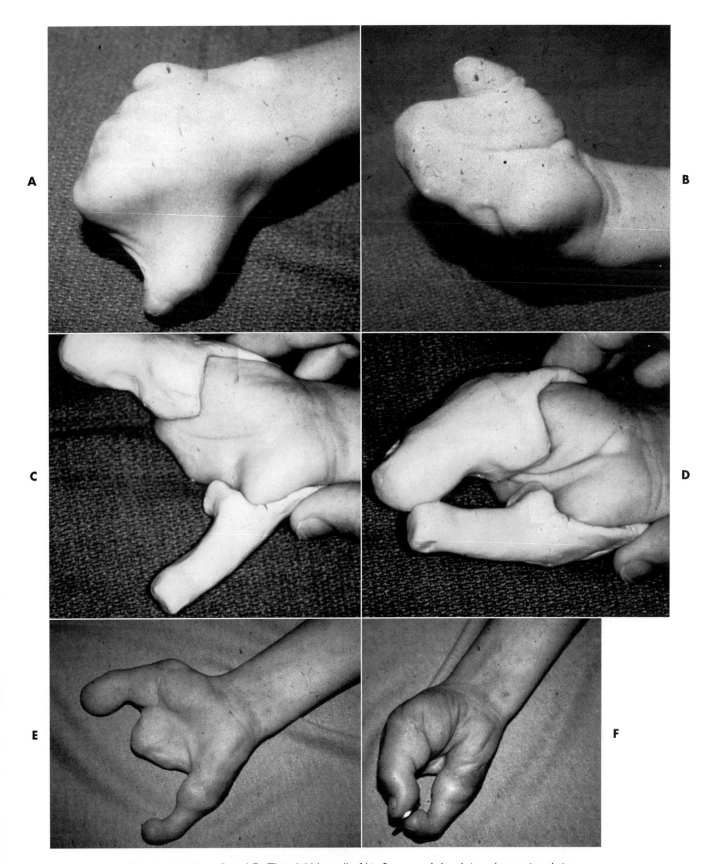

Figure 125-12. **A** and **B,** This child lost all of his fingers and thumb in a devastating chain-saw accident. **C** and **D,** Clay models of the planned right great toe to thumb transplant and second toe to little finger position. The child and the family were able to anticipate the final result. **E** and **F,** Restoring sensation, pinch, and grasp permitted the boy to remain right-hand dominant and to participate in all sporting activities. (From Buncke HJ: *Microsurgery transplantation-replantation: an atlas text,* Philadelphia, 1991, Lea & Febiger.)

MICROVASCULAR FREE TISSUE TRANSFER DATABASE

Rev. '94/1 SIKO

NAME LAST FIRST: [   ]   AGE: [   ]

CHART NUMBER: [   ]   SEX: ○ MALE   ○ FEMALE

ADMISSION DATE: [   ]   DATE OF SURGERY: [   ]

DX: [   ]

ETIOLOGY:

○ UNKNOWN   ○ ACQUIRED IDIOPATHIC
○ CONGENITAL   ○ ACQUIRED INFECTIOUS
○ POST SURGICAL   ○ FAILED FREE FLAP
○ POST TRAUMA WORK   ○ POST RADIOTHERAPY
○ POST TRAUMA NONWORK   ○ BURN/COLD/CHEMICAL
○ NEUROPATHIC/DIABETIC   ○ INADEQUATE FLAP COVER
○ PERIPHERAL VASCULAR   ○ TUMOR
○ GSW   ○ OTHER

EFFECT:

○ SOFT TISSUE DEF. OPEN   ○ MISSING JOINT
○ CONTOUR DEFICIT   ○ MISSING FINGERS
○ CONTRACTURE/UNSTABLE   ○ MISSING THUMB
○ HARD TISSUE DEF. CLOSED   ○ EXPOSED FOREIGN BODY
○ OSTEOMYELITIS   ○ OPEN JOINT
○ SOFT & HARD DEF. OPEN   ○ NEUROMA
○ SENSORY DEFICIENCY   ○ OSTEORADIONECROSIS
○ MOTOR DEFICIENCY   ○ PSEUDOARTHROSIS
○ SENSORY & MOTOR DEFICIENCY ○ LYMPHEDEMA

PREVIOUS TREATMENT: [ ]

FLAP ISCHEMIA TIME: [   ]

DONOR SITE:

○ BIEF   ○ RIB   ○ ADDUCTOR
○ DCIA   ○ SCALP   MAGNUS
○ DELTOPECTORAL   ○ SCAPULAR   ○ ULNAR
○ DORSALIS PEDIS   ○ SECOND TOE   FOREARM
○ EXTENSOR DIGIT. BREVIS ○ SERRATUS ANTERIOR   ○ 4TH TOE
○ FIRST WEB SPACE   ○ SERRATUS ANTERIOR & RIB
○ FIBULA   ○ TEMPOROPARIETAL FASCIA
○ GRACILIS   ○ TENSOR FASCIA LATA
○ GREAT TOE   ○ TOE PULP - N.V. ISLAND
○ GROIN   ○ TRANSFER DIGIT FROM HAND
○ LATERAL ARM   ○ COMBINED LATISSIMUS/SERRATUS
○ LATERAL THORACIC   ○ FREE JOINT/TOE
○ LATISSIMUS DORSI   ○ FREE JOINT/HAND
○ OMENTUM   ○ RETRANSPLANT SECOND TOE
○ PARASCAPULAR   ○ SECOND TOE & DORSALIS PEDIS
○ PECTORALIS MAJOR   ○ POSTERIOR THIGH FLAP
○ RADIAL FOREARM   ○ BOWEL
○ RECTUS ABDOMINIS   ○ A-V FISTULA
○ TRAM   ○ COMPOSITE
○ OSTEO ISLAND/HAND   ○ EN BLOC TOES
○ FIRST WEB SPACE   ○ OSTEO ISLAND/DIGIT

Figure 125-13. A copy of our data sheets for microvascular transplants. *Continued*

MFTTD PAGE 2.

ADDITIONAL TISSUE A:

○ SKIN
○ FASCIA
○ FAT
○ BONE
○ TENDON
○ NERVE
○ JOINT
○ CARTILAGE
○ MUSCLE

ADDITIONAL TISSUE B:

○ SKIN
○ FASCIA
○ FAT
○ BONE
○ TENDON
○ NERVE
○ JOINT
○ CARTILAGE
○ MUSCLE

HOSPITAL & ATTENDINGS INIT.

RECIPIENT SITE:

○ HEAD AND NECK
○ BACK
○ CHEST
○ ABDOMEN
○ UPPER ARM/SHLD
○ ELBOW
○ FOREARM
○ HAND

○ LUMBOSACRAL
○ GENITALIA
○ THIGH
○ KNEE
○ LEG TIB/FIB
○ FOOT/ANKLE
○ LOWER LIMB STUMP
○ UPPER LIMB STUMP

○ PELVIS
○ BUTTOCK

PAST HISTORY A:

○ SMOKING
○ PERIPHERAL VASCULAR (VEN.)
○ PERIPHERAL VASCULAR (ART.)
○ DIABETES
○ MALIGNANCY
○ HYPERTENSION

○ CARDIAC
○ PREVIOUS REPLANT/REVASC
○ RADIATION
○ CLOTTING DISORDER
○ CURRENT REPLANT/REVASC
○ ASTHMA

PAST HISTORY B:

○ SMOKING
○ PERIPHERAL VASCULAR (VEN.)
○ PERIPHERAL VASCULAR (ART.)
○ DIABETES
○ MALIGNANCY
○ HYPERTENSION

○ CARDIAC
○ PREVIOUS REPLANT/REVASC
○ RADIATION
○ CLOTTING DISORDER
○ CURRENT REPLANT/REVASC
○ ASTHMA

MULTIPLE FREE FLAPS:

○ NEITHER   ○ SIMULTANEOUS   ○ SEQUENTIAL   ○ SIMULTANEOUS AND SEQUENTIAL

ANGIO DONOR SITE ▫   ANGIO RECIPIENT SITE ▫

DIAGNOSIS DURATION IN MONTHS:

DIAGNOSIS DURATION IN DAYS:

TIBIAL FRACTURE CLASSIFICATION:

○ I   ○ III/a

○ II   ○ III/b

             ○ III/c

Figure 125-13, cont'd.   A copy of our data sheets for microvascular transplants.   *Continued*

MFTTD PAGE 3.

ETIOLOGY OF TIBIAL FRACTURE:

- ○ UNKNOWN
- ○ MOTORCYCLE
- ○ MVA
- ○ FALL
- ○ GSW
- ○ POSTOP
- ○ PEDESTRIAN/MVA

- ○ EXPLOSION
- ○ BICYCLE/MVA
- ○ SKI
- ○ CRUSH AT WORK
- ○ SHARP
- ○ SURGICAL
- ○ OTHER

CURRENT METHOD OF FIXATION:

- ○ NONE
- ○ PLATE
- ○ SCREWS
- ○ EXTERNAL FIXATOR
- ○ INTRAMEDULLARY ROD

- ○ THREADED PINS
- ○ TRACTION
- ○ IMPACTION/PEG
- ○ UNKNOWN
- ○ OTHER

OF DEBRIDEMENTS: [ ]   # OF SURGERIES: [ ]

OF NERVE REPAIRS: [ ]   # OF NERVE GRAFT: [ ]

LENGTH OF NERVE GRAFT: [ ]   # OF ARTERIAL REPAIRS: [ ]

RECIPIENT ARTERY:

- ○ ANTERIOR TIBIAL
- ○ DORSALIS PEDIS
- ○ POSTERIOR TIBIAL
- ○ PERONEAL
- ○ POPLITEAL
- ○ SUPERFICIAL FEMORAL
- ○ DEEP FEMORAL
- ○ RADIAL
- ○ DORSAL RADIAL
- ○ ULNAR
- ○ MEDIAN
- ○ DIGITAL
- ○ FACIAL
- ○ THYROID

- ○ OCCIPITAL
- ○ BRACHIAL
- ○ SUPERFICIAL TEMPORAL
- ○ FREE FLAP ARTERY
- ○ SUPERIOR TEMPORAL
- ○ TRANSVERSE CERVICAL
- ○ INFERIOR EPIGASTRIC
- ○ ANTERIOR INTEROSSEOUS
- ○ CAROTID
- ○ INTERNAL MAMMARY
- ○ AXILLARY
- ○ SUBCLAVIAN
- ○ THORACOACROMIAL
- ○ OTHER

- ○ EXTERNAL CAROTID
- ○ COMMON DIGITAL
- ○ MEDIAL FEMORAL CIRCUMFLEX
- ○ INFERIOR GLUTEAL
- ○ THORACODORSAL

ARTERIAL ANASTOMOSIS TECHNIQUE:

- ○ END TO END
- ○ END TO SIDE
- ○ GRAFT END TO SIDE

- ○ GRAFT END TO END
- ○ END TO END TO GRAFT
- ○ END TO SIDE TO GRAFT

- ○ END TO END TO FLAP
- ○ END TO SIDE TO FLAP

LENGHT OF A GRAFT: [ ]   A GRAFT PLAN: [ ]

OF VEIN REPAIRS: [ ]   RECIPIENT VENOUS SYSTEM:

○ SUPERFICIAL   ○ DEEP   ○ BOTH

VEIN ANASTOMOSIS TECHNIQUE:

- ○ END TO END
- ○ END TO SIDE
- ○ GRAFT END TO SIDE

- ○ GRAFT END TO END
- ○ END TO END TO GRAFT
- ○ END TO SIDE TO GRAFT

Figure 125-13, cont'd. A copy of our data sheets for microvascular transplants. *Continued*

MFTTD PAGE 4.

LENGTH OF VEIN GRAFT: V GRAFT PLAN:

OPERATIVE TIME:

OSSEOUS FIXATION:

- ○ WIRE LOOP
- ○ K-WIRE
- ○ PLATE
- ○ SCREWS
- ○ MIXED

- ○ EXTERNAL FIXATOR
- ○ CUSTOM TRAY
- ○ K-WIRE/EXTERNAL FIXATOR
- ○ IMPACTION/PEG
- ○ PLATE & SCREWS

- ○ K-WIRE/WIRE LOOP
- ○ ROD
- ○ OTHER

WOUND CLOSURE RECIPIENT:

○ PRIMARY   ○ SECONDARY   ○ LOCAL FLAP   ○ MESH   ○ MIXED

WOUND CLOSURE DONOR:

○ PRIMARY   ○ SECONDARY   ○ LOCAL FLAP   ○ MESH   ○ MIXED

RESULT:

- ○ SUCCESS
- ○ FAILURE

- ○ BOTH/FLAP SUCCESS   LOSS OF LIMB
- ○ UNKNOWN

POSTOPERATIVE DAYS: STAY (DAYS) :

DISPOSITION:

○ HOME   ○ REHAB. FLOOR   ○ OTHER HOSPITAL   ○ GUEST ACCOMMODATION   ○ DIED

CONSULTATIONS A:

- ○ INFECTIOUS DISEASE
- ○ GENERAL/CARDIOLOGY
- ○ PSYCHIATRY
- ○ PEDIATRIC
- ○ NEUROLOGY/NEUROSURGERY
- ○ ORAL SURGERY

- ○ ORTHOPAEDIC
- ○ ENT
- ○ DERMATOLOGY
- ○ OPHTALMOLOGY
- ○ VASCULAR SURGERY
- ○ GENERAL SURGERY

- ○ HEMATOLOGY
- ○ UROLOGY
- ○ OBGYN

CONSULTATIONS B:

- ○ INFECTIOUS DISEASE
- ○ GENERAL/CARDIOLOGY
- ○ PSYCHIATRY
- ○ PEDIATRIC
- ○ NEUROLOGY/NEUROSURGERY
- ○ ORAL SURGERY

- ○ ORTHOPAEDIC
- ○ ENT
- ○ DERMATOLOGY
- ○ OPHTALMOLOGY
- ○ VASCULAR SURGERY
- ○ GENERAL SURGERY

- ○ HEMATOLOGY
- ○ UROLOGY
- ○ OBGYN

CONSULTATIONS C:

- ○ INFECTIOUS DISEASE
- ○ GENERAL/CARDIOLOGY
- ○ PSYCHIATRY
- ○ PEDIATRIC
- ○ NEUROLOGY/NEUROSURGERY
- ○ ORAL SURGERY

- ○ ORTHOPAEDIC
- ○ ENT
- ○ DERMATOLOGY
- ○ OPHTALMOLOGY
- ○ VASCULAR SURGERY
- ○ GENERAL SURGERY

- ○ HEMATOLOGY
- ○ UROLOGY
- ○ OBGYN

Figure 125-13, cont'd. A copy of our data sheets for microvascular transplants. *Continued*

MFTTD PAGE 5.

WOUND PROBLEMS RECIPIENT A:

- ○ PARTIAL LOSS <25%
- ○ PARTIAL LOSS 25-50%
- ○ PARTIAL LOSS 50-75%
- ○ LOSS OF MESH GRAFT
- ○ HEMATOMA/BLEEDING
- ○ SEROMA
- ○ DEHISCENCE
- ○ POSTOP INFECTION

- ○ RECIPIENT DEMARCATION
- ○ PARTIAL LOSS UNDERMINED
- ○ INCOMPLETE COVER
- ○ PRESSURE ULCER
- ○ BLISTERING
- ○ TOURNIQUET COMPLICATION
- ○ INFECTED STSG
- ○ CONGESTION

WOUND PROBLEMS RECIPIENT B:

- ○ PARTIAL LOSS <25%
- ○ PARTIAL LOSS 25-50%
- ○ PARTIAL LOSS 50-75%
- ○ LOSS OF MESH GRAFT
- ○ HEMATOMA/BLEEDING
- ○ SEROMA
- ○ DEHISCENCE
- ○ POSTOP INFECTION

- ○ RECIPIENT DEMARCATION
- ○ PARTIAL LOSS UNDERMINED
- ○ INCOMPLETE COVER
- ○ PRESSURE ULCER
- ○ BLISTERING
- ○ TOURNIQUET COMPLICATION
- ○ INFECTED STSG
- ○ CONGESTION

WOUND PROBLEM DONOR:

- ○ HEMATOMA/BLEEDING
- ○ SEROMA
- ○ POSTOP INFECTION
- ○ DEHISCENCE
- ○ UNDERMINED SKIN NECROSIS

- ○ TRACTION INJURY
- ○ INCOMPLETE COVER
- ○ PRESSURE ULCER
- ○ BLISTERING
- ○ TOURNIQUET COMPLICATION
- ○ INFECTED STSG

PREOP HB: [   ]

PREOP PLATELET: [   ]

POSTOP HB: [   ]

POSTOP PLATELET: [   ]

DISCHARGE HB: [   ]

DISCHARGE PLATELET: [   ]

HIGHEST PLATELET: [   ]

DIAGNOSIS OF FAILURE:

- ○ ARTERIAL
- ○ VENOUS
- ○ COMBINED

- ○ RELATIVE INSUFFICIENCY
- ○ TECHNICALLY IMPOSSIBLE
- ○ UNKNOWN

POSTOP DAY (IF HOUR THEN FRACTION DAY): [   ]

FINDINGS:

- ○ NOT TAKEN BACK
- ○ CLOT AT ANASTOMOSIS
- ○ TWISTED VESSELS
- ○ MISMATCH VESSEL SIZE
- ○ BLEEDING SIDE BRANCH
- ○ TIGHT CLOSURE
- ○ MIXED VESSELS
- ○ INJURED VESSELS

- ○ TECHNICAL PROBLEM NOT I.D.
- ○ DEAD
- ○ AVULSION OF PEDICLE
- ○ HEMATOMA
- ○ POSITIONAL
- ○ NO PROBLEM FOUND
- ○ SMALL VESSELS
- ○ SPASM

- ○ RECIPIENT VEIN HYPERTENSION

Figure 125-13, cont'd. A copy of our data sheets for microvascular transplants. *Continued*

MFTTD PAGE 6.

TREATMENT A:

○ NO TREATMENT
○ REDO OF ANASTOMOSIS
○ GRAFT
○ NEW RECIPIENT VESSEL
○ SYMPATHETIC BLOCK
○ ADVENTITIAL RELEASE
○ LEECH

○ DEBRIDEMENT
○ POSITION CHANGE
○ HEPARIN
○ THROMBECTOMY
○ THROMBOLYTICS
○ HBO
○ MILKING/FOGARTHY

TREATMENT B:

○ NO TREATMENT
○ REDO OF ANASTOMOSIS
○ GRAFT
○ NEW RECIPIENT VESSEL
○ SYMPATHETIC BLOCK
○ ADVENTITIAL RELEASE
○ LEECH

○ DEBRIDEMENT
○ POSITION CHANGE
○ HEPARIN
○ THROMBECTOMY
○ THROMBOLYTICS
○ HBO
○ MILKING/FOGARTHY

RESULT OF ABOVE: ○ SUCCESS   ○ FAILURE   ○ FAIL WITH IMMEDIATE FLAP

TAKE BACKS:

ANTIBIOTICS: ○ NONE   ○ SIMPLE   ○ COMPLEX

ANTIBIOTICS NAME AND GIVEN FROM - TO:

ANTIBIOTIC 1:   FROM: TO:
ANTIBIOTIC 2:   FROM: TO:
ANTIBIOTIC 3:   FROM: TO:
ANTIBIOTIC 4:   FROM: TO:
ANTIBIOTIC 5:   FROM: TO:
ANTIBIOTIC 6:   FROM: TO:
ANTIBIOTIC 7:   FROM: TO:
ANTIBIOTIC 8:   FROM: TO:
ANTIBIOTIC 9:   FROM: TO:
ANTIBIOTIC 10:   FROM: TO:

DURATION ON ANTIBIOTICS:

ASA: ◻   DOSAGE OF ASA:

DURATION ON ASA: TIMING OF ASA: ○ PREOP
                                                      ○ POSTOP

DEXTRAN: ◻   TIMING OF DEXTRAN: ○ PREOP
                                                    ○ INTRAOP
                                                    ○ POSTOP

DURATION ON DEXTRAN:

HEPARIN: ◻   TIMING OF HEPARIN: ○ PREOP
                                                    ○ INTRAOP
                                                    ○ POSTOP

DURATION ON HEPARIN:

Figure 125-13, cont'd.   A copy of our data sheets for microvascular transplants.   *Continued*

MFTTD PAGE 7.

REASON FOR HEPARIN A:

○ CRUSH INJURY
○ INCREASED PLATELETS
○ TECHNICAL DIFFICULTY
○ PROLONGED ISCHEMIA
○ SPASM

○ ASSOCIATED REPLANT
○ DECREASED FLOW
○ CLOTTED VESSEL
○ NONE
○ VEIN GRAFT

REASON FOR HEPARIN B:

○ CRUSH INJURY
○ INCREASED PLATELETS
○ TECHNICAL DIFFICULTY
○ PROLONGED ISCHEMIA
○ SPASM

○ ASSOCIATED REPLANT
○ DECREASED FLOW
○ CLOTTED VESSEL
○ NONE
○ VEIN GRAFT

OTHER DRUGS A:

○ VASODILAN
○ HYPERBARIC OXIGEN
○ SYMPATHETIC BLOCKADE
○ NITROPASTE
○ MINIPRESS

○ STEROID
○ INDERAL
○ PAPAVERINE
○ PERSANTINE
○ OTHER

○ THORASINE
○ NIFEDIPINE
○ CARAFATE
○ DIGOXIN
○ CHLORPROMAZIN

OTHER DRUGS B:

○ VASODILAN
○ HYPERBARIC OXIGEN
○ SYMPATHETIC BLOCKADE
○ NITROPASTE
○ MINIPRESS

○ STEROID
○ INDERAL
○ PAPAVERINE
○ PERSANTINE
○ OTHER

○ THORASINE
○ NIFEDIPINE
○ CARAFATE
○ DIGOXIN

OTHER DRUGS C:

○ VASODILAN
○ HYPERBARIC OXIGEN
○ SYMPATHETIC BLOCKADE
○ NITROPASTE
○ MINIPRESS

○ STEROID
○ INDERAL
○ PAPAVERINE
○ PERSANTINE
○ OTHER

○ THORASINE
○ NIFEDIPINE
○ CARAFATE
○ DIGOXIN

MONITORING A:

○ EXTERNAL DOPPLER
○ FLUORO
○ OXIMETER
○ XENON WASHOUT

○ PH MONITORING
○ LASER DOPPLER
○ BLEEDING

MONITORING B:

○ EXTERNAL DOPPLER
○ FLUORO
○ OXIMETER
○ XENON WASHOUT

○ PH MONITORING
○ LASER DOPPLER
○ BLEEDING

DURATION OF MONITORING:

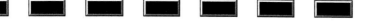

Figure 125-13, cont'd. A copy of our data sheets for microvascular transplants. *Continued*

MFTTD PAGE 8.

COMPLICATIONS NOT RELATED TO THE OP:

○ MEDICAL   ○ COLITIS
○ SURGICAL   ○ MIGRAINE
○ PSYCHIATRIC   ○ OTHER

COMPLICATIONS NOT RELATED TO THE OP:

○ MEDICAL   ○ COLITIS
○ SURGICAL   ○ MIGRAINE
○ PSYCHIATRIC   ○ OTHER

BLOOD USE:

○ NONE   ○ DONOR   ○ DONOR DESIGNATED   ○ AUTOLOGOUS   ○ BOTH

UNITS: _____   DRAIN DONOR SITE: ☐   DRAIN RECIPIENT SITE: ☐

COMMENT:

Figure 125-13, cont'd.   A copy of our data sheets for microvascular transplants.

THE DAY OF SURGERY

The two surgical teams—one each for the hand and foot—should have preliminary discussions, particularly if any unusual anatomic or medical findings are anticipated. The primary surgeon meets with the patient and family members to answer any final questions and to make sure they understand the operative plan. Arrangements are made to give progress reports to family members during these long procedures. We advise family members to stay in touch with our office, which is in the hospital, or to contact the operating room directly for status reports. If problems do develop that will prolong the surgery, a member of the surgical team will contact family members and allay their concerns. Most of our patients are from out of town and their family members stay in guest accommodations in the hospital; often they are more comfortable waiting in these quarters than in the windowless surgical waiting room.

Once the patient is brought to the operating room, the anesthesiologist takes over and the equipment is properly positioned. The donor and recipient fields are prepped simultaneously. Tourniquets that have been pretested for accuracy are placed on the arm and the leg. The anesthesiologist keeps a record of tourniquet time and advises each team as every half hour passes. It is our custom to stop at 2 hours of tourniquet time, deflate the tourniquet, and revascularize the extremity for at least 10 minutes. How long the dissection procedures take can vary considerably, from less than an hour to 2 or more hours, depending on the degree of previous injury, anatomic variations, vascular anomalies, and the experience of the operating teams. The recipient team maintains a list of the vital structures needed (e.g., extensor and flexor tendons, nerves, arteries, and veins) and advises the donor team of the critical lengths required as measured from the proposed synostosis. The "menu" of these measurements is kept on the recipient team's back table.

If a significant branch is encountered while dissecting the vascular pedicles on the venous and arterial sides, a few millimeters of this branch between the clip and the main vessel should be preserved so that the clip can be removed at a later time if problems develop at the anastomosis. This side branch can be used to access catheters to instill heparin, papaverine, or Fogarty balloon catheters.

A member of the original dissecting team from each area must be present on the recipient team once the part is transferred. Personnel changes during surgery are frequent on a teaching service in which everyone is anxious to participate. As with any sort of organized venture, be it an operation, construction job, or a watch at sea, information must be carefully transferred from one individual to another during these changes. The required length of each structure is marked with a dye pen or clip before it is transected. Spots of dye are placed on the upper surface of the arterial and venous pedicles at 1-cm intervals, with the vessels in situ to avoid twisting the pedicle before it is anastomosed. Twisting is seldom a problem on the venous side because it unfolds or unwinds itself as it fills with blood once the arterial side is completed and open. Rotation of the arterial pedicle can create a disaster and may happen under the best of circumstances. Proper rotation must be checked before the first stitch is placed. In addition to noting the dye markings, the surgeon can check for rotation by placing gentle traction on the arterial pedicle. If it rotates in one direction or another, it indicates that the pedicle is twisted. Digital massage and moisture will help to straighten out the pedicle before the anastomosis. A twisted pedicle will usually fill instantly after the repair with no evidence of a problem. However, the twist tightens and migrates distally with each pulsation and finally closes off at the first fixed spot, usually the edge of the wound as the vessel enters the toe.

The bony synostosis is performed before the vascular repairs. The dangling vascular pedicles and other structures must be protected from power tools during the maneuver by wrapping the toe in a moist gauze or lap pad so that only the bony end is exposed. Others recommend placing the toe in a surgical glove and exposing the bone through a small hole. Hand tools are often safer to use and as effective with much of the bone work. Pins are inserted in a retrograde fashion, carefully protecting all structures, and then driven proximally into the recipient bone. A smaller, oblique pin may be added to prevent rotation. The ideal situation exists when the base of the toe can be hollowed out and the remnant of proximal phalanx or metacarpal is placed inside the cortical canal of the great-toe transplant. If the articular cartilage is preserved on the thumb metacarpal or distal joint of the thumb in which only the distal phalanx is being transplanted, a compound joint of toe and thumb can be created. Even though the articular surface of the toe might be larger than the thumb, the contours are almost anatomically perfect. Such compound joints function well.

Once the synostosis is complete, arterial repair commences, with the surgeon again ensuring that the vascular pedicle has not rotated. A moderate amount of tension is acceptable because most vessels elongate once they become filled with blood; this is particularly noticeable on the venous side. However, if there is any unusual tension, an interpositional graft is safer than a procedure performed under tension. In some situations, it may be technically easier to repair the flexor tendon before the arterial repair. The flexor tendon repair should be performed as far away as possible from the level of replantation to prevent secondary scarring. The flexor tendon can be cut well back in the sole of the foot or picked up at the medial malleolus, where it is the most posterior structure. This dissection may be difficult because the tendon is not only posterior but also deeply situated behind neurovascular structures. Occasionally, the surgeon will not be able to pull the flexor pollicis tendon out of the foot. This indicates that juncturae are present between the long flexor and the common toe flexors. When this occurs, these juncturae must be cut blindly with long scissors while placing traction on the totally immobilized toe. Because flexor and extensor tendon lengths are seldom a problem, Pulvertaft weaves or similar repairs can be performed, which permit early active and passive motion. Stellate blocks help to prevent vascular spasm and also permit early mobilization of joints and tendons without pain. The fibrin clot that forms between the tendon sheath and joint capsules can be quite firm with the block. It should be broken loose on the first day postoperatively after a block to hasten the mobilization process. Once the vascular and tendon structures have been approximated, the nerves are repaired with precision because restoration of sensory function is so important. As mentioned earlier, wound closure must be accomplished without tension. Ideally, skin flaps should be adjusted so that they cover the vascular repairs and pedicles, but skin grafts can be used freely over vascular grafts and pedicles, if necessary.

The postoperative wound dressing must be loose and splinting must be simple to keep the transplant in an apposed, abducted position.

The major intraoperative problems are vascular spasm, intravascular platelet agglutination, clot formation, and failure to get a completed vascular circuit. A meticulously completed repair should not leak. If the repair does leak, it is better to replace the vascular clamps and carefully note the position of the leak, and then insert additional stitches. Operating on a leaking vessel without clamps in a bloody field is difficult, and inaccurate suture placement may result.

Should platelet clots or intravascular clotting occur, the anastomosis must be taken down or a side branch opened to permit removal of the clots with the smallest Fogarty catheter, a #2 French, which is 0.67 mm in diameter. When inflated with the recommended 0.2 ml of fluid, the balloon has a diameter of 4 mm. With small vessels, the balloon size must be reduced to permit a pulling force of 0.5 pounds or less. Care must be taken to prevent distal propagation of the clots into the transplant on the arterial side by clamping the vessel proximal to the clot. If appreciable problems are encountered, it is wise to flush the transplant with streptokinase or urokinase to clean out any fibrin or platelet clots that may have slipped into the transplant and to help to clear out the stagnant capillary bed. Streptokinase comes in various concentrations. We prefer the 250,000-unit vial, which is reconstituted with 5 ml of saline, or approximately 50,000 units/ml. One milliliter of this is diluted in 10 ml of saline to provide 5000 units/ml. Five to 10 ml are infused slowly into the transplant, depending on its size. Once in a general circulation, the 25,000 to 50,000 units have a minimal systemic effect but are very effective locally within the transplant.[2] Urokinase comes in a similar 250,000-unit vial, which must be reconstituted with sterile water for injection before dilution to 5000 units/ml with saline. Situations may develop where flow cannot be reestablished and long interpositional grafts are needed on both the arterial and the venous sides of the pedicle. It is difficult to explain these problems physiologically, but on several occasions transplants and replants have been salvaged using long grafts.

It is our present regimen to place a 1-mm Doppler probe on the cardiac side of the venous anastomosis so that continuous outflow from the transplant can be monitored.[14,24] This Doppler is held on the vessel wall with a cuff

of Vicryl mesh that is loosely clipped in a tubular fashion with small Hemoclips. The 1-mm Doppler is passed through a hole created in a 1-cm square of Vicryl mesh with a micro forceps. The hole tends to contract so that the Doppler probe does not fall out easily. The mesh is folded around the vein in a tubular fashion and loosely clipped with two small Hemoclips. Once this probe is properly aligned and a good signal is established, the small wires are sutured in several spots in the wound, brought out proximally, and secured to the skin, looping the wires and stapling them securely to the proximal extremity. The Doppler probe must be placed so that the venous signal is not dampened or overpowered by an adjacent arterial signal. When these probes function properly, they provide secure, continuous monitoring of the circulation that gives the patient, nursing staff, and all others involved a sense of security. When the signal disappears, the staff must check all connections before going immediately back to the operating room to explore the repairs and solve the problem. We have used these probes in over 100 cases and have been able to salvage 80% of cases that had to go back for additional surgery. Before use of the probe, the salvage rate for additional surgery was 50%.

The postoperative orders for all patients who undergo replant and/or transplant surgeries are similar and are designed to prevent platelet agglutination and clotting with dextran and aspirin (Figure 125-14). When complications develop, intravenous heparin is added at 500 to 1000 units/hour as a continuous drip and modulated by the partial thromboplastin time (PTT), which we like to have at twice the normal rate. Optimally, with the PTT in the range of 50% to 100% of normal, minimal bleeding occurs at the wound site. Unfortunately, heparin is a double-edged sword. It has a strong vasoplegic effect in addition to its anticlotting qualities. However, bleeding at all wound surfaces may develop, necessitating repeated transfusions. In addition, once the patient is placed on heparin for a complication, this must be continued for 7 to 10 days. In some cases, the patient is prescribed warfarin sodium to take at home after discharge. All patients are sent to the critical care unit (CCU) for a day or two after replant or transplant surgery so they can receive one-on-one supervision. The rooms must be kept warm. A heating pad is placed over a sterile towel on the transplant.

When all goes well, the patient is moved to a step-down unit on the second day and then to the regular floor on the third day. The dextran is discontinued after 5 days in uncomplicated cases, and the patient is mobilized and ambulatory by 7 to 10 days.

Vascular spasm, as we have repeatedly mentioned, is a problem more severe in young children and women. This is a natural response to injury, and the body's protective devices must be modified to keep these small vessels open. We use chlorpromazine to tranquilize the patient and for its antiserotonin effect.[3] Unfortunately, this tends to lower blood pressure. Additionally, rare central nervous system idiosyncratic responses can be quite bizarre and alarming in nature, such as spiking fevers and personality changes.

SURGICAL PROCEDURE: #1 _____

#2 _____

#3 _____

AFTER RECOVERY, PATIENT TO GO TO: ☐ CRITICAL CARE ☐ FLOOR

DIET/I&O/DRAINS

☐ NPO   ☐ NPO, ADVANCE TO _____

☐ RECORD I&O Q8 HRS × _____ DAYS.

☐ FOLEY TO GRAVITY   D/C FOLEY: ☐ NOW   ☐ IN AM

☐ RECORD DRAIN OUTPUTS Q8HRS.

☐ DRAIN #1: TYPE _____ LOC _____ TO _____ SUCTION

☐ DRAIN #2: TYPE _____ LOC _____ TO _____ SUCTION

☐ DRAIN #3: TYPE _____ LOC _____ TO _____ SUCTION

☐ DRAIN #4: TYPE _____ LOC _____ TO _____ SUCTION

☐ OTHER DRAIN _____

VITAL SIGNS/ACTIVITY/POSITIONING

V/S PER   ☐ POST-OP PROTOCOL   ☐ CCU PROTOCOL   ☐ Q _____ H

☐ BEDREST   ☐ BEDREST-BRP W/ASSIST   ☐ BEDREST-COMMODE W/ASSIST

☐ UP IN CHAIR W/ASSIST   ☐ UP AD LIB

☐ ELEVATE _____ ON PILLOWS ABOVE HEART LEVEL AT ALL TIMES.

CHECKS

☐ CHECK COLOR, TEMP, TURGOR, CAPILLARY REFILL TO _____

Q1H × 24H, THEN Q _____ H.

☐ FLUORESCEIN CHECK TO _____

☐ Q2H × 24H, Q4H × 48H   OR   ☐ Q _____ H

☐ DOPPLER CHECK TO _____

☐ Q2H × 24H, Q4H × 48H   OR   ☐ Q _____ H

☐ CALL MD IF URINE OUTPUT < 30CC/HR × 2 CONSECUTIVE HRS.

☐ CALL MD IF TEMP > 38^5, P < 60 OR > 120, SBP < 100 OR DBP > 100.

☐ OTHER CHECK _____

SPECIAL INSTRUCTIONS

☐ KEEP PT. WARM, OUT OF DRAFTS AND NO OPEN WINDOWS AT ALL TIMES.

☐ INSTRUCT NO SMOKING/SMOKE EXPOSURE.

☐ COUGH AND DEEP BREATHE Q1H WHILE AWAKE.

☐ INCENTIVE SPIROMETER AT BEDSIDE.

☐ OTHER _____

DRESSINGS

☐ STERILE TOWEL AND K-PAD OVER DRESSING.

☐ DO NOT CHANGE DRESSING.

☐ CHANGE DRESSING TO _____ W/ _____ Q _____ HR.

☐ HEPARIN SOAKED SPONGE TO NAILBED Q _____ HR.

☐ HEAT LAMP/DRYER TO SPLIT THICKNESS SKIN GRAFT DONOR SITE × 15 MIN Q2 HR UNTIL DRY.

☐ OTHER _____

✚ DAVIES MEDICAL CENTER

MICROSURGERY POST-OP ORDERS

NUR-120 (3/4/95)

Figure 125-14. A copy of our postoperative orders.   *Continued*

LABS/RADIOLOGY

CBC   □ IN PAR   □ IN AM   □ QD × 3 DAYS

CHEM 7   □ IN PAR   □ IN AM   □ QD × 3 DAYS

□ PLASMA PTT QD WHILE ON HEPARIN.

□ X-RAY _____

□ OTHER _____

IV THERAPY

□ 10% DEXTRAN 40/D5W 500 CC AT _____ CC/HR (In adults, 25cc/hr. Otherwise 8-10cc/kg/24 hrs.)

□ D5/0.45% NACL 1000 CC AT _____ CC/HR

□ D5/0.45% NACL 1000 CC WITH _____ MEQ KCL AT _____ CC/HR

□ LAC. RINGERS 1000 CC AT _____ CC/HR

□ HEPARIN 25,000 U/D5W 500 CC AT _____ U/HR OR □ TITRATE TO PTT.

□ OTHER IV_____

□ TKO IV WHEN TOLERATING PO FLUIDS WELL.

□ HEPLOCK IV WHEN TOLERATING PO FLUIDS WELL.

MEDICATION

□ FLUORESCEIN 10% 1 ML IV   □ Q2 HR × 24 HR, Q4 HR × 48 HR   OR   □ Q_____ HR

□ FLUORESCEIN 10% 0.5 ML IV   □ Q2 HR × 24 HR, Q4 HR × 48 HR   OR   □ Q_____ HR

□ MORPHINE SO4 INJ _____ TO _____ MG, SLOW IV, Q2-3 HR, PRN, PAIN

□ MORPHINE SO4 INJ _____ TO _____ MG, IM, Q2-3 HR, PRN, PAIN

□ SEE PCA ORDER SHEET

□ VICODIN 5-500 MG, 1-2 TABS, Q4-6 HR, PRN, PAIN

□ ACETAMINOPHEN 300 MG + COD .30 MG, 1-2 TABS, Q3-4 HR, PRN, PAIN

□ PROCHLORPERAZINE 10 MG, Q6H, IM or PER RECTUM, PRN, NAUSEA

□ CHLORPROMAZINE _____ (10 mg, PO or IM, q8h in adults)

□ ASA   □ 325 MG, PO or PR, QD   □ 81 MG, PO or PR, QD

□ DOCUSATE SODIUM 100 MG, PO, BID

□ RESTORIL 15-30 MG, PO QHS, PRN, SLEEP

□ CEFAZOLIN 1 GM, IV MINI, Q8H

□ OTHER MED _____

CONSULTS

□ OT/HAND THERAPY EVAL. AND TREAT. START _____ / _____ / _____ .

□ SOCIAL SERVICES CONSULT

□ CHECK WITH DR. _____ FOR:

    □ INSULIN MANAGEMENT

    □ CARDIAC MEDS

    □ RESPIRATORY MEDS

    □ SPECIFIC DIET

    □ OTHER_____

SIGNATURE: _____ , M.D.   DATE _____ / _____ / _____ .

Figure 125-14, cont'd. A copy of our postoperative orders.

SECONDARY PROCEDURES

The most common secondary procedure after toe transplantation is tenolysis. Osteotomies to improve position of the transplant are also not uncommon. Secondary neurolysis and nerve grafts are occasionally needed if satisfactory, useful sensation does not return.

OUTCOMES

The functional results of toe transplants for thumb reconstruction are usually very good.[7] We believe it is one of the most useful and satisfactory reconstructive microsurgical procedures we perform. The recent survival rate for all great-toe transplants is 98%. Sensation of a useful, protective nature is restored with two-point touch of 8 mm or less in 80% of cases. Flexion of the distal interphalangeal joint, which is so important for grip and grasp, varies from 10 degrees to 90 degrees and is most successful in patients who have had the compound toe–thumb joint capsule reconstruction. Most patients are able to return to their previous activity and work with restoration of 80% of grip on the dominant or nondominant side.[26] For patients who have had multiple injuries in addition to loss of the thumb, rehabilitation counseling and retraining are often necessary.

As we have mentioned repeatedly, loss of the toe does not compromise foot function, with the exception of specialized maneuvers needed for activities such as rock-climbing, professional skating, and professional dancing. Many patients return to their previous type of sport and work activities. Some of our patients have competed professionally in various sports after successful transplantation. One such patient, an Ecuadorian student who played for Ecuador's national soccer team, later went on to medical school and is now a practicing surgeon.

Patient satisfaction is high. However, we have had one instance in which a patient failed to develop useful function and had persistent pain in spite of excellent anatomic structures and surgical results. With all such reconstructive procedures, psychological problems may be encountered. Careful preoperative evaluation may alert the surgeon to the type of individual who is not a candidate for this type of surgery.

ACKNOWLEDGMENTS

This manuscript was sponsored by Mr. Frank Hoffman and by the Microsurgical Transplantation Research Foundation.

We wish to thank Matina Coulouris, Executive Academic Secretary, for her assistance in preparing the manuscript.

REFERENCES

1. Acland R: Notes on the handling of ultrafine suture material, *Surgery* 77:507-511, 1975.
2. Belkin M, Belkin B, Bucknam CA, et al: Intra-arterial fibrinolytic therapy: efficacy of streptokinase vs. urokinase, *Arch Surg* 121:769-773, 1986.
3. Buncke HJ, Blackfield HM: The vasoplegic effects of chlorpromazine, *Plast Reconstr Surg* 31:353-362, 1963.
4. Buncke HJ, Buncke CM, Schulz WP: Immediate Nicoladoni procedure in the Rhesus monkey, or hallux-to-hand transplantation, utilising microminiature vascular anastomoses, *Br J Plast Surg* 19:332-337, 1966.
5. Buncke HJ, McLean DH, George PT, et al: Thumb replacement: great toe transplantation by microvascular anastomosis, *Br J Plast Surg* 26:194-201, 1973.
6. Buncke HJ, Schulz WP: Total ear reimplantation in the rabbit utilising microminiature vascular anastomoses, *Br J Plast Surg* 19:15-22, 1966.
7. Buncke HJ, Valauri FA, Buncke GM: Great toe-to-hand transfer. In Meyer VE, Black MJM (editors): *Microsurgical procedures: the hand and upper limb,* New York, 1991, Churchill Livingstone.
8. Campbell Reid DA: Reconstruction of the thumb, *J Bone Joint Surg* 42B:444-465, 1960.
9. Cobbett JR: Free digital transfer: report of a case of transfer of a great toe to replace an amputated thumb, *J Bone Joint Surg* 51B:677-679, 1969.
10. Davis JE: Toe to hand transfers (pedochyrodactyloplasty), *Plast Reconstr Surg* 33:422-436, 1964.
11. Gordon L, Rosen J, Alpert BS, Buncke HJ: Free microvascular transfer of second toe ray and serratus anterior muscle for management of thumb loss at the carpometacarpal joint level, *J Hand Surg [Am]* 9:642-644, 1984.
12. Hing DN, Buncke HJ, Alpert BS: Applications of the extensor digitorum brevis muscle for soft tissue coverage, *Ann Plast Surg* 19:530-537, 1987.
13. Kelleher JE, Sullivan JG: Thumb reconstruction by digit transplantation, *Plast Reconstr Surg* 21:470-478, 1958.
14. Kind GM, Buncke GM, Newlin L, et al: Implantable, absorbable Doppler probe monitoring of microvascular tissue transplants. In *Plastic Surgery Forum* (65th Annual Scientific Meeting of American Society of Plastic and Reconstructive Surgeons, Plastic Surgery Educational Foundation and American Society of Maxillofacial Surgeons), Chicago, 1996, The Society.
15. Littler JW: Neurovascular pedicle method of digital transposition for reconstruction of the thumb, *Plast Reconstr Surg* 12:303-319, 1953.
16. Littler JW: Neurovascular pedicle transfer of tissue in reconstructive surgery of the hand, *J Bone Joint Surg* 38A:917, 1956.
17. McDonald HD, Buncke HJ, Goodstein WA: Split-thickness skin grafts in microvascular surgery, *Plast Reconstr Surg* 68:731-736, 1981.
18. Morrison WA, O'Brien BMC, MacLeod AM: Thumb reconstruction with free neurovascular wraparound flap from the big toe, *J Hand Surg [Am]* 5:575-583, 1980.
19. Nicoladoni C: Daumenplastik und orgaischer ersatz der fingerspitze: Anticheiroplastik und daktylo-plastik, *Arch Klin Chir* 61: 606, 1900.
20. Östrup LT, Berggren A: The Unilink instrument system for fast and safe microvascular anastomosis, *Ann Plast Surg* 17:521-525, 1986.
21. Poppen NK, Mann RA, O'Konski M, Buncke HJ: Amputation of the great toe, *Foot Ankle* 1:333-337, 1981.
22. Roullet J: Translocoflan d'une main. In Tubiana R (editor): *Traité de Chirurgie de la Main,* Paris, 1980, Masson.
23. Schreiber GB, Busch MP, Kleinman SH, et al: The risk of transfusion-transmitted viral infections: the retrovirus epidemiology donor study, *New Engl J Med* 334:1685-1690, 1996.

24. Swartz WM, Jones NJ, Cherup L, et al: Direct monitoring of microvascular anastomoses with the 20-mHZ ultrasonic Doppler probe: an experimental and clinical study, *Plast Reconstr Surg* 81(2):149-161, 1988.

25. Thurston JB, Buncke HJ, Chater NL, et al: A scanning electron microscopy study of microarterial damage and repair, *Plast Reconstr Surg* 57:197-203, 1976.

26. Valauri FA, Buncke HJ: Thumb reconstruction: great toe transfer, *Clin Plast Surg* 16:475-489, 1989.

27. Wilson CS, Buncke HJ, Alpert BS, et al: Composite metacarpophalangeal joint reconstruction in great toe-to-hand free tissue transfers, *J Hand Surg [Am]* 9:645-649, 1984.

CHAPTER

Pollicization

126

Nicolas Sastre
Hector Arambula

INDICATIONS

OVERVIEW

The mechanics of the human thumb distinguish man from other classifications of life because of its ability to oppose the other fingers. Thumb opposition and the superiority of man's intelligence are responsible for our advanced civilization. An opposable thumb allows the human hand to assume two prehensile working postures known as *power grip* and *precision grip,* which are required in many types of work. A mutilating thumb injury poses a significant problem because the lack of opposing hand function eliminates the ability to grasp large and small objects. Thus thumb reconstruction represents an important challenge for surgeons who practice hand surgery. As defined by most insurance companies, a hand deprived of the thumb loses approximately 40% of its function and corresponds to a total body loss of 22%, which in terms of disability is similar to the loss of an eye.[48]

In the past, thumb reconstruction was considered a miracle, but today it is possible to replace the thumb's form and function. Many surgeons have been inspired to direct their skills toward the goal of enabling a patient to return to work and social life.

There are two types of thumb loss: *congenital* and *traumatic.* Blauth[2] classified congenital hypoplasia according to five grades, and pollicization is the preferred treatment for grades three, four, and five. There are two categories of traumatic thumb loss: loss of intermediate thumb segments and amputation at different levels. The loss of intermediate segments usually requires some kind of flap coverage and bony reconstruction with corticocancellous bone grafts to restore stability and length. The loss of thumb length from amputation can significantly interfere with hand function. Emergency replantation should be considered for all thumb amputations proximal to the base of the distal phalanx. Digital arteries and veins distal to this level are difficult to identify. Replantation may also be impossible when a thumb has been severely crushed or avulsed, with accompanying injury to long segments of the digital arteries and nerves. The surgeon should discuss thumb reconstruction with the patient within the first days or weeks after an injury if immediate replantation cannot be successfully accomplished. If a patient begins to accept the loss of a thumb, incorporating a new thumb into his or her body image will be difficult and may compromise the outcome of later reconstruction.

Several methods of thumb reconstruction may be used if replantation is impossible or fails. The surgeon must be aware of these various methods, including the benefits and drawbacks of each procedure. Thumb reconstruction can be accomplished by progressive elongation of the first metacarpal (distraction),[19] osteoplastic reconstruction with a retrograde osteocutaneous forearm flap,[21] pollicization,[3,27,28,46,49] and microsurgical transfer of a toe.[7,15,29]

Pollicization was first performed a century ago by Guermonprez, a French surgeon who introduced the concept of transposition pollicization of a digit after initial studies on monkeys.[16] He used a multistage technique involving retained skin bridges, which strictly limited the arch of transposition. The technique obviously did not maintain the integrity of tendons, muscles, and nerves. Nicoladoni,[40] an Austrian surgeon, pioneered osteoplastic reconstruction of the thumb with a pectoral skin flap and bone graft at the turn of the century. The procedure was considered unsuccessful because it resulted in poor sensation and circulation. Nicoladoni subsequently suggested the use of a second toe transplant as a flap. In 1900 he reported two successful pedicle toe transfers for thumb reconstruction.[41]

In 1918 Joyce[23] performed thumb reconstruction in three patients by transferring the contralateral ring finger as a cross-hand pedicle flap. In 1919 Noesske[42] transferred an index finger to the thumb position without disturbing its intact muscles and nerves. He described an operative technique not found in the literature at that time. In the same year Kleinschmidt,[25] from Germany, described another method involving parts of unneeded or disabled fingers from the damaged hand. His method reported the delayed transfer of a damaged long finger to the thumb remnant of the same hand. In 1923 Dunlop[11] successfully transferred a disabled index finger into the thumb position, but the functional result would have been better if he had used a more normal index finger. In 1931 Bunnell[8] published a case of thumb reconstruction involving a second metacarpal, the proximal phalanx, and its neurovascular pedicle. This new thumb was perhaps the first to have good sensation and acceptable function.

In 1937 Iselin[22] emphasized that "transposition of the adjacent digit into a thumb position is the preferable method for thumb restoration but the finger of choice for transfer must be determined by the general condition of the hand." Gosset,[13] influenced by Iselin and Bunnell, converted the index finger transfer into a true island flap, but amputated the distal phalanx rather than the proximal metacarpal skeleton to adjust length. Hilgenfeldt[20] treated patients with thumb injuries sustained during World War II and chose to reconstruct them with a transfer of the long finger. After World War II, Bunnell,[9] Littler,[30] and others[4,5] progressively developed digital transfers by the neurovascular pedicle method for traumatic and congenital thumb loss. These authors described a very clear and sophisticated operative technique that typically involved transfer of the index finger. Some authors also consider pollicization worthwhile as an elective method for restoring a lost thumb.*

In selected cases, pollicization remains a good method for restoring thumb function in adults after injury. Thumb reconstruction aims to obtain, within a reasonable time, a thumb with an aesthetic appearance and function that are as close to normal as possible, with minimum donor-site morbidity. The appearance of the hand after reconstruction is a secondary consideration to its function. However, the restoration of an opposing thumb provides the damaged hand with a better image.

The arguments in favor of index finger pollicization, as proposed by Littler,[30,31] are very convincing, and the procedure is particularly recommended in cases of congenital absence. Children with a congenital absence of the thumb have a natural tendency to attempt opposition using their index finger against the three remaining fingers. Transfer of part of the intrinsic muscles may be possible by saving the metacarpophalangeal (MCP) joint and transforming it into a carpometacarpal joint. Buck-Gramcko[4,5] used a modification of this procedure in cases of congenital absence, based on the aforementioned arguments.

This generally accepted method of pollicization has undergone several modifications.[31,34] Many surgeons prefer index finger pollicization for treatment of congenital absence.[5,12,18,26] Others have developed alternative techniques that involve the transposition of other fingers in place of the index finger. Kelleher[24] transferred the fifth digit; Gosset[14] and Langlais[27] used the ring finger; Weinzweig[49] transposed the middle or the ring finger, and Merle[37] performed long-finger pollicization. However, pollicization of the index finger has remained a first choice for reconstruction for many years. This procedure is advantageous because a neighboring digit is used (which provides more normal sensation, motion, and strength) and also because loss of the index finger causes less of a donor-site problem.[30] Pollicization can be performed in selected patients, even in emergency situations, but this technique requires good knowledge of reconstructive hand surgery.[46]

---

*References 3, 27, 28, 37, 38, 46, 49.

A traumatic thumb amputation that affects one or more hand structures (including bone, muscle, skin, and vascular elements) requires the surgeon to make the following diagnostic considerations:

1. If vascular injury is suspected, an angiogram should be performed to determine the extent of vessel damage. A Doppler venous study can give a false impression because blood flow into the finger may be present from the palmar intermetacarpal arteries rather than from the common digital artery originating from the palmar arch. Venous access must made be through the femoral artery—never through direct puncture of the brachial artery—to avoid further compromise of the local circulation during this diagnostic procedure.

2. Severe crush injuries or burns may result in loss of skin and/or subcutaneous tissue in the first web space. This can result in an adduction contracture of the first ray, which decreases thumb function. The first web space may require release, including release of the adductor pollicis muscle, and the soft tissue defect may require reconstruction with a flap or split-thickness skin graft before thumb reconstruction. Lister[28] reported that 37% of 19 pollicizations required transposition of a groin flap to provide adequate soft tissue before thumb reconstruction.

3. Flexion of the new thumb may depend on the muscle strength of the index flexor profundus tendon. Lister[28] reported only 47% active motion, compared with the opposite, "normal" side, after index pollicization because of a lack of tendon excursion. To improve motion, he suggested that the profundus tendon of the transposed distal index finger be divided and connected at the wrist level to the flexor pollicis longus (FPL) of the thumb. This procedure gives more strength and better flexion and retains cerebral cortex orientation during flexion of the new thumb.

When patients are seen after an acute injury with a healed partial or complete thumb amputation, the surgeon is given time to reflect and develop the best reconstructive plan. Three fundamental factors that must be appreciated because they play a decisive role in the final outcome include: (1) amputation level, (2) the state of the remaining digits, and (3) the condition of the patient.

AMPUTATION LEVEL

The thumb includes the entire first ray. The treatment plan for reconstruction is different when the amputation is at the level of the phalanx rather than through the metacarpal base. Regardless of the technique that is chosen, the movements of abduction, adduction, flexion, and extension, and the combinations of these motions that allow opposition must be recovered.

We separate thumb amputations into two categories: *subtotal* and *total* (Figure 126-1). A thumb amputation is considered subtotal when it is through the distal first metacarpal or distal to that level. Such amputations may be in the diaphysis or distal metaphysis, proximal to the MCP joint,

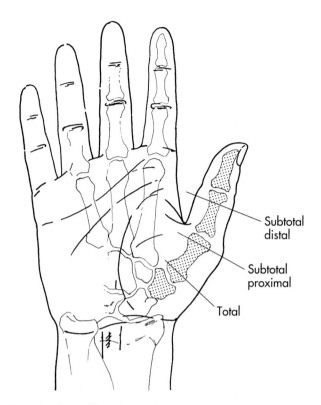

Figure 126-1. Three levels of amputation best suited for finger pollicization. In cases of total amputation, no functional thenar muscles are available to create opposition.

in the joint itself, or through the proximal phalanx distal to the MCP joint. The intrinsic thumb muscles, the first web space, and the carpometacarpal (CMC) joint are preserved. A thumb amputated at this level is not functional; patients with such amputations find it impossible to grasp small objects (e.g., pick up a button or pin or other small item). The patient's ability to grasp larger objects depends on the quality of the skin cover and the amount of scar tissue present. If good skin cover is present, it is possible to elongate the first ray and/or deepen the first web space to create a prehensile digit and space against which the fingers can grasp larger objects. The distance over which the thumb can be lengthened by distraction depends on the amount and quality of the remaining bone and the quality of the soft tissue coverage.

An amputation is considered total when it involves the base of the metacarpal or the CMC joint. None of the thenar eminence muscles, which confer stability and rotation to the thumb, are present. This kind of injury is similar to a congenital thumb deformity.

It is important to emphasize that it is not necessary for a thumb to have normal length to be useful. It must be stable and painless, and ideally it should be covered by glabrous skin with normal tactile sensation. A thumb with an amputation at the distal phalanx may be useful in some workers if fine precision pinch is not necessary. The more proximal the amputation, the more serious the injury. Thus during the emergency care of a patient with a thumb amputation it is important to save even a very short stump of the first metacarpal and as much as possible of the thenar musculature.

Littler[33] states that "sacrifice of a normal finger for a phalangeal-only thumb loss is extravagantly injudicious. The one-stage composite toe osteoplastic method of reconstruction is now the procedure of choice." Most amputated thumbs are amputated distal to the MCP joint. When reconstruction at this level is deemed worthwhile, index-finger pollicization is not a first choice unless there is concomitant injury to the index finger that is likely to result in less than optimal function; in such cases part or all of the index finger may be available for thumb reconstruction. Some type of thumb reconstruction is generally considered appropriate for amputations proximal to the middle portion of the proximal phalanx. Throughout the history of hand surgery many reconstructive techniques have been proposed for such amputations, including procedures to elongate the first ray with bone grafts or by means of sliding osteotomy, procedures involving weeks of distraction followed by secondary bone grafting into the gap, and classic osteoplastic reconstruction with a tubed pedicle flap and bone grafts. Currently two main techniques are used for thumb reconstruction: great or second toe-to-thumb transfer and pollicization of a normal finger.

Amputations through or distal to the MCP joint involve loss of only the extrinsic flexor and extensor tendons. More proximal amputations result in loss of intrinsic muscle insertions and/or their muscle bellies, leaving only the abductor pollicis longus (APL) attached to the base of the first metacarpal. Digital pollicization of the index finger brings with it six motor units that can largely replace all lost muscle function. Toe-to-hand transfers only restore the lost extrinsic muscles. When the CMC joint of the thumb is destroyed, pollicization is the only procedure that can restore that joint, because the hyperextended MCP joint of the transposed finger functions well as a basal joint. Thus it is important to determine the functional capacity of all residual thumb elements, including the intrinsic muscles of the thenar eminence, and the quality of skin cover before choosing the best method of reconstruction.

Pollicization of the index finger is preferred because it can be performed without a palmar scar. The flexor and extensor tendons usually shorten by themselves and do not require repair. The digital nerves and vessels are dissected intact and do not require the risk of microvascular anastomoses. Many authors believe that a damaged or partially amputated finger should be used for thumb reconstruction when other normal or less-injured fingers are present.[28,30,49] The damaged finger can be used because the thumb is shorter than all the other fingers, and although mobility is important at the trapeziometacarpal joint, it is less important at the MCP and interphalangeal (IP) joint levels (Figure 126-2). Occasionally, satisfactory index-finger function is preserved after damage or partial amputation of the long or ring fingers, making those fingers the best candidates for transposition. Pollicization of injured long- or ring-finger remnants has not received much attention in the literature. These comparatively useless digital stumps can be sacrificed without significant functional deficit to the rest of the hand and may be used to create a thumb with satisfactory function during a single operation.

A, B

C

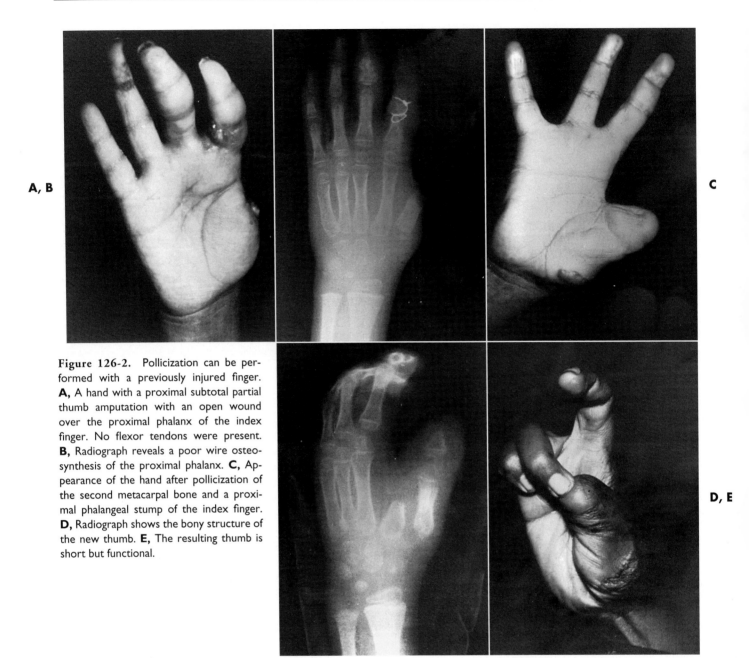

D, E

Figure 126-2. Pollicization can be performed with a previously injured finger. **A,** A hand with a proximal subtotal partial thumb amputation with an open wound over the proximal phalanx of the index finger. No flexor tendons were present. **B,** Radiograph reveals a poor wire osteosynthesis of the proximal phalanx. **C,** Appearance of the hand after pollicization of the second metacarpal bone and a proximal phalangeal stump of the index finger. **D,** Radiograph shows the bony structure of the new thumb. **E,** The resulting thumb is short but functional.

PATIENT CONSIDERATIONS

The patient's occupation, aesthetic desires, and functional requirements are very important and must be considered when choosing the best option for thumb reconstruction. Narrowing of the hand after a pollicization procedure may pose a problem for a manual worker, and loss of a great toe after a thumb reconstruction involving a toe-to-hand transfer may pose a problem for an athletic patient. Age is also a factor that greatly influences the choice of reconstruction. Young patients with open epiphyses ideally require a procedure with growth potential; thus whole-toe transfer or pollicization is preferred.

Loss of a thumb deprives the hand of refined prehension and opposition. The major aim of any reconstruction is to create a new thumb that functions as normally as possible and is aesthetically acceptable. It is important to present to the patient the possible options for reconstruction, including the risks and benefits of each procedure, and to know the patient's opinion of each approach. We are currently very enthusiastic about performing toe-to-thumb reconstruction. However, a patient with a thumb amputation may not wish to lose a toe and, consequently, we must offer pollicization as a secure, predictable, and functional alternative.

Selection of a method for reconstruction, according to Gu,[15] is based on age, patient activities, the degree and nature of thumb damage, the level of the amputation, and the general local condition of the remaining hand structures. The vascular supply to the foot is evaluated clinically by Doppler and/or arteriographical studies. An

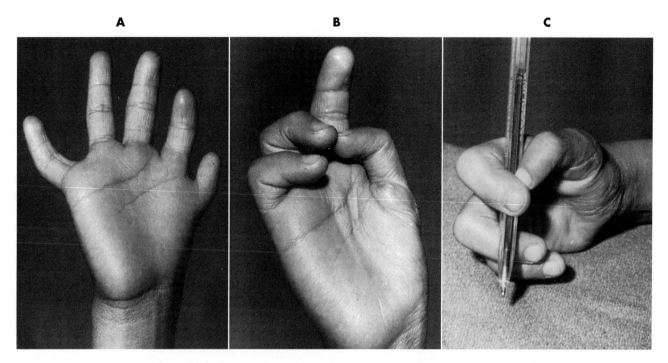

Figure 126-3. A, A thumb with congenital Blauth level-III hypoplasia. The skin of the thumb remnant is preserved for closure. **B,** The tip pinch and opposition are possible to the lateral border of the other fingers after pollicization. **C,** Distal phalanx flexion is possible for tip pinch for writing and fine pinch for picking up small objects.

Allen's test of the hand can identify occlusion of the radial or ulnar arteries and the need for arteriography of the injured hand. Microvascular toe-to-hand transfers are discussed in Chapter 125.

Pollicization and first metacarpal lengthening were popular until the late 1970s, when microsurgical techniques involving partial or total toe transfers became the best option. The description of microsurgical techniques for toe transfers by Buncke[6] in 1966 and the first reported clinical success[10] made microsurgery the method of choice for patients with thumb amputations who required reconstruction.[7,15,29] Currently transposition and microsurgical techniques each have their own role and also have become complementary.[45] The ideal surgical method of thumb reconstruction has lasting long-term or lifetime results; can be reproduced by other surgeons and surgical services; provides good function, sensation, and strength in a well-shaped, reconstructed thumb; and causes minimal functional impairment of the donor site.

Children with a hypoplastic or aplastic thumb can become very skillful in using their thumbless hands. They grasp objects with the lateral edges of their fingers and do not make contact with the pulp. They adapt their more radial finger to gain limited partial opposition that, in some circumstances, is good enough for weakly grasping large and small objects. This natural adaptation must be considered during selection of a reconstruction technique. The index finger in these patients generally has the best abduction and some rotation and is the logical finger to transpose when a four-finger hand is present (Figure 126-3).

Controversy exists regarding the ideal age of the patient undergoing index pollicization. Buck-Gramcko[5] and others[28,36] have suggested that the ideal time for the procedure is during the first year of life, when the child has not learned substitution patterns. Others believe that the best time is between 18 months and 3 years of age, when the child is not yet in school but is gaining neuromuscular maturity. The hand structures also are larger at this stage, making the procedure easier and less risky and the patient more cooperative.[47] It is important for the physician to inform a child's parents that a finger will never become a true thumb because anatomically it cannot satisfy all functions of a thumb. The new CMC joint, formerly the MCP joint, does not have the surfaces necessary for the normal rotation or movement of a thumb. Moreover, the shape of a pollicized finger is different from that of a thumb, and there are no thenar muscles.

OPERATIONS

Currently there are several reconstruction options. The technique of choice must be adapted to each patient after consideration of all of the factors previously described. This section addresses three major issues for didactic purposes: an overview of surgical management is followed by sections regarding congenital loss of the thumb and traumatic amputations of the thumb.

OVERVIEW

Different segments along the transposed digital ray may be used for pollicization, including the following:

1. The second metacarpal can be used even at the level of a metacarpal stump near the MCP joint.
2. The second metacarpal with a normal digit associated with congenital absence of the first ray can be used, with the MCP joint assuming the role of the CMC joint of the new thumb.
3. The second metacarpal with a partially amputated index finger can be sectioned to a proper length and fused with the first metacarpal to make a new thumb of appropriate length.
4. The proximal phalanx of the index finger can be fixed to the first metacarpal at a distal level. The proximal interphalangeal (PIP) joint of the index finger becomes the MCP joint of the new thumb.

Creation of a thumb with excessive length, as noted after many early attempts, detracts both functionally and aesthetically from the result of the procedure.

Basilar joint stability is essential, either through the integrity of an intact CMC joint under control of some intrinsic musculature or through fusion of the transferred digit to the metacarpal or carpus. Some authors prefer to use as much of the second metacarpal bone as necessary to place the transferred index MCP joint in the position of a thumb MCP joint so that tendons of the index interosseous muscles can be sutured to the intrinsic muscles of the thumb.[3] In such cases the distal phalanx of the transferred finger should be amputated, as in the old Gosset technique.[13] The new thumb has a normal size, only two phalanxes, one extrinsic flexor, a normal insertion to the muscles of the thumb, and no nail. If length reduction is required when transposing a finger, we believe it is preferable to resect a basal segment rather than the more important distal phalanx. The proximal phalanx or the second metacarpal head of the transferred finger can be joined to the carpus when there is a total loss of the first metacarpal.

CONGENITAL LOSS OF THE THUMB

In his large published series of pollicizations in patients with congenital thumb loss, Buck-Gramcko[5] demonstrated that the procedure, when correctly performed, achieves excellent functional and aesthetic results. All surgeons must strive to achieve the following four objectives when treating patients with congenital thumb loss:

1. Provide adequate length and proper positioning for pinch and grasp functions
2. Provide good soft tissue cover and avoid excessive scars
3. Provide or restore skin sensation
4. Provide proper muscular balance to maximize thumb function

Providing Adequate Length and Proper Positioning

An index finger used for pollicization must be shortened in most cases. This is accomplished by resection of almost all of the metacarpal so that the head with the distal epiphysis acts as the new trapezium and the PIP joint becomes the MCP joint of the new thumb. The saddle shape of the index MCP joint is different from the normal shape of the trapeziometacarpal joint. The normal rotational movement of the basilar joint cannot be reproduced with a pollicization.

The metacarpal epiphysis should be ablated if no further growth is desired.[18] The pollicized index finger also must be rotated approximately 120 degrees on its major axis to adequately achieve grasping pulp-to-pulp opposition. If the finger is rotated less than 100 degrees, the grasp of fine objects will be made between the tip of the new thumb and the lateral border of the neighboring finger, as when one holds a key. This type of pinch is less efficient and weaker than direct pulp-to-pulp opposition.

The new thumb must have both palmar and radial abduction movement. This is achieved by fixing the remaining metacarpal fragment on the scaphoid. This fixation provides a radial abduction of 20 degrees and a palmar abduction of 35 degrees during opposition of the new thumb.

Providing Good Soft Tissue Coverage and Avoiding Excessive Scars

Thumb reconstruction for congenital loss usually requires resection of a large amount of metacarpal, which leaves sufficient skin to obtain primary closure of the web space if the incisions are planned correctly. The technique must preserve the dorsal veins of the index finger because they provide the primary drainage after transposition. An ideal dissection also should leave a wide interdigital first space, with sufficient soft tissue to prevent scar contraction and permit direct closure without the placement of skin grafts. The final scars must be along the lateral edge of the transposed index ray and should not cross perpendicular to its folds. If skin grafts are required for closure, the planning was inadequate and the original skin flaps were misplaced.

Providing or Restoring Sensation

Precise and careful handling of neurovascular pedicles is vital for the short-term success of the procedure. To achieve this, a careful dissection is made to preserve the radial digital artery to the middle finger, leaving the first dorsal metacarpal artery and the radial digital artery of the index finger to be transposed exclusively with the index digit. The pedicles must be dissected carefully because in congenital cases of thumb loss vascular anomalies may be present in the index ray that can create technical problems during transposition. In some cases the finger must be transposed entirely on a single vascular pedicle.

The common digital nerve to the index and long fingers must be separated proximally, leaving intact fascicles to each digit. This is best achieved under magnification, which enables a better separation of the fascicular groups. More proximal dissection also reduces tension when the finger is transposed into its new position.

Providing Proper Muscular Balance to Maximize Thumb Function

The surgeon must take advantage of existing muscles to achieve good stability of the new thumb. The first dorsal interosseous muscle is not present in patients with thumb aplasia. The index abductor muscle can be identified, dissected, and separated for subsequent insertion into the distal part of the index finger proximal phalanx, where it functions as the abductor pollicis brevis (APB). The palmar interosseous muscle acts as the adductor pollicis (AP). The flexor digitorum profundus (FDP) and flexor digitorum superficialis (FDS) muscles shorten after transposition and usually do not require additional shortening. However, extensor muscles of the index finger must be shortened during the operation. It is important to remember that stability of the pollicized index finger is more important than its mobility.

Surgical Technique

INCISIONS. The first incision is made around the base of the index finger and is directed distally on the radial side toward the level of the IP joint. The skin of a rudimentary thumb, when present, can be used for additional skin cover. A triangular flap is outlined proximal to the base of the thumb, and the incision must reach the wrist proximally (Figure 126-4).

DISSECTIONS. The resulting flaps from the aforementioned incisions must be wide and elevated very carefully. The dissection of the dorsal veins also must be performed carefully, and small vein branches must be cauterized to preserve the larger major veins draining the index finger. The neurovascular bundles on the palmar side must be identified and carefully preserved. It is important to protect them during dissection of the muscles, using vascular retractors, a Penrose drain, or vessel loupes. The palmar interosseous muscles and the index abductor are identified, separated from the second metacarpal, and cut at their distal insertion. The flexor tendons are

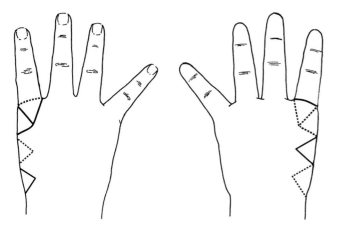

Figure 126-4. Volar and dorsal incisions mark dorsal and volar flaps used when reconstructing a thumb in a case of congenital hypoplasia. The dorsal index flap permits an easy dorsal vein dissection.

identified, and the A1 and A2 pulleys are divided. Littler[31] states that the best position for the new thumb is achieved when the MCP joint becomes the CMC joint, and that the thumb has a better working angle when the proximal phalanx is moved to the first metacarpal position. The palmar plate is visualized and the transverse metacarpal ligament is divided, freeing the first ray and making the final vascular and nerve dissection easier. The extensor tendons are isolated and the extensor digitorum communis (EDC) and extensor indicis proprius (EIP) are cut proximally. The neurovascular bundles are identified, and the radial bundle is dissected proximally to its vascular origin from the palmar arch. The ulnar digital bundle is dissected proximally to identify the proper digital artery to the long finger, which is divided. The fascicles to the ulnar digital nerve to the index finger are separated proximally from the common digital nerve in the palm. The index metacarpal is divided at a length necessary to preserve the MCP joint, which becomes the new CMC joint. The dissected neurovascular bundles must be carefully protected during bone transection, rotation to the first ray position, and final bone fixation.

Part of the second metacarpal must function as the trapezium if the latter is not present. The metacarpal is fixed in 20 degrees of pronation, with 35 degrees of palmar flexion and 20 degrees of radial abduction, to allow positioning of the proximal phalanx of the index finger in opposition to the third digit. Buck-Gramko[5] believes the MCP joint of the index finger should be hyperextended before it is attached to the carpus to increase the flexion arch of the joint and to provide a more natural-looking resting position. He places the head of the metacarpal in a partially palmar-flexed position to facilitate subsequent hyperextension, which increases the new thumb's functional range of motion. Bone fixation is achieved with two crossed Kirschner wires (K wires) (Figure 126-5).

MUSCLE FIXATION. The new thumb must be stable to allow use of the intrinsic and extrinsic flexor muscles and the extensor muscles. The abductor indicis, if present, is advanced into the radial lateral band of the transposed index finger to simulate an APB. Patients with congenital thumb loss may have loss of various intrinsic or extensor muscles. If the abductor indicis is not present in such cases, the EDC tendon can be advanced distally and anchored to the mid-shaft of the proximal phalanx to provide active abduction of the new thumb. The palmar interosseous muscle is dissected free and fixed into the ulnar lateral band to provide adduction. Other types of tendon transfers have been used to motor the pollicization, including transfers of the ring finger's FDS, abductor digiti quinti (ADQ), and extensor digiti quiniti proprius (EDQP), depending on the deficit. The flexor tendons, which are loose after transfer, adjust and shorten with time and growth of the digit and usually do not require adjustment.

Manske and McCaroll believe that the extensor musculotendinous units also shorten on their own, but most authors recommend shortening the extrinsic extensor tendons (extensor indicis proprius (EIP) and EDC) by the length of the

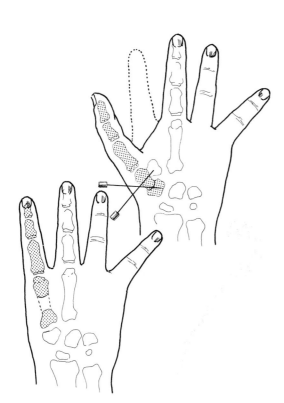

Figure 126-5. Schematic representation of a metacarpal bone resection of the index finger and osteosynthesis of the base of the first ray onto the carpal bones. The MCP joint of the index finger becomes the new CMC joint.

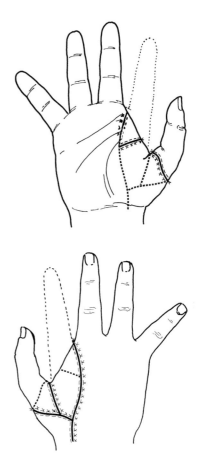

Figure 126-6. Schematic view of the hand after the last incisions are sutured on the dorsal and volar surfaces. The triangular flap allows the first web space to be closed without the danger of scar contractures.

metacarpal resection, to prevent extensor lag. Despite the surgeon's best efforts to balance the new thumb's tendon functions during the initial procedure, secondary tendon transfers, as described by Manske,[35] are sometimes necessary to improve flexion, abduction, or opposition.

CLOSING OF SKIN FLAPS. Skin adjustments must be made in almost all cases. The incisions should be planned and the skin should be closed to prevent scars in the first web space, which can produce a contracture. Any remnant thumb muscles are sutured to the transferred muscles to further balance the new digit. The incisions must be sutured with an adequate eversion technique applied to the wound edges to ensure healing by primary intention. Edges with any degree of vascular impairment after deflation of the tourniquet should be excised to achieve primary healing (Figure 126-6).

POSTOPERATIVE MANAGEMENT. The hand is placed in a large bulky dressing after surgery, which should immobilize the pollicization and decrease edema. The position of the new digit is maintained with a plaster splint. The dressing is changed at 10 to 14 days, and the sutures are removed. A new plaster cast or molded splint is applied for 6 to 8 weeks. Younger patients

often are less compliant and may require cast immobilization. K wires are removed after 8 weeks or as soon as consolidation of the bone union is observed radiologically. Exercises are usually begun after 6 to 8 weeks and do not require specialized physical therapy. In our experience and that of other authors,[18] children recover motion rapidly on their own.

TRAUMATIC AMPUTATION OF THE THUMB

Traumatic thumb amputations may be classified as total or partial amputations.

Total Amputation
A total amputation occurs when the first ray, which may include the trapezium, is completely lost. Sometimes the remaining fragment of the trapezium or the first metacarpal base is so small that it cannot be used and must be removed. The amputation should be considered total when muscles of the thenar eminence are not present or they are nonfunctional.

As in congenital thumb losses, reconstruction of a CMC joint by including the MCP joint and fusing the second

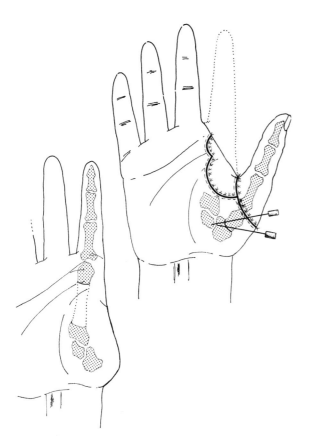

Figure 126-7. Determining the length of bone that must be resected to achieve an appropriate length for the new thumb is one of the more important considerations in pollicization. A total amputation requires transection of the metacarpal to preserve the MCP joint, which becomes the new basilar joint.

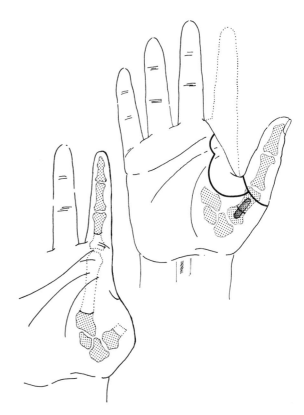

Figure 126-8. A proximal subtotal thumb amputation through the metacarpal requires both IP joints of the index finger and a segment of the proximal phalanx.

metacarpal to the scaphoid may be necessary. When the basilar joint is intact and a part of the first metacarpal remains, the proximal phalanx of the index finger should be fixed to the remaining metacarpal. The length of the proximal phalanx should be adjusted to create a thumb length that is as close to normal as possible (Figure 126-7).

Few intrinsic muscles of the thenar eminence provide opposition and therefore a secondary tendon transfer using the ring finger's FDS or ABDQ is sometimes required to improve opposition.

Partial Amputation

An amputation is considered partial when only a part of the thumb is lost. Injuries in this category range from those that result in loss of pulp only to those involving amputations through the middle third of the metacarpal. Partial thumb amputations may be categorized as proximal or distal to the MCP joint.

Morrison et al[39] described their preferred methods of thumb reconstruction at different levels of amputation. A specific type of surgical management is recommended for each level of amputation. This chapter does not discuss segmental or partial thumb loss, but discusses only the treatment of patients

with proximal amputations and loss of the MCP joint who require pollicization. These patients have lost enough length to make the thumb useless for opposition or prehension, which typically occurs with losses proximal to the proximal third of the proximal phalanx.

It is essential to restore a thumb that has two phalanges and one metacarpal. When the MCP joint of the first ray remains, a thumb pollicization requires fusion of only the middle phalanx of the index finger to the proximal phalanx of the first ray. The middle phalanx becomes the new proximal phalanx, and the distal interphalangeal (DIP) joint becomes the new IP joint of the thumb (Figure 126-8).

A subtotal amputation proximal to the MCP joint of the first ray requires a bone union between the proximal phalanx of the transposed digit and the first metacarpal. The PIP joint of the transposed index finger becomes the MCP joint of the new thumb, the middle phalanx becomes the proximal phalanx, and the DIP joint becomes the new IP joint (Figure 126-9).

Objectives of Pollicization

The characteristics of a thumb that are partly or completely lost after an amputation include positioning, stability, strength, length, movement, sensation, and appearance. Thus transposi-

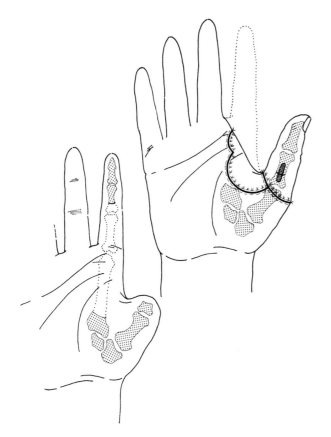

Figure 126-9. A more distal thumb amputation, which preserves the thumb MCP joint, requires only the distal phalanx and a portion of the index middle phalanx.

tion of a digit to the thumb position should address the following objectives.

POSITIONING. The position of the thumb in a hand is very important. Normal thumb opposition starts from an intermediate position between total abduction and complete adduction at approximately 45 degrees to the index axis and in 90 degrees of radial pronation. All rotation, flexion, and opposition movement is initiated beginning at this point, which is the desired resting position for a pollicization. If properly positioned, even an immobile post can function as a means to grasp objects and is better than a hand with no thumb.

STABILITY. The new thumb must be stable to resist the strength of the rest of the fingers during all of their prehensile and grasping movements, including those involving ulnarly deviating and extension vectors. The MCP joint must be firmly stabilized for flexion of the distal joint to be effective. An unstable MCP joint is prone to hyperextension during pinch, an example of which occurs in patients with ulnar nerve paralysis (Froment sign).

STRENGTH. Thumb strength during pinch and grasp is determined by the intrinsic thenar and first web-space muscles and by the extrinsic thumb flexor. Loss of muscle function from nerve injury, scarring, or surgical technique decreases

thumb and hand function and may require subsequent reconstruction with tendon transfers.

LENGTH. The length of a thumb after reconstruction should approximate that of a normal thumb. The length is adjusted to bring the thumb tip 10 to 15 mm proximal to the PIP-joint flexion crease of the long finger when the pollicization is adducted in a palmar plane.

MOVEMENT. The range of motion of a normal thumb at the basilar, MCP, and IP joints is rarely achieved by the pollicization of a digit. The goal for a thumb reconstruction is sufficient flexion to oppose the fingers and sufficient abduction and extension to grasp large objects.

SENSATION. Some authors[28] consider sensation less important than stability or motion. A patient who uses the hand mainly for grasping larger objects may not require the quality of sensory return needed by a patient who uses the new thumb for fine grasping. However, the better the quality of sensation, the better the function. Some sensation is necessary to manipulate small objects and to protect the reconstruction from external trauma such as that caused by hot, cold, or sharp objects.

APPEARANCE. The final appearance of a reconstructed thumb is related to its overall shape, placement of scars, fingernail configuration, and the appearance of the rest of the hand. The appearance of the hand and reconstructed thumb is more important in adolescent patients who suffer traumatic thumb loss and is less of a concern in cases of congenital thumb loss in which the patient has "grown up" with the deformity. However, we believe that performing an aesthetic reconstruction to achieve the best appearance possible should always be our goal.

General Considerations

Any finger can be transposed to the thumb position on a neurovascular pedicle; however, some characteristics of the index finger make it an advantageous choice. The index finger is the closest digit to the thumb and consequently has the shortest distance to move. The dorsal veins can be preserved and easily redirected, thus guaranteeing drainage of the transposed finger. When other fingers are pollicized, the dorsal veins cannot always be redirected, which can lead to venous congestion and loss of soft tissue. Sometimes a microsurgical venous anastomosis of a dorsal digital vein to a dorsal vein of the hand is required. Use of the index ray allows simpler surgical approaches with better exposure of important elements through a single incision. The index finger has a shorter distance to move to a thumb position and the neurovascular pedicles and tendons do not have to cross elements of the remaining fingers. A different incision is required in the palm of the hand when a finger other than the index is pollicized and the flexor tendons and neurovascular pedicle must be transposed across the palm. A pollicization of the long or ring finger leaves the donor metacarpal intact and preserves palmar width but is less aesthetic and may allow small objects to fall out of the palm.

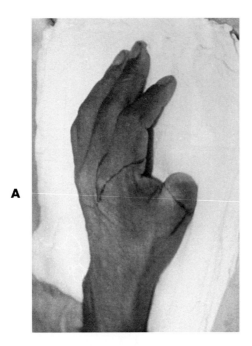 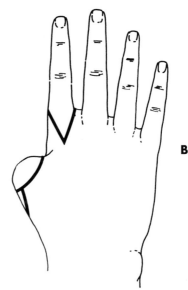

Figure 126-10. **A,** Dorsal incisions. **B,** Schematic of the dorsal incision, which creates a V flap on the dorsum of the index finger over the MCP joint.

Because the index finger has relatively independent movement of its flexor tendons, it usually is not necessary to shorten them after pollicization (unlike the extensor tendons, which should be shortened). If the flexor system does require subsequent adjustment, it is often best to join the distal flexor profundus tendon of the pollicized index finger to the FPL in the distal third of the forearm to avoid adhesions and to increase excursion. This adjustment also improves the cortical representation of thumb flexion of the distal phalanges. All pollicizations using the long or ring fingers require shortening of the flexor tendons or use of the FPL as an extrinsic motor unit to obtain independent motion and strength.

For all of the aforementioned reasons, we prefer to pollicize the index finger, even when there is a partial loss of the second ray. Another digit may be used to reconstruct the thumb if it is already injured or partially amputated. However, we believe that overall the index finger has sufficient advantages to be considered the best option for thumb reconstruction by pollicization in the majority of cases.

Technical Specifications

The vascularity of the index finger must be determined before pollicization is attempted. An injury to the thumb can harm the radial vascular pedicle of the index finger. The vascular flow in both digital vessels of the index finger must be determined with a Doppler flow probe. The index finger may be transferred on only one vascular pedicle, but this procedure demands a more careful dissection of the remaining pedicle. Angiography is recommended when vascular uncertainty is present. We have transferred several index fingers on only one vascular pedicle and one index finger on the first dorsal metacarpal artery.

INCISIONS. The Littler technique[30] is considered the best method for rearranging skin in the first web space during pollicization. This technique has undergone several modifications; we use the modification described in 1976 by Araico.[1]

The classic Littler approach is based on two incisions: an elliptical incision around the amputation stump, and one at the base of the index finger. The latter incision is rounded on the palmar side and triangular on the dorsal side. A diagonal line unites the apex of the dorsal triangle of the index finger with the most palmar point of the stump ellipse; this produces two triangular flaps—one with a dorsal base and one that is palmar. These flaps are elevated to allow an easier approach to the involved structures. In some traumatic cases scars may be present that preclude the use of these incisions and require individual variations in flap design. Distant flap coverage, such as that provided by a groin or distally based radial forearm flap, may be necessary in some cases to achieve primary closure.[45]

The Araico modification[1] involves the use of three incisions. The first is circular around the amputation stump of the first ray and extends with a proximal linear incision on the radial side of the first metacarpal. The second incision, around the base of the index finger, is circular on the palmar side and slightly triangular to the distal base on the dorsal side (Figure 126-10). A bilobed third incision joins the two previous incisions on the surface of the palm, beginning on the radial edge of the index finger and extending to the first ray. This union results in a dorsally based bilobed flap, which provides excellent exposure to all important structures. Moreover, after the incisions are closed, no scar occurs within the first interdigital space, which is covered by healthy skin (Figure 126-11).

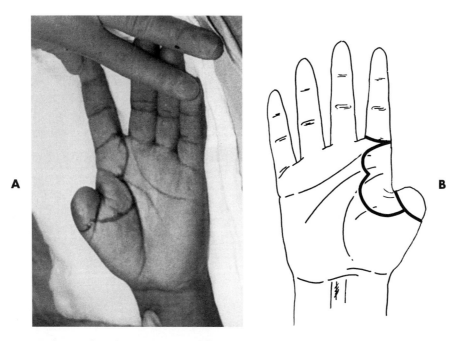

Figure 126-11. Our skin incisions are different from the Littler technique. **A,** Volar incisions. **B,** Schematic of the volar incisions shows the advantage of having only one bilobed, dorsally based flap.

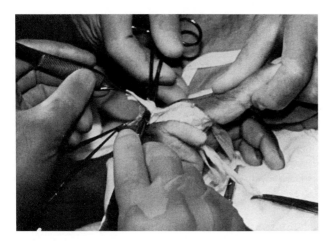

Figure 126-12. Dissection of the veins and extensor tendons by the dorsal approach.

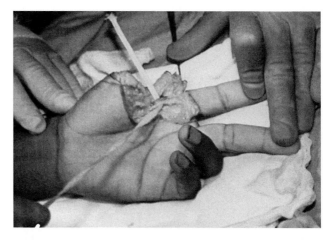

Figure 126-13. Volar cutaneous flap allows adequate exposure of the neurovascular bundles and flexor tendons.

DISSECTION. The flaps are dissected and elevated at the level of the intrinsic muscle fascia, and the appropriate structures are identified. It is best to start the dissection on the back of the index finger and to carefully identify the dorsal veins and radial sensory nerve, which must be dissected out of the dorsal flap. Some subcutaneous tissue must remain to surround the veins and preserve the lymphatics. The extensor tendons are subsequently exposed for identification of the radial EDC and the ulnar EIP, which are separated and retracted off the second metacarpal. The first dorsal interosseous muscle is also identified, including its tendon insertion into the base of the proximal phalanx. The junctura tendinea between the common extensor of the index and middle fingers is divided (Figure 126-12).

We continue on the palmar side by carefully dissecting the neurovascular pedicles (Figure 126-13). This is best achieved with loupe magnification (×3.5) or with the operating microscope. The vertical septa of the palmar aponeurosis are released, freeing the radial side structures and the flexor tendons. Next the common digital artery is dissected to its union with the first dorsal interosseous artery. The A1 and A2 pulleys are subsequently dissected to free the flexor tendons and easily uncover the palmar plate of the MCP joint. The septum of the palmar fascia, which separates the second palmar interosseous from the dorsal interosseous, is opened longitudinally to free those muscles. The interosseous artery is identified and the intermetacarpal ligament between the second and third metacarpal is divided. The common digital artery to the index and long

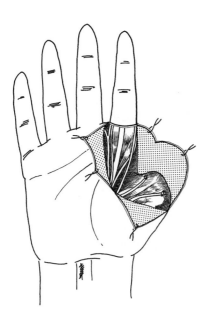

Figure 126-14. Schematic view of the volar approach shows digital arteries, digital nerves, and flexor tendons. These important elements must be dissected and preserved.

fingers is dissected proximally and the radial digital artery to the long finger is carefully cut and ligated. The common digital nerve is dissected proximally, under magnification, separating the fascicles to the index finger from those to the radial side of the long finger (Figure 126-14).

The first dorsal interosseous muscle is separated from its wide insertion onto the radial base of the proximal phalanx. This separation exposes the sagittal band of the central extensor tendon, the extensor hood, and the radial collateral ligament of the joint. The first dorsal interosseous tendon is subsequently separated from its connection to the radial lateral band, thus exposing the base of the proximal phalanx.

The origins of the dorsal and palmar interosseous muscles are elevated in a subperiosteal plane off the second metacarpal at the level of the planned osteotomy. The osteotomy is performed at a level that enables the surgeon to create a thumb of the desired length. A normal adult thumb is 9 to 11 cm long,[33] and, as mentioned, should be reconstructed so that the tip is placed within 10 to 15 mm of the PIP-joint flexion crease of the long finger. The ideal length can be determined from the contralateral normal thumb, if it is present. The osteotomy can be made in the proximal phalanx, if all or part of the first metacarpal is present, or along second metacarpal to include the MCP joint, if the first metacarpal is missing.

After the ideal length is determined, we proceed to perform an osteosynthesis (Figure 126-15, *A*). There are two types of osteosynthesis. The first involves the classic Littler[33] technique, in which a central bone peg is designed on the end of the first metacarpal, which is fit into a hole in the index proximal phalanx. The bone peg can be taken as a bone graft

from the second metacarpal, which is subsequently discarded. The index finger is rotated 90 degrees to place it into opposition and the peg fixation is secured with crossed K wires. This type of osteosynthesis requires 6 to 8 weeks of immobilization to achieve bone healing. The other technique involves the use of rigid plate fixation, with a minimum of four holes and two bicortical screws on either side of the osteosynthesis. This type of fixation is very stable and permits earlier motion, as soon as it is safe to move the tendon repairs.

TENDON ADJUSTMENT. An adjustment of the extensor is usually required if the pollicized finger has been shortened more than 5 cm. The extensors of the transposed index finger are sutured to the long extensor of the thumb, which is usually found in the proximal end of the vertical stump incision (Figure 126-15, *B*). If the long extensor of the thumb is not easily found because it has retracted or has been destroyed during the original trauma, the extensors of the index finger itself must be used. We dissect the extensor communis and suture it to the extensor indicis proprius distally in the area of the MCP joint and adjust the tension on the indicis proprius proximally. Transfer of the EIP to the extensor pollicis longus (EPL) is a method commonly used for restoring thumb extension after injury or rupture.

The flexor mechanism must be adequately freed and redirected toward the thumb position. Most authors, including Buck-Gramko,[5] agree that no adjustment of the flexor tendons is necessary because the extrinsic flexors shorten on their own. The flexor sheath is opened over the proximal phalanx to free the flexor tendons and provide access to the bone for later osteotomy or fixation.

It is important to restore thumb opposition. An incomplete amputation, which has preserved the thenar muscles, allows reattachment of the APB tendon to the base of the pollicized middle phalanx. This reattachment allows adequate rotation for opposition. When no muscle mass is present, the new thumb must be placed in an opposed position; if opposition is inadequate, a tendon transfer can be performed, most commonly using the sublimis of the ring finger.

When all muscles of the thenar eminence are absent, the first dorsal interosseous muscle is dissected and may be used as an adductor of the new thumb if it is attached to the base of the middle phalanx on the ulnar side. If the palmar interosseous muscle is in good condition, it functions as an adductor of the new thumb. The first dorsal interosseous may be used to support the long finger and is inserted into the tendon of the second dorsal interosseous on the radial side of the digit. This procedure adds extra support to the long finger during pinch.

FINAL REPAIR AND FOLLOW UP. The remaining skin in the palm must be dissected to create flaps that can be closed without tension. Skin grafts are generally not required if the skin flaps have been properly planned. In our experience, the triangle technique described by Littler[30] makes closing the base

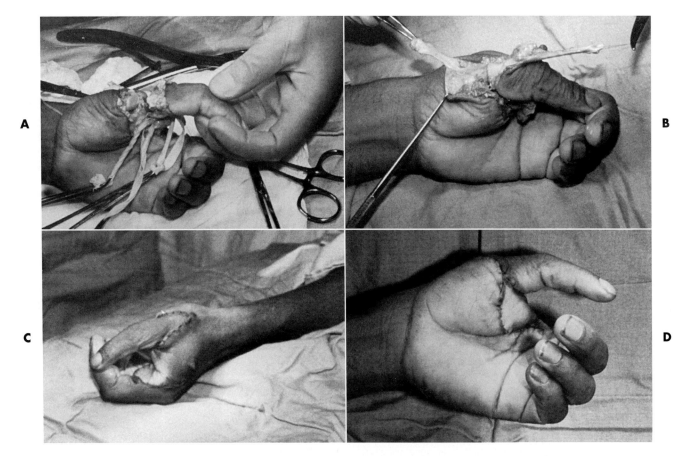

Figure 126-15. **A,** After adequate bone resection, the index finger is moved over the first ray stump and is ready for bone fixation. **B,** After bone fixation, the extensor tendons are adjusted to a new functional length. **C,** The skin is closed easily without tension. The new thumb position is radially rotated to assure opposition. **D,** The volar incision is also closed without tension.

of the transposed finger difficult, particularly when reconstruction of a large portion of the first ray is required. We use the Araico technique[1] because the bilobed flap is always loose and the incisions can be sutured without any tension (Figure 126-15, *C* and *D*).

The skin edges should be everted to promote primary healing. The neurovascular pedicles must be carefully observed before skin closure. They are always redundant and must be placed in a gentle curve to avoid kinking, which can occlude blood flow.

The pollicized digit is immobilized with a splint, which maintains the wrist in slight extension and the new digit in the same position achieved during surgery. The hand is dressed in a bulky dressing and splinted to avoid tension in the bandage. The digit is immobilized for 6 to 8 weeks if K wires were used for bone fixation, and for 3 to 4 weeks if rigid plate fixation was performed.

With time the patient's use of the digit improves and the digit assumes the overall appearance of a thumb. If flexion is weak after 1 year, we may perform a secondary flexor tendon repair in the distal forearm, uniting the proximal FPL with the distal FDP of the pollicized index finger.

OUTCOMES

We have never lost a pollicized finger because of vascular impairment. We are not aware of any reported cases of acute loss of a pollicized digit because of vascular compromise. Pollicization also provides near normal sensation. The intraneural direction necessary to isolate the nerve fascicles entering the pollicized digit produces only a temporary neuropraxia and patients usually recover fully within 6 months.

To appropriately evaluate outcomes of pollicization, we must separate the patients who underwent the procedure to correct congenital problems from those who underwent reconstruction of traumatic amputations.

CONGENITAL APLASIA OF THE THUMB

Many authors have evaluated the long-term functional results of pollicization in patients with a congenitally deficient thumb. Some have primarily evaluated the resulting range of motion[12] or pinch and grip strength,[44] and others have

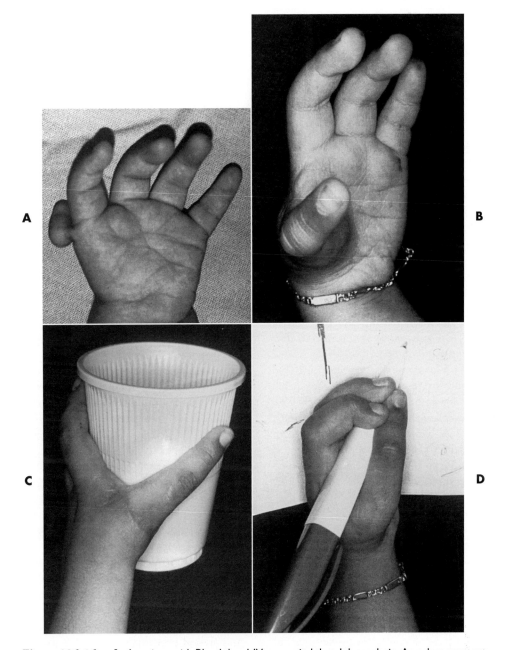

Figure 126-16. **A,** A patient with Blauth level-IV congenital thumb hypoplasia. A useless remnant of the thumb remains. **B,** Two years after pollicization of the index finger, the new thumb's position and tip rotation allow it to face the other fingers. **C** and **D,** Good opposition allows the patient to grasp both large and small objects.

calculated a functional score based on cosmetic appearance, sensation, mobility, opposition, and pinch and grip strength.[43] Free tissue transfer of a toe has been an effective treatment for patients with a traumatic thumb amputation, but for patients with congenital thumb abnormalities it has been a less appropriate alternative than index-finger pollicization (Figure 126-16).

The Manske report[36] on index finger pollicization for the treatment of a congenitally deficient thumb indicated an average total active range of motion of 98 degrees in the pollicized digit, or approximately half that of a normal thumb. The average values for grip strength and lateral, tripod, and tip pinch strength ranged from 21% to 25% of normal values. The pollicized digit was used in a manner similar to that of a normal thumb in 92% of patients handling large objects and in 77% of patients handling small objects. The time required to perform activities with the pollicized hand averaged 22% longer than with a normal hand. These results were not influenced by the age of the patient at the time of operation.

Although younger children adapt more effectively to operative procedures, surgeons should not be discouraged from performing pollicizations in older children. Manske[36] reported that children younger than 4 years of age who had previous pollicization subsequently underwent more secondary procedures than did patients who were at least 4 years of age at the time of thumb reconstruction. He noted no age-related differences in the ability of patients to regain motion or obtain maximum thumb function. Secondary operative procedures after pollicization, including opponensplasty, extensor tendon shortening, and arthrodesis, improved function of the transposed digits.

Morrison[39] reported that two-point discrimination remained normal in patients who underwent index pollicization for treatment of congenital absences, and that no problems with cerebral misrepresentation followed transposition. Among patients with congenital aplasia who underwent index pollicization (with an average 9-year follow-up), Kozin[26] reported that palmar pinch and lateral pinch strength ranged from 56% to 60% compared with the normal contralateral hand. Grip strength was 67% and manual dexterity averaged 70% compared with normal standards defined according to age and sex. However, 5% of the patients used side-to-side pinch and, in those patients, the pinch performance averaged 54% of normal, compared with 93% of normal for patients who used tip-to-tip pinch for normal prehension. In this study, values for grip and pinch strength were lower in the pollicized hand than in the contralateral hand. The differences reflect the difficulty of thumb reconstruction without appropriate intrinsic and extrinsic muscles.

Despite muscle transfers, the pollicized digit and hand remain weaker than normal. Many of the Kozin's[26] patients performed opposition pinch on request but opted for side-to-side pinch when stressed. Manske[36] believes that patients will change their technique of prehension only when the pollicized digit allows more effective function than was possible before surgery.

Percival[43] created a point scoring system for evaluating the results of pollicization, whereby fine pinch with the tip of the fingers (tip pinch), when normal, is given four points; pulp-to-pulp pinch is given two points; opposition, three points; grip strength of a tennis ball and ping pong ball and its strength, a maximum of three points; the effectiveness of movement, three points; sensation, three points; and cosmetic appearance, three points. Patients with normal thumbs typically score a total of 22 points. Results of pollicization are considered excellent when patients with reconstructed thumbs score more than 20 points. Results are considered good in patients who receive 16 to 19 points, fair in patients who receive 12 to 15 points, and poor in patients who score less than 12.

Sykes[47] used the Percival method[43] to evaluate 30 patients with congenital thumb loss who underwent pollicization of the index finger; 73% had results that were graded excellent or good, 17% had fair results, and 10% had poor results. A total of 36% required secondary surgical revision to achieve a better final outcome.

The cosmetic appearance is highly subjective and is not subject to objective standards of measurement. The overall cosmetic appearance of the hand is generally improved by pollicization. A hand with a thumb and three fingers is a less noticeable deformity than a four-fingered hand without a thumb. Manske[36] reported that his patient's parents agreed with surgeons that pollicization improved the cosmetic appearance of the hand. It is difficult to make a finger look like a thumb, but he believes that designing good skin flaps that allow the web space to join the pollicized digit at the PIP joint is also an important cosmetic principle.

THUMB AMPUTATION

Langlais[27] evaluated 15 manual workers who underwent pollicization using an undamaged ring finger after an isolated thumb amputation at or proximal to the MCP joint. The results were better when compared to patients who had thumb reconstruction by microsurgical transfer of the second toe. Pollicization in his series was reliable and produced an early return to work (which averaged 5 months), a greater range of active motion (60 degrees compared with 30 degrees), pulp-pinch and key pinch that averaged 54% of normal, a hand-grasp of 70% of normal, two-point discrimination of 5 mm, less cold intolerance, and no discomfort in the donor site of the transplanted digit.

From a functional point of view, Hentz[17] believes that lengthening the first ray is a good method for thumb reconstruction, if in the end the patient is able to make contact with the other fingers. Thus some pollicization techniques for treatment of a traumatically injured finger, such as use of a metacarpal with a fragment of a phalanx, may be appropriate for patients with an amputated first metacarpal, to restore length with a vascularized bone fragment where there is adequate skin cover and sensation (Figure 126-17).

Pollicization is the surgical treatment of choice for an amputation proximal to the MCP joint when four or even three fingers are present. It is also the easiest and safest operation, with the best outcome with regard to motor and sensory function. The primary indication for pollicization by digital transfer is total or near total loss of the thumb ray, especially when accompanied by loss of the thenar muscles. Despite isolated reports documenting the use of microvascular free toe transfers to treat patients with total traumatic loss or congenital absence, pollicization remains the procedure of choice because transfer of a toe (including the metatarsal) requires skin cover on the hand, and the loss of the first metatarsal bone in the foot produces a gait disturbance. Pollicization is described by several authors as the method of choice when there is loss of the first ray, including the CMC joint.[28,29,32,38] Sastre et al[45] reported a 50% loss of strength during pressing and squeezing in patients who required a metacarpal bone transfer for support (Figure 126-18).

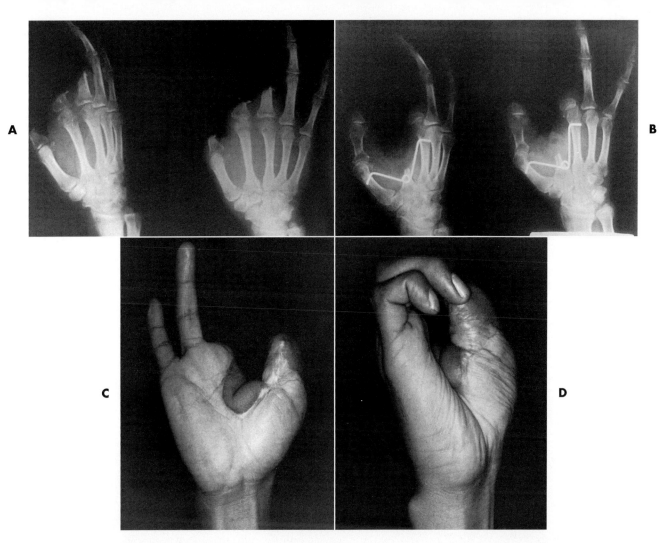

Figure 126-17. A metacarpal stump can be pollicized when there is partial loss of other fingers. **A,** Radiograph of a hand reveals amputation of the thumb, index, and middle fingers at the proximal phalangeal level. **B,** Radiograph taken after pollicization of the phalangeal stump. An internal splint was used to keep the first web space open. **C,** The new thumb is short but deepening of the first web space improves its appearance. **D,** The opposition to the other two fingers is adequate for grasping objects.

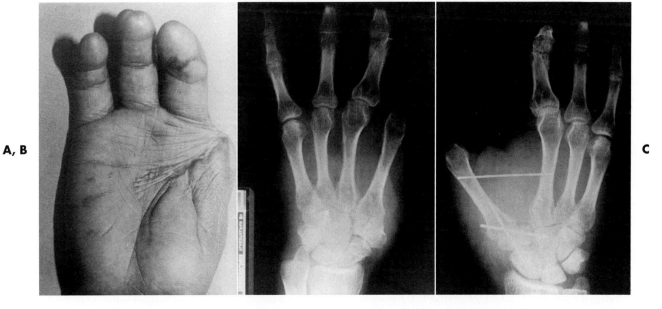

Figure 126-18. **A,** A right hand with total absence of the first ray, the index finger, and the distal phalanges of the middle and ring fingers. **B,** A radiograph shows that the trapezium and second metacarpal bones are intact. **C,** Radiograph taken after pollicization of the second metacarpal bone and fixation with three K wires.

Continued

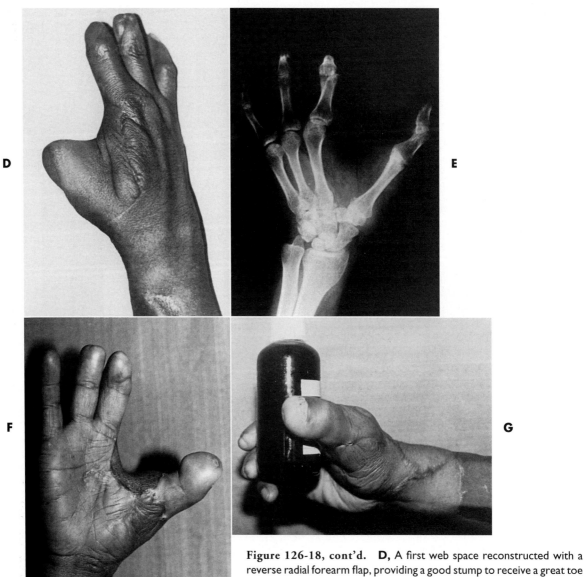

Figure 126-18, cont'd. **D,** A first web space reconstructed with a reverse radial forearm flap, providing a good stump to receive a great toe transfer. **E,** A radiograph shows the final bone structure of the new thumb. **F,** The hand after a great-toe transfer. The vessels were anastomosed to reverse the flow of the radial vessels. **G,** The resulting thumb is good and provides adequate function. (From Sastre N, Caravantes MI, Mayoral-Garcia C: *J Reconstr Microsurg* 12:431-437, 1996.)

SUMMARY

The disadvantages of pollicization include reduction of grasp leverage by 50% and reduction of grip strength by 20%, which are caused when the removal of one digital ray narrows the hand.[28] The narrowness of the hand is of minor cosmetic importance, but the potential for associated disability may cause manual workers to reject this solution. Theoretically, only one procedure is involved, but often this does not prove to be the case; in the Lister series,[28] 74% of patients required secondary operations for tenolysis, rotational osteotomy, or web-space deepening. The loss of a finger is better thought of as a strategic redeployment. The least desirable aspect of this procedure is that the hand has only three fingers.

The advantages of pollicization include a good appearance, the potential for motion at all joints in the new thumb, and good sensation. Two-point discrimination ranges between 5 to 7 mm in different series. The overriding benefit offered by pollicization and no other procedure is the reconstruction of a basal joint when it has been eliminated. Moreover, the operation is not difficult to perform (Figure 126-19). The advantages of index finger pollicization include the preservation of better phalangeal joint function, the preservation of venous flow through the dorsal veins, maintenance of normal sensation, sufficient length to accommodate any degree of thumb loss, and sufficient motor units to provide forceful movement and stability, particularly in the cardinal planes of extension–abduction and flexor–adduction (Figure 126-20).

A, B

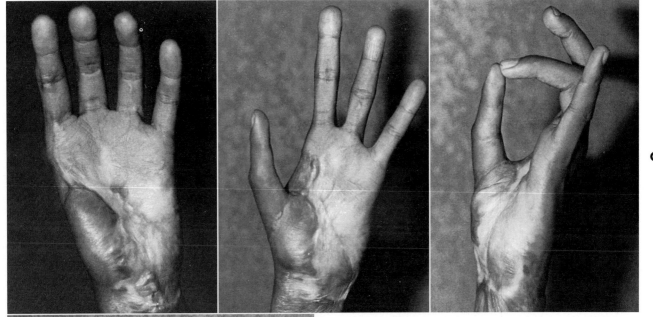

C

D

Figure 126-19. A patient who sustained a total first ray amputation of her left hand after an electrical burn. **A,** Volar view of the hand shows some scar tissue. **B,** Index finger pollicization provides a new thumb with adequate rotation and length. **C,** The fine opposition is perfect. **D,** This quick and easy procedure obtains an excellent outcome when the other hand is lost.

A

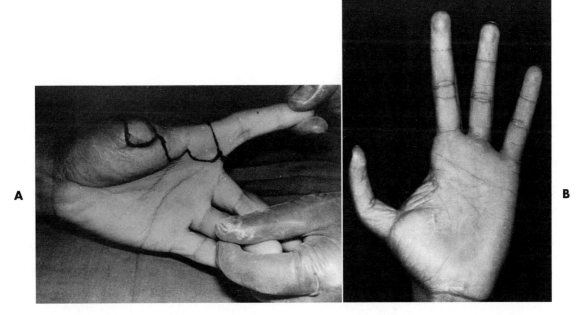

B

Figure 126-20. Proximal subtotal thumb amputation. **A,** The skin incision. **B,** The new thumb is of suitable length.

Continued

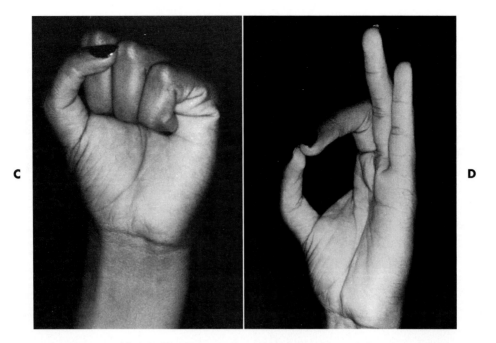

Figure 126-20, cont'd. C, The fist with the new thumb in front of the other three fingers. **D,** The new thumb in opposition.

REFERENCES

1. Araico J, Rivero A, Andrade F: Pulgarizacion con tecnica modificada, *Rev Med IMSS* 15:51, 1976.
2. Blauth W: Der hypoplastische Daumen, *Arch Orthop Unfall Chir* 62:225, 1967.
3. Brunelli GA, Brunelli GR: Reconstruction of traumatic absence of the thumb in the adult by pollicization, *Hand Clin* 8:41, 1992.
4. Buck-Gramcko D: Daumenrekonstruktion bei aplasie und hipoplasie, *Klin Med* 21:325, 1966.
5. Buck-Gramcko D: Pollicization of the index finger: method and results in aplasia and hypoplasia of the thumb, *J Bone Joint Surg* 52A:1605, 1971.
6. Buncke HJ, Buncke CM, Schulz WP: Immediate Nicoladoni procedure in Rhesus monkey or hallux-to-hand transplantation utilizing microminiature vascular anastomoses, *Br J Plast Surg* 19:332, 1966.
7. Buncke HJ, McLean DH, George PT, et al: Thumb replacement: great toe transplantation by microvascular anastomoses, *Br J Plast Surg* 26:194, 1973.
8. Bunnel S: Physiological reconstruction of a thumb after total loss, *Surg Gynecol Obstet* 52:245, 1931.
9. Bunnell S: Digit transfer by neurovascular pedicle, *J Bone Joint Surg* 34A:772, 1952.
10. Cobbett JR: Free digital transfer: report of a case of transfer of a great toe to replace an amputated thumb, *J Bone Joint Surg* 51:677, 1969.
11. Dunlop J: Use of index finger for thumb, *J Bone Joint Surg* 5:99, 1932.

12. Egloff DV, Verdan CL: Pollicization of the index finger for reconstruction of the congenitally hypoplastic or absent thumb, *J Hand Surg [Am]* 8:839, 1983.
13. Gosset J: La pollicisation de l'index, *J Chir* 65:403, 1949.
14. Gosset J, Sels M: Technique, indication et resultats de la pollicisation du 4° doigt, *Ann Chir* 18:1005, 1964.
15. Gu YD, Gao-meng Z, De-shong C, et al: Free toe transfer for thumb and finger reconstruction in 300 cases, *Plast Reconstr Surg* 91:693, 1993.
16. Guermonprez F: *Notes sur quelques resections et restaurations du pouce,* Paris, 1887, Asselin.
17. Hentz VR: Conventional techniques for thumb reconstruction, *Clin Orthop* 195:129, 1985.
18. Hentz VR: Congenital anomalies of the thumb. In McCarthy J (editor): *Plastic surgery: the hand,* Philadelphia, 1990, WB Saunders.
19. Hette K, Lemke T, Knaepler H: Die destraktion des ersten Mittelhandknochens zur Daumenerstazbildung, *Unfallchirurg* 95:294, 1992.
20. Hilgenfeldt O: *Operativer daumenersatz,* Stuttgart, 1950, Ferdinand Enke Verlag.
21. Hu W, Martin D, Baudet J: Reconstruction of the traumatic thumb: reconstruction of the thumb by osteocutaneous flaps of the forearm, *Ann Chir Plast Esthet* 38:381, 1993.
22. Iselin M: Reconstruction of the thumb, *Surgery* 2:619, 1937.
23. Joyce JL: A new operation for the substitution of a thumb, *Br J Surg* 5:499, 1918.
24. Kelleher JC, Sullivan JG: Thumb reconstruction by fifth digit transposition, *Plast Reconstr Surg* 21:470, 1958.

25. Kleinschmidt O: Ueber daumenplastik unter verwendung des unbrauchbaren mittelfingers, *Brun's Beitr Klin Chir* 120:589, 1920.

26. Kozin SH, Weiss AA, Weber JB, et al: Index finger pollicization for congenital aplasia or hypoplasia of the thumb, *J Hand Surg [Am]* 17:880, 1992.

27. Langlais F, Renaud B, Fourastier J: Reconstruction des amputations traumatiques isolees du pounce: place de la pollicisation de l'annulaire (15 cas), *Rev Chir Orthop* 79:385, 1993.

28. Lister GD: The choice of procedure following thumb amputation, *Clin Orthop* 195:45, 1985.

29. Lister GD, Kalisman M, Tsai TM: Reconstruction of the hand with free microvascular toe-to-hand transfer: experience with 54 toe transfers, *Plast Reconstr Surg* 71:372, 1983.

30. Littler JW: Neurovascular pedicle method of digital transposition for reconstruction of the thumb, *Plast Reconstr Surg* 12:303, 1953.

31. Littler JW: Restoration of the amputated thumb. In Littler JW, Cramer LM, Smith JW (editors): *Symposium on reconstructive hand surgery,* St Louis, 1974, CV Mosby.

32. Littler JW, Michon J, Merle M, et al: Discussion of functional comparison between pollicization and toe-to-hand transfer for thumb reconstruction, *J Reconstr Microsurg* 1:111, 1984.

33. Littler JW: Finger pollicization for traumatic loss. In McCarthy J (editor): *Plastic surgery: the hand,* vol 8, Philadelphia, 1990, WB Saunders.

34. Malek R, Grossman JA: The skin incision in pollicization, *J Hand Surg [Am]* 10:305, 1985.

35. Manske PR, McCaroll HR: Index finger pollicization for congenital absent or nonfunctioning thumb, *J Hand Surg [Am],* 10:606, 1985.

36. Manske PR, Rotman M, Dailey LA: Long-term functional results after pollicization for the congenitally deficient thumb, *J Hand Surg [Am]* 17:1064, 1992.

37. Merle M: La reconstruction du pouce ampute: vingt ans d'evolution des techniques et des indications, *Bull Acad Natl Med* 180:195, 1996.

38. Michon J, Merie M, Bouchon Y, Foucher G: Functional comparison between pollicization and toe-to-hand transfer for thumb reconstruction, *J Reconstr Microsurg* 1:103, 1944.

39. Morrison W, O'Brien B, MacLeod A: Experience with thumb reconstruction, *J Hand Surg [Br]* 9:223, 1984.

40. Nicoladoni C: Daumenplastik, *Wien Klin Wochenschr* 10:663, 1887.

41. Nicoladoni C: Daumenplastik und organischer ersatz der fingerspitze (anticheiro-plastik und daktyloplastik), *Arch Chir* 6:606, 1900.

42. Noesske H: Ueber ersatz des bamt metakarpus verlorenen daumens durch operative umstellung des zeige-fingers (mit lichtbildern), *Munch Med Wochenschr* 16:465, 1920.

43. Percival NJ, Sykes PJ, Chandra PT: A method of assessment of pollicization, *J Hand Surg [Br]* 16:141, 1991.

44. Roper BA, Turnebull TJ: Functional assessment after pollicization, *J Hand Surg [Br]* 11:399, 1986.

45. Sastre N, Caravantes MI, Mayoral C: Two-stage toe-to-hand reconstruction in pollicized second metacarpal and useless fingers, *J Reconstr Microsurg* 12:431, 1996.

46. Schoofs M, Leps P, Lambert F, De-Gref C: Forum: reconstruction of the traumatic thumb: Pollicization in the traumatic thumb reconstruction, *Ann Chir Plast Esthet* 38:392, 1993.

47. Sykes PJ, Chandraprakasam T, Percival NJ: Pollicization of the index finger in congenital anomalies, *J Hand Surg [Br]* 16:144, 1991.

48. Verdan C: The reconstruction of the thumb, *Surg Clin North Am* 48:1083, 1968.

49. Weinzweig N, Chen L, Chen ZW: Pollicization of the mutilated hand by transposition of middle and ring finger remnants, *Ann Plast Surg* 34:523, 1995.

PART XI

ARTHRITIS OF THE HAND AND WRIST

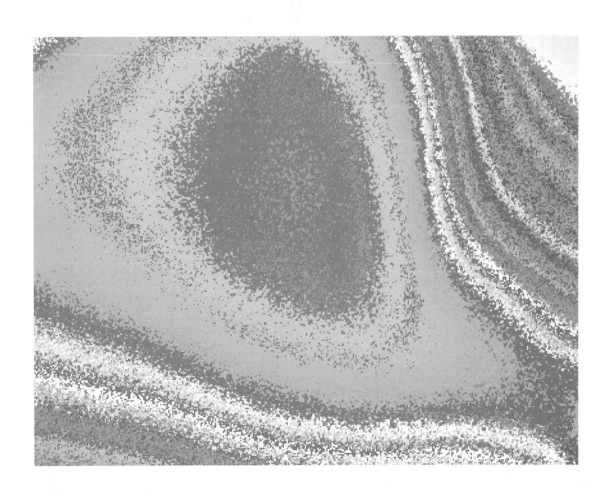

Degenerative Arthritis

127

Michael S. Bednar
Terry R. Light

DISTAL INTERPHALANGEAL JOINT ARTHRITIS

INDICATIONS

Osteoarthritis affects the distal interphalangeal (DIP) joint more frequently than any other joint in the hand (Figure 127-1, *A*). However, osteoarthritis of the DIP joint, although cosmetically unappealing, rarely is functionally disabling or painful.

Indications for treatment of the DIP joint depend on a patient's symptoms. A mucous cyst may develop from an osteophytic spur. Such cysts develop eccentrically because they originate either radially or ulnarly to the course of the terminal tendon across the DIP joint. A mucous cyst most often expands subcutaneously, compressing the underlying germinal matrix of the nail, which leads to longitudinal deformity, grooving of the nail distal to the mass, and thinning of the skin over the mass. Because the cyst communicates directly with the joint and is covered by thinned skin, aspiration should not be performed. Excision is recommended for cysts when they are painful or about to rupture, or when they affect the skin or nail cosmetically.

Osteophytes of the DIP joint are termed *Heberden's nodes.* Rarely, they may produce pain and require debridement. When a patient has pain, deformity, and instability of the joint that is severe enough to interfere with function and these symptoms cannot be alleviated by conservative measures such as splinting and the use of antiinflammatory agents, arthrodesis of the joint is indicated. The loss of DIP flexion is not functionally disabling. Implant arthroplasty rarely is recommended in the DIP joint because of the potential for implant failure accompanied by recurrent instability and pain. Implant arthroplasty may be performed in selected patients with isolated disease who specifically require motion of the DIP joint.

OPERATIONS

Mucous Cyst Excision

The incision for excision of a mucous cyst is begun in the midline over the distal third of the middle phalanx. It is angled radially or ulnarly at the DIP joint to pass over the cyst. The incision should be 3 to 4 mm from the nail as it approaches the eponychium, to preserve blood supply to the skin. A rotation flap can be designed over the middle and distal phalanges to cover the defect when the skin is particularly thin over a large area. Dissection is extended down to the cyst, with care taken to preserve at least half of the terminal extensor tendon. The joint capsule and osteophyte from which the cyst arises are identified and excised. The DIP joint is splinted for 1 week after surgery. Range-of-motion exercises subsequently are initiated and patients are allowed to return to normal activities.

Arthrodesis

Arthrodesis of the DIP joint is usually accomplished through a transverse incision over the dorsum of the joint.[2] Proximal and distal incisions may be extended from the radial and ulnar ends of the transverse incision in an H shape to provide better visualization. Care is taken not to disrupt the germinal matrix of the nail. The terminal extensor tendon is transected proximal to its insertion, and the dorsal joint capsule is opened. A small scalpel is placed in the joint space and passed proximally around the middle phalangeal head and neck to release the collateral ligaments from their insertions into the middle phalanx. When both collateral ligaments are completely incised, the joint should open like a shotgun, permitting full visualization of the articular surfaces of the middle and distal phalanges. The articular cartilage and subchondral bone is excised with a rongeur or oscillating saw to allow the two cancellous bone surfaces to make contact. The recommended

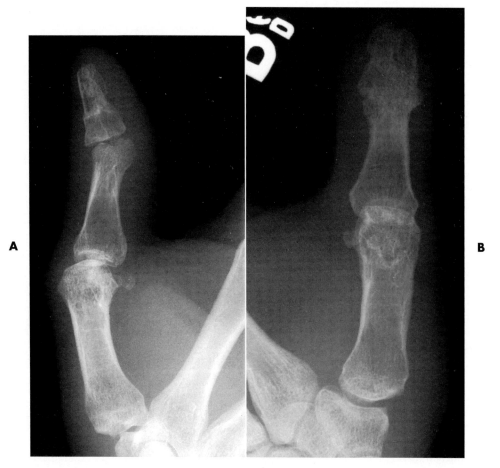

Figure 127-1. **A,** Degenerative arthritis of the IP joint of the thumb. **B,** Arthrodesis of the IP joint of the thumb after removal of K wires.

angle of fusion, which is up to 20 degrees of flexion, must be considered when the bone is removed. Full extension is the angle of choice unless the patient requires DIP flexion for some activity, such as playing a string instrument. Alignment of the fingernail with the middle phalanx ensures slight flexion of the fusion.

Fixation of the arthrodesis is accomplished with Kirschner wires (K wires) if flexion is required. If the joint is fused in full extension, use of a compressive screw, such as the Herbert or Acutrak screw, is preferable.[28] The Herbert screw may be too large for the small finger in women and too small for the interphalangeal (IP) joint of the thumb (see Figure 127-1, *B*). K wires should be used in these digits. The first K wire is inserted retrograde to the distal phalanx, exiting the tip of the finger just under the nail plate. The second K wire is inserted retrograde and angled to exit the phalanx radially or ulnarly. This wire is started eccentrically in the distal phalanx to ensure that the K wires do not cross at the arthrodesis site. Wires are advanced antegrade across the compressed arthrodesis site. Pins are left outside the skin for easier removal and to prevent tip tenderness, which may persist for a long time after the removal of buried pins.

When the Herbert screw is used for fixation, the small drill is first passed retrograde through the center of the distal phalanx and through the pulp. The drill is subsequently passed antegrade through the distal phalanx and into the middle phalanx. The distal phalanx is overdrilled antegradely with a larger drill, and the screw is placed antegrade. A screw length of 22 to 26 mm is usually required to allow the leading threads of the screw to extend to the cortical isthmus of the middle phalanx and the trailing threads to be lodged within the distal phalanx. Care is taken to ensure that proper rotational alignment is established when the screw is tightened.

The DIP joint is splinted for 2 to 6 weeks after surgery, depending on the rigidity of fixation. Active range of motion of the PIP joint is encouraged to prevent proximal stiffness. Patients may resume full activity when the fusion is confirmed by radiographs.

OUTCOMES

The most common complication after excision of a mucous cyst is recurrence, which is usually secondary to incomplete excision of the neck of the cyst and the osteophyte. Care should be taken to remove the pathology that has produced the cyst.

The most common complications after DIP arthrodesis are nonunion (12%), infection (4%), and malunion (3%).[21] Minor complications include dorsal skin necrosis, cold intolerance, permanent proximal interphalangeal (PIP) joint stiffness, paresthesias, superficial infections, and prominent hardware in the case of screw fixation. Nonunion, defined as the absence of bone bridging after 6 months, is most commonly caused by inadequate bone preparation, inadequate bone stock, or infection. Subjectively, patients note an improved appearance and hand function after DIP arthrodesis.

PROXIMAL INTERPHALANGEAL JOINT ARTHRITIS

INDICATIONS

The PIP joint is not commonly involved in cases of osteoarthritis. Degenerative changes affecting this joint are more commonly caused by posttraumatic arthritis. Restricted motion of the DIP joint has little effect on hand function, but restricted PIP-joint motion significantly compromises grip.

Treatment of PIP-joint arthritis should be conservative for as long as possible. Occasionally an osteophyte may interfere with function and may require excision. When symptoms persist because of pain or deformity, surgical treatment alternatives include arthrodesis and arthroplasty. Controversy surrounds the choice between these two procedures. Proponents of arthroplasty claim that the procedure is indicated for painful degenerative arthritis with destruction or subluxation of the joint and stiffness that cannot be effectively treated with soft tissue reconstruction alone. Arthroplasty requires adequate bone stock, an intact flexor mechanism to permit bending of the joint, and muscle/tendon balance of the flexors and extensors. Implant arthroplasty is indicated for treatment of isolated disease of the ring- or small-finger PIP joints because of their importance in the grasping of small objects. The PIP joint of the index finger should be fused to provide a solid post for lateral pinch. The PIP joint of the middle finger may be replaced if the index finger is normal or if an abnormal index PIP joint has been fused.

OPERATIONS

Arthroplasty

Silicone implant arthroplasty may be accomplished through a palmar, lateral, or dorsal approach. The dorsal approach involves the use of a curvilinear incision over the joint.[14] The extensor mechanism is opened between the central slip and one lateral band. The collateral ligaments and palmar plate are released proximally to allow dislocation of the joint. The lateral approach involves the use of a mid-lateral incision over the ulnar side of the joint.[15] The ulnar neurovascular bundle is protected and the ulnar lateral band is displaced dorsally. The ulnar collateral ligament and palmar plate are released proximally to dislocate the joint. The palmar approach provides exposure through a zigzag incision made over the proximal and middle phalanges.[13] The flexor sheath is opened between

the A2 and A4 pulleys. The palmar plate and accessory collateral ligaments are divided proximally to allow the joint to hyperextend.

After the joint is visualized, the articular surface of the middle phalanx is removed with care, to protect the central slip. The articular surface of the proximal phalanx is excised to the metaphyseal flare. Osteophytes are removed, and the medullary canals are reamed with rectangular rasps. The largest implant that can be accommodated without buckling should be used. The tips of the implant may be trimmed to prevent buckling. The radial collateral ligament is repaired by sewing it back to the proximal phalanx through a drilled hole.

Active motion is encouraged the day after surgery. The finger is protected from radial or ulnar deviating stress for 6 weeks. Extension splints may be used at night if an extensor lag is noted. Passive motion is initiated 3 weeks after surgery. Care must be taken to focus rehabilitation efforts on the PIP joint.

Other PIP-joint arthroplasty procedures, including surface replacement, cemented joint replacement, and perichondral arthroplasty have been reported.[14,20]

Arthrodesis

Fusion of the PIP joint is accomplished through a dorsal approach. The articular cartilage and subchondral bone are excised to metaphyseal, cancellous bone. Bone is contoured to allow coaptation of the surfaces at a proper angle of fusion. The PIP joint should be fused at 40 degrees in the index finger, at 45 degrees in the middle finger, at 50 degrees in the ring finger, and at 55 degrees in the small finger.

Fixation may be accomplished with one of several techniques. Two interosseous wire loops may be placed 90 degrees to each other (90–90 wires). For this technique, a 0.035-inch K wire is drilled in a medial-to-lateral and a dorsal-to-palmar direction 3 mm from the end of the prepared bones. A 20-gauge needle is placed in the drilled hole in the proximal phalanx and a 24- or 26-gauge wire is inserted in the needle. The wire is retrieved through the middle phalanx in the opposite direction, forming a loop. The wires are tightened dorsally and on the noncontact side of the finger (ulnarly on the index, middle, and ring fingers; radially on the thumb and small finger).

The tension band technique involves the use of a 0.035-inch K wire to make a medial-to-lateral hole 8 mm distal to the prepared bone surface of the middle phalanx (Figure 127-2). A 24- or 26-gauge wire is passed through the hole. Two 0.035-inch K wires are placed parallel to one another in the radial and ulnar surfaces of the middle phalanx and are drilled antegradely through the middle phalanx, across the DIP joint, through the distal phalanx, and out of the tip of the finger. The joint is reduced and the pins are drilled retrogradely into the proximal phalanx and out of the dorsal cortex. The pins are grasped proximally with the drill and removed until they are proximal to the DIP joint. The tension band wire is crossed over the dorsum of the joint, passed around the protruding K wires, and tightened. The K wires are cut, bent, and buried in the bone or soft tissue (Figure 127-2, *B*).

Active range of motion of the metacarpophalangeal (MCP) and DIP joints may begin after 1 week if fixation is firm. When

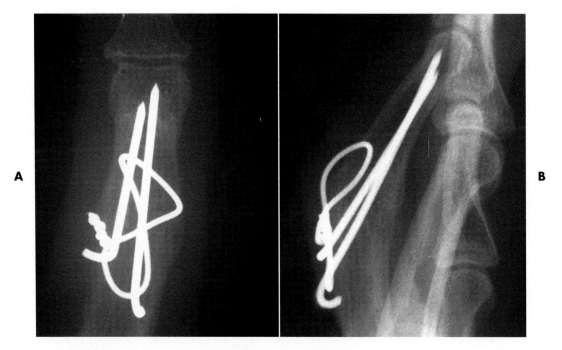

Figure 127-2. AP and lateral radiographs of a tension band arthrodesis of the PIP joint.

fixation is tenuous, the PIP joint is splinted until fusion is confirmed by radiographs, usually in 4 to 6 weeks.

OUTCOMES

PIP-joint arthroplasty dependably relieves pain and preserves some motion. The expected range of motion after the procedure is −10 to 0 degrees of extension and 30 to 70 degrees of flexion. Lin et al[13] reported 69 silicone arthroplasties in 36 patients, all of which were performed with a palmar approach. The average extensor lag improved from 17 to 8 degrees, but the average flexion did not increase (44 to 46 degrees). The average follow-up time was 3.4 years. Follow-up revealed that five implants had fractured.

Complications of PIP-joint fusion include nonunion, malunion, prominent hardware, and infection. Most authors emphasize that careful bone preparation is the most important step in attaining fusion.

ARTHRITIS OF THE CARPOMETACARPAL JOINT OF THE THUMB

INDICATIONS

The carpometacarpal (CMC) joint of the thumb is the second most common site of degenerative arthritis in the hand (Figure 127-3). The restraint of the trapeziometacarpal joint is dependent on the deep palmar "beak" ligament.[17,18] This ligament arises from the palmar–ulnar apex of the metacarpal

and limits dorsal translation of the thumb's metacarpal. Degenerative arthritis of the thumb's CMC joint has been anatomically correlated with degeneration or stretching of the beak ligament. Degeneration of the metacarpal usually begins at the palmar joint margin adjacent to the beak ligament and extends dorsally. Trapezial degeneration originates in the central palmar slope and spreads centrifugally with more advanced disease.

Radiographic findings correspond to the degree of pathology. Four radiographic stages have been defined to describe the degree of joint degeneration.[7] Eaton stage I is characterized by normal articular contours. Slight joint-space narrowing may be present because of effusion or ligament laxity. Eaton stage II is characterized by slight narrowing of the CMC joint and minimal subchondral sclerosis. Osteophytes smaller than 2 mm are present. Eaton stage III is characterized by CMC joint-space narrowing, subchondral sclerosis, and marked cyst formation. Osteophytes larger than 2 mm are present. Degenerative changes also are noted at the scaphotrapezial joint in Eaton stage IV.

Patients with arthritis in the thumb's CMC joint complain of pain that is present with activities that require lateral pinch or full abduction (e.g., pulling on pants or forcefully holding objects such as a large mixing spoon). Although many patients may have restricted range of motion and a cosmetic deformity, these rarely cause concern.

Conservative therapy often relieves the symptoms of arthritis. In one study, a forearm-based spica thumb splint improved symptoms after 6 months in 67% of patients with Eaton stages I or II disease and in 54% of patients with Eaton stages III or IV disease.[22] Some patients complain that a forearm-based splint is too restrictive for daily activities. A hand-based spica thumb splint worn during the day is well tolerated and also

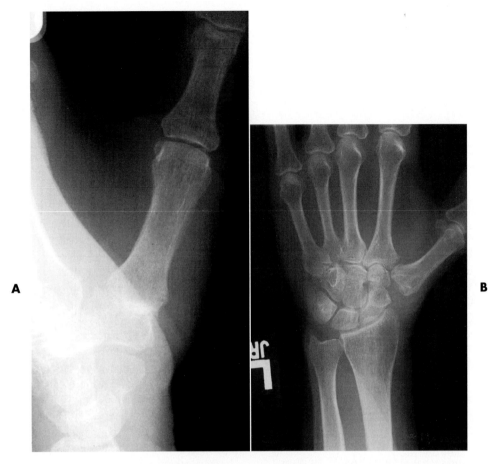

Figure 127-3. **A,** Degenerative arthritis of the CMC joint of the thumb, Eaton stage III. **B,** Trapezial excision, ligament reconstruction, and tendon interpositional arthroplasty.

provides symptom relief. A cortisone injection into the CMC joint may be effective if symptoms persist despite splinting and use of antiinflammatory agents. Patients whose symptoms are unrelieved by conservative measures are candidates for surgical intervention.

OPERATIONS

Several procedures may be used to reconstruct the thumb's CMC joint. The basic principles common to all of these procedures are removal of the degenerated joint and creation and maintenance of a space between the thumb metacarpal and the scaphoid.

Silicone implant arthroplasty is no longer recommended for the treatment of degenerative arthritis in the thumb's CMC joint.[19] Implant fragmentation and foreign-body synovitis with osteolysis caused by shear stresses on the implant were reported in long-term studies. Consequently, other reconstructive options currently are considered for this condition.

Our preferred method for treating arthritis in the thumb's CMC joint involves trapezial excision and interposition arthroplasty (Figure 127-3, *B*).[4] The flexor carpi radialis (FCR) tendon serves to recreate a beak ligament tether and provides

substance for interposition arthroplasty. The joint is approached either palmarly or dorsally. The incision begins with the palmar approach, over the FCR tendon, 2 cm proximal to the wrist crease. It extends distally for 4 cm and subsequently follows the thumb metacarpal until it is 1 cm proximal to the thumb's MCP joint. This approach avoids the dorsal sensory branch of the radial nerve and provides full visualization of the FCR tendon during excision of the trapezium. The dorsal approach involves the use of an incision dorsal to the tendons of the first dorsal compartment. Care is taken to protect the dorsal sensory branches of the radial nerve. The radial artery is visualized and protected with this approach.

The trapezium is excised piecemeal, taking care to protect the surrounding soft tissues. Some authors recommend excision of only the distal half of the trapezium if there are no degenerative changes affecting the scaphotrapezial joint, but we usually remove the entire trapezium. The FCR tendon is divided 8 to 10 cm proximal to the wrist crease. Either half or all of the FCR tendon may be used, but we prefer to use the entire tendon. Care is taken to mobilize the FCR tendon proximal to its insertion on the index metacarpal. The FCR tendon is passed through a drill hole in the base of the thumb's metacarpal. The drill hole begins on the dorsum of the metacarpal, 1 cm proximal to the articular surface. The hole exits the articular surface of the thumb's metacarpal one third of the distance from the palmar beak. Alternatively, the articular surface and subchondral bone of the metacarpal are removed and the hole exits through the cancellous metaphyseal canal. The FCR tendon is passed from proximal to distal, and the tendon is pulled tight and sutured to the metacarpal. The remaining tendon is brought back into the space between the thumb's metacarpal and scaphoid bones. The tendon is rolled in a coil and sewn to itself to create a soft tissue spacer between the metacarpal and scaphoid bones.

If the FCR tendon is not available, the abductor pollicis longus (APL) tendon may be used (Thompson suspension-plasty).[23] The entire dorsal slip of the APL tendon is divided at its musculotendinous junction through a dorsal approach. The tendon is left attached to the base of the thumb metacarpal. Excision of the trapezium and placement of the drill hole in the thumb metacarpal is the same as described previously. The APL tendon is passed through the thumb metacarpal, and a second drill hole is made through the index metacarpal base in a radiopalmar-to-dorsoulnar direction. The tendon is passed through the second drill hole and woven through the extensor carpi radialis brevis tendon.

The hand is immobilized in a short-arm spica thumb cast for 4 weeks. A spica thumb splint is worn intermittently for the next 4 weeks while range-of-motion exercises are initiated. Strengthening exercises are begun at 8 weeks.

An arthrodesis of the CMC joint is preferred in young patients with isolated CMC-joint arthritis who expect to return to heavy manual labor. Arthrodesis is contraindicated in the presence of pantrapezial arthritis or stiff MCP or IP joints. The joint is approached dorsally by incising the joint capsule to bone. The angle of fusion is set at 15 to 20 degrees of extension and 40 to 50 degrees of abduction. To attain these angles, the fingers are placed in full flexion and the distal phalanx of the thumb is placed on the dorsum of the middle phalanx of the index finger. Fixation is attained with either 0.0625-inch K wires or a 2.0- or 2.7-mm condylar blade plate. Bone graft harvested from the distal radius is used to fill bony gaps. The hand is placed in a forearm-based spica thumb splint for 2 weeks after surgery, followed by a hand-based spica thumb splint until fusion is confirmed by radiographs.

OUTCOMES

Burton and Pelligrini[4] reported that 92% of patients who had ligament reconstruction and tendon interposition arthroplasty enjoyed excellent pain relief and were subjectively satisfied with their thumb 2 years after surgery. Objectively, 28% could not touch the thumb tip to the base of the small finger, but overall grip and pinch strength improved 19% compared with preoperative values. Patients were able to resume work requiring repetitive or strenuous hand use, such as operating a punch press, performing assembly line work, and performing the duties of a dental hygienist.

Tomaino et al[24] examined the patients in Burton and Pelligrini's original study 9 years after surgery. Ninety-five percent had excellent pain relief and were satisfied with their

outcome. Grip strength had improved 93% compared with preoperative values and pinch strength improved 65%. The height of the arthroplasty space had decreased 13%, an increase from 11% seen in earlier follow-ups. However, the loss of height did not predict an unsatisfactory outcome. The authors noted that function of the thumb continues to improve for 6 years after surgery, and they emphasized the prolonged time required to attain maximum recovery.

Hanel and Condit[8] followed 30 patients who underwent fusion of the thumb's CMC joint. All patients who were manual laborers returned to work. Pinch strength was 90% and grip strength was 100% of the contralateral side. Most patients were able to bring their thumb to within 1 cm of the base of the small finger. The only consistent limitation noted after the procedure was the patients' inability to lay the hand flat on a table. The hand is usually unable to clear spaces that are less than 2 inches wide.

Bamberger et al[1] reviewed 39 CMC-joint fusions. Fixation was accomplished with K wires or staples. Five delayed unions progressed to union by 23 weeks. Three were fixed with staples and two with K wires. Three fusions developed a nonunion (no healing by 9 months). Two were fixed with staples and one was fixed with K wires. Twenty-four of these patients were followed an average of 4 years. An average 72% reduction in the adduction/abduction arc and an average 61% reduction in the flexion/extension arc were noted. Despite the decrease in motion, there were few subjective complaints. Eleven patients stated that they had no pain, seven had pain with repeated pinch or heavy use, five had pain with any activity, and one had constant pain. Four patients with fair results and one with a poor result had secondary gain (workers compensation or litigation). The authors stated that CMC-joint fusion is their procedure of choice for young laborers and older patients with degenerative arthritis.

CARPOMETACARPAL ARTHRITIS: INDEX/MIDDLE CARPAL BOSS

INDICATIONS

Degenerative arthritis can occur at the base of the metacarpals of the index and/or middle fingers (Figure 127-4). The firm, nonmobile mass may irritate the extrinsic extensor tendons, particularly with radial or ulnar deviation of the wrist. A ganglion also may arise from a carpal boss, increasing the size of the mass. A carpal boss is more commonly seen in women than in men (2:1), most often during the third and fourth decades of life. Clinical examination is aimed at determining whether the visible carpal boss is the cause of the patient's pain. Radiographic examination is facilitated by the use of a *carpal boss view*, or a lateral radiograph taken in 30 to 40 degrees of supination and 20 to 30 degrees of ulnar deviation.

Conservative treatment consists of splint immobilization, the use of antiinflammatory medications, and a steroid injection. If symptoms persist, surgical excision is indicated.

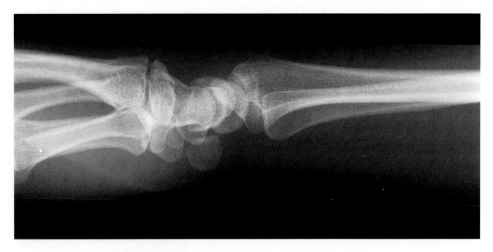

Figure 127-4. Carpal boss of the middle finger CMC joint.

OPERATIONS

The boss is approached through a longitudinal or transverse incision, and care is taken to preserve dorsal sensory branches of the radial nerve. The extensor tendons are retracted and a longitudinal incision is made over the boss. The lesion is exposed through a subperiosteal dissection. A part of the extensor carpi radialis brevis (ECRB) often is elevated from the bone with this dissection. The boss is excised with an osteotome until normal articular cartilage is seen, which usually requires excavation deep to the surface of the metacarpals of the index and middle fingers.

OUTCOMES

Inadequate excision of the carpal boss, resulting in persistent pain and swelling, is the most common complication after excision.[6] Thus it is important to excise the entire boss, exposing the CMC joint in the process. Another complication occurs when a ganglion arising from a carpal boss is confused with a routine dorsal carpal ganglion, which is excised without resection of the carpal boss. As with any procedure around the wrist, dorsal sensory branches must be carefully identified and protected. An adequate surgical approach and excision provide most patients with a significant improvement in symptoms.

PISOTRIQUETRAL ARTHRITIS

INDICATIONS

Pisotriquetral degenerative arthritis is characterized by pain over the palmar ulnar aspect of the wrist. Patients experience an exacerbation of their symptoms during activities in which the hand rests against a hard surface, such as writing or using a computer mouse. Careful palpation elicits tenderness over the

ulnar aspect of the pisotriquetral joint. The pisiform is a sesamoid bone; thus passive flexion of the wrist relaxes the flexor carpi ulnaris (FCU) and permits side-to-side or radioulnar sliding of the articular surface of the pisiform on the palmar articular surface of the triquetrum. Simultaneous compression and side-to-side shucking of the pisiform elicits pain in patients with symptomatic pisotriquetral osteoarthritis. Physical examination should allow the examiner to distinguish pisotriquetral degenerative arthritis from lunotriquetral synovitis and from FCU tenosynovitis. The pain of lunotriquetral instability is usually present over the dorsal carpus and is exacerbated by pushing the pisiform dorsally while pushing on the lunate palmarly. Patients with FCU tenosynovitis have pain at the proximal pole of the pisiform, which is made worse with flexion and ulnar deviation of the wrist against resistance.

If a fractured pisiform heals with an articular step off, degenerative change is a frequent consequence.[16] The pisotriquetral joint is not well visualized on simple anteroposterior (AP) and lateral radiographs of the wrist. The joint may be seen by obtaining a 30-degree supinated oblique view tangential to the pisiform. A standard carpal tunnel view further defines the joint. Lateral tomography also may enhance visualization of the pisotriquetral joint. Radiographs may reveal an osteochondral loose body emanating from the joint. As with all types of degenerative arthritis, a bone scan will be positive at the site of cartilage loss. If pain localization remains imprecise, injection of a local anesthetic into the pisotriquetral joint may be helpful to isolate the source of pain.

The pisiform forms the ulnar border of Guyon's canal; thus patients with osteoarthritic osteophytes emanating from the pisotriquetral joint may develop concomitant ulnar neuropathy. Symptoms of pisotriquetral degenerative arthritis may be diminished by steroid injection into the pisotriquetral joint and splinting of the wrist in slight flexion. If the patient's symptoms are unrelieved, pisiform excision should be considered.

OPERATIONS

Pisiform excision is carried out through a longitudinal palmar incision that crosses the wrist crease obliquely. The incision is radial to the readily palpable pisiform. The ulnar nerve should be decompressed. Occasionally a small branch of the ulnar nerve will transverse a trough in the pisiform. The periosteum of the pisiform is incised longitudinally and the FCU tendon is peeled off the bone. The pisiform is excised, tendon edges are approximated, and a soft dressing is applied. The patient is encouraged to mobilize the hand and wrist after the first dressing change within the first week. Patients resume full activity when comfortable, typically 4 to 8 weeks after surgery.

OUTCOMES

Coyle and Carroll[5] reported an 85% success rate in 65 procedures. Palmier[16] reported effectiveness in 21 patients who underwent pisiform excision. Belliappa and Burke[3] reported complete relief of symptoms in 7 of 9 patients who underwent pisiform excision; however, one patient reported residual symptoms around the ulnar styloid that were aggravated by forearm rotation, and another complained of residual cold intolerance.

Pisiform excision is a successful method of treating pisotriquetral arthritis that remains symptomatic after conservative care.

INTERCARPAL ARTHRITIS: SCAPHOID, TRAPEZIUM, AND TRAPEZOID

INDICATIONS

Isolated arthritis of the joint between the scaphoid, trapezium, and trapezoid (STT) may be highly symptomatic (Figure 127-5). Watson et al[26] demonstrated that isolated STT arthritis was present in 27% of 400 wrist radiographs. Watson has proposed that the term *triscaphe* be used to refer to the articulation between the trapezium, trapezoid, and scaphoid.[25] Because STT arthritis is often associated with arthritis in the thumb's CMC, it is important to determine whether symptoms are emanating from one joint or both joints. Patients often complain of pain at the base of the thumb, as do patients with arthritis in the thumb's CMC. Activities such as lifting heavy objects or wringing out a cloth cause pain.

During examination, patients with CMC arthritis have the most pain at the base of the thumb metacarpal, which is most easily palpated over the dorsal aspect of the thumb. In contrast, patients with STT arthritis experience the most pain over the distal pole of the scaphoid, which is most easily felt palmarly over the scaphoid tubercle and the distal extent of the FCR tendon. FCR tendonitis, which produces pain in response to palpation along the distal tendon, also should be considered in the differential diagnosis of STT arthritis.

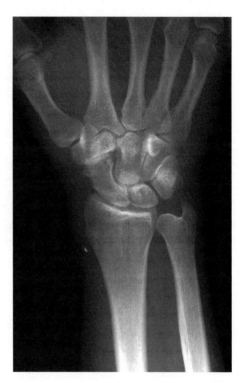

Figure 127-5. Schapho-trapezio-trapezoid degenerative arthritis.

Conservative treatment involves the use of a short-arm spica thumb splint, nonsteroidal antiinflammatory drugs, and activity modification. A cortisone injection in the mid-carpal joint may be given if symptoms persist. This is most easily placed through the radial mid-carpal arthroscopy portal of the wrist, located in the lunotriquetral joint in line with Lister's tubercle of the radius. Surgery is considered for patients who do not receive symptomatic improvement with conservative care.

OPERATIONS

STT arthrodesis aims to eliminate pain and motion in these intercarpal joints while preserving the normal three-dimensional relationship between the carpal bones. In many joint arthrodesis procedures the articular cartilage and subchondral bone are resected and the adjacent metaphyseal surfaces are approximated and coapted to provide contact between well-vascularized metaphyseal bones. This strategy is effective in achieving early bony union, but the attendant shortening of the radial side of the carpus in an STT arthrodesis distorts intercarpal relationships and subjects adjacent joints to abnormal load forces. Thus we favor the use of bone grafts to preserve radial carpal height when performing an STT fusion.

The wrist is approached through a longitudinal or transverse incision. The extensor pollicis longus (EPL) and extensor carpi radialis longus (ECRL) tendons are identified and retracted. The STT joint capsule is incised transversely. The scaphotrapezial, scaphotrapezoid, and trapezium-trapezoid joints are visualized. Articular cartilage and subchondral bone are resected with care, to preserve as much of the carpal bone as possible.

Bone graft is harvested from the ipsilateral distal radius. The

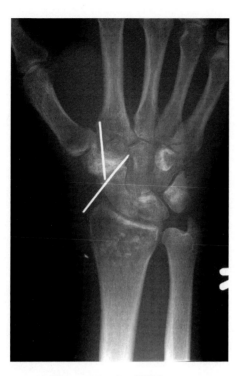

Figure 127-6. STT fusion.

proximal portion of a longitudinal skin incision allows exposure of the donor site; however, if a transverse incision is used, a second transverse incision will be required. A cortical window is created in the distal radius between the brachioradialis and ECRL or between the EPL and extensor digitorum longus. Drill holes are made in an oval pattern approximately 8 × 12 mm. An osteotome connects the holes and the cortical window is elevated. A curette is used to obtain a cancellous bone graft from the distal radial metaphysis.

K wires are inserted in the carpal bones either by retrograding the pins out from the resected articular surfaces or more commonly by inserting the pins through one of the carpal bones and into the fusion site. Care is taken to protect the dorsal sensory branch of the radial nerve when placing the pins from the radial side of the wrist. The skin should be incised and a drill guide should be placed on the bone before the pins are inserted. Pins are advanced to ensure that they engage the adjacent surface. Cancellous bone graft is meticulously packed into the interval between the resected bone surfaces. Cortical graft is carefully locked under the dorsal lips of adjacent carpal bones; to ensure normal carpal alignment and orientation, pins are advanced across the arthrodesis site. Pin depth is adjusted to obtain firm fixation in both bones but to avoid fixation across periarthrodesis articulations. Intraoperative use of fluoroscopy facilitates appropriate carpal orientation and precise pin placement. Pins are trimmed beneath the skin. A long-arm spica thumb dressing is used to securely immobilize the hand, wrist, and elbow. The dressing is changed in 2 to 5 days and a long-arm spica thumb cast is applied for 4 to 6 weeks. Subsequently a short-arm cast replaces the long-arm cast, for a total of 12 weeks of immobilization. Pins are removed when union is documented by radiographs (Figure 127-6).

OUTCOMES

Watson reported that the best results are achieved with a triscaphe fusion.[26] The nonunion rate in his series was 1% to 3%. He stated that infection, hematoma, and transient neurapraxias associated with this procedure are exceedingly rare. Watson also reported a 1.5% incidence of radioscaphoid arthritis after triscaphe fusion, which necessitated a scaphoid excision and lunate–capitate–triquetrum–hamate fusion (SLAC reconstruction). Watson routinely performed a radial styloidectomy in conjunction with triscaphe fusion after 1987.

Kleinman and Carroll[11] reported significantly more complications with triscaphe fusion. They performed 47 STT fusions in 46 patients during a 10-year period and had a complication rate of 52%. Nonunion occurred in 15% of patients, progressive carpal arthrosis in 19%, pin-tract infections in 8%, osteomyelitis in 4%, radial styloid impingement in 4%, and intractable pain despite normal radiographs in 6%. To reduce complications, the authors recommended performance of a radial styloidectomy, allowing the pins to remain subcutaneous rather than protruding through the skin, and careful removal of sufficient subchondral bone to expose cancellous bone.

The authors concluded that patients should be informed of all possible complications associated with an STT fusion when such fusion is indicated for the treatment of STT arthritis.

ARTHRITIS SECONDARY TO CHRONIC INTERCARPAL INSTABILITY

INDICATIONS

Early diagnosis and treatment of scapholunate ligament disruption is clearly preferable to treating the consequences of abnormal carpal kinematics resulting from scapholunate instability. Watson and Ballet have outlined the sequence of degenerative changes that typically result from scapholunate dissociation.[25] In radiographs, degenerative changes first appear between the scaphoid and radius as a sharp, elongated point on the radial styloid, then progress to involve the radioscaphoid joint (Figure 127-7). The capitate drives between the scaphoid and lunate with time, resulting in lunocapitate arthritis. Degenerative changes also may be seen at the hamate–lunate articulation because of the concentric relationship between the lunate and the lunate facet of the radius. The radiolunate joint surface remains uninvolved.

After degenerative changes are present, conservative treatment may partially relieve symptoms. Surgical treatment is based on the patient's symptoms and radiographic findings. Proximal row carpectomy is effective when the degenerative change is confined to the radioscaphoid articulation. When mid-carpal degenerative changes are seen between the capitate and the lunate in addition to radioscaphoid degenerative change, a proximal row carpectomy is not recommended. Surgical options in such advanced cases include mid-carpal

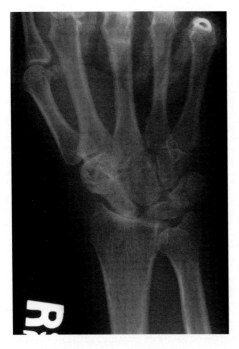

Figure 127-7. SLAC wrist.

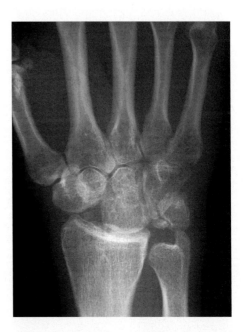

Figure 127-8. Proximal row carpectomy; note the capitate seated in the lunate fossa.

arthrodesis with scaphoid excision (SLAC reconstruction or total wrist fusion.

OPERATIONS

Proximal Row Carpectomy

The wrist is approached through a longitudinal incision. The ECRB, EPL, extensor digitorum communis (EDC), extensor indicis proprius (EIP), extensor digiti quinti (EDQ), and extensor carpi ulnaris (ECU) tendons are isolated. A transverse capsulotomy is made, both radial and ulnar to the EDC tendons. The scaphoid, lunate, and triquetrum are identified. The articular surface of the head of the capitate is inspected before any bone is resected; proximal row carpectomy may be contraindicated if this surface is compromised. The scaphoid is excised first, the triquetrum second, and the lunate last. Resection of the carpal bones may be facilitated by placing a K wire in each bone requiring resection. K wires may be used as a joystick to expose, manipulate, and excise each bone. It is essential to preserve the radioscaphocapitate and long radiolunate ligaments while the scaphoid is resected.

After the carpal bones have been completely resected, the wrist is collapsed. The capitate head is seated in the lunate fossa of the radius and the wrist is radially deviated. A limited radial styloidectomy is performed if impingement exists between the radial styloid and the trapezium. Care is taken to protect the radiocarpal ligaments. The head of the capitate should naturally shift proximally into the lunate fossa of the distal radius (Figure 127-8). The wrist capsulotomy is closed with care, to avoid excessively tightening the dorsal capsule. A bulky dressing incorporating a plaster splint is used for 5 to 7 days, and a volar

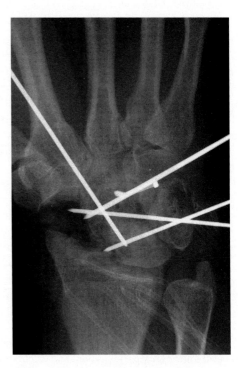

Figure 127-9. Scaphoid excision and four-corner arthrodesis shown on an intraoperative radiograph.

wrist splint is used for support during the first few weeks after surgery. Patients are encouraged to regain digital flexion and extension. Patients may begin range-of-motion exercises for the wrist a few weeks after surgery, but strengthening exercises and heavy lifting should be delayed for at least 3 months.

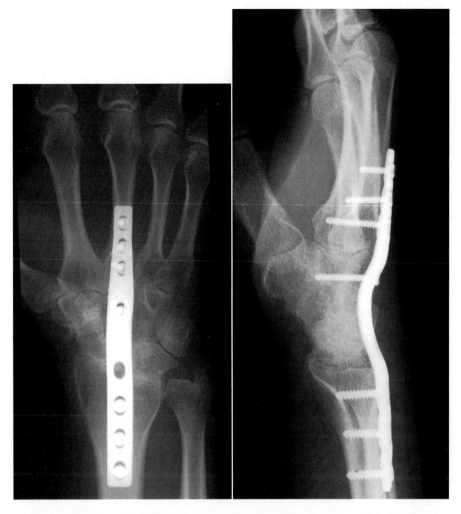

Figure 127-10. AP and lateral radiographs of a wrist arthrodesis with fusion plate.

Four-Corner Fusion With Scaphoid Excision (SLAC Reconstruction)

A central longitudinal incision is used to approach the wrist. The extensor retinaculum is opened through the third dorsal compartment, and, while maintaining protection of the tendons, a transverse incision is made at the mid-carpal joint. The scaphoid is excised while protection of the radiocarpal ligaments is maintained. The articular cartilage and subchondral bone are removed from the lunate, triquetrum, hamate, and capitate in the mid-carpal joint. Pins are placed into the capitate, hamate, and triquetrum. Cancellous bone graft harvested from the distal radius is packed into the defect. To reduce the dorsiflexed posture of the lunate, a K wire is placed into it and rotated distally, which displaces the capitate palmarly. Pins are placed between the capitate and lunate, hamate and lunate, triquetrum and capitate, and triquetrum and lunate (Figure 127-9). A long-arm splint is replaced after 1 week by a long-arm cast, which is worn for 4 to 6 weeks. A short-arm cast is worn until 12 weeks after surgery, and the pins are removed when fusion can be verified radiographically.

Total Wrist Fusion

A central, longitudinal incision is used to approach the wrist, and the extensor retinaculum is opened through the third dorsal compartment. The EPL tendon is transposed radially. An incision to bone is made over the metacarpal of the middle finger, longitudinally across the wrist, and onto the distal radius through the third dorsal compartment. Wrist capsular flaps are elevated with periosteal flaps from the metacarpal and radius. The distal radioulnar joint is not opened. The articular cartilage and cancellous bone are removed from the radioscaphoid, radiolunate, lunocapitate, scaphocapitate, and middle finger CMC joints. The CMC joint of the index finger also may be fused. Lister's tubercle and the middle finger carpal boss are removed. Cancellous bone graft, taken from either the radial metaphysis or the iliac crest, is packed into the fusion site. An AO wrist fusion plate is subsequently applied. Screws (2.7 mm) are placed into the metacarpal of the middle finger, and subsequently 3.5-mm screws are placed into the radius (Figure 127-10). The capsular and periosteal flaps are closed over the plate. A short-arm cast is worn for comfort, followed by a short-arm splint until radiographic union is seen, usually in 6 to 8 weeks.

OUTCOMES

Several studies have compared proximal row carpectomy with SLAC reconstruction. Wyrick et al[27] compared the results of 17 cases of SLAC reconstruction with those of 11 cases of proximal row carpectomy (PRC). The total arc of motion averaged 95 degrees in the SLAC group and 115 degrees in the PRC group and represented range of motion that was 47% and 64%, respectively, that of the opposite wrist. Grip strength was 74% compared with that in the opposite wrist in the SLAC group and 94% that of the opposite wrist in the PRC group. Three SLAC reconstructions failed and were converted to total wrist fusions. No failures occurred in the PRC group. The authors recommended PRC only for patients without capitate arthritis.

Krakauer et al[12] also compared SLAC reconstruction with PRC. Their SLAC group retained 54 degrees of motion, compared with 71 degrees in the PRC group. They recommend SLAC reconstruction in patients with capitolunate arthritis and PRC when the capitate is normal.

Imbriglia[10] reviewed the results of PRC 4 years after surgery. Postoperative pain relief was achieved in 26 of 27 patients. Range of motion matched or surpassed preoperative values, and grip strength improved to 80% of that of the contralateral side. Moreover, the results did not seem to deteriorate over time.

Hastings[9] outlined the complications that occurred after wrist fusion by the AO plate technique. The nonunion rate was 2%, mostly at the middle finger CMC joint. Hastings indicated that nonunion could be avoided by complete decortication of the dorsal 80% of the CMC joint down to cancellous bone. Tenderness caused by the 3.5-mm plate was present in 19% of patients, mostly at the metacarpal level. Twelve percent of patients required plate removal. Use of the new plate with 2.7-mm screws over the metacarpal may lower the rate of irritation caused by the plate. Flexor or extensor tendon adhesions occurred in 3.5% of patients. Flexor tenosynovitis typically resulted from screws that were too long and extensor tenosynovitis was caused by irritation from the plate. When tenosynovitis was not resolved after a cortisone injection, the plate was removed after a solid arthrodesis was achieved. Carpal tunnel syndrome after fusion occurred in 4% to 10% of patients; thus patients undergoing wrist fusion should be screened for carpal tunnel syndrome to prevent aggravation of the condition after surgery. Iliac crest complications occurred in 1.7% of patients and consisted of iliac crest fracture, hematoma, neuroma, hernia, or palpable deformity. The complication rate was lower if minimal stripping of the crest was performed and only cancellous bone was removed.

POSTFRACTURE DEGENERATIVE ARTHRITIS OF THE SCAPHOID

INDICATIONS

Scaphoid nonunion advanced collapse (SNAC) of the wrist, like the wrist after SLAC, also progresses in a predictable pattern (Figure 127-11). With SNAC, arthritis develops in the wrist between the distal fragment of the scaphoid and the radius. The proximal pole of the scaphoid, like the lunate, remains free of degenerative changes.

Bone grafting and fixation of the scaphoid should be performed if the wrist has not developed significant degenerative changes. A vascularized radial bone graft may improve blood flow if avascular necrosis of the proximal pole is seen at the time of surgery. After degenerative changes are present, treatment depends on the location and extent of the arthritis. A radial styloidectomy may be performed if the scaphoid fracture is distal to relieve the impingement between the rotated distal pole and the radius. Some surgeons have recommended distal scaphoid excision, recognizing that the proximal pole of the scaphoid and the rest of the proximal row subsequently will rotate into dorsiflexion. When none of these operations is possible, as in cases of SLAC wrist, a proximal row carpectomy or scaphoid excision, mid-carpal fusion, or total wrist fusion is performed.

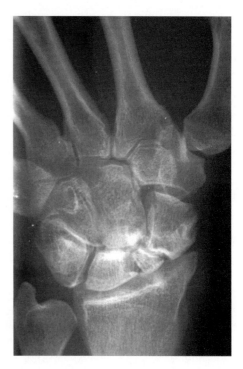

Figure 127-11. SNAC wrist; note the scaphoid nonunion and degenerative changes between the scaphoid and radius.

OPERATIONS

Radial Styloidectomy

A longitudinal incision is made over the radial styloid, dorsal to the tendons of the first dorsal compartment. Care is taken to protect the dorsal sensory branch of the radial nerve. The radiocarpal joint capsule is opened, and the radial styloid is excised to the level of the radioscaphocapitate ligament. The wrist is splinted for comfort postoperatively, and range-of-motion exercises are begun.

Distal Pole Excision

The approaches are the same as those used for treatment of CMC arthritis. Care is taken in excising the distal pole, to protect the palmar radiocarpal ligaments. The wrist is splinted for comfort postoperatively, and range-of-motion exercises are begun.

OUTCOMES

Radial styloidectomy and distal pole excision are not definitive procedures. Periods of pain relief typically are followed by degenerative changes that may require proximal row carpectomy, SLAC reconstruction, or total wrist fusion. Outcomes for these operations are discussed in preceding sections.

POSTTRAUMATIC RADIOCARPAL DEGENERATIVE ARTHRITIS

INDICATIONS

Degenerative arthritis that occurs simultaneously between the radius and scaphoid and between the radius and lunate typically is the result of an intraarticular fracture of the distal radius. Arthrodesis should be considered when posttraumatic arthritis is unresponsive to conservative methods. Radiocarpal arthrodesis is possible when mid-carpal alignment and articular surfaces are normal and preserve mid-carpal motion.

OPERATIONS

Radiocarpal Arthrodesis

The extensor retinaculum is opened through a central, longitudinal approach to the wrist, into a third dorsal compartment. The EPL tendon is transposed radially, and a transverse incision is made in the radiocarpal joint. The articular surfaces and subchondral bone of the radius, scaphoid, and lunate are removed. Cancellous bone is removed from the radial metaphysis and packed into the fusion site. K wires maintain fixation between the radius and lunate, radius and scaphoid, and scaphoid and lunate. A long-arm cast is applied until radiographic fusion is seen, usually in 6 to 8 weeks.

OUTCOMES

Radio-scaphoid-lunate fusion is highly successful in relieving pain and maintaining approximately 50% of wrist motion. Grip strength after the procedure is 75% to 80% of the contralateral side. Adequate bone preparation is required, as with any fusion, to prevent nonunion. The ulnotriquetral joint must be inspected during resection of the joint surface for ulnocarpal impingement; if the latter is present, the triquetrum should be excised.

REFERENCES

1. Bamberger HB, Stern PJ, Kiefhaber TR, et al: Trapeziometacarpal joint arthrodesis: a functional evaluation, *J Hand Surg [Am]* 17:605-611, 1991.
2. Bednar MS: Distal interphalangeal joint fusion, *Atlas of Hand Clin* 3:1-16, 1998.
3. Belliappa PP, Burke FD: Excision of the pisiform in pisotriquetral osteoarthritis, *J Hand Surg [Br]* 17:133-136, 1992.
4. Burton RI, Pelligrini VD, Jr: Surgical management of basil joint arthritis of the thumb. Part 2: Ligament reconstruction with tendon interposition arthroplasty, *J Hand Surg [Am]* 11:324-332, 1986.
5. Coyle MP, Carroll RE: Dysfunction of the pisotriquetral joint: treatment by pisiform excision, *J Hand Surg [Am]* 7:421, 1982.
6. Cuono CB, Watson HK: The carpal boss: surgical treatment and etiological considerations, *Plast Reconstr Surg* 63:88-93, 1979.
7. Eaton RG, Glickel SZ: Trapeziometacarpal arthritis: staging as a rationale for treatment, *Hand Clin* 3:455-469, 1997.
8. Hanel DT, Condit DP: Thumb metacarpal joint fusion with plate and screw fixation, *Atlas of Hand Clin* 3:41-59, 1998.
9. Hastings H II, Weiss APC, Quenzer D, et al: Arthrodesis of the wrist for post-traumatic disorders, *J Bone Joint Surg* 78A:897-902, 1996.
10. Imbriglia JE, Broudy AS, Hagberg WC, McKernan D: Proximal row carpectomy: clinical evaluation, *J Hand Surg [Am]* 15:426-430, 1990.
11. Kleinman WB, Carroll C, IV: Scapho-trapezio-trapezoid arthrodesis for treatment of chronic static and dynamic scapholunate instability: a 10-year perspective on pitfalls and complications, *J Hand Surg [Am]* 15:408-414, 1990.
12. Krakauer JD, Bischop AT, Cooney WP: Surgical treatment of scapholunate advanced collapse, *J Hand Surg [Am]* 19:751-759, 1994.
13. Lin HH, Wyrick JD, Stern PJ: Proximal interphalangeal joint silicone replacement arthroplasty: clinical results using an anterior approach, *J Hand Surg [Am]* 20:123-132, 1995.
14. Linscheid RL, Murray PM, Vidil MA, Beckenbaugh RD: Development of a surface replacement arthroplasty for proximal interphalangeal joints, *J Hand Surg [Am]* 22:286-298, 1997.

15. Lipscond PR: Synovectomy of the distal two joints of the thumb and fingers in rheumatoid arthritis, *J Bone Joint Surg* 49A:1135-1140, 1967.

16. Palmieri TJ: The excision of painful pisiform bone fractures, *Orthop Rev* 11(6):99-103, 1982.

17. Pelligrini VD, Jr: Osteoarthritis of the trapeziometacarpal joint: the path of physiology of articular cartilage degeneration. I. Anatomy and physiology of the aging joint, *J Hand Surg [Am]* 16:967-974, 1991.

18. Pelligrini VD, Jr: Osteoarthritis of the trapeziometacarpal joint: the path of physiology of articular cartilage degeneration. II. Articular wear patterns in the osteoarthritic joint, *J Hand Surg [Am]* 16:975-982, 1991.

19. Pelligrini VD, Jr, Burton RI: Surgical management of basil joint arthritis of the thumb. Part 1: Long term results of silicone implant arthroplasty, *J Hand Surg [Am]* 11:309-324, 1986.

20. Seradge H, Tutz LA, Einert HE, et al: Pericondral resurfacing arthroplasty in the hand, *J Hand Surg [Am]* 9:880-886, 1984.

21. Stern PJ, Folton DB: Distal interphalangeal joint arthrodesis: an analysis of complications, *J Hand Surg [Am]* 17:1139-1145, 1992.

22. Swigart CR, Eaton RG, Glickel SZ, Johnson C: Splinting and the treatment of arthritis of the first carpometacarpal joint, *J Hand Surg [Am]* 24:86-91, 1999.

23. Thompson JS: Suspensionplasty, *J Orthop Surg Techniques* 4:1-13, 1989.

24. Tomaino MM, Pelligrini VD, Jr, Burton RI: Arthroplasty of the basil joint of the thumb: long-term follow-up after ligament reconstruction with tendon interposition, *J Bone Joint Surg* 77A:346-355, 1995.

25. Watson HK, Ballet FL: The SLAC wrist: scapholunate advanced collapse pattern of degenerative arthritis, *J Hand Surg [Am]* 9:358-365, 1984.

26. Watson HK, Weinzweig J: Intercarpal arthodesis. In Green DP, Hotchkiss RN, Pederson WC (editors): *Green's operative hand surgery*, ed 4, New York, 1999, Churchill Livingstone.

27. Wyrick JD, Stern PJ, Kiefhaber TR: Motion-preserving procedures in the treatment of scapholunate advanced collapse wrist: proximal row carpectomy versus four-corner arthrodesis, *J Hand Surg [Am]* 20:965-970, 1995.

28. Wyrsch B, Dawson J, Alfrank S, et al: Distal interphalangeal joint arthrodesis comparing tension band wire and Herbert screw: a biomechanical and dimensional analysis, *J Hand Surg [Am]* 21:438-443, 1996.

Rheumatoid Arthritis of the Hand and Wrist

128

Forst E. Brown
E. Dale Collins
Alan Scott Harmatz

INTRODUCTION

Rheumatoid arthritis is a chronic systemic inflammatory disease of unknown etiology that involves an autoimmune antigen–antibody mechanism. The presentation of a relevant antigen to an immunogenetically susceptible host is believed to trigger the disease. A variety of arthritogenic stimuli may be responsible for activating the immune response. Significant attention has been focused on the role of infectious agents.

Harris[26] describes five stages of rheumatoid disease as determined by the pathologic process. During the first stage, macrophages or dendritic cells in the synovial membrane ingest, process, and present foreign protein antigens to T lymphocytes. These initiate a cellular immune response and stimulate the differentiation of B lymphocytes into plasma cells that secrete antibody. During the next stage, the increased number of T cells in the synovial membrane causes B-cell proliferation and differentiation and the production of antibodies in an environment characterized by angiogenesis and an increased number of synovial cells. Cytokines produced by the synovial cells and lymphocytes increase and perpetuate joint inflammation. Large numbers of activated neutrophils are chemoattracted into the synovial fluid and subsequently release proteinases, arachidonic acid metabolites, and reactive oxidants. The complement system and clotting cascade are activated, and vascular permeability increases. The production of the major proteinases, collagenase, and stromelysin by synovial cells is induced by cytokines, and these proteolytic enzymes are subsequently activated by plasmin. The inhibitors of these enzymes become saturated, allowing free enzymes to destroy articular cartilage, bone, and ligaments. In response, antibodies to collagen appear and amplify the destructive arthritis. The patient subsequently becomes symptomatic and experiences malaise, joint stiffness,

and swelling. During the third stage, examination reveals warm, swollen joints that exhibit synovial proliferation and effusion, limited movement, and occasionally rheumatoid nodules.

During stage four, the synovial pannus invades cartilage, subchondral bone, ligaments, and tendons, producing irreversible damage. Fassbender[21] has described tumorlike proliferative aggregates in this synovial tissue. The proteolytic enzymes produced by the synovium destroy the matrix proteins of articular cartilage and bone. More pronounced swelling and early instability of the joints are noted. Radiographic evidence of periarticular osteopenia may be obtained. Magnetic resonance imaging (MRI) reveals proliferative joint pannus and tendon invasion. By stage five, invasion of the cartilage and tendon by synovium, erosion of subchondral bone (Figure 128-1), and ligament damage have produced joint destruction and instability, contractures, and tendon ruptures (Figure 128-2). Radiographs reveal bony erosions, narrowed and irregular joint surfaces, and dislocated joints.

A number of secondary changes follow. Bony irregularities may cause tendon rupture, including rupture of the extensor digiti quinti (EDQ) and extensor digitorum communis (EDC) tendons by the distal ulna (Figure 128-3), and rupture of the flexor pollicis longus (FPL) and flexor digitorum profundus (FDP) tendons by the distal pole of the scaphoid.[39] Contact between altered joint surfaces produces degenerative cartilage and bone damage. Vasculitis and atrophy from disuse lead to muscle weakness. Increased joint volume and ligament laxity result in a failure to counteract the application of normal force vectors on the joints. The carpus translates volarly and supinates, and the metacarpophalangeal (MCP) joints demonstrate ulnar drift. Proximal joint position affects the alignment of the next distal joint, resulting in a zigzag deformity (Figure 128-4). Synovial swelling also compresses nerves and/or interferes with tendon gliding.

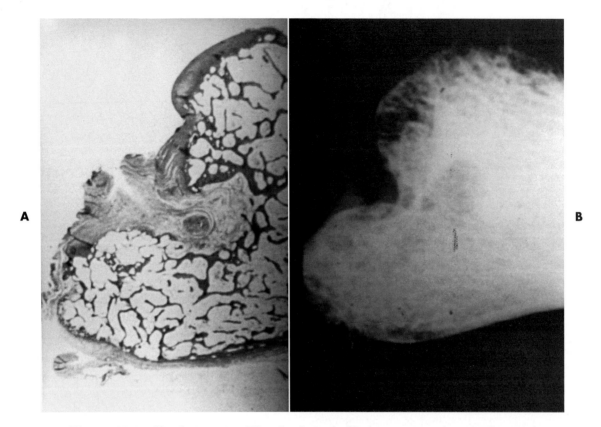

Figure 128-1. Histologic section **(A)** and radiograph **(B)** demonstrating rheumatoid synovial invasion of subchondral bone.

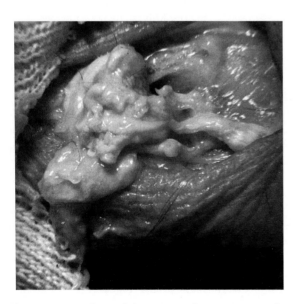

Figure 128-2. Synovial destruction of an extensor tendon.

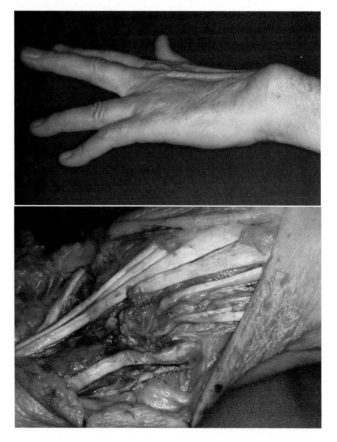

Figure 128-3. Dorsal positioning of a damaged distal ulna produces attenuation and disruption of the EDQ and EDC IV and V.

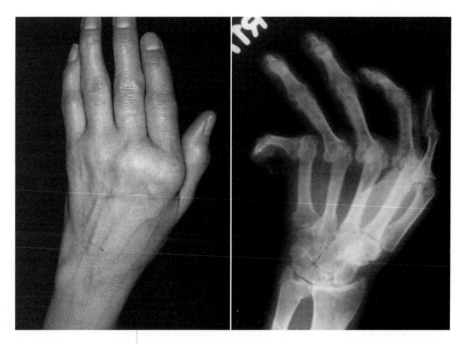

Figure 128-4. Typical zigzag deformity seen in patients with rheumatoid arthritis.

INDICATIONS

The diagnosis of rheumatoid arthritis must be made on clinical grounds. Revised criteria for diagnosis were published in 1988[2]; these have a 91% to 94% sensitivity and 89% specificity and include morning stiffness; soft tissue swelling; swelling of the proximal interphalangeal (PIP), MCP, and/or wrist joints; symmetric arthritis; subcutaneous nodules; a positive rheumatoid factor (present in 70% to 80% of patients); and radiographic evidence of erosions or osteopenia. Rheumatoid arthritis is suspected when the first four symptoms have been present for 6 or more weeks. Differential diagnoses include psoriatic arthritis, gout, pseudogout, systemic lupus erythematosus, ankylosing spondylitis, scleroderma, Reiter's syndrome, and Sjögren's syndrome.

Rheumatoid arthritis is usually accompanied by a nonspecific decrease in serum hemoglobin and a variable elevation in erythrocyte sedimentation rate (ESR), but the use of laboratory tests alone is not adequate for making a conclusive diagnosis. Quantitative measurement of C-reactive protein typically exhibits a pattern that parallels the ESR and that may correlate with the appearance of destructive arthritis in stage four. An increase in serum neutrophils, eosinophils, and thrombocytes also may occur during the active disease process. Disease-specific measurements, as of rheumatoid factor (IgM antibodies against IgG), help in the differential diagnosis but also indicate a less favorable prognosis. The significance of other immunoglobulins, such as antikeratin antibodies (99% specificity) and antiperinuclear factor, in patients with rheumatoid arthritis is currently under evaluation. Technology involving tissue-specific markers is available for use in research studies but is not yet clinically useful.[75] The same is true for technology involving genetic information (HCA-DRB1). The radiological grading of rheumatoid joints using the Larson index provides the best clinical measure of the stage and progression of rheumatoid arthritis.[36]

NONSURGICAL TREATMENT

The mainstays of treatment for rheumatoid arthritis include patient instruction, diet, rest, exercise, splinting, and medications. Non-weight-bearing exercises are used to help maintain muscle tone. Because the inflamed joint is particularly vulnerable to the effects of motion, splinting is used to rest affected joints and to counteract the effect of deforming force vectors on these joints. However, the disease has been proven to progress despite splinting and exercise programs. Nonsteroidal antiinflammatory drugs, including aspirin, are the foundation of drug therapy for rheumatoid arthritis; they serve to counteract the products of inflammation that drive the synovial proliferative response into stage four of the disease. A pyramid of treatment has been used, beginning with nonsteroidal drugs, advancing through second-line drugs such as the antimalarial medications, and culminating in the use of antimetabolites such as methotrexate and cyclosporine. Numerous studies suggest that this pyramid should be inverted to inhibit the progressive course of the disease as early as possible.[11] Low-dose steroids and intraarticular steroid injections may benefit certain patients with little risk of morbidity, but the benefit of their long-term use is difficult to prove. The surgeon must know which medications a patient is taking because they may have significant side effects. We have not recommended discontinuing rheumatoid medications in anticipation of surgery because patients have been more comfortable with their perioperative use and we have not seen an associated increase in complications. In a recent prospective study that supports this program, no difference in wound healing occurred among patients who discontinued methotrexate 1 week before surgery compared with patients who continued therapy.[55]

SURGICAL TREATMENT

The traditional role of the surgeon in the care of rheumatoid patients is to perform reconstructive or salvage surgery.[23] Improvement in function can be obtained with such treatment, but extensive joint and tendon damage limits its potential benefit. In 1959 Vaughn-Jackson advocated early prophylactic surgery.[68] In 1992 Stanley reported that early conservative surgery is a more effective way of directing surgical treatment toward the appropriate patient at the most effective time.[57] The goals of surgery include pain control, retardation of disease progression, restoration or improvement of function, and cosmetic improvement. The risks associated with complications and failure to achieve the surgical goal must be considered. Function takes precedence over appearance because a deformed hand in a rheumatoid patient may have acceptable function. Surgical goals are best achieved when the hand surgeon serves as a member of a multidisciplinary team that determines the appropriate timing for surgical intervention and can evaluate the effectiveness of various treatments.

Rheumatoid Nodules

Nodules occur in approximately 20% to 25% of patients with rheumatoid arthritis and are associated with strong seropositivity and aggressive disease. They are located on the posterior surface of the forearm and olecranon, as well as on the volar and dorsal surfaces of the fingers. They are tender to pressure, may compress digital nerves, and are unsightly. The typical histologic picture is that of a necrotic center, a surrounding wall of palisading histiocytes, and peripheral vascular connective tissue. Steroid injection can cause the nodules to regress but also can produce ulceration. Surgical removal is indicated for relief of symptoms and less frequently for cosmesis. We advise our patients that recurrence is common.

Tenosynovitis

Rheumatoid arthritis is a disease of synovial tissues that frequently involves tendons and tendon sheaths. Savill[56] reported that the incidence of tenosynovitis was 50% among patients with chronic disease; Brewerton[12] reported an incidence of 64%. Rheumatoid synovium invades and destroys collagen fibrils. The attrition of tendons is also caused by irregular bony prominences[68] and interference with blood supply. Approximately 50% of patients who undergo prophylactic tenosynovectomy have been found to have tendon invasion, a precursor to tendon rupture.[4,5,13] Impending rupture is difficult to diagnose because it can occur in the presence of minimal swelling. A history of previous tendon rupture, weakness of the involved tendons, and a change in local pain can indicate future rupture. Movement of the synovial mass with flexion and extension of the fingers signifies tendon adhesion and possible invasion (Figure 128-5). MRI studies reveal tendon invasion and rupture (Figure 128-6). Real-time ultrasound also holds promise as a helpful diagnostic tool. Because of the difficulty associated with predicting tendon rupture, most authors currently recommend prophylactic tenosynovectomy when synovial swelling persists after 4 to 6 months of appropriate medical therapy. Moreover,

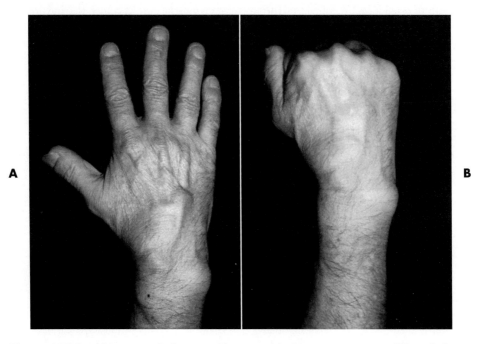

Figure 128-5. Movement of the synovial mass with finger in extension **(A)** and flexion **(B)** indicates fixation to the extensor mechanism and possible tendon invasion.

because the incidence of carpal tunnel syndrome precipitated by flexor tenosynovitis may be as high as 65%,[7] flexor tenosynovectomy performed before irreversible nerve changes occur can clear this neuropathy. Flexor tenosynovectomy also corrects restricted motion and triggering as the tendons pass through the tight confines of the carpal tunnel and digital sheaths. Local steroids can reduce the inflammatory process and swelling, but they do not influence synovial invasion or attrition of the tendons. Informing the patient and treating rheumatologist about preventing tendon rupture and permanent nerve damage has helped to facilitate early conservative surgery.

Tendon Ruptures and Transfers

The rupture of a tendon typically is clinically evident. Ulnar subluxation of the extensor tendons off the metacarpal head and posterior interosseous nerve compression may simulate extensor tendon rupture. Distal extension of the MCP joints with passive wrist flexion indicates intact tendons. Interference with tendon glide in the digital sheaths and carpal tunnel symptoms may suggest flexor-tendon rupture. Surgery is indicated for the rupture of most tendons because it is has been our experience that a subsequent tendon rupture frequently follows on the heels of the first. The inciting mechanism for the rupture or impending rupture can be eliminated and improved function can be provided with an appropriate

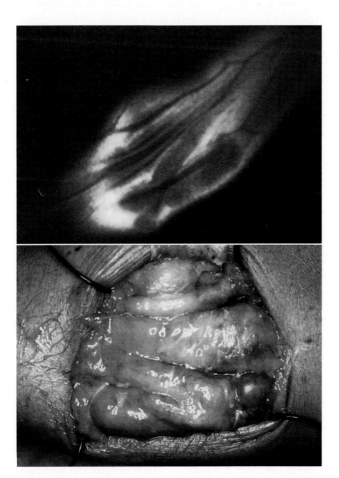

Figure 128-6. MRI evaluation helps determine the degree of synovial tendon involvement.

tendon transfer. Splinting, in some situations, provides adequate joint support to partly compensate for ruptured tendons and also allows reasonable hand function.

Synovectomy

When joint surfaces are intact and soft tissues are amenable to correction, early surgical intervention is recommended. Stanley[57] has suggested that early soft tissue surgery in association with appropriate medical care preserves more function for a longer period of time. Aschan and Moberg[3] reported satisfactory results after early synovectomy of finger joints. Yet others, such as O'Brien,[51] reported that prophylactic joint synovectomy does not significantly alter the progression of joint destruction. We submit that surgical removal of the synovium eliminates the destructive pannus and associated destructive enzymes. Pressure is taken off the joint and the patient's pain is reduced. Attenuated ligaments can be reefed or reconstructed and displaced tendons can be repositioned. Arthroscopic wrist synovectomy during early stages of disease (Larson grade 3 or less) has been reported to decrease pain and improve motion and grip strength.[1] Intraarticular steroid injections reduce joint inflammation and swelling and provide pain relief, but their long-term benefit is difficult to prove, and repeat steroid injections can produce deleterious effects on joint cartilage. However, when such injections are used judiciously they can improve hand function.

Metacarpophalangeal and Interphalangeal Joint Damage

Attenuation of collateral ligaments and capsules at the MCP joints associated with ulnar drift, volar subluxation, and extensor-tendon displacement contributes to hand deformity and there is associated synovial destruction of bone and cartilage. Synovitis without radiographic evidence of joint changes is evident in stage I of the disease and can be managed medically. Intraarticular steroids and splinting are of value. Joint-space narrowing with bony erosions occurs in stage II. Surgical synovectomy to eliminate the destructive pannus is indicated when there is proliferative synovitis. Ulnar deviation and volar subluxation, as well as more advanced radiographic changes, are evident by stage III. Wood et al[76] have demonstrated that ligament reconstruction and extensor tendon reefing during this stage provide good functional results. The patient's joint can be preserved at this stage, and the need for later interpositional arthroplasty may be obviated. Reconstruction of the patient's own joint generally results in better function than an interpositional arthroplasty, and the latter results in better function than soft tissue arthroplasty. Soft tissue surgery is inadequate for treatment of stage-IV MCP-joint disease characterized by advanced joint destruction; in such cases joint reconstruction is necessary. Numerous techniques of joint reconstruction were promoted prior to the mid-1960s, including those developed by Tupper.[66] The introduction of the silicone spacer technique by Swanson[60] heralded the modern era of joint surgery as a treatment for rheumatoid arthritis. Joint resection, with or without ligament reconstruction, extensor tendon reefing, and intrinsic transfers, repositions the proximal phalanx in a more functional position and provides pain relief.

PIP-joint involvement associated with the rheumatoid process can result in stiffness and deformity. The characteristic swan-neck deformity may have multiple and varied etiologies, including a mallet deformity at the DIP joint, rupture of the volar plate and flexor digitorum superficialis (FDS) tendon with secondary hyperextension, intrinsic tightness, or a combination of these. Classification is based on the limitation of motion in relation to the position of the MCP joint, intrinsic tightness, and radiographic changes.[48] Early figure-of-eight splinting is indicated for patients with a type-I deformity, who have full passive motion. Soft tissue surgery to limit hyperextension also is of value. Intrinsic release with or without MCP joint surgery is indicated for patients with type-II deformity, who experience intrinsic tightness that causes limited PIP joint flexion when the MCP joint is extended. Flexion of the PIP joint is limited in all MCP positions in patients with type-III deformity, but the joint is preserved. Surgical treatment can include joint mobilization, lateral band release, temporary fixation with Kirschner wires (K wires), and sometimes dorsal skin release. The joint destruction associated with type-IV deformity requires joint fusion or arthroplasty. Fusion is definitely indicated in the index finger and most likely also in the border small finger. Soft tissue or silicone interpositional arthroplasty may preserve some motion but typically does not result in significant functional improvement.

A boutonniere deformity with the PIP joint in flexion and the distal interphalangeal (DIP) joint in hyperextension is secondary to synovitis of the PIP joint. The central slip of the extensor mechanism is attenuated and the lateral bands descend volar to the PIP joint's axis of rotation. The lateral bands are placed in tension, which in turn pulls the DIP joint into hyperextension. Contracture of the retinacular ligaments, volar plate, and collateral ligaments produces a fixed deformity. Disease staging according to the Nalebuff/Millender[47] format helps in the planning of treatment. Stage I is marked by synovial swelling without significant deformity or radiographic changes. Synovectomy, splinting of the PIP joint in extension, dorsal relocation of the lateral bands, and sometimes distal extensor tenotomy are the procedures of choice. During stage II, digits demonstrate a 30-to 40-degree PIP-joint flexion deformity with full passive extension and require central slip reconstruction. During stage III, the PIP-joint flexion contracture in digits is fixed and joint changes are pronounced. Arthroplasty provides an improvement in the arc of motion rather than in the total range of motion. The extensor lag persists, however, and usually increases over time.[33] Arthrodesis in a functional position is effective in relieving pain and in improving function.

The Rheumatoid Thumb

Pain, limited motion, deformity, and instability are the hallmarks of the rheumatoid thumb. The goal of surgery is to provide a pain-free stable thumb that is permitted as much motion as possible and that can adequately pinch and grip. There are three basic types of rheumatoid thumb deformities: boutonniere, swan-neck, and gamekeeper's thumb.

The boutonniere deformity is caused by attenuation of the collateral ligaments and dorsal capsule, with volar and ulnar displacement of the extensor pollicis longus (EPL). The MCP joint is flexed and volarly subluxed and the interphalangeal (IP) joint is hyperextended. Soft tissue surgery involving ligament reefing and EPL rerouting to provide proximal phalangeal extension is typically indicated in the early stages, when no significant joint damage has occurred. However, the patient should be advised that recurrence of the deformity is very likely.[64] Arthrodesis is indicated when joint destruction has occurred and when the IP and basilar joints are minimally involved. If the IP joint is unstable, fusion of this joint can be combined with MCP arthroplasty or occasionally MCP fusion. Carpometacarpal (CMC) joint function, in the latter situation, must be satisfactory and allow positioning of the thumb tip for pinch.

Swan-neck deformity of the thumb is secondary to CMC joint disease. The CMC joint becomes unstable, dorsoradially subluxed, flexed, and adducted, which leads to MCP hyperextension and IP flexion. Treatment is directed toward correcting the CMC joint deformity by arthroplasty, stabilization, and adduction release. A volar capsulodesis may be required at the MCP joint, or arthrodesis may be necessary if there is major joint damage.

Gamekeeper's thumb consists of lateral instability caused by synovial attenuation of the ulnar collateral ligament and capsule. Ligament reconstruction performed before joint damage occurs typically provides adequate stabilization.

The Rheumatoid Wrist

Synovial damage to the triangular fibrocartilage complex (TFCC) and ligamentous support of the wrist allows volar descent and supination of the carpus followed by ulnar translation. Attenuation of the volar radiocapitate and radioscapholunate ligaments results in palmar rotation of the distal pole of the scaphoid and a loss of carpal height. The extensor carpi ulnaris (ECU) ligamentous support is weakened and the tendon subluxes volar to the axis of wrist flexion/extension. Consequently the radial wrist extensors achieve a mechanical advantage, which results in radial deviation of the wrist and secondary MCP ulnar drift. Carpal collapse reduces the mechanical effectiveness of the extrinsic extensor tendons and produces a relative intrinsic plus deformity. Hyperflexion of the scaphoid produces a secondary boutonniere deformity of the thumb. Continued joint destruction by the invading synovium causes progressive collapse, spontaneous fusion, and instability, with resulting pain, deformity, and hand dysfunction. Surgery is directed toward the elimination of pain, amelioration of the secondary changes, and preservation and restoration of function. Techniques must be tailored to the stage of the disease and the type of deformity. Wrist surgery should be performed before more distal digital deformity is corrected.

The indications for wrist synovectomy have not been well established. Total wrist synovectomy is essentially impossible because the wrist is composed of multiple joints. Studies of disease progression, including one by Hindley and Stanley,[27] show early involvement of the distal radioulnar joint, ulnar styloid, and lunate fossa. The scaphoid fossa is affected less and delayed involvement occurs in the mid-carpal area. The triquetrolunate joint is the most affected intercarpal joint. The natural history of rheumatoid arthritis suggests that joint damage in the hand follows that in the wrist by 5 years. Synovectomy of the most involved areas should be of value, but no reports confirm that such surgery definitely alters the course of the disease. Studies have indicated that surgery provides dramatic pain relief and maintenance of grip strength, with varying loss of motion. Thus wrist synovectomy most likely is indicated in patients who have painful, swollen wrists with minimal radiographic evidence of change, and in whom the disease is slowly progressive despite good medical therapy for at least 6 months. Such surgery should be considered in concert with other wrist surgery.

Repositioning of the ECU and transfer of the extensor carpi radialis longus (ECRL) to the ECU readjusts the force vectors across the wrist axis and should counteract the tendency toward radial deviation of the wrist.[25] Partial wrist fusion (radiolunate or radioscapholunate) prevents further ulnar translation of the carpus and provides some pain relief; it is of value when the mid-carpal joints are minimally involved and in the absence of rapidly aggressive disease.

Total wrist fusion provides predictable stability and pain relief.[44] The fusion should be positioned to enable reasonable function, including personal hygiene. The condition of the shoulder and elbow on the side undergoing surgery must be considered. For unilateral fusion, the wrist should be placed in a neutral position, with slight ulnar deviation. When both wrists are fused, one should be in slight flexion to facilitate personal hygiene.

Total wrist arthroplasty involving the use of a silicone implant was introduced by Swanson et al[62] and appeared to provide active wrist motion and pain relief in patients with wrists severely damaged by rheumatoid arthritis. Subsequent reports indicated frequent implant fracture, subsidence, and bone resorption around the implant, as well as particulate synovitis. Salvage wrist fusion after failed implant surgery has been a major challenge. Thus total wrist arthroplasty currently is rarely performed. However, Stanley and Tolat[59] recommend this procedure when pain-free, limited mobility is required in patients with a low-demand need and relatively quiescent disease; their recommendation is based on follow-up of 50 Swanson arthroplasties after a minimum of 6 years.

Total wrist articulated implants based on hip reconstructions were introduced by Meuli[44] and Volz[71]. These implants resulted in significant problems, which included abnormal moment arms, breakage, dislocation, subsidence, infection, and difficult secondary salvage surgery. A cemented biaxial implant subsequently used at the Mayo Clinic[17] provided better results. The implant provided pain relief and the motion required for activities of daily living, and allowed an average of 30 degrees of dorsiflexion, 5 degrees of flexion, 10 degrees of radial deviation, and 15 degrees of ulnar deviation. Failure occurred in one of six implants, primarily because of distal implant loosening. The ideal wrist implant, which would result in appropriate moment arms with an uncemented prosthesis, currently is under development.

The distal radioulnar joint, when attacked by rheumatoid synovitis, demonstrates stretching of the ligaments and joint capsule. The TFCC attenuates or becomes disrupted and the joint surfaces erode. The unstable distal ulna is displaced dorsal to the supinated carpus and distal radius and can cause attrition/rupture of the extensor tendons. Synovectomy, stabilization of the distal ulna, and repositioning of the ECU have been effective in the management of early disease. Traditionally, advanced disease was treated by resection of the distal ulna, or the *Darrach procedure*.[19] This procedure provided pain relief and usually improved supination and pronation, but sometimes also resulted in instability of the distal ulna, which is difficult to treat. Removal of the distal ulnar buttress has been determined to accentuate carpal deformities. However among patients who underwent unilateral wrist operations, Nanchahal et al[50] reported no increase in carpal translation or collapse compared with the wrists that did not receive surgical treatment. The Suave-Kapandji procedure[70] or hemiresection of the distal ulna with soft tissue interposition currently are preferred for the treatment of advanced distal radioulnar disease.

OPERATIONS

Because rheumatoid arthritis is a progressive disease involving multiple structures, surgical management of the disease must be individually tailored to address the needs of each patient. The activity and progression of the disease must be considered in conjunction with the patient's overall health, activities of daily living, and ability to follow a postoperative rehabilitation program. Many patients with rheumatoid arthritis experience abnormal wound healing, hand swelling, and stiffness that can interfere with a postoperative mobilization program. Other patients may have cervical arthritis or difficulty with jaw mobilization, which can interfere with the use of general anesthesia. Lying on an operating table for a prolonged period of time often causes discomfort. We try to limit surgery to a maximum tourniquet time of 2 hours.

Rheumatoid surgery often must be staged. When joint problems are addressed, surgery should proceed in a proximal-to-distal sequence. We agree with Stanley,[57] who gives top priority to painful conditions and those involving soft tissue disease, tendon ruptures, and symptomatic nerve compression. In recent years we have found that the use of locally injected long-acting anesthetics (e.g., bupivacaine) provides significant assistance in the management of postoperative pain in patients who have undergone rheumatoid surgery.

EXTENSOR TENOSYNOVECTOMY

In extensor tenosynovectomy, the wrist is ideally approached through a straight dorsal midline incision. Curved or angled

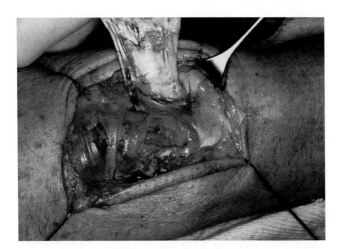

Figure 128-7. The extensor retinaculum elevated as a flap. An attempt is made to preserve the proximal quarter.

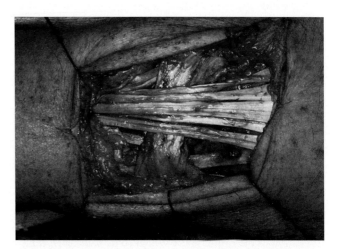

Figure 128-8. The extensor retinaculum is placed deep to the finger extensor tendons. An ulnar slip is used to reposition the ECU.

incisions can lead to skin necrosis. The dorsal soft tissues of the wrist are elevated, exposing the extensor retinaculum. The dorsal branches of the radial and ulnar nerves are identified in the subcutaneous tissue and must be protected. The longitudinally oriented veins must be preserved; however, the large crossing veins should be ligated and the smaller vessels cauterized to reduce the tendency for swelling and bleeding. The retinaculum is subsequently incised and elevated as a flap after the septa between compartments are divided. A single radially based retinacular flap typically is recommended, but we frequently incise over the fourth compartment and elevate flaps both radially and ulnarly, or over the second compartment and elevate an ulnarly based flap. It is not necessary to open the first dorsal compartment unless obvious synovial proliferation has occurred. The EPL is at risk during flap elevation because it turns radially, immediately distal to Lister's tubercle, and can be easily cut. The entire retinaculum traditionally has been elevated but we try to preserve the proximal third of the retinaculum to reduce bowstringing (Figure 128-7); we do not allow any retained retinaculum or deep fascia to interfere with completion of the tenosynovectomy. Bowstringing typically does not pose a major problem in patients with rheumatoid arthritis who have limited active motion.

Synovial resection is subsequently performed by means of sharp-scissors dissection combined with blunt curettage. When nodules are present within the tendon mass, they must be exposed and aggressively removed. We have found that retaining even one third of the cross-sectional area of the tendon preserves function and does not lead to rupture. Frayed or irregular tendons should be smoothed with a running fine monofilament suture. Tendons that appear dull, are opaque in

color, or are markedly thinned should be considered pseudotendons or evidence of a rupture in incontinuity and should be treated by tendon grafting or transfer. Distal ulna abnormalities subsequently must be corrected and radiocarpal/intercarpal wrist synovectomy also may be indicated.

We use the elevated retinacular flap to support the wrist capsule and distal radial/ulnar joint and to provide a smooth gliding surface for the extensor tendons (Figure 128-8). The proximal third of the retinaculum is brought superficial to the tendons when the entire retinaculum has been elevated and there is concern about bowstringing. Retinacular repositioning is not done after a tendon transfer, graft, or imbrication has been performed. The retinaculum is sewn loosely to prevent it from interfering with wrist flexion. A portion of the retinaculum is used to stabilize the ECU in a dorsal position. We typically release the tourniquet before skin closure to ensure adequate hemostasis. A Penrose drain is routinely placed through the incision and removed 1 or 2 days later.

Subcutaneous sutures are used when possible. When edge-to-edge skin closure is required, we alternate vertical mattress sutures with simple interrupted sutures. A volar splint is incorporated into the dressing with the wrist in neutral and the fingers extended. The dressing is usually changed within the first 3 days; subsequently, active motion is initiated. Ongoing wrist support may be necessary after a wrist synovectomy has been performed or for pain relief. We immediately initiate dynamic extensor splinting if extensor lag occurs. Splinting of the IP joints in slight flexion directs the extrinsic pull to the MCP joints.

Complications associated with this procedure include skin necrosis, bleeding, and reduced tendon glide. The patient must be observed closely during the first few weeks after surgery so

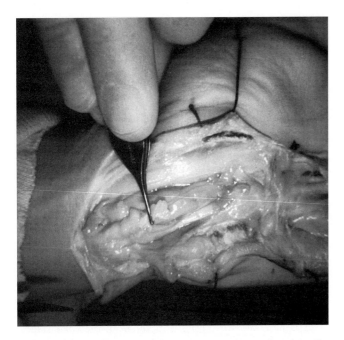

Figure 128-9. Flexor tenosynovectomy is initiated proximally, allowing early identification of the median nerve.

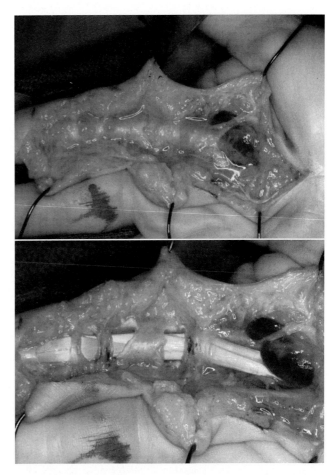

Figure 128-10. Digital flexor tenosynovectomy with preservation of the annular pulleys.

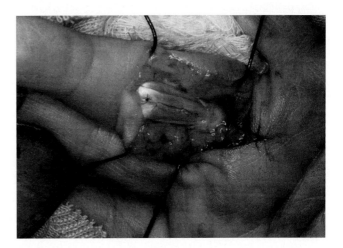

Figure 128-11. A fine monofilament suture is used to smooth the debrided tendon.

that complications are identified early. The splints must often be adjusted, and aggressive hand therapy is usually required to limit tendon-scar adhesions. If postoperative wound disruption occurs, we treat the open area with a topical antibiotic ointment in an occlusive dressing to prevent drying and suppress bacterial growth. Active motion and splinting are continued as if the wound were closed until healing occurs by secondary intention. Subsequent tenolysis may be necessary but should be deferred for several months.

FLEXOR TENOSYNOVECTOMY

Tenosynovectomy of the proximal palm and wrist incorporates the incision used for carpal tunnel release with a 3- to 5-cm zigzag extension into the proximal forearm. Bruner incisions are used for exposure of the digital sheaths. The digital and wrist incisions can be connected for total exposure of the flexor tendons. When multiple digits are involved, we usually operate on no more than two digits during one surgical procedure. Dissection must begin proximally after identification of the median nerve and its palmar cutaneous branch (Figure 128-9). The median nerve may be abnormally displaced by the proliferating synovitis and should be dissected free from the synovium, which surrounds the flexor tendons in the carpal tunnel. We divide the transverse carpal ligament longitudinally on its ulnar side, but a Z incision can be used for subsequent flap closure. The digital sheaths are markedly distended by the synovium. The annular pulleys must be retained during surgical dissection (Figure 128-10), including the A1 pulley, which is usually divided in a trigger-finger release procedure. Maintenance of the A1 pulley counteracts

the volar–ulnar torque exerted by the flexor tendons during grip. It is important to remove as much of the infiltrating synovium as possible because most flexor-tendon ruptures are caused by invasive synovitis. A tendon that is frayed after the dissection can be smoothed with a fine monofilament suture (Figure 128-11).

We routinely resect the ulnar slip of the FDS tendon because this resection provides the damaged FDP tendon with more room in which to glide. The entire FDS tendon can be sacrificed if a flexion deformity of the PIP joint is present, but we have never found this necessary. The individual FDS tendons must be freed from each other in the distal forearm and palm to provide independent motion of each digit. The FDP tendons may be enveloped in a congruent mass of tendons, synovium, and scar; it is not necessary to separate each of these, but the surgeon should remove as much of the infiltrating synovium as possible without rupturing the tendons. After synovectomy the floor of the carpal tunnel must be inspected for evidence of tendon disruption or bony irregularities. Bony spurs, if present, should be rongeured to provide a smooth surface, and exposed bone in the floor should be covered with a local flap. Passive tendon glide should be checked by applying traction to individual tendons at the wrist, which should produce unrestricted digital flexion. Any restriction of motion warrants further inspection for tendon nodules that may be impinging on the pulleys. The tourniquet subsequently should be released and all bleeding should be controlled. The skin incision edges can be infiltrated with a local anesthetic. This also provides an opportunity to check active motion in a pain-free environment if regional IV anesthesia has been used. The patient is shown the active motion that can be achieved immediately after surgery in a pain-free environment and is informed that the goal is to retain that amount of motion through hand therapy. We routinely use a Penrose or small suction drain for 1 to 2 days after surgery, at which time the dressing is replaced with one that is smaller and that allows early motion. Formal hand therapy is initiated, including individual joint stabilization to improve distal PIP-joint motion.

MANAGEMENT OF TENDON RUPTURE

Synovectomy should precede the management of extensor-tendon rupture in cases involving significant MCP-joint disease. The incision and tendon exposure are achieved with the same method as that described for extensor tenosynovectomy. The causes of tendon rupture should be eliminated before the tendons rupture, using procedures such as tenosynovectomy and distal ulna surgery. It is impossible to perform primary repair of a tendon ruptured by invasive synovitis. Occasionally, repair may be possible if the rupture is caused by attrition. Typically minimal extensor lag (20 to 30 degrees) occurs if only the EDQ is ruptured and a tendon transfer may not be required. If a single extensor tendon is ruptured, the distal stump of the ruptured tendon is debrided to healthy tissue and subsequently sewn in an interweave fashion to the adjacent tendon. We use a 3-0 or 4-0 nonabsorbable suture. It should be noted that this technique does not routinely produce full motion of the involved digit because the transferred tendon loses a percentage of its excursion owing to the angle it enters the functional tendon. Double transfers to the adjacent intact long extensor can produce an abnormal vector on the small finger, resulting in an abduction deformity.

Rupture of the tendons to the ring and small fingers can be managed by transfer of the extensor indicis proprius (EIP) tendon to the ulnar two fingers (Figure 128-12). A side-to-side transfer of the EDC III tendon to the EDC II tendon can be performed if the long extensor is ruptured. We believe it is important to repair the index extensor hood when the EIP is used because this appears to reduce the tendency for extensor lag in this finger. It is important to set the correct tension on the transferred tendons. We aim to place the fingers in 20 to 30 degrees of flexion when the wrist is moderately extended, and in neutral or slight extension when the wrist is moderately flexed. Use of the EIP is our first choice for correction of an EPL rupture (Figure 128-13). If the EIP has been used previously, the extensor pollicis brevis (EPB) can be detached from the proximal phalanx of the thumb and attached to the extensor pollicis longus (EPL) to serve as the motor for IP extension. Fusion of the IP joint is an alternative, but we have not found this to be necessary unless significant joint destruction has occurred.

It is necessary to transfer a motor from the volar side of the hand when the extensor tendons to all four fingers are

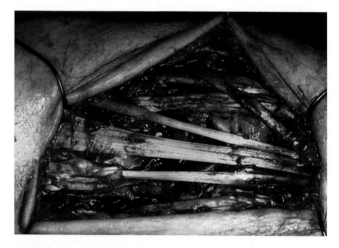

Figure 128-12. EIP transfer used as a motor for ruptured extensor tendons to the ring and small fingers.

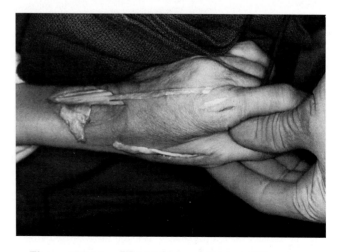

Figure 128-13. EIP transfer is used to treat EPL rupture.

ruptured. The FDS tendons to the long and ring fingers can be passed through the interosseous membrane if no significant disease or scarring is present in this area or around the radial side of the forearm.[49] An FDS transfer should not be considered when there is a digital swan-neck deformity. The wrist extensor tendons may be considered for transfer if the wrist is fused. However, because their excursion is not as great as that of the finger extensors, their use may result in reduced MCP extension. Rupture of the wrist extensors usually indicates major wrist disease; in such cases, arthrodesis typically is the procedure of choice.

We deflate the tourniquet after the transfers are completed to assess hemostasis, and more importantly, to check the tension of the transfers, which should be adjusted before skin closure. We use a drain and apply a volar splint with the wrist in slight extension and the MCP joints in slight flexion. We prefer to initiate the use of dynamic extension splints within 5 days after surgery, and to maintain passive splinting for 3 weeks. The help of a trained hand therapist is important in the postoperative management of patients who have undergone this procedure.

Ruptured flexor tendons are approached through incisions similar to those used for flexor tenosynovectomy. Tenosynovectomy and repair of any bony irregularities in the floor of the carpal tunnel are required before tendon reconstruction. Our protocol for management of an isolated FDP rupture is to ignore the tendon rupture when there is good FDS function and to stabilize the DIP joint with a tenodesis or fusion if it tends to hyperextend. No tendon surgery is required if only the FDS has ruptured. When both the FDS and FDP are ruptured in the palm or wrist, we transfer the adjacent FDS to the ruptured FDP (Figure 128-14), using a tendon graft if necessary. Moberg has reported good results using free tendon grafts to repair ruptured flexor tendons.[46] We prefer to transfer the FDS of the index finger to reconstruct a ruptured FPL; however, use of an intercalated or bridge graft or fusion of the IP joint also are good options. Rupture of both flexor tendons within the digital sheath presents a major reconstructive problem. A primary graft placed in a poor bed or a tendon transfer involving anastomosis performed within the flexor sheath typically leads to a poor functional result. A staged tendon graft with initial placement of a silicone rod should be considered in such cases. Arthrodesis of both IP joints is another option when there is severe disease.

The tourniquet should be deflated after completion of a transfer or tendon graft to obtain hemostasis and check the resulting tension. We use a drain if there is any bleeding. As with traumatic tendon lacerations, we favor early controlled motion or dynamic splinting. The suture technique should provide enough strength for the repair to withstand the stress of active flexion.

Complications after tendon transfers or grafts primarily involve inappropriate tension, disruption of the anastomosis, or scar tenodesis. Bleeding typically does not pose a problem if the tourniquet is released before wound closure and if a drain is used for 24 to 48 hours after surgery. Tenolysis, if required, should be deferred for at least 6 months. Aggressive therapy is indicated before consideration of such surgery.

METACARPOPHALANGEAL JOINT SURGERY

A longitudinal incision over the affected MCP joint is preferred when only one digit is involved, and particularly if surgery is planned for treatment of distal disease. Typically a transverse incision centered just distal to the prominence of the

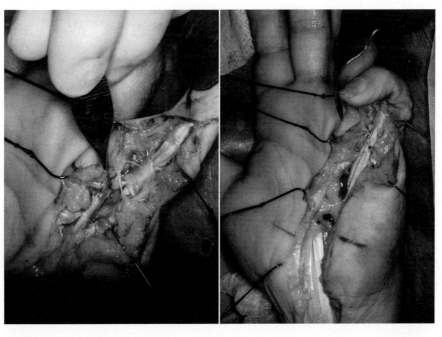

Figure 128-14. Transfer of the FDS IV tendon is our preferred technique for rupture of both small-finger flexor tendons.

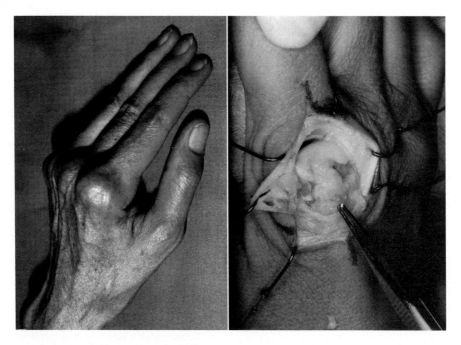

Figure 128-15. Subluxation of the MCP joints, with relative preservation of the joint surfaces.

metacarpal head is used. Skin flaps are elevated proximally and distally to expose the extensor mechanism. Care should be taken to avoid injury to the dorsal veins and sensory branches, which lie in the gutters between the metacarpal heads. The skin of patients with rheumatoid arthritis is fragile and must be handled with care. We prefer the use of fine skin hooks followed by the use of blunt retractors. We incise the extensor mechanism longitudinally, radial to the extensor tendon; other authors prefer a tendon-splitting incision or one on the ulnar side. The extensor hood is dissected free from the underlying capsule. It is easier to start distally with this dissection. If the capsule is intact, it is opened and a synovectomy is performed. Resection of the synovium deep to the collateral ligaments is difficult but necessary. Bone cysts in the metacarpal head or base of the proximal phalanx should be removed with a curette. Blunt dissection to free the volar plate is necessary to allow repositioning of the proximal phalanx in line with the metacarpal. Soft tissue reconstruction is undertaken if the joint surfaces are in reasonable condition; this involves at least intrinsic tendon release but preferably also crossed intrinsic transfers, imbrication of the radial collateral ligament, and radial positioning of the extensor tendon. The junctura tendinea also should be divided. In the intrinsic transfer the ulnar lateral band is released from the extensor mechanism, dissected proximally to its musculotendinous junction, and interweaved into the adjacent radial lateral/sagittal band mechanism. It is preferable to suture it to the radial collateral ligament in patients with a tendency toward swan-neck deformity or with very supple fingers. Oster et al[52] reported no difference in the results of these two techniques of lateral band fixation.

The transfer should be performed with enough tension to correct the ulnar drift. The abductor digiti quinti (ADQ) is divided on the ulnar side of the hand with care, to preserve the flexor digiti minimi (FDM) and the adjacent digital neurovas-

cular bundle. The capsule is subsequently reefed and the radial collateral ligament also may be tightened to reinforce the MCP joint in a neutral or radial position. When significant attenuation of the collateral ligaments and dorsal capsule has occurred, we have used a tendon or fascia lata graft to reconstruct the ligaments (Figures 128-15 and 128-16). K-wire fixation of the MCP joint in extension is necessary for 3 weeks. We prefer to bring the extensor tendon into a radial position over the metacarpal head by suturing it superficial to the radial sagittal bands in a vest-over-pants technique, using an absorbable suture. Occasionally it is necessary to incise the ulnar sagittal band to allow radial movement of the extensor tendon. Other techniques have been employed, including the suture of a distally based slip of the extensor to the radial/dorsal aspect of the proximal phalanx. Soft tissue MCP-joint reconstruction was described by Wood et al,[76] who anchored the extensor tendon to the base of the proximal phalanx with a nonabsorbable suture passed through drilled holes. As for previously described procedures, we prefer dynamic extensor splinting during the postoperative period.

Arthroplasty is indicated when significant joint destruction has occurred, using the same surgical approach to the joint. The collateral ligaments are sharply dissected off the metacarpal head, which is resected to a length that allows repositioning of the proximal phalanx. Chronic dislocation of the proximal phalanx, with the base lying volar to the metacarpal head, often results in a flattening or scooping-out of the dorsal surface of the proximal phalanx, which is evident in preoperative radiographs. Less metacarpal head is resected in such cases because the proximal phalanx must be contoured. Minimal head resection with preservation of the proximal attachment of the collateral ligaments may be necessary. All bone edges are smoothed. We palpate the bone ends before continuing, and any remaining joint synovium is subsequently removed. The

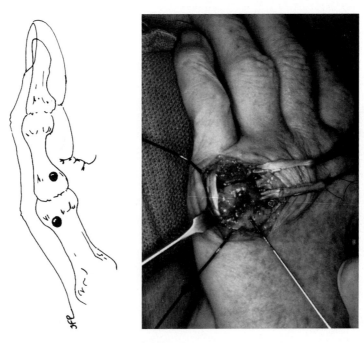

Figure 128-16. Tendon graft placed through drill holes in the metacarpal and proximal phalanges to reconstruct attenuated collateral ligaments.

remaining cartilage on the base of the proximal phalanx is removed by curettage or by means of a side-biting burr. The metacarpal is prepared for reception of the prosthesis by gentle curettage, which involves the removal of only enough bone to allow placement of the desired prosthesis. The proximal phalanx is reamed in a rectangular shape and should be held by the person drilling to avoid perforation of the bony cortex. The index finger should be held in a supinated position during reaming. Antibiotic irrigation can be used, although it is not part of our routine; we use perioperative broad-spectrum antibiotic coverage.

The prosthesis should be placed with a "no-touch" technique, using a smooth forceps. Grommets are employed only if bone support for the implants is inadequate. We reconstruct radial collateral ligament support by suturing it to the periosteum of the metacarpal or to a drilled hole in the radial end of the metacarpal. Reattachment of the ulnar ligament is not necessary, but we occasionally suture it with minimal tension to the periosteum of the metacarpal to assist in correcting any rotational deformity. We perform intrinsic transfers when the ulnar drift exceeds 30 degrees or when there is a push against the examiner's hand by the patient's small finger during finger flexion and extension.

Closure of the extensor hood and skin are the same as described for soft tissue reconstruction. A drain is used for 1 to 2 days after surgery. We incorporate a volar splint into the dressing to hold the MCP joints in extension. The dressing is replaced with a smaller one after 2 days. The therapist subsequently prepares a dynamic extension splint to hold the MCP joints in extension and slight radial deviation and to hold the PIP joints in extension. The splint is worn during most of the day but is removed once or twice for active motion exercises. A static splint that holds the wrist in a neutral position and the fingers in full extension is used at night. Close

observation is critical during the days immediately following surgery. Because reduced MCP-joint flexion in the ring and small fingers can occur, the patient must be encouraged to flex these joints. Early discontinuation of outrigger slings to these fingers may be necessary.

Potential early complications include bleeding, skin breakdown, malalignment, extensor lag, reduced MCP-joint motion, and secondary PIP-joint deformity. It should be emphasized that late implant breakage is not always an indication for surgery because subsequent function often is maintained. Late complications frequently are the result of disease progression; an associated tendency toward ulnar/volar pull on the MCP joints often results in recurrent ulnar drift and implant displacement or rupture. Particulate synovitis has not been associated with MCP implants. Secondary or salvage surgery may be necessary to preserve hand function. On occasion we have performed further metacarpal resection to allow for realignment of the proximal phalanx. When bone stock has been inadequate for implant placement we have used Tupper volar plate interpositional arthroplasty.[66]

Currently the use of silicone implants (e.g., Swanson, Sutter) provides excellent functional results. In the future endoprostheses that incorporate osseointegration may be used. In 1993, Lundborg et al[38] reported their experience with such a prosthesis.

SURGERY OF THE PROXIMAL INTERPHALANGEAL JOINT

Soft tissue reconstruction of a finger with a swan-neck deformity is performed through a dorsal hockey stick–shaped incision with a distal transverse component of the incision, which is left open at the conclusion of surgery. The lateral

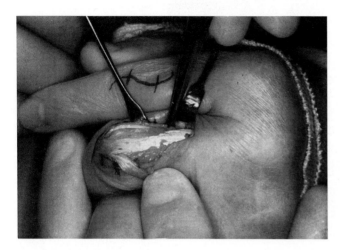

Figure 128-17. Swan-neck deformity. The lateral bands are separated from the central slip.

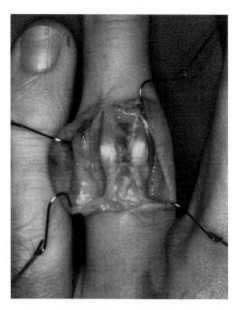

Figure 128-18. Boutonniere deformity. The lateral bands undergo dorsal mobilization and the lateral retinacular ligaments are sutured for support.

bands are separated from the central slip and are reflected volarly (Figure 128-17). The central slip is freed of any attachments to the proximal phalanx. It is usually necessary to divide the dorsal aspects of the collateral ligaments to allow the PIP joint to flex. The ulnar lateral band is divided proximally and sutured to the flexor digital sheath, which prevents recurrent hyperextension of the PIP joint. Another method involves the use of a slip of the FDS tendon, which is divided proximally and sutured to the flexor digital sheath proximal to the PIP joint, which tenodeses the joint in flexion. We check for mobility of the flexor tendons and subsequently use K wires to secure the PIP joint in flexion. Splinting may continue to be necessary when the fixation is discontinued after approximately 3 weeks. The therapist is involved in the joint mobilization program. The principal complication associated with this soft tissue surgery is that most patients achieve only a fair functional result. Moreover, this deformity tends to recur. We advise our patients accordingly.

Boutonniere deformities are approached with a slightly curved dorsal incision off the midline. The surgeon avoids as many of the dorsal veins as possible. We divide the insertion of the attenuated central slip off the middle phalanx and subsequently perform a joint synovectomy. The lateral bands are relocated dorsally; we have sutured the free ends of the divided transverse retinacular ligaments to provide support (Figure 128-18). If the hyperextension of the distal phalanx persists, a distal tenotomy over the middle part of the middle phalanx is indicated. The central slip is subsequently attached to the dorsal base of the middle phalanx with a nonabsorbable suture passed through a drilled hole. The PIP joint is splinted in extension for at least 4 weeks.

Arthroplasty or fusion is indicated when severe joint damage has occurred. We use the same slightly curved incision used for boutonniere deformities. Many authors advocate entering the joint through a tendon-splitting incision, but we prefer to free the central slip insertion and reflect the entire extensor mechanism. The collateral ligaments are elevated off the proximal phalanx, exposing the entire joint. Arthroplasty of the PIP joint is performed by resecting enough of the distal part of the proximal phalanx to allow comfortable placement of the implant without tension. The cartilage surface of the middle phalanx is removed and the two bones are reamed to accept the stems of the implant. A smooth forceps is used to handle the implant. Two drill holes are placed in the proximal phalanx and one is placed in the dorsal midline of the middle phalanx. The collateral ligaments are reattached to the proximal phalanx, using nonabsorbable sutures passed through the drill holes. The central slip is reattached to the middle phalanx with enough tension to bring the joint into extension. We prefer early dynamic splinting in the postoperative management of patients who undergo this procedure. This is alternated with static splinting of the joint in extension at night.

Arthrodesis of the PIP and DIP joints is best performed using the tension-band technique. The adjacent phalangeal surfaces are cut with an oscillating saw, with enough volar angulation to achieve the desired degree of joint flexion. The cut surfaces should be complementary and parallel K wires should be placed. A tension suture is passed through a transverse drill hole in the middle phalanx, crossed proximally, and tied around the K wires as they exit the bone. The wires are cut as close to the bone as possible and are not meant to be

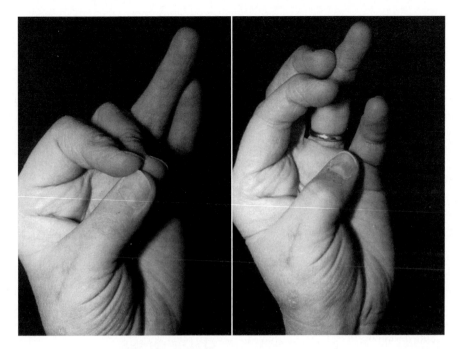

Figure 128-19. Fusion of the thumb's MCP joint provides stable pinch and reasonable mobility.

removed. Bone grafts are not necessary. Others have recommended chevron or ball and socket fusion, which are good alternatives. We provide the patient with protective splints for several weeks after surgery.

SURGERY OF THE RHEUMATOID THUMB

The Interphalangeal Joint

Arthrodesis is the procedure of choice when the IP joint is unstable or destroyed. We use the tension-band technique described earlier for PIP arthrodesis. Fusion of the IP joint provides stable pinch and no significant functional loss when the CMC and MCP joints have range of motion near normal. The IP joint is fused in slight flexion and pronation. We determine the appropriate angle by positioning the tip of the thumb against the tip of the index finger. The Herbert screw technique is also a good method for fusing the thumb's IP joint. Rarely is a bone graft indicated except in the case of arthritis mutilans. In such cases, we have used a cortical cancellous graft, typically taken from the iliac crest.

The Metacarpophalangeal Joint

We approach the MCP joint through a longitudinal midline incision. The extensor mechanism is identified and opened through a tendon-splitting incision in the EPL. The capsule is opened and a synovectomy is performed. When the joint is unstable, producing a gamekeeper's thumb, yet has good articular surfaces, we reconstruct the ligament with a segment of tendon graft as described for the MCP joint of a finger. The technique for arthroplasty also is similar to that used for the fingers. We reattach both collateral ligaments and imbricate or

reinforce the attachment of the EPB to the proximal phalanx. We place the digit in a static splint for at least the first 4 weeks after surgery because stability of the reconstruction is important. Active motion and dynamic splinting are used for the following 2 weeks. Arthrodesis, when necessary, is performed with the joint in approximately 15 degrees of flexion, 5 to 10 degrees of abduction, and 20 degrees of pronation. Supportive splinting is provided for protection and comfort. This procedure typically results in good function (Figure 128-19).

The Carpometacarpal Joint

As with swan-neck deformity of the thumb, primary disease that involves the CMC joint is treated by means of resection arthroplasty, with ligament reconstruction and soft tissue interposition rather than the use of fusion or an implant. Techniques are similar to those used for reconstruction of the typical osteoarthritic thumb MCP joint.

SURGERY OF THE RHEUMATOID WRIST

The standard approach for treating the wrist is the same as that described for extensor tenosynovectomy. Soft tissue surgery involves an interweave transfer of the ECRL to the ECU to correct radial angulation of the carpus, and repositioning of the ECU in a more dorsal position with a slip of the extensor retinaculum. A distally based slip of the ECU may be passed through the distal end of the ulna for stabilization. We do not use wrist implants and thus do not address such procedures.

The wrist capsule typically is opened by means of an inverted T-shaped incision, with the transverse component passing from the radius just distal to the TFCC. Berger[9] has designed a more anatomically oriented incision that parallels the dorsal radiotriquetral ligament and subsequently curves distally and radially to follow the course of the dorsal carpal ligament from the triquetrum to the scaphotrapezoid joint. This incision provides access to the radiocarpal and mid-carpal joints for synovectomy or bone work.

Limited arthrodesis of the radius to the lunate, as described by Chamay,[16] mimics the spontaneous fusion seen in approximately 15% of patients. We use this procedure in cases involving significant wrist pain, early ulnar translation of the carpus, and good mid-carpal joints. The scaphoid is incorporated when the radioscaphoid joint is also involved, to reduce wrist motion. The mid-carpal articular surfaces must be examined during surgery. Subsequently the opposing surfaces of the lunate and radius are debrided of cartilage. We prefer to use a rongeur and curette because power burrs can damage the subchondral bone. The lunate is reduced into the fossa and secured with a plate and screws (Figure 128-20). Staples and K wires also have been used. During fixation it is important to remember that the rim of the radius covers more than 50% of the lunate. Cancellous bone grafts from the distal radius or resected ulna are added to the fusion site. The lunate is reduced first when the scaphoid is also incorporated. We immobilize the wrist in a short-arm cast for 6 weeks or longer until bony fusion is confirmed radiographically. We expect the patient to regain only 25% to 50% of preoperative motion, but pain is significantly improved.

Total wrist fusion is usually accomplished with plate and screw fixation.[20] Opposing bone surfaces in the radiocarpal and mid-carpal areas must be denuded of bone. Newer plate models are thinner distally, to reduce the prominence beneath the extensor tendons.[58] Alternatively a Steinmann pin may be passed in a retrograde direction through the carpus until it exits between the second and third metacarpals, and subsequently tapped proximally into a previously prepared radius. This procedure places the wrist in a neutral position. The pin can be passed through the third metacarpal if the carpal bone stock is poor. Supplemental K wires or staples may be employed. Both techniques provide strong fixation and allow early discontinuation of protective splints or casts.

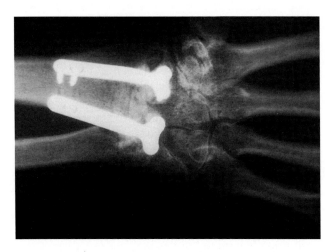

Figure 128-20. Plate fixation for radioscapholunate fusion.

We have not performed resection arthroplasties in the wrist except in the distal radioulnar joint (DRUJ). The DRUJ is approached through a longitudinal incision in the capsule that stops short of the TFCC. We perform a hemiresection of the ulnar head, preserving the most ulnar or medial portion of the head and styloid process. The collateral ligament and TFCC supports are not violated. The wrist is subsequently pronated and supinated to make certain that no bone contact occurs between the radius and ulna. Although it typically is not necessary, we usually create some local soft tissue interposition between the radius and distal ulna. We have not performed a Darrach procedure recently, and prefer a Sauve-Kapandji procedure, if indicated, for the treatment of severe DRUJ disease and the maintenance of a more normal radioulnar surface. The opposing surfaces of the radius and ulna are debrided, approximately 1 cm of the neck of the ulna is resected, and the ulna is fixed to the radius with screws.

OUTCOMES

A generous body of literature on surgical treatment of the rheumatoid hand and wrist has been produced. Most reports are retrospective case series and technical descriptions of procedures. Although many of these clinical reports stand up well when examined in isolation, difficulties arise when the reports are compared. Critical review of these reports is made difficult by the lack of uniformity in data collection, analysis of results, and reporting styles. Nonetheless, much can be gleaned from the work of these surgical investigators. This section provides an overview of surgical outcomes of various procedures, critically analyzes reported evidence, and suggests areas where more work is needed.

SYNOVECTOMY AND TENOSYNOVECTOMY

Synovitis that does not respond to medical management is the most common indication for surgical intervention. Synovectomy and tenosynovectomy are believed to slow the progression of disease and relieve associated pain and swelling. Results of flexor and extensor tenosynovectomy support the use of tenosynovectomy for safe and effective treatment of medically recalcitrant synovitis.[14] Complications are infrequent and are often related to infection or wound-healing complications. The disease may recur, in which case further surgery is an option. A tenolysis rarely may be required if active motion is impaired significantly. Three recent reports have described outcomes following tenosynovectomy (Table 128-1).[13,65,73]

Joint synovectomy often is performed in conjunction with other indicated procedures, such as wrist fusion or MCP-joint replacement. Independent reporting of outcomes for synovectomy is uncommon and no studies confirm that joint synovectomy alters the effects of the disease on that joint.

Adolfsson and Nylander[1] reported the results of arthroscopic synovectomy of the wrist in 16 patients with rheumatoid arthritis. Follow-up took place an average of 6 months after surgery and revealed no complications. All patients reported some subjective improvement in function; objective results indicated that 81% of patients had improved grip strength and 21% had improved motion.

TENDON RUPTURE

The outcomes after surgical correction of tendon ruptures may vary greatly because of the combinations of ruptures that may occur, the varying degrees of underlying joint disease, and the number of reconstructive options. Less favorable outcomes are expected when there are multiple ruptures

Table 128-1.
Outcomes After Extensor Tenosynovectomy

	BROWN AND BROWN[13]	TOLAT ET AL[65]	WHEEN ET AL[73]
Procedure	Flexor and extensor synovectomy	Flexor synovectomy	Flexor synovectomy
Indications	Synovitis, tendon rupture, limited active motion, carpal tunnel syndrome	Synovitis, tendon rupture, limited active motion, carpal tunnel syndrome	Synovitis, tendon rupture, limited active motion
Number of patients	90	43	15
Mean follow-up time (years)	5.8	5.6	4
Complications			
Recurrence	8%	8%	31%
Tendon rupture	6%	2%	0
Infection		4%	0
Pain evaluation	NR	VAS* Preoperative 0.4 Postoperative 7.5	NR
Patient satisfaction	NR	VAS† Postoperative 2.2	72% satisfied
Function	NR	NR	Patient report: 22% restored 59% improved 6% no change
Postoperative ROM	NR 33% poor 22% fair 14% good 31% excellent	J and P Criteria‡ 16% poor 23% fair 43% good 18% excellent	Modified J and P Criteria‡
Grip strength	NR	Unreliable measurements	NR

NR, Not reported; ROM, range of motion; VAS, visual analogue scale.
*Huskisson[28] visual analogue scale for pain (0 = no pain, 10 = severe pain).
†Huskisson[28] visual analogue scale for patient satisfaction (0 = full satisfaction, 10 = complete dissatisfaction).
‡Active motion evaluations based on Jackson and Paton[30] grading system.

and for those that occur in the digits, compared with ruptures in the palm or wrist. Patients with severe underlying joint disease and associated upper extremity limitations also have poorer outcomes. Early synovectomy, as noted previously, may retard or prevent tendon ruptures by decreasing synovial invasion of the tendons, and the correction of bony deformities may delay or avoid ruptures secondary to attrition.

METACARPAL-JOINT ARTHROPLASTY

The outcomes of MCP-joint arthroplasty are well documented in terms of range of motion, extensor lag, ulnar drift, infection, and implant fracture. Beevers and Seedhom[8] reviewed these results and compared prostheses used for MCP-joint arthroplasty. Recent long-term follow-up studies[34,40,74] provide critical information about the change in range of motion and recurrent ulnar drift over time (Table 128-2). Arthroplasty produces little effect on the total range of motion of the MCP joints, but the arc of motion after surgery appears to be more functional. Correction of ulnar drift brings the fingers into a better position for grasp and pinch. Results of Kirschenbaum's series indicate no significant worsening of the arc of motion, extensor lag, or ulnar drift with time.[34] Other authors suggest that patients are less satisfied with time because of a decreasing range of motion. Early gains in strength are not maintained but pain typically does not recur. Late silicone implant fracture is often demonstrated radiographically but does not appear to affect function; this indicates that the implant functions primarily as a spacer.

The effects of MCP-joint arthroplasty on overall hand function and activities of daily living are not as well documented. Study questionnaires have been used to assay patients' impressions regarding pain relief, functional improvement, cosmesis, and the ability to perform the activities of daily living; however, these questionnaires were not standardized or validated. Patient satisfaction decreased with time but was also associated with disease progression and other joint problems. Rothwell et al[54] used the Baltimore quantitative upper-extremity function test before surgery and as many as 3 to 4 years after surgery in an attempt to determine the effect of MCP-joint arthroplasty on the ability to perform everyday tasks. Rapid improvement in hand function occurred during the first 6 weeks after surgery and remained virtually unchanged at all subsequent intervals. Long-term functional change must be documented with such standardized testing.

REPAIR OF THE WRIST

The wrist is severely damaged in the terminal stages of rheumatoid arthritis. The end-stage wrist is typically supinated and volarly dislocated and also exhibits destruction of the carpus and complete dissociation of the radiocarpal joint. Numerous procedures are used in an attempt to prevent or treat the progression of disease. The outcomes of selected techniques are discussed by joint in the following sections.

Radiocarpal Joint
Swanson introduced a silicone radiocarpal joint replacement in the mid-1970s that remains the most commonly used

Table 128-2.
Outcomes After MCP Arthroplasty

	MAURER ET AL[40]	WILSON ET AL[74]	KIRSCHENBAUM ET AL[34]
Number of patients	105	77	27
Number of implants used	446	375	144
Mean follow-up time (years)	8.9	9.6	8.5
ROM arc (degrees)	39	Early 46 Late 29	Early 41-55 Late 36-50
Extension deficit (degrees)	9	Early 9 Late 21	Early 7-19 Late 14-21
Ulnar drift percentage (degrees)	16 (10-25)	13 (>20)	Early 1-6 Late (4-11)
Postoperative fractures (%)	15% polymer 8% high performance	3.2% require removal	15% polymer 10% high performance

ROM, Range of motion.

prosthesis.[61,62] However, popularity of the implant has waned recently because long-term studies have noted a significant incidence of associated silicone synovitis and higher rates of associated prosthetic failures and fractures than were reported previously. The implant remains in use but indications for its use are currently more limited. Use of the implant is superior to arthrodesis in preserving some motion, which is necessary for the performance of daily living activities. The severity of disease, the patient's need for motion, and the patient's activity demands must be evaluated before a decision between arthroplasty and arthrodesis can be made. Tables 128-3 and 128-4 summarize recent reports on the outcomes and complications that occur after silicone wrist arthroplasty.

Table 128-3.
Outcomes After Silicone Wrist Arthroplasty

REFERENCE	NUMBER OF WRISTS	MEAN FOLLOW-UP (years)	OVERALL RESULTS	POSTOPERATIVE ROM (mean values)	POSTOPERATIVE PAIN
Vicar et al[69]	70	6.8	22% poor/fair 78% good/ excellent	Flexion 32 degrees Extension 29 degrees	93% none/mild
Capone[15]	44	2.5	NR	No significant difference from preoperative values	91% with pain relief
Fatti et al[22]	39	5.8	75% poor/fair 25% good/ excellent	Similar to preoperative values	41% mild, 50% moderate/ severe
Jolly et al[32]	15	1.9	52% poor/fair 48% good/ excellent	Flexion 39 degrees Extension 6 degrees	65% none/mild 35% moderate/ severe
Stanley and Tolat[59]	50	8	34% poor/fair 66% good/ excellent	Flexion 31 degrees Extension 25 degrees	Mean VAS* 1.7

NR, Not reported; ROM, range of motion; VAS, visual analogue scale.
*Huskisson[28] visual analogue scale for pain (0 = no pain, 10 = severe pain).

Table 128-4.
Complications After Silicone Wrist Arthroplasty

REFERENCE	% IMPLANT FRACTURE	% IMPLANT FAILURE	% SILICONE SYNOVITIS	% WOUND INFECTION	% HEMATOMA
Vicar et al[69]	8	5	—	—	5
Capone[15]	5	10	—	—	—
Fatti et al[22]	21	23	26	5	—
Jolly et al[32]	52	30	—	—	—
Stanley and Tolat[59]	22	14	0	6	—

Table 128-5.
Outcomes After Total Wrist Arthrodesis

REFERENCE	NUMBER OF WRISTS	MEAN FOLLOW-UP (years)	OVERALL RESULTS	FUSION METHOD (TIME TO FUSION)	POSTOPERATIVE PAIN
Craigen and Stanley[18]	11	6.8	NR	Steinmann pin* or AO plate† (not reported)	100% relief
Howard et al[28]	17	4.3	NR	AO plate* (10 weeks) Bone plate and screws (13.6 weeks)	Mean pain on 5-point scale: AO plate, 1.2; bone plate and screws, 1.1
Kobus and Turner[35]	87	6.0	3% poor 97% good or excellent§	Steinmann pin‡ (10.8 weeks)	100% mild or no pain
Pech et al[53]	29	1.7	NR	L plate (10.7 weeks)	NR
Vicar and Burton[69]	33	6.8	13% poor/fair 87% good or excellent§	Steinmann pin‡ (Not reported)	Mean VAS 1.7 of 10

NR, Not reported; VAS, visual analogue scale.
*Technique as described by Stanley et al.[58]
†Technique as described by Dick.[20]
‡Technique as described by Millender and Nalebuff.[45]
§Overall result determined by methods described by Vicar and Burton.[69]

Total wrist arthrodesis was for many years the treatment of choice for progressive radiocarpal disease in the patient with rheumatoid arthritis. It remains the treatment of choice for severely damaged wrists and for patients with high activity demands. Limited arthrodesis may be appropriate in earlier stages of rheumatoid disease, when some preservation of motion is expected. Tables 128-5 and 128-6 summarize recent reports on outcomes and complications following total wrist arthrodesis. Although surgeons continue to perform fusions using Steinmann pin fixation, more are moving toward plate and screw fixation. Plate fixation allows earlier return of hand motion and results in fewer implant complications.

Distal Radioulnar Joint

Distal ulnar head excision in conjunction with synovectomy and reconstruction of the TFCC is cited by Feldon et al[24] as the procedure of choice for the treatment of caput ulna syndrome. These authors base their recommendations on the procedure's reliable improvement of pain and range of motion. The most common complication associated with the procedure is painful forearm rotation, which may respond to prolonged splinting. If nonsurgical measures do not improve the pain, a secondary soft

tissue stabilization of the distal ulna may be performed. Some authors recommend stabilization at the time of resection to prevent this problem. Tables 128-7, 128-8, and 128-9 summarize five recent reports on the Darrach procedure.

Hemiresection of the distal ulna with soft tissue interposition preserves the ulnar styloid and its attachments. This method was first described by Bowers in 1985.[10] Watson et al[72] have suggested a matched distal ulnar hemiresection as a treatment for DRUJ derangement. These procedures are only indicated when the TFCC is intact or can be repaired. Reports on outcomes after use of these techniques[6,10,72] indicate that most patients have pain relief, are satisfied with their results, and have improved motion.

The Sauve-Kapandji procedure, which involves fusion of the DRUJ in conjunction with resection of a segment of the distal ulna, has recently resurfaced as an option for the treatment of DRUJ derangements, especially in younger patients. This procedure has resurfaced because it is believed to preserve ulnocarpal support and forearm rotation, and to improve the appearance and stability of the wrist. Table 128-10 summarizes recent reports on the outcomes and complications associated with this procedure.

Table 128-6.
Complications After Wrist Arthrodesis

REFERENCE	WOUND INFECTION (%)	DELAYED HEALING (%)	NONUNION (%)	CARPAL TUNNEL SYNDROME (%)	REQUIRING HARDWARE REMOVAL (%)	HEMATOMA (%)
Craigen and Stanley[18]	NR	NR	NR	NR	NR	NR
Howard et al[28]	6	—	—	—	6	—
Kobus and Turner[35]	0	3	2	6	13	—
Pech et al[53]	3	—	0	—	—	—
Vicar and Burton[69]	—	—	0	9	—	3

NR, Not reported.

Table 128-7.
Indications, Pain Relief, and Complications for Resection of the Distal Ulna

REFERENCE	NUMBER OF WRISTS	MEAN FOLLOW-UP (years)	INDICATIONS	POSTOPERATIVE PAIN (%)	COMPLICATIONS (%)
Brumfield et al[14]	102	11	Synovitis	83 with less pain	Recurrent synovitis (15); tendon rupture (5)
Ishikawa et al[30]	43	11	Tendon rupture, synovitis, pain, functional limitations	88 with no pain; 12 with mild pain	Recurrent synovitis (4)
Leslie et al[37]	26	3.5	Caput ulnae pain, deformity	85 with no pain; 15 with mild or moderate pain	NR
Nanchalal et al[50]	40	6.4	Pain, ROM* limitation, joint disease	55% with no pain 45% improved	NR
Van Gemert et al[67]	28	6.2	Pain, ROM limitations	NR	Wound infection (7); hematoma (7); neuroma (11)

NR, Not reported; *ROM*, range of motion.

Table 128-8.
Wrist Motion After Resection of the Distal Ulna

REFERENCE	DISEASE SEVERITY (Grading System)	MEAN POSTOPERATIVE ROM* IN DEGREES (Change from Preoperative Value)	MEAN ROM FOR UNOPERATED CONTRALATERAL WRIST
Brumfield et al[14]	NR	Wrist flexion 26 (−6) Wrist extension 24 (−6)	NR
Ishikawa et al[30]	26% Grade I-II 74% Grade III-IV (Larsen's)	Wrist flexion 26 (−6) Wrist extension 24 (−6) Forearm pronation 88 (+18) Forearm supination 72 (−2)	Wrist flexion 43 Wrist extension 38 Forearm pronation 88 Forearm supination 68
Leslie et al[37]	NR	Wrist flexion 42 (+3) Wrist extension 40 (+2) Forearm pronation 85 (+10) Forearm supination 65 (+10)	NR

NR, Not reported; ROM, range of motion.

Table 128-9.
Radiologic Comparison With Unoperated Contralateral Wrist After Resection of the Distal Ulna

REFERENCE	NUMBER OF PATIENTS	MEAN FOLLOW-UP (years)	CARPAL COLLAPSE	ULNAR TRANSLOCATION	PALMAR SUBLUXATION
Ishikawa et al[30]	43	11	Similar in operated and unoperated wrists	Greater in operated wrists	Similar in operated and unoperated wrists
Nanchalal et al[50]	40	6.4	No significant difference between operated and unoperated wrists	No significant difference between operated and unoperated wrists	NR
Van Gemert et al[67]	28	6.2	NR	Similar in operated and unoperated wrists	NR

NR, Not reported.

Table 128-10.
Outcomes for the Sauve-Kapandji Procedure

REFERENCE	NUMBER OF WRISTS	MEAN FOLLOW-UP (years)	RA PATIENTS ONLY	MEAN POSTOPERATIVE ROM IN DEGREES (Change from preoperative value in degrees)	PATIENT SATISFACTION	COMPLICATIONS
Rothwell et al[54]	28	4	No	>80 degrees rotation in 70%	NR	Nonunion in 21%
Taleisnik[63]	17	5.8	No	94% with full forearm rotation	NR	Delayed healing (6); infection (6); ulnar instability (5)
Vincent et al[70]	21	3.3	Yes	Wrist flexion 36 (+9) Wrist extension 47 (+2) Forearm pronation 78 (0) Forearm supination 62 (−26)	100% would have surgery again	Ulnar instability (5)

NR, Not reported; *ROM*, range of motion.

A distal ulnar silicone implant was developed by Swanson,[60] who advocates its use for patients who have rheumatoid arthritis with DRUJ involvement. Many surgeons have abandoned this technique because of numerous associated complications, including silicone synovitis, bone resorption, and implant failure.[41]

RECOMMENDATIONS FOR FUTURE RESEARCH

Emphasis on quality of life and patient satisfaction are central to outcomes research. There can be no more appropriate application of these measures than in studies of patients with rheumatoid arthritis. Our standard measures of motion and strength often do not accurately reflect the benefits of surgical intervention. Any surgeon who has performed MCP-joint replacements or a wrist arthroplasty is aware that although objective tests, such as grip strength and range-of-motion measurements, may indicate little change, patients often note marked improvement in pain, function, and satisfaction. Thus clinical studies of surgical treatment of

rheumatoid arthritis should place a greater emphasis on patient-reported measures of pain, satisfaction, and physical functioning.

A number of well-validated instruments, or panels of standardized questions, have been developed in recent years that are appropriate for evaluating outcomes in patients with rheumatoid arthritis. Currently the many questionnaires available make it difficult to determine which are most appropriate. A few recommended tests and questionnaires are presented in Table 128-11 to serve as a guide for clinical investigators who are studying the outcomes of surgical treatments for rheumatoid arthritis.

Patient Assessment of Pain and Satisfaction
Visual analogue scales for pain were popularized by Huskisson during the 1970s.[29] Classically, pain is depicted on a continuum of "no pain" to "pain as bad as it can be." A 10-cm horizontal scale is typically used,[43] but the scale can be formatted vertically or with a scale numbered from 1 to 10. The horizontal scale has been used most frequently in surgical reports on rheumatoid arthritis. Alternatively, the Arthritis

Table 128-11.
Recommended Tests and Questionnaires

DISEASE MEASURE	METHOD OF ASSESSMENT
Patient's assessment of pain	Horizontal visual analogue scale (10 cm) of patient's current level of pain
Patient's global assessment of physical functioning	Horizontal visual analogue scale (10 cm) of patient's current level of global functioning
Patient's assessment of satisfaction	Horizontal visual analogue scale (10 cm) of patient's current level of satisfaction
Physician's assessment of function	Horizontal visual analogue scale (10 cm) of patient's current level of satisfaction

Impact Measurement Scale (AIMS) captures pain in one of its subscales.

PATIENT ASSESSMENT OF PHYSICAL FUNCTIONING, GLOBAL HEALTH STATUS, AND QUALITY OF LIFE

AIMS is a 45-item questionnaire that assesses mobility, physical activity, dexterity, activities of daily living, pain, depression, and anxiety.[42] It was designed, as the name implies, for use in clinical research in arthritis patients and has been applied widely. It is reliable, well validated, and sensitive to changes that occur with clinical trials on rheumatoid arthritis patients. Specific subscales may be selected if only particular aspects are to be evaluated in a given study.

Physician Assessment of Physical Function

Routine objective measures of hand function, such as pinch and grip strength and range of motion, may be influenced by the rheumatoid patient's concomitant disease in other joints and soft tissues. Motion and strength are usually improved after surgery but are rarely normal. The Jebsen and Minnesota tests for manipulation provide more information about how well the patient functions in daily tasks.

SUMMARY

The goals of rheumatoid hand surgery are to alleviate pain, restore function and stability, slow the progression or consequences of disease, and improve or correct the associated deformities. The purpose of clinical investigations is to serve as the basis for medical decision making. Thus the most important outcome of any investigation for rheumatoid surgery of the hand is information on the following: pain, function, quality of life, stability, alignment, appearance, and alteration of the disease process. These factors should be the focus of future outcome studies.

REFERENCES

1. Adolfsson L, Nylander G: Arthroscopic synovectomy of the rheumatoid wrist, *J Hand Surg [Br]* 18:92-96, 1993.
2. Arnett F, Edworthy S, Bloch D, et al: The American Rheumatism Association 1987 revised criteria for classification of rheumatoid arthritis, *Arthritis Rheum* 31:315-324, 1988.
3. Aschan W, Moberg E: A long-term study of the effect of early synovectomy in rheumatoid arthritis, *Bull Hosp Joint Dis* 44(2):106-121, 1984.
4. Backdahl M, Strandberg D: The treatment of nodose tendinitis in the rheumatoid hand, *Acta Rheumatol Scand* 11:145-160, 1965.
5. Backhouse K, Kay A, Coomes E, Kates A: Tendon involvement in the rheumatoid hand, *Ann Rheum Dis* 30:236-242, 1971.
6. Bain GI, Pugh DM, MacDermid JC, Roth JH: Matched hemiresection interposition arthroplasty of the distal radioulnar joint, *J Hand Surg [Am]* 20(6):944-950, 1995.
7. Barnes C, Curry H: Carpal tunnel syndrome in rheumatoid arthritis: a clinical and electrodiagnostic survey, *Ann Rheum Dis* 26:226-233, 1970.
8. Beevers D, Seedhom B: Metacarpophalangeal joint prostheses: a review of the clinical results of past and current designs, *J Hand Surg [Br]* 20(2):125-136, 1995.
9. Berger R, Bishop A, Bettinger P: New dorsal capsulotomy for the surgical exposure of the wrist, *Ann Plast Surg* 35:54-59, 1995.
10. Bowers W: Distal radioulnar joint arthroplasty: the hemiresection–interposition technique, *J Hand Surg [Am]* 10:169-178, 1985.
11. Breedveld F, Dijkmans B: Differential therapy in early and late stages of rheumatoid arthritis, *Curr Opin Rheum* 8:226-229, 1996.
12. Brewerton D: The rheumatoid hand, *Proc R Soc Med* 59:225-228, 1966.
13. Brown F, Brown M-L: Long-term results after tenosynovectomy to treat the rheumatoid hand, *J Hand Surg [Am]* 13:704-708, 1988.
14. Brumfield R Jr, Kuschner SH, Gellman H, et al: Results of dorsal wrist synovectomies in the rheumatoid hand, *J Hand Surg [Am]* 15(5):733-735, 1990.

15. Capone R: The titanium grommet in flexible implant arthroplasty of the radiocarpal joint: a long-term review of 44 cases, *Plast Reconstr Surg* 96:667-672, 1995.

16. Chamay A, Della Santa D, Vilaseca A: Radiolunate arthrodesis factor of stability for the rheumatoid wrist, *Ann Chir Main* 2:5-17, 1983.

17. Cobb T, Beckenbaugh R: Biaxial total-wrist arthroplasty: *J Hand Surg [Am]* 21(6):1011-1021, 1996.

18. Craigen MA, Stanley JK: Distal ulnar instability following wrist arthrodesis in men, *J Hand Surg [Br]* (2):155-158, 1995.

19. Darrach W, Dwight K: Derangements of the inferior radioulnar articulation, *Med Rec* 87:708, 1915.

20. Dick H: Wrist arthrodesis. In Green D (editor): *Operative hand surgery,* vol 1, ed 3, New York, 1993, Churchill Livingstone.

21. Fassbender H: *Joint destruction in various arthritic diseases: articular cartilage biochemistry,* New York, 1986, Raven Press.

22. Fatti JF, Palmer AK, Greenky S, Mosher JF: Long-term results of Swanson interpositional arthroplasty: part II, *J Hand Surg [Am]* 16:432-437, 1991.

23. Feldon P: Rheumatoid arthritis. In ASFSOTHU Committee Hand Surgery Update, Aurora, Colo, 1996, American Academy of Orthopedic Surgeons, pp 173-181.

24. Feldon P, Millender LH, Nalebuff EA: Rheumatoid arthritis in the hand and wrist. In Green D (editor): *Operative hand surgery,* vol 2, ed 3, New York, 1993, Churchill Livingstone.

25. Ferlic D, Clayton M: Tendon transfers for radial rotation in the rheumatoid wrist, *J Bone Joint Surg* 55:880-888, 1973.

26. Harris ED Jr: Rheumatoid arthritis: pathophysiology and implications for therapy, *New Engl J Med* 322:1277-1289, 1990.

27. Hindley C, Stanley J: The rheumatoid wrist: patterns of disease progression, *J Hand Surg [Br]* 16(3):275-279, 1991.

28. Howard AC, Stanley D, Getty CJ: Wrist arthrodesis in rheumatoid arthritis: a comparison of two methods of fusion, *J Hand Surg [Br]* 18(3):377-380, 1993.

29. Huskisson EC: Measurement of pain, *Lancet* 2:1127-1131, 1974.

30. Ishikawa H, Hanyu T, Tajima T: Rheumatoid wrists treated with synovectomy of the extensor tendons and wrist joint combined with a Darrach procedure, *J Hand Surg [Am]* 17:1109-1117, 1992.

31. Jackson IT, Paton KC: The extended approach to flexor synovitis in rheumatoid arthritis, *Br J Plast Reconstr Surg* 26:122-131, 1973.

32. Jolly SL, Ferlic DC, Clayton ML, et al: Swanson silicone arthroplasty of the wrist in rheumatoid arthritis: a long-term follow-up, *J Hand Surg [Am]* 17(1):142-149, 1992.

33. Kiefhaber T, Strickland J: Soft tissue reconstruction for rheumatoid swan-neck and boutonniere deformities: long-term results, *J Hand Surg [Am]* 18(6):984-989, 1993.

34. Kirschenbaum D, Schneider L, Adams D, Cody R: Arthroplasty of the metacarpophalangeal joints with use of silicone-rubber implants in patients who have rheumatoid arthritis, *J Bone Joint Surg* 75A(1):3-12, 1993.

35. Kobus RJ, Turner RH: Wrist arthrodesis for treatment of rheumatoid arthritis, *J Hand Surg* 15(4):541-546, 1990.

36. Larson A, Dale K, Eck M, Pahle J: Radiographic evaluation of rheumatoid arthritis by standard reference films, *J Hand Surg* 8:667-669, 1983.

37. Leslie BM, Carlson G, Ruby LK: Results of extensor carpi ulnaris tenodesis in the rheumatoid wrist undergoing a distal ulnar excision (published erratum appears in *J Hand Surg [Am]* 16(1):132, 1991), *J Hand Surg [Am]* 15(4):547-551, 1990.

38. Lundborg G, Branemark P, Carlsson I: Metacarpophalangeal joint arthroplasty based on the osteointegration concept, *J Hand Surg [Br]* 18:693-703, 1993.

39. Mannerfelt L, Norman O: Attrition ruptures of flexor tendons in rheumatoid arthritis caused by bony spurs in the carpal tunnel: a clinical and radiological study, *J Bone Joint Surg* 51B: 270, 1969.

40. Maurer R, Ranawat C, McCormack R, et al: Long-term follow-up of the Swanson MCP arthroplasty for rheumatoid arthritis, *J Hand Surg [Am]* 15(5): 810-811, 1990.

41. McMurtry RY, Paley D, Marks P, Axelrod T: A critical analysis of Swanson ulnar head replacement arthroplasty: rheumatoid versus nonrheumatoid, *J Hand Surg [Am]* 15(2): 224-231, 1990.

42. Meenan R, Mason J, Anderson J, et al: AIMS 2: the content and properties of a revised and expanded Arthritis Impact Measurement Scales health status questionnaire, *Arthritis Rheum* 35:1-10, 1992.

43. Melzack R: The McGill pain questionnaire: major properties and scoring methods, *Pain* 1:277-299, 1975.

44. Meuli HC: Arthroplasty of the wrist, *Clin Orthop* 149:118-125, 1980. 45. Millender L, Nalebuff E: Reconstructive surgery in the rheumatoid hand, *Orthop Clin North Am* 6:709-732, 1975.

45. Moberg E: Tendon grafting and tendon suture in rheumatoid arthritis, *Am J Surg* 109:325-326, 1965.

46. Nalebuff E, Millender L: Surgical treatment of the boutonniere deformity in rheumatoid arthritis, *Orthop Clin North Am* 6(3):753-763, 1975.

47. Nalebuff E, Millender L: Surgical treatment of the swan neck deformity in rheumatoid arthritis, *Orthop Clin North Am* 6(3):733-752, 1975.

48. Nalebuff E, Patel M: Flexor digitorum sublimis transfer for multiple extensor tendon ruptures in rheumatoid arthritis, *Plast Reconstr Surg* 52:530-533, 1973.

49. Nanchahal J, Sykes P, Williams R: Excision of the distal ulna in rheumatoid arthritis: is the price too high? *J Hand Surg [Br]* 21(2):189-196, 1996.

50. O'Brien E: Surgical principles and planning for the rheumatoid hand and wrist, *Clin Plast Surg* 23(3):407-420, 1996.

51. Oster L, Blair W, Steyres C: Crossed intrinsic transfers, *J Hand Surg [Am]* 14:963-971, 1989.

52. Pech J, Sosna A, Rybka V, Pokorny D: Wrist arthrodesis in rheumatoid arthritis: a new technique using internal fixation, *Br J Bone Joint Surg* 78(5):783-786, 1996.

53. Rothwell A, Cragg K, O'Neill L: Hand function following silastic arthroplasty of the metacarpophalangeal joints in the rheumatoid hand, *J Hand Surg [Br]* 22(1):90-93, 1997.

54. Sany J, Anaya JM, Canovas F, et al: Influence of methotrexate on the frequency of postoperative infectious complications in patients with rheumatoid arthritis, *J Rheumatol* 20(7):1129-1132, 1993.

55. Savill D: Some aspects of rheumatoid hand surgery. In *La Main Rheumatismale*, Paris, 1966, L'Expansion Scientifique Francaise, pp 2-29.

56. Stanley J: Conservative surgery in the management of rheumatoid disease of the hand and wrist, *J Hand Surg [Br]* 17:339-342, 1992.

57. Stanley J, Gupta S, Hullin M: Modified instruments for wrist fusion, *J Hand Surg [Br]* 11(2):245-249, 1986.

58. Stanley J, Tolat A: Long-term results of Swanson silastic arthroplasty in the rheumatoid wrist, *J Hand Surg [Br]* 18:381-388, 1993.

59. Swanson A: Silicone rubber implants for replacement of arthritic or destroyed joints in the hand, *Surg Clin North Am* 54A:1113-1127, 1968.

60. Swanson A: Flexible implant resection arthroplasty in the hand and extremities, St. Louis, 1973, Mosby.

61. Swanson A, Swanson G, Maupin B: Flexible implant arthroplasty of the radiocarpal joint: surgical technique and long-term study, *Clin Orthop* 187:94-106, 1984.

62. Taleisnik J: The Sauve-Kapandji procedure, *Clin Orthop* 275:110-123, 1992.

63. Terrono A, Millender L, Nalebuff E: Boutonniere rheumatoid thumb deformity, *J Hand Surg [Am]* 15:999-1003, 1990.

64. Tolat AR, Stanley JK, Evans RA: Flexor tenosynovectomy and tenolysis in longstanding rheumatoid arthritis, *J Hand Surg [Br]* 21(4):538-543, 1996.

65. Tupper J: The metacarpophalangeal volar plate arthroplasty, *J Hand Surg [Am]* 14(2):371-375, 1989.

66. Van Gemert AML, Spauwen PHM: Radiological evaluation of the long-term effects of resection of the distal ulna in rheumatoid arthritis, *J Hand Surg [Br]* 19:330-333, 1994.

67. Vaughan-Jackson O: Attrition ruptures of tendons as a factor in the production of deformities in the rheumatoid hand, *Proc R Soc Med* 52:132-134, 1959.

68. Vicar AJ, Burton RI: Surgical management of the rheumatoid wrist: fusion or arthroplasty, *J Hand Surg [Am]* 11:790-797, 1986.

69. Vincent K, Szabo R, Agee J: The Sauve-Karpanji procedure for reconstruction of the rheumatoid distal radioulnar joint, *J Hand Surg* 16(6):978-983, 1993.

70. Volz RG: The development of a total wrist arthroplasty, *Clin Orthop* 116-209, 1976.

71. Watson H, Ryu J, Burgess R: Matched distal ulnar resection, *J Hand Surg [Am]* 11:812-817, 1986.

72. Wheen DJ, Tonkin MA, Green J, Bronkhorst M: Long-term results following digital flexor tenosynovectomy in rheumatoid arthritis, *J Hand Surg [Am]* 20(5):790-794, 1995.

73. Wilson Y, Sykes P, Niranjan N: Long-term follow-up of Swanson's silastic arthroplasty of the metacarpophalangeal joints in rheumatoid arthritis, *J Hand Surg [Br]* 18(1):81-91, 1993.

74. Wollheim F: Established and new biochemical tools for diagnosis and monitoring of rheumatoid arthritis, *Curr Opin Rheum* 8:221-225, 1996.

75. Wood V, Ichertz D, Yahiku H: Soft tissue metacarpophalangeal reconstruction for treatment of rheumatoid hand deformity, *J Hand Surg [Am]* 14:163-174, 1989.

PART XII

TUMORS

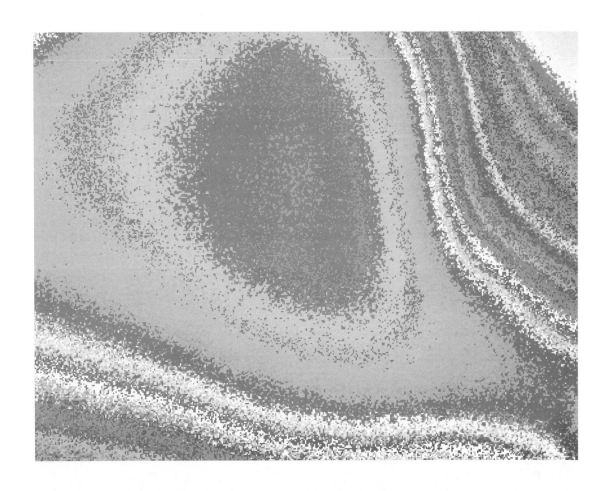

CHAPTER 129

Benign Soft Tissue Tumors

George L. Lucas

INTRODUCTION

Hand surgeons see patients with tumefactions of the hand almost every day, but the overall incidence of hand tumors in the population at large is quite small. Moreover, although humans are subject to a large variety of neoplasms,[5,25] most hand tumors are benign. In a review of a large hand practice, Leung[11] determined that less than 3% of new patients had tumors and that 92% of these were benign soft tissue tumors. Thus the ratio of 100 benign neoplasms for every 1 malignant soft tissue neoplasm found in the human body most likely also is a reasonable estimate for the hand.[6] Any tissue (e.g., skin, muscle, bone, nerve, vessel) can be the site of origin of a tumor in the hand, but it is perhaps simpler to classify tumors as those involving either bone or soft tissue. This chapter deals with benign soft tissue tumors, all of which can be grouped according to their tissue of origin or according to the predominant tissue type within the lesion (e.g., fibrous, vascular, synovial, or fibrohistiocytic). Some lesions are difficult to classify and some overlap may exist between categories of lesions; for example, some lesions are quasimalignant (e.g., desmoid) and others are very slowly growing malignancies that are biologically more similar to benign lesions. The most common lesions of the hand, such as ganglion cysts and epidermoid inclusion cysts that typically are classified as tumors, are not true neoplasms. Such lesions are reactions to injury or secondary tumefactions but are not truly "new growths." Therefore I believe it is more useful to describe the lesions that are likely to be encountered in practice than to review the extensive list of different histologic possibilities.

The hand is such a compact, tightly integrated structure that any deviation in form is usually recognized fairly quickly by a patient. Any mass that is exerting pressure on a nerve, stretching the skin, or interfering with function may be brought to the patient's awareness by observation, palpation, or pain. Most benign soft tumors concern patients more because of the mass or "bump" than because of pain or interference with function; although patients aren't likely to admit it, they are often concerned that the newly discovered lump is a cancer. When evaluating and advising patients about these lumps, physicians should reassure the patient that the mass is far more likely to be benign than malignant. Patients rarely appear with what looks like a malignancy from the outset. In cases involving malignancy, the tenor of discussion between physician and patient must be changed appropriately, but such situations occur very rarely, even for hand surgeons.

INDICATIONS

Physical examination of the hand should follow a consistent pattern regardless of the presenting complaint, but evaluation of a lump should involve consideration of its duration, location, size, mobility, tenderness, discoloration, and deformability. A palmar mass on the digit or palm, for example, should suggest the possibility of an epidermoid inclusion cyst, whereas a dorsal wrist mass typically is a ganglion. A small, tender mass along the course of the digital nerve is most likely a neurilemoma or a posttraumatic neuroma. A ganglion or a cyst of the tendon sheath may be somewhat mobile and even compressible; in contrast, an extraabdominal desmoid has a distinctly rock-hard feel.

Imaging studies may not lead to definitive diagnoses but are nearly always advised as part of a comprehensive evaluation. A conventional two-plane radiograph should be the first imaging study ordered and may be helpful in sizing the lesion as well as demonstrating bony erosion, mineralization, or phleboliths. Magnetic resonance imaging (MRI) can accurately define the anatomy of a soft tissue tumor and identify ganglions, lipomas, hemangiomas, and chondromas; however, MRI is seldom necessary or cost effective in determining the treatment of a hand mass. Similarly, ultrasound may provide information about a lesion but seldom is necessary to guide treatment.

A confident diagnosis of a hand mass can be determined from physical examination, standard radiographs, and the patient's history. The surgeon should assure the patient that a diagnosis typically can be made by observation. Most often the patient and physician agree to remove the lesion surgically by means of excisional biopsy. Thus indications for surgery typically are based on the patient's awareness of a mass; a patient often requests removal of a mass even when he or she is not functionally compromised by it. Excisional biopsy is usually straightforward, but the compact nature of the hand's structure requires that the surgeon have a thorough knowledge of hand anatomy and respect for structures in the vicinity of the mass. Excision of a neurilemoma, for example, requires careful dissection of the lesion from the digital nerve under magnification; thorough eradication of a benign histiocytoma or a cyst of the tendon sheath requires similar attention to detail. Excision of an epidermoid inclusion cyst may require excision of a small strip of skin accompanying the cyst, and removal of a ganglion requires a search for the "stalk" of the cyst. Open excisional biopsy is appropriate treatment for lesions that are unquestionably benign, and it is the most reliable method for obtaining adequate tissue for accurate histologic confirmation. Almost all lesions classified as benign soft tissue tumors of the hand are managed by excisional biopsy. Generic information regarding surgical indications may be adequate for most lesions; exceptions are noted in this chapter where appropriate.

The hand is an intricate, compact, sensitive, and delicate structure; any deviation in contour or palpable mass typically comes to a patient's attention quite early. For this reason, patients often seek medical care for lesions that are only a few millimeters in size. Such lesions often are visible and nearly always are palpable. The mass also may be painful or tender and may interfere with function of a joint, tendon, or nerve. Such masses are always worrisome for patients. Although the overwhelming odds are in favor of the lesion being benign, the remote possibility of malignancy must be considered. When a physician suspects a malignancy, the patient evaluation and approach to the lesion must be much more cautious and may require vascular dye studies, MRI, computed tomography (CT), or ultrasound. Such studies assist in proper staging of the lesion and allow selection of the best biopsy technique, as described in Chapter 130. The patient must be informed that it is typically safe to forgo surgical removal of a benign tumor. This information must be tempered with advice that the lesion is likely to grow, albeit slowly, and that it may cause functional impairment in the future. Alternative treatments for such lesions (e.g., radiation, acupuncture, chiropractic) typically are not available, with the exception of ganglions, which can be cured by aspiration in perhaps 25% of patients. All of the lesions described in the following section (with the exception of those affecting small children) can be surgically treated with the use of regional anesthetic techniques. Anesthetics used in these procedures often are administered by the surgeon, which minimizes the expense of the surgery. Tourniquet control is essential for all such procedures.

OPERATIONS

GANGLION CYSTS

Ganglion cysts, the most frequently encountered soft tissue masses in the hand and wrist, reportedly account for 33% to 69% of all hand tumors. They can occur at several locations around the hand and wrist. Most lesions occur on the dorsum of the wrist and are specifically associated with the scapholunate ligament (Figure 129-1).[2] Less common locations include the volar wrist (20%),[8] where the lesions are associated with the scaphotrapezial joint and often with degenerative change in the basal joints of the thumb; the lateral and dorsal aspects of the digits; and the dorsum of the distal interphalangeal joint (DIP) joint, which is the location of the so-called *mucous cyst*. Cysts of the tendon sheath also can be classified as ganglion cysts because all of these lesions are histologically identical. Ganglion cysts are more common in women than in men and also are more common in the second to fourth decades of life. Patients who seek treatment for a mass typically have been aware of it for an extended period of time—sometimes for years—and often they have noted variations in the lesion's size. Some of these patients have attempted the folk remedy of "hitting it with the Bible," and some have noted that the lesion disappears temporarily if it is bumped. A ganglion cyst occasionally arises as an acute lesion after trauma to the hand or wrist; in such cases it is often difficult to convince workers' compensation insurers that such an event could occur in the course of a patient's employment.

Patients often complain of pain in the wrist or hand associated with the ganglion cysts, and the lesion itself is sometimes tender to palpation. The cyst is compressible and slightly mobile and can be transilluminated. Aspiration of synovial-like fluid confirms the diagnosis but seldom provides a lasting cure.[22] Aspiration is often accompanied by the injection of a small amount of steroid into the lesion, but this may have no particular effect. Lesions that occur distal to the wrist on the dorsum of the hand may be cysts of the tendon or

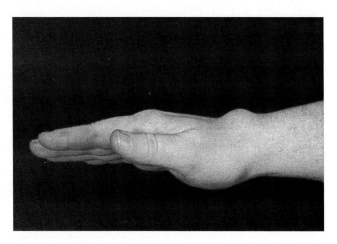

Figure 129-1. Lateral view of a modest-sized dorsal carpal ganglion.

tendon sheath. This possibility can be confirmed by observation of the movement of the mass with excursion of the extensor tendon. A mass on the proximal dorsum of the hand initially may be confused with a carpometacarpal (CMC) boss, but the latter is not compressible and is not reported to change size. Anomalous muscle bellies do change in size as they enlarge in response to gripping; these may be confused with ganglions and often are associated with a small ganglion that is intimately connected to the muscle.[13] A ganglion may arise in an intramuscular location or even in an intraneural location, thus differential diagnoses of virtually all soft tissue hand masses should include that of a ganglion cyst.

Radiographs typically are not helpful in making the diagnosis of a ganglion. However, wrist films should be obtained for acute ganglions and for small, tender lesions at the base of the thumb, which are often associated with osteoarthritis of the CMC joint of the thumb. All of these lesions have their genesis in the capsule or ligaments of the joints of the wrist or hand; the most common example is the dorsal wrist ganglion, which usually arises from the scapholunate ligament. Thus surgical treatment should involve dissection down the stalk of the lesion to its origin on the ligament or joint capsule, with excision of a modest section of the capsule to remove the origin of the stalk and any capsular cysts.

Capsular cysts are sometimes called *daughter cysts* and their retention has been suggested as a cause of recurrent ganglion cysts. Dissection should be performed bluntly, but gently, to avoid rupture of the cyst. Lister[12] has recommended opening the cyst if it adheres to the radial artery and leaving a small segment of the cyst wall attached to the artery to minimize damage to the vessel. He recommends closure of the capsular defect by suture in such cases; frequently this is also possible with dorsal ganglions if capsulectomy has not been extensive. Virtually all cysts have some venous channels or superficial nerves stretched over them that must be preserved by careful dissection. Most dorsal lesions can be approached by a transverse incision in a skin crease, with a subcuticular closure to minimize cosmetic concerns. Volar lesions should usually be approached through a longitudinal incision, which can be extended if necessary. Excised tissue should be sent to a pathologist for histologic confirmation, but cultures or other studies on the tissue are unnecessary.

Osterman[19] reported arthroscopic excision of ganglion cysts whereby the base of the ganglion is excised as a small capsular resection from within the joint. This procedure will require much wider experience before it can be recommended; however, there are several advantages to arthroscopic treatment, such as minimal scarring, and perhaps more importantly, the access to information about the wrist from inspection of intraarticular structures. Osterman, for example, found other intraarticular pathologic conditions in 42% of his patients.[19]

Recurrent carpal ganglions pose much greater difficulties during treatment. They often require scar excision or revision, involving difficult dissection through the capsule and scar and difficulty in establishing tissue planes around the cyst. This often requires extensive capsular resection and creates the potential for capsular instability. Thus serious efforts should be made to reinforce or replace the capsular defect with other local tissue and to provide extensive postoperative stabilization with a splint or cast.

Postoperative care in most other cases is rather simple. A soft dressing, including an elastic bandage, is applied at the time of surgery and is removed when the patient returns to the physician's office approximately 10 days later. No splint is required for uncomplicated cases. After removal of the bandage, active exercises are encouraged to allow restoration of wrist and finger motion. Most workers, with the exception of laborers, can return to their job activities within a few days of surgery.

Reports have suggested that the recurrence rate for ganglion cysts may be as high as 34%. Recent surgical techniques have produced fewer recurrences but have not eliminated them. Often a recurrence appears within the first several months after surgery. Keloid scars, infection, and neuromas are possible complications but are very uncommon. Instability of the carpus has been reported after wide capsular resection, which should not be indiscriminate.

Dorsal transverse incisions made in skin creases and closed with a subcuticular suture create minimal scarring, but a longitudinal volar incision will result in a modest scar. Surprisingly, local rotation flap coverage of mucous cysts almost always results in a barely visible scar on the dorsum of the digit. Thus patients whose lesions do not recur are invariably satisfied with the result.

A small subgroup of ganglions occurs on the ulnar aspect of the wrist, often stretching the dorsal cutaneous branch of the ulnar nerve.[14] These lesions arise from the pisohamate joint or the triangular fibrocartilage area. They arise rather quickly and presumably stretch the overlying nerve, creating a painful paresthesia over the dorsoulnar aspect of the hand. Consequently, careful retraction of the nerve during resection is mandatory. The capsular defect that remains after resection often is small and can be closed by scarification and suture. Histologically, such lesions are identical to other ganglions.

Cysts of the tendon sheath or volar retinacular ganglions are extremely common lesions that present as tender, BB-sized masses at the volar base of the digit. Their size (less than 1 cm), location, characteristic response to palpation, and associated tenderness provide a very reliable diagnosis. Surgical treatment is rarely necessary. Patients should receive reassurance and instructions to massage the lesion until it ruptures, which is appropriate treatment for virtually all of these lesions. Occasionally the lesion may increase in size enough to warrant puncture with a needle under local anesthesia, but surgical excision is rarely indicated. If surgery is considered, digital block anesthesia can be used. Removal of the ganglion and a small patch of the A1 pulley of the flexor tendon sheath can be achieved through an oblique incision. Simple skin closure and minimal dressing allow rapid return to activity. Similar lesions occur in association with extensor tendons and can occur within the tendinous structure of an accessory finger extensor on the dorsum of the hand.[13] Movement of the mass with tendon excursion or grip ensures an accurate diagnosis.

MUCOUS CYSTS

The so-called *mucous cyst* is appropriately considered as a ganglion because it arises from a joint and is histologically indistinguishable from any other type of ganglion or tendon sheath cyst. The mucous cyst is associated with degenerative changes in the DIP joint of the finger, and successful treatment is predicated on the recognition of this fact. A radiograph of the DIP joint typically reveals narrowing and the presence of osteophytes. Just as the stalk from a dorsal wrist ganglion can be traced down to the dorsal wrist capsule, so too can the stalk of a mucous cyst be traced to the DIP joint. The skin over the cyst is very thin, and consequently spontaneous or traumatic rupture and secondary contamination of the DIP joint can occur. Thus a mucous cyst requires surgical removal; attempted aspiration invariably is followed by recurrence.

Patients who present with a mucous cyst typically are in their sixth or seventh decade. Some have previously sought relief from a dermatologist or family physician; in some cases a dermatologist has made unsuccessful attempts at shaving or freezing the cyst. Some patients initially note a grooving of the fingernail but do not perceive the cyst that appears just proximal to the nail fold (Figure 129-2). The cyst often obliterates the nail fold, which interferes with surgical excision. Function of the digit is impaired as a consequence of the arthritis, and radiographs reveal osteophytes, joint-space irregularity, and sclerosis.

Various incisions and surgical techniques have been described. An H-shaped incision is most commonly used when there are osteophytes on both sides of the DIP joint. I prefer to remove the skin overlying the cyst, which has the potential to necrose, and to resurface the small area with a local rotation flap. This procedure is easily performed under digital block anesthesia. The cyst should be traced back to the DIP joint, which is opened and debrided; any osteophytes are removed during excision of the cyst. The capsular defect is closed with absorbable suture, and the skin flap is inset with multiple 5-0 or 6-0 nylon sutures. Care should be taken to avoid damage to the germinal nail matrix or the extensor tendon. A light dressing is applied, which is removed when the patient returns for suture removal 10 days after surgery. If the surgeon suspects that healing has not occurred, alternate sutures are removed and the remainder are left in place for another 4 to 5 days. Rarely, recurrence or infection may occur, but healing is usually uneventful and the scar from the rotated flap is barely visible. However, the patient may continue to experience some difficulty because of underlying arthritis in the joint. The patient should be reassured that the grooving in the nail gradually disappears over several months.

EPIDERMOID INCLUSION CYSTS

Epidermoid inclusion cysts are perhaps the second most common hand tumors seen in my practice.[15] These lesions present as slowly enlarging localized swelling, usually on the palmar surface of the hand (Figure 129-3). The patient often describes a previous puncture wound to the palm, which is the genesis of such lesions (Figure 129-4).[17] Any skin disruption, including a puncture, laceration, or incision can implant epidermal cell elements into the dermis and subcutaneous tissue, where continued production of keratin and other epidermal products produces a thick-walled cyst containing laminated white, cheesy, or curdy material.[15] These lesions are most common in adults who perform labor with their hands

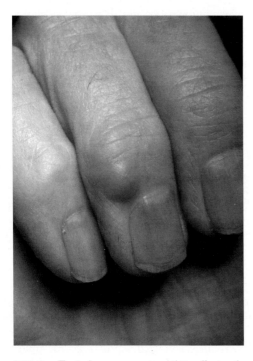

Figure 129-2. Typical mucous cyst exhibits effects of pressure on the nail plate.

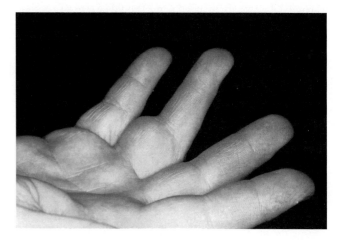

Figure 129-3. Typical appearance of an epidermal inclusion cyst on the palmar surface of a digit. (From Lucas GL: *J Southern Ortho Assoc* 8:188-192, 1999.)

(e.g., farmers, factory workers, builders) and who sustain frequent minor hand lacerations or cracks in the skin. Epidermoid inclusion cysts rarely occur in children, except after surgical procedures, which further supports the implantation theory of cyst development. Some epidermal inclusion cysts may involve bone, most often the distal phalanx; in such cases a thin shell of cortical bone may partially surround the cyst (Figure 129-5). Thus routine radiographs of the involved area should be obtained. All cystic material must be surgically removed to prevent a recurrence.

Malignant deterioration does not occur; however, one patient in my series with a verrucous epidermoid carcinoma had physical and surgical findings that were quite consistent with an epidermoid inclusion cyst. Thus all material excised should be submitted for histologic evaluation. Epidermoid inclusion cysts occasionally rupture and discharge thick, white material. Although such discharge does not yield organisms on culture, the area may become secondarily infected, prompting a visit to a physician.

Alternatives to treatment by surgical excision are not available. Moreover, these lesions must be excised completely to prevent recurrence. A careful, complete excision, often including removal of a strip of adherent skin, should limit the number of recurrent lesions. These lesions typically are superficial and thus place the nerves, vessels, or tendons at minimal risk. Surgery can be accomplished with regional anesthesia to minimize the risk to the patient. Postoperative management is simple and involves application of a light dressing and return to activity within a few days. Complications such as neuroma, troublesome scar, infection, or joint contracture are very rare but some patients may experience recurrence. Patients need to be seen only once after surgery for suture removal; during this visit they are also instructed in wound care and given advice regarding activity. Most patients are very satisfied with the outcome after surgical excision, are able to use their hand normally, and can return to their previous work activity.

GIANT CELL TUMORS

The commonly encountered giant cell tumor of the tendon sheath, like the cysts previously described, most likely is not a true neoplasm but rather a reaction to injury.[7,20] Some experts consider giant cell tumors of the tendon sheath to be the second most common benign hand lesions. I believe the name may cause confusion with giant cell tumors of bone; thus I prefer the term *benign histiocytoma* (although I recognize the potential for confusion with malignant fibrous histiocytoma and perhaps the improper implication that the lesion has a neoplastic nature). This lesion is also known by several other names, including *pigmented villonodular tenovaginosynovitis*, *xanthoma*, and *nodular tenosynovitis*.

These lesions are fairly common and seem to occur most

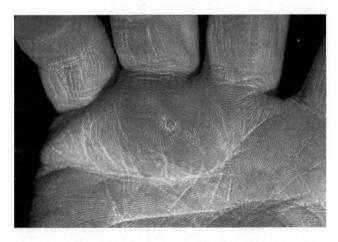

Figure 129-4. Epidermal inclusion cyst at the base of the ring finger. Note the chronic effects of the puncture wound, which most likely was the genesis of the underlying cyst. (From Lucas GL: *J Southern Ortho Assoc* 8:188-192, 1999.)

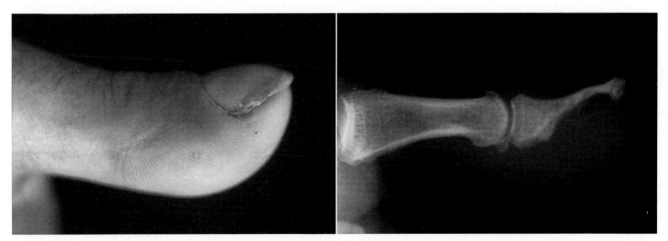

Figure 129-5. **A,** Large epidermal inclusion cyst involving the pulp of the thumb. **B,** Radiograph of the lesion reveals extensive bony erosion of the distal phalanx.

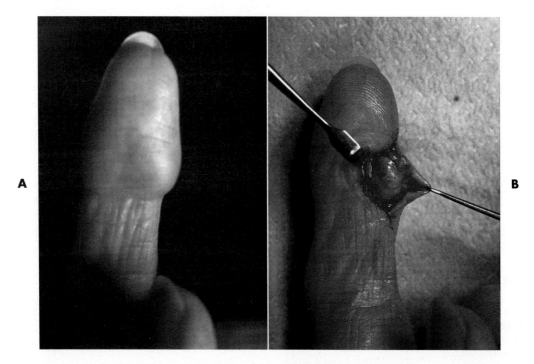

Figure 129-6. A, Slightly irregular, firm nodule on the distal segment of the finger is suggestive of a giant cell tumor of the tendon sheath. **B,** Intraoperative photo shows a firm, irregular, dark-colored, lobular lesion that extends much further than is apparent in this view. Laboratory examination confirmed the diagnosis of a histiocytoma.

frequently in women who are middle-aged or older. They do not occur exclusively along the tendon sheath but also develop at other sites where synovial fluid is produced, including joints (20% of cases) and capsular ligaments. They present as painless, irregular masses; examination typically reveals that these are more extensive than the patient realized, and surgery may reveal wide extensions (Figure 129-6). Clinically these lesions are most commonly confused with ganglion cysts, although their fixation to deeper tissues may be an aid in diagnosis. The lesions often compress adjacent bone, which can be confirmed in routine radiographs. MRI may be used to more accurately define the extent of the lesion; however, the current expense of MRI studies makes them practical only in very extensive cases. During surgery the lesions appear as irregular, multiloculated, subcutaneous masses with a variegated coloration of brown, yellow, and, less commonly, orange. Because they proliferate they may interfere with joint or tendon function; thus surgical excision must involve meticulous use of loupe magnification to avoid an incomplete excision followed by a recurrence. It is not uncommon for such lesions to essentially "wrap around" a joint, causing growth of giant cell tissue on both the flexor and extensor sides of the digit. Both dorsal and volar incisions may be necessary in such cases to remove all of the tumor. Patients should be warned that this invasive nature causes a significant recurrence rate of nearly 10%. One of my patients underwent surgery for her eleventh recurrence![1] Postoperative therapy is dictated by the extent of dissection during surgery. In most cases, early active and passive range-of-motion exercises are required to prevent tendon adhesions and to increase digital motion.

DERMATOFIBROMA

A dermatofibroma is a benign fibrous tumor of the skin and is considered the histologic counterpart to a fibrous histiocytoma. It presents as a firm, solitary or multiple, nodular lesion that is red to red-brown in color and is often painful and tender. These lesions, which are most commonly referred to dermatologists, should be excised for pathologic examination to rule out the presence of a malignancy such as malignant fibrous histiocytoma.

LIPOMAS

Lipomas are extremely common tumors of mesenchymal origin that do not occur often in the upper extremity and occur even more rarely in the hand.[10] They are believed to be more common in women. Lipomas are characteristically solid and well-defined by palpation; they are not tender but may be quite large in size and often produce symptoms caused by their mass. They tend to occur in the subcutaneous tissue, but deeper intermuscular, intramuscular, or intrafascial lesions can occur and may be more difficult to excise. An accurate diagnosis usually can be obtained clinically; however, confirmation may be achieved with radiographs, which reveal a well-defined water or fat density that produces a lucent delineation of the lesion. Occasionally, a lesion adjacent to bone may cause a pressure indentation in the bone. Patients may request removal after gradual enlargement of the mass begins to interfere with hand function. These lesions have well-defined surgical margins that allow them to be easily "shelled out" but always are attached to the fascia or other deeper structures containing the lesion's blood supply. This attachment, or vascular pedicle, must be detached and cauterized. Dissection must be performed carefully because lipomas can displace nerves or tendons and occasionally may surround a nerve or vessel.

Recurrence is very uncommon and malignant degeneration most likely does not occur. Some histologic variants, such as fibrolipomas, myxoid fibrolipomas, and angiolipomas cannot be diagnosed clinically but are determined by pathologic examination after surgery. Management after surgery is simple, and patients can resume full activity within several days of operation.

FIBROUS-TISSUE TUMORS

A wide variety of tumors that originate in fibrous tissue are uncommon in the hand (Figure 129-7). These include dermal or subdermal fibromas, fibromas of the tendon sheath, nodular fasciitis, fibrous tumors of infancy and childhood, and juvenile aponeurotic fibroma. The latter two lesions occur in children and are particularly worrisome to parents and inexperienced physicians.

Nodular fasciitis is an uncommon lesion that must be distinguished from palmar fibromatosis, which is a variant of Dupuytren's diathesis. Nodular fasciitis occurs more commonly on the forearm than in the hand and is a quasineoplastic lesion that occurs after a traumatic event in 10% to 15% of cases. It presents as a small but rapidly growing mass, which is usually less than 3 cm in diameter and often is very tender. This lesion may occur in a subcutaneous, intramuscular, or fascial location and usually can be palpated. The pathologist who receives an excised specimen must be fully informed of the clinical characteristics because histologic confusion with a fibrosarcoma can occur.

Fibromas of the tendon sheath are difficult to distinguish from tendon sheath cysts. Both lesions present as small, slightly tender nodules associated with the tendon sheath. Small fibromas can interfere with tendon function; like tendon sheath cysts, they are treated by excision of the mass and a small segment of underlying tendon sheath. Inadequate resection of the lesion may lead to recurrence. Such lesions can be histologically distinguished from giant cell tumors of the tendon sheath because they have less cellularity and do not possess giant cells.[3]

Although most soft tissue lesions of the hand require complete excisional biopsy, patients with juvenile aponeurotic fibroma require a conservative local excision that does not sacrifice essential structures. This lesion, which was first described by Keasby in 1961, presents as a rapidly growing, painless, firm, irregular mass on the sole of the foot or palm of the hand in children.[9,26] Affected children have frequent recurrences initially, but as they grow older the recurrences become less frequent and more self-limited. Thus radical excision is not indicated, although repeated subtotal resections may be necessary to contain the size of the tumor. Consider-

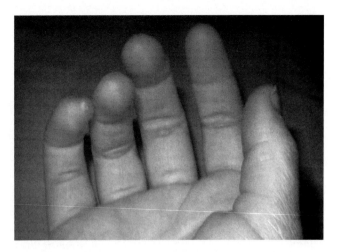

Figure 129-7. Fibroma at the tip of a child's finger.

able discipline on the part of the surgeon, bolstered by consultations with expert pathologists, is necessary to avoid a mistaken diagnosis of malignancy. Fears of malignancy are heightened by the histologic appearance of these lesions, which reveals a highly cellular proliferation of pleomorphic fibroblastic nuclei. Despite infiltration into surrounding fat and muscle, evidence of mitotic activity in the tumor does not exist. No instances of metastasis have been reported in the literature. Radiographs of this lesion are helpful because they may reveal calcification that corresponds to calcifications seen during microscopic examination of the tissue. Cutaneous scarring after one or several excisions is likely to produce some morbidity.

The so-called *recurring digital fibrous tumor of childhood* occurs as multiple smooth masses on the dorsum of the fingers and toes of infants or children and may alarm parents and physicians.[21] The masses may appear simultaneously on several digits. The multicentric nature of this lesion suggests an infectious origin—most likely that of a virus. Diagnosis depends on identification of intracytoplasmic inclusion bodies, which are easily seen with special stains. These inclusions are not seen in soft tissue sarcomas or benign fibrous lesions, and their presence supports the viral theory of origin. After the proper diagnosis has been confirmed, conservative therapy is indicated unless there is interference with function of a joint or tendon or concern about appearance (especially that of the fingernails). Distant spread has not been observed but local recurrence occurs in more than 50% of cases.

VASCULAR LESIONS

Although hemangiomas occur in the hand, they are discussed in Chapter 132. Two lesions, the vascular leiomyoma and the intraluminal endothelial hyperplasia, or *Masson's hemangioma,* are histologically related to hemangiomas and present as noncompressible, solid lesions. Treatment for both is straightforward and involves surgical excision under regional or local anesthesia.

A vascular leiomyoma or dermal angiomyoma is a small tumor that most likely arises from the tunica muscularis in the walls of small vessels and presents as a slowly enlarging, painless mass. These lesions are located in the dermis or subcutaneous layer and therefore do not interfere with the function of deeper structures. The lesions present as well-encapsulated, white, round or oval lesions at the time of excision. Microscopically they feature interlacing bundles of smooth muscle fibers surrounding multiple vascular channels. In 1997 Neviaser[18] pointed out that these lesions are not rare and occur in the hand, wrist, or forearm in as many as 30% of cases; moreover, he noted that recurrence as a malignancy was reported on at least one occasion.

Masson's hemangioma is far less common. In a large series reported by Clearkin and Enzinger,[4] this lesion appeared more often on the fingers than in any other location. It presents as a small, dark subdermal or subcutaneous lesion, and although it is histologically a vascular lesion it presents clinically as a solid mass and is therefore mentioned in this section. A recent variation presented to me as a much larger lesion on the palmar surface of the thumb in a young child. This lesion is benign despite its histologic appearance, which resembles that of an angiosarcoma (so much so that it is often called *Masson's pseudoangiosarcoma*). Differential diagnoses based on microscopic appearance include several types of benign and malignant vascular proliferative processes. If a diagnosis of angiosarcoma is returned after removal of such a lesion, additional consultation from an experienced pathologist must be obtained. Simple surgical excision of the lesion typically cures this perfectly benign condition.

FOREIGN BODY REACTIONS

Foreign body reactions commonly occur in the hand and may present as a mass that the patient cannot relate to an injury. Most patients who sustain an injury involving a wooden splinter or metal or glass penetration seek medical attention shortly after the incident. A patient is usually able to remove a foreign body from the hand without too much difficulty at the time of injury, but portions of a wooden sliver or other foreign material may be left behind and may produce a tender, painful mass. Retention of the foreign body induces the development of a foreign-body granuloma mass. Chronic inflammation associated with the granuloma can result in joint contracture or stiffness. An examining physician often can discern the presence of a foreign body within soft tissue swelling. The local area typically is very tender and erythematous (Figure 129-8). Radiographs should be obtained in multiple projections to identify retained foreign bodies. Small wood fragments are not visible on plain radiographs but may be identified by ultrasound or MRI.[24]

Surgical excision is the treatment of choice for foreign body granulomas and should include removal of a small segment of skin if a notable cutaneous scar remains from the original injury. The dissection must proceed very carefully and the surgeon must be aware of the possibility of iatrogenic nerve or

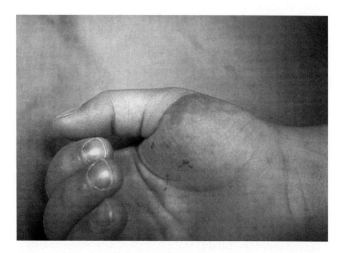

Figure 129-8. Tender swelling in the thenar eminence. Note the rather sharp protuberance just proximal to the metacarpophalangeal crease, which represents a catfish spine. The patient recalled sustaining a puncture caused by the object several weeks previously.

tendon injury. Loupe magnification is a necessity for many of the smaller lesions. Twenty-four to 48 hours of broad-spectrum antibiotic coverage is indicated. The ultimate prognosis is quite good after excision of the offending foreign body and the surrounding reaction. The physician should suspect a self-induced or factitious problem if the lesion recurs because some patients occasionally mutilate themselves with small pieces of wire or needles. Penetration by toothpicks deserves special mention. This occurs most commonly through the sole of the foot but occasionally occurs through the palmar surface of the hand. A toothpick contaminated by oral bacteria can inoculate a variety of organisms into the hand and can create a rather virulent local infection, which requires vigorous antibiotic treatment in addition to surgical excision.

LOCALIZED NODULES

Gouty tophi and rheumatoid nodules are two types of localized nodules that often occur on the hand. The diagnosis typically is not difficult in the setting of the underlying disease; however, when gout is present, an inflamed, painful tophus may be the presenting feature of the disease. Gouty tohpi and rheumatoid nodules are both firm, irregular, nodular masses of variable size. The tophus often is white and covered with thin skin, which may be eroded, allowing an extrusion of white, chalky, or pasty material and creating the clinical impression of an infection (Figure 129-9). Tophi are infrequently removed surgically; however, excision may be indicated to allow the patient to wear a ring, to control drainage and/or infection, or to decrease the urate burden on the body. The mainstay of

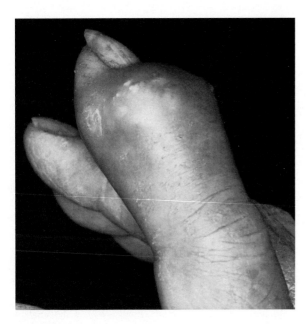

Figure 129-9. Large gouty tophus located at the DIP joint.

treatment for gout is medical management of the underlying metabolic disorder.

Unlike tophi, which are oriented around joints, rheumatoid nodules can occur at any location along the digits or along other areas of the upper extremity. Rheumatoid nodules may be somewhat tender but do not appear red or inflamed unless the thin, overlying skin has ruptured and allowed the development of a secondary infection. They may produce symptoms if they overlie a digital nerve and compromise nerve function. Patients often request removal of the nodules because of difficulty grasping or pinching, or to improve their appearance. Surgical separation of the nodule from the skin or deeper fascial structures is difficult but may be facilitated by loupe magnification. Unfortunately, recurrence of such nodules is quite common and, as with gout, medical treatment of the rheumatoid disease is essential.

PERIPHERAL NERVE TUMORS

Peripheral nerve tumors, which comprise less than 5% of all hand tumors, have a somewhat distinctive presentation.[23,27] It is important to recognize these lesions because excision of a tumor with its associated nerve can cause irreparable loss of nerve function. Such resections have occurred with obvious consequences. Posttraumatic neuromata, which are the most common peripheral nerve lesions encountered in the hand, are not true tumors and require distinct methods of treatment. Two peripheral nerve tumors, the neurilemoma and neurofibroma, deserve mention here. Neurilemomas also are known as *schwannomas* because of their origin from the Schwann cells of the neurilemma. This tumor appears as a slightly elongated swelling along the course of a nerve, which may cause some minor discomfort and even some sensory change distally. Paresthesias may be elicited by tapping on the lesion, and

patients may complain of similar symptoms with gripping or other activities that put pressure on the nerve. These lesions are seen throughout adulthood and present while they are quite small in size. Careful dissection through an adequate zigzag incision under magnification allows separation of an ovoid, firm mass from the normal fascicles of the nerve without damage to the nerve itself. Recurrence is uncommon and malignant degeneration has not been reported.

The neurofibroma, in contrast, does not shell out of the nerve easily as it is infiltrated throughout the nerve trunk. Removal of a segment of a major nerve trunk sacrifices significant nerve function and might not be justified; however, in some circumstances resection of a neurofibroma and a segment of nerve may be considered if the resulting gap can be overcome by a tension-free nerve repair. This approach is not applicable when the lesion affects a major peripheral nerve, but may be possible when the lesion arises in a digital nerve. Neurofibromas may be solitary or multiple. When they are associated with Von Recklinghausen's disease, the possibility of malignant degeneration must be considered; malignant degeneration in solitary lesions is much less common. The prognosis for lesions associated with Von Recklinghausen's disease is guarded. Age appears to influence the presence of solitary or multiple lesions; the solitary lesion is seen most often during the first decade, and most multiple lesions occur in patients older than 30 years of age. In further contrast to the neurilemoma, the neurofibroma is often associated with local pain and peripheral nerve dysfunction, which might be expected given the diffuse proliferation of neural elements seen in histologic specimens. A surgeon must not decide to excise a neurofibroma without considering the consequence of injury to the affected nerve.

GRANULAR CELL TUMOR

Brief mention must be made of a rare hand tumor called a *granular cell tumor*. On the basis of histoimmunochemical staining, some experts believe that this tumor originates from Schwann cells.[16] These lesions typically are solitary but may exist multifocally in as many as 25% of cases. They are distinctly uncommon on the hand, but as many as 20% may occur in the upper extremity. Most commonly, however, these lesions occur on the tongue. The lesions grow slowly and may become painful or pruritic with time. Skin changes associated with pseudoepitheliomatous hyperplasia may give rise to the mistaken diagnosis of various skin lesions, ranging from verrucae to squamous carcinoma. Isolated lesions may be somewhat mobile, leading to confusion with pedunculated ganglions or neurilemomas; deeper lesions are more fixed. A firm consistency may indicate malignancy; indeed, malignant change occurs in approximately 3% of reported cases. No alternatives to treatment by surgical excision are available, but excision is usually curative and recurrences are uncommon. Because these lesions often occur in the vicinity of digital nerves, nerve structures are vulnerable to injury during resection.

REFERENCES

1. Adamson BE, Lucas GL: Multiple recurrence of digital pigmented villonodular tenosynovitis: a case report, *J Hand Surg [Am]* 10:278-280, 1985.
2. Angelides AC, Wallace PW: The dorsal ganglion of the wrist: its pathogenesis, gross and microscopic anatomy, and surgical treatment, *J Hand Surg [Am]* 1:228-235, 1976.
3. Chung EB, Enzinger FM: Fibroma of tendon sheath, *Cancer* 41:1945, 1979.
4. Clearkin KP, Enzinger FM: Intravascular papillary endothelial hyperplasia, *Arch Pathol Lab Med* 100:441-444, 1976.
5. Diao E, Moy OJ: Common tumors, *Ortho Clin North Am* 23:187-196, 1992.
6. Enzinger FM, Weiss S: *Soft tissue tumors,* ed 2, St. Louis, 1988, Mosby.
7. Glowacki KA, Weiss AP: Giant cell tumors of tendon sheath, *Hand Clin* 11:245-253, 1995.
8. Greendyke SD, Wilson M, Shepler TR: Anterior wrist ganglia from the scaphotrapezial joint, *J Hand Surg [Am]* 17:487-490, 1992.
9. Keasbey LE: Juvenile aponeurotic fibroma (calcifying fibroma): a distinctive tumor arising in the palms and soles of young children, *Cancer* 6:338, 1953.
10. Leffert RD: Lipomas of the upper extremity, *J Bone Joint Surg* 54A:1262-1266, 1972.
11. Leung PC: Tumors of the hand, *The Hand* 13:169-176, 1981.
12. Lister GD, Smith RR: Protection of the radial artery in the resection of adherent ganglions in the wrist, *Plast Reconstr Surg* 1:127-129, 1978.
13. Lucas GL: An intratendinous cyst in the extensor digitorum brevis manus tendon, *J Hand Surg [Am]* 4:176-177, 1979.
14. Lucas GL: Irritative neuritis of the dorsal cutaneous branch of the ulnar nerve from underlying ganglion, *Clin Orthop* 186:216-219, 1984.
15. Lucas GL: Epidermoid inclusion cysts of the hand, *J Southern Ortho Assoc* 8:188-192, 1999.
16. Maher DP: Granular cell tumor in the hand, *J Hand Surg [Am]* 12:800-803, 1987.
17. McFarland GB: Soft tissue tumors. In Green DP (editor): *Operative hand surgery,* ed 2, New York, 1988, Churchill Livingstone.
18. Neviaser RJ, Newman W: Dermal angiomyoma of the upper extremity, *J Hand Surg [Am]* 2:271-274, 1977.
19. Osterman L: Arthroscopic treatment of wrist ganglions, *Hand Clin* 11:7-12, 1995.
20. Phalen GS, McCormack LJ, Gazale WJ: Giant cell tumor of tendon sheath in the hand, *Clin Orthop* 15:140-151, 1959.
21. Poppen NK, Niebauer JJ: Recurring digital fibrous tumor of childhood, *J Hand Surg [Am]* 2:253-255, 1977.
22. Richman JA, Gelberman RH, Engber WD, et al: Ganglions of the wrist and digits: results of treatment and cyst wall puncture, *J Hand Surg [Am]* 12:1041-1043, 1987.
23. Rinaldi E: Neurilemomas and neurofibromas of the upper limb, *J Hand Surg [Am]* 8:590-593, 1983.
24. Russell RC, Williamson DA, Sullivan JW, et al: Detection of foreign bodies in the hand, *J Hand Surg [Am]* 16:2-11, 1991.
25. Shapiro PS, Seitz WH: Non-neoplastic tumors of the hand and upper extremity, *Hand Clin* 11:133-160, 1995.
26. Specht EE, Staheli LT: Juvenile aponeurotic fibroma, *J Hand Surg [Am]* 2:256-257, 1977.
27. Strickland JW, Steichen JB: Nerve tumors of the hand and forearm, *J Hand Surg [Am]* 2:285-291, 1977.

CHAPTER 130

Malignant Soft Tissue Tumors

Hans U. Steinau
Peter M. Vogt
Heinz-Herbert Homann
Detlev Hebebrand

INTRODUCTION

Soft tissue sarcomas are rare mesenchymal malignancies that account for approximately 1% of cancers in adults and about 10% to 15% of those in children. The term *soft tissue sarcoma* is usually used in the literature as the description of a tumor entity. Extremity sarcomas, however, are a very heterogeneous group of tumors that differ in their biologic aggressiveness, response to treatment, manifestation site, and cytogenetic background.[8,9,21,24]

The accepted treatment protocol for extremity sarcomas has evolved to include limb-sparing resection of the tumor in combination with radiation and/or chemotherapy. Survival rates after limb-sparing resections are comparable to limb ablation procedures, and the patients have a better quality of life, superior function, improved self-esteem, and an intact body image.[3,14,16,26,29]

The incidence of oncologically justified limb ablation has dropped below 10% within specialized tumor centers that employ multimodality treatment. According to the literature, amputation is still a recommended surgical option, however, in cases that require the creation of a large defect. Additional indications for amputation include anaplastic tumors; early recurrence of tumor after adequate resection; infiltration of major nerves, blood vessels, and joints, as well as tumors infiltrating the femur and tibia; sarcomas of the foot; and patients presenting with severe damage caused by radiation therapy.[15,21,26,33]

The vast majority of patients with extremity sarcomas are not treated in specialized tumor centers, and in my practice we see many patients who have had inadequate tumor resection because the treating surgeon was not able to manage technical problems with defect coverage and functional loss. Local recurrence is then inevitable, and many of our patients are first seen after one or more local recurrences of tumor.

The risk of a primary or secondary amputation, the expected functional and aesthetic results, and the prognostic parameters for individual patients therefore largely depend on the technical ability of the surgical team that has been integrated into a multispecialty tumor board.

Plastic surgeons have previously been involved in the treatment of patients with soft tissue sarcomas only in cases of extensive ulcerations, multiple local recurrences, irradiation damage, wound-healing disturbances, and functional deficiencies after muscle-group resection. Clinical reports about this special area of reconstruction are therefore singular or are reported as small series.[7,11,12,22,37] Earlier monographs on the surgical treatment of soft tissue sarcomas do not routinely discuss reconstruction options because many patients were treated by primary amputation.[1,15,16,26] Today, reconstructive plastic surgical procedures are employed as part of a multidisciplinary treatment plan; a considerable amount of these earlier clinical conditions do not occur and there is less loss of function or eventual limb amputation.

OPERATIONS

RESECTION AND PRIMARY RECONSTRUCTION

The vast majority of soft tissue extremity sarcomas are usually diagnosed after excision of a slowly growing soft tissue mass. The patient's own history of the disease is rarely, if ever, helpful because more than 80% will report trauma to the region where the lesion developed. Clinical parameters that should alert the physician to the possibility of a potential malignancy are location deep to the fascia, painful infiltration of the neighboring muscle, tumor size of more than 5 cm, or a tumor mass within the groin, popliteal, or axillary fossa. An incisional or needle biopsy should be performed before surgery in all suspected cases. The surgeon should anticipate what structures will need to be resected, and the biopsy site to a suspicious soft tissue tumor should be placed within the area of the potential resection plan. The suction drains used after a definitive resection should be placed through the scar or close to the incision line. If these principles are not followed properly, the tumor-contaminated areas may necessitate an extended resection with a larger soft tissue defect that will require complex reconstructive procedures or even an amputation.[10,18,30]

Careful preoperative multidisciplinary planning plays a key role in the surgical outcome. Modern diagnostic tools, including nuclear magnetic resonance (NMR) imaging to provide three-dimensional pictures of the extent, topographic localization, and possible satellites of the sarcoma, aid in this effort.[6,16,34] In contrast to accepted principles of surgical oncology in which a two-team approach is recommended, I believe the procedure for limb malignancies should *not* be divided into resectional and reconstructive parts. Important motor branches for salvage of the remaining neuromuscular units, the dominant blood vessels for muscle or fascial flaps, and the recipient vessels for microsurgical transplantations are best identified when the plastic surgeon participates from the beginning of the operation. A careful anatomic dissection of individual structures within the proximity of the tumor, in combination with adventitial dissection of major blood vessels or removal of the perineural connective tissue, will sometimes permit the surgeon to preserve important functional structures without compromising the adequacy of the tumor resection. It is obvious that a tourniquet or temporary clamping of the femoral, iliac, or axillary vessels allows for easier dissection and identification of structures within a bloodless field. The need for a blood transfusion is also avoided by using a tourniquet.

If the deep venous system of the limbs must be sacrificed, the superficial venous and lymphatic drainage pathways must be preserved from resection. The locations of these important structures should be considered before surgery so incisional biopsies or definite surgical approaches do not result in their destruction. This is especially important in patients who will require postoperative radiotherapy, because intact venous and lymphatic outflow will diminish the amount of lymphedema and venous insufficiency. Therefore incisional biopsies should not routinely be placed directly on top of the tumor bulk, but should respect these often-neglected functional structures.

It is essential to achieve specimen margins that are free of tumor to avoid the risk of local recurrence.[2,3,14,35,41] This status is generally known as an *R0-Resection*. Microscopic residual tumor (R1) resection should not be an indication for irradiation per se. The patient's postoperative NMR scan and the operation report should be discussed at the Tumor Board, and revisional surgery (including excision of the former tumor cavity en bloc) should be recommended as a consensus. R2 resections leave viable parts of the soft tissue sarcoma and are recommended only in cases of palliative debulking procedures.

There is still debate about the extent of the resectional procedure. Although amputation is no longer accepted as a routine procedure, terms such as *radical resection* are now used without a proper definition. A *compartmental resection* includes neighboring muscle groups from origin to insertion. Convincing data from pathohistological serial sectioning have, up to now, been lacking. The field of irradiation after a compartmental resection will be extended without improving local

control. A *wide local excision* leaves an envelope of 2 to 5 cm of normal, uninvolved tissue around the tumor, which is removed en bloc. *Shelling out* of a soft tissue sarcoma results in an intolerably high local recurrence rate.[2,36,39,41] Accurate definitions of the surgical procedure, including the "minimal safety distance" within the resectional specimen, are essential if prospective randomized studies are planned to develop data about the benefit of surgery.

All information about the procedure should be placed in the patient's chart and should be updated at every restaging. There are several systems used today to rate tumors in clinical oncological procedures, but the tumor, node, metastasis, grade (TNMG) staging system is probably best for defining the sarcoma patient's risk profile. The TNMG formula defines soft tissue sarcomas smaller (T1) or larger (T2) than 5 cm; positive lymph nodes, distant metastasis, and tumor grading complete the information.[9,23]

The pathohistological investigation will give information about the grading of the sarcoma, including the mitosis counts, amount of tumor necrosis, and tumor differentiation. A second opinion from a specialized pathologist should be sought, if necessary, to determine the proper grading of the tumor. This additional information is important, especially in cases in which there is a difference of opinion on the histopathological diagnosis or when there is local tumor recurrence, to provide correct data for the patient to enter a treatment protocol.[8]

Multivariate analysis of soft tissue sarcomas demonstrates that factors such as tumor size of more than 5 cm in diameter, location deep to the fascia, high mitotic counts, frequent mitosis, large areas of necrosis, and dedifferentiation of sarcoma cells (grade 3) have the most unfavorable prognosis.[8,14,16,35,41] Certain tumor subgroups, such as rhabdomyosarcoma in adults, angiosarcoma, epithelioid cell sarcoma, and biphasic synovial cell sarcoma, are also associated with lower survival rates.

Local recurrence is more frequently observed after R1 resection in high-grade sarcomas or subtypes such as myxoid tumor variants.

Additional information about the expected long-term survival rate of a given patient can now be obtained by measuring the deoxyribonucleic acid (DNA) content of a tumor or analyzing factors representing cellular proliferation levels, such as Ki67, or the activity of energy-dependent membrane pumps (p-glycoprotein [P-Gp]). Cytogenetic analysis may be helpful in patients in which the subgroup assignment is in question. Specific chromosomal alterations, such as translocation, have to date been identified for nearly every subtype of soft tissue sarcoma.[5,24]

All of these factors are considered by the members of the Tumor Board when they are trying to determine the best overall management strategy for the patient. Another planning parameter considered by the Tumor Board is the indication or necessity of reconstructive plastic surgical procedures (Box 130-1). The vast majority of extremity sarcomas are located within the thigh and are treated by the oncological surgeon by wide local excision and primary closure.

Technical problems can arise after resection of an extended tumor mass. The excision of a large muscle mass or major

Box 130-1.
Indications for Reconstructive Plastic Surgery in Limb Oncology

PRIMARY TREATMENT PHASE
Malignancies of the hand or foot
Expected exposure or resection of bone segments, joints, tendons, or neuromuscular units
Soft tissue defects, subcutaneous cavities
Segmental amputation and salvage replantation
Palliative procedures

EARLY POSTOPERATIVE TREATMENT PHASE
Wound-healing complications
Reintervention after positive margins of the resection specimen

SECONDARY TREATMENT PHASE
Chronic wound-healing complications, osteomyelitis
Radiation sequelae (fibrosis, ulceration, lymphedema)
Functional and aesthetic deficiencies
Local recurrence (reconstructive options, limb sparing, amputation stump problems)
Palliative procedures

TREATMENT OF LONG-TERM SURVIVORS
Functional and aesthetic deficiencies
Radiation sequelae
Local recurrence, reconstructive options
Amputation stump problems
Secondary malignancies

nerve segments may leave an extremity with little function. Very thin skin flaps or those closed under tension or over a large wound cavity are prone to flap necrosis, infection, and wound breakdown. The resultant wound-healing complications can be avoided primarily, or should be treated if they occur secondarily, by covering the wound and filling the cavity with a well-vascularized muscle flap.[7,11,12,32,37]

An infection that develops several days after surgery may cause severe complications, such as tendon necrosis, fasciitis, loss of implants, and repeated fistula formation. Surgical problems are also associated with specific areas of the body. Tumors that involve the soft tissues from the elbow joint down to the mid-palm will usually require sophisticated techniques for soft tissue coverage and reconstruction, including the requirement for sensation and restoration of motor function in the upper extremity.

An analogous zone can be identified in the lower extremity extending from the knee joint to the sole of the foot. The problem areas become even larger in cases in which there has been a local recurrence that requires an even larger resection.

If the tumor is located in a finger or in the palm region, ray amputation should be performed, including tenosynovectomy and resection of the periosteum, intrinsic muscles, and joint capsules.[4,14,22,29,35] The resection of multiple digits will require sophisticated reconstruction methods. The array of available treatment modalities should at least result in the preservation or

construction of a hand with sensate grip. The patient in Figure 130-1 demonstrates a good functional result despite the fact that an extended ray amputation of the third and fourth fingers had to be done to achieve a complete tumor resection (R0). In contrast to cases involving traumatic injuries in which the intermetacarpal structures are still present, fixation of the palmar arch in tumor cases can only be achieved by use of interpositional grafts, often using digital "spare parts." Two phalanges in this case were used as a corticocancellous graft to preserve normal motion of the second and fifth rays. The technically difficult soft tissue defect was covered using filet flaps from the dorsal aspect of the amputated fingers. The patient's resultant grip strength and finger mobility permitted independent daily care and reintegration into his profession.

Patients with forearm or lower-leg tumors require a resection that leaves an envelop of 2 to 5 cm of uninvolved tissue around the tumor and usually results in functional deficiencies that can be corrected by primary tendon transfers, tenodeses, or arthrodeses. The resultant soft tissue defects are covered either with local, pedicled, or microsurgically transferred flaps, depending on the size of the deficit. Flap coverage is especially indicated in patients undergoing multimodality treatment, because preoperative irradiation, implantation of radioactive seeds (brachytherapy) and/or chemotherapy have been reported to increase the rate of wound-healing complications by up to 40%.[1,34,35,41]

Postoperative chemotherapy or radiotherapy must then be delayed until wound closure occurs by secondary intention or after a surgical revision. Well-vascularized myocutaneous flaps, however, guarantee primary wound healing and serve as a biological space filler of cavities caused by large resection sites. It is obvious that surgeons involved in surgical treatment of soft tissue sarcomas must be knowledgeable and technically capable of performing the whole spectrum of reconstructive flap procedures, tendon transfers, bone substitution techniques, vascular macrosurgery and microsurgery, and tissue transplantation (Box 130-2). Many of these cases are very complex and require broad-based knowledge of all reconstructive possibilities. All of the various reconstructive methods and techniques have been developed and employed over the years in the reconstruction of traumatically injured extremities. The first oncologic attempts at reconstruction date back to 1883 when a soft tissue sarcoma of the biceps humeri was replaced by a dog muscle with a "successful end result."[13] Today, microsurgical free tissue transfers are indicated to provide well-vascularized coverage in patients with severe irradiation damage or an otherwise high risk of infection. Despite the fact that vessel diameters of about 1.5 mm are used, these flaps will even tolerate hyperthermic perfusion, including chemotherapeutic agents, during the immediate postoperative period.

Figure 130-2 clearly demonstrates the advantage of a free microvascular flap transplantation in combination with tendon transfers. The patient was suffering from the fourth local recurrence of an epithelioid sarcoma and would have been subjected to a transhumeral amputation in earlier times. The exposed bone and tendons that were present after a wide oncologic excision could only be covered by a large microsurgi-

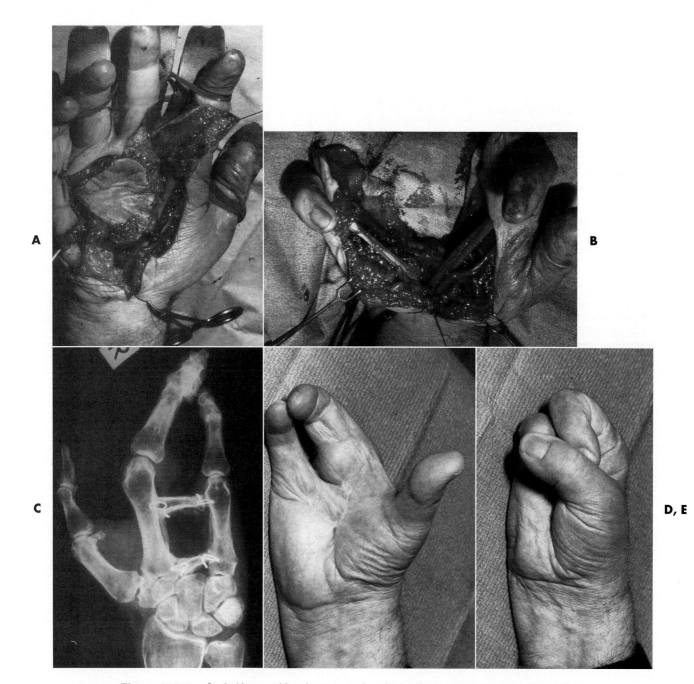

Figure 130-1. **A,** A 61-year-old male presented with the first local recurrence of a grade 2 synovial cell sarcoma of the third intermetacarpal space (T2 N0 M0 G2). **B,** An en bloc resection of the third and fourth finger rays, including the adjacent intrinsic musculature was performed, along with a tenosynovectomy of the second and fifth flexor tendon sheaths. Epineurectomies and partial resection of the median and ulnar nerves were also performed with preservation of the thumb, radial index, and little finger ulnar digital nerves. **C,** The metacarpal was stabilized by interpositioning of two second phalanges, which were stripped of their periosteum and fixed by Kirschner wires (K wires) and circumferential wires. The resultant soft tissue defect was reconstructed using local flaps harvested from the radial and ulnar aspects of the third and fourth fingers. The postoperative course was uneventful. Six weeks after surgery, regional hyperthermic perfusion of the upper extremity was performed using the cytotoxic drug Melfalan. **D** and **E,** Three years later, the hand has good grip strength and the patient uses it without problems for daily activities. There is no evidence of local recurrence or distant metastases. (From Steinau HU, et al: *Eur J Plastic Surg* 11:3-14, 1988.)

Box 130-2.
Types of Reconstructive Plastic Surgery in Limb Oncology

SKIN AND SUBCUTANEOUS TISSUE DEFECTS
Skin grafts, local flaps
Pedicled fasciocutaneous and musculocutaneous flaps
Microsurgical free tissue transfer

NEUROMUSCULAR SYSTEM DEFICIENCY
Neurovascular island flaps
Segmental nerve resection and grafting
Pedicled neurovascular muscle graft
Free neuromuscular tissue transfer
Tendon transfer, tenodesis
Arthrodesis, resection arthroplasty
Orthesis, prosthesis

BONE RESECTION AND REPLACEMENT
Cancellous, corticocancellous graft
Microvascular bone transfer
Allograft, Ilisarov's distraction
Resection arthroplasty, endoprosthesis
Elongation, atypical stump formation

BLOOD VESSELS
Adventitial dissection
Resection and interposition
Extraanatomical bypass

COMBINED PROCEDURES
Microsurgical transplantation and replantation
Osteomyocutaneous flaps
Free neurovascular flaps
Toe-to-hand transfer
Salvage replantation, spare-part use

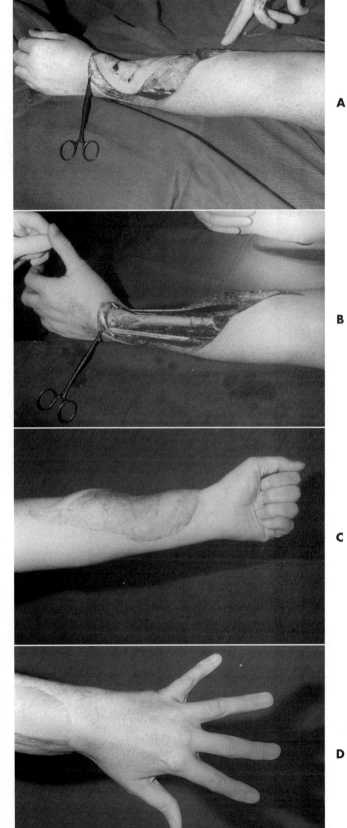

A

B

C

D

Figure 130-2. A 40-year-old patient was admitted to our unit suffering from the fourth local recurrence of an epithelioid sarcoma (T2 N0 M0 G2) within the distal radial forearm. A wide local excision, including periosteum and a portion of the radial cortex, was performed **(A)** in addition to removal of the flexor pollicis longus (FPL), extensor digitorum communis (EDC) to the long finger, the extensor pollicis longus (EPL), extensor pollicis brevis (EPB), extensor carpi radialis longus (ECRL) and brevis (ECRB), the radial artery, and the noncomitant veins was performed **(B).** Primary functional reconstruction was achieved by tenodeses of the EDC of the long finger and the EPL to the EDC of the ring finger, Pulvertaft fixation of the palmaris longus (PL) to the abductor pollicis longus (APL), and fixation of the flexor digitorum superficialis (FDS) of the long finger to the distal tendon of the FPL. The large soft tissue defect was covered by microsurgical transplantation of a myocutaneous latissimus dorsi flap. End-to-end anastomoses were done between the thoracodorsal artery and vein with the radial artery and the major concomitant vein. Six weeks later, lymphadenectomy of the right axilla and hyperthermic perfusion with cytostatic drugs did not interfere with primary wound healing. **C** and **D** demonstrate the functional result with adequate finger, thumb, and wrist joint mobility 3½ years later. Four years later, bilateral pulmonary metastases were surgically removed, with chemotherapy employed before and after surgery.

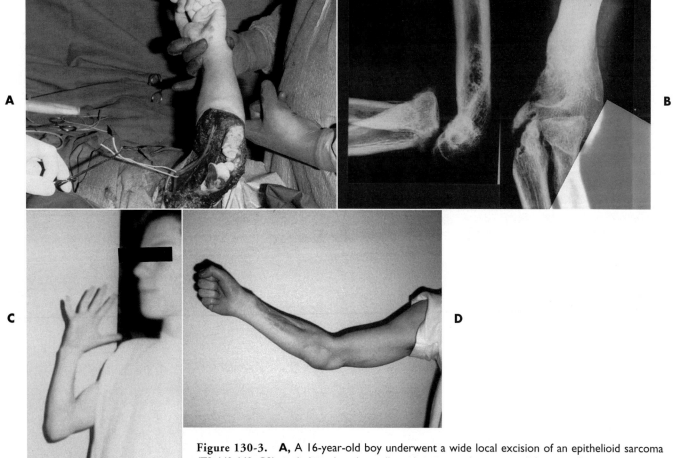

Figure 130-3. **A,** A 16-year-old boy underwent a wide local excision of an epithelioid sarcoma (T2 N0 M0 G3), including the ulnar elbow hemijoint, the proximal forearm flexors, and distal triceps muscle. The ulnar nerve was freed by epineurectomy, and the brachial artery was dissected free from the surrounding tissue. A proximally based radial forearm flap was used to cover the defect, and the ulnar collateral ligament was reconstructed with tendon grafts pulled through drill holes in the distal humerus and the proximal ulna **(B).** The remaining donor-site defect was closed with a split-thickness skin graft. After employing preoperative and postoperative chemotherapy according to the pediatric protocol, the patient demonstrates no evidence of local or systemic relapse. Six years later, the patient has pain-free elbow-joint movement and only minor hand disability **(C** and **D).**

cal free flap transfer. The patient underwent lymphadenectomy and hyperthermic perfusion of the arm 6 weeks later without compromising the viability of the microvessels and flap.

Segmental limb resection and salvage replantation or arthroplasty should be considered in patients with circumferential tumors or when there is attachment to major joints. This is analogous to the loss of a joint from trauma, or joint damage caused by a specific infection.[7,17,33,40] Figure 130-3 shows the unexpected functional result after ulnar hemiresection of the elbow joint. This 16-year-old suffered from an epithelioid sarcoma that infiltrated but did not penetrate the ulnar joint capsule and required a wide local excision. The patient had preoperative chemotherapy followed by a wide local resection with simultaneous free tendon grafts to reconstruct the ulnar collateral ligament. The large soft tissue defect was covered by a proximally based radial forearm flap. The patient also underwent postoperative chemotherapy. All of the oncological priorities were met, and the reconstructive options that were chosen were deemed to be the adequate solution for the

patient's specific problem. Six years later, the patient returned with full extension and flexion of the hand, and the elbow joint demonstrated a tolerable reduction of joint movement. It is obvious that "basic limb function" was achieved, despite the fact that important structures of the elbow joint and the surrounding musculature had been removed.

Interestingly, the upper and lower extremities tolerate a considerable loss of neuromuscular functional units. Frequently, adjuvant therapies are recommended because there is no clinical experience with limb-sparing procedures or reconstructive plastic surgical procedures because most patients in the past were treated by amputation. Patients with segmental amputations and/or replantation of the distal limb remnant will benefit from these methods because stump lengthening or stump-length preservation will result in permanent restoration of residual limb function and optimal prosthetic rehabilitation.[7,33,40]

Myoelectric prosthetic fitting in the upper extremity requires an adequate forearm stump segment covered with adequate soft tissues that allow permanent pressure distribution. Patients undergoing transhumeral amputation require stump lengths that will minimize the system of thoracic fixation belts and will result in better power control.

The quality of skin should be considered in patients who will receive multimodality treatment. An area covered by a split-thickness skin graft will not tolerate radiotherapy. Thinned flaps or grafts or insensate skin is likely to cause problems if an orthoses or prosthetic device is planned after surgery. The primary goal in these oncological cases should not be to close the defect, but to reconstruct a functionally stable, sensate soft tissue envelope that will accommodate a prosthesis.

Despite the obvious benefits of sophisticated plastic surgical procedures in limb oncology, the choice of a method that satisfies the patient's specific demands should play the key role. It is not justified, especially in patients with tumors, to perform difficult procedures if a simple local flap or a graft will solve the problem. Each patient must be considered individually, including the magnitude of his or her disease, the expected life span, and the functional goals after reconstruction.

ADJUVANT THERAPIES

Hyperfractionated high-dosage irradiation has been recommended to reduce the rate of local tumor recurrence.[34] The degree of benefit from treatment compared with the early and late complication rates still remains controversial.[41] Many patients may not experience a relapse after adequate tumor surgery alone, but they will be confronted with the complications of radiation therapy for the rest of their lives.[3] The long-term sequelae of radiation therapy were reported by Suit and Spiro[34] and included bone pathological fractures in 6% of patients, contractures in 20%, moderate to severe strength reduction in 20%, decreased range of motion in 32%, chronic infection in 9%, chronic edema in 19%, and induration in 57%.[34]

Wound-healing disturbances during the initial treatment phase have been reported in as many as 40% of cases when surgery and postoperative radiotherapy are combined.* It must be assumed that these rates of early and late complications are considerably higher in centers where this type of case is infrequently encountered by physicians less familiar with lymph-node drainage patterns and multimodality treatment plans for lesions of the distal extremities.

Intraoperative or postoperative brachytherapy employing radioactive seeds into the tumor bed after surery has been alternatively recommended to reduce the incidence of wound problems. Analyses of the patients showed improvement in local control limited to high-grade sarcomas, and local complications were reduced but not eliminated.

Radical resection and adjuvant radiotherapy results in local control without improving long-term survival rates. Numerous adjuvant chemotherapy protocols have therefore been introduced, but none have shown significant improvement in survival. An actual multicenter meta-analysis of extremity lesions

in adults resulted in an absolute increase in survival of only 7% after 10 years. There was also no clear evidence that any subgroup of patients or tumors would benefit from any present chemotherapy protocol.[36]

Hyperthermic isolated limb perfusion employing various chemotherapeutic agents has been used to treat patients with nonresectable sarcomas in an attempt to gain local control. Multicenter studies reported successful response rates of approximately 30%, partial remission rates of 50%, and a limb-salvage rate of 82%. Toxic reactions to extremity microcirculation, erythema and edema, damage to deep tissues, venous thrombosis, and neurologic deficiencies have all been observed. In most cases, the perfusion regimens should not be considered superior to surgery and radiotherapy.[25] Their clinical use is justified for patients with extensive tumors or difficult surgical anatomy.

The side effects of concomitant adjuvant therapies, such as delayed or altered wound healing, the degree of lymphedema, venous problems, subcutaneous fibrosis, muscle induration, destruction of growth plates in children, neurological deficiencies, chronic pain syndromes, and the patient's overall treatment burden, are all factors that must be considered and discussed before the treatment program begins.* Multimodality treatment protocols should therefore be restricted to institutions that compile their data about soft tissue sarcomas into a multicenter clinical study analysis. Only in this way will it be possible for us to obtain meaningful statistics and develop the best treatment protocols for future patients.

PALLIATION PROCEDURES

Patients with large ulcerated tumors and lymph node or distant metastases should be viewed as potential candidates for palliation procedures, depending on their general condition, the burden of the surgical procedure, and their estimated survival time.[33] Tumor removal or debulking cannot influence the fatal outcome, but it will improve the quality of life by reducing pain or the need for analgesics, eliminating foul odors, and making the mobility, social contacts, and daily care of these patients easier during their final months. Figure 130-4 shows a patient suffering from the eighth local recurrence of a primarily extraosseous chondrosarcoma. The design of several parallel and criss-crossing surgical incision lines clearly shows that previous attempts to remove the tumor were not performed by surgeons familiar with oncological principles. The large tumor was likely to perforate, leaving the patient with an infected cavity of football size. All options were discussed with the patient and because at the time no peripheral metastases could be observed, the patient agreed to palliative surgery.

Interscapulothoracic amputation had been advised in earlier times for every musculoskeletal tumor around the shoulder girdle. Actual internal joint-resection techniques used in primary treatment cases provide the patient with considerable residual limb function and an intact body image. In this case,

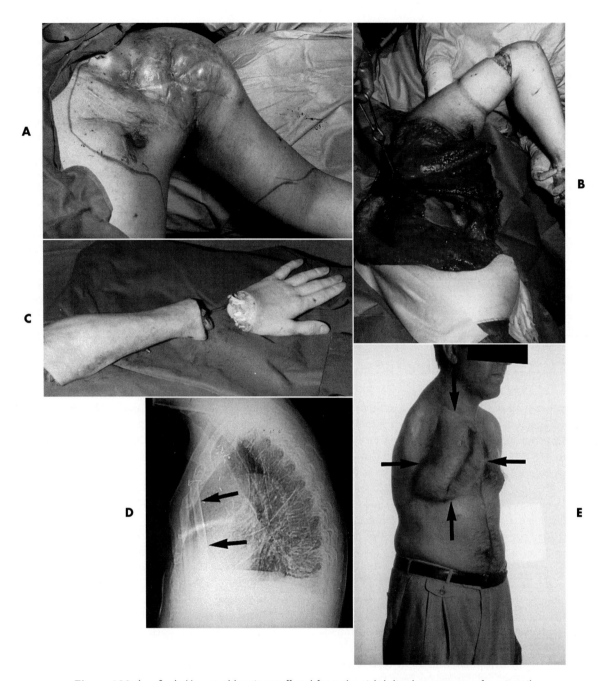

Figure 130-4. **A,** A 46-year-old patient suffered from the eighth local recurrence of a primarily extraosseous chondrosarcoma within the right pectoral region (T2 N0 M0 G2). NMR images demonstrated infiltration of the thoracic wall. The central tumor mass was likely to perforate. There was infiltration of the brachial plexus and pain with movement of the shoulder joint, necessitating the use of strong pain medication. Preoperative staging did not reveal distant metastases, and therefore palliative interscapulothoracic amputation was indicated, including three-fourths of the first to fifth ribs **(B).** The extensive defect was covered with a free forearm salvage flap from the amputated arm **(C),** keeping the radius and ulna as stabilizers of the thoracic wall. Revascularization of the flap was obtained by end-to-side anastomoses of the brachial artery to the stump of the axillary artery and two vena comitans to the external jugular vein. Sixteen days later, the patient was released with primary wound healing. **D,** A chest radiograph demonstrates the radius and ulna fixed to the rib segments by circumferential wiring. **E,** Five months after surgery, with coverage of the anterolateral chest wall by a forearm segment. An orthotic device was to used to ameliorate the shoulder contour. (From Steinau HU, et al: *Eur J Plastic Surg* 11:115, 1992.)

however, an interscapulothoracic amputation was inevitable because of infiltration of the brachial plexus and tumor spread into the thoracic wall. Local flaps could not be harvested because of the loss of all dominant vascular pedicles, so free tissue transfer of the dorsally opened complete forearm segment was done. The radius and ulna served as stabilizers of the thoracic wall (Figure 130-4, *D*); the forearm soft tissues were designed to permit later orthotic supplementation *(arrows)* (Figure 130-4, *E*).

Patients should also be considered for a palliative procedure when there are metastases present and they are in good clinical condition. A palliative procedure should be done only if a short hospital stay and adequate treatment burden can be estimated for the terminally ill patient. The treatment should address the problems of daily wound care and pain management. Even in patients with a large necrotic tumor mass, well-vascularized flaps or "spare-part" surgery after a palliative resection will almost always result in primary wound healing and early release from the hospital. Adequate flap coverage permits palliative adjuvant chemotherapy and/or radiotherapy without the risk of severe local inflammation, ulceration, or septic complications.

SECONDARY SURGICAL PROCEDURES

We have found that more radical secondary resections are necessary in patients who have undergone an inadequate primary soft tissue sarcoma removal by surgeons who are not familiar with the actual treatment requirements of these tumors. The decision to perform additional surgery on a patient who has only recently undergone a primary surgical procedure must be carefully made after considering several factors. The parameters for or against a "second-look" operation are difficult to define, but the following factors may be helpful.

1. The procedure was defined in the surgical report as "radical" despite the fact the postoperative NMR scans show normal surrounding muscle groups.
2. The operative note describes a "compartmental resection and dissection of blood vessels" but postoperative arteriography demonstrates intact branches of the main tumor vessels.
3. The histopathological report cites "multiple fragments of a soft tissue sarcoma" despite the fact the surgeon described an "en bloc resection."
4. Previous medical opinion has deemed the lesion "nonresectable" or "an indication for amputation" when NMR analysis reveals the possibility for a wide local resection, including a complex reconstructive procedure.
5. The term *radical surgery* is used in the chart, despite the fact that the surgeon describes "easy tumor removal out of the capsule."
6. No staging, grading, or safety margins are defined.
7. A "radical resection" of a malignant peripheral nerve-sheath tumor was performed, resulting in complete function of the limb.

8. Despite the description of a "wide local excision" or "compartment resection," the pathology report describes tumor cells "very close to or involving the surgical margins."
9. Incisions crossing main lymph pathways or several muscle compartments, or suction drain sites placed far from the incision line leave doubts about the adequacy of surgical resection.

All these data should be carefully analyzed and, if necessary, a second-look procedure should be performed to obtain adequate surgical margins. Free margins not only provide a lowered risk for local recurrence but also achieve a longer remission period without the necessity of repeated surgical and/or ancillary procedures.

It is still presently open to debate whether radical surgery with clear margins will influence the overall survival rate. However, it should also be considered that in modern industrial nations cancer patients will have more trouble holding their jobs if repeated courses of treatment are necessary. The patients with soft tissue sarcomas in our series had an average age of 52 years, with an overall long-term survival achieved in about 65% of cases, leaving an average of some 15 years of employment possible. A single comprehensive treatment plan is therefore preferred to allow permanent reintegration of these patients into the work force. The remaining group of high-risk patients will benefit from a useful limb and short hospital stay for the remaining months of their lives.

Control investigations that include routine postoperative oncologic clinical follow-up examinations, NMR scans, sonograms, and chest radiographs are recommended at 3- to 4-month intervals in patients with soft tissue extremity sarcomas. The degree of benefit for the patients remains controversial because to date there are no prospective studies available to prove that early detection of a recurrence will result in better long-term survival.[21] Surgical removal of pulmonary metastases will guarantee 5-year survival rates in up to 25% of the patients.[38] Routine follow-up examinations, however, run a considerable risk of identifying false positive results. Radiologists unfamiliar with complex reconstructive muscle-tendon transfers or flap transplantation may diagnose from NMR images residual masses or local recurrences when normal anatomy has been altered or if postoperative seroma, hematoma, and/or swelling are present. Patients must then endure several days of anxiety until needle biopsies aided by sonography provide a conclusive diagnosis. The plastic surgeon must therefore be integrated into the overall oncological surveillance protocol and the final decision-making process, and treatment recommendations should be made to the patients only after interdisciplinary discussion of the findings.

Reexcisions are technically difficult and are indicated as second-look operations for salvage procedures, when there are wound-healing complications, and in cases of local relapse. Recurrence rates of about 6% to 10% must be expected even when the best surgical and adjuvant therapy has been employed. Multivariate analysis defines R0-resection, high-grade sarcoma, and myxoid subtypes of tumor as the most important indicators for local control.[14,16,36,41] The very same principles of safe margins—en bloc removal and reconstructive plastic surgical procedures, especially in patients who have had previous irradiation—are followed for surgical reinterventions. The case complexity, including the creation of a large surgical defect, the need for tendon transfers, and blood vessel replacement, increases with every relapse and reexcision. The whole spectrum of reconstruction options listed in Box 130-2 should be applied again before amputation is considered. Primary treatment at institutions less familiar with the overall oncologic strategies required to treat patients with extremity sarcomas can result in the sequelae of irradiation; secondary malignancies within the field of irradiation; functional deficiencies caused by muscle, nerve, or tendon loss; and, finally, aesthetic problems with scar formation or contour deformities. The plastic surgeon will face all of these clinical conditions in long-time survivors of extremity sarcomas and must be able to develop comprehensive treatment and reconstructive options.

REHABILITATION

Careful planning of rehabilitative procedures such as physiotherapy, ergonomics, and grip training should be integrated primarily into the treatment rationale *before* surgery. The functional deficits associated with the expected resectional defect can be determined using nuclear magnetic resonance imaging (NMR) to identify the structures that must be resected.[6] Cancer patients undergoing multimodal treatment often have problems related to the extent of their illness, in contrast to patients whose surgery is trauma related. The compliance of patients who are also receiving chemotherapy and/or radiotherapy is often less than that seen in patients who have suffered a traumatic injury.

Patients with sarcomas must also shoulder the burden of the diagnosis of "cancer." They may be required to undergo repeated surgical procedures, all associated with pain. They may experience psychosocial and school-related problems, wound-healing disturbances, nausea, ulcerations of mucous membranes, adynamia, and conflicts within the family. All of these factors do not contribute to a superior functional outcome or compliance with rehabilitation. Multimodality treatment may sometimes require a two-stage procedure, especially in children, whereby reconstructive surgery is done after chemotherapy and/or radiotherapy. Reconstructive options leading to the ability of simple grip should be preferred in the treatment of elderly patients because long-lasting, intensive training programs are not likely to be accepted.

The outcome of physiotherapy and ergonomic training should be followed sequentially by the plastic surgeon responsible for the reconstructive procedure. A thorough discussion with the patient and his or her family about essential rehabilitative treatment should be done before surgery in an attempt to avoid the above-mentioned complications. The patient should be told not only about the surgical procedures and adjuvant therapies, but he or she also should be meticulously informed about the rehabilitation programs that will require consequent participation. The parents of children who are being treated for limb tumors should be aware of the importance of rehabilitation therapy as early as possible. The surgeon and the family must work together to guide the young patient in one successful direction after treatment.

OUTCOMES

Between 1978 and 1992, we treated 182 patients with soft tissue sarcomas of the extremities either by wide local excision, muscle group resection, or stump length–sparing amputations. Of the 182 patients, 106 were referred to our unit with local recurrences, of which 40 appeared with a first recurrence, 25 were having a second recurrence, and 41 were experiencing their third to eleventh recurrences. There were 147 patients who were categorized as high risk based on histopathologic tumor grading and/or other clinical parameters.

The patients ranged in age from 8 months to 78 years, with a mean age of 52 years. There were 151 patients who were treated surgically in an attempt to obtain a cure. A palliative procedure was performed in 31 patients with extensive tumor growth and high-risk conditions, including distant metastases.

Our patient population had a high incidence of local recurrence after surgery at another institution; therefore 29 patients with limb tumors received amputation or segmental resection, including three ray amputations, two above-elbow amputations, two resection arthroplasties of the shoulder joint (Tikhof-Linberg), and six interscapulothoracic resections of the upper extremity. There were three modified Chopart amputations, seven knee-joint disarticulations, four above-knee amputations, two hip-joint disarticulations, and two hemipelvectomies performed for lower-extremity tumors.

All other patients received limb-sparing and function-sparing procedures whereby extensive oncologic defects were closed in 57 cases with skin grafts and/or fascia flaps, in 36 cases with large pedicled muscle flaps, and in 44 cases with microsurgical free tissue transfers. Functional rehabilitation was achieved in 43 patients with primary tendon transfers.

None of the patients with microsurgically transplanted flaps, pedicled muscle flaps, or fascia flaps developed complete necrosis. The incidence of marginal secondary wound healing was 9%, and seroma formation 28%, which is comparable to other specialized tumor centers treating similar patients with complicated extremity tumors.

Patients undergoing stump-preservation or stump-elongation procedures were fitted with a prosthesis within the same time frame after surgery as was required for conventional amputation stumps.

We had a mean follow-up time of 53 months, during which 52 patients (28.5%) died of their disease, one died from a pulmonary embolism, and two died after complications of chemotherapy. Twenty-two patients at an average of 53 months after surgery have lymph-node or pulmonary metastases. A local recurrence of tumor developed in 11 of 151 patients who had undergone a curative tumor resection, usually within a period of 24 months after the previous surgery. Of 31 patients who had palliative surgical procedures, 10 developed a local recurrence after surgery; however, only four out of 31 patients who underwent palliative limb resection required secondary amputation.

SUMMARY

1. Limb-sparing resection in combination with adjuvant therapies produces survival rates comparable to amputation. The functional results and the potential for local recurrence depend mainly on the adequacy of the primary surgery.
2. Reconstructive plastic surgical procedures increase the rate of limb salvage by providing safe soft tissue coverage, even in patients with large oncologically created defects.
3. Conventional and free tissue transfer flap techniques will diminish the rate of wound-healing complications in patients undergoing multimodality treatment.
4. Microsurgical transplantation procedures allow spare-part surgery and salvage replantation in patients who require segmental amputation. Stump-length preservation or stump elongation will result in prosthetic supplementation that is superior to conventional amputation techniques.
5. Primary functional reconstruction should be integrated into the overall treatment plan employing tendon and muscle transfers. Free microvascular tissue transplantation or pedicled flaps can provide coverage of exposed tendons, neurovascular structures, and bones and will restore contour deformities.
6. Functional and socioeconomic rehabilitation must be primarily planned and integrated into a multimodality treatment option.
7. Reconstructive plastic surgery should be integrated primarily into sarcoma treatment protocols to obtain the optimal functional and aesthetic rehabilitation of the patient.
8. Long-term survivors often experience late sequelae such as irradiation fibrosis or ulceration, functional deficiencies, contour defects, and secondary malignancies, all of which may again require the full spectrum of reconstructive plastic surgical procedures.

REFERENCES

1. Arbeit JM, Hilaris BS, Brennan MF: Wound complications in the multimodality treatment of extremity and superficial truncal sarcomas, *J Clin Oncol* 5:480-488, 1987.
2. Bell RS, O'Sullivan B, Liu FR, et al: The surgical margin in soft-tissue sarcoma, *J Bone Joint Surg* 71A:370-376, 1989.
3. Bray PW, Bell RS, Bowen CV, et al: Limb salvage surgery and adjuvant radiotherapy for soft tissue sarcomas of the forearm and hand, *J Hand Surg* 22(3):495-503, 1997.
4. Brien EW, Terek RM, Geer RJ, et al: Treatment of soft-tissue sarcomas of the hand, *J Bone Joint Surg* 77(4):564-571, 1995.
5. Budach W, Budach V, Socha B, et al: DNA content as a predictor of clinical outcome in soft tissue sarcoma patients, *Eur J Cancer* 30A(12):1815-1821, 1994.
6. Chang AE, Matory YL, Dwyer AJ, et al: Magnetic resonance imaging versus computed tomography in the evaluation of soft tissue tumors of the extremities, *Ann Surg* 205:430-436, 1987.
7. Chen ZW: *Microsurgery,* Heidelberg, 1982, Springer.
8. Coindre JM, Trojani M, Contesso G, et al: Reproducibility of a histopathologic grading system for adult soft tissue sarcoma, *Cancer* 58:306-401, 1986.
9. Enneking WF: A system of staging musculoskeletal neoplasms, *Clin Orthop* 204:9-31, 1986.
10. Enneking WF, Maale GE: The effect of inadvertent tumor contamination of wounds during the surgical resection of musculoskeletal neoplasms, *Cancer* 62:1251-1257, 1988.
11. Evans GR, Black JJ, Robb GL, et al: Adjuvant therapy: the effects on microvascular lower extremity reconstruction, *Ann Plast Surg* 39(2):141-144, 1997.
12. Harii K: Microvascular free flaps for skin coverage: indications and selections of donor sites, *Clin Plast Surg* 10:1-12, 1983.
13. Helferich H: Ueber muskeltransplantation beim menschen, *Arch Clin Surg* 28:562-568, 1883.
14. Johnstone PA, Wexler LH, Venzon DJ, et al: Sarcomas of the hand and foot: analysis of local control and functional result with combined multimodality therapy in extremity preservation, *Int J Radiat Oncol Biol Phys* 29(4):735-745, 1994.
15. Karakousis CP: *Atlas of operations for soft tissue tumors,* New York, 1985, McGraw-Hill.
16. Keus RB, Rutgers EJ, Ho GH, et al: Limb-sparing therapy of extremity soft tissue sarcomas: treatment outcome and long-term functional results, *Eur J Cancer* 30A(10):1459-1463, 1994.
17. Malaver MM, Sugarbaker PH, Lampert M, et al: The Tikhoff-Linberg procedure: report of ten patients and presentation of a modified technique for tumors of the proximal humerus, *Surgery* 97:518-527, 1985.
18. Mankin HJ, Lange TA, Spanier SS: The hazards of biopsy in patients with malignant primary bone and soft tissue tumors, *J Bone Joint Surg* 64A:1121-1127, 1982.
19. Peat BG, Bell RS, Davis A, et al: Wound healing complications after soft tissue sarcoma surgery, *Plast Reconstr Surg* 980-987, 1994.
20. Pelton JG, Del Rowe JD, Bolen JW, et al: Fast neutron radiotherapy for soft tissue sarcomas, *Am J Clin Oncol* 9(5):397-403, 1986.
21. Pisters PWT, Leung DHY, Woodruff J, et al: Analysis of prognostic factors in 1041 patients with localized soft tissue sarcomas of the extremities, *J Clin Oncol* 14:1679-1689, 1996.
22. Rock MG, Wood MB, Fleegler EJ: Reconstruction for malignant tumors of the upper limb. In *Tumors of the hand and upper limb,* Edinburgh, 1993, Churchill Livingstone.

23. Russell WO, Cohen J, Enzinger F, et al: A clinical and pathological staging system for soft tissue sarcomas, *Cancer* 40:1542-1550, 1997.

24. Sandberg AA, Bridge JA: *The cytogenetics of bone and soft tissue tumors,* New York, 1995, Springer-Verlag.

25. Schaffordt-Koops H, Eggermont AMM, Lienard D, et al: Hyperthermic isolated limb perfusion for the treatment of soft tissue sarcomas, *Semin Surg Oncol* 14:210-214, 1998.

26. Shiu MH, Brennan MF: *Surgical management of soft tissue sarcoma,* Philadelphia, 1989, Lea & Felbinger.

27. Skibber JM, Lotze MT, Seipp CA, et al: Limb sparing surgery for soft tissue sarcomas: wound related morbidity in patients undergoing wide local excision, *Surgery* (3)102:447-453, 1987.

28. Smith RJ: Complications of surgical treatment of tumors of the hand. In Bostwick J (editor): *Complications in hand surgery,* London, 1986, WB Saunders.

29. Steinau HU, Ehrl H, Biemer E: Reconstructive plastic surgery in soft tissue sarcomas of the extremities, *Eur J Plast Surg* 11:3-14, 1988.

30. Steinau HU, Gradinger R, Claudi B, Biemer E: *Soft tissue sarcomas of the extremities: limb sparing resection and reconstruction,* PSEF instructional courses, vol 3, edited by Robert Russell, St. Louis, 1990, Mosby, pp 116-138.

31. Steinau HU, Soeder H, Schnabel G, et al: Mikrochirurgischer muskellappentransfer zur deckung ausgedehnter strahlenulcera. In Lemperle G (editor): *Chirurgie der strahlenfolgen,* Munchen, 1984, Urban und Schwarzenberg.

32. Steinau HU, Buttemeyer R, Vogt P, et al: Reconstruction and salvage of extremities. In Kroll SS (editor): *Reconstructive plastic surgery for cancer,* St. Louis, 1996, Mosby.

33. Steinau HU, Germann G, Klein W, et al: The "epaulette" flap: replantation of osteomyocutaneous forearm segments in inter-scapulothoracic amputations, *Eur J Plast Surg* 15:283-288, 1992.

34. Suit HDS, Spiro I: Role of radiation in the management of adult patients with sarcoma of soft tissue, *Semin Surg Oncol* 10:347-356, 1994.

35. Talbert ML, Zagars GK, Sherman NE, Romsdahl MM: Conservative surgery and radiation therapy for soft tissue sarcoma of the wrist, hand, ankle and foot, *Cancer* 66(12):2482-2491, 1990.

36. Tierney JF: Adjuvant chemotherapy for localized resectable soft tissue sarcoma of adults: meta-analysis of individual data, *Lancet* 350(6)6:1647-1654, 1997.

37. Usui M, Ischii S: Microsurgical reconstructive surgery following wide resection of bone and soft tissue sarcomas in the upper extremities, *J Rec Microsurg* 2:77-85, 1986.

38. Van Geel AN, Pastroino U, Jauch KW, et al: Surgical treatment of lung metastases, *Cancer* 77:675-682, 1996.

39. Walker MJ, Wood DK, Briele HA, et al: Soft tissue sarcomas of the distal extremities, *Surgery* 99(4):392-398, 1986.

40. Windhager R, Millesi H, Kotz R: Resection-replantation for primary malignant tumors of the arm: an alternative to fore-quarter amputation, *J Bone Joint Surg [Br]* 77(2):176-184, 1995.

41. Yang JC, Chang AE, Baker AR, et al: Randomized prospective study of the benefit of adjuvant radiation therapy in the treatment of soft tissue sarcomas of the extremity, *J Clin Oncol* 16(1)197-203, 1998.

CHAPTER 131

Surgical Management of Bone Tumors

Chris S. Helmstedter
Lawrence R. Menendez

INTRODUCTION

Musculoskeletal malignancies are quite rare, comprising less than 1% of all new malignant tumors.[47] There are, for example, only an estimated 1000 to 2000 new cases of osteosarcoma yearly in the United States.[7] The treatment of bone tumors has been dramatically altered in the past 20 years by advances in imaging, chemotherapy, and radiation therapy. Currently, the physician must be able to evaluate a new patient and formulate an accurate diagnosis that will allow treatment to be initiated in an efficient and cost-effective manner. The appropriate form of surgical management is selected once a bone tumor has been properly diagnosed and staged.

INDICATIONS

STAGING

A thorough knowledge of tumor staging is essential before discussing specific diagnoses and their treatment. Sarcomas were originally staged in a fashion similar to carcinomas.[28] In 1980 Enneking[13] introduced a new staging system solely for musculoskeletal tumors that was subsequently adopted by the Musculoskeletal Tumor Society (MSTS). This system allows selection of appropriate treatment, general assessment of prognosis, and the comparative evaluation of results. It can also help the surgeon select the appropriate surgical margin with or without an adjuvant treatment plan to maximize the likelihood of local control.

The most basic staging decision is to determine whether a lesion is benign or malignant. This is not always easy because more aggressive benign lesions can often mimic malignancies, and low-grade malignancies can often appear quite indolent.

The staging of benign bone tumors uses the Arabic numerals 1 through 3 (Figure 131-1). Stage 1 lesions are described as *inactive*. They may heal spontaneously and have an indolent

clinical course. These lesions are well-encapsulated, are often asymptomatic, and are commonly seen as incidental findings on radiographs taken for other reasons. Stage 2 lesions are denoted as *active*. Progressive symptomatic growth is characteristic. These lesions are well-encapsulated but may deform their boundaries, causing expansion of the cortical bone. Stage 3 lesions are termed *aggressive*. They are locally invasive and often extend beyond natural boundaries with an associated soft tissue component. In addition, some stage 3 benign tumors, such as chondroblastoma and giant cell tumor, can paradoxically metastasize to the lung.

The tumor staging system gives an indication of the biological behavior of the tumor and thus gives the treating physician guidelines with which to formulate a treatment plan. Tumors show more aggressive clinical behavior with increasing surgical stage and therefore warrant more aggressive treatment regimens. Many stage 1 benign lesions require observation only and need no surgical intervention. Stage 2 lesions, however, require surgical intervention to treat the patient's symptoms and prevent further bone destruction. These lesions can generally be treated by intralesional excision procedures and subsequent bone grafting as necessary. Stage 3 lesions warrant more aggressive intralesional procedures that utilize margin-extending adjuvants; occasionally these lesions require resection with a margin of normal tissue.

Malignant tumors are designated by Roman numerals I through III (Table 131-1). These are further subdivided with capital letters A or B, depending on whether the tumor is intracompartmental or extracompartmental. A compartment is an anatomic area whose boundaries provide a barrier to tumor penetration. These barriers are all relative and vary in quality. Good barriers against tumor penetration include articular cartilage, deep muscular fascia, joint capsules, and periosteum. Poor barriers include the loose areolar connective tissue of the popliteal or antecubital fossae, subcutaneous fatty tissue, and skeletal muscle. When a tumor originating in one compartment crosses compartmental boundaries, it becomes extracompartmental. There are also anatomic areas that are automatically designated as extracompartmental because of the lack of tissues that can act as a good barrier. The flexor fossae, groin, hands, and hindfoot are common areas that are designated as extracompartmental (Table 131-2).

The staging system represents the complex relationship between three factors: grade (G), an assessment of the biological aggressiveness of the lesion; local extent (T), consideration of the tumor site and compartmental status; and the presence or absence of metastases (M). Stage I lesions are low-grade invasive. They are histologically well-differentiated, having minimal mitoses and cellular atypia. Local recurrence is more common than metastases. Stage II lesions are histologically high grade and often contain mitotic figures, intralesional necrosis,

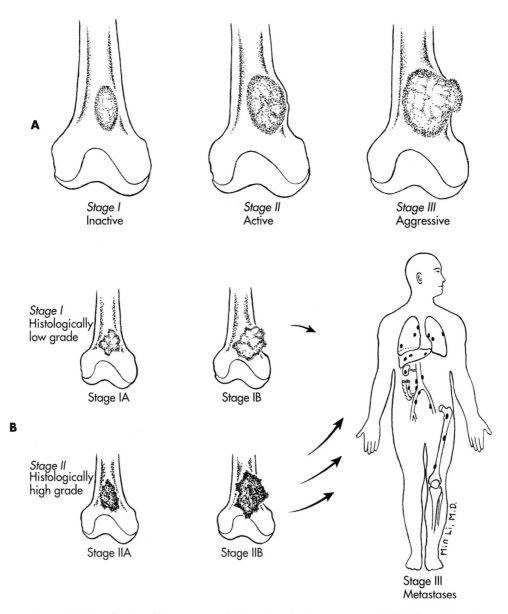

Figure 131-1. Staging of bone tumors. **A,** Histologically benign stages 1-3, (G₀). Stage 1: Inactive. Tumor may heal spontaneously with indolent clinical course; well-encapsulated. Stage 2: Active. Tumor has progressive, symptomatic growth; remains intracapsular. Although it is limited by natural boundaries, it may deform them. Stage 3: Aggressive. Tumor is locally invasive but not limited by capsule or natural boundaries. It may penetrate cortex. It has a higher rate of recurrence. **B,** Malignant stages I-III. Stage I: Histologically low grade (G₁). Tumor is well-differentiated; few mitoses; moderate nuclear atypia. Tumor tends to recur locally. Radioisotope uptake moderate. Stage IA: Intraosseous; intracompartmental. Stage IB: Extraosseous; extracompartmental, penetrates cortex. Stage II: Histologically high grade (G₂). Tumor is poorly differentiated; high cell-to-matrix ratio; frequent mitoses; much nuclear atypia, necrosis, neovascularity; permeative. Destructive. Radioisotope uptake intense. Higher incidence of metastases. Stage IIA: Intraosseous; intracompartmental. Stage IIB: Extraosseous; extracompartmental, penetrates cortex. Stage III: Metastases. Tumor is regional or remote (visceral, lymphatic, or osseous).

and neovascularity. They are often poorly differentiated and have a high incidence of metastasis. The majority of these lesions are symptomatic, rapidly growing, and present with extracompartmental (i.e., stage IIB) disease. Stage III lesions have regional or remote metastasis at presentation and can be either high or low grade.

The overall management of patients with bone sarcomas should be directed by a physician who is familiar with the treatment of these tumors. The treatment of bone sarcomas uses many modalities and often involves input from many specialties, including pathology, medical oncology, radiation oncology, surgical oncology, plastic surgery, vascular surgery, psychiatry, and physical or occupational therapy, among others. A comprehensive treatment plan can only be formulated by a physician who is readily conversant in the management of sarcomas. Therefore the surgical management of bone tumors should not be undertaken by a surgeon who has little experience in this area.

CLINICAL PRESENTATION

The diagnostic process begins with a thorough patient history and physical examination. The patient's symptoms, including their onset, duration, and severity, are noted. Pain is a common presenting feature, and details about the pain should be obtained. Information about recent illnesses or trauma and past medical problems is also critical to separate tumors from traumatic or inflammatory lesions. The patient's family history is important with reference to some diseases that have a high association with tumors and dysplasias. Malignant lesions may be associated with systemic symptoms of weight loss, appetite changes, fevers, and general malaise. Patients with metastatic disease often have a history of carcinoma. The local area of

Table 131-1.
Surgical Stages

STAGE	GRADE	SITE
IA	Low (G1)	Intracompartmental (T1)
IB	Low (G1)	Extracompartmental (T2)
IIA	High (G2)	Intracompartmental (T1)
IIB	High (G2)	Extracompartmental (T2)
III	Any (G) regional or distant metastasis	Any (T)

From Enneking WF, Spanier SS, Goodman MA: *Clin Orthop* 153:111, 1980.

Table 131-2.
Surgical Sites by Tumor Type

INTRACOMPARTMENTAL (T1)	EXTRACOMPARTMENTAL (T2)
Intraosseous	Soft tissue extension
Intraarticular	Soft tissue extension
Superficial to deep fascia	Deep fascial extension
Paraosseous	Intraosseous or extrafascial
Interfascial compartments	Extrafascial planes or spaces
Ray or hand or foot	Mid and hind foot
Posterior calf	Popliteal space
Anterolateral leg	Groin-femoral triangle
Anterior thigh	Intrapelvic
Medial thigh	Mid-hand
Posterior thigh	Antecubital fossae
Buttocks	Axilla
Volar forearm	Periclavicular
Dorsal forearm	Paraspinal
Anterior arm	Head and neck
Posterior arm	
Parascapular	

From Enneking WF, Spanier SS, Goodman MA: *Clin Orthop* 153:110, 1980.

concern should be examined only after a general physical examination has been performed. The physician who evaluates a tumor should look for other clues, such as skin changes, skeletal deformities, or lymphadenopathy, to help make the diagnosis. A palpable soft tissue mass on local examination generally indicates a more aggressive process, and the size, consistency, and mobility of the mass should be noted. Examination of the heart, lungs, spine, abdomen, breasts (women), and prostate (men) in adult patients is helpful when considering metastatic disease.

LABORATORY STUDIES

Laboratory values are helpful but are generally nonspecific and certainly are not diagnostic of any particular sarcoma. A complete blood count (CBC) and erythrocyte sedimentation rate (ESR) help evaluate the patient for a possible infection. However, both can be altered with certain malignancies, such as Ewing's sarcoma. Hematocrit levels and the platelet count must be considered when surgical options that might cause extensive blood loss are planned. Certain laboratory values are important with primary bone tumors. Approximately 50% of patients with osteosarcoma have an elevated alkaline phosphatase, and some feel there is prognostic significance associated with these elevated values.[2] Similarly, many patients with Ewing's sarcoma have an elevated lactate dehydrogenase (LDH) level. Electrolyte studies are important when developing treatment plans for adult patients. Many metastatic and hematologic malignancies are associated with hypercalcemia, which should be aggressively treated before any surgical intervention.

IMAGING STUDIES

Radiographs

At least two 90-degree orthogonal radiographic views of the involved bone are necessary for the diagnosis and management of any bone lesion. The plain radiograph is the least expensive and yet the most diagnostic study to obtain in a patient with a suspected tumor. The physician should evaluate four parameters when reviewing a radiograph of a bone lesion.[11] First, the exact anatomic location of the lesion should be defined, including whether it is central or eccentric in location in the epiphysis, metaphysis, or diaphysis. This is important because certain lesions have a propensity for specific areas of the bone. Second, the physician should describe what the lesion itself is doing to the bone structure. Is there cortical destruction or expansion of the cortical diameter? The third parameter is to define what the bone is doing to the lesion, noting reactive bone formation about the lesion or cortical hypertrophy. Periosteal reactions are generally seen about more aggressive lesions or lesions with an associated fracture. Finally, there are specific characteristics that can occasionally be seen in the matrix that can help make the diagnosis of a specific lesion. The matrix of a fibrous dysplasia, for example, may have a ground glass appearance,

or an enchondroma will have stippled calcifications. Other important aspects to note on plain radiographs are the patterns of bone destruction and the size and margination of the lesion. Larger lesions that are more poorly marginated generally are more aggressive.

Bone Scan

Staging of bone lesions often begins with a three-phase bone scan. The bone scan now plays a less important role in defining local extent of the tumor since the advent of high resolution computed tomography (CT) scanners and magnetic resonance imaging (MRI). However, many bone lesions (e.g., enchondromas, fibrous dysplasia, giant cell tumor of bone, and carcinoma metastases) can be multifocal at the initial presentation, and the bone scan offers a sensitive and inexpensive method of examining the osseous structures of the entire body. The local intensity is also helpful in determining the biological behavior of the tumor locally and adds clues to the differential diagnosis.

Computed Tomography and Magnetic Resonance Imaging

Local imaging of the primary lesion is usually accomplished with CT or MRI. Most operable lesions should be scanned in some form to more accurately define the tumor margin and aid in preoperative surgical planning. MRI is superior to CT in showing the intramedullary extent of the bone lesion, delineating any soft tissue component, and showing the adjacent neurovascular structures. A CT scan obtained with new high-resolution scanners gives excellent soft tissue detail but is not as good as MRI at delineating the marrow involvement within the bone. CT is generally superior to MRI at revealing very thin reactive rims of bone and detecting minute matrix calcification or ossification within a lesion. CT also very accurately defines the extent of cortical destruction, allowing better assessment of the structural integrity of the involved bone and the risk of pathologic fracture.

A CT scan of the chest should be obtained in patients with suspected malignant bone tumors and some aggressive benign lesions. The majority of sarcomas will have their first sign of metastasis in the lung. Knowing whether metastatic disease is present dramatically changes the patient's prognosis and may alter subsequent treatment. This knowledge allows the physician to have a better understanding of the patient's overall tumor biology and can help with patient education and counseling.

Ultrasound and Positron Emission Tomography Imaging

Further imaging modalities that are useful in certain situations are ultrasound and positron emission tomography (PET) imaging. Ultrasound is an inexpensive way of differentiating a cystic mass from a solid tumor mass, but it has largely been supplanted by MRI as an initial diagnostic study. PET scanning is beneficial in the evaluation of some carcinomas, such as hepatic carcinoma and melanoma. Its role in the evaluation of benign and malignant mesenchymal tumors, however, is still being defined.

CLASSIFICATION OF TUMORS

Classifying tumors by histologic subtype is less useful clinically but facilitates a general discussion of their basic radiographic and histologic features.

Cartilaginous Lesions

Cartilaginous lesions as a whole make up the second most common primary bone tumors after those of hematopoietic origin.[9] They are the most common primary bone tumors of the upper extremity, and benign disease is slightly more prevalent than malignant. Cartilaginous lesions are usually slow growing, with symptoms developing over months. A biopsy is usually required for definitive diagnosis to be made, but some lesions have a very characteristic radiographic appearance and do not warrant a biopsy or other surgical intervention.

Enchondroma

Enchondromas are benign cartilage lesions that can occur in any bone formed by enchondral ossification. Mirra[37] has proposed that these lesions possibly arise from misplaced islands of cartilage that are shed into the medullary substance from abnormal or dysplastic foci of cartilage within the growth plate. This is further reinforced by the fact that the lesions usually present within the second or third decade of life. They are the most common primary bone lesions of the hand, frequently involving the phalanges. Most are symptomatic, causing digital swelling and pain.[27] Other common sites are the proximal humerus, the proximal and distal metaphysis of the femur, and the foot. Enchondromas are often found as incidental findings in the long bones when radiographs are taken for minor trauma or pain from some other cause.

Enchondromas are typically central radiolucencies in the medullary canal and are metaphyseal to diaphyseal. Mild endosteal scalloping and cortical expansion with a minimal reactive rim of bone is typical. Intralesional calcification is common and described as punctate or "popcornlike" (Figure 131-2). Differential diagnoses include epidermoid cyst, fibrous dysplasia, unicameral bone cyst, chondroblastoma, and chondromyxoid fibroma.

Lesions of the hand often require treatment, whereas lesions in many other sites are treated with observation because the natural history of enchondroma is to change from an active stage 2 lesion to a latent stage 1 lesion at skeletal maturity. The risk of malignant transformation of a solitary lesion is minimal.

Multiple enchondromatosis (Ollier's disease) and enchondromatosis with associated hemangiomas (Maffucci's syndrome) usually present earlier in life than typical solitary enchondromas and have a more aggressive histology. The extent of disease is variable, but often there are leg-length discrepancies, multiple skeletal deformities, and pathologic fractures.[43] The malignant transformation rate is in the range of 30% to 50%, usually occurring after 30 years of age.

Osteochondroma

Osteochondroma is the most common benign bone tumor.[22] These lesions are thought to arise from a defect in the perichondral ring at the growth plate that gets separated and

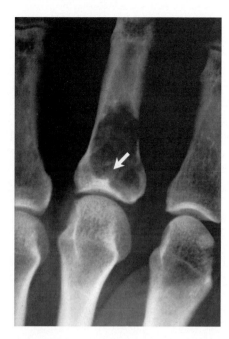

Figure 131-2. An enchondroma involving the proximal aspect of the long finger proximal phalanx. Note the small punctate calcifications *(white arrow)*.

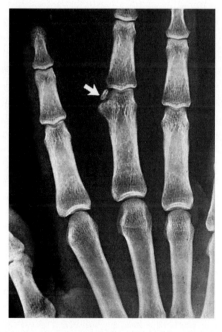

Figure 131-3. An osteochondroma involving the distal aspect of the long finger proximal phalanx *(white arrow)*. Atypically, this lesion is growing toward the adjacent articulation rather than away.

thus grows independently.[19] Growth of these lesions often stops within 1 to 2 years of skeletal maturity. Common sites include the distal femur, the proximal humerus, and the proximal tibia. Twenty percent of these lesions occur in the upper extremity; only 2% occur in the hand (Figure 131-3).[4] The peak incidence for developing an osteochondroma is in the second decade. The typical presentation is a firm, fixed, palpable mass that is usually nontender. Occasionally, soft tissue irritation of an overlying tendon or muscle causes pain. Radiographs reveal a bony excrescence (sessile or pedunculated) off the metaphyseal area of the bone that is often pointing away from the adjacent joint and epiphysis. The medullary canal of the exostosis is continuous with that of the underlying bone. Excisional biopsy is usually curative if the entire cartilaginous cap is excised. Histologically, the lesions appear similar to a growth plate, although more disordered. Multiple heritable exostosis is an autosomal dominant disorder with variable penetrance characterized by multiple osteochondromata. Patients with the disorder have a higher rate of malignant transformation and must be followed more closely.

Chondroblastoma

Chondroblastoma is a benign tumor of the chondroblastic germ cells in the epiphysis usually seen in patients less than 25 years old. It can also be found in epiphyseal-equivalent areas such as the greater trochanteric or olecranon apophysis. Common sites include the distal femur, the proximal tibia, or the proximal humerus. However, like enchondromas, chondroblastomas can affect any bone formed by enchondral ossification. Patients with this form of chondroblastoma commonly present with soft tissue swelling and pain in the area with loss of joint range of motion.

Radiographically, chondroblastomas are eccentric epiphyseal lesions surrounded with a moderately thick reactive rim of bone (Figure 131-4, A). There may be mild endosteal scalloping and cortical expansion. Small intralesional calcifications are less consistent than with enchondroma. Associated metaphyseal involvement is not uncommon. MRI often shows a significant component of edema in the surrounding bone marrow and soft tissues, which can be misinterpreted as infection.

Plump chondroblasts, when seen side by side histologically, give a characteristic cobblestone appearance. Intracellular calcification occurs as the lesion matures, leaving a thin, lacelike network of calcification between the cells reminiscent of chicken wire. Treatment of chondroblastoma is extended curettage with bone grafting or cementation.

Chondromyxoid Fibroma

Chondromyxoid fibromas are rare, eccentric, cartilaginous lesions that occur most commonly in the metaphyseal bone about the knee.[24] They are prone to form near the anterior tibial cortex, where they have a lobulated, well-defined, reactive rim of bone.

The cartilaginous component of a chondromyxoid fibroma has the appearance of fibrocartilage rather than the hyaline type seen with enchondromas. Three distinct tissue types must be present to make the diagnosis. The basophilic myxoid component often predominates, with chondroid foci being seen in variable amounts. An associate spindle cell component makes the final diagnosis.[17]

Chondrosarcoma

Chondrosarcoma is typically a low-grade malignant neoplasm resulting in cartilaginous matrix production by the malignant chondrocytes. Reactive bone may be present, but neoplastic

osteoid from malignant osteoblasts is never seen. Secondary chondrosarcomas occur in middle-aged patients with a previous benign precursor, such as an enchondroma or osteochondroma.[16] Primary chondrosarcomas occur in older patients without a benign precursor and are much more common in the axial skeleton and pelvic and shoulder girdles.[44]

It is often very difficult to distinguish histologically between benign and malignant cartilage neoplasms, making incisional biopsy frequently unreliable. The decision as to whether a cartilage lesion is malignant or benign should be made before the biopsy based on the history, physical examination, and the imaging studies. A CT scan through the lesion helps to visualize exuberant calcifications, severe endosteal scalloping, cortical hypertrophy, and possible cortical breakthrough.

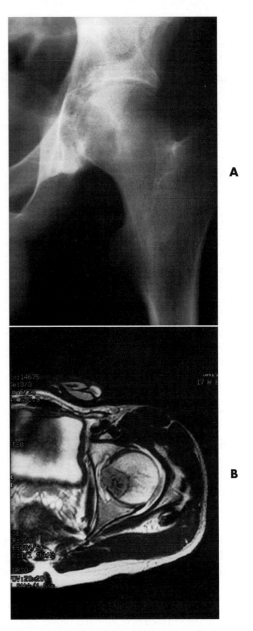

Figure 131-4. **A,** An irregular radiolucent lesion involving the femoral head of a 19-year-old boy with hip pain. **B,** The axial MRI image shows breakthrough of the medial cortex with involvement of the hip joint.

These findings, together with an associated soft tissue mass, are indicative of a malignant lesion (Figure 131-5). The surgeon in this case would proceed with incisional biopsy solely to prove the lesion cartilaginous and proceed with immediate resection. Radiation and chemotherapy are not effective adjuvant treatments for patients with chondrosarcoma, and therefore surgical excision is the treatment of choice.

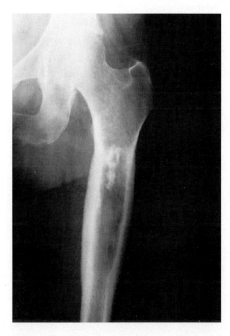

Figure 131-5. An intramedullary lesion of the proximal femoral diaphysis in a 52-year-old woman shows calcification, endosteal scalloping, and cortical thickening, all consistent with chondrosarcoma.

There are three distinct histological variants of chondrosarcoma. The rare clear cell chondrosarcoma is the malignant version of the chondroblastoma occurring in the epiphyses of younger patients. Like other chondrosarcomas, it is low grade and treated solely by surgical resection and reconstruction.[48] Dedifferentiated chondrosarcoma is a low-grade cartilage neoplasm that has associated areas of high-grade spindle cell sarcoma. The prognosis for patients with these types of tumors is quite poor, despite neoadjuvant chemotherapy and surgery. The last subtype is mesenchymal chondrosarcoma, which consists of a high-grade spindle cell neoplasm of the soft tissues that has associated islands of mature cartilage within it. These lesions are also treated with a combination of chemotherapy and surgical resection. Their prognosis, however, is somewhat better than the dedifferentiated subtype.[23]

Bone-Forming Neoplasms

OSTEOID OSTEOMA. Osteoid osteomas are small, benign bone-forming neoplasms that present most commonly in the second to third decade of life. They occur more commonly in the lower extremity, primarily in the femur and tibia. Hand and wrist lesions account for only 5% to 15% of these neoplasms, with the most common site being the proximal phalanx.[3] The majority of lesions are associated with a dull, aching, continuous pain that is often relieved by taking nonsteroidal antiinflammatory medication. Physical examination is usually specific for point tenderness directly over the lesion, with an otherwise normal examination. Radiographs typically demonstrate a marked sclerosis in the area of the lesion with a central radiolucent nidus. The nidus may only be visible on CT scan (Figure 131-6). Cancellous bone and juxtaarticular lesions are often less characteristic radiographically. Contrast-enhanced CT scans allow visualization of the nidus and assessment of its vascularity, differentiating it from a Brodie's abscess.[36] The

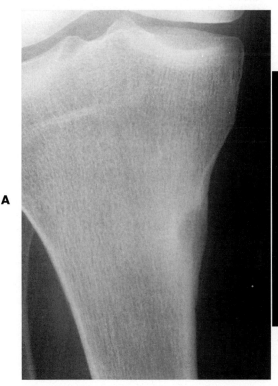
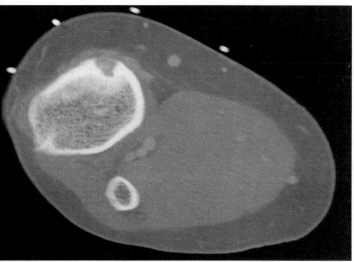

Figure 131-6. A, An osteoid osteoma involving the proximal medial tibial cortex. Note the small size of the nidus. **B,** The CT scan easily shows the central nidus with surrounding sclerosis.

specimen grossly appears pink to red in color because of the intense vascularity of the lesion. Histologically, one sees benign plump osteoblasts making seams of osteoid within a loose fibrovascular tissue.

The natural history of osteoid osteoma is to gradually resolve and become painless in 2 to 3 years. The pain is usually of such intensity, however, that most patients request surgical intervention. Previously recommended techniques have included en bloc resection or extended curettage. The current procedure of choice is extended curettage with preoperative localization using CT-guided techniques.[32] A technique of percutaneous radio frequency ablation has more recently been described.[41] Early reports have shown that most patients experience excellent relief of pain, and radiographic healing of the lesions has been seen within 3 to 6 months.[41] The local recurrence rate with this technique is not accurately known, and its use at this time is still investigational.

OSTEOBLASTOMA. Osteoblastomas are histologically very similar to osteoid osteomas but often have a markedly different radiographic appearance and clinical course.[15,5] Osteoblastomas are larger than osteoid osteomas and are typically over 2 cm. The location is different as well, with osteoblastomas occurring in the cancellous bone of the posterior column of the spine. Osteoblastomas are large radiolucent lesions radiographically, with a small thin rim of reactive bone. Histologically, osteoblasts produce osteoid in a fibrovascular stroma. In general, osteoblastoma appears slightly more aggressive, with plumper, more hyperchromatic osteoblasts about plump bars of osteoid. Some osteoblastomas are stage 3, benign, aggressive lesions termed *aggressive osteoblastoma* and have a higher local recurrence rate.

OSTEOGENIC SARCOMA. Over 80% of osteosarcomas occur in patients younger than 30 who usually present with bone pain unrelated to activity. Osteosarcoma is most common in the distal femur, followed by the proximal tibia and proximal femur. The most commonly involved bone in the upper extremity is the proximal humerus followed by the distal radius.[40] Over 90% of patients have an associated soft tissue mass and stage IIB disease at the time of presentation.

Radiographs show a mixed radiodense and radiolucent pattern in the metaphysis, and periosteal reaction is quite common, often in a sunburst pattern. MRI typically demonstrates marrow involvement that is far beyond that appreciated on plain film radiographs (Figure 131-7). Histologically, there is a malignant spindle-cell stroma with abundant mitotic figures and severe atypia that produces a lacelike network of osteoid matrix. These lesions can be primarily osteoblastic, chondroblastic, or fibroblastic, but always have a spindle-cell component. Telangiectatic osteosarcoma has a predominance of aneurysmal cystic changes within the lesion that can mimic benign aneurysmal bone cysts and must be adequately biopsied.

Treatment for osteogenic sarcoma is surgical resection with neoadjuvant multiagent chemotherapy. Greater than 90% of patients with osteogenic sarcoma can currently be treated with limb-salvage surgical techniques that avoid amputation. Patients are continued on chemotherapy after surgery that is

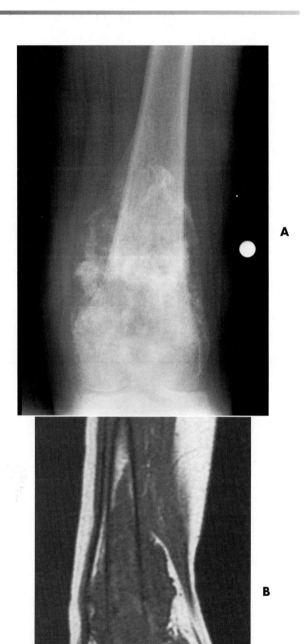

Figure 131-7. **A,** An anteroposterior (AP) radiograph of the distal femur shows a mixed destructive, radiodense lesion in the metaphysis. **B,** The MRI scan reveals additional bony involvement not seen on the plain-film radiograph, consistent with osteogenic sarcoma.

tailored to the tumor and based on the amount of necrosis observed in the resected specimen. The survival rate of patients without pulmonary metastases currently approaches 50% to 70% 5 years after diagnosis.[10,29]

Other variants of classic osteogenic sarcoma are the low-grade parosteal osteosarcoma, the intermediate-grade periosteal

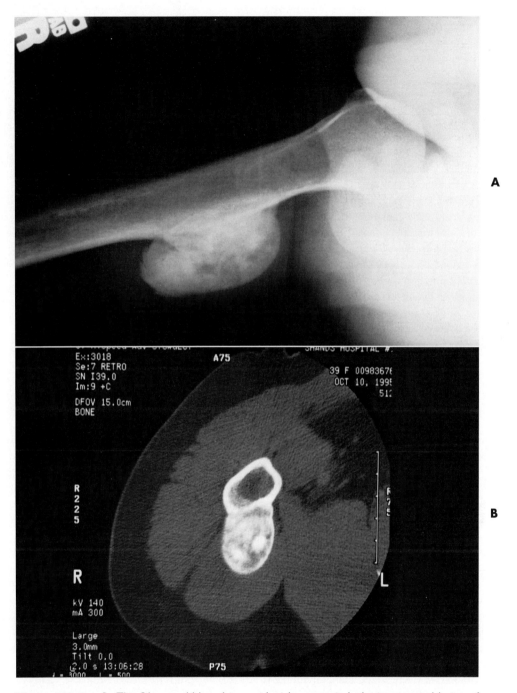

Figure 131-8. **A,** This 31-year-old bus driver with right arm pain had a juxtacortical lesion of dense bone involving the right humeral diaphysis. **B,** The CT scan confirms mineralization within the center of the lesion, making parosteal osteosarcoma the most likely diagnosis.

osteosarcoma, and the high-grade secondary osteosarcoma. The parosteal lesions less commonly require chemotherapy, and treatment is surgical resection with a minimal cuff of soft tissue (Figure 131-8).[31] Periosteal osteogenic sarcoma is more rare, and the histological grading is more variable. Chemotherapy is included in the treatment if the disease is high grade in appearance. The secondary osteosarcomas that arise from Paget's disease or after radiation have an exceptionally poor prognosis.

A recent report has documented only a 10% to 20% 5-year survival in patients who develop osteosarcomas in association with these two conditions.[20]

Reticuloendothelial Lesions
HISTIOCYTOSIS. The benign reticuloendothelioses are a disease continuum that includes eosinophilic granuloma, Hand-Schüller-Christian disease, and Letterer-Siwe disease.

These lesions were previously believed to be inflammatory in origin; however, recent studies have demonstrated clonality of the cells, which supports a neoplastic origin.[51] Eosinophilic granuloma is the most common lesion, and the predominant inflammatory cell found is the eosinophil. Aggregates of xanthomatous histiocytes dominate the histologic picture, and in most instances, solitary lesions heal spontaneously.

EWING'S SARCOMA. Ewing's sarcoma is a small, round cell tumor probably of neuroectodermal origin. These lesions usually occur in the second or third decade of life, and only 20% are found in the upper extremity, with the humerus being the most common site. Patients with Ewing's sarcoma may have symptoms that mimic osteomyelitis. The tumor infiltrates the haversian canals of the bone and exits the bone without diffuse cortical destruction. Radiographs show a mottled, permeative, radiolucent lesion with poor boundaries and an aggressive laminated or "onion peel" periosteal reaction (Figure 131-9). Most of these lesions present as stage IIB lesions with a large soft tissue mass. Monotonous sheets of small, blue, round cells with a large central nucleus and little cytoplasm are seen histologically. Patients with Ewing's tumors have been found to have the chromosome 11-22 translocation that is also present on primitive neuroectodermal tumors (PNET). Treatment of both tumors is with neoadjuvant chemotherapy and surgery and/or radiation, depending on the size and location of the primary lesion. Multiple studies have shown an advantage in local control with surgical resection.[39]

Myeloma

Myeloma is the most common primary malignancy of bone. It typically occurs in patients over 40 years of age. The majority of cases produce monoclonal immunoglobulins. The bones involved are primarily those containing red marrow, such as the vertebral bodies, ilium, scapulae, and ribs. Radiographically, the lesions are purely radiolucent with minimal reactive bone around them and are described as "punched-out" lesions. Bone scintigraphy is negative in 50% of the lesions, and therefore patients need to be staged with plain-film radiograph skeletal surveys. These lesions are usually very sensitive to chemotherapy and radiation techniques. The average long-term survival of patients with multiple bone lesions is 4 years. Surgery is generally not indicated in the management of this tumor unless there is significant risk of fracture.

METASTATIC CARCINOMA. Metastatic adenocarcinoma is the most common malignancy to involve bone. Breast and prostate carcinomas have bone metastasis rates as high as 85% in autopsy studies. Bone is the third most common metastatic site for carcinomas. The majority of metastatic lesions involve the axial skeleton, with the femur as the most common long-bone site. Upper-extremity lesions account for only 20% of metastatic lesions. Metastatic disease below the elbow is quite uncommon, and when present in the hand often mimics infection. Lung carcinoma is the most common primary disease to cause these acrometastases. Radiographs typically show an aggressive radiolucent lesion, often with a periosteal reaction

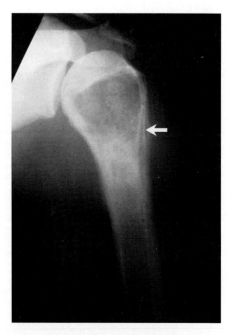

Figure 131-9. Typical radiographic presentation of a Ewing's sarcoma. Note the permeative pattern of bone destruction and the laminated or "onion peel" periosteal reaction *(white arrow)*.

and associated soft tissue mass. Breast and prostate carcinomas can, however, produce highly blastic lesions.

Histologically, most metastatic lesions are easily distinguished from sarcomas. Treatment for metastatic bone lesions is determined by multiple factors, including the patient's projected life expectancy, the extent of the metastatic disease, and the patient's functional status at the time of presentation. In general, surgical treatment for metastatic lesions is only used in cases of impending or actual fracture and is followed by postoperative adjuvant radiation therapy.

Miscellaneous Tumors

UNICAMERAL BONE CYST. A bone cyst is a cavity filled with a translucent yellow serous fluid that somewhat resembles synovial fluid biochemically. If the bone cyst had previously undergone pathologic fracture, the cyst fluid can be tainted red or brown. Simple bone cysts occur most commonly in the long bones, with greater than 90% of the lesions occurring in the proximal femur and proximal humerus. They usually present within the first to second decade of life after pathologic fracture. Early lesions will be located in the central metaphysis that abuts the physeal plate (Figure 131-10). In general, older lesions have grown away from the physis and are seen in patients older than 12.[42] They become multiloculated, and the cortex thickens. Histologically, the cavity is lined with a shiny membrane overlying a loose fibrous tissue stroma and capillary network. The membrane is thicker in mature lesions and may contain hemosiderin and cholesterol deposits.[14]

Treatment of unicameral bone cysts has typically been aspiration and injection of methylprednisolone steroid.[38] Commonly, two or three aspirations and injections are

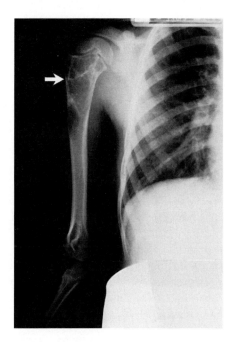

Figure 131-10. Unicameral bone cysts commonly present after pathologic fracture *(white arrow)*. This lesion abuts the physeal plate and thus has an increased risk of recurrence after treatment.

required to facilitate healing of the lesion. The natural history of bone cysts is usually that of spontaneous healing in adulthood. When fracture occurs, the callus will occasionally heal the cyst and no subsequent treatment will be needed.

ANEURYSMAL BONE CYST. Aneurysmal bone cysts are blood-filled cystic cavities that are lined by a thick, fleshy membrane that has an endothelial-like inner layer. A loose mesenchymal tissue with scattered giant cells, often with hemosiderin in their cytoplasm, is seen under the lining. Half of the lesions occur as secondary lesions in another tumor, including giant cell tumors, chondroblastoma, osteoblastoma, and some malignant lesions.[47] The secondary lesions can actually be larger than the associated primary tumor. Radiographs demonstrate a metaphyseal, expansile lesion, often with a rim of reactive bone so thin that it is only seen on axial images of a CT scan. CT and MRI studies can both reveal a fluid-fluid level caused by settling of the cyst fluid proteins. A careful biopsy is needed before curettage to rule out telangiectatic osteosarcoma or other primary tumor.

FIBROUS DYSPLASIA. Fibrous dysplasia is a congenital dysplasia of a bone that presents with pain that is secondary to either pathologic fracture, presumed microfracture, or simple skeletal insufficiency caused by lack of bone stock. It commonly presents in the 10- to 30-year-old age group, and approximately 80% of the lesions are monoostotic.[14] Radiographically, fibrous dysplasia can be quite variable. It is generally a central metaphyseal or diaphyseal lesion that causes mild cortical expansion; the central matrix often has a ground-glass appearance (Figure 131-11, *A*). Histologically,

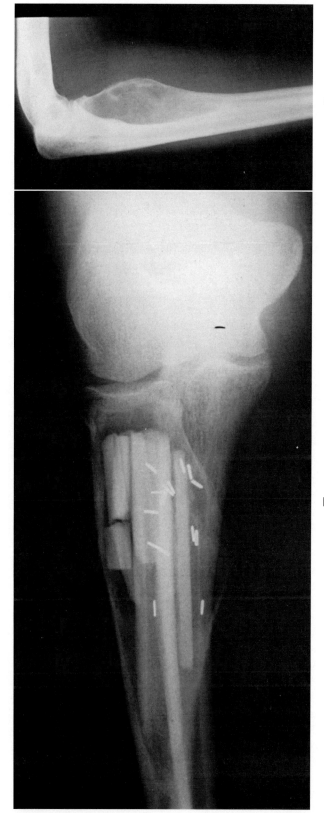

Figure 131-11. A, This proximal radius lesion shows the typical ground-glass appearance of fibrous dysplasia. The patient complained of repetitive pain, presumably from microfracture within the lesions. **B,** Treatment was with curettage and cortical strut grafting using fibular allograft.

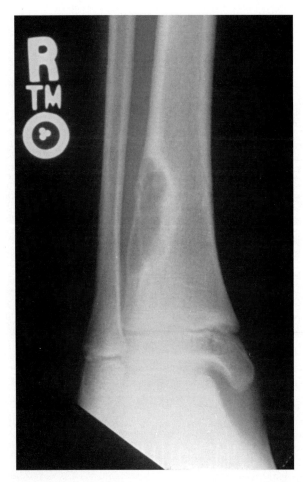

Figure 131-12. Eccentric cortical radiolucency with geographic destruction of the distal tibial bone. The site is common for nonossifying fibromas.

one sees a benign fibrous connective tissue background with small islands of immature trabeculae that resemble "commas" or "Chinese letters." There is usually no significant rim of osteoblasts lining the trabeculae, and it is believed that the matrix formation is from the mesenchymal cells themselves. Curettage of the cyst and cortical strut grafting are commonly employed when surgery is necessary (Figure 131-11, *B*).[12]

NONOSSIFYING FIBROMA. Nonossifying fibromas are localized defects in the cortex of long bones that are usually seen in the first decade of life. They are eccentric, metaphyseal lesions with a very geographic pattern of destruction (Figure 131-12). Histologically, one sees abundant immature fibroblasts replacing the bone tissue. The fibroma develops histiocytes and cholesterol slits with aging. Treatment is by observation unless there is imminent risk of developing a pathologic fracture. Most of these lesions go on to ossify at skeletal maturity.

GIANT CELL TUMORS. Giant cell tumors are uncommon lesions in the upper extremity, with the majority being found in the distal third of the radius. Most lesions in the hand and wrist area involve the phalanges or the metacarpals and tend

to develop at a younger age and have a shorter length of symptoms.[8] Giant cell tumors of the lower extremity typically occur in the distal femur and proximal tibia. Approximately one third of the lesions are aggressive stage 3 lesions with cortical breakthrough and a soft tissue component. Five percent of patients present with or develop pulmonary metastases, and less than 1% of cases are multicentric at presentation.

Radiographs typically show an eccentric radiolucent lesion that involves the epiphysis and metaphysis of the involved bone. The lesion has a distinct margin, but no significant reactive rim of bone (Figure 131-13, *A*). Histologically, numerous giant cells, which may have abundant nuclei, are littered throughout a fibrovascular stroma with numerous histiocytes. The treatment for most lesions is extended curettage and associated adjuvants, such as polymethylmethacrylate bone cement, liquid nitrogen, or phenol. If destruction of the involved bone is severe, these lesions are better treated with resection and reconstruction (Figure 131-13, *B*).

OPERATIONS

With few exceptions, surgery is the mainstay of treatment for patients with bone tumors. The goal of surgery is to achieve local control of the neoplasm, because without complete excision all malignant tumors and the majority of benign tumors will recur locally. Patients who experience a local recurrence of a sarcoma will be twice as likely to die of the disease as those who do not. Local tumor control does not guarantee that a patient with a bone sarcoma will be cured, but the converse is also true that no patient with a bone sarcoma can be cured if local control of the tumor is not achieved.

There are four basic categories of operation in the treatment of musculoskeletal oncologic conditions: (1) biopsy, (2) curettage, (3) resection, and (4) amputation. Before discussing the different surgical options, the surgeon must have a thorough understanding of surgical margins. There are only four oncologic margins that can be achieved: intralesional, marginal, wide, and radical. Each of these margins can be accomplished by either an amputation or limb-salvage surgery. The margin of a resection depends on the relative relationship between the resection plane and the tumor's reactive zone. Not all resections and amputations are therefore wide or radical excisions (Figure 131-14). If a resection or amputation is performed within the reactive zone, it is still considered a marginal surgical resection. The margin may be "radical" from a psychosocial perspective, but in oncologic terms the margin is only marginal and the likelihood of local recurrence is as great as if a curettage had been performed. All curettage procedures are by definition intralesional and should be performed meticulously and only for benign lesions.

It is imperative in treating sarcomas that the desired oncologic margin be achieved, even if this means converting a

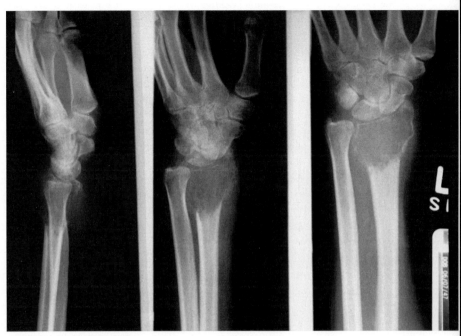
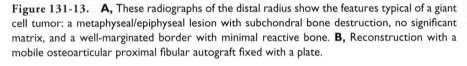
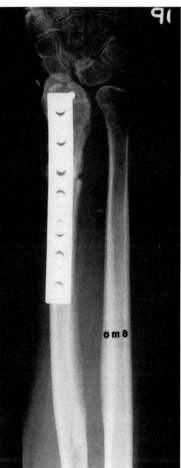

Figure 131-13. **A,** These radiographs of the distal radius show the features typical of a giant cell tumor: a metaphyseal/epiphyseal lesion with subchondral bone destruction, no significant matrix, and a well-marginated border with minimal reactive bone. **B,** Reconstruction with a mobile osteoarticular proximal fibular autograft fixed with a plate.

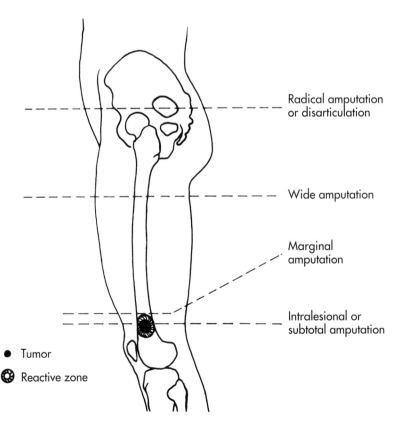

Radical amputation or disarticulation

Wide amputation

Marginal amputation

Intralesional or subtotal amputation

● Tumor

⊛ Reactive zone

Figure 131-14. The various types of amputations are shown for a theoretical lesion of the distal femur. (From Enneking WF, Spanier SS, Goodman MA: *Clin Orthop* 153:114, 1980.)

limb-salvage procedure to an amputation. The following three goals in the treatment of patients with bone sarcomas are in order of importance:

1. Save the patient's life by achieving local tumor control
2. Salvage the affected extremity
3. Maximize the function of the salvaged extremity

The oncologic margin should never be compromised in an attempt to achieve limb salvage. Whether treatment is performed by a single experienced oncologic surgeon or a team involving an oncologist, orthopedist, and plastic surgeon, the principals of oncologic surgery should be meticulously followed. Compromise of the oncologic margins usually occurs when the surgeon concentrates on the second phase of the procedure before successfully completing the first.

Adequate surgical margins for most bone tumors can be achieved with both limb-salvage surgery and amputation, but limb salvage has generally become the standard of practice in the management of bone tumors. The increased risk of local recurrence in patients with sarcomas treated by limb-salvage surgery compared with those treated by amputation is only 5% or less.[45] Most patients with bone tumors are eligible for limb-salvaging treatment, but some are not. There are several contraindications to performing a limb-salvage procedure, including inability to achieve an adequate oncologic margin or when the functional recovery of the extremity after a limb-salvage surgery is expected to be worse than after an amputation. Patients with osteogenic sarcoma of the distal tibia, for example, are best treated with a below-knee amputation rather than a limb-salvage procedure. Patients who have tumor involvement of two or more anatomic compartments and the associated neurovascular structures usually require amputation, as do those with a displaced pathologic fracture through the primary sarcoma. Local contamination is generally so extreme in this situation that it is impossible to achieve an adequate oncologic margin. A compartmental resection is also difficult in patients with an infected tumor or wound.

In practice, only a few patients with large, neglected tumors, or those who have sustained displaced pathologic fractures are not amenable to limb salvage and are best managed with ablative procedures. Limb salvage, however, should not be undertaken if it will jeopardize the patient's outcome; when necessary, the patient should be urged to proceed with amputation if indicated. Under no circumstances should a surgical margin be compromised to achieve a limb-salvage procedure which, if local recurrence develops, is certainly doomed to failure. The different types of reconstruction available are quite variable and can be as much or more technically demanding than the excision.

BIOPSY

Obtaining a biopsy is the most important diagnostic procedure in the evaluation of a bone lesion. All imaging studies should be performed before the biopsy is performed. The bleeding and inflammation caused by a biopsy will tend to obscure and complicate the analysis and interpretation of any imaging studies done after the procedure. The histologic analysis of a bone tumor should be performed only with a thorough knowledge of the patient's history and after careful review of the radiographs and imaging studies. One should never attempt to analyze the biopsy specimen without considering the other data because musculoskeletal lesions can have a similar histologic appearance but present quite different radiographic and clinical pictures. The biopsy should only be performed by a surgeon prepared to perform the definitive procedure. It should not be delegated to the most junior member of the surgical team because it is "only a biopsy."

Approximately 12% of patients referred to a surgical oncologist after biopsy are noted to have a biopsy incision that either precludes limb-salvage surgery or makes the operation more difficult.[34] Biopsies should be performed through longitudinal incisions over the tumor where it is closest to the skin. The biopsy approach should not involve a neurovascular or intermuscular plane, should not open a joint capsule, and should be transmuscular within only one anatomic compartment. The incision should be as small as possible, yet allow adequate sampling of the tumor mass. During the procedure, no sharp forceps or retractors should be used because they readily penetrate the peripheral soft tissues and can spread tumor cells beyond the tissue exposed in the wound. The retractors should also be used with the minimum amount of force necessary to provide adequate exposure. All tissue exposed at the time of biopsy should be considered contaminated and should be resected at the time of the definitive procedure. The biopsy should obtain sufficient tissue for frozen section analysis and provide additional tissue for immunohistochemical staining, cytogenic analysis, and electron-microscopic procedures as indicated. Care should be taken not to crush the tissue with forceps or clamps. Frozen section is performed at all biopsy procedures to document that representative neoplastic tissue has been obtained and to give a provisional diagnosis to the patient. Culture of the area should routinely be obtained at the time of biopsy. Fine-needle aspirates and core needle-biopsy techniques are also available. The puncture wound of a needle biopsy should be tattooed so that it can be resected during the definitive surgical procedure. The accuracy rates of needle biopsies, however, have not been universally reproduced in all centers and are very pathologist dependent. Therefore biopsies of most bone lesions should be performed using an open, incisional approach because it is more accurate and allows more tissue to be obtained, ensuring an adequate specimen for histologic staining or other diagnostic procedures.

Finally, sound closure should be performed only after meticulous hemostasis is obtained. Formation of extensive hematoma after biopsy of a malignant lesion contaminates all tissues in contact with the hematoma, and the exposed area should be resected at the time of definite procedure. An extensive hematoma that forms after an incisional biopsy of a malignant lesion can convert a limb-salvage procedure into an amputation. A drain should be left within the wound if complete hemostasis cannot be obtained; the drain should be brought out in line with the skin incision no further than 1 cm from the wound apex. The drain exit site should then be resected at the time of the definitive procedure along with the biopsy tract. A cortical window must at times be made to biopsy an intraosseous lesion. Hemostasis can then be obtained with a small plug of polymethylmethacrylate (PMMA) cement. The superficial aspect of the wound should be thoroughly irrigated before closure, and any remaining tumor debris should be removed.

CURETTAGE

Surgical treatment for most benign tumors generally consists of curettage of the lesion. Traditionally this has been accomplished with a hand-held curette, but more recently surgeons have performed "extended curettage" by utilizing high-speed burrs. The burring should be completely performed in a systematic manner to ensure that the lesion is resected completely from all sides of the cavity (Figure 131-15). Alternating burring with pulse lavage irrigation in conjunction with use of a head lamp allows excellent visualization of the cavity. Removing a bone lesion in this fashion still results in an intralesional margin from an oncologic standpoint. The rates for local recurrence tend to be less when this technique is employed.[50] It is mandatory in any bone curettage procedure that the entire cavity be inspected to remove all visible tumor. This requires the creation of an adequate cortical window. Fear or reluctance to create such a window may severely compromise the curettage and result in an early local recurrence. Visualization can at times be facilitated with use of a dental mirror.

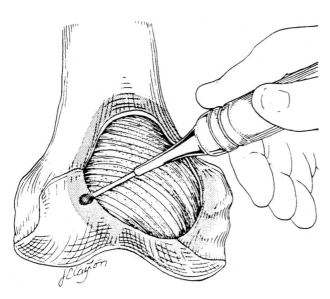

Figure 131-15. Diagram shows the method of extended curettage in which the margin of the curettage cavity is meticulously burred in a systematic fashion. (From Wilkens RM, et al: *Orthopedics* 15:704, 1992.)

Curettage is often supplemented with surgical adjuvant therapy, especially in cases of giant cell tumor. The adjuvant most commonly employed is PMMA. It is believed that this compound assists with local control by extending "tumor kill" through the heat of polymerization and by a direct cytotoxic effect of the monomer.[50] An added benefit of this material is that it provides immediate stabilization of the skeletal defect. Other advantages of cementation over bone grafting are that immobilization time is minimized and local recurrences are readily detectable around the radiographically opaque bone cement.

Liquid nitrogen has also been used as a surgical adjuvant. The liquid, at −196° C, is either poured or sprayed into the surgical defect. The defect is thawed with warmed saline and the process is repeated two more times for a total of three freeze/thaw cycles. Cell death is mediated through thermal, mechanical, and biochemical mechanisms. Liquid nitrogen achieves a margin of necrosis of 7 to 12 mm and is often used in conjunction with PMMA cement.[1] It is typically reserved for the treatment of recurrent lesions or aggressive stage 3 lesions that have a significant local recurrence rate and an increased secondary fracture rate after treatment. Other agents such as phenol and hydrogen peroxide are less commonly used.

Curettage is most commonly followed by packing the cavity with a cancellous bone graft as the method of skeletal reconstruction. It is very important to keep the bone graft harvest site free from tumor contamination. A totally separate set of instruments should be used, and all involved surgeons and scrub personnel should change gowns and gloves before working in the donor-site area.

Iliac crest autograft is considered to be the "gold standard" by which all other forms of graft material are judged. The patient with an autologous bone graft often achieves excellent results; however, the procedure requires an additional incision to harvest the graft. This is not only costly and time consuming, but also uncomfortable for the patient. In many instances, the iliac crest bone graft–harvesting site is more painful after surgery than the area into which the graft is placed.

The second most common bone graft used is allograft bone obtained from a bone bank. This material achieves less favorable results than an autologous bone graft but it is readily available and is often used to supplement autologous bone grafts when there is insufficient bone available to be harvested from the patient. There are concerns, however, regarding quality control of bone banks; *all* allograft bone should be obtained from a bone bank approved by the American Association of Tissue Banks. The remote possibility of viral disease transmission, including hepatitis C and acquired immunodeficiency syndrome (AIDS), is also of concern, although the risk is actually quite low because of sophisticated testing procedures.

The third alternative for a bone graft is the use of artificial substitutes. The three types of substitutes currently available in the United States are a coral-based product (Pro Osteon), a calcium sulfate material (Osteoset), and a demineralized human bone collagen product (Grafton). The first two substitutes provide an osteoconductive matrix on which bone can grow, but Pro Osteon remains unremodeled within the body and both have no osteoinductive capabilities. The third substitute has osteoinductive capabilities and will remodel.

Many metastatic carcinoma lesions that cause structural deficiencies to bone can be treated with curettage and cementation combined with internal fixation. Renal cell carcinoma and thyroid carcinoma both have a notorious reputation for extensive bleeding. Preoperative embolization is therefore performed to minimize intraoperative blood loss. During curettage and prophylactic internal fixation, these lesions will often continue to bleed excessively until the entire lesion is curetted from the bone. Stopping to pack and apply pressure to these wounds only results in further blood loss; once the curettage is begun, it should be completed as rapidly as possible. In general, bone grafting is contraindicated with metastatic lesions because most patients will receive postoperative radiation that will inhibit incorporation of the graft.

RESECTION/AMPUTATION

Most malignant bone tumors and some stage 3 benign aggressive bone tumors should be treated with resection or amputation. Most primary malignant bone tumors are metaphyseal in location and such resections usually require sacrifice of the adjacent joint. This naturally adds to the complexity of any reconstructive procedure. There are three components or phases to any limb-salvage procedure: tumor resection, skeletal reconstruction, and soft tissue reconstruction. Each component needs to be successfully completed or failure of the operation is likely. They are equally important and each requires close attention to detail. A surgeon, for example, may adequately resect an osteogenic sarcoma of the proximal tibia and reconstruct the bony defect with an endoprosthesis or an allograft, but he or she may fail to provide adequate soft tissue coverage of the implant. This failure could lead to wound breakdown, infection, and subsequent amputation. Alternatively, an elegant skeletal and soft tissue reconstruction can be performed after an inadequate oncologic procedure, which leads to disseminated disease and death. In this case, the surgeon salvages the limb, but at a significant price to the patient.

Phase One: Tumor Resection

The incisional biopsy tract should be completely excised at the time of resection and should include any tissue exposed at the time of biopsy. Any muscle group involved with tumor should also be removed with the surgery, and the resection plan should be through entirely normal tissue outside the reactive zone (i.e., wide margins). A greater margin of normal tissue must be resected with high-grade malignancies because these lesions often have microscopic fingerlike projections or small satellite areas extending radially from the primary tumor mass that cannot be grossly identified at the time of excision. Neoadjuvant chemotherapy or radiation administered before surgery often causes significant necrosis of the tumor mass and allows maturation of the reactive zone and some encapsulation

of the tumor mass. Most bone sarcomas shrink significantly with chemotherapy, which facilitates resection. In addition, neoadjuvant therapy may cause necrosis of the peripheral tumor projections, permitting less aggressive margins of normal tissue to be taken at the time of resection.

Amputations are still performed for 10% of patients with bone sarcomas of the extremities, when there is extensive neurovascular involvement or when resection would leave a functionally useless extremity. It is important to realize that an ablative procedure does not guarantee a wide or radical margin. Amputation often does not significantly improve surgical margins when there is involvement of the pelvic or shoulder girdle because of multiple adjacent neurovascular and visceral structures.

Phase Two: Skeletal Reconstruction

Large skeletal defects may be reconstructed by several different modalities. There is presently considerable controversy among orthopedic oncologists with regard to the optimal method of skeletal reconstruction in various anatomic locations. Obviously, with such a lack of consensus, it is clear that good and poor results can be obtained with any of these modalities. The selection of any skeletal reconstructive procedure should be based on the experience of the surgeon, the availability of the reconstructive materials, and the expectations of the patient.

Current modalities for skeletal reconstruction include Van Ness rotation arthroplasty, endoprosthetic replacement, osteoarticular allografts, allograft/prosthetic composites, and creation of a pseudarthrosis.

VAN NESS ROTATION ARTHROPLASTY. The Van Ness rotation arthroplasty is in some ways a bridge between an amputation and a limb-salvage procedure. It is most often employed for tumors about the distal femur. It involves en bloc resection of the distal femur, shortening the extremity, turning the foot 180 degrees, and performing osteosynthesis of the tibia to the remaining femur (Figure 131-16). In this fashion, the triceps surae acts as a quadriceps mechanism, and the ankle joint acts as a knee joint. The patient is then fitted with a special prosthesis for ambulation. The function of patients treated in this manner is similar to a below-the-knee amputation and is quite superior to that of patients with conventional above-knee amputations. This procedure is more widely employed in Europe than in North America, mostly because of psychosocial concerns regarding the appearance of the extremity after such a procedure.

ENDOPROSTHETIC REPLACEMENT. Currently the most common form of skeletal reconstruction involves the insertion of an endoprosthesis fabricated of metal and polyethylene plastic. These implants generally have long intramedullary stems that are fixed to the host bone with PMMA cement. The "working" end of the implant is then designed to replace the involved joint that was sacrificed as part of the tumor resection. The knee, hip, and shoulder joints are most commonly replaced. Initially these implants were fashioned on a custom basis. They have largely been replaced by modular systems that

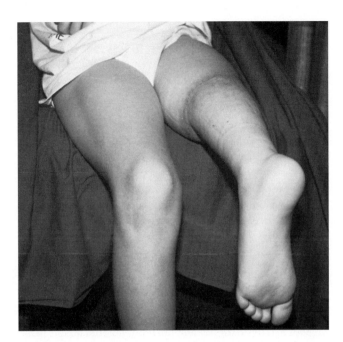

Figure 131-16. An 11-year-old boy with a well-healed Van Ness rotational arthroplasty.

are less expensive and more versatile. These implants can be assembled in the operating room and allow accurate restoration of limb length even if additional bone resection is required. These modular implants generally have an intramedullary component, an articular component, and one or more intercalary components. These implants allow joint motion and are generally well accepted and preferred by patients who desire a functional articulation. Endoprostheses have the distinct advantage of being readily stable at the time of implantation allowing more aggressive weight bearing as tolerated and physical therapy immediately after surgery.

The associated rate of infection with endoprosthetic replacement is only about 2% to 3%. The major concern regarding their use is their long-term durability. Implant loosening and breakage are of major concern. Malawer and Associates, however, have recently demonstrated the ability of these implants to survive the remaining life of patients who have high-grade sarcomas. The 5-year functional survival rate of these implants is approximately 80%, with a 10-year survival rate of about 60%.[33] Clearly, patients who are cured of their tumor will outlive these prostheses, requiring multiple revision procedures.

OSTEOARTICULAR ALLOGRAFTS. Osteoarticular allografts with articular cartilage cryopreserved in glycerol have been widely used to reconstruct skeletal defects. Donors are rigorously tested for syphilis, hepatitis, human immunodeficiency virus (HIV), and other infectious diseases, but viral transmission remains a concern, and there have been documented cases of both hepatitis C and HIV transmission with implanted allografts. Allografts preserved in this manner are fixed to the host bone with some form of osteosynthesis, and a ligamentous reconstruction is then performed, as seen in the proximal humeral allograft in Figure 131-17. The grafts allow

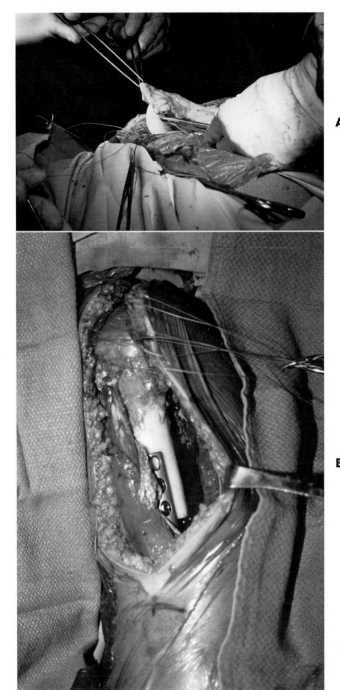

Figure 131-17. A, This proximal humeral osteoarticular allograft was fixed to the host bone with a locked intramedullary rod. The photo illustrates the meticulous repair of the rotator cuff tendons to tendons on the graft. **B,** The graft is further stabilized to the host bone with a small-fragment titanium plate. The rotator-cuff repair is completed, and the long head of the biceps has been tenodesed to the soft tissues on the allograft.

joint motion, and excellent functional results have been obtained. Joint stability, however, is less reliable than with prosthetic reconstruction. Additional problems associated with osteoarticular allografts include fracture and infection. Fractures through these allografts can be treated by traditional means, but occasionally require removal of the graft and reconstruction.

Infection rates of 15% to 20% have been reported with allografts, which generally mandates removal of the graft.[30] Salvage of the extremity is difficult and time consuming in this setting. The advantage of using an osteoarticular allograft is that it allows ligament and muscle attachment, which can improve function, especially about the knee and hip. Allografts perform better after resection of low-grade malignant tumors in which chemotherapy or radiation, which both delay graft union, will not play a role in the patient's management.

ALLOGRAFT/PROSTHETIC COMPOSITE. A combination of an allograft and endoprosthesis can be utilized at times to perform a skeletal reconstruction. Proponents of this method believe it combines the superior stability and joint function of a prosthesis with the allograft advantage of replacing bone stock. The inherent shortcomings of these two modalities—prosthetic loosening, fracture, infection, and nonunion—are not eliminated when they are used in combination. Superior results can be achieved with this method, and the proximal femur is a common site (Figure 131-18).[18]

INTERCALARY RECONSTRUCTION. An intercalary reconstruction is required in those cases in which the adjacent joint is not sacrificed as part of the tumor resection. Such a reconstruction can be accomplished by inserting an allograft or metallic implant. The allograft can be secured with an intramedullary rod or plates. The endoprosthesis can be secured with PMMA. Excellent results are generally obtained with either method.

JOINT ARTHRODESIS. Resection followed by arthrodesis plays an important role the treatment of patients who require extensive muscle resection or a strong, durable reconstruction without the worry of loosening. In patients who require strength and stability of the affected joint, an arthrodesis may be the reconstructive procedure of choice. However, stability is achieved at the expense of mobility. The arthrodesis can be achieved by application of internal fixation and massive bone

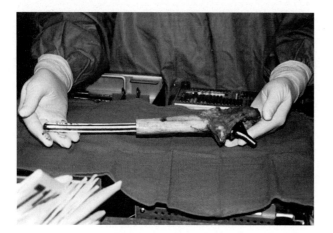

Figure 131-18. Allograft prosthesis composites are most commonly used to reconstruct the proximal femur. The long-stem hip prosthesis is cemented into the allograft on the back table.

grafts. Union of the bone graft to host bone can, at times, be difficult. An arthrodesis in certain circumstances will suit the lifestyle and expectation of the patient, minimizing the risk of subsequent revision procedures.[42]

CREATION OF A PSEUDOARTHROSIS. Occasionally, the amount of bone resection necessary to achieve an adequate oncologic margin is so extensive that an adequate skeletal reconstruction cannot be achieved. A pseudoarthrosis of the affected joint can be achieved in such cases by immobilizing the joint for approximately 6 weeks. Patients will have varied degrees of motion, stability, and pain. In general, this is not a satisfactory reconstructive procedure. It is used more often after extensive pelvic resections that involve removal of the entire innominate bone.

Phase Three: Soft Tissue Reconstruction

The aim of soft tissue reconstruction in limb-salvage cases is to provide adequate soft tissue coverage over the implant or allograft and to maximize limb function. Inadequate soft tissue coverage over an implant can lead to wound breakdown, infection, and perhaps amputation. Appropriate muscle transfer can not only provide coverage but can also contribute dynamic joint stabilization and substitute for muscle function lost as a result of tumor resection.

LOCAL MUSCLE TRANSFERS. Resection of stage IIB extracompartmental tumors often requires extensive muscle resection and subsequent soft tissue coverage procedures at the time of reconstruction. Anterior transposition of the hamstrings can assist with active knee extension in limb-salvage procedures about the knee when the quadricep muscles have been sacrificed. The gastrocnemius flap is also helpful in providing anterior leg coverage around the knee after both distal femoral and proximal tibial resections.[26] The patellar tendon can also be secured to the muscle to help reconstruct the extensor mechanism of the knee. The pectoralis major as well as the latissimus dorsi muscles can be utilized for dynamic stabilization in limb-salvage procedures about the shoulder. Intraoperative decisions must be made to select the appropriate muscle for transfer based on the extent of the tumor resection, but careful preoperative planning can provide a general plan for reconstruction that can be modified as necessary.

OBLITERATION OF DEAD SPACE. Obliteration of dead space created by tumor resection is a significant challenge that must be met to maximize the results of limb-salvage procedures. A large surgical defect will often be left after en bloc tumor resection. Vital structures, such as vessels, nerves, bone, and implants, may be exposed over long segments. Simple closure of the overlying skin may often lead to seroma formation and infection. Skin necrosis will also lead to exposure of these structures. Rotational muscle flaps or free vascularized muscle flaps are often used to fill these soft tissue defects. Skin grafts or myocutaneous flaps are also employed to provide adequate coverage.

There are certain oncologic concerns regarding the use of free vascularized flaps or even rotational flaps in limb-salvage procedures. Contamination of the donor site is foremost among these concerns. The following precautions should be observed to minimize the risk of contamination:

1. A separate set of instruments should be used to harvest the graft
2. The operating team should change gowns and gloves after tumor resection and skeletal reconstruction
3. Two teams should be utilized if possible with separate sets of instruments
4. The surgical defect should be covered while the graft is being harvested
5. Movement of the surgeon between donor and recipient sites should be avoided

If a free tissue transfer or rotational flap has been performed in a limb-salvage procedure, the donor site must be followed carefully for tumor recurrence. The donor site should be staged and evaluated not only with physical examination, but also with appropriate imaging studies. Any suspicious lesions should be biopsied.

We have now performed 50 free vascularized or rotational muscle flaps as part of limb-salvage procedures for musculoskeletal sarcomas. We have experienced two instances of donor-site contamination and tumor development despite following the appropriate precautions. Many of these procedures could not have been successfully completed without the use of these flaps, and therefore many amputations would have been required. We believe that the small risk of donor-site contamination is not a contradiction to the use of immediate free tissue transfers or rotational flaps in limb-salvage procedures for treatment of musculoskeletal sarcomas. Adherence to the above-noted precautions is mandatory when such soft tissue transfers are to be utilized.

OUTCOMES

CURETTAGE

The majority of benign intraosseous tumors treated with curettage and subsequent bone grafting versus cementation have excellent functional results. The actual functional outcome of any given case will depend on the type of lesion, its biological behavior, and, most importantly, the exact anatomic site and the degree of bone destruction present at the time of diagnosis and treatment. The articular surfaces are generally left intact with curettage procedures, and joint function approaches normal. Minor decreases in joint range of motion that are not functionally significant are the most common sequelae of these procedures. Nine patients treated for tumors about the knee with curettage, cryosurgery, and cementation all had excellent functional results according to the rating systems of the MSTS and the Hospital for Special Surgery.[1,14] There is an increased incidence of postoperative pathologic

fracture (22%) when cryosurgery with liquid nitrogen is used, which is probably related to the additional bone necrosis that occurs at the periphery of the curettage. Cryosurgery also has an increased risk of wound-healing difficulties (5% to 10%).

RESECTIONS

The outcome of resection procedures varies greatly with the size and location of the lesion. Patients with larger lesions that require resection of more soft tissue tend to have a less functional result. Multiple studies have documented the psychologic and functional benefit of limb-salvage procedures over amputations. Compartmental resections have previously had complication rates far above those of standard orthopedic procedures. Over the last 10 years, however, there has been much greater emphasis on the use of local soft tissue rotation flaps to provide soft tissue coverage for metallic prostheses and/or allograft and hardware reconstructions. The placement of soft tissue coverage allows wound closure without significant tension and prevents the marginal necrosis of the wound that was previously so common. Flap coverage has dramatically reduced the rate of infection and wound dehiscence, but the overall complication rate remains substantially higher than for more conventional orthopedic procedures.

Proximal femoral prostheses have reported survival rates of 88% at 10 years, and allograft prosthetic composites have shown survival advantages in direct comparison studies.[49,52] Bone resorption at the prosthesis-bone interface occurs secondary to stress shielding in approximately half of the cases involving femurs. It has not, however, been associated with future aseptic loosening. Instability with these reconstructions is a problem, but the dislocation rate of 2% to 14% can be minimized by using a bipolar component rather than acetabular resurfacing. In addition, the rate of acetabular component loosening has been reported to be as high as 46% of cases in short-term studies. Functional outcome of these reconstructions is variable and depends primarily on the function of the abductor muscles. Excellent or good results can be achieved in 50% to 60% of cases.

Distal femoral reconstruction using endoprostheses has achieved unparalleled success. Functional evaluations have revealed 70% to 90% good or excellent results, and complication rates of infection and fracture are far below those for allografts or composite reconstructions. Stem fatigue failures have been virtually eliminated with the use of stronger alloy metals. Polyethylene bushing failure remains a persistent late problem; however, this complication is usually easily rectified.[6] Aseptic loosening will continue to be the major problem facing young patients who survive their oncologic disease.

Proximal tibial reconstructions continue to be limited functionally by poor reconstruction of the extensor mechanism. Reconstruction with medial gastrocnemius muscle flap transfer is probably the most reliable method of reconstruction and also assists with prosthesis coverage and wound healing.[25] Use of Dacron tape to suture the residual patellar tendon to the prosthesis is inferior to the gastrocnemius transfer and commonly results in patella alta with a severe extensor lag. Proximal tibial replacements are functionally the worst of the major reconstructive sites.[33]

Function after proximal humeral replacement is highly dependent on deltoid muscle function. The prosthesis acts more as a passive spacer than a shoulder joint without the axillary nerve and deltoid muscle function. Elbow and hand function in these cases remains virtually normal. Stability can be obtained by joint reconstruction using Gortex grafts or Mersilene mesh. Malawer and Chou[33] have reported a "stable-unstable" reconstruction method that has achieved the best functional results of any of the reconstruction sites. These functional results, however, have not been duplicated by all major centers.

In general, osteoarticular allografts have not achieved the functional results and success of prosthetic replacement. Some isolated allografts have lasted over 10 years; however, the majority continue to fail either through infection or fracture after 4 to 5 years. The infection rate after an allograft implantation is higher than that of a prostheses alone, probably secondary to the additional operative time required for allograft implantation.[30] The current infection rate of prosthetic implantation is approximately 5% to 10%. There is also a greater than 15% nonunion rate at the allograft host junctions.[46] Iliac crest bone grafting of the junction is indicated if a radiographic union is not achieved within 1 year after surgery. The patient is not allowed to be fully weight bearing during this time because the junction between host and allograft bone has not completely healed. Thus the morbidity from allograft procedures is much longer than that of metal prosthetic implants, which are immediately stable. Unfortunately, the majority of patients receiving endoprostheses are quite young, and if they survive their disease they will require prosthesis longevity far beyond 10 years. The need for durable reconstructive options becomes even more critical as the survival rate for patients with bone sarcomas increases. Revision procedures are often not as durable as the original reconstruction and therefore these patients will require multiple operative procedures over their lifetime.

REFERENCES

1. Aboulafia AJ, Rosenbaum DH, Sicard-Rosenbaum L, et al: Treatment of large subchondral tumors of the knee with cryosurgery and composite reconstruction, *Clin Orthop* 307: 189-199, 1994.
2. Bacci G, Picci P, Maurizio O, et al: Prognostic value of serum alkaline phosphatase in osteosarcoma, *Tumori* 73:331-336, 1987.
3. Bednar M, Weiland A, Light T: Osteoid osteoma of the upper extremity, *Hand Clin* 11:211-221, 1995.
4. Burgess RC: Physeal osteochondroma of a phalanx, *South Med J* 83:1087, 1990.
5. Capanna R, Betteli G, Biagini R, et al: Aneurysmal cysts of long bones, *Ital J Orthop Traumatol* XI:421-429, 1985.
6. Capanna R, Morris HG, Campanacci D, et al: Modular uncemented prosthetic reconstruction after resection of tumours of the distal femur, *J Bone Joint Surg* 76B:178-186, 1994.
7. Dahlin DC: *Bone tumors: general aspects and data on 6221 cases,* ed 3, Springfield, Ill, 1978, Charles C. Thomas, pp 156-175.
8. Dahlin DC: Giant-cell-bearing lesions of bone of the hands, *Hand Clin* 3:291-297, 1987.
9. Dahlin DC, Unni KK: *Bone tumors,* ed 4, Springfield, Ill, 1986, Charles C. Thomas.
10. Eilber F, Guiliano A, Eckardt J, et al: Adjuvant chemotherapy for osteosarcoma: a randomized prospective trial, *J Clin Oncol* 5:21-26, 1987.
11. Enneking WF: *Musculoskeletal tumor surgery,* New York, 1983, Churchill Livingstone.
12. Enneking WF, Gearen PF: Fibrous dysplasia of the femoral neck, *J Bone Joint Surg* 68A:1415-1422, 1986.
13. Enneking WF, Spanier SS, Goodman MA: The surgical staging of musculoskeletal sarcoma, *Clin Orthop* 153:106-119, 1980.
14. Enneking WF, Dunham W, Gebhardt MC, et al: A system for the functional evaluation of reconstructive procedures after surgical treatment of tumors of the musculoskeletal system, *Clin Orthop* 286:241-246, 1993.
15. Frasicca F, Waltrip R, Sponseller P, et al: Clinicopathologic features and treatment of osteoid osteomas and osteoblastomas in children and adolescents, *Orthop Clin North Am* 27:559-574, 1996.
16. Garrison RC, Unni KK, Mc Leod RA, et al: Chondrosarcoma arising in osteochondroma, *Cancer* 49:1890-1897, 1982.
17. Gherlinzoni F, Rock M, Pieci P: Chondromyxoid fibroma, *J Bone Joint Surg* 65A:198-204, 1983.
18. Gitelis S, Piasecki P: Allograft prosthetic arthroplasty for osteosarcoma and other aggressive bone tumors, *Clin Orthop* 270:197-201, 1991.
19. Giudici MA, Moser RP Jr, Kransdorf MJ: Cartilaginous bone tumors, *Radiol Clin North Am* 31:237-259, 1993.
20. Healy JH, Bass D: Radiation and pagetic osteogenic sarcoma, *Clin Orthop* 270:128-134, 1991.
21. Horowitz SM, Lane JM, Healey JH: Soft-tissue management with prosthetic replacement for sarcomas around the knee, *Clin Orthop* 275:226-231, 1992.
22. Huvos AG: Osteochondromas and enchondromas. In Huvos AG (editor): *Bone tumors: diagnosis, treatment, and prognosis,* Philadelphia, 1979, WB Saunders.
23. Huvos AG, Rosen G, Dabska M, et al: Mesenchymal chondrosarcoma: a clinicopathologic analysis of 35 patients with emphasis on treatment, *Cancer* 51:1230-1237, 1983.
24. Jaffe HL, Lichtenstein L: Chondromyxoid fibroma of bone, *Arch Pathol* 45:541-551, 1948.
25. Jaureguito JW, DuBois CM, Smith SR, et al: Medial gastrocnemius transpositin flap for the treatment of disruption of the extensor mechanism after total knee arthroplasty, *J Bone Joint Surg* 79A:866-873, 1997.
26. Kotz R: Rotationplasty, *Semin Surg Oncol* 13:34-40, 1997.
27. Kuur E, Hansen SL, Lindequiest S: Treatment of solitary enchondromas in fingers, *J Hand Surg* 14B:109-112, 1989.
28. Lichenstein L: *Bone tumors,* ed 4, St. Louis, 1972, Mosby.

29. Link MP, Goorin AM, Miser AW, et al: The effect of adjuvant chemotherapy on relapse-free survival in patients with osteosarcoma of the extremity, *N Engl J Med* 314:1600-1606, 1986.

30. Lord CF, Gebhardt MC, Tomford WW, et al: Infection in bone allografts: incidence, nature, and treatment, *J Bone Joint Surg* 70:369-376, 1988.

31. Luck JV Jr, Luck JV, Schwinn CP: Parosteal osteosarcoma: a treatment oriented study, *Clin Orthop* 153:92-105, 1980.

32. Magre GR, Menendez LR: Preoperative CT localization and marking of osteoid osteoma: description of a new technique, *J Comput Assist Tomogr* 20:526-529, 1996.

33. Malawer MM, Chou LB: Prosthetic survival and clinical results with use of large segment replacements in the treatment of high-grade bone sarcomas, *J Bone Joint Surg* 77A:1154-1165, 1995.

34. Mankin HJ, Lange TA, Spanier SS: The hazards of biopsy in patients with malignant primary bone and soft-tissue tumors, *J Bone Joint Surg* 64A:1123-1127, 1982.

35. Marsh BW, Bonfiglio M, Brady LP, et al: Benign osteoblastoma: range of manifestations, *J Bone Joint Surg* 57A:1-9, 1975.

36. McGrath BE, Bush CH, Nelson TE, Scarborough MT: Evaluation of suspected osteoid osteoma, *Clin Orthop* 327:247-252, 1996.

37. Mirra JM: *Bone tumors: clinical, radiological, and pathologic correlations,* Philadelphia, 1989, Lea & Febiger, p 534.

38. Oppenheim W, Galleno H: Operative treatment versus steroid injection in the management of unicameral bone cysts, *J Pediatr Orthop* 4:1-7, 1984.

39. Ozaki T, Hillmann A, Hoffmann C, et al: Significance of surgical margin on the prognosis of patients with Ewing's sarcoma, *Cancer* 78:892, 1996.

40. Putnam M, Cohen M: Malignant bony tumors of the upper extremity, *Hand Clin* 11:265-286, 1995.

41. Rosenthal DI, Alexander A, Rosenburg AE, et al: Ablation of osteoid osteomas with a percutaneously placed electrode: a new procedure, *Musculoskeletal Radiology* 183:29-33, 1992.

42. Scarborough MT, Helmstedter CS: Arthrodesis after resection of bone tumors, *Semin Surg Oncol* 13:25-33, 1997.

43. Shapiro F: Ollier's disease: an assessment of angular deformity, shortening, and pathologic fracture in twenty-one patients, *J Bone Joint Surg* 64A:95-103, 1982.

44. Sheth DS, Yasko AW, Johnson ME, et al: Chondrosarcoma of the pelvis: prognostic factors for 67 patients treated with definitive surgery, *Cancer* 78:745-750, 1996.

45. Simon MA, Aschliman MA, Thomas N, et al: Limb-salvage treatment versus amputation for osteosarcoma of the distal end of the femur, *J Bone Joint Surg* 68:1331-1337, 1986.

46. Toni A, Neff JR, Sudanese A, et al: The role of chemotherapy in patients with nonmetastatic Ewing's sarcoma of the limbs, *Clin Orthop* 286:225-240, 1993.

47. United States Department of Health, Education, and Welfare: *Cancer patient survival report #5,* USDHEW Pub No (NIH), Washington, DC, 1976, pp 77-92.

48. Unni KK, Dahlin DC, Beabout JW, et al: Chondrosarcoma: clear-cell variant, *J Bone Joint Surg* 58A:676-683, 1976.

49. Unwin PS, Walker PS, Briggs TW, et al: Aseptic loosening in 1001 cases of cemented custom-made bone tumour replacements of the lower limb. In Campanacci M, Capanna R (editors): *Eighth international symposium on limb salvage,* Florence, Italy, 1995, p 47.

50. Willert HG: Clinical results of the temporary acrylic bone cement plug in the treatment of bone tumors: a multicentric study. In Enneking WF (editor): *Limb salvage in musculoskeletal oncology,* New York, 1987, Churchill Livingstone.

51. Williams CL, Busque L, Griffith BB, et al: Langehans' cell histocytosis (Histiocytosis X): a clonal proliferative disease, *N Engl J Med* 331:154-160, 1994.

52. Zehr RJ, Enneking WF, Scarborough MT: Allograft-prosthesis composite vs. megaprosthesis in proximal femoral reconstruction. In Campanacci M, Capanna R (editors): *Eighth international symposium on limb salvage,* Florence, Italy, 1995, p 58.

PART XIII

VASCULAR DISORDERS

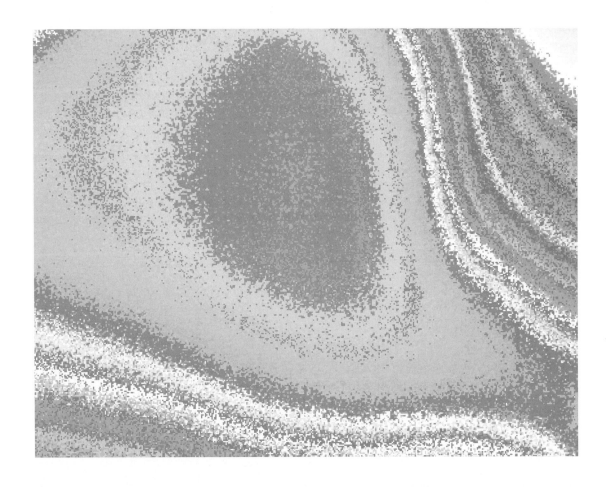

Vascular Injuries and Disorders

C. Lin Puckett
Mark T. Boschert
Matthew J. Concannon

INTRODUCTION

VASCULAR ANATOMY OF THE HAND

The ulnar and radial arteries are the dominant blood supply to the hand. They begin in the proximal forearm at the division of the brachial artery. The radial artery passes the distal end of the radius and runs in a course toward the dorsum of the hand, where it is covered by the tendons of the abductor pollicis longus (APL) and the extensor pollicis brevis (EPB). It then passes deep to the extensor pollicis longus (EPL) tendon to pass through the first dorsal interosseous muscle between the first and second metacarpals, where, in the deep portion of the palm, it ends in the deep volar arch. A volar branch of the radial artery occurs at the level of the styloid process of the radius and courses distally on the abductor pollicis brevis (APB) muscle, where it curves and usually joins the superficial volar arterial arch. This branch supplies the muscles and skin of the thumb.

The ulnar artery enters the hand through Guyon's canal with the ulnar nerve. Guyon's canal is bounded by the hook of the hamate radially and the pisiform ulnarly. The floor of Guyon's canal is formed by the pisohamate ligament; above the artery lies fascial extensions from the flexor carpi ulnaris (FCU), subcutaneous fat, and skin. A deep volar branch of the of the ulnar artery begins near the pisiform bone and then descends between the origin of the flexor digiti quinti brevis (FDQB) and abductor digiti quinti (ADQ) through the origin of the opponens digiti quinti (ODQ). It usually communicates at this point with the deep volar arterial arch. Near this branch, the ulnar artery also branches to the muscles of the hypothenar eminence. The main ulnar artery terminates as the superficial volar arch. This lies just beneath the palmar aponeurosis and communicates radially with the small superficial volar ramus of the radial artery. This classic arterial pattern is seen in Figure 132-1 and has been described in many texts and articles.[15,37] In 1961 Coleman and Anson[15] examined a large series of cadaver hands and defined the most common arterial pattern as consisting of a complete arch, which was found in approximately 79% of their study specimens. The remaining 21% had incomplete arches. Various authors, however, offer differing percentages as to the incidence of the so-called "normal" pattern, and it is appropriate to note that variations are more the rule than the exception. The textbook description of two complete arches with all contributions and branches is actually a relatively rare anatomic pattern.

LACERATIONS

OPERATIONS

Penetration and avulsion injuries to the hand may result in perforation or transection of major vessels, resulting in profuse hemorrhage. Repair of such injuries is required to restore normal blood flow to the hand or digits and to prevent serious blood loss. Transected vessels may be ligated or repaired. Small vessels in the hand and digits are best repaired using microsurgical technique. All transected vessels should be thoroughly debrided and the damaged portion of the vessel excised. Usually some length can be gained by performing a proximal and distal dissection of the vessel ends. The anastomosis should not be performed under extreme tension because this greatly increases the risk of postoperative thrombosis. If there is insufficient length for a primary anastomosis without tension, a vein graft should be used to bridge the gap.

OUTCOMES

The direct repair of a lacerated artery in the arm, hand, or finger is usually associated with a good result, particularly in the larger vessels of the arm. The introduction and wide application of microsurgical techniques have allowed direct repair of vessels at the digital level, with patency rates above

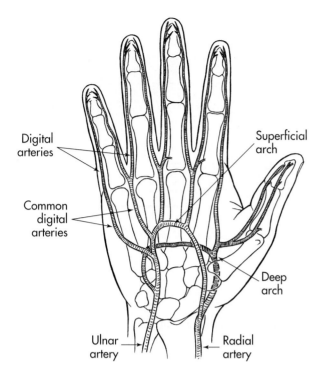

Figure 132-1. The classical arterial pattern of the hand. (From Concannon MJ: *Common hand problems in primary care,* Philadelphia, 1999, Hanley & Belfus, p 7.)

95%. Avulsion injuries that cause damage to long segments of the vessel wall have less reliable patency rates after repair. Stretching the artery causes disruption of the intima both proximal and distal to the actual transection site. Failure to completely debride this damaged section of artery, which must usually be replaced with a vein graft, will almost guarantee thrombosis at the arterial repair. The outcome of arterial repair in avulsion injuries is much poorer than in other vascular trauma because the artery may have internal damage over long segments that is not appreciated at the time of repair.

ANEURYSMS OF THE HAND

True aneurysms are rare occurrences in the hand. The most common etiologies of hand aneurysms are trauma and infection. The most frequent sites of traumatic aneurysms are the thenar and hypothenar eminences and the superficial arch.[57,74] True aneurysms are localized arterial dilations that contain all layers of the vessel wall, including the adventitia, media, and intima. These may be congenital or acquired. Aneurysms of the hand distal to the superficial and deep palmar arches are very rare, although an aneurysm of a common digital artery has been reported.[23] False aneurysms are actually pulsating hematomas and usually occur after a penetrating injury. A

traumatic hematoma surrounds the artery at the perforation site. The hematoma becomes organized, undergoes endothelial ingrowth, and eventually becomes a fibrotic, pulsating mass. Pseudoaneurysms of the radial artery are commonly seen after placement of arterial lines or punctures to obtain blood gas levels.

INDICATIONS

Patients with aneurysms of the hand most frequently complain of a pulsatile mass that may be painful or tender. Symptoms of ischemia may be present. The diagnosis of a hand aneurysm is usually suspected on the basis of physical examination. The mass may have an audible bruit and may decrease in size with proximal occlusion of the vessel. The mass may initially be difficult to differentiate from an infection or a ganglion. A wrist ganglion may pulsate when it is in close proximity to the radial artery. It can be differentiated from a true or pseudoaneurysm by transillumination. Kay et al[38] report two such cases of aneurysm that were initially considered an infection. Arteriosclerotic aneurysms of the hand are extremely rare, but Malt[45] and Thorrens et al[71] have reported cases. Mycotic aneurysms are also rare and may initially present as an infection, followed subsequently by a definitive mass.[4] Regardless of the type of aneurysm, the diagnosis should be supported by vascular studies. Noninvasive studies may be employed if available, but arteriography, coupled with digital subtraction and magnification, remains the gold standard test and provides an invaluable road map for surgical intervention.

OPERATIONS

Indications for surgical excision or repair include the risk of distal embolization, rupture, or expansion of the aneurysm, which would cause pressure on surrounding structures. Once it has been determined that excision of the aneurysm and ligation or repair of the proximal and distal vessel would produce no vascular compromise of the hand, treatment can proceed. Pseudoaneurysms of the wrist are best treated by excision and primary arterial repair. True aneurysms can be excised and the proximal and distal vessel ends ligated if prior clamping of the vessel produces no vascular compromise distally.

OUTCOMES

Russell and Steichen[64] reported a series of radial artery pseudoaneurysms that were resected and repaired with good return of distal blood flow. Rothkopf et al[63] and Harris et al[31] each reported a small series of ulnar artery aneurysms with uniformly good outcomes after resection and selective microvascular reconstruction.

ARTERIOVENOUS FISTULAE

In 1757 Hunter described congenital arteriovenous (AV) fistulae with the characteristic thrill, bruit, pulsations, and vascular dilation of these lesions. These lesions, including the traumatic variety, are rare in the upper extremity, with the exception of high-flow AV malformations.[12,47] Large AV fistulae can shunt a significant volume of blood, resulting in hemodynamic consequences such as high output failure, but this rarely occurs in AV fistulae distal to the elbow.

Szilagyi et al,[69] in a large review of peripheral congenital AV fistulae, found that the great majority became manifest in the first 10 years of life; however, 24% appeared after the age of 20. This delay in appearance may be attributed to persisting fetal vascular connections that were obliterated but later reopened.[36,69] As expected, most traumatic AV fistulae result from penetrating injuries.[47]

INDICATIONS AND OPERATIONS

A history and a physical examination that reveals a palpable mass may suggest an AV fistula. The presence of a thrill, bruit, and pulsatile dilated vessel may clinch the diagnosis, which should be confirmed by arteriography. A positive Branham's sign, with a decrease in the heart rate and elevation of blood pressure by AV fistula occlusion, would not be expected with an AV fistula in the hand. An arteriogram helps delineate the extent of the involvement and serves as a guide for possible surgical treatment. Emile Holman,[35] in the era prior to effective vascular reconstruction, defined the proper treatment of an AV fistula as quadripolar ligation of the feeding vessels. Ligation of the arterial feeding vessels alone may lead to distal gangrene because the collateral arterial flow will continue to feed the lower resistance vessels of the fistula rather than perfuse the more distal tissues. Treatment of the acquired AV fistula may or may not involve resection of the fistula in addition to quadripolar control, but resection is desirable in the case of AV malformations. Arterial reconstruction is indicated if distal blood flow from the artery feeding the malformation is necessary to maintain tissue viability.

OUTCOMES

Congenital AV fistulae of the hand were reviewed by Gelberman et al[24] in 1978 in an attempt to establish a treatment protocol. They found that fistulae with bony involvement were poorly controlled by excision and had a high recurrence rate, whereas lesions that were well-localized to a single vessel and without bony involvement responded well to excision. Diffuse digital masses with extensive involvement of the palm and adjacent digits also responded poorly to simple excision. Amputation of the affected digit

or ray along with excision of any adjacent mass was the procedure of choice in patients with intraosseous involvement or significantly decreased distal blood flow. Surgical excision was used only as a last resort in patients who had diffuse fistulae with involvement of more than one digit and with more proximal vessel dilation.

OBSTRUCTIVE DISORDERS

EMBOLI

Indications and Operations

Arterial emboli to the upper extremity are caused by either cardiac or proximal artery pathology. Cardiac causes include an arrhythmia or left-sided cardiac valvular disease that produces a mural thrombus. A proximal arterial lesion, such as an atherosclerotic plaque, a blunt or penetrating trauma, or an AV fistula can produce distal embolization of clot or arterial wall fragments. A proximal aneurysm may also produce solid elements that can embolize distally. Patients with a diseased mitral or aortic valve can develop mural thrombi or plaques that can loosen and be "showered" downstream. Severe or prolonged cardiac arrhythmia may allow blood to become stationary within the heart, forming a thrombus that can then be propagated downstream, usually when normal sinus rhythm is restored. Seventeen percent of all cardiogenic emboli involve the upper extremity, with occlusion of larger proximal vessels (10% subclavian, 22% axillary, and 64% brachial).[4,76]

Noncardiogenic emboli in the upper extremity usually lodge in the palmar arch or in digital vessels and less frequently in the ulnar or radial arteries.[76] The diagnosis is suspected by the presence of distal ischemia and confirmed by the characteristic appearance of emboli on arteriogram, which usually shows multiple filling defects (Figure 132-2). The arteriogram may also identify the proximal lesion responsible for the embolus. Treatment of upper-extremity emboli is aimed at elimination of the source and addressing the ischemic sequelae of the emboli.[76] Cardiogenic sources may require treatment by a cardiologist and/or cardiac surgeon, whereas proximal arterial lesions often require excision and vascular repair. Retrievable emboli may occasionally be removed using microvascular surgical techniques, and there may be a role for clot-lysing drugs such as urokinase or streptokinase. Heparin remains a mainstay of therapy.

Outcomes

Treatment of emboli begins with eliminating the source. The final outcome in these cases depends on the degree of tissue lost secondary to ischemia from the emboli. Those patients who present with multiple emboli and diffuse areas of ischemia will obviously have a worse outcome than those who present earlier with less ischemic injury. The goal is to establish a diagnosis and to treat the problem before massive or prolonged embolization causes distal tissue necrosis and permanent injury.

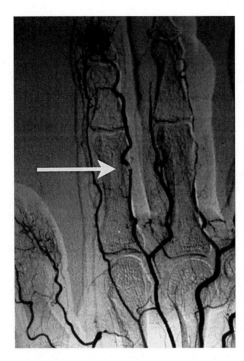

Figure 132-2. This arteriogram shows an embolus lodged within the digital artery seen at the point of the arrow.

THROMBOSIS

Ulnar artery thrombosis was first recorded by Von Rosen[75] in 1934. The etiology of this condition was blunt injury to the palm of the hand. In 1970 Conn et al[16] coined the term *hypothenar hammer syndrome* to describe ulnar artery thrombosis within the Guyon's canal, and they believed that repetitive trauma was the most common cause. Numerous reports have identified activities such as baseball, handball, and hockey, and the use of vibrating power tools as a causative agent.[6,16] An important contributing factor seems to be the use of tobacco products. The anatomic position of the ulnar artery in Guyon's canal certainly predisposes it to contusion when the heel of the hand is repeatedly driven against a firm object. The condition is therefore common in males engaged in manual labor, such as a mechanic or builder who occasionally uses the ulnar side of the hand as a hammer to turn a wrench or strike a board.

Indications

The most common presenting symptoms of ulnar artery thrombosis are hand pain, cold intolerance, and numbness, usually in the ulnar digits. There is usually a history of repetitive mild hand trauma. Physical signs of vascular insufficiency may be present and even small distal trophic ulcers in chronic cases. Ulnar nerve irritation may be demonstrated in Guyon's canal, and a Tinel's sign may be elicited. The diagnosis can be confirmed by a positive Allen's test or Doppler examination, in which occlusion of the ulnar artery can be indicated by manually occluding the radial artery.[40] The diagnosis is further refined by arteriography to define the limits and exact location of the occlusion.

Operations

Preventive measures should obviously be considered for workers and athletes whose hands are more subject to repetitive trauma.[6] Conservative treatment for patients with existing cases consists of cessation of nicotine products and limiting exposure to cold. Surgery is indicated if these measures do not provide relief. In 1937, Leriche[42] reported his experience with excision of the ulnar artery occlusion in a concept analogous to his treatment of aortoiliac insufficiency. The resultant localized sympathectomy was believed to be important in accomplishing vascular dilation and improved collateral flow. In 1964 Koman[40] advocated the use of microvascular arterial reconstruction of the artery and local and regional sympathectomy. Most authors now believe that resection of the thrombosed segment, with the resultant localized sympathectomy, is an integral component of therapy, regardless of whether reconstruction of the vessel is accomplished.[27]

Hypothenar hammer syndrome is certainly the most common and best understood example of vascular thrombosis in the hand, but occlusion of the radial artery can also cause symptoms. A common cause of radial artery thrombosis is iatrogenic injury that occurs during cannulation of the artery for arterial pressure monitoring or blood sampling. These cases can have devastating sequelae when inadequate evaluation before the cannulation failed to reveal a preexisting ulnar artery occlusion or inadequate hand perfusion from the ulnar artery alone. A properly performed Allen's test should eliminate this problem, but patients with radial artery thrombosis can be symptomatic even in the face of a patent ulnar artery, and a therapeutic approach analogous to that adopted for ulnar artery thrombosis may be required.[40,59] Restoration of blood flow by excision of the thrombosed segment and direct repair or the use of a venous interpositional graft may be required to restore distal blood flow. Less common causes of arteriothrombosis, such as atherosclerosis, have been reported, but are rare.[7,14,70]

Digital ischemia secondary to thrombosis of a persistent median artery has been described by Aulicino.[3] He reports that a persistent median artery is involved with the superficial palmar arch in 1.1% to 16.1% of these cases. Thrombosis of this median artery has also been documented as a cause of carpal tunnel syndrome.[46]

Outcomes

In 1978 Given et al[27] compared patients treated predominantly with a sympathectomy approach with those in whom arterial reconstruction was also employed. This study concluded that arterial reconstruction plus sympathectomy offered a significantly improved outcome over sympathectomy alone. Therefore most hand surgeons today would advocate not only resection of the thrombosed segment with its attendant localized sympathectomy but also vascular reconstruction, as long as adequate runoff allows a reasonable opportunity for maintenance of patency (Figure 132-3).

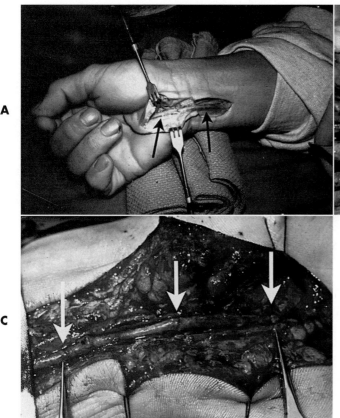

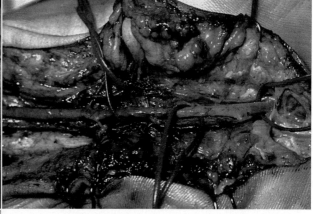

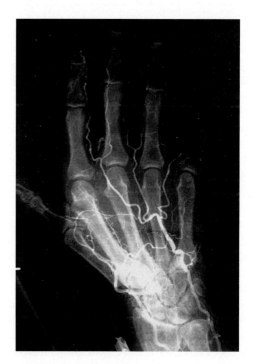

Figure 132-3. **A,** The thrombosed ulnar artery is indicated by the arrows. **B,** The ulnar artery is isolated and is seen surrounded by vessel loops. **C,** The thrombosed segment of artery has been replaced with a vein graft, indicated by the white arrows. The anastomoses are seen at the points of the jeweler's forceps.

BUERGER'S DISEASE

Indications

Buerger's disease, or thromboangiitis obliterans, has been defined as an idiopathic, segmental, inflammatory, and recurrent occlusive disease that primarily affects the small or medium-sized arteries and veins of the extremities (Figure 132-4). This disease was first described by Buerger in 1908 and is seen primarily in the extremities of young male smokers.[39,48] The pathogenesis is not completely known, although in 1983 Adar[2] described cellular and humoral immune reactivity to collagen in a high percentage of patients with Buerger's disease. Classically, Buerger's disease begins before the age of 40. Its first clinical manifestations are trophic changes followed by spontaneous ischemic pain at rest and venous thrombosis. This venous thrombosis is often superficial, but can be quite profound in some cases.[73]

Persistent evolution of the disease was observed in a review by Van der Stricht et al[73] of patients who continued to smoke and was characterized by a progressive inflammatory invasion of the distal arteries. The progression of this disease process is significantly slowed after total suppression of cigarette smoking. Although this measure avoids the extension of the disease, it has no impact on the ischemic manifestations that have already occurred. Surgical management includes local debridement of necrotic tissue and wound care. Sympathectomy may

Figure 132-4. This arteriogram of a patient with Buerger's disease reveals the segmentally constricted areas of the digital vessels.

be useful to increase distal vasodilation. It should be noted that sympathectomy does not change the evolution of the arterial lesion or protect against the harmful effect of nicotine exposure.[73] Repeated blunt trauma to the hand or fingers plays some role in the development of the disease, and care should be taken not to injure the hands or fingers through occupation or athletics.[32]

Outcomes

The most important aspect in the treatment of Buerger's disease is patient education of the relevance of cigarette smoking to the pathogenesis of this disease. Cessation of nicotine exposure is significantly more important than any other medical or surgical therapeutic approach in these patients. Most patients will see a significant improvement in symptoms, or at least failure of progression of the disease, if nicotine can be totally avoided. A direct digital sympathectomy may also offer palliation or further improvement.[20] Occasionally, although the circumstances are quite rare, vascular reconstruction by bypassing an occluded segment may be feasible. These measures may be helpful, but are viewed as salvage efforts.

THE VASOSPASTIC DISORDERS

INDICATIONS

Vasospastic disorders of the hand are caused by a variety of conditions. Environmental factors, including occupational trauma (such as from exposure to vibrating tools), may lead to digital vasospasm.[29,49] Exposure to certain drugs and toxins, such as ergotamine (commonly used in the treatment of migraine headaches) and sympathomimetic drugs, may also induce digital vasospasm. Other disease processes may also lead to digital vasospasm, such as connective tissue diseases or neurovascular compression syndromes (e.g., thoracic outlet syndrome or carpal tunnel syndrome). An interesting group of patients may develop vasospastic symptoms after a frostbite injury. Any of these conditions can lead to a set of symptoms referred to as *Raynaud's phenomenon.* This condition consists of digital ischemia caused by exposure to cold or other sympathetic stimuli such as pain or emotional stress. The affected digits become cool and blanch for a short period. This is followed by a period of vasodilation with a tuberous appearance of the digit, which can be associated with dysesthesias. Maurice Raynaud[61] first published his paper on "Local Asphyxia and Symmetrical Gangrene of the Extremity" in 1862. The term *Raynaud's disease* is reserved for those patients who have the symptoms of intermittent digital vasospasm (Raynaud's phenomenon) in the absence of any identifiable organic cause.

Evaluation of patients with chronic digital ischemia secondary to vasospasm may be done by noninvasive techniques such as duplex scanner examination or by angiogram (Figure 132-5). Radioisotopes, such as technetium 99, may also be used to visualize the perfusion of the digits with radionucleotide tagged cells, but resolution is imprecise. Cold

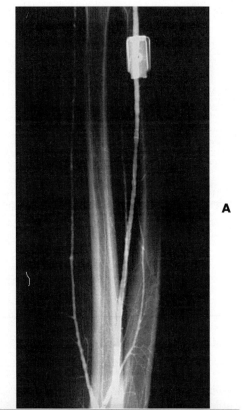

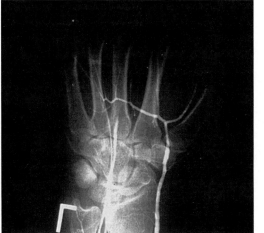

Figure 132-5. The angiograms in **A** and **B** show the arteries of the forearm and hand with the "bumpy" appearance secondary to vasospasm.

stress testing by exposing the hand to cold water, as described by Wilgis,[77] may help reproduce the symptoms. A sympathetic block with local anesthetic may allow evaluation of the sympathetic contribution to the production of ischemia in the digit.

Treatment of vasospasm begins with behavior modification. A large number of these patients are smokers, and complete cessation of exposure to all nicotine products and cold environments is mandatory. Many patients with Raynaud's phenomenon are improved by moving to a warmer climate and stopping the use of nicotine and are able to resume a normal life. Results

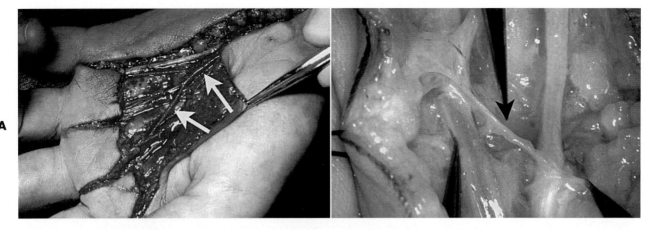

Figure 132-6. **A,** The ulnar artery is exposed within the palm of the hand, seen at the end of the arrows. **B,** The digital nerve, with the small digital nerve branch, is seen at the point of the arrow extending over to the ulnar artery.

of drug treatment for vasospasm have been inconsistent and have included the use of calcium channel blockers, a serotonin receptor blocker (Ketanserin), topical nitroglycerin, and alpha-adrenergic blockers such as Reserpine.[8] Of these, Reserpine has been proven to be the most valuable and some encouraging results have followed intraarterial injection. Biofeedback has been shown to have benefit for some patients in achieving a reduction of reported symptoms.[22]

OPERATIONS

Surgical intervention, when indicated, has been directed toward interruption of the sympathetic innervation. The results after cervicothoracic sympathectomy have been disappointing, with only short-term improvement. More distal sympathectomy has seemed to provide greater specificity and longevity.[49] This may be because the sympathetic fibers join the vessels quite distally.

Flatt[20] points out that the radial artery receives sympathetic filaments from the radial nerve and the lateral cutaneous nerve of the forearm. The ulnar artery receives three branches from the ulnar nerve and a branch from the medial cutaneous nerve of the forearm. The superficial palmar arterial arch receives nearly a dozen branches from the common digital nerves, and the deep palmar arch receives branches from the ulnar and median nerves. The digital arteries themselves are said to receive anywhere from three to 12 sympathetic nerve twigs.[20,78]

The sympathetic fibers to the digital arteries ramify within the adventitia; therefore adventitial stripping offers an effective sympathectomy distal to the point of adventitial removal. Flatt recommends that at least a 3- to 4-mm longitudinal segments should be cleared. The depth to which one removes the adventitia remains variable, but the more thorough the removal, the greater the likelihood of complete sympathectomy. Flatt, Wilgis, and others have proposed various incisions, but we have preferred a J-shaped incision, with extensions

as necessary into the web spaces (Figure 132-6). Healing is a concern, and avoidance of distally based flaps is important.

OUTCOMES

Results have been best when the pathology is pure vasospasm, with less dramatic results in patients who have obstructive or collagen vascular disease. Even so, sympathectomy may well result in some improvement in patients with scleroderma, and may result in more distal digital salvage.[32,53]

VASCULAR TUMORS AND MALFORMATIONS

HEMANGIOMAS

Mulliken and Glowacki's publication in 1982 and their subsequent text on vascular birthmarks have done much to create a more reasonable interpretation in what was previously a confusing array of descriptions of congenital vascular tumors.[52] Mulliken's efforts have made terms such as *cavernous hemangioma* and *capillary hemangioma* archaic. Instead, two new entities have evolved, with the designations of *hemangioma* versus *vascular malformation*. Hemangiomas are quite specific entities that usually appear within 2 weeks after birth, grow rapidly during the first year of life, and subsequently involute to a significant degree (Figure 132-7). All hemangiomas involute and many do so completely. In contrast, vascular malformations do not "grow" other than by hemodynamic enlargement, and none of them involute. The so-called *strawberry* lesion is the typical hemangioma. The diagnosis is usually apparent from history and examination. Growth of these lesions actually encompasses cellular proliferation, and the bulk of the tumor can increase significantly in size.

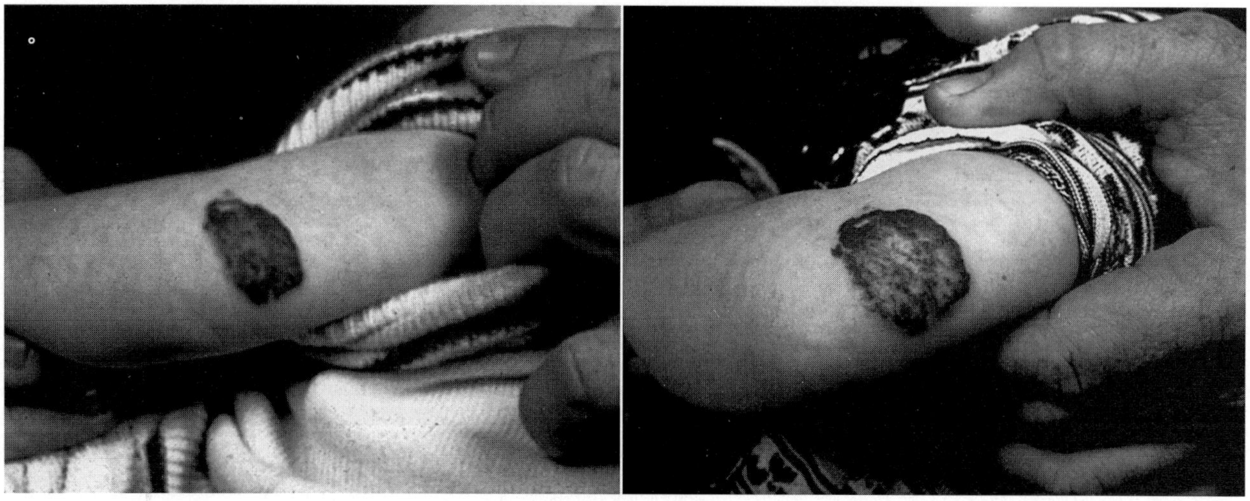

Figure 132-7. A, A hemangioma on the left arm of a child, with a raised ruborous appearance. **B,** There is significant diminution of the hemangioma in the same child 1 year later, with visible areas of epithelium within the previously raised lesion.

Treatment

The majority of hemangiomas will require no treatment other than careful observation. Education of the parents to the probable course of rapid growth followed by involution is the responsibility of the treating surgeon. One often spends more effort in this educational process, avoiding surgery, than would have been expended to simply proceed with surgical extirpation. Early laser treatment of a "herald spot," thereby destroying the potential for early growth, has been reported by Achauer et al[1] but the study lacks a nontreated control group. The vast majority of patients, however, do not require surgery. Only those hemangiomas in dangerous positions should be considered for surgical removal. Obstruction of an orifice or interference with vision are indications for removal of large facial hemangiomas. Treatment indications in the upper extremity are more likely to be for those lesions that are easily traumatized, frequently bleed, or ulcerate. Avoidance or surgical delay is clearly to the patient's advantage and in keeping with the maximum preservation of normal function and appearance. Light compressive wraps can be used to slow growth and speed resolution in established cases. Occasionally, the residual scar will have a negative cosmetic effect and can be improved by resection, but this effort can be reserved for later in life. When resection is necessary, it should be performed under tourniquet control and incorporate a cuff of normal skin to avoid leaving tumor behind.[18,52] We emphasize again, however, that these circumstances will be exceptional.

Outcomes

The result of nonoperative treatment of extremity hemangiomas is usually quite good, with complete resolution expected in most patients by the age of 10. Functional impairment from these lesions is rare in the upper extremity, unlike the face, in which obstruction of the visual axis or airway may demand urgent treatment. The parents of most patients need reassurance that the lesion will spontaneously regress.

VASCULAR MALFORMATIONS

Any part of the vascular tree can be involved in a vascular malformation. It is therefore possible to have capillary malformations termed *port wine stains*; *venous malformations,* composed predominantly of venous channels; *AV malformations,* containing elements of artery, vein, and capillaries and often associated with some degree of AV shunting; and even *lymphatic malformations.*[72] AV malformations are further designated as either low-flow or high-flow lesions. High-flow AV malformations contain multiple AV fistulae and are treated as previously discussed (see p. 2325).[72]

Capillary malformations are important from a cosmetic sense, especially when they occur on visible areas, such as the hands and face. They have no hemodynamic significance, and resection is indicated in most circumstances for aesthetic improvement. The development of laser technology now permits treatment of those lesions on an outpatient basis, with minimal scarring.[25] Venous malformations are characterized by the bluish discoloration of the swelling and by the common characteristic of decompression with elevation and filling or tensing with dependency of the extremity. AV malformations generally do not decompress with elevation, and some high-flow lesions may have a bruit and pulsate. Lymphatic malformations in the hand and upper extremity are extremely rare and may present primarily with intermittent episodes of infection. Surgical excision may be indicated in patients with recurring infections.

Outcomes

Treatment of low-flow AV and venous malformations is primarily undertaken for correction of the cosmetic deformity

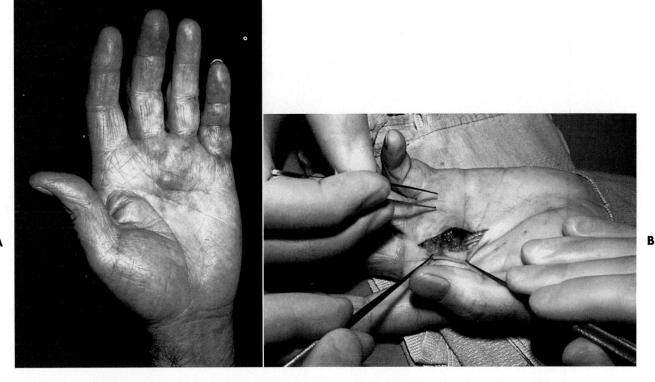

Figure 132-8. **A,** The patient's left hand is seen with the bluish, discolored appearance of the skin overlying a venous vascular malformation. **B,** The vascular malformation exposed at the time of surgery.

(Figure 132-8). Other than appearance, these lesions often cause no symptoms except that venous malformations are occasionally predisposed to have localized thromboses, which can be painful.[72] Resection of these lesions is often unrewarding because a radical approach cannot be justified in light of their benign nature, and consequently there is often tumor left behind. Occasionally, nerve compression associated with one of the vascular malformations may be an indication for surgery. Treatment of vascular malformations should, in general, be conservative. Surgical ablative therapy may be indicated for specific reasons, including improving the appearance, but resectional therapy may be disappointing because of the necessity to leave behind significant portions of the tumor.

GLOMUS TUMORS

INDICATIONS

Glomus tumors account for approximately 1% of all hand tumors. They are more common in women, usually appear between the ages of 30 and 50, and approximately 50% occur in the subungual area.[56]

Characteristically, glomus tumors are exquisitely tender and functionally limit the activity of the patient. Most patients present with an isolated lesion, but a multiple glomus tumor syndrome has been described that may be transmitted in an autosomal-dominant inheritance pattern. Glomus tumors contain solid masses of glomus cells that arise from the normal neuromyoarteriovenous glomus. The normal glomus unit appears to act as a micro AV shunt, which most likely has a thermoregulatory function.[34,56]

Patients who develop a glomus tumor usually present with a triad of symptoms including pain, tenderness, and cold sensitivity. Occasionally, tumors may have no symptoms. A bluish discoloration of a nail bed or of the skin overlying the tumor may be visible, but in many cases there is no apparent lesion. Distortion of the nail by the tumor is a helpful diagnostic clue when present (Figure 132-9, *A*).[18,56] Reproduction of pain by cold stimulation, such as a cold-water immersion test, is usually diagnostic.

OPERATIONS

There is no valuable nonsurgical treatment of glomus tumors. The surgical treatment is usually straightforward. Subungual lesions are approached by removing the nail plate, incising the nail bed, and shelling out the tumor (Figure 132-9, *B* and *C*). The nail bed should then be repaired anatomically with fine absorbable sutures; the nail plate should be replaced over the incision repair to facilitate nail-bed healing without scar.

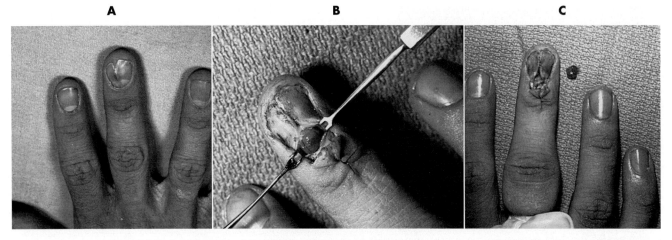

Figure 132-9. **A,** An underlying glomus tumor caused a nail-plate deformity of the long finger. **B,** The glomus tumor is seen at the time of surgical exposure. **C,** The glomus tumor after excision.

Tumors in other areas can usually be excised with a simple bilenticular incision.

OUTCOMES

There is some suggestion that glomus tumors are neoplasms, but they are not prone to recur after complete resection. Patients usually have complete resolution of symptoms without recurrence.[9,10,18,56]

PYOGENIC GRANULOMA

Pyogenic granuloma is a strange disorder that often presents after relatively trivial trauma. It represents an exuberant accumulation of granulation tissue that grows rapidly, producing a violacious-appearing mound of convoluted vessels. It is usually easily diagnosed, although its appearance and coloration may be suggestive of more sinister lesions, such as melanoma. Treatment consists of simple debridement and/or cauterization of the base with a silver nitrate stick. Healing by secondary intention occurs in most cases without sequelae.

MALIGNANT VASCULAR TUMORS

ANGIOSARCOMA

Indications

Angiosarcoma is an aggressive, high-grade neoplasm. The treatment of choice is wide excision and adjuvant chemotherapy. A distinctive variant is epithelioid angiosarcoma, a high-grade neoplasm that usually arises in the intramuscular soft tissue. This entity mimics an epithelial tumor both morphologically and immunohistochemically, and may be easily mistaken for an epithelial neoplasm.[21]

Outcomes

The largest series of these cases (72 patients) reported a 12% 5-year survival rate; half of the patients died within 15 months of diagnosis.[33] The most important factor in determining prognosis was the size of the initial lesion. Patients with tumors that were less than 5 cm in diameter had a significantly better prognosis than those with larger lesions.[44] Factors such as patient gender and location and histological grading of the lesion do not affect the prognosis or outcome.[33] Death occurs either by local extension of tumor or by metastasis. Typically, recurrences and metastases are noted within 2 years of diagnosis.

KAPOSI'S SARCOMA

Indications

Kaposi's sarcoma (KS) is classified into classic (sporadic), endemic, and acquired immunodeficiency syndrome (AIDS)–related (epidemic) forms. The classic form of the disease occurs primarily in males (90%) between the ages of 50 and 70 years. Classic KS tumors present as one or more asymptomatic red, purple, or brown patches, plaques, or nodular skin lesions. The disease is often limited to single or multiple lesions localized to one or both lower extremities.

Approximately 30% of AIDS patients have KS. Its clinical course is not relentlessly progressive, and regressions sometimes take place. Early lesions have a peculiar inflammatory appearance and are often multicentric. The exact nature of this entity has been controversial, but KS is now believed to be a multifocal reactive vascular hyperplasia rather than a neoplasm.[5] It is suggested that KS in patients with AIDS results from the enhanced secretion of immune-modulating factors with angiogenesis-promoting activity by cells attempting to correct or compensate for an immune disorder.[43] There appears to be no fundamental difference in the histological appearance of KS among the various clinical groups.[19]

Outcomes

KS typically runs a relatively benign, indolent course for decades, with slow enlargement of the original tumors and the gradual development of additional lesions. Venous stasis and lymphedema of the involved lower extremity are frequent complications. Up to one third of the patients with classic KS develop a second primary malignancy, most often non-Hodgkin's lymphoma.[62,65,66]

LYMPHEDEMA

INDICATIONS

Lymphedema of the upper extremity, with the exception of the postmastectomy variety, is uncommon. Lymphedema results from an inadequacy or obstruction of lymphatics and the accumulation of interstitial fluid. The primary function of the lymphatics appears to be the removal of macromolecules that do not easily reenter capillaries. Accumulation of these giant molecules in the interstitial space results in an oncotic pressure gradient with a fluid shift that produces edema (Figure 132-10). Two varieties of lymphedema are recognized, congenital and acquired. Congenital lymphedemas are caused by an inadequate or insufficient number of lymphatics that may appear at birth or early life, around the time of puberty (precox), or in adulthood (tarda). These are all very difficult to treat. Acquired or obstructive lymphedema results when once normal-functioning lymphatics are blocked or removed, often after a surgical procedure, a disease process such as filariasis, or radiation. Some authors believe that time is the only differential in the arbitrary designation of congenital and acquired lymphedema, and that the fundamental problem in all forms is an inadequacy of lymphatic regeneration. This would explain why some individuals develop lymphedema after lymphatic resection (as with a mastectomy or lymphadenectomy) and others do not.

The diagnosis of lymphedema is usually apparent from history and physical examination and by the elimination of other causes of edema. Some key diagnostic points include edematous involvement of the digits (venous insufficiency edema rarely involves digits), rare pigmentation or coloration changes, and rare ulceration of the skin. Lymphangiograms are diagnostic, but are rarely indicated and, if done with lipiadol, may cause further injury to the lymphatics.

Treatment of upper-extremity lymphedema is almost exclusively conservative or medical in nature, with only rare indications for surgery. Elastic compression and elevation are the mainstays of therapy, coupled with careful education of the patient in these techniques, good hygiene, and quick treatment of any infection with antibiotics. Mild and moderate degrees

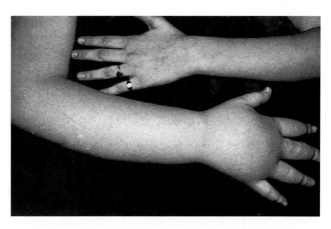

Figure 132-10. Lymphedema of the upper extremity.

of swelling can be readily controlled by elastic compression and elevation. More severe cases may require use of one of the intermittent positive-pressure devices (Lymphopress) on a regular basis. Occasionally, diuretics may be indicated, and there remains some interest in the value of the benzopyrones, which seem to work by breaking down the macromolecules and facilitating their removal.[13]

OPERATIONS

The surgical procedures for treatment of lymphedema have evolved along two lines: (1) ablative procedures designed to surgically remove the edematous tissue or (2) procedures intended to augment lymph flow or egress from the lymphedematous area. Ablative procedures have been advocated by Charles,[11] Sistrunk,[68] Miller,[50,51] and others in recent years. These operations remove the subcutaneous layer of the extremity and cover the muscle with skin grafts or skin flaps. Although functional improvement accompanies the removal of the heavy edematous subcutaneous tissue, cosmetic results have usually been dismal. Miller's main contribution of using thin skin flaps for coverage has produced a more acceptable cosmetic outcome.

Many of the procedures proposed to improve lymph flow have incorporated the use of flaps transplanted into the edematous area from a healthy origin,[26] transfer of omentum,[28] use of suture wicks,[30,67] and various forms of lymphaticovenous communications.[17,41,54,55,58] Initially lymph node/venous anastomoses were proposed and later truncal lymphaticovenous anastomoses were proposed along with anastomosis of dermal lymphatics. Lymphaticovenous anastomosis, as reported by O'Brien et al and others has been successful in some cases in decreasing hand and forearm edema. The criticism of this procedure is that when the elevated lymphatic pressure decreases as the interstitial fluid is drained from the extremity flow across a patent lymphaticovenous anastomosis may be reversed when the lymphatic pressure falls below the normal venous pressure, resulting in clotting and subsequent fibrosis.[60]

OUTCOMES

Surgery is reserved for only those cases that are progressive in the face of an appropriate medical regimen. The tissue ablative techniques probably have longer duration of improvement, but in most cases should be viewed as palliative because edema almost always recurs. Enthusiasm for lymphaticovenous anastomosis for the treatment of lymphedema has waned in recent years. Some cases have shown dramatic improvement after various forms of lymphovenous anastomosis but with time recurrence of edema is probable. A diligent medical regimen of elastic support, elevation, and positive pressure devices is certainly the mainstay of therapy.

REFERENCES

1. Achauer BM, Vanderkam VM: Strawberry hemangioma of infancy: early definitive treatment with an Argon laser, *Plast Reconstr Surg* 88:486-489, 1991.

2. Adar R, Papa MZ, Halpern Z, et al: Cellular sensitivity to collagen in thromboangiitis obliterans, *N Engl J Med* 308:1113-1116, 1983.

3. Aulicino PL, Klavans SM, DuPuy TE: Digital ischemia secondary to thrombosis of a persistent median artery, *J Hand Surg [Am]* 9:820-823, 1984.

4. Baird RJ, Lajos TZ: Emboli to the arm, *Ann Surg* 160:905, 1964.

5. Bayler AC, Lucas SB: Kaposi's sarcoma or Kaposi's disease? A personal reappraisal, In Fletcher CDM, McKee PH (editors): *Pathology of soft tissue tumours,* Edinburgh, 1990, Churchill Livingstone.

6. Cabrera JM, McCue FC III: Nonosseous athletic injuries of the elbow, forearm, and hand, *Clin Sports Med* 5:681-700, 1986.

7. Caffee HH, Master NT: Atherosclerosis of the forearm and hand, *J Hand Surg [Am]* 9:193-196, 1984.

8. Campbell PM, LeRoy EC: Raynaud phenomenon, *Semin Arthritis Rheum* 16(2):92-103, 1986.

9. Carlstedt T, Lugnegard H: Glomus tumor in the hand: a clinical and morphologic study, *Acta Orthop Scand* 54:296-302, 1983.

10. Carroll RE, Berman AT: Glomus tumors of the hand: review of the literature and report on twenty eight cases, *J Bone Joint Surg* 54:691-703, 1972.

11. Charles RH: Elephantiasis scroti. In Latham A, English TC (editors): *A system of treatment,* vol 3, London, 1912, Churchill-Livingstone.

12. Clarke SW: Congenital arteriovenous fistula of the hand, *Proc R Soc Med* 59:855-856, 1966.

13. Clodius L, Pillar NB: Conservative therapy for postmastectomy lymphedema, *Chirurgia Plastica* 4:193, 1978.

14. Coffman JD, Davies WT: Vasospastic diseases: a review, *Prog Cardiovasc Dis* 18:123-146, 1975.

15. Coleman SS, Anson BJ: Arterial patterns in the hand based upon a study of 650 specimens, *Surg Gynecol Obstet* 113:408-424, 1961.

16. Conn J Jr, Bergan JJ, Bell JL: Hypothenar hammer syndrome: posttraumatic digital ischemia, *Surgery* 68:1122-1128, 1970.

17. Degni M: New technique of lymphatic-venous anastomosis (buried type) for the treatment of lymphedema, *Vasa* 3:479-483, 1974.

18. Diao E, Moy OJ: Common tumors, *Orthop Clin North Am* 23:187-196, 1992.

19. Enzinger FM, Weiss SW: Malignant vascular tumors. In Enzinger FM, Weiss SW (editors): *Soft tissue tumors,* ed 2, St. Louis, 1988, Mosby.

20. Flatt AE: Digital artery sympathectomy, *J Hand Surg [Am]* 5:550-556, 1980.

21. Fletcher CD, Beham A, Bekir S, et al: Epithelioid angiosarcoma of deep soft issue: a distinctive tumor readily mistaken for an epithelial neoplasm, *Am J Surg Pathol* 15:915-924, 1991.

22. Freedman RR: Physiological mechanisms of temperature biofeedback, *Biofeedback & Self Regulation* 16:95-115, 1991.

23. Freiberg A, Fish J: Aneurysm of a common digital artery: case report and literature review, *Can J Surg* 31:254-255, 1988.

24. Gelberman RH, Goldner JL: Congenital arteriovenous fistulae of the hand, *J Hand Surg [Am]* 3:451-454, 1978.

25. Geronemus RG: Pulsed dye laser treatment of vascular lesions in children, *J Dermatol Surg Oncol* 19:303-310, 1993.

26. Gilles Sir H, Fraser FR: Treatment of lymphoedema by plastic operation, *Br Med J* 1:96, 1935.

27. Given KS, Puckett CL, Kleinert HE: Ulnar artery thrombosis, *Plast Reconstr Surg* 61:405-411, 1978.

28. Goldsmith HS: Long term evaluation of omental transposition for chronic lymphedema, *Ann Surg* 180:847-849, 1974.

29. Greenstein D, Parkin A, Maughan J, Kester RC: Perfusion defects in vibration white finger: a clinical assessment using isotope limb blood flow, *Cardiovascular Surg* 2(3):354-358, 1994.

30. Handley WS: Lymphangioplasty: a new method for the relief of the brawny arm of breast cancer and for similar conditions of lymphatic oedema, *Lancet* 1:783, 1908.

31. Harris EJ Jr, Taylor LM Jr, Edwards JM, et al: Surgical treatment of distal ulnar artery aneurysm, *Am J Surg* 159:527-530, 1990.

32. Hirai M, Shionoya S: Arterial obstruction of the upper limb in Buerger's disease: its incidence and primary lesion, *Br J Surg* 66:124-128, 1979.

33. Holden CA, Spittle MF, Jones EW: Angiosarcoma of the face and scalp, prognosis and treatment, *Cancer* 59:1046-1057, 1987.

34. Hollins PJ: Multiple glomus tumors, *Proc R Soc Med* 64:806, 1971.

35. Holman E: *Abnormal arteriovenous communications,* ed 2, Springfield, Ill, 1968, Charles C. Thomas.

36. Hurst LN, Rankin RN, Antonyshyn OM: Arteriovenous fistulae after replantation surgery, *Plast Reconstr Surg,* 77:664-667, 1986.

37. Ikeda A, Ugawa A, Kazihara Y, Hamada N: Arterial patterns in the hand based on a three-dimensional analysis of 220 cadaver hands, *J Hand Surg* 13:501-509, 1988.

38. Kay PR, Abraham JS, Davies DR, Bertfield H: Ulnar artery aneurysms after injury mimicking acute infection in the hand, *Injury* 19:402-404, 1988.

39. Kimura T, Yoshizaki S, Tsushima N, et al: Buerger's colour, *Br J Surg* 77:1299-1301, 1990.

40. Koman LA, Urbaniak JR: Ulnar artery insufficiency: a guide to treatment, *J Hand Surg [Am]* 6:16-24, 1981.

41. Laine JB, Howard JM: Experimental lymphaticovenous anastomosis, *Surgical Forum* 14:111, 1963.

42. Leriche R, Fontaine R, Dupertuis SM: Arteriectomy: with follow-up studies on 78 operations, *Surg Gynecol Obstet* 64:149-155, 1937.

43. Levy JA, Ziegler JL: Acquired immunodeficiency syndrome is an opportunistic infection and Kaposi's sarcoma results from secondary immune stimulation, *Lancet* 2:78-81, 1983.

44. Maddox JC, Evans HL: Angiosarcoma of skin and soft tissue: a study of forty-four cases, *Cancer* 48:1907-1921, 1981.

45. Malt S: An arteriosclerotic aneurysm of the hand, *Arch Surg* 113:762-763, 1978.

46. Maxwell JA, Kepes JJ, Ketchum LD: Acute carpal tunnel syndrome secondary to thrombosis of a persistent median artery: case report, *J Neurosurg* 38:774-777, 1973.

47. May JW Jr, Atkinson R, Rosen H: Traumatic arteriovenous fistula of the thumb after blunt trauma: a case report, *J Hand Surg [Am]* 9:253-255, 1984.

48. McKusick VA, Harris WS, Ottesen OE, et al: Buerger's disease: a distinct clinical and pathologic entity, *JAMA* 181:5-12, 1962.

49. Miller LM, Morgan RF: Vasospastic disorders: etiology, recognition, and treatment, *Hand Clin* 9(1):171-187, 1993.

50. Miller TA: Surgical management of lymphedema of the extremity, *Ann Plast Surg* 1:184-187, 1978.

51. Miller TA, Wyatt LE, Rudkin GH: Staged skin and subcutaneous excision for lymphedema: a favorable report of long-term results (with discussion), *Plast Reconstr Surg* 102:1486-1501, 1998.

52. Mulliken JB, Glowacki J: Hemangiomas and vascular malformations in infants and children: a classification based on endothelial characteristics, *Plast Reconstr Surg* 69:412-422, 1982.

53. O'Brien BM, Kumar PA, Mellow CG, Oliver TV: Radical microarteriolysis in the treatment of vasospastic disorders of the hand, especially scleroderma, *Br J Hand Surg* 17:447-452, 1992.

54. O'Brien BM, Shafiroff BB: Microlymphaticovenous and resectional surgery in obstructive lymphedema, *World J Surg* 3:3-15, 1979.

55. O'Brien BM, Sykes P, Threlfall GN, Browning FS: Microlymphaticovenous anastomoses for obstructive lymphedema, *Plast Reconstr Surg* 60:197-211, 1977.

56. Palmieri TJ: Common tumors of the hand, *Orthop Rev* 16:367-378, 1987.

57. Poirier RA, Stansel HC Jr: Arterial aneurysms of the hand, *Am J Surg* 124:72-74, 1972.

58. Politowski M, Bartkowski S, Dynowski J: Treatment of lymphedema of the limbs by lymphatic-venous fistula, *Surgery* 66:639-643, 1969.

59. Puckett CL, Major B, Werner R: Remember the allen test! *Mo Med* 76:81-83, 1979.

60. Puckett CL, Jacobs GR, Hurvitz JS, Silver D: Evaluation of lymphovenous anastomoses in obstructive lymphedema, *Plast Reconstr Surg* 66:116-120, 1980.

61. Raynaud M: *Local asphyxia and symmetrical gangrene of the extremities: selected monographs translated by T. Barlow,* London, 1888, New Sydenham Society, pp 121:1.

62. Reynolds WA, Winkelmann RK, Soule EH: Kaposi's sarcoma: a clinicopathologic study with particular reference to its relationship to the reticuloendothelial system, *Medicine* 44(5):419-443, 1965.

63. Rothkopf DM, Bryan DJ, Cuadros CL, May JW Jr: Surgical management of ulnar artery aneurysms, *J Hand Surg [Am]* 15:891-897, 1990.

64. Russell RC, Steichen JB, Zook EG: Radial artery pseudoaneurysms: diagnosis, prevention and treatment, *Ortho Rev* 8:49-54, 1979.

65. Safai B, Good RA: Kaposi's sarcoma: a review and recent developments, *Clinical Bulletin* 10(2):62-69, 1980.

66. Safai B, Mike V, Giraldo G, et al: Association of Kaposi's sarcoma with second primary malignancies: possible etiopathogenic implications, *Cancer* 45(6):1472-1479, 1980.

67. Silver D, Puckett CL: Lymphangioplasty: a ten year evaluation, *Surgery* 80:748-755, 1976.

68. Sistrunk WE: Further experiences with the kondoleon operation of elephantiasis, *JAMA* 71:800, 1918.

69. Szilagyi DE, Smith RF, Elliott JP, Hageman JH: Congenital arteriovenous anomalies of the limbs, *Arch Surg* 111:423-429, 1976.

70. Taylor LM Jr, Bauer GM, Porter JM: Finger gangrene caused by small artery occlusive disease, *Ann Surg* 193:453-461, 1981.

71. Thorrens S, Trippel OH, Bergan JJ: Arteriosclerotic aneurysms of the hand: excision and restoration of continuity, *Arch Surg* 92:937-939, 1966.

72. Upton J, Coombs C: Vascular tumors in children, *Hand Clin* 11:307-337, 1995.

73. Van der Stricht J, Goldstein M, Flamand JP, Belenger J: Evolution and prognosis of thromboangiitis obliterans, *J Cardiovasc Surg* 14:9-16, 1973.

74. Von Kuster L, Abt AB: Traumatic aneurysms of the ulnar artery, *Arch Pathol Lab Med* 104:75-78, 1980.

75. Von Rosen S: Ein fall von thrombose in der arteria ulnaris nach einwirkung von stumpfer Gewalt, *Acta Chir Scandinav* 73:500-506, 1934.

76. Whelan TJ Jr: Management of vascular disease of the upper extremity, *Surg Clin North Am* 62:373-389, 1982.

77. Wilgis EF: Evaluation and treatment of chronic digital ischemia, *Ann Surg* 193(6):693-698, 1981.

78. Wilgis EF: Digital sympathectomy for vascular insufficiency, *Hand Clin* 1:361-367, 1985.

CHAPTER 133

Reflex Sympathetic Dystrophy

Wyndell H. Merritt

INTRODUCTION

Reflex sympathetic dystrophy (RSD) remains the most frustrating of all hand disorders because of our profound confusion about its cause and treatment. Also called *complex regional pain syndrome (CRPS), algoneurodystrophy, causalgia,* and over 40 other terms, this perplexing medical disorder is best characterized as a peculiar, painful state that seems out of proportion to the injury or condition and may become associated with dystrophic change. No comprehensive explanation exists for this disorder, nor is there any universally successful method of treatment.

Because the course of this disorder seems to be unpredictable and it develops with little or no warning, the clinician may initially underrate the consequence of disproportionate pain and later be confronted with an atrophied, dystrophic, functionless hand, which is now easily diagnosed as reflex dystrophy. Unfortunately, once diagnosis becomes easy, treatment is less likely to succeed because dystrophic changes are difficult, if not impossible, to reverse. The etiology, pathophysiology, and definition of this disorder all remain obscure, but it is imperative that those who manage hand problems develop the sensitivity necessary to recognize the problem early and to intervene to try to prevent the full-blown stages of this devastating condition. This is difficult because there are no specific diagnostic tests for RSD, thus it remains ultimately a clinical diagnosis. Thermography,[89,181] plethysmography,[223] and radioisotopic bone scan[170,199] are useful tests to assist in diagnosis; however, none are definitive.[167,219] Response to sympathetic block was used at one time as a definitive criterion for diagnosis,[30,191] but blocks are not uniformly successful[1,289,291,333] and are no longer required.[167,219] We must therefore rely on clinical judgment to make the diagnosis, which makes study of the topic difficult. As a result, even the term *reflex sympathetic dystrophy* evokes controversy and reflects misunderstanding. There is confusion about most aspects of this syndrome, including its name, definition, pathophysiology, and even the process of diagnosis. This disorder has such a wide spectrum of precipitating causes, a remarkable variety of treatment

techniques, and an unpredictable variation in clinical manifestations and responses that its basic cause must be multifactorial. It is presently best defined as a complex, unpredictable response, producing pain that is out of proportion to the inciting event, condition, or expected healing response, that is usually associated with an inflammatory or sympathetic change (e.g., edema, stiffness, temperature abnormality) that may eventuate into dystrophic change. Because its unknown cause is thought to be multifactorial, RSD is best described as a *syndrome.*[334]

This chapter reviews much of what is known of the disorder, hypothesizes etiologic mechanisms, reviews outcomes of popular treatment techniques, and proposes 10 principles for management within our current limited knowledge of this perplexing subject.

DEFINITIONS, CLASSIFICATIONS, AND TERMINOLOGY

It is hard to define a clinical entity with no standardized diagnostic criteria and no clear understanding of its origin. Therefore we should not be surprised that the criteria for diagnosis and classification of RSD are confusing and controversial. Indeed, controversy begins with its name, there being at least 50 medical disorders describing symptoms that include disproportionate pain and autonomic nervous system–type dysfunction. Box 133-1 lists 50 such disorders that may vary somewhat in anatomic location, severity, tissues affected, and autonomic manifestations, but all of which may be classified as RSD or CRPS.

In 1991 Amadio et al[7] reported the conclusions of a committee appointed to better define this disorder. The committee selected three basic criteria for diagnosis:
1. Disproportionate pain
2. Interference with function
3. Autonomic-type abnormality (e.g., swelling, temperature change, sweating, skin discoloration, osteoporosis)

Box 133-1.
Different Terms Used for Reflex Sympathetic Dystrophy Syndromes

Acute atrophy of bone
Algodystrophy
Algoneurodystrophy
Causalgia
Complex regional pain syndrome (types I and II)
Chronic segmental arteriospasm
Chronic traumatic edema
Erythralgia
Major causalgia
Mimocausalgia states
Minor causalgia
Neurodystrophic syndromes
Neurotrophic rheumatism
Painful osteoporosis
Peripheral neuralgia
Postinfarction sclerodactyly
Posttraumatic arterial spasm
Posttraumatic arthritis
Posttraumatic dystrophy
Posttraumatic edema
Posttraumatic neurovascular pain syndrome
Posttraumatic osteoporosis
Posttraumatic pain syndrome
Posttraumatic spreading neuralgia
Posttraumatic sympathalgia
Posttraumatic sympathetic dystrophy (dysfunction)
Posttraumatic trophoneurosis
Posttraumatic vasomotor syndrome (disorder)
Ravaut's neurotrophic rheumatism
Reflex atrophy
Reflex dystrophy
Reflex hyperemic deossification
Reflex nerve atrophy
Reflex nervous dystrophy
Reflex neurovascular dystrophy
Reflex sympathetic dystrophy
Regional migratory transient osteoporosis
Shoulder-hand syndrome
Steinbrocker syndrome
Sudeck's atrophy (syndrome)
Sudeck's osteoporosis
Sympathalgia
Sympathetic dystrophy
Sympathetic neurovascular dystrophy
Sympathetically maintained pain
Thalamic syndrome
Traumatic angiospasm
Traumatic edema
Traumatic reflex osteodystrophy
Traumatic vasospasm

tion) and allodynia (marked pain from a usually nonnoxious stimulation), and it is usually constant, although it varies in intensity. Even though the initial inciting event may seem minor, the amount of distress caused by reflex dystrophy pain is profound and should never be underestimated, nor belittled.

There is no single test that will consistently diagnose early reflex dystrophy, and diagnostic criteria vary widely among authors. Although all agree that pain is the predominant feature, there is no consensus regarding the degree or extent of autonomic, dystrophic, or inflammatory change needed to secure the diagnosis. Indeed, some authors require only the presence of the unique hyperpathia and allodynia pain patterns and the associated distress to justify diagnosis.[267,311] The value of this approach recognizes that earlier treatment may improve the prognosis.[139,167,173,218] Unfortunately, most patients are usually symptomatic more than 6 months before the true nature of the disorder is recognized and diagnosed, having often been misdiagnosed as malingerers or psychoneurotics in the interval.[318] On the other hand, the opportunity to classify any undiagnosed pain as RSD has created cynicism about its overuse. Many clinicians now believe RSD has lost its usefulness as a designation because of this indiscriminate use, causing the diagnosis to no longer convey a clear meaning.[157] Therefore the administrative and legal implications of a diagnosis of RSD, combined with less motivation to seek other possible diagnostic explanations for unexplained pain, have led to some reluctance to use the term *reflex sympathetic dystrophy* as a diagnosis.

The International Pain Nomenclature Group task force introduced the term *complex regional pain syndrome (CRPS)* in 1996 to replace *reflex sympathetic dystrophy (RSD)*.[39,301] CRPS describes a variety of painful conditions that develop after injury that appear regionally and exceed the degree and duration of pain expected from the inciting event. This syndrome usually results in significantly impaired function, with variable progression over time.

CRPS is divided into two major categories and three types of disorders: (1) sympathetically maintained pain syndrome (SMPS), types I and II, and (2) sympathetically independent pain syndrome (SIPS), type III. SMPS is subcategorized into two types. Type I (classically described RSD) has the following criteria:

1. Follows an initiating noxious event
2. Continuous pain or allodynia/hyperpathia occurs that is not limited to the territory of a single peripheral nerve(s) and appears disproportionate to the inciting event
3. There is or has been evidence of edema, skin blood-flow abnormality, abnormal pseudomotor activity, and motor dysfunction disproportionate to the inciting event
4. This diagnosis is excluded by the existence of conditions that would otherwise account for the degree of pain and dysfunction

SMPS type II (classic *major causalgia*) criteria include the following:

1. Develops after a nerve injury
2. Is usually a more regionally confined presentation (but not necessarily), limited to the territory of the involved nerve(s)

One could argue that other disorders, such as severe Raynaud's phenomenon with sclerodactyly, fulfill these criteria. However, it is the peculiar nature of the disproportionate pain that distinguishes RSD from all other disorders. This pain is characterized by hyperpathia (prolonged pain after stimula-

3. Spontaneous pain or allodynia/hyperalgesia is usually limited to the area involved but may spread variably distally or proximally, not in the territory of a dermatologic or peripheral nerve distribution

4. Evidence of edema, blood-flow abnormality, or abnormal pseudomotor abnormality that is or has been shown in the region of pain subsequent to the inciting event, or motor dysfunction disproportionate to the inciting event

5. This diagnosis is excluded by conditions that would otherwise account for the degree of pain and dysfunction

The CRPS type III *(sympathetically independent pain)* classification identifies cases of disproportionate pain and sensory change with motor and tissue change that do not characteristically respond to sympathetic block. These are not typically subclassified.

One advantage of this new classification system is to acknowledge that chronic pain syndromes exist that do not consistently respond to sympathetic blocks. Another advantage is to avoid the prejudicial designation of an RSD diagnosis, with its legal and administrative connotations. However, one should not mistakenly infer that this new classification system implies any new proof that this disorder is caused or "maintained" by the sympathetic nervous system, nor that any new treatment regimens exist. There are no new objective criteria, and in some respects the new designation adds to the confusion by implying a new understanding.

In 1972 Sunderland[308] stated his objection to defining any disorder based on response to a treatment as follows: "To define a certain type of pain by reference to its response to one form of treatment, namely sympathetic interruption, is artificial... and unreasonable." It would be as though we subclassified rheumatoid arthritis as steroid-maintained rheumatoid arthritis (SMRA) for responders, and steroid-independent rheumatoid arthritis (SIRA) for nonresponders, with some implication that the steroid played a role in the origin of the disease. We must avoid defining as complex an entity as reflex dystrophy by treatment response alone.

A standardized criterion was initially proposed for CRPS that was based on the use of phentolamine blocks.[53] This was done in a controlled fashion, utilizing a placebo to identify which patients had subjective pain relief from a placebo, which had response to phentolamine, and which had no response. This subclassified patients as placebo-responders, those with sympathetically maintained pain, and those with sympathetically independent pain. Unfortunately, phentolamine is presently not available for this intravenous test in the United States. Furthermore, the criteria did not clarify how one would classify patients who had variable response to sympathetic block, as do many patients with RSD. This classification system also does not include the 10% to 30% of patients who spontaneously develop reflex dystrophy and do not fulfill the criteria of an "initiating noxious event." Therefore this newer classification system has advantages and limitations, with continued need for better definition and classification.

An older classification system by Lankford[173] that utilized precipitating causes as a means to classify RSD into five clinical types remains popular with many clinicians.[297] Lankford classified RSD as *minor causalgia, minor traumatic dystrophy, shoulder-hand syndrome, major traumatic dystrophy,* and *major causalgia.*

Minor causalgia is described as an injury involving a purely sensory nerve in the distal portion of the extremities (e.g., injury to the superficial palmar branch of the median nerve after carpal tunnel surgery).

Minor traumatic dystrophy is described as the most common clinical form of RSD initiated by an injury that does not involve damage to any specific nerve, such as crushed fingers, sprains, and phalangeal fractures.

Shoulder-hand syndrome is usually caused by a proximal trauma or painful visceral lesion, with manifestations initiated in the shoulder and eventually involving the whole upper extremity. Examples include shoulder or neck injury, cervical disk pathology, heart attack, stroke, Pancoast's tumor, or stomach ulceration. However, any distal reflex dystrophy in the hand may progress to shoulder-hand syndrome. Characteristically, in this disorder the shoulder has limited motion and may become "frozen." Recognition of this classification is important, because it may be a heralding manifestation of ovarian or pancreatic carcinoma, or other occult visceral disorders.

Major traumatic dystrophy involves major trauma to the hand, such as severe crush injuries or Colles' fracture, but does not involve a specific nerve injury.

Major causalgia is the classic disorder described by Mitchell[227] involving a partial injury to a major mixed nerve in the proximal part of the extremity, such as a high-velocity gunshot wound through the arm. This is the group of patients most likely to benefit from sympathetic interruption.

Unfortunately, neither of these classification systems gives insight into the fundamental cause of this disorder, nor do they offer prognostic information or direction for treatment. Currently, the classification systems for RSD serve only to better communicate descriptions of the disorder and sometimes confuse our knowledge of the cause.

Much of the medical community feels that RSD is over-diagnosed and used as a catchall label for any patient complaining of pain.[235] Some clinicians argue reflex dystrophy should not be considered a single entity and should *never* be diagnosed.[58] Ochoa[244] claims that patients diagnosed with RSD are either misdiagnosed or remain undiagnosed. Well-meaning clinicians are concerned that the diagnosis of RSD may give a false sense of security, creating neglect for further investigation of the patient's complaints. In response to this hazard, Amadio suggested that excessive, nonanatomic, or other abnormal patterns of pain be categorized as "pain dysfunction syndrome" rather than RSD.[6] The misconception that RSD is a well-defined, explicable entity may have precipitated the administrative and legal actions that cause clinicians to become timid about its use as a diagnosis. Nonetheless, it is only by early recognition and intervention that we are likely to improve the patient's outcome.

HISTORICAL PERSPECTIVES AND ETIOLOGIC HYPOTHESES

During the American Civil War, Mitchell et al[228] identified and carefully recorded symptoms in certain Yankee soldiers who had a peculiar quality, duration, and response to pain after nerve damage caused by musket-ball injuries of the extremities. Their careful description of the unusually distressing complaints remains unparalleled. They describe a severe burning pain that could be aggravated by simple environmental stimuli such as a slightest breeze, temperature change, gazing upward, light touch, motion of the extremity, touching objects of different textures such as a slick bed sheet, unexpected noise, emotional change, or even the sound of certain words. Many found relief only while the extremity was wrapped in moist, cool cloth, and Mitchell noted that the intensity of pain "varied from the most trivial burning to a state of torture," noting that the patients were never completely free of discomfort. This burning sensation could evolve into dystrophic change in the cutaneous tissue and muscle. Mitchell et al reported that even in cold weather some soldiers would fill their boots with cold water and place their injured feet into them to try and relieve the burning pain. Others would wrap cold, wet towels around an injured upper extremity. These patients had partial, major, mixed-nerve injury (causalgia) with symptoms that are otherwise indistinguishable from those developing in nonnerve injury reflex dystrophy. Impressed with this burning nature of the pain, years later Mitchell[227] coined the term "causalgia" for this disorder, originating from the Greek *kausas* (heat) and *algos* (pain), to denote the burning pain described by his patients. It is interesting to note that many of his patients with dystrophy did not recover. Mitchell's son, John, described treating some of his father's patients who had causalgia 30 years after the end of the War of Northern Aggression.[226] The first extant record of similar pain after a gunshot nerve injury was by Demark,[68] whose patient was wounded in the arm at the storming of Badajoz in 1812. Because of persistent burning pain and dystrophic change, Denmark eventually amputated the patient's arm at the midhumeral level. On examination of the arm, he found a pellet embedded in the nerve.

Non-nerve injury that produces symptoms otherwise indistinguishable from causalgia was probably first described by Ambrose Paré (1510-1590) after he performed a simple blood-letting procedure on the arm of his ruler, Charles IX, King of France, as a treatment for fever.[60] The procedure was followed by an immediate intense burning pain and loss of function that no doubt greatly frustrated this renowned French military surgeon. It was not, however, until over 300 years later that Evans[93] coined the term *reflex sympathetic dystrophy* specifically to differentiate this syndrome that is without major nerve trauma from Mitchell's term *causalgia*, which does include major proximal nerve injury. Evans' patients had less apparent cause for the disorder, frequently presenting with sprains or minor fractures, although their symptoms eventually

became equally as severe as those of the nerve-injured patients. The fact that RSD and causalgia are two distinctly separate entities with similar manifestations is often overlooked and causes confusion. In 1900 Sudeck described radiologic signs of the disease, demonstrating acute bone atrophy and osteoporosis associated with pain. He believed inflammation caused these changes, later known as *Sudeck's atrophy*. A year later, Keinböck[158] described similar findings that occur after trauma.

In 1916 Leriche[184] suggested that stress provoked a reflex arc that follows the root of the sympathetic nervous system, which he believed was largely responsible for the disorder. Later he introduced the use of sympathetic blocks for diagnosis and treatment, diagnosing his patients as "post-traumatic painful osteoporosis." The same year Spurling[299] described the successful use of sympathectomy for causalgia in a bootlegger whose symptoms derived from a gunshot wound.

In 1942 Lewis[187] believed causalgia was due to the release of pain-producing vasodilator substances from nerve endings into the tissues of the skin as a result of antidromic impulses set up from cutaneous sensory fibers at the injury site. Livingston[192] in 1943 proposed a central reflex mechanism for this disorder at the spinal cord level, adopting the "internuncial pool theory" previously advanced in 1938 by Lorente de No.[193] Then the "artificial synapse theory" was proposed by Doupe et al,[74] suggesting the creation of a synapse by trauma or nerve damage between sympathetic efferent fibers and afferent sensory fibers to form a kind of short circuit at the site of nerve injury. The gate control theory of Melzack and Wall[216] was proposed in 1965 to explain the multiple factors in sensory and emotional experience we recognize as pain. They proposed a careful balance of large-and small-fiber input to the central nervous system (CNS) that could be disrupted by injury to a body area and create a self-perpetuating pain cycle. Roberts[274] proposed the concept of "sympathetically maintained pain" that has become widely accepted by most pain centers. He hypothesized that the primary pathology begins with sensitization of wide-dynamic-range (WDR) neurons of the spinal cord by hyperactive nociceptors in the periphery, which are continuously activated by sympathetic efferent stimulation that need not be hyperactive.

In recent years, there has been increasing recognition that neurotransmitter substances beyond the traditional autonomic nervous system concept of sympathetic release of noradrenaline and parasympathetic release of acetylcholine must play a significant role in the inflammatory or sympathetic manifestations of this disorder. Other mediators are found in autonomic fibers and in nociceptor pain fibers, including a host of neurotransmitter peptides such as substance P, neurokinin, somatostatin, neuropeptide Y, calcitonin gene-related peptide, serotonin, dopamine, gamma aminobutyric acid, adrenocorticotropic hormone (ACTH), angiotensin, cholecystokinin, and many others.[28] It is well appreciated that some of these neurotransmitter substances are capable of mediating peripheral inflammatory response and central pain, and they are important in an understanding of RSD.[219] Indeed, many authors now question the importance of the sympathetic nervous system in the origin and perpetuation of this disorder.*

Another factor less considered in most hypotheses is the importance of the CNS endogenous pain control system. This system provides a defending mechanism that can selectively monitor and modulate activity in pain-transmitting neurons via inhibitory systems within the dorsal horn of the medulla.[5] Although the precise role of this opioid system is not yet understood in reflex dystrophy, it is undoubtedly important.

INCIDENCE

Fortunately, RSD is not common. Unfortunately, it is certainly not rare. The exact incidence will be impossible to accurately assess until there is uniform terminology and agreement on diagnostic criteria. At present the diagnosis remains clinical, with only supporting objective criteria; thus the standard for diagnosis depends on the view of the observer. It is understandable that the proportion of cases varies greatly with different observers. For example, in his review of nerve injury cases, Sunderland[308] found that reports of causalgia varied from less than 1%[55] to 16%.[308] In a review by Veldman et al[326] of 829 cases of CRPS, 1% to 2% of patients developed the syndrome after fracture and 2% to 5% after peripheral nerve injury. Interestingly his series showed a range of 1% to 26% with no identifiable precipitating cause. Plewes[258] estimated that RSD occurred in one of every 2000 accidents, whereas Hartley[134] reported one in 20 after trauma. Overall, it appears that most reports find about a 5% incidence after likely precipitating causes, such as a sprain, elective surgery, or fracture. Thus the more common injuries and surgery, such as Colles' fracture and carpal tunnel syndrome, have the highest frequency of cause.

Incidence rates are as frequent as 40% to 70% in some conditions, such as reflex dystrophy associated with hemiplegia of vascular or traumatic origin, and are characterized by shoulder-hand syndrome, or shoulder-elbow-hand syndrome.[78] Furthermore, in some reported series, 10% to 30% of patients have spontaneous occurrence with no evident precipitating cause or condition.[75,169,212,326] The condition is most commonly found in the upper and lower extremities, but orofacial RSD has been reported after maxillofacial surgery,[163] head injury,[318] and dental procedures,[33,206] and after vascular surgery in the neck.[9] This group of patients does not appear to develop the dystrophic change commonly seen in the extremities[9,148] and appears to have a better prognosis.[9] Rare cases are described in the hip,[65,77] usually associated with pregnancy, and in the spine.[69,76]

Some reports show greater frequency in women[84,260] and others men.[54] However, in most reports the disorder seems to occur equally in the two sexes and with no predisposition for the dominant extremity.[165,169,191] Rothschild[276] makes the interesting observation that there appears to be a 3:1 female predominance if no trauma is present and a 3:1 male predominance when trauma is the precipitating cause.

Most age ranges involved are from 30 to 60 years, with the mean in the late 40s. Children were initially thought to be exempt from this disorder, but there have been increasing reports and awareness of childhood involvement.[254] Diagnosis may be more difficult in children, because over half develop the syndrome without an identifiable traumatic incidence,[27] suggesting to some authors that psychogenic problems and stress response may play an etiologic role.[288,337] Others conclude that psychologic manifestations are the effect and not the cause of the disorder.[196,284] Children typically have a shorter duration, a better prognosis, and less incidence of dystrophic change than adults.[27,97,162,272,279]

RSD is therefore a polymorphic condition that may well occur more frequently than reported, in all ages, in both sexes, and either spontaneously or precipitated by a wide variety of causes such as trauma.

PROGNOSIS AND OUTCOME OF TREATMENT

There is a widespread misconception that reflex dystrophy always spontaneously improves and "burns out" with time. It is probable that observation of the rare patient with causalgia after nerve injury led to this generalization. Causalgia generally involves partial injury to a major mixed nerve that will usually improve spontaneously and may completely resolve.[308] However, numerous authors have observed that complete remission is rare.[142,226,260,277] Shumaker,[290] for example, reported only three spontaneous remissions in 90 reflex dystrophy patients he followed. Indeed, long-term cases are at risk of suicide.[142]

Surgical efforts to treat reflex dystrophy were well summarized by Sunderland[308] in 1972 as having an initial interval of seeming success, only to later have "a disheartening tendency for the pain to recur...."

Nath et al[235] provide an excellent overview of reflex dystrophy treatment results among the three most popular management methods, and their findings seem bizarre. By reviewing the reported results of stellate ganglion block, intravenous sympathetic blockade, and surgical sympathectomy, they found an astonishing variation in results among all three. For example, of 25 reports using stellate ganglion block, results varied from 100% failure rate in 75 patients in one study[321] to 100% success rate in 30 patients in another.[264] With use of sympathetic blockade in 15 studies reviewed, results varied from 100% good in 38 patients[249] to a 93% failure rate in 15 patients.[38] Surgical sympathectomy results were just as varied among 19 studies reviewed, with results ranging from 99% good in 70 patients[321] to 95% failure in 27 patients.[123,124] This is a disgraceful spectrum that initially

---

*References 73, 218, 243-245, 281, 299, 323, 324.

seems inexplicable, with success and failure rates ranging from zero to 100% in all three treatment methods. However, the authors noted that among all 59 studies, only seven had 1-year or greater follow-up, and only seven were prospective randomized studies (not the same seven). Most reports gave no definitive length of follow-up and were retrospective nonrandomized by design. Subbarao and Stillwell[306] shed some light on why these reports might vary. In their long-term follow-up of 125 patients more than 1 year after treatment (average 14.5 months), they found treating physicians reported 77% satisfactory to excellent progress 3 months after treatment, whereas late follow-up revealed that 87% of these patients still complained bitterly about pain or stiffness, only 25% had resumed full activity, and only one patient of the series reported complete relief of symptoms. Add to the follow-up and control problems the variable and objective criteria used for diagnosis by the different authors, and such a wide range of results from different, honest researchers becomes explicable.

Overall review of the literature gives the impression that for most treatment methods, approximately one third of patients receive excellent to good relief from symptoms, approximately one third note some improvement, and approximately one third experience no improvement or they worsen. Wang's[333] 3-year study of sympathetic block results, however, suggests that if treated within 6 months the good to excellent group might be increased to approximately two thirds. However, there is no good long-term study of recurrence rates or evolution into other chronic pain conditions. In our own series of patients, we thought our good to excellent results in established cases of reflex dystrophy were 67%, until on review we included the patients who had been lost to follow-up because they did not complete treatment or did not return. If these were regarded as failures (which they likely were), then our results fell into the one third range, similar to the other studies.

In general, one should expect that patients with this disorder may continue to have some degree of chronic pain. If we can but help them cope with the pain and resume their usual function and activity, this would be an adequate and realistic goal.

PRECIPITATING CAUSES

There is an incredible array of reported precipitating causes for reflex dystrophy that are as widely varied as the spectrum of names given the disorder. Traumatic causes vary from a paper cut on the finger to spinal-cord injury, and nontraumatic conditions causing the disorder are as varied as ovarian carcinoma, shingles, myocardial infarction, stroke, and use of phenobarbital.

Because virtually any trauma or incident can apparently lead to reflex dystrophy, the most common hand operations, such as carpal tunnel surgery, and the most common injuries,

such as Colles' fractures, share blame as the most common precipitating events. For example, reflex dystrophy is reported to occur after as many as 2%[197] to 5%[189] of carpal tunnel operations and after as many as 11%[168] to 37%[13-15] of Colles' fractures. In most reports, soft tissue trauma is the most common precipitating cause, with fracture a close second. Together, these represent 45% to 55% of the precipitating cause in some series of reflex dystrophy.[93,171,298,318]

Nontraumatic causes represent quite a spectrum, with cardiac origin a common systemic cause in 5% to 20% of cases,[171] minor trauma in approximately 10% to 14% of cases,[93] and elective surgery in 10% to 16% of some reported series.[197] Less frequent causes include dental extractions,[33,205,206] ovarian[214] and pancreatic[222] carcinoma, stroke,[318] myocardial infarction,[52] spinal cord injury,[75-80] myelogram,[230] diabetic neuropathy,[75] herpes zoster,[318] facial fracture,[163] carotid surgery,[9] degenerative disk disease,[154] meningococcal meningitis,[213] cervical rib resection,[142] phenobarbital,[75] and venipuncture and intramuscular injection of pain medication.[142] In many reports, no apparent cause for onset was seen at all in as many as 30% of cases.[75,169,212]

This disorder clearly can have any type precipitating cause or no apparent cause at all. It therefore seems unfair that physicians have frequently been held liable for causing the disorder, because its onset seems so ubiquitous and potentially spontaneous. Certainly the variety of causes, some of which obviously originate in the CNS, leads to suspicion that cortical function plays a major role in the etiology of RSD.

CLINICAL MANIFESTATIONS, STAGES, AND FORMS

CHARACTERISTIC PAIN

The peculiar unremitting pain of reflex dystrophy is its most distinguishing clinical feature, and we should develop the sensitivity to recognize it. Clinical presentations vary widely, but all patients experience persistent pain of unusually distressing character that is way out of proportion to what one would expect from typical somatic pain. Indeed, patients with reflex dystrophy will exclaim that the degree of this pain is unlike any of their prior experience. The distinguishing characteristics are hyperpathia and allodynia, along with severe anguish and distress. The pain is usually constant, not completely relieved by rest, and aggravated by motion, activity, or temperature change. Although reflex dystrophy may arise in a typical nerve distribution, it often progresses to a wider and more diffuse area than that supplied by the nerve and may develop "mirror image" pain in the contralateral extremity, or progress to distant extremities.[156]

Looking and listening carefully to the patient's behavior and pain description provides our best opportunity for early diagnosis. This requires the busy surgeon to patiently pause and endure what sometimes seems to be an endless, detailed description of disproportionate pain with an unexplained pattern and degree of distress. These patients frequently describe constant, diffuse, "deep ache," "burning," "tearing," or "cutting" pain, with "intense," "shooting," "electric" episodes that are usually aggravated by motion, but may occur spontaneously. The pain usually interferes with work and sleep and tends to radiate to nonanatomic peripheral nerve distributions, although rarely it may remain confined to a single digit. Evidence of "mirror image" advancement into the contralateral extremity is reported in as many as 25% of patients.[169,291] In my experience, such migration is more common in patients with a CNS-related cause, such as stroke, than in those with a hand injury. Hand therapists may note that situational stress or the emotional state influence these episodes, even though the patients seem unaware of these influences. Questionnaires answered by the patients will deny emotional influence causing or being caused by reflex dystrophy, in spite of data showing life stress is a significant factor.[109] This seems to be due to a high incidence of alexithymia (inability to verbalize one's emotions; thought to be caused by lack of awareness; thus patient has no perception of mood) among patients with reflex dystrophy.[317] Although they can describe their symptoms in every detail, patients will rarely acknowledge any emotional response, and often become annoyed when depression, anxiety, or psychiatric assessment is suggested.

Observation of the patient's behavior is as important as the pain description in making an early diagnosis. Patients with reflex dystrophy seem to be less able to cope with their circumstance than are other patients with hand injuries, and they are less able to trust their physicians, both during examination or when receiving reassurance. They tend to fearfully withdraw from the examiner's touch (Figure 133-1), and repeat strained, anxious questions, demanding an explanation for their distress in sometimes an accusatory fashion. Patients with chronic reflex dystrophy may indict all previous treatment efforts, former physicians, and previous therapists. Although they may deny emotional distress, these patients appear more dismayed, angry, and desperate about their dilemma than similar, even more severely hand-injured patients. Patients with RSD quickly feel rejected and resentful when well-meaning but impatient surgeons point out their relative lack of physical findings. The surgeon must be wary of his or her negative countertransference that easily occurs when dealing with the demanding repetitive questions, desperate request for immediate relief, elaborate description of how compliance is impossible, and the look and demand of unfulfilled dependency that are often expressed by these patients. Many seek a magical operation or instant cure, and the clinician must resist the patient's lust for surgery, which at best usually offers only temporary relief. Even though these patients are provided greater attention than others, they are quick to anger and develop feelings of rejection if one tries to abbreviate their pain litany. Unless the diagnosis is made early, gaining their confidence requires great patience, and I find that hand therapists are better at providing this needed compassion.

Even though a patient's extremity may appear anatomically capable, functional activity is often impaired by the pain and

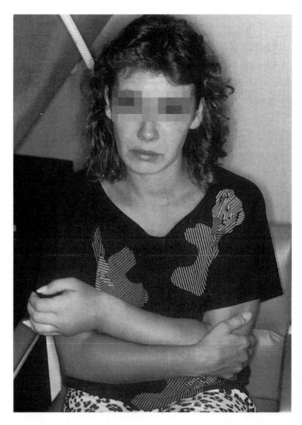

Figure 133-1. 29-year-old woman with stage I RSD 3 months after work injury, protecting her hand from examination.

the patient develops avoidance patterns. Any unexpected withdrawal response in a hand-injured patient, such as when removing sutures, should alert the surgeon to provide immediate additional investigation and support. Until later dystrophic changes occur, pain remains the dominant functional limitation. Study of patients even 3 to 9 years after onset of pain demonstrated that it was still the predominant clinical factor limiting function.[109,110]

Finally, it is a provocative fact that the peculiar quality of reflex dystrophy pain shares similar features to those originating from known primary lesions or dysfunction in the CNS. Central pain syndromes arising from anterior spinal artery syndrome (ASAS); cortical, thalamic, and brainstem strokes; syringomyelia; and central dysesthesia syndrome in spinal cord injury, cause pain described as unlike any other pain in the patient's experience. It is depicted as "intractable," "constant," and "burning," with allodynia that may be triggered by cold, heat, or touch, and often hyperalgesia characterized as spontaneous pain with an overreaction to external stimuli. Like those with reflex dystrophy, most patients with CNS-related injuries have measurable changes in their thresholds for hot and cold sensation. They do not, however, have the other dystrophic changes and the edema of reflex dystrophy unless there is paresis. It is curious that only a small percentage of the patients with CNS injuries develop these pain syndromes (e.g., only one third of patients with spinal cord injuries[26] and 8% of the stroke population).[8] As with RSD patients, persons who suffer from pain caused by injuries to the CNS and who later become asymptomatic remain at risk for recurrence. Examples include patients whose central pain was rekindled many years later by some innocuous or, on the surface, unrelated procedure or event.[26,176] It seems likely that the mechanisms causing the pain of reflex dystrophy and CNS-related pain syndromes will prove to be similar once they are ever understood. For the present, a careful history with meticulous characterization of the pain and observation of the patient's emotional response remain the best tools for early recognition and diagnosis of reflex dystrophy.

PHYSICAL FINDINGS AND STAGES

The first noticeable physical finding in reflex dystrophy is the patient's avoidance of touch or use of the affected extremity because of pain, with tremor present in 50% of cases and involuntary movement present in 35%.[326] However, the first measurable objective changes may be characterized as being from either low-grade inflammation or autonomic activity.

Box 133-2.
Clinical Stages and Findings in Reflex Sympathetic Dystrophy

STAGE I (EARLIEST FINDINGS)
Burning, aching, throbbing pain, with varying intensity that is always present and seems disproportionate
Decreased function caused by pain
Allodynia: pain from usually nonnoxious stimuli (light touch)
Hyperpathia: persistent pain following a stimulus
Trigger points with referred pain
Protective posture to avoid examination
Anxiety and depression
Increased temperature and inflammatory appearance about joints

STAGE II (NEUROINFLAMMATORY OR SYMPATHETIC FINDINGS)
Edema or induration from edema
Hyperhidrosis (early) or dryness (late)
Color change, redness (early) or cyanosis (late)
Increased hair growth
Temperature increase (early) or decrease (late)
Joint or extremity swelling and pain
Active decreased motion

STAGE III (DYSTROPHIC FINDINGS)
Thin, glossy, atrophic skin
Osteoporosis: patchy (early) or generalized (late)
Dense fibrosis
Ankylosis
Stiffness
Muscle atrophy
Decreased hair growth
Contractures
Disuse

Edema is often the first-noted abnormality associated with RSD and may be either pitting or nonpitting. Mottled color change, often redness or cyanosis, is also seen early, sometimes without edema. Temperature change is usually present, with warmness more common early and coolness later in the course of the disorder, and there may be either sweating or dryness. Joint swelling may be seen, and there is usually decreased range of motion that is more pronounced than would be expected from the degree of swelling. Cyanosis is sometimes noted at the joint flexion creases.

The pattern is of vasomotor abnormality, with low-grade inflammatory change and disproportionate pain. Results of synovial tissue testing have been controversial, but biopsy has revealed mild inflammatory changes compared with control tissue[108,171] and hyperplasia of synovial tissue.[207] However, the degree of subjective pain seems to be too great to derive from these mild synovial changes. Some authors[30,117,150] believe reflex dystrophy represents exaggeration of a normal universal inflammatory response. Patients without reflex dystrophy show a diminution of inflammatory response with time, whereas patients with reflex dystrophy progress to more pronounced inflammatory symptoms and possibly later trophic change.

Most surgeons agree with Betcher's[30] classification of reflex dystrophy clinical features into three progressive stages (Box 133-2). However, it must be understood that patients exhibit enormous variation in presenting symptoms, duration, and mixture of characteristics in each stage. Many never progress beyond stage I for years or throughout the course of their disease, whereas others may rapidly progress to the dystrophic stage III within 3 to 6 months. Because of this individualized response and course, these stages have no great clinical value other than a convenient means of describing the degree of clinical change and its prognostic implications. Therefore the stages refer to the amount of clinical change rather than a

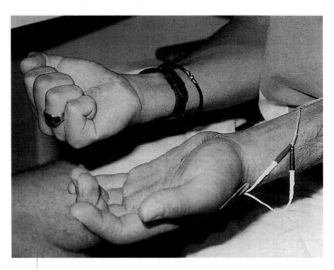

Figure 133-2. Hands of a 26-year-old male with stage I RSD of one hand 10 weeks after bilateral carpal tunnel release. Edema and pain interfere with flexion. He eventually responded to sympathectomy, but 6 years later developed "mirror-image" RSD in the previously uninvolved hand.

chronology of this disorder. These stages may be summarized as *acute* (stage I), with mild autonomic and inflammatory change; *subacute* (stage II), with marked autonomic and inflammatory change; and *chronic* (stage III), with permanent dystrophic change. In all three stages, pain remains the predominant feature.

Acute, or *stage I,* symptoms are dominated by constant burning or aching pain that varies in intensity and may radiate. This is an inexplicably intense pain that interferes with function and usually with motion. Aggravation by normally nonpainful stimuli (allodynia) is evident, and the patient may avoid even the soft touch of an examiner. Physical signs are variable, but they are largely vasomotor, with swelling and edema, redness, mottled cyanosis or other changes in color, increased warmth or coolness, and increased sweating or possibly dryness (Figure 133-2).[174] Although studies show increased blood flow in patients with acute reflex dystrophy, there appears to be impaired oxygen extraction, with a paradoxical tissue hypoxia that has led some investigators to

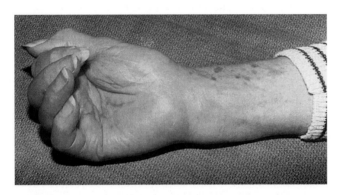

Figure 133-3. Hand of a 49-year-old woman with stage I RSD 5 weeks after surgery for Dupuytren's contracture of the ring finger; patient is unable to flex all four digits. She responded to sympathetic blocks, steroids, and prolonged stress-loading hand therapy.

suspect that inflammatory free radicals are responsible.[322] Limited joint motion, present in over half of the patients, is largely caused by pain; proximal muscle trigger points that refer distally are present in over one half of the patients (Figure 133-3).[93,218-220,322] Some early trophic changes may occur, such as ridging of the nails, increased or decreased hair growth, pigmentation change, and obliteration of fat planes. Bone scintigraphic studies reveal changes as early as 6 weeks after injury. The acute stage lasts approximately 3 months, and the findings are sufficiently subtle that these patients are often misdiagnosed as malingerers or hysterics until second-stage characteristics appear.[318]

Subacute, or *stage II,* reflex dystrophy may characteristically last 9 to 12 months, and the symptoms are still dominated by constant pain that reaches maximum intensity.[174] The diagnosis is now more obvious because trophic changes become evident, with atrophy of skin and subcutaneous tissue causing glossy, thin skin; decreased hair growth; and loss of wrinkling and fingertip pads or "pencil pointing" of involved digits (Figure 133-4). If the syndrome progresses, Raynaud's phenomenon may develop, with previous redness now giving way to a cyanotic, cold-intolerant extremity that maintains a reduced resting temperature. Brawny edema may be present, and restricted joint motion that was previously an active response to pain now becomes permanent because of capsular remodeling and ankylosis. A curious association is the occasional development of palmar fasciitis, thickening of palmar fascia, and Dupuytren's nodules in many patients.[174,302] Mottled, patchy, subchondral osteoporosis may be evident on routine radiographs, and muscle atrophy may become evident. Many of these patients will demonstrate trigger points over muscles proximal to the primary area of discomfort, and the signs and symptoms may progressively spread to adjacent areas if not brought under control.[93,322]

Chronic, or *stage III,* reflex dystrophy still has a dominant symptom of chronic intractable pain. However, now the

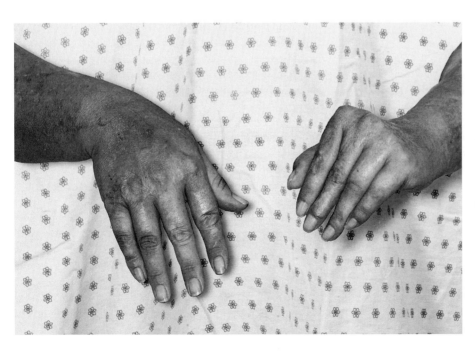

Figure 133-4. A 35-year-old woman with stage II RSD of the left hand 9 months after carpal tunnel surgery. She has tapered fingers; smooth, shiny skin; and diffuse changes seen on radiographs, all of which are characteristic of stage II RSD. (Courtesy Robert C. Russell, MD.)

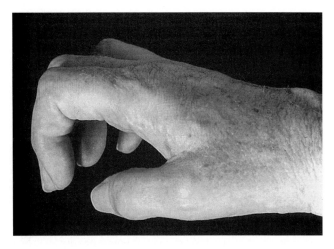

Figure 133-5. Patient with stage III RSD 6 years after injury and chronic causalgia.

physical appearance corresponds to the symptoms, with a pale, cool, dry extremity that has thinly stretched skin and progressive muscle atrophy. Often there is a fixed flexion or extension joint contracture with fibrous ankylosis and loss of the thumb web space (Figure 133-5). Hair growth is diminished. Osteoporosis may change from spotty to a generalized demineralization. At this stage patients may persuade surgeons to attempt amputation to control the pain of their functionless extremity. Although it may appear a reasonable request, amputation should be avoided. In the late stage of reflex dystrophy, the intractable pain involves reflex patterns at the cortical level. Efforts to rid the patient of pain in this fashion will generally offer only temporary benefit, if at all. Therefore amputation may lead only to pleas for additional, higher amputations. Individuals with stage III disease are chronically depressed and may become suicidal.[142]

CLINICAL FORMS

The current classification symptoms of reflex dystrophy do not have much practical value because virtually any inciting injury, or even no apparent injury at all, may lead to reflex dystrophy, and the severity and duration have no correlation with the site or nature of onset and do not imply different outcomes, origins, or treatment techniques. However, three clinical forms do seem so distinct that they warrant separate discussion because of their specific clinical manifestations and therapeutic implications. These forms are causalgia, shoulder-hand syndrome, and Sudeck's osteoporosis.

Causalgia

Major causalgia is the most distinct form of reflex dystrophy, if indeed it should even be included. Causalgia is distinguished by (1) its cause, which is a specific partial injury to a proximal major mixed nerve; (2) its onset, which is usually immediate; (3) its course, which usually includes some degree of

spontaneous improvement; and (4) its superior response rate to sympathetic blocks and sympathectomy, compared with other forms of reflex dystrophy.

As originally described, first by Denmark in the War of 1812 and then by Mitchell in the American War of Northern Aggression, this disorder has a specific onset associated with penetrating wounds that partly injure major nerves. Causalgia is distinguished from other forms of reflex dystrophy by its specific known nerve injury. The International Association for the Study of Pain Subcommittee on Taxonomy describes causalgia as "a syndrome of sustained burning pain after traumatic nerve lesion, combined with vasomotor and pseudomotor dysfunction and later trophic change."[45] Of all of the hand-pain dystrophic syndromes, causalgia has the most obvious peripheral irritation to the nervous system. It is usually caused by nerve injuries situated above the elbow and knee, most often caused by high-velocity missile wounds, in which the nerves have been subjected to rapid and violent deformation, with partial injury. The median nerve is most commonly involved in the upper extremity, and most patients report the onset of pain immediately or soon after being wounded. In one series of war casualties, the incidence of causalgia was 5.8%, with symptom onset in less than 6 hours in 75% of the patients. Sympathectomy corrected all of the cases in this series.[152]

Although the injury is usually above the knee or elbow, causalgia pain remains confined to the distal part of the extremity more often than other types of reflex dystrophy, although it does not remain restricted to the involved nerve distribution.[156] Trophic changes associated with causalgia appear early, and because of the associated nerve injury permanent change is more likely to occur. However, in most patients the neurologic deficit and pain gradually improve to a variable degree, especially in the first 6 months.[88,228,308] Numerous reports indicate the symptoms rarely ever completely disappear.[219,277,290] Sympathetic nerve block is usually dramatic in its temporary relief of causalgia, and repeated blocks may produce sustained relief in some cases.[165] When only temporary relief consistently results, surgery is indicated. Sympathectomy remains the treatment of choice, with excellent response reported in 70% to 100% of patients[152]; however, isolated reports of success with phenoxybenzamine and guanethidine suggest that pharmacologic nerve block may also prove effective.[111,126] Neurotomy, periarterial sympathectomy, and even posterior rhizotomy have been discredited as ineffective methods of treating causalgia.[122,152] Sunderland[308] points out that true causalgia is rare in civilian practice, and he suggests that the combat conditions of emotional stress may be as important as the high-velocity wound in the etiology of this disorder.

There has been debate over whether reflex dystrophy and causalgia are the same disorder.[311] When Evans[93] introduced the term *reflex sympathetic dystrophy* in 1947, he pointed out these patients had previously been diagnosed as having *causalgia* because of their chief symptom—an agonizing burning pain. In his series of 57 reflex dystrophy patients, none had major nerve injury and most had only minor trauma or sprain. Tahmoush's 1981 study[311] demonstrated that the pain of causalgia is indistinguishable from other forms of reflex dystrophy. However, causalgia is a very specific form among the clinical presentations of reflex dystrophy, and the term *causalgia* should be reserved for cases in which major nerve injury has occurred.[318] The cause and onset of other reflex dystrophies are less well understood, and even though they have similar pain manifestations, these other forms often respond well to a program of only exercise and edema control,[1,250] a regimen that cannot usually be carried out by the causalgia patient unless sympathetic nerve block or sympathectomy is first done to control the pain.

Shoulder-Hand Syndrome

When the pain of reflex dystrophy originates in the shoulder, it should be separately identified because this may represent a proximal inciting cause. Any reflex dystrophy of the finger, hand, wrist, or forearm may progress proximally to include the shoulder and become *shoulder-hand syndrome*. However, when the symptoms originate in the shoulder and rapidly progress distally to involve the hand, the clinician must be alert to the possibility of a visceral disease such as ovarian,[214] pancreatic,[222] or breast[218-220] carcinoma, heart attack,[90] gastric ulcer, Pancoast's tumor,[174] and stroke.[66] These systemic causes seem as common as other proximal initiating causes of shoulder-hand syndrome, such as shoulder or neck injury and cervical disk disorders.[154] Therefore when there is no obvious distal or proximal source for shoulder-hand syndrome, a thorough medical workup is necessary. "Mirror image" involvement of the contralateral extremity is more common in shoulder-hand syndrome than in other forms of reflex dystrophy, perhaps because of the more frequent association of systemic or CNS origin.

The response of patients with shoulder-hand syndrome to treatment is similar to that of other forms of reflex dystrophy; however, physical therapy measures are emphasized because they appear to be particularly beneficial in this disorder (Figure 133-6).[154] When addressing attention to the more apparent pain and edema of reflex dystrophy that originates in the hand, it is important not to overlook subtle, progressive stiffness that may develop in the shoulder and become shoulder-hand syndrome. Therapy sometimes seems to require proximal success first, and attention must be given to the stiff shoulder before significant improvement can be achieved in the involved hand.

Sudeck's Osteoporosis

Sudeck's osteoporosis or atrophy is diagnosed because of the apparent skeletal involvement seen on radiographs. It is worthwhile to identify separately, however, because it frequently responds to intramuscular calcitonin treatment. No other particular features distinguish it from other forms of reflex dystrophy, and the initial radiographic pattern is of patchy, mottled demineralization, especially in the juxtaarticular areas, and it resembles the osteoporosis of disuse.[108] However, the onset of osteoporosis is much more rapid than can be explained by simple disuse, with findings as early as 4 to

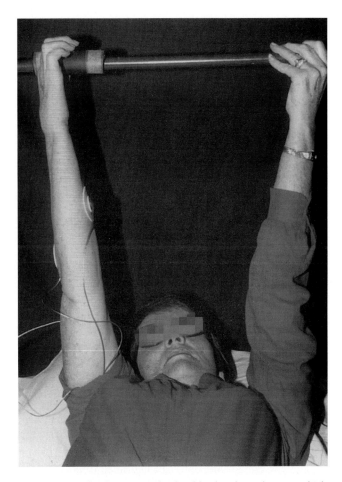

Figure 133-6. Patient with shoulder-hand syndrome, which improved with TENS and hand therapy.

6 weeks after onset of symptoms and changes that would characteristically take as long as 10 years of disuse. This may occur with only minor changes in motor function, and the patients may still be using their extremities as the changes occur. Any form of reflex dystrophy may eventually develop this characteristic osteoporosis, with incidence reported as high as 30% to 70%.[169] Using fine-detail radiography, Genant et al[108] identified the following five types of bone resorption associated with reflex dystrophy:

1. Irregular absorption of trabecular bone in the metaphysis, creating a patchy appearance
2. Subperiosteal bone resorption
3. Intracortical bone resorption
4. Endosteal bone resorption
5. Surface erosions of subchondral juxtaarticular bone

Although treatment and results in Sudeck's osteoporosis are similar to those in other forms of dystrophy, their separate identification is warranted to attempt calcitonin therapy, which may reverse the osteoblastic activity and the pain in Sudeck's osteoporosis.[243]

Myofascial Dysfunction

Although most reports on RSD or CRPS do not include myofascial dysfunction trigger points among clinical findings, several authors document their frequent presence. Indeed, in his original 1947 treatise, Evans observed multiple trigger points in 36 of his 57 patients (63%), and I have noted a 67% incidence among my patients.[219] Knowledge about myofascial dysfunction trigger points and their treatment can be useful in the management of reflex dystrophy. This clinical feature may be overlooked because of confusion and doubt about its pathophysiology and significance. Like reflex dystrophy, myofascial dysfunction is a clinical diagnosis without definitive laboratory criteria, and also like reflex dystrophy, there are those who even question its existence.[40]

Unfortunately, myofascial dysfunction is grouped with disorders of even less-clear criteria, such as fibromyalgia; however, the clinical findings of myofascial trigger points appear more distinct and have some interesting correlation with reflex dystrophy. Myofascial dysfunction is characterized by specific proximal trigger points arising in muscle or fascia that elicit immediate referred pain or numbness at distant sites and sometimes produce autonomic change. The term *trigger* is used because, like pulling the trigger of a gun, palpation of a trigger point, for example in the forearm, projects pain or numbness to a distant target in the zone of referral, such as the wrist. The trigger point itself is a hyperirritable locus in a taut band of skeletal muscle and usually is found as a palpable "lump." Pressure over this nodule causes pain that is perceived in the distal extremity. It may vary from mild discomfort to intolerable pain. In rare instances it causes autonomic change, such as vasoconstriction, sweating, and color change. In my experience, patients are usually totally unaware of their trigger points and are surprised by the discovery, with findings that are convincing. The relationship of trigger points to their zone of referral is predictable, although they do not follow any neurologic or segmental patterns and most commonly refer to the region where the muscle inserts. Long ago, Kellgren[159] noted that painful injection of muscle results in perceived pain at the region of insertion rather than the site of injection. These referral zones are characterized for each muscle by Trevell and Simons.[319] For example, when a trigger point of the extensor carpi radialis longus (ECRL) muscle is activated over the humeral lateral condyle it will predictably refer pain or tingling to the radiodorsal region of the hand and wrist. Trevell and Simons offer the following eight criteria to identify active trigger points of myofascial dysfunction:

1. A history of sudden-onset of pain after injury or acute overload stress
2. Characteristic patterns of pain referred from specific muscular trigger points
3. Weakness and restriction in the stretch range of motion of affected muscles
4. A taut, palpable band or nodule in the affected muscle
5. Exquisite focal tenderness to digital pressure in the band or nodule of taut muscle
6. A local twitch response elicited through snapping, palpation, or needling of the trigger point spot

7. Reproduction of the patient's pain complaint by pressure against or needling of the trigger point
8. Elimination of symptoms by treatment specifically to the affected muscle trigger-point site

These findings have been challenged by study of various clinicians' ability to specifically identify trigger points of myofascial dysfunction and distinguish them from fibromyalgia.[340] However, recognition of these sites of pain are important in the diagnosis and treatment of patients with a complex chronic pain syndrome such as reflex dystrophy. Specific treatment is beneficial. Trevell and Simons[319] contend that in the absence of treatment, trigger points become a chronic condition that does not spontaneously resolve and may progress to involve adjacent musculature, resulting in stiffness and muscular weakness.

Debate on the etiology of myofascial trigger points ranges from the concept of a local "rheumatism" by Virchow in 1852 to a central neurologic dysfunction,[160,161,344] or psychiatric disorder.[40] As in reflex dystrophy, the overwhelming symptom of myofascial dysfunction is unexplained pain, with lowered threshold, so that the pain may be caused by factors such as minimal muscle activity, temperature change, or even emotional stress. The pain may persist long after stimulation of the trigger-point site. However, patients with myofascial dysfunction that is not associated with reflex dystrophy differ in that they will have pain-free intervals, and relief occurs with rest, such as when splinted. In both myofascial dysfunction and reflex dystrophy, use and muscular activity usually aggravate pain.

Treatment for myofascial dysfunction varies, but the use of muscle stretch and vasocoolant spray or icing to inactivate the trigger points have been popularized by Trevell and Simons. Other reported treatment techniques include heat[229]; injection of trigger points with local anesthetic,[25] steroid,[345] or saline[105]; "ischemic" compression by prolonged digital pressure[266]; massage[339]; ultrasound[345]; biofeedback; transcutaneous electrical neural stimulation (TENS); and a variety of pharmacologic agents used to control insomnia, depression, pain, and inflammation.[319]

The goal of therapy in dealing with patients who have the common combination of reflex dystrophy and myofascial trigger points that refer should be to inactivate the hyperirritable trigger points before activities such as strengthening exercises or work simulation, or even range-of-motion exercise in the painful referral zone. Unfortunately, the use of vasocoolant spray or ice is rarely tolerated by the patient with reflex dystrophy, who usually has cold intolerance. Measures such as massage, ultrasound, pressure, TENS, or injection must frequently be employed to gain control of these trigger points. It is important for any patient with myofascial trigger points to utilize a program of eccentric (stretch) strengthening exercise to avoid recurrence of the trigger points once they are under control. This will be compatible with the usual stress-loading program that is utilized for reflex dystrophy. The importance of gaining control over these irritable muscle foci before more aggressive distal therapy is emphasized.

BIOLOGIC MECHANISMS CAUSING TROPHIC CHANGES: NEUROGENIC INFLAMMATION

One of the most perplexing features of RSD is the apparent physiologic and anatomic changes that occur without apparent peripheral cause. Even though the original injury seems minor, or there was no injury at all, these dystrophic changes can become dramatic, with permanent stiffness, atrophy, osteoporosis, tapered fingertips, and tight, shiny skin. This functionless, chronically painful state leads some patients to request amputation and contemplate suicide.

The mechanisms for these dramatic physiologic changes remain unclear. Disuse is a widely accepted explanation; however, anyone witnessing the sometimes rapid alteration in blood flow, temperature change, mottled appearance, edema, rapid osteoporosis, and joint inflammation in these patients cannot accept such a simple explanation. At this time, other explanations remain hypothetical, but warrant review. There is an increasing understanding of the complex internal neurogenic pain-neurotransmitter systems and intrinsic physiologic pain-inhibition mechanisms, which someday may explain the changes associated with reflex dystrophy.

NEUROGENIC INFLAMMATION: THE ROLE OF SUBSTANCE P AND OTHER NEUROPEPTIDES

When noxious external mechanical and thermal stimulation, such as cuts or burns, activate peripheral unmyelinated afferent pain fibers, we expect a characteristic pain and inflammatory response. These afferent fibers are responsive to a variety of internal chemical stimuli, with local inflammation enhanced through the release of vasodilating mediators (histamine, bradykinin, and prostaglandin) from damaged tissues. These afferent fibers are also modified and mediated by centrally produced neuropeptides. Whereas a noxious stimulus is mediated to the CNS via nociceptive afferents, simultaneous conduction occurs in the same fibers away from the CNS in response to the stimulus. This backflow, known as *axon reflux* results in the release of vasoactive neuropeptide substances, such as substance P (SP), calcitonin gene-related peptide (CGRP), bradykinin, serotonin, somatostatin, neurokinin, and others. Some investigators have regarded reflex dystrophy as a manifestation of chronic neuropathic pain,[121,149,218-220] whereas others point to local prolonged and sustained regional inflammation as the primary source, and a comprehensive explanation remains lacking.

Over 50 years ago Lewis[187,188] hypothesized that primary afferent pain receptors released substances that cause inflammation. Today more than 20 neuropeptide neurotransmitter substances are being characterized,[180] many of which are known to be inflammatory mediators.[186] Therefore the most provocative possible source of inflammation in reflex dystrophy may be the afferent receptors themselves. These unmyelin-ated, bidirectional, afferent pain receptors not only respond to produce pain centrally, but are also capable of releasing inflammatory mediators peripherally in response to either peripheral or central stimulation. It is interesting that the highest concentrations of these endings are in the hands, feet, and face—the most common locations for reflex dystrophy. For example, afferent neurons are known to synthesize and release the neurotransmitter substance P in the CNS, where it is believed to mediate pain transmission,[180] but up to 90% of this neuropeptide is actually transmitted from the cell body to the peripheral terminals of these afferent fibers, from which it can be released to contribute to inflammation.[186] Experimentally, substance P is known to cause physiologic changes associated with inflammatory response when injected directly into peripheral tissues[101,182] or by stimulation of peripheral nerves at an intensity known to release substance P.[34,151] These changes from substance P injection or stimulation include vasodilatation, increased vascular permeability, pavementing of leukocytes in venules, stimulation of phagocytosis by polymorphonuclear leukocytes, degranulation of mast cells, and a host of other characteristic inflammatory changes. Substance P even has inflammatory immunologic properties that are largely stimulatory, such as stimulation of T lymphocytes,[255] increased production of IGA,[300] elicitation of mononuclear leukocyte chemotaxis,[278] and release of lysosomal enzymes with generation of thromboxane.[135] Furthermore, this neurotransmitter has been shown to enhance proliferation of fibroblasts and smooth muscle cells,[241] tending toward fibroplasia. Among the neurotransmitters, substance P is the most attractive to implicate in reflex dystrophy because it appears to generate such a profound generalized inflammatory response and it has been the most studied (the first neurotransmitter identified and purified).[186] Several substance-P antagonists have been developed, but thus far show neither high affinity nor selectivity.[101] Although substance-P antagonists show some inhibition of inflammatory response, each seems to only inhibit a part of the response, such as those that inhibit histamine release and others that inhibit thermally induced edema in the rat. Capsaicin (the "hot pepper" substance) is not an antagonist, but acts to deplete afferent nociceptive neurons of substance P and other neuropeptides, and appears to reduce axoplasmic transport of neuropeptide. Its action is not completely understood, but repeated application results in desensitization to inflammatory agents without tactile loss of pressure or temperature sensation.

Studies suggest substance P could be an important direct or indirect mediator of neurogenic inflammation, but other neurotransmitter substances known to be released from unmyelinated afferent pain endings are also capable of eliciting various inflammatory responses. Two that are known to coexist with substance P in the afferent neurons are CGRP and neurokinin A. CGRP is a potent vasodilator that has been used therapeutically to prevent vasoconstriction in Raynaud's syndrome.[220] CGRP is released from perivascular nerves. It also can produce a wheal and flare reaction in human skin, but is less potent than substance P. It differs from substance P in that the vasodilatation is of slow onset and longer lasting (more than 4 hours) and is not inhibited by antihistaminics, indicating a different mechanism of action. CGRP does not cause increased vascular permeability that might cause edema but is nonetheless synergistic with other mediators that do cause vascular permeability. Neurokinin A does increase vascular permeability and cause vasodilatation and is also a very potent bronchoconstricting agent. There are numerous other neurotransmitter substances that are undoubtedly important in the mediation of neurogenic inflammation, such as the neuropeptides present in the sympathetic (e.g., neuropeptide Y and norepinephrine) and parasympathetic (vasoactive intestinal peptides and acetylcholine) nervous systems, as well as cyclooxygenase, which is known to be present in the midbrain and is a key enzyme in the synthesis of the prostaglandin system forming prostaglandins, prostacyclin, and thromboxane A_2. It is the prostaglandin system that appears to be inhibited by aspirin and nonsteroidal antiinflammatory drugs (NSAIDS).[141] Proinflammatory cytokines, such as interleukin-1 (IL-1) and interleukin-6 (IL-6), and tumor necrosis factor-A (TNF-A) are known to be synthesized in the brain and are released in the inflammatory tissues with sensitization of the afferent receptors, producing local hyperalgesia.[64] It is believed that these free cytokines may modulate nociception via the prostaglandin system. Interplay between the sensory system neurotransmitters and prostanoid system undoubtedly occurs; PGE-2 or PGI-2 exposure is known to potentiate capsaicin-evoked release of substance P for cultured rat sensory neurons. Furthermore, substance P can evoke release of prostaglandin E-2.[322]

The extent to which this complicated neurotransmitter system may function independently of external stimuli remains questionable. As currently conceived, afferent nociceptive impulses are followed by simultaneous axon reflex release of neurotransmitter substances capable of causing and maintaining various inflammatory responses. This must involve a complex regulatory system and it is conceivable that dysregulation of this neuropeptide system could result in inappropriate quantity and length of neuropeptide secretion. This might explain the enormous variability in patient response, and selective neurotransmitter release may be responsible for individual differences observed in the objective "sympathetic" manifestations in patients with reflex dystrophy.

Schott[282] hypothesized that in patients with reflex dystrophy, substance P and CGRP are involved in the inflammatory reaction and the accompanying motor and sensory disturbance. Indeed, analysis of blood samples obtained from 61 patients with reflex dystrophy showed significantly increased systemic levels of bradykinin and CGRP compared with 21 controls.[36]

Role of the Sympathetic Nervous System

The majority of reports on RSD/CRPS/algodystrophy assume abnormal sympathetic activity to be the predominant etiologic factor.[167,171] Yet the major proof of this conclusion remains the clinical response to sympathetic block, which is sufficiently

variable that it is no longer a requirement for diagnosis.* Concluding etiologic cause by response to treatment is a treacherous approach, especially when there is such varied response among different patients, and even in the same patient on different occasions.[95,218-220,244-246]

To clarify which patients have pain from sympathetic origin, the phentolamine block test was developed to identify patients with "sympathetically maintained pain,"[53] a concept first proposed by Roberts.[274] This concept holds that the aspect of pain relieved by regional block of the sympathetic ganglia for the painful area is the sympathetically maintained pain. Many authors now contest the original hypothesis of an abnormal sympathetic short-circuitry reflex arc (e-phase), initially suggested by Leriche and now others.[61,95,281,301] Experimental findings, however, do not show hyperactivity of the sympathetic nervous system.[18,282,283] In fact, in the early stages of reflex dystrophy, there appears to be sympathetic hypofunction, with increased arterial flow, rather than sympathetic overactivity and vasoconstriction.[59] Proponents for sympathetically maintained pain point out evidence that although there is no increased sympathetic secretion, the afferent pain nociceptors become hypersensitized to normal sympathetic norepinephrine release,[53] and the sustained release leads to secondary hyperalgesia.[164] Under the influence of a sympathetic block, norepinephrine is no longer released to activate nociceptors and the central sensitization is reversed. Others suggest the mechanism is by means of polymodal C-fibers that do not belong to the sympathetic nervous system but often travel with the sympathetic nerves. This might explain the success of sympathetic blocks.[28] Study of experimental arthritis in rats suggests that sympathetic efferents may in fact be able to modify the inflammatory response. Sympathectomy and sympathetic blocks in rats with experimental arthritis significantly reduce the inflammatory response.[186]

There are now a growing number of investigators who question the role of the sympathetic nervous system in any way other than a modulatory fashion.[28,219,244-246,283,322] Unfortunately, most reported series of sympathetic blocks are not placebo controlled, and patients with reflex dystrophy/CRPS are known to be heavy placebo responders.[244-246] Indeed, several placebo-controlled studies showed sympathetic block to be no more effective than the placebo.[244-246] An additional confounding factor is recognition of the analgesic effect produced by simple use of the tourniquet alone.[95,236,237]

Many of the initial clinical findings of RSD do appear to involve sympathetic manifestations, with abnormalities of temperature, skin color and appearance, hair growth, sweat pattern, and edema. It is just as possible these are mediated via neurogenic secretion from the afferent nociceptors as the sympathetic efferents, but surely these two systems must both be implicated to ultimately understand this disorder. If proinflammatory neuropeptide secretion from these afferent sensory nerve terminals is largely responsible for the inflammatory and autonomic changes associated with RSD, it becomes

---

*References 6, 149, 166, 218, 260, 299, 323.

understandable how antiinflammatory drugs such as steroids and DMSO, drugs that produce pharmacologic block, and local anesthetic sympathetic nerve blocks may all reduce the peripheral neurotransmission in some cases in which the sympathetic modification is great. However, these measures may all prove ineffective in other patients in which the sympathetic modification is minimal. When the primary reflex or stimulus for neurotransmitter release is at a higher cortical level, CNS modulators (e.g., TENS, biofeedback therapy, antiepileptic medication, antidepressant drugs, acupuncture, dorsal root stimulation, and hypnosis) may prove to be of greater benefit. These methods likely rely on the endogenous CNS pain-control neurotransmitter system (enkephalin-endorphin) rather than peripheral modification of afferent response. Endorphin inhibition of substance P from the spinal cord, spinal trigeminal nucleus, and primary sensory neurons in culture has been documented experimentally and may account for the success of these central treatment techniques in reflex dystrophy and also the frequency of placebo effect.[180] The debate whether this disorder is primarily mediated from the sympathetic versus the afferent nociceptor system becomes moot if one recognizes that this is likely to vary, depending on the higher cerebral neuropeptide dysregulation.

ETIOLOGY

There is no current unifying hypothesis that adequately explains the disproportionate pain associated with vasomotor, inflammatory, and dystrophic changes we call RSD/CRPS/algodystrophy. The fact that the disorder arises from such an outrageous spectrum of differing precipitating causes truly suggests RSD to be a syndrome rather than a specific entity, with multiple etiologic factors expressed in similar symptomology. Theories for etiologic mechanisms characteristically focus on one of three levels in the nervous system: peripheral, spinal cord, and cerebral, in the search for an anatomic, physiologic, or psychologic explanation. There remains the need for a unifying concept.

PERIPHERAL ANATOMIC BASIS: E-PHASE THEORY

Over 50 years ago Doupe et al[74] proposed that injury permitted artificial synapses (E-phases) to develop at the injury site so that efferent sympathetic nerves could activate afferent fibers. Thus innocent impulses, such as temperature, might cross directly into a fiber system that records the experience as painful in the CNS. Although this was proposed to explain causalgia pain after major nerve injury, other authors suggested similar cross stimulation might occur with non-nerve injury, with E-phases from sympathetic efferent fibers to sensory nociceptor afferent fibers.[70] Current proponents of this

theory suggest abnormal sensitization and spontaneous ectopic discharge.

SPINAL CORD LEVEL: INTERNUNCIAL POOL THEORY

Livingston[192] and Lorente de No[193] proposed that peripheral nerve stimulation could activate the interconnecting internuncial neural pool at the segmental level of the spinal cord, and this increased activity could spread to involved nearby sympathetic neurons. This produced a cyclical, self-perpetuating impulse. The concept was expanded by Roberts,[274] who suggested that peripheral trauma activates unmyelinated peripheral nociceptors initially, leading to excitation of wide-dynamic-range (WDR) neurons on the spinal cord. Thusly activated, WDR neuron activity summates to become responsive to all afferent input, continuing to respond even after stimulation ceases or injury heals. Adjacent sympathetic activity is increased, which lowers the threshold of mechanoreceptors. Under these circumstances, mild stimulation in the periphery can precipitate a pronounced sympathetic neurovascular response. More recent considerations are that inhibitory mechanisms fail at the spinal cord level and can be replaced by pharmacologic agents, such as NMDA (n-methyl-d-aspartate) and neurokinin receptors.[22,71,334]

PSYCHOPHYSIOLOGIC MECHANISMS

None of the theories offered for peripheral synapse or spinal cord origin of reflex dystrophy explain why an estimated 95% to 98% of patients with soft tissue injury do not develop this disorder. Furthermore, these theories cannot account for those patients who develop the syndrome after stroke, myocardial infarction, or ovarian cancer, or those who acquire it spontaneously, with no known injury or precipitating factor at all. This has led some to theorize that there may be a predisposing psychologic makeup playing a role in the etiology of RSD/CRPS in some, if not all, cases.

PSYCHOLOGICAL FINDINGS

The first question to be answered is whether patients with RSD/CRPS are significantly different psychologically from other patients with hand injuries. Based on his personal observations, Bunnell[51] stated his opinion that patients with RSD have "emotional and vasomotor instability and are subject to neuroses." He suggested that their mental state was to some extent responsible for the persistence of the disorder.

Hardy et al[132] compared psychologic test results in patients with reflex dystrophy with others who had hand injuries. She used a blind evaluation in 17 patients with rigid criteria for the reflex dystrophy diagnosis. Diagnostic criteria included characteristic pain and at least three objective changes, such as a temperature difference of at least 4 degrees, volume change greater than 10 ml, abnormal ninhydrin test, osteoporosis, and other measurable criteria. Psychologic tests included intelligence, body concept, personal control, and the Hopkins symptom checklist, which rates five primary dimensions: somatization, obsessive/compulsive traits, interpersonal sensitivity, depression, and anxiety. This study showed significant differences in the psychologic profile of patients with reflex dystrophy in four of the tests, using the one-way Analysis of Variance test for significance. The patients with reflex dystrophy tested significantly higher than controls in anxiety, depression, interpersonal sensitivity, and somatization. One test, body cathexis, approached significance (P=0.58) with the dystrophy patients testing lower than controls. Intelligence, concepts of personal control, and obsessive/compulsive features were not different in the two groups of patients (Table 133-1). Thus a patient with reflex dystrophy might be described as someone more anxious and depressed than other patients with hand injuries, and with more frequent complaints of somatic distress and less ability to relate interpersonally. The study also suggests that they are more dissatisfied with their bodies.

It has been suggested that the difference in personality traits in patients with reflex dystrophy are due to the fact that they experience greater pain because of a lower threshold.[89] Hardy also attempted to answer this question and determined that the difference was not due to a lower pain threshold because visual linear analog scale testing[270] and ischemic ratio pain test[303] did not show any difference in pain threshold or overall pain complaints in the two groups. However, review of precipitating causes in this series did demonstrate that the reflex dystrophy group appeared to have less serious injuries overall than those in the control group, in spite of equivalent pain. Crush injury was common among controls, and digital fractures and soft tissue injuries were common among those with reflex dystrophy. None of the patients in this series had causalgia from major mixed-nerve injury. Thus it appears that non-nerve–injured reflex dystrophy patients do have a significantly different psychologic makeup compared with that of other patients with hand injuries. I suspect it to be a predisposing characteristic. Now there is widespread acceptance that patients with reflex dystrophy do have significantly greater anxiety, depression, and possibly other psychologic differences. However, the majority of investigators believe these psychologic differences are a result, rather than a cause, of reflex dystrophy.[167]

Psychiatric evaluation of 34 of our patients with RSD revealed that most were from dysfunctional backgrounds, enduring difficulty such as parental alcoholism, death of parents, rape, and other childhood abuse. Furthermore, all but four fulfilled clinical criteria for a diagnosis of alexithymia. Although the psychiatrist, Dr. Janaki Theogaraj, was blinded insofar as each patient's diagnosis, the evaluation was clinical and did not include psychologic testing for alexithymia.[317] This testing is now available in the form of the Toronto Alexithymia Scale. In this series of patients there were more women than men, they generally had an excellent work history up until the injury, and most had been in abusive marital relationships.

While only Theogaraj has observed the prevalence of alexithymia in patients with RSD, others have recognized the increased incidence of chronic pain syndrome among alexithymic patients and have identified increased sympathetic

Table 133-1.
Results of Psychologic and Pain Tests, Comparing RSD/CRPS Patients and Hand-Injured Controls

TEST/FEATURE	RESULTS IN RSD/CRPS	SIGNIFICANCE
Pain level (threshold)	No significant difference	
Visual analog scale		P = 0.500
Ischemic ratio tourniquet test		P = 0.300
Obsessive/compulsive	No significant difference	P = 0.257
Locus of control	No significant difference	P = 0.519
Intelligence	No significant difference	P = 0.310
Self-cathexis	No significant difference	P = 0.080
Body cathexis (body satisfaction)	Approaches significantly less	P = 0.058
Somatization	Significantly greater	P = 0.005
Interpersonal sensitivity	Significantly greater	P = 0.023
Depression	Significantly greater	P = 0.022
Anxiety	Significantly greater	P = 0.044

response to experimental stress, its relationship to anxiety and depression, and the recognition that alexithymia may contribute to chronic pain by means of sympathetic arousal.[103]

Alexithymia, literally translated, means "a lack of words for mood or emotion." Formulated by Nemiah and Sifneos[238] in the 1970s, discussion of this construct is found predominantly in the psychosomatic literature to depict a personality profile marked by an inability to verbalize one's feelings and an inability to discriminate between feelings and physical sensation. These patients are unable to recognize or differentiate their emotional state and are characterized by a paucity of dreams and fantasies and a tendency to think in a concrete, utilitarian manner (Box 133-3). They may be described as being "blind to their emotional feeling," but in psychiatric studies these patients clearly have great sensitivity and response to the emotions of other people. In the psychosomatic literature, alexithymia has been of clinical interest primarily because of its association with somatic symptoms and a lack of response to conventional psychotherapy.[146,185] These patients are described as having an "externally oriented cognitive style" and there is now strong suggestion that early traumatic childhood experiences and abuse play a significant role in its etiology.[168] Furthermore, there is suggestion that certain physiologic abnormalities, such as peptic ulceration, are risk factors in patients with alexithymia.[106] In her psychiatric evaluation of 203 consecutive patients with reflex dystrophy, Didierjean[72] described them in a fashion that is consistent with alexithymia: "Their speech is rather a flat narrative, with few references to fantasy."

It is recognized that alexithymic patients do not respond to conventional psychotherapy, which may be due to the fact that alexithymic patients never developed or matured any conscious awareness of their own emotion, and much of conventional psychotherapy relies on cognitive release of suppressed emotion. One might imagine how the child of alcoholic or foster parents may "learn not to feel" as a method of coping with unpredictable parental or authority-figure behavior. In such an environment, expression of joy or anger might be followed by unpredictable parental response. In this fashion, the child grows up emotionally undeveloped, without an awareness of his or her feelings, and with a continuum of unfulfilled dependency needs, a quick sense of rejection, and often unconsciously suppressed anger. Studies of alexithymic patients suggest that disassociation from traumatic events during childhood may play a role in its etiology. Emotional stress in

---

Box 133-3.
Characteristics of Alexithymia

Difficulty identifying and describing feelings
Difficulty distinguishing between feelings and the bodily sensations of emotional arousal
Constricted imagined processes (e.g., a paucity of fantasies)
Externally oriented cognitive style

---

such individuals who are "blind to their emotions" goes unrecognized and may be transmitted at the midbrain level as physical stress, possibly stimulating neuropeptide reflex in the CNS. Unfortunately, at present there has been no study utilizing the Toronto Alexithymic Scale, which currently provides the best-recognized testing mechanism for diagnosis. Treatment of alexithymia is largely by general psychiatric support because the disorder probably represents a fundamental developmental problem, not easily altered by psychotherapy.

Any patient who complains of disproportionate pain after a minor injury or operation and who seems obviously anxious and depressed should immediately be treated by compassionate, intensive hand therapy to try to obviate any further development of this problem. This is especially true when patients are prone to give endless, detailed, concrete descriptions of their physical manifestations and seem oblivious to their anger, depression, or other emotions. The worst possible approach is to try and minimize the patient's plea for support by appearing nonchalant and belittling the symptoms. These patients already have unfulfilled dependency needs and feel easily rejected. Although they are relatively unaware of their own emotions, they are quite sensitive to the suspicion and negative countertransference that so often occurs in dealing with a patient who complains of great somatic distress and has minimal objective findings.

ROLE OF THE OPIOID PAIN-CONTROL SYSTEM

Much research has identified an intrinsic pain-inhibiting system represented at descending levels in the midbrain, medulla, and spinal cord. The role of this modulating system in reflex dystrophy has not been described, but in a disorder with unexplained pain as its dominant feature, this system must surely be important and warrants attention.

Early evidence of an endogenous pain-control system was by electrical stimulation of the midbrain of animals to produce anesthesia for surgery.[209,271] Soon afterward, a relationship was identified with naturally occurring endogenous morphine-like neuropeptides (enkephalins and endorphins), which had receptors in the brain and spinal cord.[145] Naloxone, a specific opiate or morphine antagonist, blocks the analgesia produced by brainstem stimulation at levels of the midbrain, medulla, and spinal cord,[20] indicating the importance of this endorphin system in CNS control of pain. Furthermore, experiments suggest control requires transmission from above the spinal cord along the dorsal part of the lateral funiculus to pathways of interconnection at the spinal level, where pain inhibition occurs.

Endorphins appear to have a direct inhibitory effect on the production and release of the pain-producing neuropeptide substance P at these levels.[180] When released at afferent terminals, substance P is known to produce inflammatory change in the periphery and pain at the cerebral level.

Reflex dystrophy patients are known to have a high response rate from placebo treatments, as high as one third from placebo blocks.[46] *Placebo effect* is a term describing relief of pain or other symptoms after a sham treatment, and it is thought largely to be derived from expectation of benefit from the supposed medication or treatment. For many years this response was regarded with contempt by clinicians, until the endogenous opioid pain system offered a physiologic explanation. Indeed, study of the opioid system in patients treated with placebo suggests the significant role endorphins play in producing pain relief.[120] However, there is general consensus that patient confidence and expectation of relief are essential requirements for activating the CNS endogenous pain-inhibition system.[99] Thus the critical importance of a positive, confident, compassionate, and consistent approach to all patients with reflex dystrophy may have a rational scientific basis, as well as a humanitarian one, but this would seem to be especially true when using central treatment methods such as acupuncture, biofeedback, TENS, dorsal column stimulation, stress loading, antiepileptic medication, and physical therapy.

If, indeed, central endogenous pain control is required for coping with reflex dystrophy, the hopeless attitude found among those who have had the disorder more than 6 months, have difficulty with interpersonal relationships, and who have complicated and antagonistic interpersonal relationships would certainly complicate their successful treatment. This may explain why late treatment is so difficult.

PSYCHOPHYSIOLOGIC ETIOLOGY

Any theory about the etiology of RSD must reconcile the vast array of differing precipitating causes, the wide unpredictable variation of clinical manifestations, the variable successes and failures of profoundly differing treatment techniques, and the contradictory research results, which together suggest mechanisms at three different levels of the sensory and/or autonomic nervous systems. The pathogenesis must be multifactorial because it is so highly variable from one patient to the next. To that extent *reflex sympathetic dystrophy* might better be described as *reflex dystrophy syndrome*, with common manifestations of pain and circulatory change in response to very different precipitating factors (the basic criteria for a syndrome). If there are predisposing personality characteristics for reflex dystrophy patients, afferent unmyelinated pain endings may release neuropeptides that cause persistent inflammation, and expectation of relief may be able to activate a descending system of opioids that can inhibit the neuropeptides that cause pain and inflammation. How these findings can be etiologic factors is open to speculation, but an attractive unifying hypothesis is that a varying CNS bias may lead to dysregulation of the neuropeptide system reflex. This speculation requires a departure from conventional capitalized western thought. Descartes is held responsible for defining the human as a creature with a mind "entirely separate" from the body, and the growth of psychiatry as a distinct specialty reflects this western concept.[23] Unfortunately, physicians and their patients envision these reflex dystrophy disorders as either only in the head or only the hand. Somehow, the idea that a pain

disorder might arise from predominantly cerebral mechanisms is looked on contemptuously by western society. However, relationships between personality characteristics, psychologic stress, and somatic illness are accepted in certain other illnesses, such as peptic ulcer disease. We do recognize that physiologic manifestations of stress occur via the autonomic nervous system,[48] and study of normal subjects reveals very consistent but very different individualized patterns of sympathetic response for each person. Certain neuroses are known to have somatic consequences.[48,92,145,293] Therefore it is distinctly possible that personality characteristics (such as alexithymia), unusual conditions of stress at the time of injury (such as combat), or the nature of neural insult (such as high-velocity nerve wounding or midbrain stroke) may bias the CNS toward dysregulation of the complex mediators of pain and neurogenic inflammation.

Electrical stereotactic brainstem stimulation in 198 conscious patients with either chronic dystrophic pain or somatic pain from carcinoma revealed reproduction of the characteristic burning pain only in those with dystrophic pain.[313] This suggests some fundamental alteration has occurred at the midbrain level to cause pain with electrical stimulation that distinguishes these patients from those with somatic peripheral pain. It is not unreasonable to postulate that mesencephalic reticulothalamocortical circuits at this level are similarly sensitive to innocent afferent neural input, causing inappropriate pain neuropeptide release at this cortical level. Thus in some patients the pain of reflex dystrophy may be a distinct entity from somatic pain, arising from alteration of the CNS at the midbrain level that, once established, persists despite removal of the original peripheral stimulus.

If such a central mechanism exists, those with alexithymia would be expected to be at greater risk of having central misrepresentation of emotional stress and minor injury. In a controlled study, Gertzen et al[110] confirmed Hardy's earlier findings that patients with reflex dystrophy have significantly greater depression and were more "emotionally unstable" than controls. In addition, he found that 80% of these patients had a recent stressful "life event" compared with 20% of the controls, suggesting that stress was a major etiological factor in his series. Van Houdenhove,[325] in an uncontrolled psychiatric evaluation of patients with RSD, reported that nearly all had a major stressful life event within a significant timeframe of developing the syndrome.

Other factors that could bias the CNS toward this hypersensitivity could include circumstances surrounding an injury and the psychologic makeup of the patient and his or her characteristic response to stress. Sunderland[309] noted that causalgia occurs more frequently under stressful battle conditions than civilian settings. Work-related injury in which there is some type of antagonistic relationship with the employer and adverse relationships with previous physicians certainly seem to prevail in patients with RSD. If stressful circumstances in patients with predisposed personalities produce alteration in the CNS, then with whatever treatment is used it behooves physicians and therapists to also permit expression of the fear and anger these circumstances have caused, in hopes of reducing this central hypersensitivity. This may take great patience in dealing with those who have alexithymia and tend to speak concretely with great detail. Such a biased CNS midbrain could initiate pain-causing descending excitation, ultimately releasing neuropeptide inflammatory mediators that might cause the inflammatory and sympathetic response seen in reflex dystrophy. Furthermore, it is conceivable that the confident, reassured, and optimistic patient may be able to counter this process with the descending endogenous enkephalin-endorphin system, which is known to be able to inhibit pain and substance P at the spinal cord level.

The importance of a centrally mediated system with varying mechanisms causing midbrain dysregulation could explain the wide variation in precipitating cause and patient response, with some having predominantly neurogenic insult leading to the disorder, such as stroke and major mixed-nerve injury, and others having a central bias that makes them highly susceptible with minor injury or no injury at all.

DIAGNOSTIC TECHNIQUES

There is no objective laboratory study that is specific for reflex dystrophy. Although numerous objective studies are useful to support the diagnosis, it remains ultimately clinical. In fact, laboratory studies are sometimes erroneously used to make reflex dystrophy a diagnosis of exclusion, ruling out other disorders. This approach overlooks the fact that reflex dystrophy has been associated with a variety of disorders, such as diabetes, herpes infection, carcinoma, heart disease, thyroid disease, arthritis, and stroke; abnormal lab studies therefore should not exclude the diagnosis (see Precipitating Causes, p. 2342). However, typical patients with reflex dystrophy have a normal sedimentation rate, C-reactive protein, leukocyte count, and other acute-phase reactants in spite of an appearance of inflammation.[207] The need for early diagnosis led researchers to explore several areas for possible objective diagnostic signs. Parameters of the sympathetic nervous system were most frequently studied and included temperature, skin conductance, blood flow, and radioisotope uptake in bone. Functional measurement parameters, such as sweat testing, sensation, strength, range of motion, fine manipulation, and endurance were also tested.

RADIOGRAPHY

Radiologic studies have been the most definitive objective test for reflex dystrophy, with some reports showing regional osteopenia on plain radiographs in as high as 80% of cases.[13,108] The classic Sudeck's atrophy radiologic finding that is diagnostic on plain film is patchy demineralization, with periarticular osteopenia, subchondral erosion and/or cysts, and endosteal cortical bone resorption. Although changes are most easily first visualized in the metaphyseal areas, quantitative testing confirms that the actual resorption of cortical and cancellous bone is equivocal, simply becoming more visible first in the least dense cancellous region.[15] Unfortunately, considerable demineralization is necessary for osteopenia to become visible on standard anteroposterior (AP) and lateral radiographs,[12] which places the patient in a later stage with a worse prognosis by the time diagnosis is made on routine radiographs. Use of radionuclide bone scanning will show these changes earlier.

RADIONUCLIDE BONE SCAN

Radionuclide scintigraphic studies using three-phase technetium-labeled diphosphonate bone scanning provide an important diagnostic tool, with abnormal scans reported in approximately 60% of patients with reflex dystrophy.[170] Although the increased uptake is not constant, it is very useful because it will appear before any radiographic change. Mackinnon and Holder[199] refined this technique with specific criteria, noting that diffuse uptake of tracer in the delayed image (phase 3) correlates well with the diagnosis of reflex dystrophy. They reported a 96% diagnostic success. However, their reflex dystrophy diagnostic criteria included later trophic manifestations, and there were already routine radiographic changes on plain radiographs in 65% of their patients. Doury[78] points out that children, and in rare cases adults, will actually show a decrease in uptake. Investigators who use bone scan as a required diagnostic prerequisite classify patients with decreased uptake as "pseudodystrophy."[82] Our greatest need is for a diagnostic test that permits early detection, and with our current methods a negative bone scan does not rule out the diagnosis.[167] A "positive" scan has high specificity but poor sensitivity; however, it remains one of the most useful diagnostic techniques because changes occur before standard radiographic change.[336] It is important to recognize that a "positive" test is not a prerequisite for diagnosis, but when a "positive" test is present, calcitonin treatment may be a practical therapeutic consideration.

Quantitative scintigraphy has also been utilized and permits assessment of bone mineral content and density. However, the findings do not correlate well with the outcome of treatment. In addition, the severity of the changes seen on routine radiographs are quite slow to improve after successful treatment.[175] The greatest differences on quantitative bone study were found in those patients with the longest disease duration. The degree of bone loss in reflex dystrophy over a few months is what might be expected in 10 years in the course of uncomplicated osteoporosis,[31] whereas normal bone mass is restored by 19 weeks after uncomplicated fracture at cortical sites and by 31 weeks in trabecular bone.[207] Therefore the rapidity of bone resorption in reflex dystrophy is far greater than that seen with disuse osteoporosis and reflects marked regional hyperemia, with evidence of microvascular hyperpermeability.[207] On occasion, the abnormal bone turnover may be confined to a single digit, but may later progress to include a ray, or most commonly become diffuse throughout the hand.[166] Although bone scan remains one of the most useful diagnostic tools in reflex dystrophy assessment, at present it should not be held as a prerequisite for early diagnosis and will not afford prognostic information, although it may provide an indication for calcitonin therapy.

MAGNETIC RESONANCE IMAGING

Changes that can be seen on magnetic resonance imaging (MRI) do occur early in reflex dystrophy, but they are too nonspecific to be diagnostic and they change according to the stage of the disease.[78,207] Early changes reveal a mild articular effusion, bone-marrow edema, and a weak T1 signal, with an increased T2 signal of the affected bone area without precise limits, probably indicating transient bone-marrow hyperemia.[207] These modifications may regress later, with a normal MRI or a few cases of "Swiss-cheese" signal. Edema and hyperemia may be enhanced by the use of gadolinium, but in later stages there is no edema, and the MRI findings in the dystrophic stage are minimal.[207]

THERMOGRAPHY

Temperature measurement is reflected by thermography, which is done by measuring the natural infrared emission of human body heat by means of an infrared sensitive camera (Figure 133-7). This test is appealing because it is noninvasive and safe.[136] Thermography is regarded by some to be the most sensitive test in the diagnosis of reflex dystrophy,[139] but studies

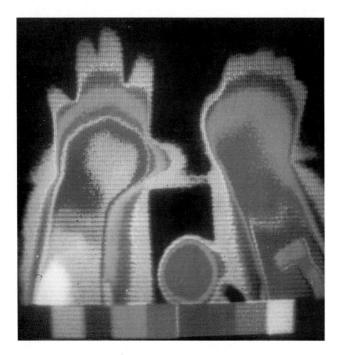

Figure 133-7. Thermography demonstrating RSD of the left hand.

show such a spectrum of temperature variability in reflex dystrophy that its value is limited.[138,211,291] For example, in one study, 32% of pain patients had a temperature in the affected side that was 1° Fahrenheit or more warmer than in the uninvolved hand, whereas 68% had a temperature that was cooler in the affected side by less than 1° Fahrenheit or more. In most chronic cases of reflex dystrophy, the affected hand has a cooler temperature, whereas in early cases the affected hand is generally warmer than the uninvolved hand. Presumably, there is an interval in between in which the temperatures may be equal! Even enthusiasts of this technique acknowledge that, in early stages, thermography may show confusing results.[139] Because of this temperature variability, the diagnostic value of thermography is questionable, and we find it easier to simply measure the temperature of the patient's involved extremity compared with that of the other hand at the time of clinic visits. However, infrared thermography may be useful to help the clinician communicate with the patient regarding the illness and to monitor progress.

OTHER DIAGNOSTIC TESTS

Galvanic skin conductance is reported to be abnormal in patients with reflex dystrophy.[63,311] It is interesting that the large concentration of eccrine sweat glands of the palms of hands and soles of feet respond to emotional stress rather than to increased temperature. Electrodes on the affected palm can detect a subtle change in electrical conductance before any visible sweating, and the results are compared with those of the unaffected side. The method requires tedious understanding of the equipment and is useless if there is bilateral involvement, nerve injury, or if the patient is on medication. It is therefore useful only as an early diagnostic indicator.

Quantitative sweat response (QSART) has been popularized by Lowe[194] and is especially useful in patients with fibroneuropathy because it quantitates sweat response to thermoregulatory testing. Lowe has noted abnormalities in patients with reflex dystrophy.

Capillary blood velocity (CBV), determined with microscopic epiillumination of digital skin, combined with *laser Doppler flux (LDF)* offers a sensitive assessment of skin blood flow.[94,248] Koman[167] points out the importance of using stress, such as cold stress, to afford reproducible dynamic response patterns. He points out that in reflex dystrophy increased flow may be accompanied by decreased nutrition as a result of arteriovenous shunting or a decrease in microvascular flow. It is necessary to simultaneously analyze digital temperature, laser Doppler flux, microvascular perfusion, and nutritional flow by vital capillaroscopy to obtain an overall view of these dynamics. These methods represent exciting research techniques that may offer insight into therapeutic response but at present they are not universally available, and their precise role in the diagnosis and treatment of reflex dystrophy is yet to be determined.

Electromyographic and *nerve conduction* studies show no specific abnormality associated with reflex dystrophy, although abnormality may be found when there is known nerve damage, such as in causalgia.[171]

Response to sympathetic block is regarded by many to be the best criterion for reflex dystrophy diagnosis. However, recognition that this response is variable among patients and may be absent in as many as 30% of patients has led to CRPS diagnosis designations, with subclassification of *sympathetically maintained pain* for those who respond to blocks. Other patients are subclassified as having *sympathetically independent pain.* The precise role of the sympathetic nervous system remains controversial; however, the value of a positive sympathetic block response remains a valuable indicator of therapy options.

FUNCTIONAL ASSESSMENT

It is important to clarify precisely which changes are most responsible for interfering with function in patients with reflex dystrophy. This helps the patient focus on measures to gain control of the specific problem. For example, if cold stimulates increased pain and decreased function, temperature biofeedback therapy and methods of cold avoidance should be stressed, whereas in a different patient edema control may be a more important variable. Although sophisticated diagnostic instrumentation and tests of autonomic function exist, from a practical point of view most patients need simple functional assessment by a physician and hand therapist, with simple reproducible measurements to monitor progress. These include volumetric displacement measurement of swelling; direct temperature measurement with comparison of fingers on the affected hand and those of the unaffected extremity; ninhydrin sweat testing; color and appearance observation; range of motion; strength; fine manipulation testing; sensory testing with two-point discrimination, moving two-point discrimination, and Semmes Weinstein monofilament testing; temperature cold recovery time (length of time for temperature to return to baseline after cold exposure); and pain assessment using a visual analog scale and a pain diagram drawn by the patient. These simple tests afford an easily reproducible method to monitor success in the therapeutic effort and offer the patient an important feedback for therapeutic intervention.

DIFFERENTIAL DIAGNOSES

CONNECTIVE TISSUE DISORDERS

Early manifestations of connective tissue disease may mimic symptoms of reflex dystrophy. For example, patients with scleroderma or mixed connective tissue disease usually have vasomotor disturbance, frequent joint swelling and inflammation, pain, possible trophic change, and apprehension. Manifestations of reflex dystrophy, however, differ in that the pain is constant and not only when there are vasospastic episodes or when using the inflamed extremity. Pain in reflex dystrophy is usually more diffuse and not well localized. Allodynia and

hyperpathia are also present, along with greater distress, apprehension, and pain out of proportion to the physical findings. In patients with connective tissue disease, a trial of rest and splints will usually relieve discomfort of joint inflammation, and calcium channel blockers may control vasospasm, but these measures are not as effective for reflex dystrophy. Serum studies for uric acid level, rheumatoid factor, and sedimentation rate are usually negative in most patients with reflex dystrophy. However, one must remember that reflex dystrophy can occur in association with connective tissue disease.

PSYCHIATRIC DISORDERS

Three psychiatric disorders may be confused with reflex dystrophy: malingering, factitious disorders, and conversion disorders.

Malingering is a conscious misrepresentation of symptoms for a personal reason, most frequently to avoid work or increase compensation. Because malingerers are consciously untruthful, their affect may betray them. They tend to be withdrawn, observant, and seem less distressed than patients with reflex dystrophy. Their physical findings will usually vary to an extent that their lack of honesty becomes apparent (Figure 133-8). Sensory measurements, such as the Semmes-Weinstein

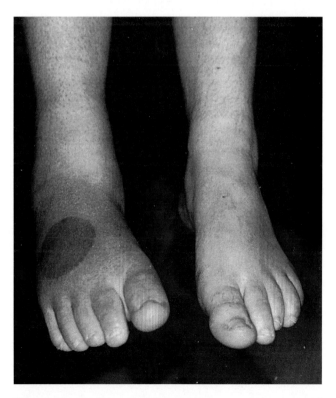

Figure 133-8. Feet of 24-year-old woman seen for reported "RSD" 1 year after dropping a box at work on her leg. She developed a first-degree circular burn "spontaneously" the morning of evaluation, and has a telltale circular tourniquet ankle indentation above the level of edema. Litigation was pending.

monofilament or two-point discrimination test, often will not correlate with the patient's ability to do fine manipulation on Moberg or similar tests. Grip-strength measurements taken at sequential resistance settings may confirm the examiner's suspicion that the malingerer's efforts are fraudulent when the measurements do not result in a bell-shaped curve and there is more than 20% difference in the measurement. Rapid alternating grip measurements may show a much greater strength than the patient's average, deliberate, conscious strength measurements. When the effort is genuine, rapid alternating grip should approximate the same maximum grip strength achieved when done more slowly. It is advisable not to confront patients considered to be malingerers, no matter how obvious their lack of integrity becomes. Litigation may be pending and the surgeon may be accused of taking sides on issues in which he or she desires no involvement. Furthermore, no useful purpose is served by arguing with the patient about findings and complaints that are manifestly not genuine.[267] Rather, it is important to clearly document that the patient's symptoms and findings are inconsistent. Let others pass judgment.

Factitious wounding, especially when there is no apparent secondary gain, is a serious psychiatric disorder that can be difficult to diagnose. In true factitial disorders, the patient seems unaware that the injury is self-inflicted and often has supportive family members who share in the denial.[267] Such a case is difficult to diagnose, even after one suspects its presence, because the patient will always deny the possibility and has to be shown by use of a cast, direct observation on an in-patient basis, or some other means that the edema, nonhealing ulcer, or other manifestation is self inflicted. One pathognomonic finding is the inability of the patient to tolerate an Unna boot, casting, or any other measures that prohibit access to the wound. This is a most useful way to make the diagnosis. Sometimes, self-inflicted injury causes apparent peritendinous fibrosis on the dorsum of the hand, as described by Secretan[285] in 1901. Unfortunately, simple confrontation does little or nothing to help patients with factitious disorders, who will simply take their symptoms elsewhere, unless they are somehow persuaded to undergo intensive psychotherapy.

Conversion disorders, or hysteric neuroses, are signs and symptoms of physical disorders that originate from psychiatric conflict. These are not deliberate, conscious, or understood by the patient, and have no explicable physical disorder associated with them. Two examples are hysterical paralysis and clenched-fist syndrome. Physical examination will reveal the sincerity of the patient and the absence of findings appropriate for the bizarre symptoms. Complete loss of sensation will often follow nonanatomic patterns, such as stocking/glove anesthesia. The patient does not seem terribly concerned about these dramatic findings. These patients do not appear to be as distressed or in as much pain as are those with reflex dystrophy. Simmons and Vasile[294] suggested that clenched-fist syndrome may be symbolic of the patient's suppressed anger. These patients usually respond favorably to psychotherapeutic inter-

vention. However, on occasion clenched-fist syndrome may also be associated with reflex dystrophy.[218-220]

MYOFASCIAL DYSFUNCTION

Myofascial dysfunction is pain of inapparent cause that is occasionally associated with autonomic change. The fact that trigger points of myofascial dysfunction are reported in over half of the patients with reflex dystrophy makes one wonder if the two disorders may have common etiologic features.[218-220] Like reflex dystrophy, the pain in myofascial dysfunction seems disproportionate, with no apparent cause until the trigger points that reproduce the referred pain are identified. This differs from reflex dystrophy in that myofascial dysfunction pain may be relieved by rest, such as by use of a splint, or may be relieved by injection of the trigger points.

When myofascial dysfunction is associated with reflex dystrophy, the latter symptoms predominate. In treatment, however, it becomes important to inactivate the proximal trigger points as part of effective therapy for reflex dystrophy.

VOLKMANN'S ISCHEMIC CONTRACTURE

Volkmann's ischemic contracture is a response to partial or complete vascular compromise, such as by a displaced supracondylar humeral fracture that compresses the brachial artery, or a compartment syndrome, such as occurs after a burn or crush injury. Volkmann himself attributed the cause to ischemia from tight bandaging.[330] The condition can be caused by arterial spasm, small-vessel occlusion, venous congestion, compartment syndrome, or all of the above.[320] This condition may cause ischemic contracture of the forearm flexors or intrinsic muscles after trauma, especially if a cast becomes too tight. The ultimate result—progressive fibrosis, contracture, and ankylosis—looks like late stages of reflex dystrophy. It is therefore easy for legal advisers to confuse the two disorders by misinterpreting the symptoms of the patient with reflex dystrophy as the result of having had a cast too tight. However, the onset and findings are quite distinct, even though either condition may arise as a sequel to trauma and immobilization. One particularly confusing group of patients is those who are on dialysis and sustain a vascular steal at the time of access shunting, resulting in neurologic loss and immediate pain. These patients are distinguished by a gradual recovery of sensation and function after takedown of the shunt.

The classic symptoms of arterial compromise that can progress to a Volkmann's ischemic contracture are "the five Ps": paresthesia, pallor, pulselessness, pain with finger extension, and paresis. Their presence indicates immediate need for release of dressings or cast, better stabilization of fractures, escharotomy, fasciotomy, or whatever it takes to correct the vascular compromise. If the condition progresses, contracture and necrosis of the involved muscles develop, usually in the finger flexors of the forearm and intrinsic muscles of the hand. When the process arises in the forearm, there is progressive contracture of the fingers and progressive neurologic loss that can be stopped, and sometimes sensation improved, by extensive neurolysis, placing the median and ulnar nerves in a subcutaneous position.[256] There is no fully satisfactory treatment for established Volkmann's ischemic contracture of the forearm muscles, but flexor slide procedure[320] and free microvascular muscle replacement[204] have been used to correct established contracture and replace the lost flexors.

Volkmann's ischemic contracture of the intrinsic muscles is not as easily recognized as is forearm flexion contracture, and it may look more like reflex dystrophy. However, the early manifestations include intrinsic tightness and pain when the "intrinsic test" is performed (i.e., placing the metacarpophalangeal [MCP] joint in extension and assessing whether tight intrinsic muscles now cause the interphalangeal [IP] joints to remain extended and resist flexion). Early intrinsic tightness secondary to increased intrinsic compartment pressures is best handled by intrinsic fasciotomy.

Although the late dystrophic hand of Volkmann's ischemic contracture is similar in appearance to a hand in the late stages of reflex dystrophy, the pain characteristics are distinct. The patient with reflex dystrophy complains bitterly of persistent pain that interferes with sleep, whereas the patient with late Volkmann's ischemic contracture develops progressive anesthesia and paralysis of the hand. Although both reflex dystrophy and Volkmann's ischemic contracture begin with symptoms of pain and may benefit from loosening dressings, it is important to distinguish between them. Although fasciotomy can be of great benefit to prevent Volkmann's ischemic contracture, it is usually contraindicated in reflex dystrophy, in which any early operation may further aggravate and complicate the pain syndrome.

LOCAL NERVE IRRITATION

Certain persistent nerve irritation or inflammation, such as may occur with atypical carpal tunnel syndrome or painful neuroma, appears to mimic or precipitate reflex dystrophy. Patients with acute carpal tunnel syndrome (not associated with trauma), incomplete carpal tunnel release, or neuroma formation from severance of the palmar sensory branch of the median nerve may demonstrate exaggerated pain, edema, and vasomotor instability, often with proximal trigger points and pain in the entire upper extremity. Clinicians should be dissuaded from performing a surgical search for the "precipitating irritant" causing reflex dystrophy until the inappropriate degree of pain is controlled by nonsurgical means. In my experience, preoperative control of diffuse inappropriate manifestations of pain allows a smoother course after surgery. Early surgery in the midst of an acute pain syndrome may accelerate pain manifestations. However, the exceptions are patients with acute carpal tunnel syndrome associated with Colles' fracture or similar trauma in which immediate surgical release is necessary to relieve symptoms that will otherwise worsen.

TREATMENT TECHNIQUES AND RESULTS

The wide spectrum of treatment methods and varying reported results for reflex dystrophy is as perplexing as the myriad of names given the disorder and the array of precipitating causes. This treatment spectrum ranges from psychotherapy to sympathectomy, with enthusiastic proponents for a host of differing methods. All techniques are directed at interrupting the reflex pain cycle, but the fact that so many different methods exist is testimony that none are universally successful.[173] Assessment of treatment results is confusing, with each major treatment technique showing a high percentage of success in some reports and poor results in others (see p. 2341).

Four important factors are probably responsible for the dramatic discrepancies in reported treatment results: (1) the lack of controls, (2) the absence of long-term follow-up, (3) the absence of objective criteria for diagnosis or any uniform criteria for treatment success, and (4) the great variability among patients with this disorder. In their excellent overview of results among the most frequent treatment techniques, Nath et al[235] document the paucity of studies with controls and long-term follow-up. Reflex dystrophy patients are highly susceptible to the placebo effect.[95,96] In fact, placebo effect may be the important factor in many successful treatment techniques, if one accepts that cerebral factors play an important role in etiology. Placebo effect is thought to be mediated via the endogenous opioid system and involves expectation of relief. This factor must be controlled to be convinced the treatment studied is better than similar sham treatment. Many favored techniques, such as intravenous phentolamine and guanethidine blocks, have not passed this test.

Long-term follow-up is lacking in most studies. Subbarao and Stillwell[306] showed that although treating physicians were convinced that two thirds of their patients had resolved reflex dystrophy symptoms before discharge, late questionnaire evaluation actually found the opposite, with most patients still symptomatic and only one having no residual symptoms. In Wang's study of late result from sympathetic block,[333] only a little more than one third of the patients were improved 3 years after treatment. However, an important observation in their study was that those treated within 6 months of onset had a significantly better result, with two thirds remaining improved at 3 years after treatment, documenting that early intervention appears to give better long-term results.

By far the best treatment for RSD is prevention.[205,219] Although it is impossible to prove someone would have developed the disorder, I am convinced that many patients who show disproportionate pain, anxiety, dissociation, and greater swelling and stiffness than anticipated might develop the persistent, exaggerated inflammatory response and unrelenting pain of this disorder were it not for intervention. This intervention can only be achieved by prompt presumptive diagnosis of "early signs of reflex dystrophy." Any patient who appears to have an undue response to injury or surgery, such as exaggerated pain and fear on suture removal or excessive and irrelevant anxious questions, should be followed carefully and given whatever additional support and encouragement he or she needs to resume confident use of his or her hand. Hand therapists can be an enormous help in the treatment of these patients because they can provide the additional time and reassurance so often needed to achieve functional use in these more anxious patients. However, some patients develop the disorder in spite of our intense efforts.

Patients with established, easily diagnosed reflex dystrophy also need support, but by this stage they are often suspicious, depressed, resentful, and pessimistic; these are characteristics not inclined toward expectation of relief. These patients often request surgery or some other dramatic intervention. They also represent a profound therapeutic challenge, and a variety of treatment options may be necessary to find one that offers benefit. The surgeon must remain optimistic and positive in outlook with these late cases, but communicate the realistic knowledge that no magic cure is available. The overall treatment goal will be to help these patients cope and live with their condition, with gradual functional improvement achieved from treatment. In each case of reflex dystrophy, the physician must make a strenuous effort to (1) gain the confidence of the patient, (2) make the patient understand the surgeon's sincere desire to help, and (3) communicate the belief that with the patient's cooperation satisfactory rehabilitation is a possibility.[290] Although there is no consensus regarding the best treatment, there is general agreement that the earlier any treatment is instituted, the better the prognosis. We must be honest with the patients and ourselves that predicting the course and result of treatment in this disorder is a lot like predicting the weather. We have some idea of what to expect, but are not surprised to be wrong. To that extent, the clinician must be willing to individualize treatment with as many modifications and changes as are needed to find a treatment regimen that offers benefit. Indeed, the principal generalization in treatment should be the willing individualization of treatment to fit each patient's different manifestations, needs, and clinical course. The following treatment methods vary greatly, but should be selected according to the specific symptoms. Generally, starting with the least invasive and morbid technique and gradually adding new methods until a regimen succeeds while attempting to maintain a positive, constructive outlook is the best course of action (see Practical Principles in The Treatment of Reflex Dystrophy, p. 2369).

SURGICAL TREATMENT

With certain exceptions, efforts to seek surgical solutions for reflex dystrophy should be discouraged. Sunderland[308] well summarized surgical treatment results as follows: "Operations have been performed for pain at nearly every possible site in the pathway from the peripheral receptors to the sensory cortex. At every level, the story is the same—some encouraging results, but a disheartening tendency for the pain to recur.... We should remember, however, that many procedures for the relief of pain have had their crowded hour of general enthusiastic adoption, only to fade gradually into oblivion. Results were claimed at first for neurotomy, amputation, and posterior rhizotomy, which experience could not confirm."

Sympathectomy

Although many surgical techniques, such as periarterial sympathectomy,[152] posterior rhizotomy (dorsal root section),[309] cordotomy (spinothalamic transection), neurolysis, and neurectomy[1,122] have proved of little value in the treatment of reflex dystrophy, sympathectomy has remained useful in selected patients. Leriche[184] introduced the concept in 1916 and Spurling[299] popularized the operation in 1930. Sympathectomy is of greatest value in cases with proximal nerve injury, such as causalgia, and is generally less useful in the slowly developing dystrophy caused by minor trauma or CNS origin, such as stroke.[152] When the pain reflex arc originates more centrally, the peripheral modulation by sympathectomy is less valuable.

The patient most likely to benefit from sympathectomy is one who obtains repeated, dramatic, temporary relief from sympathetic blocks, but for whom the relief never lasts longer than the duration of the anesthetic, and for whom there is no placebo effect using saline for the block. Patients with no response to sympathetic blocks are not likely to respond to sympathectomy, and another treatment should be attempted.[1,93] Unfortunately, one popular recommendation is that sympathectomy be reserved for patients who are refractory to all other treatments, including sympathetic blocks. This recommendation should not be followed and may be punitive to the patient.

The reported results of sympathectomy in the treatment of reflex dystrophy vary widely. For example, in the 19 studies of sympathectomy reviewed by Nath et al,[235] the results range from a 99% good result in 70 patients[321] and 93% good in 30 patients[4] to failure rates of 95% in 27 patients[123,124] and 83% failure in 15 patients.[201] These findings reflect the wide spectrum of reported results seen throughout study of all methods of treatment.

Failure of sympathectomy to relieve reflex dystrophy symptoms may be due to technical problems because adequate sympathectomy requires complete denervation of the sympathetic fibers from the lower half of the sympathetic ganglion through the first four thoracic ganglia.[52,152,203,211] However, the fact that many patients with successful sympathectomy later develop recurrent symptoms is thought by some to be due to secondary upregulation of distal receptors, which may produce supersensitivity to circulating or endogenous catecholamine with recurrence of symptoms. However, I have seen some patients after sympathectomy who not only developed recurrent symptoms in the involved extremity, but also advancement to involve the other extremity (the "mirror effect"), suggesting central phenomena that cannot be explained on a technical basis.

Although sympathectomies may be useful, they have significant morbidity and should be done only after adequate trial of nonsurgical management. In fact, sympathectomy itself is known to precipitate localized dystrophic pain and Horner's syndrome, which occurs in approximately 14% of patients.[280] The recent use of endoscopic ganglionectomy has reduced the morbidity of sympathectomy somewhat.[286] Causalgia is the one form of reflex dystrophy that is most likely to be improved by sympathectomy. Bonica's review[44] of 500 patients treated with surgical sympathectomy for causalgia found that 84% experienced excellent pain relief, 12% fair relief, and only 4% no improvement. However, an initial trial of serial nerve blocks, with either anesthetic or pharmacologic agents, is still warranted in causalgia patients and many times will prove adequate without surgery. Sympathectomy for other forms of reflex dystrophy does not have such an encouraging rate of success.[93,167]

Transaxillary Decompression of the Subclavian Vein

Wilhelm[338] observed clinical and neurogenic similarities between patients with thoracic outlet syndrome and those with RSD. He studied 21 patients with reflex dystrophy over a 7-year interval and reported stenotic changes in the subclavian vein with "greater or lesser impairment of venous flow" in 20 of these patients on venogram study. In nine patients who proved refractory to conservative management, decompression was performed, with resection of the first rib, along with sympathectomy. With an average 7-year follow-up, Wilhelm reported an 88% good to excellent result in this small series of patients, all of whom had stage II disease, with the exception of one patient who had stage III. It should be pointed out that successful response by sympathetic block was a prerequisite for surgical consideration, and sympathectomy was also done along with the subclavian vein decompression.

Wilhelm hypothesizes that some degree of subclavian flow impairment, generally caused by compressing structures such as the anterior scalene muscle, Sibson's fascia, the subclavian muscle, and the costoclavicular ligament, may be a predisposing factor to the development of reflex dystrophy, with the edema that is commonly found in these patients caused by venous congestion and impaired arterial flow. He explains the disorder in patients who have myocardial infarction or stroke as being associated with immobility. One might question whether the benefit of surgery was due to the sympathectomy in patients who already demonstrated response to blocks, or whether this procedure will fall into the category described by Sunderland (see p. 2341), with transient popularity but recurrent disorder. However, Boome[47] described similar

successful results doing a decompression by means of the supraclavicular pathway. This may be an oversimplification of a complex disorder, but their series is interesting, and further study is needed.

Surgical Control of Peripheral Nerve Irritants

Many patients with reflex dystrophy have an associated identifiable peripheral nerve irritant ("dystrophic focus") that seems disproportionately painful and could be considered for elective surgical correction. Examples are painful neuromas, neuromas in continuity, intraneural fibrosis, stiff joints, fracture malunions, carpal instability, and previous carpal tunnel release. We must protect the patient from our desire to find a simple surgical solution for reflex dystrophy. The wary surgeon will gain control of the inappropriate symptom complex *before* elective surgery, so that the continuous pain, edema, withdrawal, and hyperesthesia are all well controlled and the patient's symptoms have narrowed to what one would consider to be an appropriate level characteristically seen with the problem. This may be accomplished by pharmacologic treatment, a goal-oriented hand-therapy program using desensitization techniques,[133] autonomic blocks, and the other measures utilized for reflex dystrophy. I have reviewed many litigation cases in which surgeons arduously and heroically attempted operation after operation—even amputation—to try and solve these patients' desperate complaints, usually resulting in only temporary relief that is soon obviated by recurrent symptoms. Just because one can find an abnormality that will lend itself to surgery does not mean the symptom complex will be resolved. In fact, without prior control of the disproportionate pain, surgery can result in a worsening status, with a disappointed and sometimes litigious patient.

An exception to delay and conservative management is acute carpal tunnel syndrome or similar acute compression syndromes that occur after trauma or Colles' fracture. The timing and progressive nature of this problem indicates the need for immediate surgery to avoid a chronic pain syndrome.[155]

Once the patient with reflex dystrophy has control of pain, it is no longer continuous (e.g., relief achieved with splinting), and it remains under control for weeks or months, consideration for elective surgery can be entertained. This could include resection or repair of superficial radial nerve neuromas, palmaris brevis turnover flap for carpal tunnel median nerve adherence, fracture nonunion correction, or capsulotomies and tenolyses for treatment of resulting stiff joints. In these circumstances, the surgeon should be aware of the significant risk for exacerbation of symptoms and should have a long-acting block or continuous-block anesthetic before surgery, even if a general anesthetic is used, to avoid redevelopment of a reflex cycle with the CNS.

Implanted Electrical Stimulation

Use of implantable neurostimulation systems for treatment of chronic pain has gained increasing popularity at pain management centers as newer electrode technology allows a more widespread and flexible pattern of stimulation. Implantable stimulation devices have been placed at various sites throughout the nervous system from the grey matter,[143,343] dorsal column,[177,234] and spinal cord[172,273] to the peripheral nerve level.[119] When painful peripheral nerves are treated, improvement using peripheral nerve block is a prerequisite, along with some temporary success with transcutaneous nerve stimulation.[62] Theories for the efficacy of this treatment are based on the gate control theory, with stimulation of large, myelinated fibers blocking pain transmission through the spinal cord; alternatively, there may be release of endogenous opioids by stimulation as well.

Caution should be exercised in this area, however, because most of the reports of success do not separate patients with reflex dystrophy/causalgia/CRPS, with some exceptions.[17,177] I agree with Cooney,[62] who believes this treatment should be confined to patients whose pain is "somatically" derived and not from "sympathetic overstimulation/reflex sympathetic dystrophy." His results showed over 80% success in 2-year follow-up in a group of patients without reflex dystrophy. I have been impressed in a few patients followed after implant placement that, like other procedures, the initial results seem promising but they are followed by the disappointment of recurrent symptomology and, in one case, mirror-image disease.

STELLATE GANGLION AND OTHER NERVE BLOCKS

Percutaneous stellate ganglion sympathetic nerve block has remained the most widely accepted form of treatment for reflex dystrophy in the United States. In fact, many early investigators believed that successful sympathetic nerve blocks should be a prerequisite for diagnosis.[30] However, blocks are not uniformly successful and are no longer required for diagnosis, although they are widely utilized to distinguish sympathetically maintained pain classification of types I or II CRPS.[167] Percutaneous sympathetic block must be regarded as only one of the many treatment possibilities and it is usually best suited for those patients whose subjective manifestations seem predominantly sympathetic, such as abnormal skin color, temperature, and sweat. Kasdan and others[58,157] point out that the most favorable scenario for successful treatment with sympathetic block is a patient who is treated within the first 6 months of onset for an afflicted limb that is warmer than its counterpart, the usual stage I change.

Percutaneous sympathetic block is most successful (at least for the duration of the block) in the nerve-injured causalgia form of reflex dystrophy (CRPS type II), and it is this group of patients that is also most likely to benefit from sympathectomy.[1,290] In other groups, sympathetic block may fail in more than one third of patients.[58,290,333] Ochoa[244-246] is convinced that sympathetic blocks afford no relief, or only relief attainable because of the placebo response. Indeed, patients with reflex dystrophy are heavy placebo responders[327] and most blocks are not placebo controlled. However, if the patient

obtains relief it may be a successful treatment, whether it is caused by the placebo effect or the pharmacologic agent used. When blocks are done as a prerequisite to sympathectomy, it is important to alternate the anesthetic agent from a short-acting agent to a long-acting agent without informing the patient. By this means, one might rule out the placebo effect; if relief corresponds to the known length of the anesthetic, one can be more confident that a sympathectomy will likely afford benefit.

If neuropeptide dysfunction is an important mechanism in many cases of reflex dystrophy, it can be understood how sympathetic modification of the afferent pain endings could prove beneficial in some patients, especially those with a predominantly peripheral insult, and not in others whose stimulus may be a more firmly established central cycle. Reflex pain firmly established at the central level is more likely to respond to methods that activate the endogenous opioid internal pain control system, which is known to interfere with pain neurotransmitter (substance P) production and secretion.[180] This endogenous control might explain why "placebo blocks" are frequently successful in as many as 30% of patients.[21,42,244-246]

Reported results of stellate ganglion block treatment vary greatly, from 100% failure rate in 75 patients in one study[321] and an 86% failure in another[340] to a 100% success rate reported by others.[140,264] Wang et al[333] studied 3-year follow-up results of percutaneous sympathetic nerve blocks and found that only 40% of the patients had good to excellent results, in contrast to reports with more optimistic findings but shorter follow-up. However, these researchers made note that in patients treated within 6 months of onset of their disease, there was a 70% success rate after 3 years, underlining the importance of early treatment.

Most authors use serial blocks to obtain sustained relief,[44,165] but a few patients have experienced complete relief after a single percutaneous stellate ganglion block combined with an active hand-therapy program.[1,290] When using serial sympathetic blocks, most clinicians prefer to use daily or alternate-day blocks for 3 to 5 days as a trial.[1] If this is successful, pain relief should progressively outlast the duration of the anesthetic. Use of long-acting and short-acting anesthetic agents, without informing the patient, can assess the placebo effect. As long as the duration of pain relief is increasing and the severity of the recurrent pain is decreasing, the blocks should be continued, although at lesser intervals.

It is important that during the block treatments patients should be encouraged to perform activities that previously were painful, usually under the supervision of a hand therapist. The importance of making frequent, active use of the extremity as their condition improves should be stressed to patients. The therapist or physician can use a brachial plexus block to determine if a patient's stiffness is due to pain or fibrosis by assessing the passive range of motion of the digits while they are anesthetized and paralyzed. Sometimes patients obtain improvement with brachial plexus blocks and not stellate ganglion blocks.[86] When repeated sympathetic blocks offer consistent benefit, but only for the duration of the short- or long-acting agent, sympathectomy or other oral or topical blockers should be considered.[1]

Some clinicians prefer use of continuous blockade for several days as a method to break the pain cycle.[29,137,191] This may be done by continuous infusion of a local anesthetic over the area of the stellate ganglion or paravertebral ganglia or along the brachial plexus. This is usually done in the hospital with observation of the patient's tolerance and has proven successful in selected patients.[191]

Some authors contend that failure of percutaneous stellate ganglion blocks is usually due to technical error resulting in incomplete block of the sympathetic nervous system. Lankford[174] points out that the stellate ganglion and upper two or three dorsal sympathetic ganglia must be included and if complete block of the upper portion of the stellate ganglion is achieved, a Horner's syndrome will be noted, including ptosis (eyelid drooping), myosis (pupil constriction), enophthalmos, and dilation of conjunctival vessels. Other authors believe that the only benefit from sympathetic block actually is due only to the anesthetic effect on the adjacent somatic nervous system and not the sympathetic nervous system at all! Certainly the role of the sympathetic nervous system and sympathetic block in reflex dystrophy has become more controversial, but in certain patients it nonetheless seems beneficial, especially in those whose manifestations are predominantly autonomic change. Patients with minimal sympathetic abnormality but characteristic pain often respond to an active program of hand therapy alone, with nerve blocks being reserved for use if hand therapy fails.[1,250]

Local regional nerve block may be useful in patients whose symptoms have become confined to a specific region, such as that supplied by the superficial radial nerve or an amputation stump with a painful digital neuroma. Local long-acting nerve blocks can be quite beneficial in breaking the pain cycle.

Intravenous Regional Infusion

Use of intravenous medication infused into an extremity isolated by arterial tourniquet for anesthetic purpose was described by Bier in 1908 and is commonly known as a "Bier block." Pharmacologic sympathetic block using this technique seems attractive and was introduced by Hannington-Kiff in 1974.[126] This has been a popular treatment technique, especially in England, although the drug they used was never approved for this purpose in the United States.[41,98,127] The block using guanethidine lasts only 15 to 20 minutes, but the duration of response seems longer than characteristic stellate ganglion blocks because there is a 5-day half-life for displacing norepinephrine in the postganglionic system.[41,342]

Other pharmacologic agents used for reflex dystrophy in this fashion include reserpine,[24,118] phentolamine,[11] bretylium tosylate,[140] and steroids.[261] Currently, reserpine and phentolamine have been taken off the commercial market in the United States for parenteral use, and only bretylium tosylate and steroids remain available. Parenteral use of bretylium tosylate is approved for cardiac ventricular arrhythmias. It has activity similar to guanethidine, with inhibition of norepi-

nephrine release and uptake, and there are reports of successful use and minimal side effects in patients with reflex dystrophy. Steroids are often used with bretylium.[85,100,128]

Results of intravenous guanethidine sympathetic blocks in 15 reports varied from 100% good to 93% failure.[38,98,235] Although earlier controlled studies suggested guanethidine gave better pain relief than placebo,[113] more recent randomized, double-blind comparison of intravenous guanethidine, reserpine, and saline showed equal improvement at 30 minutes and still no difference at 24 hours.[38] A similar study using phentolamine showed no advantage over placebo.[244-246] Whether the benefit of intravenous sympathetic block is predominantly a placebo response or the result of modulation of the afferent pain system by sympathetic controls remains unknown, but the many reports of its successful use, especially when utilized early in the patient's course, maintain its worth as a treatment option. Generally, sequential blocks (three to five) are utilized, although lasting relief has been obtained by single intravenous infusion in some reports.

Transcutaneous Electrical Nerve Stimulation

The successful use of transcutaneous electrical nerve stimulation (TENS) has been reported in reflex dystrophy.[221,272,304,332] Its mechanism is hypothesized to be activation of the endogenous opioid analgesic system to release endorphins[257] that may inhibit pain at the level of the spinothalamic tract.[177,257] Animal and human studies using high-intensity, low-frequency TENS suggest such a mechanism.[102]

Although TENS has been reported as a sole effective treatment for reflex dystrophy, I have generally found it more useful as an adjunctive therapy to assist with pain control while other measures, such as hand therapy, stellate ganglion block, and pharmacologic treatment, are utilized. TENS may be particularly useful when there are minimal inflammatory or autonomic changes and pain is the predominant manifestation. Like all other methods of treatment, TENS is reported as most effective when initiated early after the onset of symptoms and may be of minimal value, or only adjunctively valuable, after the pain reflex is firmly established.

Acupuncture

Acupuncture using electrodes and/or transdermal needles has been used to treat reflex dystrophy with varying results. It is of interest that the most successful series reported by Chan and Chow[57] was in Chinese patients in Hong Kong. They reported excellent results using electroacupuncture in patients who did not respond to hand therapy and analgesic treatment. Their technique varied from standard use of Chinese loci, in that they chose loci in the region of maximal discomfort in the affected limb and followed known innervation patterns. Chan and Chow reported excellent results in 70% and improvement in 90% of their patients, but pointed out that these were Chinese patients with confidence in acupuncture, whose expectation of relief may have played a role in activating the release of endorphin pain inhibitors in the CNS. In experimental subjects, acupuncture has been reported to be blocked by naloxone, a morphine antagonist, suggesting the importance of the endogenous pain-control system in acupuncture success.[210,251]

In the west, this technique has usually been employed as an adjunctive measure without as much success, possibly because patients have less confidence in the method and thus less activation of the endogenous pain-control system.

Biofeedback Therapy

More than 30 years ago, Miller and others found that autonomic function, such as temperature control, can be "trained."[224] We found that temperature biofeedback is a useful adjunctive treatment for patients who have pronounced temperature change in their clinical manifestations. In patients capable of biofeedback training, control of the temperature difference appears to be associated with control or better tolerance of their pain.[133] It usually takes one to four sessions to determine if a patient is a candidate for this type of training, in which they engage in self-hypnosis maneuvers by imagining themselves in an environmental temperature situation that favorably alters their skin temperature while they monitor visual or audio readings. Voluntary control of this autonomic function provides pain control and is a provocative observation that awaits explanation. After 12 treatment sessions of approximately 45 minutes each, most successful biofeedback patients are able to accurately estimate their involved digital temperature within one or two degrees.

Although we have used biofeedback as only an adjunctive measure with hand therapy, pharmacologic therapy, blocks, or other treatment techniques, there are reports of biofeedback as a primary treatment[3,19,35,38,125] and as other self-hypnosis techniques.[107] Biofeedback therapy is best suited for patients with pronounced temperature change early in the course of their reflex dystrophy.

Pharmacologic Medical Treatment

As it does in all other aspects of this disorder, controversy exists regarding which types of medications are effective for treatment of reflex dystrophy. To some extent, pharmacologic choices are dictated by each clinician's concept of etiophysiologic mechanisms and to some extent by the individual patient's clinical manifestations. The United States Food and Drug Administration (FDA) has to date approved no single pharmacologic agent as safe and effective for treatment of reflex dystrophy or CRPS, although several agents may be classified as "possibly effective." Therefore, there is *no one drug of choice*.

Review of the huge spectrum of reported pharmacologic treatment regimens for reflex dystrophy is beyond the scope of this chapter. However, it is important to review the different classifications of treatment for differing etiological concepts, with examples of each, so that the clinician can shop among them for the one agent that might benefit a particular patient.

The choices differ according to whether one believes a particular patient's problem is predominantly from overactivity or increased sensitivity of the sympathetic nervous system, a chronically exaggerated inflammatory response, a predominantly CNS-mediated reflex, or principally a peripheral vascular disorder. Clearly, these mechanisms are not independent of one another, but opinions differ regarding which is most etiologically important, and medications should be directed to those manifestations that seem to prevail in an individual patient, with ready flexibility to switch to others as needed.

Furthermore, Mackin[198] points out the importance of offhand, deliberate, upbeat comments about specific medications when writing prescriptions in the presence of patients in a section he entitles *Zen and the Neglected Subtle Art of Effective Prescription Writing*. He implies that this method indirectly increases the medication's effectiveness and tolerance. Whether this is by placebo effect or not is irrelevant to the patient if it works.

Sympatholytics

The development of newer, more specific alpha-adrenergic blocking agents raised hopes of simpler methods and increased efficiency for sympathetic blockade than with the older, nonspecific alpha and beta blockers. Unfortunately, many of the oral agents still result in such prohibitive side effects that they are not tolerated, especially by what Mackin characterizes as the "self-diagnosed *medication-sensitive*" individual that seems to be common among patients with reflex dystrophy.

Clonidine (Catapres) is among the most useful of the sympatholytics. It is an alpha-2-adrenergic agonist that is active in the dorsal horn and brainstem to suppress CNS noradrenergic activity and peripheral sympathetic tone.[262] In our experience this is most useful in its transdermal patch form as an adjunctive treatment along with hand therapy and other measures. It may also be administered by intravenous, epidural, and oral routes. Oral clonidine may be given in doses of 0.1 to 0.4 mg daily, and may be particularly useful for weaning narcotic-addicted patients by blocking withdrawal effects.[198] Although listed as a sympatholytic medication, clonidine also clearly has CNS overtones and seems promising in its topical application.

Phentolamine (Regitine) is a postsynaptic alpha-1 antagonist and a presynaptic alpha-2 antagonist and should be well suited to produce a favorable chemical sympathectomy. It has been widely utilized intravenously as a diagnostic test for sympathetically maintained pain (CRPS types I and II) but is no longer commercially available for parenteral use in the United States. Its value has been questioned by placebo-control study that suggested its benefit was the placebo effect and not via specific drug action.[327] Oral use has been poorly tolerated and is not well studied.

Prazosin (Minipress) is a selective alpha-1-adrenergic antagonist generally used as an antihypertensive. Its benefit in causalgia has been reported but control studies are not yet available.[2] Orthostatic hypotension is a frequent complication; therefore the first dose should be no more than 1 mg, and then increased 1 mg per day over 1 to 2 weeks until the maximum of 10 to 12 mg per day is reached. Farcot et al[96] have pointed out that at beneficial dosages these side effects become a significant clinical problem.

Phenoxybenzamine (Dibenzyline) is a combined alpha-1/alpha-2 antagonist and has been reported as a successful oral sympathetic blocker for reflex dystrophy treatment, but its nonselective features cause widespread side effects.[111] Although it benefits by blocking alpha-adrenergic receptors in the afflicted extremity, it also blocks vasoconstriction in the rest of the body, causing dizziness from orthostatic hypotension, reflex tachycardia, nasal stuffiness, myosis, and inhibition of ejaculation.[114] A starting dose of 10 mg per day is gradually increased by 10 mg every 2 or 3 days until there is either pain relief or too much postural hypotension, with an average dose of 80 mg per day.

Propranolol (Inderal) is a beta-adrenergic receptor blocker that has been studied longer than other oral sympathetic blocking agents, with reports of successful use in reflex dystrophy by its pronounced ability to reduce peripheral vein and artery response to sympathetic stimulation.[295,305,329] The usual oral dosage is 40 mg three to four times per day, but it must be used cautiously in patients with cardiac disease, and it is contraindicated in patients with asthma. Interestingly, propranolol, along with another beta-blocker, pindolol, has received more general use in France than in the United States.[10]

Calcium channel blockers, such as *nifedipine,* are not true sympathetic blockers, but function to decrease sympathetic smooth muscle tone and improve blood flow, warming digits by preventing calcium release after stimulation of adrenergic receptors. These are beneficial in patients with reflex dystrophy selected because of "cool" extremities,[153,265] and they reduce vasoconstriction by actually "stabilizing" rather than physiologically "blocking" the so-called "slow" l-type membrane calcium channels to impede intracellular calcium ion movement and reduce smooth muscle contractility.[231] Verapamil, diltiazem, amlodipine, and nifedipine are the principal calcium antagonists available; however, verapamil has a predominantly cardiac effect and is not useful for reflex dystrophy. Nifedipine (Procardia, Adalat) has been most widely utilized for reflex dystrophy at dosages of 30 to 60 mg per day.[153,265] Many patients who develop headache and dizziness on nifedipine are better able to tolerate diltiazem (Cardizem) in dosages of 90 to 180 mg per day.[220] Nifedipine and verapamil have a negative effect on SA and AV nodal conduction and myocardial contractility, and caution should be exercised with use in cardiac-impaired patients.[104] Amlodipine (Norvasc) is a better choice for these patients because it has little or no effect on the SA and AV nodal conduction and may be equally effective in preventing peripheral vasoconstriction.[242]

Antiinflammatory Medications

Corticosteroids have long been recognized as beneficial in some patients with reflex dystrophy.[171] More recent interest in the etiological hypothesis that reflex dystrophy is due to an exaggerated neuropeptide-induced inflammatory tissue response caused by free radicals has led to recent use of free radical scavengers and neuropeptide suppressants as well.

NSAIDs such as ibuprofen are of questionable value in the treatment of reflex dystrophy without convincing studies either

for or against their use. Much of their benefit is thought to be due to inhibition of prostaglandins, which are proinflammatory mediators.[323] Specifically, it is known that these drugs can inhibit the enzyme cyclooxygenase, which is responsible for the conversion of arachidonic acid to the terminal prostaglandins that promote inflammation and can excite or sensitize various neurons in producing pain.[81,259,324] I favor use of NSAID medications as an adjunct in any patient who finds them subjectively beneficial, generally first offering ibuprofen at 600 mg three times a day. The patients most likely to benefit are those who are at stage I.[239]

Corticosteroids have long proven beneficial in some patients with reflex dystrophy, either using a short-term high-dose method[171] or long-term use.[112] Control study with placebo confirms steroid benefit in reflex dystrophy.[59] However, Kozin[169] observed that steroid response in patients who have predominantly pain without inflammatory or autonomic findings is not as good. He uses a "burst" of oral prednisone, starting with 15 mg four times a day for 3 to 4 days, then 10 mg four times a day for another 3 or 4 days, then tapering by using morning dosages of 30 mg, 20 mg, 15 mg, 10 mg, and 5 mg for 3 days each. Others have described successful use of intravenous steroids with a Bier block, and this may be used in conjunction with intravenous bretylium.[261] Biopsies of synovium in patients with reflex dystrophy have shown mild inflammatory change,[108,171] and steroids seem most useful in those patients with marked edema; erythematous, swollen, painful, and stiff joints; and other symptoms of inflammatory or autonomic response.

Free radical scavengers such as intravenous mannitol and dimethyl sulfoxide (DMSO) are proposed for acute reflex dystrophy.[322] Control study of topical DMSO showed significantly better results than placebo.[117] In severe acute reflex dystrophy, intravenous mannitol is given (10%, 1 liter per day) for 1 week to patients with normal renal function; subsequently, 50% DMSO cream is applied to the afflicted area five times a day for 2 or 3 months. Less severe cases are given only the DMSO.[322]

Capsaicin, a naturally occurring alkaloid, quiets nociceptive cutaneous C-fiber afferents by first stimulating and then blocking them by depleting the neuropeptide substance P, which reduces membrane excitability and blocks axon transport. Its use for chronic pain has been contradictory,[195,316] and its use for reflex dystrophy is limited by the availability of only low-concentrate (0.075%) topical cream (Axsain), which causes initial discomfort at the site of application. Use of capsaicin can be attempted in selected patients with very localized symptoms.

"Central-Acting" Pharmacologic Agents

ANTICONVULSANTS. Antiepileptic drugs are among the most interesting and provocative group of pharmacologic medications for reflex dystrophy and other neuropathic pain syndromes. It is puzzling that although phenobarbital, one of the oldest and most widely-used anticonvulsants, is known to sometimes cause reflex dystrophy,[78] the anticonvulsant gabapentin (Neurontin) is one of the "hottest" new drugs for pain control.[198] The central change by which antiepilepsy drugs can "cause" or "correct" reflex dystrophy is certainly a provocative question. Unfortunately, in the high dosages used for epilepsy, most of these drugs can cause sedation, confusion, diplopia, vertigo, and ataxia. Fortunately, those who benefit from the use of these drugs to treat neuropathic pain may usually do so at lower dosages.

Gabapentin is marketed as a treatment for refractory seizure disorders; however, it is shown to significantly benefit patients with neuropathic pain syndromes in a randomized, double-blind, placebo-controlled, multicenter study.[16] Gabapentin is structurally related to γ-aminobutyric acid (GABA), a neurotransmitter that plays a role in pain transmission and modulation. Its precise mechanism of action is not understood because it is not converted to GABA, is not a GABA-antagonist, and does not inhibit GABA uptake.[240] It does alter GABA synthesis and release and blood serotonin levels.[315] Unlike GABA, gabapentin does cross the blood-brain barrier and is eliminated by renal excretion, so it must be used carefully in patients with renal insufficiency, especially with a creatinine clearance of less than 60 ml per minute.[87,331] It has been used successfully for treatment of reflex dystrophy, but experience is still limited.[215] The most frequent side effects are dizziness and somnolence,[16] and although the optimal dosage for reflex dystrophy has yet to be established, Mackin recommends starting low at 100 mg once or twice a day and increasing slowly to three daily dosages for a total of 900 to 1200 mg per day. If patients report no benefit at 1 g per day, Mackin believes that higher dosages (up to 3600 mg) are unlikely to prove beneficial.

Phenytoin (Dilantin) and *carbamazepine (Tegretol)* both function as Na$^+$ channel antagonists to block Na$^+$ influx across cell membranes. This is thought to reduce the afferent excitability that may be a source of pain and has been reported to benefit patients with reflex dystrophy.[287]

Clonazepam (Klonopin) is a benzodiazepine that facilitates binding of the inhibitory neurotransmitter GABA to its specific channel receptors, and it has been used successfully to treat allodynia in patients with chronic pain syndromes.

Valproic acid (Depakene) also increases activity of the neurotransmitter GABA, though its specific mechanism remains unknown.

ANTIDEPRESSANTS, ANXIETY, AND SLEEP MEDICATIONS

On psychiatric testing, patients with reflex dystrophy are found to be significantly depressed and anxious. It is difficult to distinguish between depression and anxiety, even for experts, and the psychiatric literature suggests that the best diagnostic indicator is the response to antidepressant medication.[275] In reflex dystrophy, sleep disturbance is usually present. Although the pattern of disturbance is usually characteristic of depression (awakening in the early morning hours), these alexithymic-prone patients almost always deny depression, even though their demeanor seems otherwise.

They generally need medication for sleep and, when tolerated, I find the tricyclic antidepressant amitriptyline (Elavil) to be the most useful for this purpose.

Tricyclic antidepressants have been the most widely used antidepressants for neuropathic pain patients.[167,198,218-220,314] This is probably due to their adjunctive effects, rather than primary antidepressive features, because in much lower dosages than needed to treat psychotic depression, sleep-promoting effects and some degree of analgesia occur, and the onset of action is earlier than the 2 to 3 weeks needed for depression treatment.[225] Amitriptyline (Elavil) is the prototype and most generally effective,[198] with its pharmacologic effect attributed to blocking of CNS monoamine pumps, thereby inhibiting neurotransmitter reuptake at nerve terminals, especially serotonin and norepinephrine. It takes approximately 2 to 3 weeks to adequately deplete these terminals for severe depression control in a dosage of up to 300 mg per day; however, for the sleep disturbance associated with reflex dystrophy, only 10 to 25 mg per night may be needed. Conceivably, other neurotransmitter substances may be inhibited that carry pain and inflammation. Unfortunately, while tertiary tricyclic antidepressants seem the most effective for neuropathic pain (amitriptyline, imipramine, and doxepin) they have a higher incidence of anticholinergic side effects (e.g., sedation, confusion, blurred vision, dry mouth, tachycardia, constipation, sexual dysfunction, and weight gain), especially at higher dosages. Secondary monoamine tricyclic antidepressants, such as desipramine and nortriptyline (Pamelor) have less anticholinergic activity and may be better tolerated, especially by the elderly or those who seem to be "medication sensitive." These medications have less serotonergic activity than the tertiary monoamines, however desipramine (Norpramin) has been as effective as amitriptyline in a placebo-controlled study to assess its use as a treatment for painful diabetic neuropathy.[208] Amitriptyline must be used with care in the elderly and in patients with heart disease, narrow-angle glaucoma, prostatism, and seizure disorders.[198] When this medication is used in an adjunctive fashion with other measures of treatment for reflex dystrophy it is important to start dosages low (10 to 25 mg at bedtime) and titrate a slow increase until good rest is achieved. When high dosages of amitriptyline are needed for psychotic levels of depression, psychiatric assistance is recommended because overdosage can cause life-threatening cardiac arrhythmias and there is a 2- to 3-week delay in the primary benefit for depression. It is therefore valuable to use caution concerning quantities and refills prescribed to patients with major depression who are at risk for suicide.

Nontricyclic antidepressants, including serotonin reuptake inhibitors, have been increasingly popular as adjunctive measures over the past decade because of fewer side effects. Generally there are fewer reports supporting their use for symptoms of reflex dystrophy. Because most of these have "activating" effects, they are administered early in the day to avoid insomnia, and they are not as useful as the tricyclic antidepressants for treatment of common sleep-disturbance complaints.

Selective serotonin reuptake inhibitors (SSRI) are a new class of relatively safe medications that are widely used in the treatment of other conditions but have been the subject of only scant research as a treatment for reflex dystrophy. Popular examples include *sertraline (Zoloft), fluoxetine (Prozac),* and *paroxetine (Paxil).* These drugs bind to the presynaptic serotonin carrier in the CNS to inhibit serotonin reuptake, and paroxetine has been shown to reduce diabetic neuropathy pain.[296] Chambliss[56] points out that the combination of amitriptyline (Elavil) at 25 mg per day and fluoxetine (Prozac) at 20 mg per day may offer more benefit than either drug alone.

Certain nontricyclic, nonserotonin reuptake inhibitor antidepressants have been tried for treatment of chronic pain despite scarce data, including *trazodone (Desyrel), venlafaxine (Effexor), nefazodone (Serzone),* and *maprotiline (Ludiomil).* Among these, venlafaxine might be the most promising because it strongly inhibits both serotonin and norepinephrine reuptake.[198]

Anxiety and sleep medications must be chosen carefully for use by patients with reflex dystrophy. For example, phenobarbital can actually cause reflex dystrophy,[75-80] and other tranquilizers, such as other barbiturates and meprobamate, have antianalgesia effects.[239] *Diazepam (Valium)* has been recommended in the past,[165,173] but although it is a useful antianxiety medication it is not as effective against depression, and patients with reflex dystrophy may develop antianalgesia response and physical dependence after long use.[239] When amitriptyline cannot be tolerated for sleep, a mild medication such as an antihistamine should be chosen. Poor rest is known to create hyperirritable muscle response, and patients with reflex dystrophy need rest to avoid developing the trigger points of hyperirritable muscle foci.

Opioid use has become popular in pain management centers in the United States because available long-acting opioids permit normal daily activity in many patients with chronic pain. Addiction is reported in fewer than 2% of those who use preparations such as MS-Contin every 8 to 12 hours; methadone and levorphanol every 8 hours; and slow-release oxycodone, hydromorphone, and hydrocodone combinations.[252] However, I and others[198] caution that patients with reflex dystrophy should not be grouped with those who suffer from chronic back and other types of pain for this treatment. Data on these patients do not separate the reflex dystrophy group, and I have seen the sorrowful state of unrelenting reflex dystrophy pain compounded with addiction after this treatment approach. If one accepts the concept of an internal opioid pain-control mechanism in humans, it could be expected to function as other internal organ systems; the thyroid decreases output when exogenous thyroid is given, the adrenal gland does the same when ACTH is given, the pancreas also reduces output when insulin is given, and so on. Use of exogenous opioids would conceivably inhibit production of the internal endorphin system and therefore interfere with treatment programs believed to activate the endorphin internal pain-control system (e.g., TENS, implanted electrical stimulation, acupuncture, and stress loading). Although these

mechanisms are hypothetical, I suspect narcotic treatment for reflex dystrophy is a better treatment for the doctor than the patient, and the more time-consuming and troublesome techniques to help these patients to slowly gain control of their pain is a better approach in all but the absolute treatment failures. We should therefore exhaust other techniques of treatment before resorting to chronic narcotic usage. Certainly short-acting opioid preparations, such as propoxyphene (Darvocet), hydrocodone (Tylox), meperidine (Demerol), and pentazocine (Talwin), are to be avoided for chronic use in patients with reflex dystrophy because they can cause CNS toxicity and addiction with long-term use.[252]

CALCITONIN

Calcitonin is a hormone in a separate category. Its success for treating reflex dystrophy was totally unexpected, with benefits that were unforeseeable other than antiosteoclastic properties. It has become the most frequently used treatment method in France and various other European countries for over 20 years subsequent to its introduction by Eisinger et al[91] in 1973 in a series of 46 cases.[10,67,233] In Doury's double-blind, placebo-controlled study[80] (using 100 U/day of salmon calcitonin) there was significant subjective benefit at 2 weeks, but no difference at 1 month after treatment. It has been found that only high dosages have been beneficial. Currently, recombinant human calcitonin is generally given at a dose of 0.5 g to 1 g per day using intramuscular injections daily for 2 weeks for phase I reflex dystrophy, with better tolerance than that achieved with salmon calcitonin. Intramuscular injections daily for 2 weeks is the usual regimen for phase I reflex dystrophy, and better results are reported when patients are treated soon after onset.[10] Side effects of calcitonin treatment include flushes, nausea, and malaise during the hour after injection, but this usually lasts only 2 to 3 hours. They are unpleasant side effects, but not serious. Efforts at nasal administration have been disappointing.[32] The mechanism by which the calcitonin reduces the pain and edema of reflex dystrophy remains unknown and cannot be explained by its antiosteoclastic activity alone, but it probably has some regulatory effect on the microcirculation and seems best suited for those patients with evidence of Sudeck's osteoporosis on three-phase bone scan.

OTHER MISCELLANEOUS PHARMACOLOGIC AGENTS

Baclofen (Lioresal) is a strong GABA receptor agonist, and seems particularly useful for lancinating pain and ongoing muscle spasms and cramps. It is best initiated slowly at 5 mg twice a day, then increased by 5 to 10 mg every 3 to 4 days, with a thrice-daily regimen of up to 40 to 60 mg a day.[198]

Tramadol (Ultram) is a CNS-active analgesic, neither nonsteroidal nor true opioid, that inhibits reuptake of serotonin and norepinephrine, and weakly binds to μ-opioid receptors.[83,268,269] It has been used as a nonnarcotic pain medication after surgery in the elderly, but seems beneficial as a supplemental pain medication for chronic nociceptive pain, comparable to a weak narcotic. At dosages of 50 to 100 mg three to four times a day, some patients suffer side effects similar to those caused by narcotics (e.g., somnolence, confusion, constipation, and nausea).[198] When tolerated, it seems a better choice than opioids for reflex dystrophy pain.

Mexiletine (Mexitil) blocks Na^+ membrane channels and is thought to stabilize cell membranes to reduce the abnormally excitable nerve discharges. Patients with no electrocardiographic evidence of conduction abnormality must be selected. Tolerance is limited, with significant side effects. Controlled study of neuropathic pain associated with diabetic neuropathy demonstrated significant benefit at 10 mg/kg/day; however, serious drug reactions are possible, including a lupus-like syndrome, abnormal liver function, blood dyscrasias, and impotence.[130,167]

HAND THERAPY

I believe that hand therapy itself is the foundation of treatment for most patients with reflex dystrophy, whereas TENS, pharmacologic intervention, nerve blocks, biofeedback, and/or surgery serve as the adjunctive measures. Busy hand surgeons usually find patients with reflex dystrophy burdensome because of their excessive demands for time and the commitment required by the surgeon for long-term treatment of this usually nonsurgical problem. Hand therapists can supply this demand for time and commitment. Unfortunately, the health care insurance system in place in the United States today often complicates this already difficult problem with "benefit limitations" that cannot be successfully appealed or overridden in a timely fashion.

Whatever treatment method is chosen, it is imperative to establish baseline measurement criteria to monitor progress. This includes ninhydrin sweat testing; sensory testing with Semmes Weinstein monofilaments; moving and static two-point discrimination tests; measurement of vibration sense, resting temperature, grip and pinch strength, and range of motion; volumetric measurement of edema, assessment of response to cold (cold recovery time), pain assessment, and a hand function test such as the Perdue pegboard, Jebsen, or Moberg tests. Often the patient will sense slow improvement only when shown improvement by these objective parameters.

The knowledgeable hand therapist individualizes treatment according to each patient's status and needs, choosing measured criteria as goals for improvement. For example, if temperature change and weakness are predominant findings, a program of biofeedback therapy and strengthening exercises may be initially chosen, with change of program if no objective improvement occurs. "Rest and motion"[10] are principles of management that indicate the need for partial rest in a splinted functional position, and frequent physical activity, pressure, and motion to the fullest extent that does not cause pain. Heat can be valuable to relax muscle spasm and improve joint

motion. However, heat with dependency in a whirlpool should be avoided in patients with edema because this will likely aggravate swelling.[173]

Muscle trigger points of myofascial dysfunction must be treated, but the usual methods of ice, massage, and cold spray are often intolerable in patients with reflex dystrophy, and warm massage, stretch exercises, and injection of trigger points may be utilized instead.

Desensitization is often needed in patients with reflex dystrophy who have hypersensitivity and disuse patterns. A graded program organized on the basis of objective measurements and a series of objective goals is used, starting with tuning-fork stimulation and working through battery and electrical vibratory stimulation, identification of textures, object identification, and, finally, work simulation.[133] In patients with reflex dystrophy, this program must be administered by a supportive therapist working closely with the patient, as opposed to other hand-injured patients who often seem to be able to conduct the program on their own at home. In preoperative patients, such as those with disproportionately painful neuromas, desensitization should precede surgical correction to avoid exacerbating a pain syndrome.[218]

Techniques such as *ultrasound* over the stellate ganglion[115] or the involved peripheral nerves,[263] *biofeedback*,[35] *desensitization*,[133] and *stress loading*[335] all involve intense personal support by the therapist. No single modality or method succeeds in all patients, and individualization and flexibility are essential. The importance of psychological support or encouragement cannot be overemphasized and may be an essential feature of treatment success; it therefore seems valuable to have the same therapist work with a particular patient once good rapport is established.

Work simulation is an important part of any reflex dystrophy therapy program, especially for worker's compensation cases. Many patients with the chronic pain of reflex dystrophy take pride in achieving these work-simulation objective goals and returning to healthy functional use, even though many will still acknowledge pain on a visual analog scale. It seems that the program allows them to better adjust or cope with the discomfort. For some reason, the anxiety and activity of work return seems to precipitate recurrent symptoms in many patients. The reassurance of having successfully completed work activity while being encouraged and supported in an understanding therapy environment will do much to allay the patient's fear and permit smooth transition when returning to the workplace.

PSYCHOTHERAPY

Reflex dystrophy is not a psychiatric disorder[167] nor is it a peripheral anatomic entity that is separate from CNS and psychogenic effect. Psychiatric literature identifies this as a medical problem that might be mistakenly diagnosed as psychogenic and should be referred to the surgeon,[89] whereas many surgeons believe patients with reflex dystrophy need psychotherapy and should be referred to a psychiatrist.[42,134,138,247] This paradox acknowledges that neither specialty is comfortable with this disorder, which fits into neither discipline well. Most cases of reflex dystrophy are not surgical, but the patients certainly do not regard their symptoms and findings as emotional and do not easily accept psychotherapy or even psychiatric evaluation. I have found that the easiest solution is to use a psychiatric consultant in the hand therapy arena who is introduced as a supportive person there to help the patient deal with the emotional impact of losing hand function. Most patients are comfortable with this explanation and cooperative with the psychiatrist, who can explore etiologic patterns and assist with current conflicts regarding the patient's personal and family life and the need for psychotropic medications.

Because most of these patients seem to be alexithymic,[317] they are resistant to the "central" psychoanalytic approach; however, because they do have an apparent peripheral problem, a more "peripheral" form of psychotherapeutic support is possible. This is accomplished with standard hand-therapy technique and support along with "cognitive behavioral therapy," which provides the patient with skills and pacing activities used in minimizing pain.[303] The patient may learn to extinguish pain behavior (even though still experiencing some pain) and develops a personal sense of control over the pain, rather than feeling like its victim.[239] Psychiatric consultation is also helpful in deciding whether tranquilizers or antidepressant drugs may benefit a particular patient, but in most cases low doses of amitriptyline (10 to 50 mg at night) are given for sleep disturbance.

There are a few isolated reports of successful treatment of reflex dystrophy by psychotherapy alone, and these stress the importance of helping the patient feel responsible and in control.[3,190,289,291] However, whether it is a psychiatrist, psychologist, surgeon, internist, or hand therapist that is the major provider of treatment, the importance of consistent psychologic support, sympathy, reassurance, and stubborn encouragement for these patients cannot be overestimated. Generally, the support from a psychiatrist or psychologist is beneficial, provided the primary caregiver continues to provide support as well.

PRACTICAL PRINCIPLES IN THE TREATMENT OF REFLEX DYSTROPHY

Any arrogance about treatment of this disorder must be held suspect in the absence of a unifying hypothesis or distinctive diagnostic criteria and in the presence of such an incredible array of inciting causes (sometimes no apparent cause at all) and remarkable spectrum of different treatment techniques (none universally successful). However, until we have better understanding of the mechanisms underlying this disorder the following 10 principles are offered as a practical approach to these patients. Any physician willing to undertake manage-

ment of patients with reflex dystrophy must search his or her soul and muster compassion for these difficult patients to manage each on an individual basis, altering the treatment regimen as necessary to patiently assist them in coping with this devastating disorder.

1. *The best treatment is prevention.* Take seriously any patient whose pain complaints seem disproportionate and who anxiously asks extensive, detailed questions, often repeating the same inquiries and requiring additional physician attention and reassurance. Similarly, the postoperative patient who seems to withdraw and disassociate from the physician because of pain needs additional therapeutic support. This is usually best provided by hand therapy, in which parameters such as volume, temperature, sweat, sensation, and strength are monitored and nonpainful mobilization activities are encouraged (Figure 133-9). Certainly, if the patient improves, you will never be able to demonstrate that this would have evolved into reflex dystrophy. However, most clinicians and therapists believe that additional support and early intervention have prevented the development of full-blown reflex dystrophy. In an attempt to prospectively study psychological factors several years ago, Maureen Hardy, MS, RPT, CHT, found that none of her prospective candidates developed reflex dystrophy after surgery or injury during 3 years of study. She finally resorted to established cases of reflex dystrophy to fulfill her strict diagnostic criteria for the study.[132] Hardy explains that many patients appeared to develop disproportionate pain with some minimal change of temperature or edema, but they responded to early, intense intervention and did not go on to fulfill her strict diagnostic criteria for reflex dystrophy. She believes that early therapeutic intervention likely obviated development of the diagnosis in these prospective candidates.

The worst possible therapeutic approach is to belittle or minimize the patient's complaint because of the lack of objective findings. If Hardy's study is correct, these are sensitized patients who are already significantly anxious, depressed, have poor self-image, and easily feel rejected but somatize their anger. To minimize their complaints may add fuel to the stress-related features that likely play a role in the etiology of this disorder. One may see this reflected in the bitterness many patients express about their previous care. The clinician should not presume the patient is exaggerating his or her symptoms. To quote Sunderland,[308] "to adopt such an attitude is, in fact, to commit a grievous error; apart from the serious mistake in diagnosis, a great injustice is being done to the patient in attempting to lay upon him both the blame for being ill and the responsibility for curing himself. The patient is the only witness we have, and if he says he has pain, there are no grounds on which we can contradict him." In today's managed care environment, providing this very important, early, intense support based on the intuition of the clinician will prove increasingly difficult.

2. *The earlier the treatment, the better the prognosis.* With a few exceptions, most authors agree that RSD becomes increasingly recalcitrant to therapeutic efforts after 6 months. One of the most provocative studies supporting this conclusion was by Wang et al,[333] whose study of long-term response

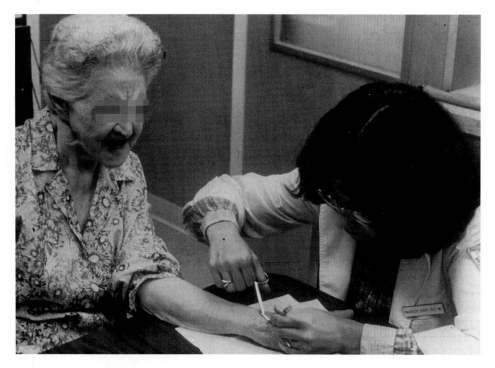

Figure 133-9. Exaggerated pain response at the time of suture removal, an indication for additional support and therapy. (Courtesy Maureen Hardy.)

to sympathetic block 3 years after treatment saw only 40% of patients with good to excellent results, and 38% with poor results. However, when the patients had received sympathetic blocks within 6 months of the onset of their disease, 70% acknowledged successful treatment 3 years later, indicating that this treatment, as are others, is most successful when instituted early.

3. *Individualize treatment methods to the particular patient's manifestations.* By utilizing objective parameters of their symptoms, patients can be characterized as having manifestations that are predominantly sympathetic, inflammatory, or central (when the peripheral response is minimal). Clinicians should use sympathetic blocks, for example, if sympathetic symptoms predominate, such as changes in temperature, color, and sweat. Temperature biofeedback treatment should be attempted when the only major change is in the temperature of the affected area. If inflammatory symptoms predominate, such as stiffness, joint discomfort, swelling, and pain with joint motion, antiinflammatory agents, such as a short-term burst of steroids, should be used. Central stimulation, such as TENS, Neurontin, hypnosis, acupuncture, and stress loading, should be used if central pain predominates. All treatment techniques should include regular hand therapy support with monitoring of objective parameters.

4. *Start with the least invasive and morbid treatment techniques.* By use of objective monitoring, gradually alter and try new treatments until one of these regimens shows objective improvement. The clinician should maintain a positive outlook throughout the course of treatment and reassure the patient that there are many different treatment methods and they will be explored until one demonstrates improvement. Do

not expect much subjective improvement in the patient's pain manifestation until you can demonstrate objective measured improvement to the patient (which may instill some hope and confidence needed for the patient to control his or her pain). These patients rarely think they are better until they are shown to be. Objective improvement usually precedes subjective improvement, and the physician must maintain stubborn optimism with compassionate honesty about the goal to help patients cope with their pain.

5. *Minimize stressful situations.* This group of patients seems to be particularly prone to conflict, usually feeling victimized and poorly understood, and they often express distress that no one understands or believes their degree of suffering. It is easy to become impatient with their complaints, but it is important to patiently listen and to help modify any stress-producing situations, when possible, to minimize rather than aggravate their problem.

6. *Encourage litigation settlements as soon as possible.* Unrealistic unconscious expectations of dramatic cure, wealth from litigation settlement, or revenge against an employer or spouse create additional progressive disappointment, resentment, and depression unless these expectations are recognized by the treating clinician and gently eliminated whenever possible. It may be that these expectations arise from unfulfilled childhood dependency needs and tend to be immature and unrealistic, but they are also unconscious. There is no conventional psychotherapy that will resolve this, so the patient must be encouraged to avoid measures that will additionally complicate and increase stress. Much of this will be accomplished by listening to the patient vent his or her frustrations and anger and requires the patience of a saint

(generally hand therapists have greater potential for sainthood than hand surgeons). Unfortunately, litigation increases stress and encourages victimization, with an implication that the worse the problem is, the better the settlement potential. Often, a healthier therapeutic environment exists after settlement, but the problem of reflex dystrophy usually persists.

7. *Control the disproportionate pain and other marked symptoms of reflex dystrophy before elective surgery.* Do not expect surgery to control disproportionate pain. There is a popular misguided belief that most reflex dystrophy is altogether due to a single peripheral cause or irritant, possibly because a precipitating cause can frequently be identified. One should avoid a surgical search for such a cause, at least until the disproportionate pain is controlled. Usually there is temporary relief of pain after surgery, then exacerbation or worsening pain and requests for additional surgery, and the surgeon may be held responsible for worsening the symptoms. Amputation will not likely rid the patient of the pain, although it certainly will of their extremity.

When surgery is done on a patient with reflex dystrophy who has developed control of the pain or in any patient with a history of reflex dystrophy, long-acting blocks should be used during surgery, even if the patient has a general anesthetic, to avoid exacerbating reflex dystrophy. It appears that if one can keep the brain blind to the stimulation during surgery, this may avoid recreating the pain cycle.

There are two situations in which surgery is a beneficial treatment for reflex dystrophy. One is when sympathetic block relieves pain to the time limits of the block and sympathectomy can be particularly recommended. Another is when acute reflex dystrophy is associated with acute traumatic carpal tunnel syndrome after a Colles' fracture, in which case immediate surgical release of the carpal tunnel is indicated.[155]

8. *Regard the patient with reflex dystrophy as an impaired individual with a chronic illness.* Paul Brand pointed out that we must regard the patient with chronic pain with the same compassion as we would patients with rheumatoid arthritis or diabetes.[49] Unfortunately, the patient with reflex dystrophy is usually not appreciative of our efforts at compassion because he or she is frustrated by our inability to adequately explain or quickly correct the problem that the patient certainly does not regard as a chronic illness. We should provide a positive, optimistic outlook designed to instill confidence and the expectation of improvement, but not imply a greater understanding or ability than is actually present. It is not easy to acknowledge our ignorance to our patients and at the same time remain optimistic and supportive. We do not understand the basic underlying problem and therefore cannot confidently solve it. We can only help the patient cope by assuring them of our compassion and continued support, much as we do when dealing with patients with connective tissue disease and other chronic disorders. Some patients will get well, others will only become better able to cope with the disorder, and others will just disappear. We must recognize that some of these patients may "need their pain" although they desperately cry for relief. These patients many times complicate their treatment plan with noncompliant behavior and intolerance to drug and other

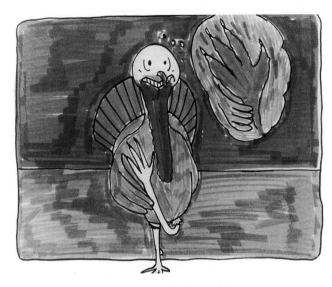

Figure 133-10. Patients should not be called "turkeys" out of compassion for the patient and respect for the Meleagris gallopavo, the noble American Wild Turkey.

treatment regimens. Retaining a positive outlook and diluting the responsibility by a team approach with the hand therapist and psychologic counseling is helpful in managing these difficult patients.

9. *Never discharge the patient with reflex dystrophy.* Patients with reflex dystrophy are recognized to be at risk for redevelopment of the syndrome, usually at a new location. The complex psychophysiologic features and the etiology of this disorder may relate to unfulfilled dependency needs in some patients, and an important therapeutic feature may be the opportunity to return annually to express their current status to their caregivers. Those who do not need to return will not, but others seem to appreciate the opportunity to express how they have coped with their difficulties, and one suspects it may afford a benefit to prevent recurrence.

10. *Do not call these patients "turkeys."* The compassion needed to comprehend and successfully manage patients with reflex dystrophy is incompatible with such a rude designation and, furthermore, shows a profound disrespect for the Meleagris gallopavo, the noble American wild turkey (Figure 133-10).

SUMMARY

Can you prevent reflex dystrophy? Certainly not always, because some highly predisposed patients apparently develop the disorder spontaneously. However, empiric observation has convinced many of us that on recognition of the earliest signs (e.g., disproportionate pain, swelling, vasomotor instability, increased anxiety, and fear of function), immediate therapeutic intervention seems to obviate development of the disorder in some patients. It is impossible to prove what percentage of these patients would have progressed to the full-blown disorder without such attention. At present, we certainly cannot identify those at risk, and the disorder is unpredictable, with no correlation between severity of injury and degree of reflex dystrophy. At our hand center, as in others, we see very few patients who develop reflex dystrophy while being treated. However, we see many referrals with the established disorder who usually complain bitterly about a lack of attention and failure to have their symptoms taken seriously by their previous caregivers.

We cannot expect to prevent such a poorly understood disorder; however, there are six measures that may reduce the possibility of reflex dystrophy:

1. As early as 1942 Miller suggested that a significant preventive factor was the importance of communication with the patient, expressing reassurance of support and assistance for relief of his or her anxiety and pain.[50]
2. The earliest possible active motion and function within the patient's pain threshold should be encouraged. Newer methods of management, such as relative motion splinting that will permit immediate active motion after long extensor repair, or secure plate fracture fixation that allows immediate active motion, will do much to discourage the victimization that accompanies immobilization and reflex dystrophy.
3. Whenever possible, prolonged use of external fixation should be avoided.[283] One report noted the development of reflex dystrophy in 9.8% of patients after radiometacarpal external fixation of distal radius wrist fractures and a 5.5% incidence after external minifixation of the hand. However, an even higher incidence was suggested in patients with distraction external fixation.
4. Remove any cast or splint that the patient believes is too tight or is causing pain. In general, reflex dystrophy is more common in patients who are immobilized and a sense by the patient that a tight cast is causing their symptoms is frequent, even though the clinician finds no evidence on physical inspection. Nonetheless, the cast should be removed and replaced as often as necessary to rid the patient of burning, incessant pain. If unrelenting pain continues, it is appropriate to abandon immobilization completely (other than perhaps a soft dressing) after thorough communication with the patient regarding the need to control his or her pain. One must also be certain there is no other explanation for the pain, such as acute carpal tunnel syndrome, infection, or ischemia. As soon as the patient has subjective relief, the immobilization can be gently replaced. The patient will likely have better function in spite of a nonunion or tendon rupture than he or she will with the disaster of reflex dystrophy. In my experience, these patients actually kept their extremities protected until the pain was sufficiently relieved to permit reimmobilization. This reasoning must be discussed with the patient, explaining that relief of pain is more important than success of the procedure. This allows the patient to establish a sense of control. It is very important to conduct this discussion with compassion and not hostility. I have no explanation

for why this temporary departure from immobilization, first shown to me by Dr. Earl E. Peacock, Jr., many years ago, seems to provide relief.

5. Avoid any measures that increase inflammation. For example, avoid painful, forced, passive range-of-motion therapy or the use of dynamic splints until the acute postoperative inflammation subsides. Pain must be the indication to limit passive forced motion, which must remain within a relatively pain-free range. Antiinflammatory medication may benefit symptoms of inflammation. Although it is important to keep the extremity elevated to reduce edema, motion must still be encouraged.
6. Be wary of patients with a history of reflex dystrophy, recognizing that they are at greater risk. When surgery is necessary in a patient with previous reflex dystrophy, a long-acting block of the operative area should be performed before making an incision, even when the patient is having a general anesthetic. Try to keep the CNS unaware of the procedure as long as possible to avoid recreation of the "reflex" or "cycle" that can recur. The incidence of recurrent reflex dystrophy is reported to be as high as 15%,[123,124] but it is probably even higher, and it usually recurs at a different site. We notice that many patients whose hand reflex dystrophy treatment seemed controlled will return after having developed subsequent pain in the back or neck or another painful disorder.

In situations in which physicians cannot predict who is predisposed or under what circumstances patients may develop this disorder, it seems patently unfair there are so many negligence litigation cases against physicians. We have no more control or understanding of this disorder than we do of rheumatoid arthritis, scleroderma, Raynaud's syndrome, and a host of other inflammatory, vasoactive, connective tissue conditions. It therefore seems absurd that physicians are so frequently held responsible for causing this one. However, the American litigation system has seen opportunity when science cannot prove that a management technique or agent *did not* cause a disorder. This is illustrated by successful litigation against the manufacturers of silicone breast prostheses, which were alleged to have caused connective tissue disorders, in spite of no scientific evidence to support this claim. If our observations are accurate that many patients with reflex dystrophy may have suppressed, unconscious anger and unfulfilled dependency needs, we cannot be surprised by the frequency with which they may embrace litigation. We need to try to understand the complex and abstruse psychologic makeup in each patient to support him or her as best we can while providing the objective goals for improvement in this disorder. Unfortunately, litigation often accuses physicians of delay in diagnosis or improper treatment without recognition that there is no uniform diagnostic criteria and no uniformly successful treatment method and that prognosis is not predictable. Indeed, stress factors such as pending litigation aggravate symptoms of reflex dystrophy and direct attention away from needed time for therapy.

Our best bet to reduce the incidence of this disorder and the litigation associated with its unsuccessful treatment is immediate psychologic and hand-therapy support for patients who appear unduly anxious and depressed and have disproportionate pain. This is now frustrated by a system of managed care that often limits or delays hand-therapy benefits and is not presently held liable.

The study of reflex dystrophy brings into sharp focus our recognition of the large amount of cerebral cortex dedicated to hand activity and our profound ignorance of the mechanisms involved in the interrelationship of the CNS physiology and hand function. Once these are understood, we may discover that Pulvertaft's belief that the hand is the "mirror of man's emotion" is true, and we may even someday assess the patient's emotional state by measuring the neurotransmitter substances associated with reflex dystrophy.[267]

REFERENCES

1. Abram SE: Pain of sympathetic origin. In Raj P (editor): *Practical management of pain,* New York, 1986, Yearbook Medical.

2. Abram SE, Lightfoot RW: Treatment of long-standing causalgia with prazosin, *Reg Anesth* 6:79-81, 1981.

3. Alioto JT: Behavioral treatment of reflex sympathetic dystrophy, *Psychosomatics* 22:539-540, 1981.

4. Allbritten FF, Maltby GL: Causalgia secondary to injury of the major peripheral nerves, *Surgery* 38:407, 1946.

5. Allmay BGL, Johansson F, von Knorring L, et al: Endorphins in chronic pain: differences in CSF endorphin levels between organic and psychogenic pain syndromes, *Pain* 24:297-311, 1986.

6. Amadio PC: Pain dysfunction syndromes, *J Bone Joint Surg* 70A: 944-949, 1988.

7. Amadio PC, Mackinnon SE, Merritt WH, et al: Reflex sympathetic dystrophy syndrome: consensus report of the ad hoc committee of the American Association for Hand Surgery on the definition of reflex sympathetic dystrophy syndrome, *J Plast Reconstr Surg* 87:371-375, 1991.

8. Andersen G, Vestergaard K, Ingman-Nielsen M, et al: Incidence of central post-stroke pain, *Pain* 61:187, 1995.

9. Arden RL, Bahu SJ, Zuazu MA, Berguer R: Reflex sympathetic dystrophy of the face: current treatment recommendations, *Laryngoscope* 108:437-442, 1998.

10. Arlet J, Maziéres B: Medical treatment of reflex sympathetic dystrophy, *Hand Clin* 13(3):477-483, 1997.

11. Arnér S: Intravenous phentolamine tests: diagnostic and prognostic use in reflex sympathetic dystrophy, *Pain* 46:17-22, 1991.

12. Arriagada M, Arinoviche R: X-ray bone densitometry in the diagnosis and follow-up of reflex sympathetic dystrophy syndrome, *J Rheumatol* 21:498-500, 1994.

13. Atkins RM, Duckworth T, Kanis JA: Algodystrophy following Colles' fracture, *J Hand Surg [Br]* 14:161-164, 1989.

14. Atkins RM, Duckworth T, Kanis JA: Features of algodystrophy after Colles' fracture, *J Bone Joint Surg* 72:105-110, 1990.

15. Atkins RM, Tindale W, Bickerstaff D, Kanis JA: Quantitative bone scintigraphy in reflex sympathetic dystrophy, *Br J Rheumatol* 32:41-45, 1993.

16. Backonja M, Beydoun A, Edwards KR, et al: Gabapentin for the symptomatic treatment of painful neuropathy in patients with diabetes mellitus: a randomized, controlled trial, *JAMA* 280:1831-1836, 1998.

17. Barolat G, Schwartzmann R, Woo R: Epidural spinal cord stimulation in the management of reflex sympathetic dystrophy, *Appl Neurophysiol* 50:442-443, 1987.

18. Baron R, Blumberg H, Jänig W: Clinical characteristics of patients with complex regional pain syndrome in Germany, with special emphasis on vasomotor function. In Jänig W, Stanton-Hicks M (editors): *Reflex sympathetic dystrophy, a reappraisal: progress in pain research and management,* Seattle, 1996, IASP Press.

19. Barowsky EI, Zweig JB, Moskowitz J: Thermal biofeedback in the treatment of symptoms associated with reflex sympathetic dystrophy, *J Child Neurol* 2:229-232, 1987.

20. Basbaum AI, Fields HL: Endogenous pain control mechanisms: review and hypothesis, *Ann Neurol* 4:451, 1978.

21. Beecher HK: *Measurement of subjective responses,* New York, 1959, Oxford University Press.

22. Bennett GJ: Neuropathic pain. In Wahl PD, Melzack R (editors): *Textbook of pain,* Edinburgh, 1994, Churchill-Livingstone.

23. Benson H: *The mind-body effect,* New York, 1979, Simon & Schuster.

24. Benzon HT, Chomka CM, Brunner EA: Treatment of reflex sympathetic dystrophy with regional intravenous reserpine, *Anesth Analg* 59:500-502, 1980.

25. Berges PU: Myofascial pain syndrome, *Postgrad Med* 53:161, 1973.

26. Beric A: Neuropathic pain syndromes: central pain and dysesthesia syndrome, *Neurol Clin* 16(4):899-917, 1998.

27. Bernstein BH: Reflex neurovascular dystrophy in childhood, *J Pediatr* 93:211, 1978.

28. Berthelot JM, Glemareck J, Guillot P, et al: Algodystrophy (reflex sympathetic dystrophy syndrome) and causalgia: novel concepts regarding the nosology, pathophysiology, and pathogenesis of complex regional pain syndromes: is the sympathetic hyperactivity hypothesis wrong? *Revue du Rhumatisme* (English edition) 64(7-9), 481-491, 1997.

29. Betcher AM, Bean G, Casten DF: Continuous Procaine blocks of paravertebral sympathetic ganglions, *JAMA* 151:288-292, 1953.

30. Betcher AM, Casten D: Reflex sympathetic dystrophy: criteria for diagnosis and treatment, *Anesthesiology* 16:994, 1955.

31. Bickerstaff DR, Charlesworth D, Kanis JA: Changes in cortical and trabecular bone in algodystrophy, *Br J Rheum* 32:46-51, 1993.

32. Bickerstaff DR, Kanis JA: The use of nasal calcitonin in the treatment of posttraumatic algodystrophy, *Br J Rheum* 30:291, 1991.

33. Biggs JT, Miranda FJ: Dental causalgia: a chronic oral pain syndrome, *Quintessence Int* 14:595, 1983.

34. Bill A, Stjernschantz J, Mandahla, et al: Substance P: release on trigeminal stimulation: effects in the eye, *Acta Physiol Scand* 101:371, 1979.

35. Blacker HM: Volitional sympathetic control, *Anesth Analg* 59:785-788, 1980.

36. Blair SJ: Role of neuropeptides in pathogenesis of RSD. In Prog. and Abst. RSD. Brussels, p. 18, 1996.

37. Blanchard EB: The use of temperature biofeedback in the treatment of chronic pain due to causalgia, *Biofeedback Self Regul* 4:183-188, 1979.

38. Blanchard J, Ramamurthy S, Walsh N, et al: Intravenous regional sympatholysis: a double-blind comparison of guanethidine, reserpine, and normal saline, *J Pain Symptom Manage* 5:357-361, 1990.

39. Boas RA: Complex regional pain syndromes: symptoms, signs, differential diagnosis. In Jänig W, Stanton-Hicks M (editors): *Reflex sympathetic dystrophy: a reappraisal,* Seattle, 1996, IAST Press.

40. Bohr TW: Fibromyalgia syndrome and myofascial pain syndrome: do they exist? *Neurol Clin* 13(2):365-384, 1995.

41. Bonelli A, Conoscente F, Moveilia PG, et al: Regional intravenous guanethidine versus stellate block in reflex sympathetic dystrophies: a randomized trial, *Pain* 16:297-307, 1983.

42. Bonica JJ: *Pain,* Philadelphia, 1953, Lea & Febiger, p. 913.

43. Bonica JJ: Causalgia and other reflex sympathetic dystrophies, *Postgrad Med* 53:143, 1973.

44. Bonica JJ: Causalgia and other reflex sympathetic dystrophies, *Adv Pain Resther* 3:141-166, 1979.

45. Bonica JJ: The need of a taxonomy, *Pain* 6:247-252, 1979.

46. Bonica JJ, Butler SH: The management and function of pain centers. In Swerdlow M (editor): *Relief of intractable pain,* New York, 1978, Excerpta Medica Foundation.

47. Boome R: Presented at the IFSSH meeting. Vancouver, May 1998.

48. Branch C: *Aspects of anxiety,* Philadelphia, 1965, JB Lippincott.

49. Brand P, Yancey P: *Pain: the gift nobody wants,* New York, 1993, Harper Collins.

50. Bruehl S, Carlson CR: Predisposing psychological factors in the development of reflex sympathetic dystrophy: a review of the empirical evidence, *Clin J Pain* 8:287-299, 1992.

51. Bunnell S: Trophic and vascular conditions. In Boyes JH (editor): *Bunnell's surgery of the hand,* ed 5, Philadelphia, 1978, JB Lippincott.

52. Burch GE, Giles TD: Cardiac causalgia, *Arch Intern Med* 125:809, 1970.

53. Campbell JN, Raja SN, Seilig DK, et al: Diagnosis and management of sympathetically maintained pain, *Prog Pain Res Manage* 1:85-100, 1994.

54. Carron H, Weller R: Treatment of post-traumatic sympathetic dystrophy, *Adz Neurol* 4:485, 1974.

55. Carter HS: On causalgia and allied painful conditions due to lesions of peripheral nerves, *J Neurol Psychopath* 3:1, 1922.

56. Chambliss ML: Are serotonin uptake inhibitors useful in chronic pain syndrome such as fibromyalgia or diabetic polyneuropathy? *Arch Fam Med* 7(5):470-471, 1998.

57. Chan CS, Chow SP: Electroacupuncture in the treatment of posttraumatic sympathetic dystrophy (Sudeck's atrophy), *Br J Anesth* 53:899, 1981.

58. Chelimsky TC, Lowe PA, Naessens JM, et al: Value of autonomic testing in reflex sympathetic dystrophy, *Mayo Clin Proc* 70:1029-1040, 1995.

59. Christensen K, Jensen EM, Noer I: The reflex dystrophy syndrome: response to treatment with systemic corticosteroids, *Acta Chir Hand* 148:653, 1982.

60. Clark G: Causalgia: a discussion of the chronic pain syndromes in the upper limb. In Hunter JM (editor): *Rehabilitation of the hand,* St. Louis, 1978, Mosby.

61. Cooke ED, Ward C: Vicious circles in reflex sympathetic dystrophy: a hypothesis, discussion paper, *J R Soc Med* 83:96-99, 1990.

62. Cooney WP: Electrical stimulation and the treatment of complex regional pain syndromes of the upper extremity, *Hand Clin* 13(3):519-526, 1997.

63. Cronin KD, Kirsner RLG: Diagnosis of reflex sympathetic dysfunction: use of skin potential response, *Anesthesia* 37:848, 1982.

64. Cunha FQ, Poole S, Lorenzetti BB, Ferreira SH: The pivotal role of tumor necrosis factor α in the development of inflammatory hyperalgesia, *Br J Pharmacol* 107:660-664, 1992.

65. Curtiss PH, Kinald WP: Transitory demineralization of the hip in pregnancy: a report of three cases, *J Bone Joint Surg* 41A:1327-1332, 1959.

66. Davis S, Petrillo C, Eichberg R, Chu D: Shoulder-hand syndrome in hemiplegic population: 5-year retrospective study, *Arch Phys Med Rehabil* 58:353, 1977.

67. De Bastiani G, Nogarin L, Perusi M: Tratamento della syndromi algodistrofiche con la calcitonina, *Minerva Med* 69:1485-1495, 1978.

68. Denmark A: An example of symptoms resembling tic douloureux produced by a wound in the radial nerve, *Med-Chir Trans* 4:48, 1813.

69. Dequeker J, Gusen SP, Verstaeten A, et al: Vertebral crush fracture syndrome in reflex sympathetic dystrophy, *Bone* 7:89-94, 1986.

70. De Takats G: Sympathetic reflex dystrophy, *Med Clin North Am* 49:117, 1965.

71. Dickenson AH, Chapman V, Green GM: The pharmacology of excitatory and inhibitory amino acid-mediated events in the transmission and modulation of pain in the spinal cord, *Gen Pharmacol* 28:633-638, 1997.

72. Didierjean A: Psychological aspects of algodystrophy, *Hand Clin* 13(3):363-366, 1997.

73. Dotson RM: Causalgia–reflex sympathetic dystrophy– sympathetically maintained pain: myth and reality, *Muscle Nerve* 16:1049-55, 1993.

74. Doupe J, Cullen CH, Chance GQ: Posttraumatic pain and causalgia syndrome, *J Neurol Psych* 7:33, 1944.

75. Doury PC: Reflex sympathetic dystrophy (algodystrophy), *Int Med Special* 6:67, 1985.

76. Doury PC: L'algodystrophie du rachis, *Rev Rhum Ed Fr* 56:697-701, 1989.

77. Doury PC: L'algodystophie de la grossesse ou du post-partum, *Semaine Des Hôpitaux* 72:117-124, 1996.

78. Doury PC: Algodystrophy: a spectrum of disease, historical perspectives, criteria of diagnosis, and principles of treatment, *Hand Clin* 13(3):327-337, 1997.

79. Doury PC, Dirheimer Y, Pattin S: *Algodystrophy: diagnosis and therapy of a frequent disease of the locomotor apparatus,* New York, 1981, Springer Verlag.

80. Doury P, Pattin S, Delahaye RP, et al: La calitonine dans l'algodystrophie sympathique réflexe, *Nouv Presse Med* 7: 3156, 1975.

81. Dray A, Urban L: New pharmacological strategies for pain relief, *Annu Rev Pharmacol Toxicol* 36:253-280, 1996.

82. Driessens E: Infrequent presentations of reflex sympathetic dystrophy and pseudodystrophy, *Hand Clin* 13(3):413-422, 1997.

83. Drissen B, Ryman W: Interaction of the central analgesic, tramadol, with the uptake and release of 5-hydroxytryptamine in the rat brain in vitro, *Br J Pharmacol* 105:147-151, 1992.

84. Drucker W, Hubay C, Holden W, Bukovnic J: Pathogenesis of post-traumatic sympathetic dystrophy, *Am J Surg* 97:454, 1959.

85. Duncan KH, Lewis RC, Racz G, Nordyke MD: Treatment of upper extremity reflex sympathetic dystrophy with joint stiffness using sympatheticolytic Bier blocks and manipulation, *Orthopedics* 11:883-886, 1988.

86. Durrani Z, Winnie AP: Diagnostic and therapeutic brachial plexus blocks for RSD, unresponsive to stellate ganglion block, *Anesth Analg* 74(suppl):77, 1992.

87. Dyck PJ, Litchy WJ, Lehman KA, et al: Variables influencing neuropathic endpoints: the Rochester diabetic neuropathic study of healthy subjects, *Neurology* 45:1115-1121, 1995.

88. Echlin F, Owens FM Jr, Wells WL: Observations on major and minor causalgia, *Arch Neurol Psychol* 62:183, 1949.

89. Ecker A: Reflex sympathetic dystrophy: thermography in diagnosis: psychiatric considerations, *Psych Ann* 14:787, 1984.

90. Edeiken J: Shoulder-hand syndrome following myocardial infarction, with special reference to prognosis, *Circulation* 41:14, 1957.

91. Eisinger J, Acquaviva P, d'Omevony, et al: Traitement des algodystrophies par la calcitonie: resultats préliminaires, *Marseille Médical* 110:373-376, 1973.

92. Enelow A: *Depression in medical practice,* West Point, Penn, 1970, Merrick, Sharp, and Dohme.

93. Evans J: Sympathetic dystrophy: report of 57 cases, *Ann Intern Med* 26:417, 1947.

94. Fagrell B, Froneck A, Intaglietta M: A microscope television system for dynamic studies of blood flow velocity in human skin capillaries, *Am J Physiology* 233(2):H318-321, 1977.

95. Farcot JM, Gautherie M, Foucher G: Regional intravenous sympathetic nerve blocks, *Hand Clin* 13(3):499-517, 1997.

96. Farcot JM, Grasser C, Foucher G, et al: Tratements locaux intravenieux des algodystrophies de la main: buflomedil versus guanéthidine, suivi á long terme, *Ann Chir Main Memb Super* 9:296-304, 1990.

97. Fermaglich D: Reflex sympathetic dystrophy in children, *Pediatrics* 60:6, 881, 1977.

98. Field J, Monk C, Atkins RM: Objective improvements in algodystrophy following regional intravenous guanethidine, *J Hand Surg Br* 18:339, 1993.

99. Fields HL, Levine JD: Placebo analgesia: a role for endorphins? *Trends Neurosci* I:271, 1984.

100. Ford SR, Forest WH Jr, Eltherington L: The treatment of reflex sympathetic dystrophy with intravenous regional bretylium, *Anesthesiology* 68:137-140, 1988.

101. Foreman JC, Jordan CC, Piotrowski W: Inner action of neurotensin with the substance P receptor mediating histamine release from rat mast cells and the flare in human skin, *Br J Pharmacol* 77:531, 1982.

102. Frederickson RCA, Geary LE: Endogenous opioid peptides; review of physiological, pharmacological, and clinical aspects, *Prog Neurobiol* 19:19, 1982.

103. Friedlander L, Lumley M, Farchione T, Doyal G: Testing the alexithymia hypothesis: physiological and subjective responses during relaxation and stress, *J Nerv Ment Dis* 185(4):233-239, 1997.

104. Frishman WH, Sonnenblick EH: Calcium channel blockers. In Hearst JW (editor): *The heart,* New York, 1990, McGraw-Hill.

105. Frost FA, Jessen B, Siggard-Anderson J: A controlled, double blind comparison of mepivacaine injection versus saline injection for myofascial pain, *Lancet* 1:499, 1980.

106. Fukunishi I, Kaji N, Hosaka T, et al: Relationship of alexithymia and poor social support to ulcerative change on gastrofiberscopy, *Psychosomatics* 38:20-26, 1997.

107. Gainer MJ: Hypnotherapy for reflex sympathetic dystrophy, *Am J Clin Hypn* 34:227-232, 1992.

108. Genant HK, Kozin F, Bekerman C, et al: The reflex sympathetic dystrophy syndrome, *Radiology* 117:21-32, 1975.

109. Gertzen JH: Reflex sympathetic dystrophy: outcome and measurement, *Acta Orthop Scand* (suppl 279)69:1-3, 1998.

110. Gertzen JH, de Bruijn HP, de Bruijn Kofman AT, et al: Reflex sympathetic dystrophy: early treatment and psychological aspects, *Arch Phys Med Rehabil* 75:442-446, 1994.

111. Ghostine SWY, Comair YG, Turner DM, et al: Phenoxybenzamine in the treatment of causalgia, *J Neurosurg* 60:263, 1984.

112. Glick EN, Helal B: Posttraumatic neurodystrophy: treatment by corticosteroids, *Hand* 8:45, 1976.

113. Glynn CJ, Basedow RW, Walsh JA: Pain relief following post-ganglionic sympathetic blockade with IV guanethidine, *Br J Anaesth* 53:297, 1981.

114. Goodman AG, Goodman LS, Gilman A: *The pharmacological basis of therapeutics,* ed 6, New York, 1980, Macmillan Publishing Co.

115. Goodman CR: Treatment of shoulder-hand syndrome: combined with ultrasonic applications of stellate ganglion and physical medicine, *NY State J Med* 71:559, 1971.

116. Goris RJ: Reflex sympathetic dystrophy: model of a severe regional inflammatory response syndrome, *World J Surg* 22(2):197-202, 1998.

117. Goris RJ, Dongen LM, Winters HA: Are toxic oxygen radicals involved in the pathogenesis of reflex sympathetic dystrophy? *Free Radic Res Commun* 3:13-18, 1987.

118. Gorsky BH: Intravenous perfusion with reserpine for Raynaud's phenomenon, *Reg Anaesth* 2:5, 1977.

119. Gould JS: Treatment of the painful injured nerve in continuity. In Gelberman RH (editor): *Operative nerve repair in reconstruction,* Philadelphia, 1991, JB Lippincott.

120. Gracely RH, Dubner R, Wolskee PJ, Deeter WR: Placebo and naloxone can alter post-surgical pain by separate mechanisms, *Nature* 306:264, 1983.

121. Gracely RH, Lynch SA, Bennett GJ: Painful neuropathy: altered central processing maintained dynamically by peripheral input, *Pain* 51:175-194, 1992.

122. Greenberg RP, Price DD, Becker DP: Complications of persistent postoperative pain. InGreenfield LJ (editor): *Complications in surgery and trauma,* Philadelphia, 1983, JB Lippincott.

123. Greipp ME: Reflex sympathetic dystrophy syndrome: a retrospective pain study, *J Adv Surg* 15:1452, 1990.

124. Greipp ME, Thomas AF: New thoughts on reflex sympathetic dystrophy syndrome, *J Neurosci Nurs* 22:313-316, 1990.

125. Grunert BK, Divine CA, Sanger JR, et al: Thermal self-regulation for pain control and reflex sympathetic dystrophy syndrome, *J Hand Surg [Am]* 15:615-618, 1990.

126. Hannington-Kiff JG: Intravenous regional sympathetic block with guanethidine, *Lancet* 1:1019-1020, 1974.

127. Hannington-Kiff JG: Pharmacologic target blocks in hand surgery and rehabilitation, *J Hand Surg [Br]* 9:29-36, 1984.

128. Hanowell LH, Kanefield JK, Soriano SG III: A recommendation for reduced lidocaine dosage during intravenous regional bretylium treatment of reflex sympathetic dystrophy (letter), *Anesthesiology* 71:811-812, 1989.

129. Hans G, Darvar G: Recent advances in the pharmacology of nerve-injury pain, *Neurol Clin* 16(4):951-965, 1998.

130. Hardman JG, Limbird LE, Molinoff TB, Ruddon RW, Gilman AG (editors): *Goodman and Gilman's, the pharmacological basis of therapeutics,* ed 9, New York, 1996, McGraw-Hill.

131. Hardy MA, Merritt WH: *A model to study sympathetic dystrophy: psychological testing and biofeedback results,* presented at the Plastic Surgery Research Council annual meeting, Hershey, Penn, 1982.

132. Hardy MA, Merritt WH: Psychological evaluation and pain assessment in patients with RSD, *J Hand Ther* 1:155-164, 1988.

133. Hardy MA, Moran CA, Merritt WH: Desensitization of the traumatized hand, *VA Med J* 109:134, 1982.

134. Hartley J: Reflex hyperemic deossification (Sudeck's atrophy), *J Mount Sinai Hosp* 22:268, 1955.

135. Hartung HP, Toyka KV: Activation of macrophages by substance P: induction of oxidative burst and thromboxane release, *J Pharmacol* 89:301, 1983.

136. Hendler N, Uematsu S, Long D: Thermographic validation of physical complaints in "psychogenic pain" patients, *Psychosomatics* 23:283, 1982.

137. Hobelmann CF Jr, Dellon AL: Use of prolonged sympathetic blockade as an adjunct to surgery in the patient with sympathetically maintained pain, *Microsurgery* 10:151-153, 1989.

138. Holden WD: Sympathetic dystrophy. *Arch Surg* 57:373, 1948.

139. Hooshmand H: *Chronic pain: reflex sympathetic dystrophy: prevention and management,* Boca Raton, Fla, 1993, CRC Press.

140. Hord AH, Rooks MD, Stephens BO, et al: Intravenous regional bretylium and lidocaine for treatment of reflex sympathetic dystrophy: a randomized, double-blind study, *Anesth Analg* 74:818-821, 1992.

141. Hori T, Oka T, Hosoi M, Aou S: Pain modulatory actions of cytokines and prostaglandin E2 in the brain, *Ann NY Acad Sci* 840:269-81, 1998.

142. Horowitz SH: Brachial plexus injuries with causalgia resulting in trans-axillary rib resection, *Arch Surg* 120:1189, 1985.

143. Hosobuchi Y: Subcortical electrical stimulation for control of intractable pain in humans: report of 122 cases (1970-1984), *J Neurosurg* 64:543-553, 1986.

144. Houston B: Control over stress: locus of control and response to stress, *J Pers Social Psych* 21:249, 1972.

145. Hughes J, Smith TW, Kosterliz HW, et al: Identification of two related pentapeptides from the brain with potent opiate agonist activity, *Nature* 258:577, 1975.

146. Irwin HJ, Melbin-Helberg EB: Alexithymia and dissociative tendencies, *J Clin Psych* 53(2):159-166, 1997.

147. Jadad AR, Carroll D, Glynn C, et al: Intravenous regional sympathetic blockade for pain-relief in reflex sympathetic dystrophy: a systemic review and a randomized double-blind crossover study, *J Pain Symptom Manage* 10:13, 1995.

148. Jaeger B, Singer E, Kroening R: Reflex sympathetic dystrophy of the face: a report of two cases and review of the literature, *Arch Neurol* 43:693, 1986.

149. Jänig W: Experimental approach to reflex sympathetic dystrophy and related syndromes (editorial), *Pain* 46:241-245, 1991.

150. Jänig W: The puzzle of "reflex sympathetic dystrophy:" mechanisms, hypothetics, open questions. In Jänig W, Stanton-Hicks M (editors): *Reflex sympathetic dystrophy: a reappraisal: progress in pain research and management,* Seattle, 1996, IASP Press.

151. Jansco N, Jansco-Gabor A, Szolesanyi J: Direct evidence for direct neurogenic inflammation and its prevention by denervation and by pretreatment with capsaicin, *Br J Pharmacol* 31:138, 1967.

152. Jebara VA, Saade B: Causalgia: a wartime experience: report of 20 treated cases, *J Trauma* 27:519, 1987.

153. Jensen NH: Accurate diagnosis and drug selection in chronic pain patients, *Postgrad Med J* 67(suppl):2-8, 1991.

154. Johnson EW, Pannozzo AN: Management of shoulder/hand syndrome, *JAMA* 195:108, 1966.

155. Jupiter JB, Seiler JG, Zienowicz R: Sympathetic maintained pain (causalgia) associated with demonstrable peripheral nerve lesions, *J Bone Joint Surg* 76A:1376-1384, 1994.

156. Karklin J, Chenoweth A, Murphy F: Causalgia: A review of its characteristics, diagnosis and treatment, *Surgery* 21:321, 1947.

157. Kasdan ML, Johnson AL: Reflex sympathetic dystrophy, *Occup Med* 13(3):521-531, 1998.

158. Keinböck R: Uber akute Knockenatrophie bei Entzundung-processen an den Extremataten (falchlich sagenannate inactivi-tats atrophie der Knochen) und ihre Diagnose nach dem Rouetegen-Bilds, *Wien Med Wochenschr* 5:1345, 1901.

159. Kellgren JH: Observations on referred pain arising from muscle, *Clin Sci* 3:175, 1938.

160. Kelly M: The nature of fibrositis. I. The myalgic lesion and its secondary effects: a reflex theory, *Ann Rheum Dis* 5:1, 1945.

161. Kelly M: The relief of facial pain by procaine injections, *J Am Geriatr Soc* 11:586, 1963.

162. Kesler RM, Saulsbury FT, Miller LT, et al: Reflex sympathetic dystrophy in children: treatment with transcutaneous nerve stimulation, *Pediatrics* 82:728-732, 1988.

163. Khoury R, Kennedy SF, MacNamara TE: Facial causalgia: report of case, *J Oral Surg* 38:782, 1980.

164. Kinman E, Levine JD: Involvement of the sympathetic postganglionic neurons in capsaicin-induced secondary hyper-algesia in the rat, *Neuropsy* 65:283-291, 1995.

165. Kleinert H, Cole N, Wayne L, et al: Post-traumatic sympa-thetic dystrophy, *Orthop Clin North Am* 4:917, 1973.

166. Kline SC, Holder LE: Segmental reflex sympathetic dystrophy: clinical and scintigraphic criteria, *J Hand Surg [Am]* 18:853-859, 1993.

167. Koman LA, Poehling GG, Smith TL: Complex regional pain syndrome: reflex sympathetic dystrophy and causalgia. In Green DP, Hotchkiss RN, Pederson WC (editors): *Green's operative hand surgery*, ed 4, New York, Churchill-Livingstone.

168. Kooiman CG, Spinhoven P, Trijsburg RW, Rooijmans HG: Perceived parental attitude: alexithymia and defense style in psychiatric outpatients, *Psychother Psychosom* 67(2):81-87, 1998.

169. Kozin F: Reflex sympathetic dystrophy syndrome, *Bull Rheum Dis* 36:1, 1986.

170. Kozin F, Genant H, Bekerman C, McCarty D: The reflex sympathetic dystrophy syndrome. II. Roentgenographic and scintigraphic bilaterality and of periarticular accentuation, *Am J Med* 60:332, 1976.

171. Kozin F, McCarty DJ, Sims J, Fenant H: The reflex sympathetic dystrophy syndrome. I. Clinical and histological studies: evidence for bilaterality, response to corticosteroids and articular involvement, *Am J Med* 60:321, 1976.

172. Kumar K, Nath R, Wyant GM: Treatment of chronic pain by epidural spinal cord stimulation: a ten-year experience, *J Neurosurg* 75:402-407, 1991.

173. Lankford LL: Reflex sympathetic dystrophy. In Green DP (editor): *Operative hand surgery*, vol I, New York, 1982, Churchill-Livingstone.

174. Lankford LL: Reflex sympathetic dystrophy. In Green DP (editor): *Operative hand surgery*, vol III, New York, 1993, Churchill-Livingstone.

175. Laroche M, Redon-Dumolard A, Mazieres D: An x-ray absorptiometry study of reflex sympathetic dystrophy, *Rev RhumEngl Ed* 64(2):106-111, 1997.

176. Lauterbach E: Fluoxetine withdrawal and thalamic pain, *Neurology* 44:983, 1994.

177. Law JD: Spinal cord stimulation for intractable pain due to reflex sympathetic dystrophy, *CNI Rev* 17-22, 1993.

178. Lee KH: Transcutaneous nerve stimulators inhibit spinotha-lamic tract cells, *Adv Pain Res Ther* 9:203, 1985.

179. Lee MHM, Ernst M: The sympatholytic effect of acupuncture as evidenced by thermography: a preliminary report, *Orthop Rev* 12:67-72, 1983.

180. Leeman SE, Gamse R, Lackner D, Gamse G: Effect of capsaicin pretreatment on capsule evoked release of immuno-reactive somatostatin and substance P from primary sensory neurons, *Naunyn Shmiedebergs Arch Pharmacol* 316:38, 1981.

181. Lehman EPJ: Traumatic vasospasm: a study of four cases of vasospasm in the upper extremity, *Arch Surg* 29:92, 1934.

182. Lembeck F, Gamse R, Juan H: Substance P and sensory nerve endings. In Von Euler US, Pernow B (editors): *Substance P, presented at the 37th Noble Symposium, Stockholm, 1976,* New York, 1977, Raven Press.

183. Leo KC: Use of electrical stimulation and acupuncture points for treatment of reflex sympathetic dystrophy in a child: a case report, *Phys Ther* 63:957-959, 1983.

184. Leriche R: De la causalgie envisagé comme une nérvite du sympathique et son traitement par la dénudation et l'excision des plexus nerveux péri-artériels, *Pres Med* 24:178, 1916.

185. Lesser IM: A review of the alexithymia concept, *Psychosom Med* 43:531-543, 1981.

186. Levine JD, Goetzl, Basbaum AI: Contrast of the nervous system to pathophysiology of rheumatoid and other poly-arthritides, *Rheum Dis Clin North Am* 13:369, 1987.

187. Lewis R: *Pain,* New York, 1942, McMillan, p 124.

188. Lewis T: The blood vessels of the human skin and their responses, London, 1927, Shaw.

189. Lichtman DM, Florio RL, Mack GE: Carpal tunnel release under local anesthesia: evaluation of the outpatient procedure, *J Hand Surg* 4:544, 1979.

190. Lidz T, Payne RL: Causalgia: report of recovery following relief of emotional stress, *Arch Neurol Psych* 53:222, 1945.

191. Linson MA, Leffert R, Todd DP: The treatment of upper extremity reflex sympathetic dystrophy with prolonged contin-uous stellate ganglion blockade, *J Hand Surg* 8:153, 1983.

192. Livingston WK: *Pain mechanisms,* New York, 1943, Mac-millan.

193. Lorente de No R: Analysis of the activity of the chains of the internuncial neurons, *J Neurophysiol* 1:207, 1938.

194. Lowe PA, Caskey PE, Tuck RR, et al: Quantitative sudomotor axon reflex test in normal and neuropathic subjects, *Ann Neurol* 14:573-580, 1983.

195. Lowe PA, Opfer-Gehrking TL, Dyck PJ, et al: Double-blind, placebo-controlled study of the application of capsaicin cream in chronic distal painful polyneuropathy, *Pain* 62:163-168, 1995.

196. Lynch ME: Psychological aspects of reflex sympathetic dystrophy: a review of adult and pediatric literature, *Pain* 49:337-347, 1992.

197. Macdonald RI, Lichtman DM, Hanlon JJ, Wilson JN: Complications of surgical release for carpal tunnel syndrome, *J Hand Surg* 3:70, 1978.

198. Mackin GA: Medical and pharmacologic management of upper extremity neuropathic pain syndromes, *J Hand Ther* 10:96-109, 1997.

199. Mackinnon SE, Holder LE: The use of three-phase radionuclide bone scanning in the diagnosis of reflex sympathetic dystrophy, *J Hand Surg* 9:556, 1984.

200. Mackinnon SE, Holder LE: Reflex sympathetic dystrophy in the hands: clinical and scintigraphic criteria, *Radiology* 152:517, 1984.

201. Mailis A, Meindok H, Papagapiou M, et al: Alterations of the three-phase bone scan after sympathectomy, *Clin J Pain* 10:146, 1994.

202. Mailis A, Wade J: Profile of women with possible genetic predisposition to reflex sympathetic dystrophy: a pilot study, *Clin J Pain* 10:210, 1994.

203. Manart FD, Sadler Jr TR, Schmitt EA, Ranier WG: Upper dorsal sympathectomy, *Am J Surg* 150:762, 1985.

204. Mankeltow RT, McKee NH: Free muscle transplantation to provide active finger flexion, *J Hand Surg* 3:416, 1976.

205. Markoff M, Farole A: Reflex sympathetic dystrophy syndrome: case report with review of the literature, *Oral Surg* 661:23, 1986.

206. Massler M: Dental causalgia, *Quintessence Int* 12:341, 1981.

207. Masson C, Audran M, Pascaretti C, et al: Further vascular, bone, and autonomic investigations in algodystrophy, *Acta Orthop Belg* 64(1):77-87, 1998.

208. Max MB, Lynch S, Muir J, et al: Effects of desipramine, amitriptyline, and fluoxetine on pain in diabetic neuropathy, *Engl J Med* 326:1250-1256, 1992.

209. Mayer DJ, Liebeskind JC: Pain reduction by focal electrical stimulation of the brain: an anatomical and behavioral analysis, *Brain Res* 68:73, 1974.

210. Mayer DJ, Price DD, Rafii A: Antagonism of acupuncture analgesia in man by the narcotic antagonist naloxone, *Brain Res* 121:36, 1977.

211. Mayfield FH, Divine JW: Causalgia, *Surg Gynecol Obstet* 80:631, 1945.

212. McCarty DJ: *Arthritis and allied conditions*, ed 9, Philadelphia, 1979, Lea & Febiger, p 1111.

213. McLelland J, Ellis SJ: Causalgia as a complication of meningococcal meningitis, *Br Med J* 292:1710, 1986.

214. Medsgar TA Jr, Dixon JA, Garwood VF: Palmar fasciitis and polyarthritis associated with ovarian carcinoma, *Ann Intern Med* 96:424, 1982.

215. Mellick GA, Mellicy LB, Mellick GB: Gabapentin and the management of reflex sympathetic dystrophy, *J Pain Symptom Manage* 10:265-266, 1995.

216. Melzak R, Wald PD: Pain mechanisms: a new theory, *Science* 150:971, 1965.

217. Merrill RL: Orofacial pain mechanisms and their clinical application, *Dental Clin North Am* 41(2):167-187, 1997.

218. Merritt WH: Complications of hand surgery and trauma. In Greenfield LJ (editor): *Complications in surgery and trauma*, Philadelphia, 1984, JB Lippincott.

219. Merritt WH: Reflex sympathetic dystrophy. In McCarthy JG (editor): *Plastic surgery*, vol 7, Philadelphia, 1990, WB Saunders.

220. Merritt WH: Comprehensive management of Raynaud's syndrome, *Clin Plast Surg* 24(1):133-159, 1997.

221. Meyer GA, Fields HL: Causalgia treated by selective large fiber stimulation of peripheral nerve, *Brain* 95:163, 1972.

222. Michaels RM, Sorber JA: Reflex sympathetic dystrophy as a probable paraneoplastic syndrome: case report and literature review, *Arthritis Rheum* 27:1183, 1984.

223. Miller DS, DeTakats G: Post-traumatic dystrophy of the extremities: Sudeck's extremity, *Surg Gynecol Obstet* 125:558, 1941.

224. Miller NE: Learning of visceral and glandular responses, *Science* 163:434-445, 1969.

225. Mindham RHS: Tricyclic antidepressants and amine precursors. In Paykel ES (editor): *Handbook of affective disorders*, New York, 1982, Oxford University Press.

226. Mitchell JK: Remote consequences of injuries of nerves and their treatment, Philadelphia, 1895, Lea.

227. Mitchell SW: Causalgia. In *Injuries of nerves and their consequences*, Philadelphia, 1872, Lea Brothers & Company.

228. Mitchell SW, Moorehouse GR, Keen WW: *Gunshot wounds and other injuries of nerves*, Philadelphia, 1864, JB Lippincott.

229. Modell W, Trevell J: The treatment of painful disorders of skeletal muscle, *NY State J Med* 48:2050, 1948.

230. Morettin LB, Wilson M: Severe reflex algodystrophy (Sudeck's atrophy) as a complication of myelography: report of two cases, *Am J Roentgenol* 110:156, 1970.

231. Moriau M, Lavenne-Pardonge E, Crasborn L, et al: Treatment of Raynaud's phenomenon with piracetam, *Drug Res* 43:526-535, 1993.

232. Moriwaki K, Yuge O, Tanaka H, et al: Neuropathic pain and prolonged regional inflammation as two distinct symptomological components in complex regional pain syndrome, with patchy osteoporosis: a pilot study, *Pain* 72:277-282, 1997.

233. Munzenberg KL: Therapie des Sudeck syndrom mit calcitonin, *Dtsch Med Wochenschr* 103:26-29, 1978.

234. Nashold BS, Friedman H: Dorsal column stimulation for control of pain, *J Neurosurg* 36:590-597, 1972.

235. Nath RK, Mackinnon SE, Stelnicki E: Reflex sympathetic dystrophy: the controversy continues, *Clin Plast Surg* 23(3):435-446, 1996.

236. Nathan PW: Involvement of the sympathetic nervous system in pain. In Kosterlitz HW, Terenius LY (editors): *Pain and society*, Dahlam konferenzen weinheim, verkag, chemie Gmbh, 1980.

237. Nathan PW: Pain and the sympathetic system, *J Auton Nerve Syst* 7:363-370, 1983.

238. Nemiah JC, Sifneos PE: Affect and fantasy in patients with psychosomatic disorders, *Psychosom Med* 2:26-34, 1970.

239. Neumann M: Nonsurgical management of pain secondary to peripheral nerve injuries, *Orthop Clin North Am* 19:165, 1988.

240. Neurontin prescribing information. In *Physician's Desk Reference*, Montvale, NJ, 1995, Medical Economics Co.

241. Nilsson J, von Euler AM, Dalsgaard CJ: Stimulation of connective tissue cell growth by substance P and substance K, *Nature* 315:61, 1985.

242. Norvasc: In *Physician's Desk Reference,* Montvale, NJ, 1996, Medical Economics Data.

243. Nuti R, Vattimo A, Martini G, et al: Carbocalcitonin treatment in Sudeck's atrophy, *Clin Orthop Rel Res* 215:217-222, 1987.

244. Ochoa JL: Reflex sympathetic dystrophy: a tragic error in medical science, *Hippocrates Lantern* 3:1-6, 1995.

245. Ochoa JL: Reflex? Sympathetic? Dystrophy? Triple questioned again, *Mayo Clin Proc* 70:1124-1126, 1995.

246. Ochoa JL, Verdugo RJ: Reflex sympathetic dystrophy: a common clinical avenue for somatoform expression, *Neurol Clin* 13:351-363, 1995.

247. Omer G: Management of pain syndromes in the upper extremity. In Hunter JM (editor): *Rehabilitation of the hand,* St. Louis, 1978, Mosby.

248. Ostergren IR, Fagrell B, Stranden E: Skin microvascular circulation in the sympathetic dystrophies evaluated by video photometric capillaroscopy and laser Doppler fluxmetry, *Eur J Clin Invest* 18:305-308, 1988.

249. Owens JC: Causalgia, *Am Surg* 23:636, 1957.

250. Pak J, Martin GM, Magness JL, Kavanaugh GJ: Reflex sympathetic dystrophy: review of 140 cases, *Minn Med* 53:507, 1970.

251. Panerai AE, Martini A, Abbate D, et al: ß-endorphin, met-enkephalin and ß-lipotropin in chronic pain in electro-acupuncture, *Adv Pain Res Ther* 5:543-547, 1983.

252. Pappagallo M, Campbell JN: The pharmacologic management of chronic back pain. In Frymoyer JW (editor): *The adult spine: principles and practice,* ed 2, Philadelphia, 1997, Lippincott-Raven.

253. Paré A: *Les Oeuvres d'Ambroise Paré,* Paris, 1968, Gabrien Buon, p 401.

254. Parrillo SJ: Reflex sympathetic dystrophy in children, *Ped Emerg Care* 14(3):217-220, 1998.

255. Payan D, Goetzl E: Modulation of lymphocyte function by sensory neuropeptides, *J Immunol* 135:783(suppl), 1985.

256. Peacock EE Jr: *Wound repair,* ed 3, Philadelphia, 1984, WB Saunders.

257. Peets JM, Pomeranz B: Acupuncture-like transcutaneous electrical nerve stimulation analgesia is influenced by spinal cord endorphins, but no serotonin: an intrathecal pharmacological study, *Adv Pain Res Ther* 9:519, 1985.

258. Plewes LW: Sudeck's atrophy in the hand, *J Bone Joint Surg* 38:195, 1956.

259. Polisson R: NSAIDs: practical and therapeutic considerations in their selections. *Am J Med* 100:315-365, 1996.

260. Pollock LJ, Davis L: *Peripheral nerve injuries,* New York, 1933, Paul B. Hobber.

261. Poplawski ZJ, Wylie AM, Murray JS: Posttraumatic dystrophy of the extremities: a clinical review and trial of treatment, *J Bone Joint Surg* 65A:642-655, 1983.

262. Portenoy RK: Neuropathic pain. In Portenoy RK, Kanner RN (editors): *Pain management: theory and practice,* Philadelphia, 1996, Davis.

263. Portwood MM, Lieberman JS, Taylor RG: Ultrasound treatment of reflex sympathetic dystrophy, *Arch Phys Med Rehab* 68:116, 1987.

264. Procacci P, Francini F, Zoppi M, et al: Cutaneous pain threshold changes after sympathetic block in reflex dystrophies, *Pain* 1:167, 1975.

265. Prough DS, McLeskey CH, Poehling GG, et al: Efficacy of oral nifedipine in treatment of reflex sympathetic dystrophy, *Anesthesiol* 62:796-799, 1985.

266. Prudden B: *Pain erasure: the Bonnie Prudden way,* New York, 1980, M. Evans & Co.

267. Pulvertaft RG: Psychological aspects of hand injuries, *Hand* 7:93, 1975.

268. Raffa RV, Fridericks E, Reimann W, et al: Complimentary and synergistic antinociceptive interaction between enantiomers of tramadol, *J Pharmacol Ther* 267:331-340, 1993.

269. Rauck RL, Rouff GE, McMillan JI: Comparison of tramadol and acetaminophen with codeine for long-term pain management in elderly patients, *Curr Ther Res* 55:1417-1431, 1994.

270. Revill SI, Robinson JO, Rosen M, Hogge M: The reliability of a linear analog scale for evaluating pain, *Anesthesia* 31:1191, 1976.

271. Reynolds DV: Surgery in the rat during electrical analgesia induced by focal brain stimulation, *Science* 164:444, 1969.

272. Richlin DM, Carron H, Rowlingson JC, et al: Reflex sympathetic dystrophy: successful treatment by transcutaneous nerve stimulation, *J Pediatr* 93:84, 1978.

273. Robaina FJ, Dominquez M, Diaz M, et al: Spinal cord stimulation for relief of chronic pain and vasospastic disorders of the upper limbs, *Neurosurg* 24:63-67, 1989.

274. Roberts WJ: An hypothesis on the physiological basis for causalgia and unrelated pain, *Pain* 24:297-311, 1986.

275. Roth M, Mountjoy CQ: The distinction between anxiety states and depressive disorders. In Paykel ES (editor): *Handbook of affective disorders,* New York, 1982, Oxford University Press.

276. Rothschild B: Reflex sympathetic dystrophy, *Arthr Care Res* 3:144-153, 1990.

277. Rowlingson JC: The sympathetic dystrophies, *Int Anesthesiol Clin* 21:117, 1983.

278. Ruff MR, Wahl SM, Pert CB: Substance P receptor-mediated chemotaxis of human monocytes, *Peptides* 6(suppl):107, 1985.

279. Ruggeri SB, Athreya BH, Doughty R: Reflex sympathetic dystrophy in children, *Clin Orthop* 163:225-230, 1982.

280. Schott GD: Mechanisms of causalgia and related clinical conditions: the role of the central and the sympathetic nervous system, *Brain* 109:771, 1986.

281. Schott GD: Visceral afferents: their contribution to "sympathetic dependent" pain, *Brain* 117:397-413, 1994.

282. Schott GD: An unsympathetic view of pain, *Lancet* 345:634-636, 1995.

283. Schuind F, Burny F: Can algodystrophy be prevented after hand surgery? *Hand Clin* 13(3):455-476, 1997.

284. Schwartzman RJ, McLellan TL: Reflex sympathetic dystrophy: a review, *Arch Neurol* 44:555-561, 1987.

285. Secretan H: Oedeme dur et hyperplasie tramatique du metacarpe dorsal, *Rev Med Suisse Romande* 21:409, 1901.

286. Sharony R, Saute M, Uretzky G: Video assisted thoracic surgery: our experience with 102 patients, *J Cardiovasc Surg* 35:173-176, 1994.

287. Shaturvedi S: Phenytoin and reflex sympathetic dystrophy, *Pain* 36: 379-380, 1989.

288. Sherry DD, Weisman R: Psychologic aspects of childhood reflex sympathetic dystrophy, *Pediatrics* 81:572-578, 1988.

289. Shumaker Jr HB: Causalgia: a general discussion, *Surgery* 28:485, 1948.

290. Shumaker Jr HB: A personal overview of causalgia and other reflex dystrophies, *Ann Surg* 201:278, 1985.

291. Shumaker Jr HB, Seigel IJ, Upjohn RH: Causalgia. II. The signs and symptoms with particular reference to vasomotor disturbance, *Surg Gynecol Obstet* 86:452, 1948.

292. Sifneos PE: The prevalence of "alexithymic" characteristics in psychosomatic patients, *Psychother Psychosom* 22:255-262, 1973.

293. Silverman S: *Psychological aspects of physical symptoms,* East Norwalk, Conn, 1968, Appleton-Century-Crofts.

294. Simmons B, Vasile R: The clenched fist syndrome, *J Hand Surg* 5: 420, 1980.

295. Simpson G: Propranolol for causalgia and Sudeck's atrophy, *JAMA* 227:327, 1974.

296. Sindrup SH, Gram LF, Brosen K, et al: The selective serotonin reuptake inhibitor paroxetine is effective in treatment of diabetic neuropathy syndromes, *Pain* 42:135-144, 1990.

297. Soucacos PN, Diznitsas L, Beris A, et al: Reflex sympathetic dystrophy upper extremity: clinical features in response to multimodal management, *Hand Clin* 13(3):339-354, 1997.

298. Spebar MJ, Rosenthal D, Collins GJ Jr, et al: Changing trends in causalgia, *M J Surg* 142:744, 1981.

299. Spurling RG: Causalgia of the upper extremity, treatment by dorsal sympathetic ganglionectomy, *Arch Neurol Psychol* 23:784, 1930.

300. Stanisz AM, Defus D, Bienenstock J: Differential effects of vasoactive intestinal peptides, substance P, and somatostatin on immunoglobulin synthesis and proliferation of lymphocytes from Peyer's patches, mesenteric lymph nodes, and spleen, *J Immunol* 136:152, 1986.

301. Stanton-Hicks M, Jänig W, Hassenbusch S, et al: Reflex sympathetic dystrophy: changing concepts in taxonomy, *Pain* 63:127-133, 1995.

302. Steinbrocker O: Shoulder-hand syndrome: present perspective, *Arch Phys Med Rehabil* 49:388, 1968.

303. Sternbach RA: Recent advances in psychologic pain therapy, *Adv Pain Res Ther* 7:251, 1984.

304. Stilz RJ, Carron H, Saunders DB: Case history #96: reflex sympathetic dystrophy in a 6-year-old: successful treatment by transcutaneous nerve stimulation, *Anesth Analg* 56:438, 1977.

305. Stjarne L, Brundin J: Beta-2 adrenoceptors facilitating noradrenaline secretion from human vasoconstrictor nerve, *Acta Physiol Scand* 97:88, 1978.

306. Subbarao J, Stillwell GK: Reflex sympathetic dystrophy syndrome of the upper extremity: analysis of total outcome management of 125 cases, *Arch Phys Med Rehab* 62:549, 1981.

307. Sudeck P: Ueber die akute entzundliche Knochenatrophie, *Arc Klin Chir* 62:147, 1900.

308. Sunderland S: *Nerve and nerve injuries,* Edinburgh, 1972, Churchill-Livingstone, p 441.

309. Sunderland S: Pain mechanisms in causalgia, *J Neurol Neurosurg Psychiatry* 39:471, 1976.

310. Sunderland S, Kelly M: The painful sequelae of injuries to peripheral nerves, *Aust NZ J Surg* 18:75, 1948.

311. Tahmoush AJ: Causalgia: redefinition as a clinical pain syndrome, *Pain* 10:187, 1981.

312. Tahmoush AJ, Malley J, Jennings JR: Skin conductance, temperature, and blood flow in causalgia, *Neurol* 33:1483, 1983.

313. Tasker RR, Organ LW, Hawrylyshyn P: Deafferentation and causalgia. In Bonica JJ (editor): *Pain,* New York, 1980, Raven Press.

314. Taub A, Collins Jr WF: Observations on treatment of denervation, dysesthesia with psychotropic drugs: postherpetic neuralgia: anesthesia dolorosa peripheral neuropathy, *Adv Neurol* 4:309, 1974.

315. Taylor CP, Gee NS, Su PV, et al: A summary of mechanistic hypotheses of gabapentin pharmacology, *Epilepsy Res* 29:233-249, 1998.

316. The Capsaicin Study Group: Treatment of painful diabetic neuropathy with topical capsaicin: a multi-center, double-blind, vehicle-controlled study, *Arch Int Med* 151:2225-2229, 1991.

317. Theogaraj J, Merritt WH: *Psychological evaluation of patients with RSD.* Presented at the first annual meeting of the American Society for Peripheral Nerve, Charlottesville, Virginia, 1990.

318. Thompson JE: The diagnosis and management of post-traumatic pain syndromes (causalgia), *Austr NZ J Surg* 49:299, 1979.

319. Trevell JG, Simons D: *Myofascial pain and dysfunction: the trigger point manual,* Baltimore, 1983, Williams & Wilkins.

320. Tsuge K: Management of established Volkmann's contracture. In Green DP (editor): *Operative hand surgery,* New York, 1982, Churchill-Livingstone.

321. Ulmer JL, Mayfield FN: Causalgia: a study of 75 cases, *Surg Gynecol Obstet* 83:789, 1946.

322. Van der Laan L, Goris RJ: Reflex sympathetic dystrophy: an exaggerated regional inflammatory response? *Hand Clin* 13(3):373-385, 1997.

323. Vane JR: Inhibition of prostaglandin synthesis as a mechanism of action for the aspirin-like drugs, *Nature (New Biol)* 231:232-235, 1971.

324. Vane JR, Botting RM: Mechanism of action of antiinflammatory drugs, *Int J Tissue React* 20(1):3-15, 1998.

325. Van Houdenhove B: Algoneurodystrophy: a psychiatrist's point of view, *Clin Rheum* 5:399-406, 1986.

326. Veldman PHJM, Reynen HM, Artz IE, Goris RJA: Signs and symptoms of reflex sympathetic dystrophy: prospective study of 829 patients, *Lancet* 342:1012-1016, 1993.

327. Verdugo RJ, Ochoa JL: Sympathetically maintained pain. I. Phentolamine block questions the concept, *Neurology* 44: 1003-1010, 1994.

328. Virchow R: Ueber Parenchymatose entzundung. *Arch Pathol Anat* 4:261, 1852.

329. Visitsunthorn U, Prete P: Reflex sympathetic dystrophy of the lower extremity: a complication of herpes zoster with dramatic response to propranolol, *West J Med* 135:62, 1981.

330. Volkmann R: Die ischaemishchen Muskellah-mungen und Kontrachturen, *Zentralbl Chir* 8:801, 1881.

331. Vollmer KO, Von Hodenberg A, Kolle EU: Pharmakinetics and metabolism of gabapentin in rat, dog and man, *Arzneimittelforschung* 36:830-839, 1986.

332. Wall PD, Sweet WH: Temporary abolition of pain in man, *Science* 155:108, 1977.

333. Wang JK, Johnson KA, Ilstrup DM: Sympathetic blocks for reflex sympathetic dystrophy, *Pain* 23:13, 1985.

334. Wasner G, Backonja M, Baron R: Traumatic neuralgias: complex regional pain syndrome (reflex sympathetic dystrophy in causalgia): clinical characteristics, pathophysiologic mechanisms and therapies, *Neurol Clin* 16(4):851-868, 1998.

335. Watson HK, Carlson L: Treatment of reflex sympathetic dystrophy of the hand with an active "stress loading" program, *J Hand Surg [Am]* 12:779, 1987.

336. Werner R, Davidoff G, Jackson D, et al: Factors affecting the sensitivity and specificity of the three-phase technetium bone scan in the diagnosis of reflex sympathetic dystrophy syndrome in the upper extremity, *J Hand Surg [Am]* 14:520-523, 1989.

337. Wilder RT, Berde CB, Wolohan M, et al: Reflex sympathetic dystrophy in children, *J Bone Joint Surg* 74:910-919, 1992.

338. Wilhelm A: Stenosis of the subclavian vein: an unknown cause of resistant reflex sympathetic dystrophy, *Hand Clin* 13:(3): 387-411, 1997.

339. Williams HL, Elkins EC: Myalgia of the head, *Arch Phys Ther* 23:14, 1942.

340. Wirth FP, Rutherford RB: A civilian experience with causalgia, *Arch Surg* 100:633, 1970.

341. Wolfe F, Simons D, Fricton J, et al: The fibromyalgia in myofascial pain syndromes: a preliminary study of tender points and trigger points in persons with fibromyalgia, myofascial pain syndrome, and no disease, *J Rheumatol* 19:944, 1992.

342. Woosley RL, Niews AS: Drug therapy: guanethidine, *Engl J Med* 295:1053, 1976.

343. Young RF, Chambi VI: Pain relief by electrical stimulation of the periaqueductal and periventricular grey matter: evidence for a non-opioid mechanism, *J Neurosurg* 66:364-371, 1987.

344. Yunus M: Towards the model of pathophysiology of fibromyalgia: aberrant central pain mechanisms with peripheral modulation, *J Rheumatol* 19:846, 1992.

345. Zohn DA, Mennell J: *Musculoskeletal pain: principles of physical diagnosis and physical treatment,* Boston, 1976, Little, Brown & Co, p 126.

PART XIV

THERMAL INJURY

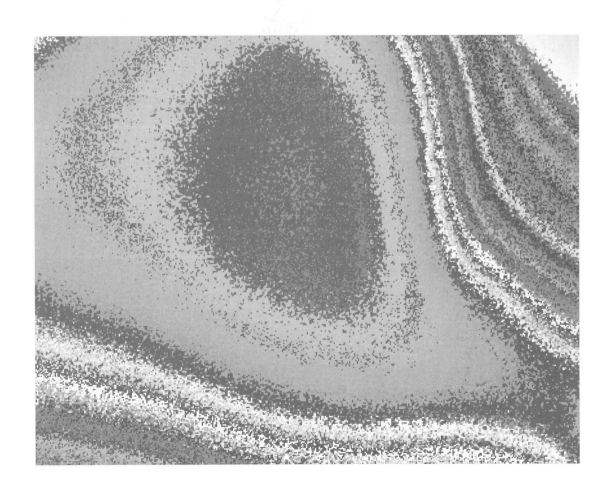

CHAPTER 134

Burns

John O. Kucan

INTRODUCTION

Surgical treatment of the burned patient begins shortly after the traumatic event and has become a major element in modern management of burn wounds. The "sine qua non" of burn care is closure of the burn wound because it represents the visual and tangible conclusion of a broad spectrum of care that is initiated in the immediate postburn period. Attainment of this goal presents numerous challenges, and the gamut of operative procedures employed to achieve this end ranges from relatively simple to highly complex and potentially life threatening. These procedures may become necessary at any time within the postburn period: in the acute, intermediate, chronic, or rehabilitative phases, or perhaps many years after the initial injury.

The hands are the most commonly burned area of the body. Although they comprise only about 5% of the total body surface area, the human hands are unique by virtue of their functional importance. For this reason, the American Burn Association has categorized hand burns as "major thermal injuries."[1] Such a classification may at first be viewed as an exaggeration, but closer scrutiny permits an appreciation of the singular importance of the hand and the functional consequences of thermal injury. Hand burns require specialized care to maximize the potential for optimal functional outcome.

The spectrum of burn injuries to the hands is broad when viewed from the perspectives of etiology and severity. Bilateral injuries are quite common. In 1963 Moncrief[51] reported that 75% of patients treated at Brooke Army Medical Center had sustained hand burns, and 80% of those were bilateral. In the civilian population of burn patients, the incidence of hand burns exceeds 50%. The frequency of such injuries, coupled with a variety of etiologies and severities, produces a wide array of functional impairments. A basic philosophy that guides treatment from the outset is to "circumvent the need for future reconstruction and rehabilitation." Incorporation of this tenet as the foundation of all treatment for burned hands optimizes the functional outcome. Therefore the primary goal of treatment is the attainment of stable, pliable soft tissue coverage, through which preservation and/or restoration of optimal function can be realized (Box 134-1).

Numerous factors and concerns, many uncontrollable, must be considered when the surgeon contemplates performing a surgical procedure on a burn patient. Clinical experience, sound judgment, breadth of knowledge, technical skill, and a clear understanding of the particular individual's needs are fundamental to a successful outcome. The medical and surgical challenges that characterize this group of traumatized patients are among the most daunting in surgical practice. The preservation of the patient's life, though of primary importance, is no longer the solitary measure of successful treatment, but serves as the basis for the process of restoring the patient to optimal function and appearance. The focus of this chapter is the surgical care of the patient who has sustained burns to the hand, culminating in a closed burn wound with preservation and restoration of maximal function. The primary goal of this chapter is to present a rational and organized approach to the surgical management of the thermally injured hand that is within the context of total patient care and can serve as a basis for appropriate decision making and surgical care.

INDICATIONS

THE PROBLEM

After successful fluid resuscitation, healing the burn wound becomes the most important goal in the patient's care. This attitude was present before the era of surgical excision of the burn wound, but the practical necessities inherent to successfully employing this mode of treatment were neither clearly defined nor technically available. The last three decades, however, have witnessed a gradual but inexorable revolution in wound care that is characterized by timely, efficient removal of devitalized tissue and prompt wound closure with autografts, skin substitutes, or biologic dressings.* These advances, in conjunction with similarly dramatic and efficacious developments in the area of critical care medicine, topical and systemic antimicrobial therapy, and nutritional and immunologic support, have favorably altered treatment outcomes in burn

---

*References 3, 4, 5, 9, 10, 27.

apeutic processes. Multiple variables influence the priority, extent, and timing of surgical excision and grafting, as well as the need for alternative wound-closure methods. It is within this complex of variables that the care of the burned hand is undertaken (Box 134-2).

ANALYSIS OF THE PROBLEM

Successful treatment of the burned hand requires a correct analysis of the problem and the development of an organized and systematic treatment plan. A complete patient history is the first component of this process. In addition to the patient's medical history, it should include a thorough recounting of the history of the injury, with emphasis on the mechanism of injury. Hand dominance, occupation, special activities or hobbies, and the age of the patient should be recorded. A complete, thorough physical examination and physiological stabilization of the patient are essential.

The burns should be carefully examined to determine as accurately as possible the extent and depth of injury, keeping in mind that a progression in the depth of the burn wound in the immediate 24 to 48 hours after injury is inevitable. The burns should be mapped and attention should be directed to the specific areas involved. An appreciation of the mechanism of injury may be of great importance in helping to ascertain the magnitude of injury. The essential elements of this evaluation are listed in Box 134-3.[42]

ABNORMAL ANATOMY

Burn depth is determined by the thickness of the dermis that has been damaged or destroyed by heating and, ultimately, by the viability of the epidermal appendages from which reepithelialization of the burn wound may occur. First-degree burn injuries damage only the epidermis, resulting in pain, erythema, desquamation, and scarless healing within 5 to 7 days. Second-degree burns involve only a partial-thickness of the dermis but are subdivided into two distinct categories: superficial and deep.

patients.* A surgical approach to the burn wound, however, has exerted a profound effect on the incidence of invasive burn-wound sepsis and has altered the character of septic episodes.[59,75,76] Surgical excision and grafting result in earlier closure of the burn wound and in large measure contribute to improved survival and functional results in burn patients.†

The primary determinants of wound management are the depth and extent of the burn injury. Premorbid and comorbid factors, however, include a wide array of complex and potentially life-threatening problems that continually impose an additional measure of difficulty in the decision-making and ther-

*References 8, 11, 12, 13, 30, 43, 49, 52.
†References 11, 37, 48, 49, 52, 59.

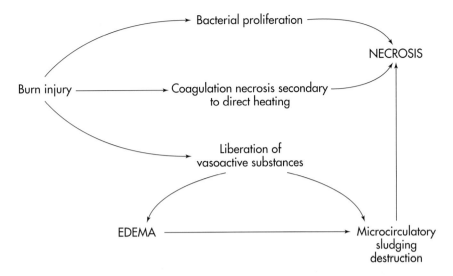

Figure 134-1. Elements contributing to tissue destruction after burn injury.

Superficial partial-thickness injuries are characterized by blister formation and pain; if protected from infection, dessication, or additional external trauma, scarless healing takes place within 7 to 14 days. An excellent cosmetic and functional outcome is generally anticipated. Deep partial-thickness burns, however, are more like full-thickness injuries, often requiring lengthy healing times that may exceed 3 or 4 weeks. Such wounds are relatively insensate and may have some blistering, but they are more likely to be covered by variable amounts of eschar. When permitted to heal spontaneously, these wounds do so at a very slow rate and often result in hypertrophic scars, with their attendant cosmetic and functional sequelae. Deep partial-thickness wounds should be managed in the same fashion as full-thickness wounds—by prompt excision and closure.

Full-thickness, or third-degree, burns have no potential for spontaneous healing except from the unburned periphery. Excisional debridement and wound closure by skin grafts are therefore necessary to achieve permanent wound closure. The option of allowing spontaneous healing by the processes of contraction and epithelialization from the edges is occasionally a consideration, but only if a secondary contracture deformity is unlikely.

Fourth-degree burns involve not only the skin but extend into and beyond the subcutaneous plane and involve deeper structures such as muscle, bone, and tendon. Treatment of these injuries requires extensive deep debridement, sometimes resulting in exposure of important structures. Closure of such wounds may be possible with skin grafts; however, in many patients complex wound-closure methods with pedicled or free flaps provide the only means of stable and reliable wound closure. Amputation is often necessary in the management of these devastating injuries.

Thermal injury causes cellular death and injury both directly and indirectly as injured cells liberate numerous vasoactive products that produce edema, vasoconstriction, and ultimately tissue necrosis (Box 134-4). Bacterial colonization, with subse-

> **Box 134-4.**
> **Vasoactive Substances Liberated From Damaged Cells**
>
> - Histamine
> - Serotonin
> - Kinins
> - Thromboxane
> - Prostaglandins
> - Free oxygen radicals
> - Lipid peroxides

quent proliferation and overgrowth, may further contribute to tissue destruction (Figure 134-1).

Burn eschar, which is in fact an open wound, is a major obstacle to wound healing. Left untreated, it serves as a fertile pabulum for bacterial proliferation and the egress of fluids, electrolytes, and serum proteins. It does not constitute a physiologic barrier of any kind and must be totally absent from the burn wound before wound closure can occur. Burn eschar plays a dominant role in altered homeostasis, hemostasis, immunocompetence, formation of vasoactive substances, and in the development of sepsis and distant organ dysfunction. Excision of burn eschar in conjunction with prompt wound closure, either by permanent autologous skin grafts or temporary wound closure methods, significantly reduces the aforementioned physiologic alterations.[75] The mechanical effects of the burn eschar in the immediate postburn period may also result in an extremity compartment syndrome or severe limitations in chest-wall excursion and ventilation. Prompt decompression is of paramount importance in achieving limb salvage and may be life saving in patients who have circumferential, nonyielding burn wounds of the chest wall (Figure 134-2).

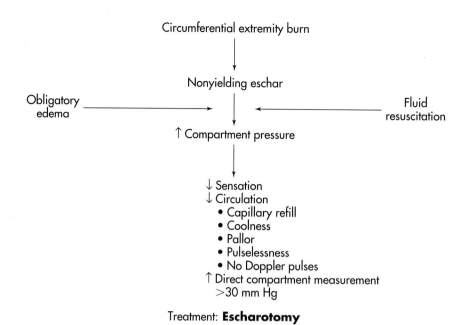

Figure 134-2. Schema of pathophysiology, diagnosis, and treatment of upper-extremity compartment syndrome.

ACUTE TREATMENT OF THE BURNED HAND

Treatment of the burned hand is founded on the following basic principles established by Salisbury[65]:

1. Protection from further injury
2. Maintenance of circulation
3. Prevention of infection
4. Attainment of expeditious wound closure
5. Preservation of motion
6. Achievement of functional rehabilitation

The nature of the treatment provided to the patient with burned hands depends primarily on the degree of injury. First-degree burns require only symptomatic outpatient treatment. Patients with small, circumscribed, partial-thickness and full-thickness burns of the upper extremities may be admitted to the hospital at the physician's discretion. All patients with burns of the hands and upper extremities, except for minor injuries, are best treated in the hospital setting. Hospitalization of patients with bilateral hand burns is generally mandatory.[15,42]

Conceptually, burn wounds consist of three specific zones: (1) the "zone of coagulation," an area of irreversible injury; (2) the "zone of stasis," the intermediate region of damaged but potentially salvageable cells; and (3) the "zone of hyperemia," the peripheral, transiently affected area that is destined to heal. Cooling of the burn wound within the first 30 minutes after injury may help to limit the amount of tissue within the "zone of stasis" that can progress to cell death. Prevention of wound maceration or desiccation is essential. Blisters should be aspirated or debrided to remove the fluid, which contains high levels of thromboxane and other vasoactive substances known to be deleterious to the microcirculation within the "zone of stasis."[29,42]

Control of edema is imperative and can be achieved to some degree by elevating the injured upper extremity above the level of the heart.[2,42] The circumferentially burned hand and upper extremity must be observed for the development of a compartment syndrome. Because the clinical signs and symptoms of compartment syndrome may be misleading, delayed, misinterpreted, or sometimes ignored, direct compartment measurement employing a hand-held, portable compartment-measuring device (Stryker) provides accurate, reliable, and meaningful information. Measurements of the forearm compartment pressures (anterior and posterior) and the pressures within the intrinsic muscles of the hand are required. These may be performed serially to evaluate both the need for and the efficacy of decompression.[42] Prompt decompression by surgical or chemical escharotomy is indicated when compartment pressures exceed 30 mm Hg (Figure 134-3).

Surgical escharotomy is performed by incision of the offending circumferential eschar, thus achieving decompression of the hand and/or arm. This procedure requires meticulous hemostasis to prevent potentially significant hemorrhage. Lysis of the eschar by application of proteolytic enzymes may be effective in selected patients and avoids placement of surgical incisions. Enzymatic escharotomy offers certain advantages over surgical escharotomy, including avoidance of surgical incisions, decreased morbidity, improved estimation of burn-wound depth, and earlier preparation of the wound for definitive wound closure. Chemical escharotomy using the papain-urea ointment Accuzyme may be effective in some patients, but monitoring of compartment pressures during treatment is imperative. This treatment modality should not be employed in the presence of charred full-thickness burns, high-voltage electrical injuries, when compartment pressures are elevated, or when

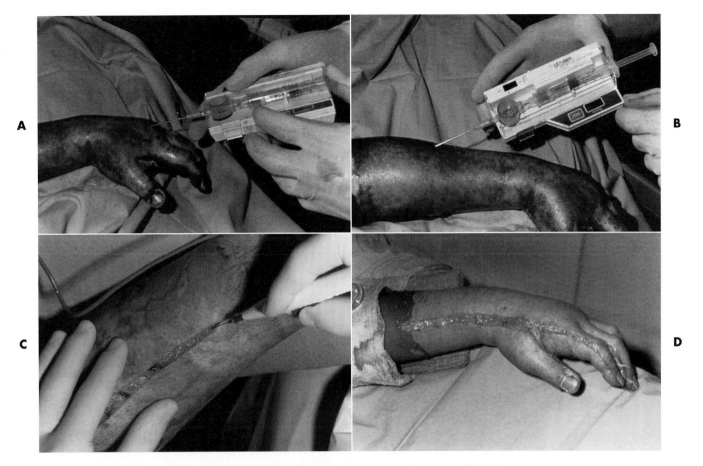

Figure 134-3. **A,** Direct intrinsic muscle compartment measurement. **B,** Direct intracompartment pressure measurement of dorsal forearm with Stryker device. **C,** Surgical escharotomy employing electrocautery. Note intact veins in subcutaneous fat. **D,** Completed surgical escharotomy. Note the incorrect placement of incisions on thumb and index finger which should be on the "nondominant" sides of the digits.

more than 4 to 6 hours have elapsed from the time of burn injury.[42]

Infection of the burned hand, although uncommon, is nonetheless possible. During the initial edema phase, inactivation of antistreptococcal fatty acids of the skin may increase the likelihood of developing streptococcal cellulitis. Administration of a specific antistreptococcal drug such as penicillin or erythromycin during the edema phase may be indicated. Topical antimicrobial therapy is indicated in deep partial-thickness and full-thickness burns to control bacterial proliferation and prevent burn-wound sepsis. Silver sulfadiazine cream is most commonly used for this indication. It can be incorporated in a semiocclusive hand dressing or can be used in conjunction with Gore-Tex bags, which permit motion but prevent maceration.*

Autologous skin is the only permanent wound cover. Adequate, durable, stable, supple cover is essential to normal hand function. Prompt closure of the burn wound offers several important benefits, such as a decrease in wound infection rate, scar formation, and contractures, and a marked reduction in pain and length of hospitalization. Likewise, therapy and rehabilitation can be initiated earlier, and the potential need for additional reconstructive procedures is substantially reduced.

INFORMED CONSENT

Informed consent for patients about to undergo surgical treatment of their burn wounds may be a complex matter. The variability of burn patients and their injuries in terms of causation; patient age; depth, extent, and location of the burns; premorbid and comorbid factors; and psychological and socioeconomic factors must be considered. These factors and many others will directly affect the informed-consent process. The patient's age or physical and mental status, for example, may preclude the possibility of direct communication with or consent by the patient, thereby placing the entire decision-making responsibility on others. The broad array of psychosocial and medicolegal ramifications of such circumstances may

*References 38, 42, 47, 50, 60, 71, 73, 74.

be complex and potentially treacherous. Furthermore, when the mode of injury arouses the suspicion of abuse or neglect, strict adherence to the legal guidelines for reporting and obtaining consent for any necessary surgical procedures is imperative.

The process of informed consent requires a clear, accurate, complete, and sometimes graphic description of the operation, risks, benefits, complications, and alternatives to treatment, and the overall prognosis for the patient's recovery. Broad generalizations and excessive optimism and enthusiasm should be avoided despite the desire to buoy the spirits of the patient and family members. The patient and family members must be provided with an overall explanation and description of the treatment plan and the specific role of surgical intervention in this process. Providing specific information about the procedure is essential and should include descriptions of what will be done and an explanation of why it should be done. Recruiting former burn patients as volunteers to help answer the patient's or family's questions regarding both immediate and long-term concerns may be of great benefit. Providing procedure-specific audiovisual materials (e.g., videotapes) can also be very helpful in providing a better degree of understanding to the burned patient and his or her family members.

A description of the operation and subsequent donor-site care should be discussed if autograft closure of the burn wound is to be performed. If temporary closure of the wound will be required, necessitating additional operative procedures to achieve final wound closure with autografts, this information must be clearly transmitted to all concerned parties. The possibility of blood transfusions, infection, hematoma, graft loss, donor-site conversion, reoperation, postoperative hemorrhage, respiratory dysfunction, and possible death must be addressed. If amputation appears imminent, preparation of the patient and family for this eventuality is imperative. Additional opinions from uninvolved consultants may be of great value in providing additional objective support for the necessity of amputation and addressing potential medicolegal concerns and implications. The potential for long-term or even life-long sequelae and the need for additional surgical procedures, both immediately and in the future, should be discussed.

The influence of the patient's premorbid and comorbid factors on the treatment plan and overall prognosis must be presented. Clarity, candor, caution, consistency, completeness, and concern should be the hallmarks of the informed-consent process. Patients in whom the likelihood for surgery appears low initially should nevertheless be prepared for this possibility if wound healing is delayed, which can occur when burn-wound depth is underestimated or when other factors interfere with the timely and predicted healing of the burn wound. Surgery should be recommended to those patients in whom it is obvious that spontaneous healing of the burn wound is not possible within 10 to 14 days. This approach offers the greatest potential for reducing the likelihood of septic burn-wound complications, hastening functional recovery, improving cosmetic results, and potentially decreasing the length and cost of hospitalization. Unless emergent surgical decompression or

> **Box 134-5.**
> **Systemic Effects of the Burn Wound**
>
> - Coagulopathy, thrombocytopenia
> - Alterations in red blood cell life span, deformability
> - Immune alterations
> - Impairment of neutrophil function
> - Hepatic dysfunction
> - Myocardial dysfunction
> - Endocrinopathy
> - Renal dysfunction
> - Decreased splanchnic blood flow
> - Pulmonary dysfunction
> - Catabolism

management of a potentially life-threatening condition is needed, excision and grafting of the burn wound should proceed 3 to 5 days after injury. A small, well-defined wound, however, can be addressed within 24 to 48 hours after the patient is hospitalized, thereby hastening the overall care regimen.*

The expectant treatment of deep dermal burns has become the exception rather than the rule in modern burn care. No longer is it appropriate or acceptable to treat such injuries by waiting for the occurrence of spontaneous eschar separation, with its attendant pain, suffering, septic episodes, delayed healing, severe scarring, metabolic abnormalities, protracted hospitalization, and high mortality rates. Modern burn care is based on surgical treatment of the burn wound. The elimination of a lengthy inflammatory phase of wound healing and the restoration of cutaneous integrity have yielded substantial benefits to patients (Box 134-5).†

OPERATIONS

EVOLUTION OF SURGICAL TECHNIQUES

The last 25 years have witnessed a dramatic improvement in burn care, not the least of which has been an aggressive surgical approach to the burn wound. Despite a general awareness of the deficiencies related to the expectant treatment method of burn-wound care, philosophic, practical, and technologic constraints severely restricted early aggressive surgical management of the burn wound. Before the "era of excision," burn wounds were managed in direct contrast to the fundamental principle applied to other traumatic wounds (i.e., the prompt elimination of all devitalized tissue). Only those patients with trivial burn wounds were managed by true surgical therapy. Patients with extensive burn injuries were routinely managed

---

*References 9, 11, 14, 20, 60, 64.
†References 27, 30, 31, 49, 52, 75, 76.

by the "expectant" method, with the major expectation that all patients would suffer from a bout of local or systemic sepsis as a result of early bacterial colonization of the burn wound. Physiologic monitoring was essentially nonexistent, pathophysiology of the burn wound was a mystery, and nutritional and physiologic support were severely lacking. Equally absent were effective topical antimicrobial agents, systemic antibiotics, power dermatomes, physiotherapy, and the technologic and basic science support that are present in abundance today.[52]

The introduction of topical antibacterial preparations in the early 1960s heralded a major advance in burn treatment and served as a potent catalyst for the investigation of burns and their treatment.[50] These new discoveries were rapidly incorporated into the clinical care of burn patients. The development of reliable power dermatomes, mesh expanders and expansion techniques, safe antibiotics, and monitoring equipment and techniques, along with the development of critical care as a distinct medical discipline resulted in major improvements in the care of the burned patient. An aggressive surgical approach to the burn wound, originally championed by Janzekovic, gradually gained acceptance and replaced the nonsurgical approach used for decades.[30,31,37,75,76]

AVAILABLE TECHNIQUES

Wound-closure options for burns of the hand are primarily determined by the depth of the burn wound and consist of the following[41]:

1. Spontaneous healing (<14 days)
2. Early wound excision and split-thickness autografting
3. Delayed spontaneous healing (>14 days)
4. Delayed split-thickness skin grafting (>14 days)
5. Delayed excision and split-thickness skin grafting

Superficial burn wounds that are expected to heal within 14 days should be protected from desiccation. These wounds generally require no topical antimicrobials and may be effectively treated by emollient-impregnated, nonadhering gauze dressings (Xeroform, Xeroflo); skin substitutes (Biobrane); biologic dressings (cadaver homograft, porcine xenograft); or calcium alginate dressings.* The primary management requirements of these patients are pain control and the maintenance of an active range of motion. Uncomplicated healing and full functional recovery can be expected (Figure 134-4).

Patients with burn wounds that are not expected to heal completely by 14 days and all third-degree burns should be treated by surgical excision and skin grafting. Exceptions to this approach include small burns in patients with severe coexisting disease, or small circumscribed burns that may heal spontaneously without resultant functional disturbance, most notably burn-scar contractures. Direct excision of small, deep, partial-thickness or full-thickness burns is occasionally possible

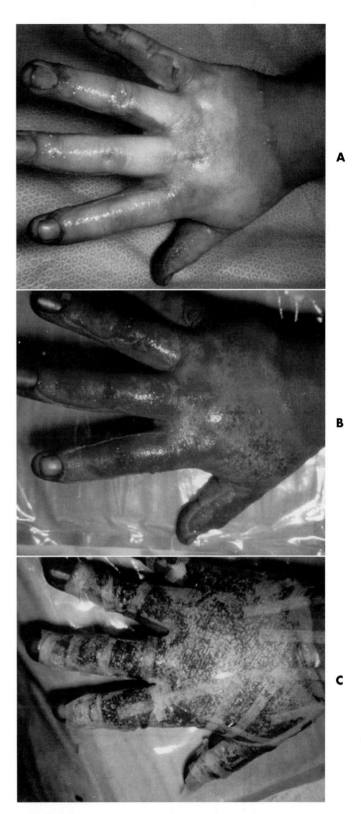

Figure 134-4. **A,** Partial thickness burn of the hand. **B,** After enzymatic debridement, with evidence of punctate bleeding. **C,** Biosynthetic membrane (Biobrane) applied to the debrided burn wound.

---

*References 18, 26, 38, 39, 42, 74.

in areas of skin laxity, such as small areas on the dorsum of the hand or forearm.

Deep partial-thickness and full-thickness burns of the hands are best managed by early surgical excision and skin grafting. Burn-wound depth is the primary determinant of healing time, thus the earlier the wound depth can be determined, the sooner definitive treatment can be initiated. Although numerous methods of determining burn-wound depth have been described, investigated, and clinically evaluated, there exists no single universally accepted, reliable tool that accomplishes this task. The judgment of an experienced surgeon, coupled with a thorough history of the injury and a clinical examination, continues to be the best means for determining the depth of the burn injury. Early enzymatic debridement by eliminating a significant amount of devitalized tissue may also provide additional useful information and may increase the accuracy of the estimation of burn-wound depth.[42]

When the severity of burn injury to a digit or extremity precludes functional salvage, or when the burned part jeopardizes the well-being of the patient, amputation may be required. Consideration should be given to providing the most functional amputation possible, being mindful of the overall limitations that the remainder of the burn injuries may impose on the patient and the functional capabilities of modern prosthetic devices.

EXCISION AND GRAFTING

The majority of patients treated in burn centers do not have life-threatening injuries. The average burn size treated in these facilities is less than 20% of the body surface area. Fewer than one third of patients have burn injuries that exceed 30% of the body surface area. Therefore the overall survival and success rates of surgical attempts at burn-wound closure are generally high.[49]

Deep partial-thickness and full-thickness burn wounds of the hands that are believed to require surgical excision and grafting can be treated by either tangential excision or excision to the deep investing fascia. Patients with an obvious charred full-thickness burn with subcutaneous tissue involvement are best managed by excision to the fascia and sheet grafts of split-thickness skin. This technique provides a viable bed for autografting, but the resultant edema and cosmetic defect secondary to loss of the subcutaneous tissue may be problematic, especially when such excision involves the forearm and proximal arm. Patients with deep partial-thickness or full-thickness burns of the upper extremities with minimal subcutaneous tissue damage are usually treated by tangential excision of the burn wound. The technique of intradermal debridement is more tedious than fascial excision but is most commonly employed and overcomes the aforementioned shortcomings of excision to the fascia. The intradermal debridement technique serially removes successive, thin layers of nonviable tissue (8/1000ths of an inch) with either guarded knives or dermatomes until the entire eschar is removed and completely viable tissue is encountered. A rotary dermabrader can be used to debride small, hard-to-reach areas, such as the web spaces or the hands of small children (Figure 134-5).[22]

Excision of the burn wound is generally undertaken from 1 to 5 days after injury. Several days' delay may be required before undertaking the procedure in those instances in which the depth of the wound is not obvious initially. A number of techniques have been employed to determine the depth of the burn wound, but none of these methods provide a universally applicable and reliable means of determining burn-wound depth. What is universally true, however, is that the

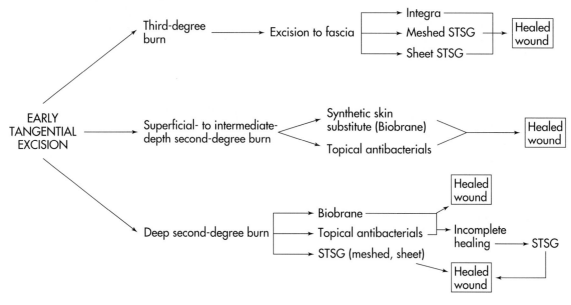

Figure 134-5. Guidelines for surgical management of the burned hand. *STSG,* Split-thickness skin graft.

burn wound will become deeper during the succeeding hours after injury and will always be deeper than when it was initially seen.[8,42]

Excision of the burn wound is not an innocuous procedure. This operation can be associated with prodigious blood loss. Preoperative preparation and operative execution should therefore focus on techniques to minimize intraoperative hemorrhage and the subsequent need for blood transfusions (Box 134-6).[8,13] Pneumatic tourniquets should be routinely employed, but exsanguination of the extremity before inflation should be avoided because the pooled blood within the dermal and subdermal plexus may serve as a reliable guideline in determining the depth and adequacy of excision. Additional hemostatic techniques are routinely employed and include application of a dilute epinephrine spray or epinephrine solution–saturated Telfa pads (1:300,000 dilution), topical thrombin, and firm compression wraps and pressure dressings before tourniquet deflation.[42] The dressings should be left in place for a minimum of 10 minutes, then removed carefully after gentle moistening of the dressing with a misting of epinephrine solution. Dressing removal should be from proximal to distal to overcome the potential venous congestion and excess bleeding that may be caused by a proximal tourniquet effect of tight compression wrapping. Electrocautery and suture-ligation of bleeding points will help to control residual hemorrhage. Application of autografts or skin substitutes/biologic dressings should only be performed when absolute hemostasis has been achieved (Box 134-7). In the event that bleeding persists despite vigorous attempts at hemostasis, sterile, moist dressings should be applied to the wounds, the wounds should be firmly dressed, and the patient should be returned to the operating room in 24 hours for delayed wound closure of a hemostatically secure wound bed (Figure 134-6).

Once complete hemostasis has been accomplished, the excised burn wound is covered with sheet grafts of split-thickness autograft of approximately 12/1000ths of an inch thickness, meshed unexpanded autografts (1.5:1 expansion ratio), and biologic dressings or synthetic skin substitutes, depending on the dictates of the situation. The wound coverings are secured to the wound bed with surgical staples or absorbable sutures. Grafts to the dorsum of the hand should be applied with the wrist in volar flexion to maximize the amount of skin that is placed onto the surgical defect. Conversely, grafts to the palmar surface of the hand or the volar wrist region should be placed with the wrist in maximal dorsiflexion to place as much skin as possible into the surgically excised burn wound. A concerted effort should be made to avoid placement of graft edges in straight lines along the ulnar or radial aspects of digits or the hand and wrist. Interposition of the skin graft edges in the form of interdigitating "darts" along any potential site of linear scar contracture is an important consideration. Sheet grafts provide a somewhat better cosmetic appearance after healing than meshed autografts on the dorsum of the hand, but there is no difference in the rate of "take" between the two types of grafts. Meshed split-thickness autografts are quite acceptable on more proximal regions of the forearm and hand, do not result in an untoward cosmetic appearance, and should be used when donor-site availability is an important consideration.

The newly placed skin grafts are then dressed with a single layer of nonadhering gauze (Xeroform, N-terface, Adaptic) and are then secured with a wrap of Kling. Absorbent gauze dressings are then placed and wrapped with additional Kling wrap or elastic tubular stretch gauze. Joints and other areas of potential motion are immobilized as needed by the application of splints constructed of either plaster or heat-malleable material (Orthoplast). Sufficient dressing material must be present between the plaster splint and skin surface to prevent thermal burns secondary to the exothermic reaction of plaster splint material. The interstices of the meshed autografts must be protected from desiccation and infection. This is best

---

Box 134-6.
Presurgical Patient Preparation

SYSTEMIC FACTORS
- Platelet count, PT, PTT
- WBC count
- Hgb, Hct
- Electrolytes, glucose, BUN, creatinine
- Serum protein, albumin
- Arterial blood gases, pH
- Urinalysis
- Cardiac output, CVP, PCWP, EDV*
- Normovolemia*
- Stable on ventilator*
- Tidal volume*

WOUND (LOCAL) FACTORS
- Bacteriologic status of wound
  - Wound biopsy
  - Semiquantitative surface cultures
- Perioperative antibiotics
- Wound inspection

BUN, Blood, urea, nitrogen; *CVP*, central venous pressure; *EDV*, end-diastolic volume; *Hct*, hematocrit; *Hgb*, hemoglobin; *PCWP*, pulmonary capillary wedge pressure; *PT*, prothrombin time; *PTT*, partial thromboplastin time; *WBC*, white blood cell.
*Mandatory for patients on ventilators/inhalation injury patients.

Box 134-7.
Grafting the Burned Hand

- Complete escharectomy → viable bed
- Sheet grafts whenever possible
- Provision of maximal amount of skin
- Complete hemostasis
- Immobilization/splinting
- Rapid mobilization/ROM exercises

ROM, Range of motion.

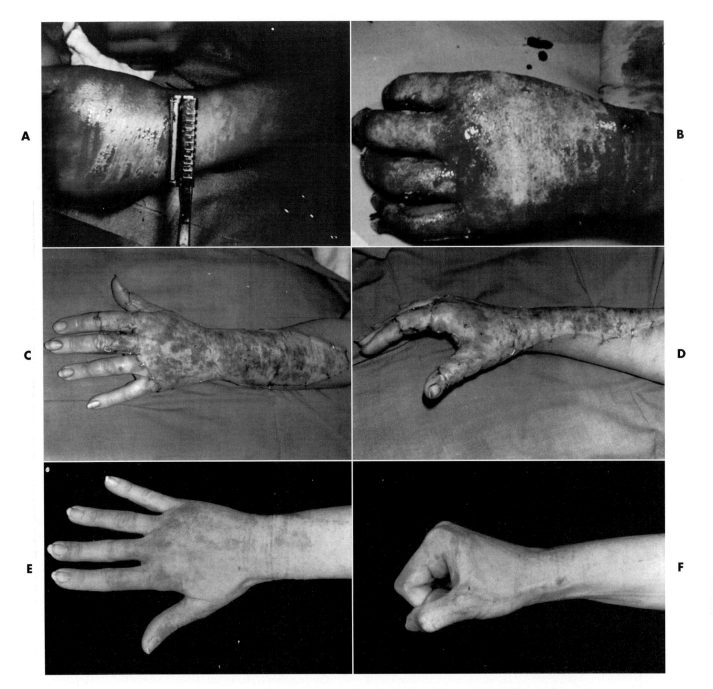

Figure 134-6. **A,** Intradermal debridement (tangential excision) of dorsal hand burn employing a Weck blade. **B,** Appearance of wound after completion of excision. **C,** Sheet grafts in place. Note transverse orientation of grafts (postoperative day 3). **D,** Lateral view of hand and forearm after skin grafts. **E,** Appearance of the grafts 4 months after surgery. **F,** Postoperative range of motion at 4 months after surgery.

accomplished by soaking the dressings with 5% Sulfamylon solution, which is the only topical antibacterial agent approved for use with meshed autografts. The dressings are remoistened every 6 to 8 hours as needed.

Deep partial and full-thickness burn injuries to the palmar hand surfaces are less common than injuries to the dorsum. Palmar wounds are much more difficult to excise and graft than dorsal hand burns, and the functional outcome after these types of injuries is frequently less successful than those after

dorsal hand burns (Figure 134-7). Similarly, circumferential hand burns provide considerable therapeutic challenges and are characterized by relatively poor functional outcomes and the near-universal need for secondary reconstructive procedures. There is a dearth of information in the published literature regarding the optimum treatment of these injuries. The application of full or thick partial-thickness skin grafts to the palmar surface and maintenance of the palmar breadth and thumb abduction are critical components in achieving a

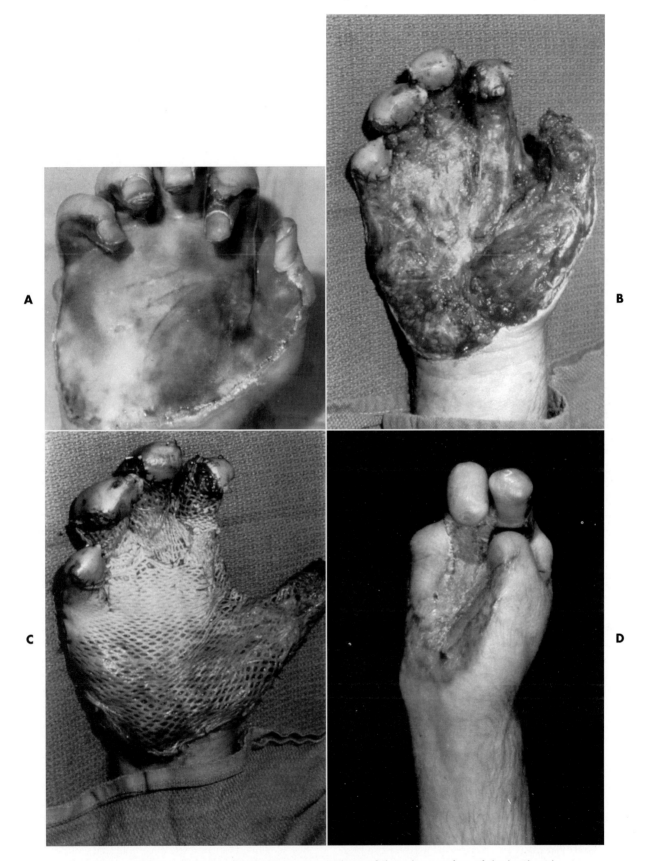

Figure 134-7. **A,** Severe fourth-degree contact burn of the palmar surface of the hand, with charring and flexion deformity of the digits. **B,** Appearance of the wound after initial excision and debridement, with partial amputation of involved digits. **C,** Meshed autograft in place. **D,** Marked functional deformity occurring in the early postoperative period.

satisfactory outcome. Such grafts provide a superior quality skin and greater resistance to the contractile forces of the palmar region than thin split-thickness skin grafts.[67] The qualitative results of early intervention, the use of thick grafts, careful and correct postoperative splinting, and early initiation of hand therapy produce results that are superior to those observed in similar wounds managed by delayed grafting onto a granulating, contracting wound bed.

The majority of hand burns occur on the dorsal surface. Until recently, the optimal treatment of these wounds was somewhat controversial. However, recent data founded on fundamental biologic responses to wounding and wound healing, along with well-controlled clinical studies and observations, solidify the concept of early excision and grafting as the most appropriate and acceptable method for the treatment of deep dermal and full-thickness dorsal hand and arm burns. This aggressive surgical approach results in a high degree of functional success while substantially reducing pain, length of hospitalization, and the frequency of secondary revisional procedures.*

Excision to fascia and subsequent skin grafting should be performed in those cases where the subcutaneous tissues have sustained a substantial injury and the viability of the subdermal fat and its ability to support a split-thickness skin graft is in question. Excision to the fascia can be performed more quickly and with considerably less blood loss than intradermal debridement. The major objection to this approach is related to the rather prominent and unsightly contour deformity that occurs at the junction of the unburned skin and the excised burn wound and the potential for secondary distal edema resulting from the disruption of lymphatic drainage. It may be very difficult, however, to confidently identify viable fat in burns that extend into the subcutaneous plane. Autograft loss as a result of such an error in judgment is unacceptable, and in those situations where there is uncertainty about the viability of the recipient bed it is far more preferable to perform excision to the level of the investing fascia. This maneuver will maximize the likelihood of achieving a viable recipient bed and a thoroughly debrided burn wound and minimize blood loss. The junction of the fascial excision and unburned or less deeply burned skin may be the source of considerable postoperative bleeding from the transected ends of blood vessels along the cut dermal edge or contiguous subdermal fat. These vessels should be secured before wound closure and the application of dressings to minimize the need for premature or emergent dressing removal in the immediate postoperative period.

Fourth-degree burns of the hand and upper extremity resulting from thermal trauma or high-voltage electrical injury are infrequent but devastating injuries. Wound closure with skin grafts is often not possible because there is involvement of subcutaneous structures such as tendon, bone, joints, nerves, or blood vessels that frequently dictates the need for complex, challenging, and innovative wound-closure methods. Flap coverage is often necessary, with regional pedicled flaps or free tissue transfers serving as the primary reconstructive tools.

Primary or delayed amputations are frequently required. The overall functional outcomes, however, are considerably better than those of a few decades ago because of advances in reconstructive surgical techniques, especially reconstructive microsurgery.[56,66,68,73]

Partial-thickness burn wounds involving the palmar surface of the hand are infrequently excised because most heal spontaneously as a result of the greater thickness of the palmar skin. If, however, excision is indicated and undertaken, the task is made far more difficult by the absence of a defined surgical plane. Complete hemostasis before graft application is essential, as is correct splinting in the antideformity position. Effective early mobilization, proper splinting, edema control, and a carefully orchestrated hand-therapy program are necessary for success.

To be successful, skin grafting of the burned hand should be carried out in accordance with the following established guidelines:

1. The recipient bed must be viable and devoid of eschar or infection
2. Hemostasis must be complete
3. Sheet grafts should be employed whenever possible
4. The maximum amount of skin should be provided by placing the hand in extreme positions, thereby accentuating the defect
5. Immobilization and splinting must be used to prevent mechanical disruption of the skin graft from the recipient bed
6. "Darting" or interposition of skin grafts with other grafts or unburned skin should be performed to diminish the likelihood of linear contractures or syndactyly formation

The incidence of bacteremia in conjunction with wound manipulation is considerable (20% to 25%). Therefore perioperative antibiotic prophylaxis for both gram-positive and gram-negative organisms is recommended. Aminoglycoside or cephalosporin antibiotics are most commonly employed, with dosing schedules sufficient to achieve a therapeutic blood level in the immediate perioperative period, but are not extended beyond 8 to 12 hours postoperatively. Antibiotic prophylaxis can be limited to the initial preoperative dose in patients with small total body surface area burns (<10% total body surface area).

The operating time itself should not exceed 2 hours. The total area excised, including the hands, during a single procedure should not exceed 20% of the total body surface area. Adherence to these guidelines will minimize interoperative blood loss, transfusion requirements, and physiologic stresses imposed on the patient. This approach maximizes surgical treatment while decreasing the incidence of potential problems that are seen in protracted, one-stage procedures performed on critically ill patients. The priority for excision and closure in patients suffering from critical burns (>50% total body surface area) is to achieve the greatest reduction in burn size and the best likelihood for complete uncomplicated graft "take" as fast as possible. The treatment of hand burns is a secondary concern in these patients. However, the primary functional areas should be excised and grafted first in burn patients in whom a high mortality rate is not the predominant concern to aid in accelerating functional recovery.[6,8,12,13,20]

---

*References 17-19, 23, 40, 46, 47, 52.

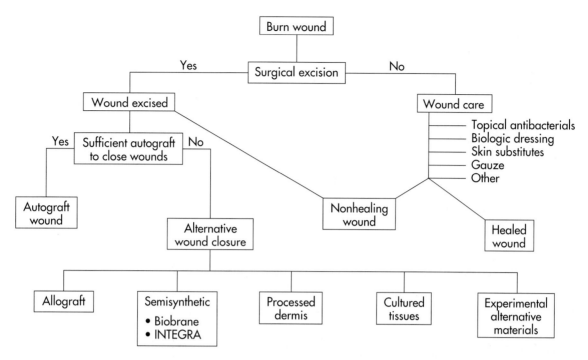

Figure 134-8. Algorithm for management of the burned hand.

The dressings that have been placed over skin grafts of temporarily closed wounds should be examined daily. They should be left in place for 3 to 5 days in the absence of obvious problems such as bleeding, a foul smell or discharge, and fever. Meticulous cleansing, inspection, and necessary debridement or trimming are performed at the initial graft inspection, and the wounds are then redressed in the same fashion. Subsequent inspections are carried out at 1-or 2-day intervals depending on the appearance of the wounds at the preceding inspection and according to the preference and judgment of the surgeon. Generally, by the seventh to tenth postoperative day, sufficient graft incorporation should have occurred to permit mobilization and motion. It is important in the first few days after initiation of motion to inspect skin grafts or skin substitutes daily to ensure they remain intact. Light dressings or elastic support material (Tubigrip) are used to protect the grafts. Light nonadhering dressings should be employed in the case of meshed autografts until complete closure of the mesh interstices has occurred.[42,66,78]

GENERAL GUIDELINES FOR EXCISION

Staged excision of the burn wound is necessary in patients whose burns exceed 30% to 40% of the total body surface area. The deepest burns should be excised first. The primary goal in massive injuries should be the rapid and maximal reduction in the total size of the burn wound as quickly and safely as possible. Functional and cosmetic areas, such as the hands, should be given treatment priority in patients whose burns are not life threatening. If joint involvement is present, excision and immobilization by internal fixation may be necessary. Wounds should not be excised unless definitive skin grafting or alternative wound coverage with biologic, biosynthetic, or

synthetic dressings can be performed because freshly excised wounds will become contaminated or desiccated if not covered, resulting in a more complex situation (Figure 134-8).*

COMPLEX COVERAGE

The overwhelming majority of hand and upper-extremity burns are amenable to closure by skin grafts after surgical debridement, but this approach may not be possible in certain situations. Involvement of deep structures (as occurs in fourth-degree burn injuries, high-voltage electrical injuries, or deep burns occurring in areas devoid of subcutaneous tissues) presents unique and challenging problems that are not amenable to closure by simple skin grafting. The need for more complex coverage is dictated by several factors: the size, depth, and location of the burn wound; the nature and functional importance of subjacent structures; the short-and long-term morbidity resulting from failure to provide effective and timely coverage; and the adequacy of the blood supply of the excised wound to support a skin graft. Additional considerations include motion, long-term durability, and preservation or restoration of function. Flap coverage is required when underlying bone, tendon, nerve, joint, or major blood vessels are involved.

Flap selection is dictated by several important considerations, including the location and size of the wound, the quality and availability of local tissue, and the age and overall condition of the patient. Local or regional cutaneous, fascial, fasciocutaneous, muscle, or myocutaneous flaps may be employed if required and available (Figure 134-9). In certain instances, however, coverage, preservation, or salvage can only be attained by the use of a free tissue transfer. These situations require

*References 30, 31, 46, 47, 48, 49, 52.

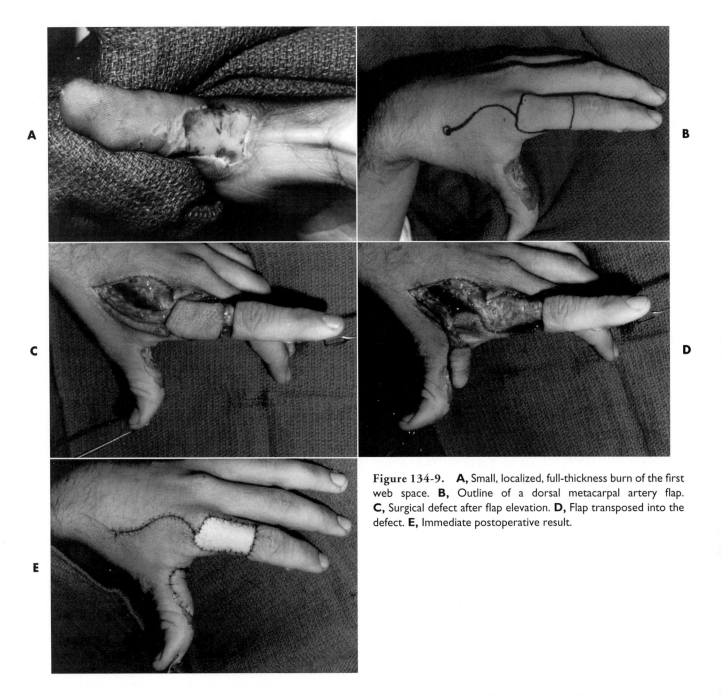

Figure 134-9. **A,** Small, localized, full-thickness burn of the first web space. **B,** Outline of a dorsal metacarpal artery flap. **C,** Surgical defect after flap elevation. **D,** Flap transposed into the defect. **E,** Immediate postoperative result.

considerable planning and ingenuity—the hallmarks of modern reconstructive microsurgery. The issues of donor-site selection morbidity, postoperative care, and the long-term benefits to the patient must be considered. Patient selection and the immediate and long-term goals and consequences of such procedures merit considerable thought and discussion.[42,73,77,80]

WOUND COVERAGE

The immediate coverage of excised burn wounds is mandatory. Autografts, either sheet or meshed, provide the only reliable means to achieve permanent wound closure. However, alternative wound-closure methods may be required to achieve temporary wound closure when autografting of the burn

wounds is not achievable or is contraindicated after excision. Adherence to the same exacting criteria that are used to ensure complete "take" of autografts is essential for successful and consistent results when employing the various types of skin substitutes. These materials function poorly in the presence of hematoma, infection, inadequately debrided recipient sites, or unrestricted motion before adherence, the same factors that prevent successful incorporation of autograft skin.[42]

Although fresh cadaver allograft is the "gold standard" of biologic dressings (Figure 134-10), its usefulness is limited by a lack of availability, rigorous processing and storage requirements, limited shelf life, and the potential for disease transmission. These limitations have stimulated the development of several effective skin substitutes. The two commonly employed materials are Biobrane and Integra. The composi-

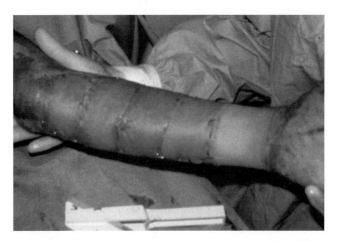

Figure 134-10. Cadaver homograft temporary wound closure after burn-wound excision.

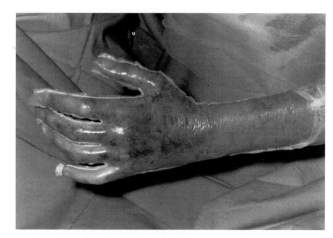

Figure 134-11. Biobrane glove coverage of burned hand and forearm.

tion of both materials is conceptually similar in that they both consist of a silicone epidermal analogue and a collagen-peptide–based dermal equivalent. Biobrane requires a minimum of 24 hours after placement to achieve good initial adherence. Once incorporated into the burn wound, it may be left in place for extensive periods of time (>90 days) but must be removed completely before the application of autograft skin (Figure 134-11). Removal may be very difficult when Biobrane has been in place for longer than 2 to 3 weeks and may require a modified reexcision of the wound to achieve total removal. Integra, by contrast, takes much longer to incorporate into the wound, and the dermal equivalent undergoes transformation into a permanent neodermis. The Silastic epidermal equivalent is removed at 14 to 21 days after initial placement of the material, and the neodermis is then covered with very thin epidermal autografts (3/1000ths to 4/1000ths of an inch). These biosynthetic materials are good alternatives to cadaver allograft and function well on freshly excised wounds. They are far less tolerant of bacterial contamination, however, than either autograft or allograft.*

Cultured epidermal autografts are essentially useless in the treatment of hand burns. Cultured epidermal autografts perform much better when placed on a viable dermal bed than when placed on a dermis-devoid excised wound; however, it is very difficult to conceptualize a situation in which they could be recommended for the treatment of burned hands.†

PATIENT PREPARATION AND PLANNING

Patient selection for excision and grafting is based on the previously discussed guidelines. The timing of the operation is dictated by numerous factors, including the patient's overall condition and response to resuscitation and the presence of an inhalation injury and respiratory failure. Before subjecting the patient to a potentially life-threatening surgical procedure, the systemic and local factors that may influence the surgical outcome must be addressed. Surgery should be postponed until the patient's physiologic status is sufficiently restored to withstand the stresses imposed by general anesthesia and surgical intervention. This cannot be achieved in some patients, and they never undergo an operative procedure. If the abnormalities are being caused by burn-wound sepsis, however, prompt debridement in conjunction with appropriate supportive and therapeutic measure is mandatory to correct the problem. Grafting is usually delayed in these situations.

An organized surgical plan is essential before beginning in the operating room. The sites, extent, and type of excision should be chosen. Donor sites should be selected and specific equipment and logistical needs addressed. The particular operative requirements, such as personnel, blood products, dressing materials, and other equipment needs, should be clearly identified, reviewed, and arranged in advance. Likewise, patient transport issues, both before and after surgery, must be considered and properly managed to expedite transport to and from the operating suite.

ANESTHETIC CONSIDERATIONS

An experienced anesthesiologist who understands the unique requirements and systemic responses of a burned patient is vital to the safe and uneventful performance of the surgical procedure. The anesthesiologist must provide adequate personnel to address the numerous physiologic needs of the anesthetized burn patient. These include the maintenance of proper room and patient core temperatures, rigorous fluid volume control, strict respiratory and metabolic support, and continuous monitoring of vital signs, urine output, cardiac rhythm and function, and tissue oxygenation. Effective communication throughout the surgical procedure between the surgical team leader and the anesthesiologist is necessary to ensure optimal patient care.

Vigilant observation of the volume and rapidity of blood loss and the prompt correction of any abnormality are critical

---

*References 26, 28, 32-35, 44, 55, 71.
†References 3, 6, 21, 26, 36, 54, 57, 81.

to performing safe surgical excision and grafting procedures. Close monitoring of the patient's physiologic responses to rapid volume changes and the ability to anticipate and minimize these fluxes are important elements in performing uncomplicated surgery. Sound surgical technique aimed at achieving an expeditious removal of the eschar while minimizing blood loss is the keystone of safe excisional surgery.

DONOR SITES

Primary emphasis is placed on effective management of the burn wound, but split-thickness skin graft donor sites must also be managed appropriately, especially in patients who suffer from major life-threatening injuries. Permanent wound closure depends on the availability of an adequate amount of autograft skin. Therefore considerable attention should be given to the donor sites to optimize healing. Autografts should be harvested before excision or manipulation of the burn wound to avoid donor-site contamination and/or potential infection with subsequent conversion of the donor sites. Skin grafts should be harvested with skill and precision. If the dermatome is not working properly, another machine should be obtained immediately. Dermatome blades should be replaced as soon as they become dull. Hemostasis should be pursued vigorously to minimize both intraoperative blood loss and to diminish postoperative donor-site problems. There is no ideal donor-site dressing, but donor sites should be dressed in a manner that will protect them from external trauma and contamination, minimize the patient's discomfort, prevent dessication, and reduce the likelihood of infection while providing an environment that may hasten the rate of reepithelialization. Donor sites merit regular inspection so that any problems can be addressed promptly and effectively.[6,8,69]

POSTOPERATIVE MANAGEMENT

Postoperative positioning, splinting, and bed requirements are determined by the body locations that were treated. Hands that have received skin grafts must be elevated higher than the heart to minimize postoperative edema and venous congestion. All special equipment needs must be anticipated before the patient departs the operating room. The patient's bed should be readied and the patient transferred directly onto the bed to eliminate any unnecessary movements that may jeopardize skin grafts or other wound dressings. Information regarding the patient's condition and pertinent details of the surgical procedure should be conveyed to all personnel who will care for the patient during the postoperative period. Specific concerns and requirements should be clearly communicated and accurately recorded. Nursing considerations assume primary importance when the patient arrives in the postanesthesia recovery area or intensive care unit. These include airway management, fluid and electrolyte balance, hemodynamic status, pain control, mental status, and thermoregulation. Once the patient's immediate postoperative status is deemed stable, vital signs and other physiologic parameters are monitored, and

periodic laboratory tests are performed. The patient's family is notified of his or her status and given a report regarding the operative procedure. Wound-care observation for inordinate edema formation and bleeding, proper immobilization, and splinting are performed. The schedule for dressing changes and the specific elements of wound care depend on the individual needs and circumstances of each patient.

PRESERVATION OF MOTION

Proper splinting and positioning of the hands must be initiated as quickly as possible after a burn injury to preserve motion. Elevation of the injured part to minimize edema formation cannot be overemphasized. Gentle, active range-of-motion exercises of the joints in the hand, wrist, elbow, and shoulder should be encouraged under the supervision of a hand therapist as soon as the grafts have taken. The hand should be splinted in the intrinsic-plus "position of safety" with the wrist in mild dorsiflexion, metacarpophalangeal (MCP) joints flexed (70 to 80 degrees), and the interphalangeal (IP) joints in extension. The thumb should be abducted and slightly circumducted into the palm. In situations in which deep burns overlie joints, minimal motion or immobilization in the safe position, either by splinting or internal fixation, should be considered to reduce the likelihood of joint exposure or extensor tendon rupture.[2,42,61,62]

Gentle, active range-of-motion exercises are usually initiated on the fifth or sixth day after excision. Active assisted and passive range of motion is initiated in a progressive and graded fashion. Long-term splinting and the employment of continuous passive motion machines may be helpful in achieving full motion (Figure 134-12).[61,62,82] Range of motion of all joints in the burned extremity should be measured and regularly documented. Failure to note substantive progress after the initiation of therapy should prompt careful reexamination of the grafts and reappraisal of the postoperative therapy program. The return of optimal hand function is a primary goal of treatment, but the final result will not become apparent immediately after wound closure because complete wound healing and scar softening and maturation require many months to reach completion. During this time, close supervision, scar compression with elastic gloves and sleeves, range-of-motion exercises, scar massage, and edema control are critical. The degree of functional recovery must be based on objective measurements and observation of the patient's ability to perform specific tasks. Functional capacity testing and work evaluation are frequently necessary to determine the degree and permanency of the disability. Recent data suggest that the use of a commercially available computer-assisted impairment evaluation system may provide a useful and accurate adjunct in the total rehabilitative process because of ease of operation, reproducibility, and reduced examination times. The implementation of a personalized, comprehensive, and closely supervised hand-therapy program is essential to maximize rehabilitation. The rehabilitation process is initiated shortly after the patient's admission and generally is not completed until many months, and in some cases years, after discharge.[68,83]

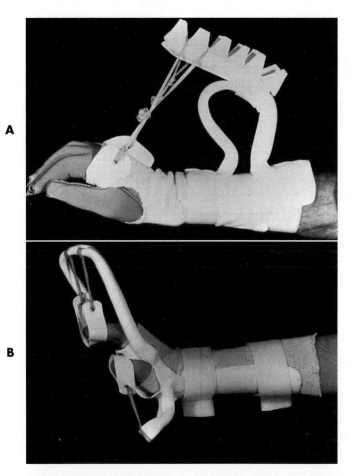

Figure 134-12. A, Dynamic traction appliance to improve wrist extension. **B,** Dynamic traction splinting for established flexion contractures of digits.

RECONSTRUCTION OF THE BURNED HAND

Reconstruction of the burned hand often presents a formidable challenge. The need for reconstruction is the result of several contributing factors acting independently or in concert. They include the severity of the initial injury; involvement of specific structures; adequacy of initial care; prior management of the burn wound, including operative treatment and postoperative care; the quality of hand therapy; and the motivation and reliability of the patient and caregivers. Reconstruction must often address established deformities and their functional consequences. The ultimate success or failure of reconstructive procedures also depends on all of these factors.

The global goals of reconstructive surgery are the restoration of form and function. In the hand, this translates into power, delicacy, mobility, dexterity, and tactile sensibility. The hand must operate in concert with the more proximal regions of the upper extremity; thus proximal defects must also be addressed and successfully managed to optimize hand function.

There is a broad spectrum of deformities and problems requiring reconstruction that vary in both preservation and severity (Box 134-8). Some can be corrected by straightforward methods, whereas others may defy satisfactory resolution. A

---

thoughtful, stepwise assessment of the deformities, the involvement of subjacent structures and tissues, and a thorough determination and documentation of function are necessary before any reconstructive effort. Photographic documentation, radiographs, neurologic and vascular studies, and range-of-motion measurements must be assessed before a plan for reconstruction can be initiated. A thorough and realistic discussion with the patient and his or her family members, employer, and, frequently, the insurance carrier is necessary. Once the deformities and functional deficiencies have been identified, a reconstructive plan can be outlined and refined.[73] The ability of the surgeon to correct the problem must be considered, and the wishes and priorities of both the patient and surgeon must be in accord.

A stable and durable skin cover is the first priority because this surface must be able to endure the functional demands of everyday life. Wounds that were permitted to heal spontaneously, or those treated by the application of thinly or widely meshed split-thickness skin grafts, may not be adequate to provide the required dorsal hand-skin coverage. These types of dorsal hand-skin covers are frequently subject to serious problems, including itching, contracture, and scar hypertrophy, along with repeated episodes of skin breakdown (Figure 134-13). In severe cases in which conservative therapy has proven inadequate, the requirements of durable and functional dorsal skin coverage are generally met by removal of the entire scar and inadequate skin grafts, release of contractures, and resurfacing of the entire area with full or thick split-thickness sheet grafts. Flap coverage may be necessary if there are exposed extensor tendons or joints present or when nerve or vascular reconstruction is required. The use of fascial or fasciocutaneous flaps, such as the radial forearm flap, lateral arm flap, or the temporalis fascia flap, provide excellent dorsal hand coverage and generally achieve the reconstructive goals. Fixed deformities of deep structures, both soft and hard, may require releases, bone fusions, amputations, transpositions, or grafts (Figure 134-14).*

Sheet graft coverage should be employed whenever possible. The grafts should be applied transversely, with the wrist in moderate flexion, the MCP joints at 90 degrees, and the IP joints in full extension. Motion is avoided for 5 to 7 days after surgery. Once initiated, it is generally accompanied by night splinting, active daytime therapy, and the use of compression

---

*References 7, 24, 25, 41, 45, 58, 70, 72, 77, 80.

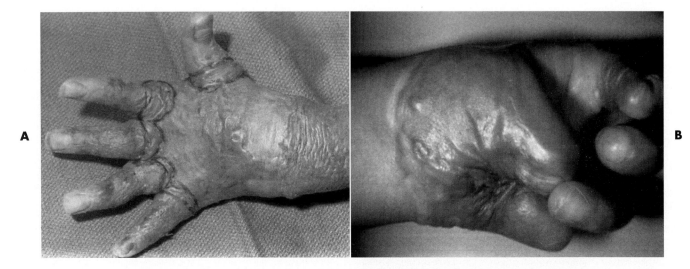

Figure 134-13. **A,** Hypertrophic scarring and dorsal burn-scar contracture after inadequate provision of skin and postoperative splinting. **B,** Severe palmar contracture after hand burn in a child.

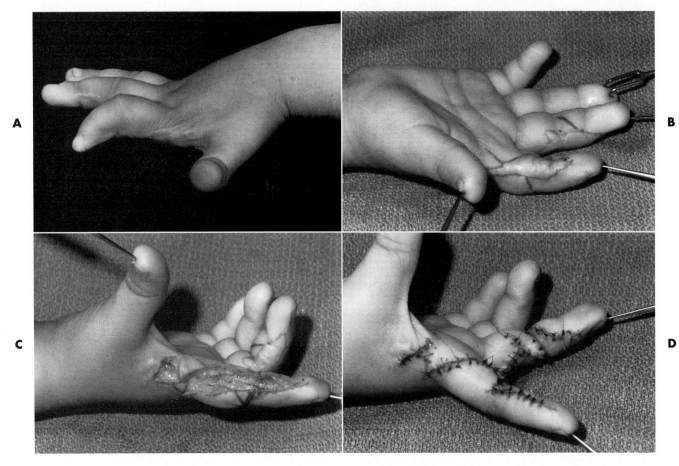

Figure 134-14. **A,** Contracture of index finger. **B,** Thick, contracted palmar scar of index and long fingers. **C,** After excision of restrictive scar. **D,** Z-plasty lengthening and wound closure.

garment therapy. Occasionally, the use of continuous passive motion therapy may be of significant value in achieving long-term success.[63,68]

The wide array of problems and the many techniques described to deal with them are beyond the scope of this chapter.

Nevertheless, a number of basic guidelines are applicable, including the following:

1. Adhere to the reconstructive ladder, from simple to more complex
2. Choose the best reconstruction for the patient

3. Plan alternatives and "second options" in advance
4. Review the options with the patient and permit the patient to participate in the decision-making process
5. Do not let personal bias or goals distort the objective
6. Amputation of a part may be a reasonable and necessary treatment option
7. The most simple solution may not be the best solution
8. Always be cognizant of the patient's needs in terms of the activities of daily living, occupation, and underlying psychological and psychosocial criteria

Peripheral compression neuropathies involving the median and ulnar nerves have been described in as many as 30% of burned patients. These problems occasionally resolve with conservative treatment. However, if there is no evidence of progressive resolution documented by appropriate neurologic studies, surgical decompression should be performed. Occasionally, cutaneous or digital neuromas may form after excision, grafting, or amputation and require treatment.[73]

The correction of burn syndactyly is most frequently accomplished by the use of local flaps, Z-plasties, skin grafts, or a combination of these modalities.[7,41] Nail-bed complications, which can be quite problematic, include deformities, grooving, and nonadherence. Concomitant bacterial or fungal infections are frequent, and dermatologic consultation is often needed to achieve resolution. Surgical approaches to nail-bed problems include obliteration, split-thickness skin grafts, split nail-bed grafts, and reverse dermal grafts, but these procedures should be not performed until 6 to 8 months after wound closure.[72,73]

The development of Volkmann's ischemic contracture after burn injury is rare because of increased awareness and improved monitoring techniques, but intrinsic muscle ischemia and fibrosis remain common sequelae in burned upper extremities despite the performance of surgical escharotomy. A postmortem study conducted by the U.S. Army Institute of Surgical Research showed ischemic intrinsic muscle necrosis in two thirds of patients with burned upper extremities thought to be adequately decompressed by surgical escharotomy. Direct intrinsic compartment measurement provides the only means to accurately assess intracompartmental pressure, but this evaluation is performed infrequently. Decompression of the intrinsic muscles is accomplished by incision of the investing fascia through dorsal incisions in the first web space and between the metacarpals.[42]

Tendon complications involving the extensor tendons are much more common than those involving flexor tendons. The most common extensor-tendon problems are tendon rupture or adhesion. Joint deformities frequently occur concomitant with the tendon problems, and successful reconstruction must address both problems in a single operative approach. This has prompted the use of a number of sophisticated and complex reconstructions, including reverse ulnar-artery island flaps, reverse dorsometacarpal flaps, distal radial-artery flaps, pedicled intercostal cutaneous perforator flaps, and composite tendinocutaneous flaps.*

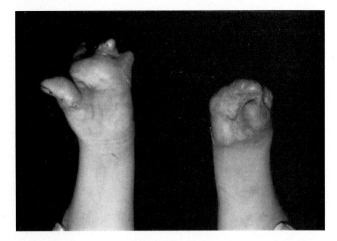

Figure 134-15. Bilateral "mitten-hand" deformities after burns of the hands.

Tenolysis is usually unsuccessful because the adhesions consist of burn scar, which encases the tendon throughout the entire extent of the healed burn wound. Good quality skin coverage is the essential prerequisite for successful tendon reconstruction.

Heterotopic ossification occurs in approximately 10% to 13% of patients who have sustained burns of the upper extremities. The most common site is the elbow, with posterior involvement more common in adults and anterior involvement more common in children.[16,42] Although paraarticular calcification occurs most often when the area surrounding the elbow has been burned, it may also occur when the burned area is at a distance from the elbow. Management depends on early recognition of this entity, although radiographic changes may not appear until 6 to 10 weeks after the burn injury.[16,42] It is interesting to note that once the burn wound has healed and the patient has recovered, the ability to form this ectopic bone vanishes.

Complex, challenging reconstructions are necessary in those situations in which the burn injury and subsequent treatment resulted in loss of part or all of the digits and/or thumb. These may include metacarpal stacking, advancement pollicization, creation of a web space, flap resurfacing, or microvascular toe-to-thumb or toe-to-finger transfer (Figure 134-15).[73]

The application of moisturizing agents to a scarred or grafted area helps to control dryness, itching, and fissure formation, thereby improving patient comfort, skin pliability, and, ultimately, function. The use of splints, pressure garments, custom inserts, or silicone gel sheeting may also help minimize the frequency or severity of scar formation and its sequelae. Inclusion of intermittent mechanical compression therapy in the rehabilitative regimen of patients suffering from chronic recalcitrant edema of the upper extremity after burn injury and its subsequent treatment can provide variable degrees of benefit (Figure 134-16).*

*References 24, 45, 58, 73, 77, 80.

*References 2, 17, 19, 60, 61, 82, 83.

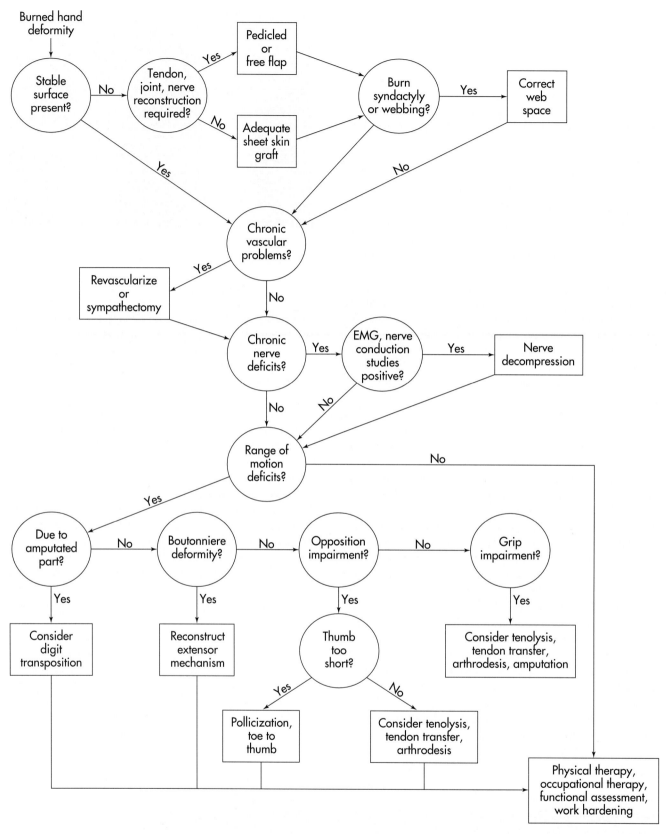

Figure 134-16. Algorithm for reconstruction of the burned hand. (From Strock LL, McCauley RL, Smith, DJ, Robson MC: Reconstruction of the burned hand. In Herndon DN [editor]: *Total burn care*, Philadelphia, 1996, WB Saunders.)

OUTCOMES

The major complications associated with excisional surgery can be assigned to one of two categories: systemic or local. Systemic complications involve major organ systems and include coagulopathy, fluid and electrolyte disturbances, acid-base derangements, respiratory failure, pneumonia, atelectasis, sepsis, cardiac dysfunction, or renal, neurologic, and endocrine disorders. Local complications consist primarily of wound-related problems, such as graft disruption and loss, unrecognized hematoma or postoperative bleeding from the operated sites, infections, and donor-site complications. Successful management, as with all complications, is more likely if these problems are recognized early and managed promptly.

Most burn patients do not suffer from life-threatening injuries. The average burn size of patients treated in burn centers in the United States is less than 20% of the total body surface area, and survival rates approach 98%. Death in these patients is predominantly caused by inhalation injury and its complications or comorbid factors such as advanced age and accompanying age-related systemic diseases. Ample donor sites are present in the vast majority of these patients, which permits one-stage wound debridement and definitive closure. Few patients in this group suffer from physiologic derangements of sufficient magnitude to prohibit early operative treatment. Therefore delay in treating these patients is generally unlikely, and patients suffering from such relatively limited injuries should undergo surgical excision and skin grafting within a few days of the injury. Skin graft "take" is normally excellent, resulting in prompt, uncomplicated wound closure that is achieved by one or, in rare instances, two surgical procedures. This translates into a significant reduction in pain, shortened hospitalization, diminished cost of treatment, and a more rapid initiation of motion and functional rehabilitation.

Does complete early surgical wound closure in patients with burned hands, in whom survival is not an issue and a protracted effort to save the patient's life does not interfere with the initiation of early rehabilitation, produce superior cosmetic and functional results when compared with similar wounds in which wound closure may be delayed for 2 weeks or more? Prospective randomized studies have shown no significant long-term difference in function when aggressive hand therapy was initiated and continued in wounds allowed to heal spontaneously, despite healing times approaching 30 days. However, the two key variables—quality and duration of therapy—are pivotal to the outcome. The success in such a regimen is therefore invariably dependent on the availability and quality of therapy. More commonly, however, this degree of hand therapy may not be provided with the same dedication and commitment as occurs when this activity is the integral part of an ongoing study. Furthermore, these studies were performed long before the era of managed care and the clear delineation and acceptance of early excision and grafting as a viable treatment modality. There is now ample evidence that early excision, when performed by an experienced surgeon, is a safe and effective procedure that does in fact reduce hospitalization when performed in patients suffering from less than 25% total body surface area burns, and this procedure should be recommended to patients. Prompt excision and autografting favorably influence the quality of the cosmetic result by greatly shortening the inflammatory and fibroplastic phases of wound healing. The grafted skin is more supple and more durable than a thin epidermal covering resulting from spontaneous healing in deep dermal burns. Although hypertrophic scarring cannot be completely eliminated after excision and grafting, it is far more likely to occur only along the edges of the skin grafts where they abut each other or at the unburned or spontaneously healed wound edges. This problem is far less pronounced and more easily managed than a thick, nonyielding cicatrix, which is common after spontaneous healing of a deep dermal upper-extremity burn.[17,18,19,23,31]

It is also evident that as the area of the total body surface that is burned increases, the advantages attributed to early excision progressively diminish, including cost reduction and length of hospitalization. Factors other than the burn wound itself invariably influence the type, duration, and ultimately the cost of treatment. Staged surgical wound excision and closure are required, and the initiation of treatment may be delayed beyond the first 3 to 5 days because of physiologic abnormalities that may make surgical intervention dangerous or impossible. Early total excision within 24 to 48 hours of injury has been effectively abandoned. The notion that elimination of the burn wound in the immediate post-burn period would yield significant improvement in survival and hasten recovery has not come to fruition.

A recent retrospective analysis of 1047 acute hand burns in which the treatment plan emphasized prompt sheet autograft wound closure, the selective use of axial pin fixation and flap reconstruction, and aggressive splinting and range-of-motion exercises, reported normal function in 97% of those patients with superficial injuries and 81% of patients with deep dermal and full-thickness injuries requiring surgery. However, only 9% of individuals with injuries involving the extensor mechanism, joint capsule, or bone had normal hand function, although 90% of these patients were able to independently perform activities of daily living.[68] Another study that evaluated outcomes of 35 fourth-degree hand burns in 25 patients demonstrated the importance and utility of flap reconstruction in the management of these devastating injuries when compared with patients treated with delayed closure employing prolonged immobilization and delayed autografting.[56]

Innovative and aggressive hand therapy and rehabilitation have proven to be extraordinarily important components in the overall management of burned hands. The dedicated and frequently novel approaches to the functional rehabilitation of patients with burns in general, and hand burns in particular, have contributed greatly to improved outcomes. The application of various techniques in this era of cost-containment, such as out-patient grafting of hand burns and Unna's bandage application, continually challenges all members of the burn-care team to strive for excellence in results despite the fiscal and administrative obstacles that may confront them.

Substantial progress has been made in the care of burned patients over the last half-century. This progress is the result of the synergy between basic science investigation, technologic innovation, and the insatiable desire on the part of caregivers of burn patients to improve the lot of their charges. Further improvements in the care of the burn patient will undoubtedly continue, but perhaps more slowly than in the recent past. These advances will most likely occur as a result of the improved treatment of pulmonary injury, pulmonary failure, and improved wound coverage materials. These advances will come at a high cost, but will society be willing to underwrite this cost? Burn reconstruction and functional preservation and rehabilitation, which have received less attention than acute care issues, will undoubtedly come to the forefront of burn research and clinical application because they offer a genuine hope for a significant improvement in the quality of burn victims' lives.

Surgical treatment of the burn wound is an early and important step in the continuum of care that is required to achieve timely coverage of the burn wound, minimize morbidity, and achieve an optimal functional outcome. It is an essential component of modern burn care that has as its ultimate goal the return of the patient to a fulfilling, unimpeded, and productive life.

REFERENCES

1. American Burn Association: Guidelines for service standards and severity classifications in the treatment of burn injury, *American College of Surgeons Bulletin* 69:10, 1984.
2. Ause Elias KL, Richard R, Millerm SF, Finley RK: The effect of mechanical compression on chronic hand edema after burn injury: a preliminary report, *J Burn Care Rehabil* 15(1):29-33, 1994.
3. Burke JF: Observations on the development of an artificial skin: presidential address, 1982 American Burn Association Meeting, *J Trauma* 23:543-551, 1983.
4. Burke JF, Bondoc CC, Quimby WC: Primary burn excision and immediate grafting: a method shortening illness, *J Trauma* 14(5):389-395, 1974.
5. Burke JF, Quimby WC, Bondoc CC: Primary excision and prompt grafting as routine therapy for the treatment of thermal burns in children, *Surg Clin North Am* 56:477-494, 1976.
6. Carucci DJ, Pearce SC, Innes DJ, et al: Evaluation of hemostatic agents for skin graft donor sites, *J Burn Care Rehabil* 5:321-323, 1984.
7. Chang LY: Reverse dorsometacarpal flap in digits and web-space reconstruction, *Ann Plast Surg* 33(3):281-289, 1994.
8. Cullen JJ, Murray DJ, Kealey GP: Changes in coagulation factors in patients with burns during acute blood loss, *J Burn Care Rehabil* 10:517-522, 1989.
9. Deitch EA: A policy of early excision and grafting in elderly burn patients shortens the hospital stay and improves survival, *Burns* 12:109-114, 1985.
10. Deitch EA, Clothier J: Burns in the elderly: an early surgical approach, *J Trauma* 23:891-894, 1983.
11. Demling RH: Improved survival after massive burns, *J Trauma* 23:179-183, 1983.
12. Demling RH: Effect of early burn excision and grafting on pulmonary function, *J Trauma* 24:830-834, 1984.
13. Desai MH, Herndon DN, Broemeling L, et al: Early burn wound excision significantly reduces blood loss, *Ann Surg* 211:753-762, 1990.
14. Donoff RB, Burke JF, Altobelli DE, et al: Excision of burns of the face, *Plast Reconstr Surg* 77:744-751, 1986.
15. Drueck C: Emergency department treatment of hand burns, *Emerg Med Clin North Am* 11(3):797-809, 1993.
16. Edlich RF, Horowitz JH, Rheubanks H, et al: Heterotopic calcification and ossification in burn patients, *J Burn Care Rehabil* 6:363-368, 1985.
17. Edstrom LE, Robson MC, Macchiaverna JR, Scala AD: Management of deep partial thickness dorsal hand burns, *Orthop Review* 8:27-33, 1979.
18. Edstrom LE, Robson MC, Macchiaverna JR, Scala AD: Prospective randomized treatments for burned hands: nonoperative vs. operative, *Scand J Plast Reconstr Surg* 13(1):131-135, 1979.
19. Engrav LH, Heimbach DM, Reus JL, et al: Early excision and grafting vs. nonoperative treatment of burns of indeterminate depth: a randomized prospective study, *J Trauma* 23:1001-1004, 1983.
20. Foy HM, Pavlin ED, Heimbach DM: Excision and grafting of large burns: operation length not related to increased morbidity, *J Trauma* 26:51-53, 1986.
21. Gallico GG, Compton CC, O'Connor NE: New approaches to skin coverage. In Morris PJ, Tilner NJ (editors): *Progress in transplantation,* vol 2, London, 1985, Churchill Livingstone.
22. Gonzalez R, Heiss WH, Viebeck B: Twelve years' experience with the abrasion method for the management of burn wounds in children, *J Ped Surg* 21:200-201, 1986.
23. Goodwin CW, Maguire MS, McManus WF, Pruitt BA: Prospective study of burn wound excision of the hands, *J Trauma* 23:510-517, 1983.
24. Grobbelaar AO, Harrison DH: The distally based ulnar artery island flap in hand reconstruction, *J Hand Surg [Br]* 1997; 22(2): 204-211, 1997.
25. Hallock GG: Homodigital flaps: especially for treatment of the burned hand, *J Burn Care Rehabil* 16(5):503-507, 1995.
26. Hansborough JF: *Wound coverage with biologic dressings and skin substitutes,* Austin, Texas, 1992, RG Lendes, pp 13-115.
27. Hara M, Peters WJ, Douglas LG, Morris SF: An early surgical approach to burns in the elderly, *J Trauma* 30:430-432, 1990.
28. Heck EL, Bergstresser PR, Baxter CR: Composite skin graft: frozen dermal allografts support the engraftment and expansion of autologous epidermis, *J Trauma* 25:106-112, 1985.
29. Heggers JP, Ko F, Robson MC, et al: Evaluation of burn blister fluid, *Plast Reconstr Surg* 65:798-803, 1980.
30. Heimbach DM: Early burn excision and grafting, *Surg Clin North Am* 67:93-107, 1987.

31. Heimbach DM, Engrav LH: *Surgical management of the burn wound,* New York, 1984, Raven Press, pp 146-152.

32. Heimbach DM, Luterman A, Burke J, et al: Artificial dermis for major burns, *Ann Surg* 208:313-320, 1988.

33. Herndon DN, Parks DH: Comparison of serial debridement and autografting and early massive excision with cadaver skin overlay in the treatment of large burns in children, *J Trauma* 26:149-152, 1986.

34. Herndon DN, Rutan RL: Comparison of cultured epidermal autograft and massive excision with serial autografting plus homograft overly, *J Burn Care Rehabil* 13:154-157, 1992.

35. Herndon DN, Rutan RL: Use of dermal templates and cultured cells for permanent skin replacement, *Wounds* 4:50-53, 1992.

36. Jaksic T, Burke JF: The use of artificial skin for burns, *Annu Rev Med* 38:107-117, 1987.

37. Janzekovic Z: The burn wound from the surgical point of view, *J Trauma* 15:42-61, 1975.

38. Jostkleigrewe F, Brandt KA, Flechsig G, et al: Treatment of partial thickness burns of the hand with the preshaped, semipermeable Procel Burn Cover, *Burns* 21(4):297-300, 1995.

39. Kneafsey B, O'Shaughnessy M, Condon KC: The use of calcium alginate dressings in deep hand burns, *Burns* 22(11):40-43, 1996.

40. Krizek TJ, Flagg SV, Wolfort FG, Jabaley ME: Delayed primary excision and skin grafting of the burned hand, *Plast Reconstr Surg* 51:524-529, 1973.

41. Krizek TJ, Robson MC, Flagg SV: Management of burn syndactyly, *J Trauma* 14:587-593, 1974.

42. Kucan JO: Burn injuries. In Manske PR (editor): *Hand surgery update,* Englewood, Colo, 1994, American Society for Surgery of the Hand, pp 42(1)-42(7).

43. Kucan JO, Smoot EC: Five percent mafenide acetate solution in the treatment of thermal injuries, *J Burn Care Rehabil* 14:158-163, 1993.

44. Lattari V, Jones LM, Varcelotti JR, et al: The use of permanent dermal allograft in full-thickness burns of the hand and foot: a report of three cases, *J Burn Care Rehabil* 18(2):147-155, 1997.

45. Lee KS, Park SW, Kim HY: Tendinocutaneous free flap transfer from the dorsum of the foot, *Microsurg* 15(12):882-885, 1994.

46. Levine BA, Sirinek KF, Peterson HD, Pruitt BA: Efficacy of tangential excision and immediate grafting of deep second degree burns of the hand, *J Trauma* 9:670-673, 1979.

47. McHugh TP, Robson MC, Heggers JP, et al: Therapeutic efficacy of Biobrane in partial and full thickness thermal injury, *Surgery* 100:661-664, 1986.

48. McManus WF, Mason AD, Pruitt BA: Excision of the burn wound in patients with large burns, *Arch Surg* 124:718-720, 1989.

49. Monafo WW, Bessey PQ: Benefits and limitations of burn wound excision, *World J Surg* 16:37-42, 1992.

50. Monafo WW, West MA: Current treatment recommendations for topical burn therapy, *Drugs* 40:364-373, 1990.

51. Moncrief JA: The treatment of hand burns, *Mil Med* 128:50, 1963.

52. Muller MJ, Nicolai M, Wiggins R, et al: Modern treatment of a burn wound. In Herndon D (editor): *Total burn care,* Philadelphia, 1996, WB Saunders.

53. Munster AM, Smith-Meek M, Sharkey P: The effect of early surgical intervention on mortality and cost-effectiveness in burn care, 1978-1991, *Burns* 20:61-64, 1994.

54. Munster AM, Weiner SH, Spence RJ: Cultured epidermis for the coverage of massive burn wounds: a single center experience, *Ann Surg* 211:676-680, 1990.

55. Murphy GF, Orgill DP, Hancock WW, et al: Morphological reconstitution of the skin by use of biodegradable polymeric graft, *Lab Invest* 54:45, 1986.

56. Nuchtern JG, Engrav LH, Nakamura DY, et al: Treatment of fourth degree hand burns, *J Burn Care Rehabil* 16:36-42, 1995.

57. O'Connor NE, Gallico GG, Compton CC: The role of tissue cultured epithelial cells in acute burn care, *Proc American Burn Assoc* 18:164, 1985.

58. Onishi K, Maruyama Y, Yoshitake H: Transversely designed dorsal metacarpal v-y advancement flaps for dorsal hand reconstruction, *Br J Plast Surg* 49(3):165-169, 1996.

59. Pietsch JB, Netscher DT, Nagaraj HS: Early excision of major burns in children: effect on morbidity and mortality, *J Pediatr Surg* 20:754-757, 1985.

60. Pruitt BA, McManus AT: The changing epidemiology of infection in burn patients, *World J Surg* 16:57-67, 1992.

61. Richard R, Schall S, Staley M, Miller S: Hand burn splint fabrication: correction for bandage thickness, *J Burn Care Rehabil* 15(4):369-371, 1994.

62. Richard R, Staley M, Daugherty MB, et al: The wide variety of designs for dorsal hand burn splints, *J Burn Care Rehabil* 15(3):275-280, 1994.

63. Robson MC, Smith DJ, Vander Zee AJ: Making the burned hand functional, *Clin Plast Surg* 19(3):663-671, 1992.

64. Saffle JR, Larson CM, Sullivan J, Shelby J: The continuing challenge of burn care in the elderly, *Surgery* 108:534-543, 1990.

65. Salisbury RE, Levine NS: The early management of upper extremity thermal injury. In Salisbury RE (editor): *Burns of the upper extremity,* Philadelphia, 1976, WB Saunders.

66. Sanford S, Gore D: Unna's boot dressings facilitate outpatient skin grafting of the hands, *J Burn Care Rehabil* 17(4):323-326, 1996.

67. Schwanholt C, Greenhalgh DG, Warden GD: A comparison of full thickness versus split thickness autografts for the coverage of deep palm burns in the very young pediatric patient, *J Burn Care Rehabil* 14(1):29-33, 1993.

68. Sheridan RL, Hurley J, Smith MA, et al: The acutely burned hand: management and outcome based on a ten year experience with 1047 acute hand burns, *J Trauma* 38(3):406-411, 1995.

69. Sherman ST, Demling RH, Lalonde C, et al: Growth hormone enhances re-epithelialization of human split thickness skin graft donor sites, *Surg Forum* 40:37-39, 1989.

70. Simpson RL, Flaherty ME: The burned small finger, *Burn Rehab Reconstr* 19:673-682, 1992.

71. Smith DJ, McHugh TP, Phillips LG, et al: Biosynthetic compound dressings-management of hand burns, *Burns* 14:405-408, 1988.

72. Stern PJ, Neale HW, Graham TJ, Warden GD: Classification and treatment of postburn proximal interphalangeal joint flexion contractures in children, *J Hand Surg [Am]* 12:450-453, 1987.

73. Strock LL, McCauley RL, Smith DJ, Robson MC: Reconstruction of the burned hand. In Herndon DN (editor): *Total burn care,* Philadelphia, 1996, WB Saunders.

74. Terrill PJ, Kedwards SM, Lawrence JC: The use of GORE-TEX bags for hand burns, *Burns* 17:161-165, 1991.

75. Thompson P, Herndon DN, Abston S: Effect of early excision on patients with major thermal injury, *J Trauma* 27:205-207, 1987.

76. Tompkins RG, Burke JF, Schoenfeld EA, et al: Prompt eschar excision: a treatment system contributing to reduce burn mortality, *Ann Surg* 204:272-282, 1986.

77. Upton J, Rogers C, Durham-Smith G, Swartz WM: Clinical applications of free temporoparietal flaps in hand reconstruction, *J Hand Surg [Am]* 11:475-483, 1986.

78. Ward RS, Reddy R, Brockway C, et al: Uses of Coban self-adherent wrap in management of postburn hand grafts: case reports, *J Burn Care Rehabil* 15(4):364-369, 1994.

79. Watson SB, Miller JG: Optimizing skin graft take in children's hand burns: the use of silastic foam dressings, *Burns* 19(6):519-521, 1993.

80. Weinzweig N, Chen L, Chen ZW: The distally based radial forearm fasciosubcutaneous flap with preservation of the radial artery: an anatomic and clinical approach, *Plast Reconstr Surg* 94(5):675-684, 1994.

81. Yahnas IV: What criteria should be used for designing artificial skin replacements and how well do the current grafting materials meet these criteria? *J Trauma* 24:S29-S39, 1984.

82. Yotsuyanagi T, Yokoi K, Omizo M: A simple and compressive splint for palmar skin grafting in young children with burns, *Burns* 20(1):55-57, 1994.

83. Zeller J, Sturm G, Cruse CW: Patients with burns are successful in work hardening programs, *J Burn Care Rehabil* 14:189-196, 1993.

CHAPTER 135

Frostbite

Nicole Zook Sommer

INTRODUCTION

The peril of nature's cold elements on the ill-prepared and unsheltered have been well documented throughout history. The majority of cold-weather injuries in modern times have been recorded during military campaigns. Improper clothing, poor hygiene, insufficient shelter and training, and limited access to health care while on duty condemned a multitude of ground soldiers to the often fatal or mutilating consequences of cold injury.

The writings of Baron Larrey, General Surgeon-in-Chief of the Napoleon Grand Army, are particularly well known for their detailed description of frostbite injury. In 1812 Napoleon set out with 385,000 French Grand Alliance soldiers for Russia. The troops were drawn deep into the Russian countryside as the Russian soldiers retreated. Three thousand French soldiers survived the first winter to subsequently retreat back to France, a journey only approximately 300 would eventually survive.[13,39]

Many ground troops were lost during World War I to the sequelae of cold injury.Similarly, the consequences of cold exposure in World War II and the Korean Conflict accounted for 10% of the total casualties.[13] American soldiers suffered 55,000 cold injuries in World War II and 8000 in Korea. World War II pilots were exposed to high-altitude frostbite injury, which caused a rapid tissue freezing different from the usual slow freeze experienced by ground troops.[13] Today, civilian frostbite injuries are often reported during inclement weather or major disasters.

Cold injury has varying manifestations depending on the temperature, environment, and type and duration of exposure. Systemic cold injury, known as *hypothermia,* is defined as a body temperature significantly below 98.6° F (37° C) and is classified as mild, moderate, and severe. Localized cold injury has been divided into four categories: trench foot, frostnip, chilblains, and frostbite. *Trench foot,* also called *cold immersion foot,* occurs after prolonged exposure, usually lasting several days, to wet, cool conditions at approximately 1° to 10° C (35° to 50° F) without actual tissue freezing. This condition was seen in military ground troops forced to spend days in deep trenches with their feet immersed in cold puddles and mud.[19,39,43] Trench-foot injury causes painful and erythematous extremities that later turn pale and edematous, often developing blisters. *Frostnip* is a mild cold injury that presents as blanched, numb skin. This is often seen in individuals exposed to cold, fast-moving air.[39] *Chilblains* is a severe, nonfreezing injury found commonly on the dorsum of the fingers, toes, heels, nose, and ears. It is associated with above-freezing temperatures accompanied by high humidity. Common symptoms include erythema, pruritus, and causalgia. The natural history of trench foot, frostnip, and chilblain injuries is, for the most part, uneventful, expectant healing.

Frostbite injury results in local tissue destruction after exposure to extreme cold, commonly in tissues with low blood flow or in exposed areas of skin that are unprotected. Frostbite has a greater morbidity and mortality than a nonfreezing cold injury such as trench foot because of the severity of the injury, the increased risk of general hypothermia, and the overall increase in tissue loss.[13] Frostbite injury has been compared with that of thermal injury in developing Jackson's three zones of tissue injury.[29] Immediately after injury there is a central zone of coagulation representing irreversible cell death. Surrounding this area is the zone of stasis, which may progress to coagulation and cell death secondary to vessel thrombosis, or may resolve with cell survival. The microcirculation in this area is initially open after rewarming but may gradually become occluded and collapse. The third and outermost area of injury is termed the *zone of hyperemia,* in which spontaneous recovery of the tissue will occur in less than 10 days.[17,29]

Tissues most often injured by frostbite include, in descending order, toes, fingers, the tip of the nose, and the ears.[12] The middle finger and thumb often escape the worst injury because of their protection by the other digits. The thumb is protected by the thenar muscles and its proximity to the radial artery. Feet are more frequently injured than hands, often bilaterally. Various tissues within the extremities are affected to different degrees by cold injury. The least cold-sensitive tissues in decreasing order include ligaments, tendons, bone, and cartilage. The most cold-sensitive tissue is bone marrow, followed by nerve and muscle. Blood vessels and skin appear to fall somewhere in between.[36] Fortunately, a large majority of cold injuries are of a superficial nature, with skin the only tissue injured. Skin acts as a protective barrier by shielding the deeper structures from cold injury. Bone and cartilage are spared unless injury is of a severe degree or duration.

Boswick[5] described the epidemiology of cold injuries in a study of 843 civilian patients seen over a 10-year period. The patients ranged from 1 to 93 years of age, and 76% of the injuries occurred in patients between 30 to 60 years old. There appeared to be a 1:1 male to female ratio. Injury to the lower extremity was more common than the upper extremity, and 44% of lower-extremity injures were bilateral. Approximately 10% of the patients experienced upper- and lower-extremity injury. Eighty percent of injured children suffer from upper-extremity injuries in a bilateral glovelike pattern. Children wearing gloves sustained a cold injury only to the lower extremity. The severity of injury was less in children than adults. Greater than 50% of the patients studied were under the influence of alcohol at the time of cold injury. Forty percent required surgical debridement and/or amputation, and 20% needed a second procedure.[5]

INDICATIONS

ETIOLOGY

Multiple factors determine an individual's susceptibility to cold injury. The major factors include the absolute ambient temperature, duration of cold exposure, wind velocity, moist/wet conditions, immobility, lack of proper clothing, and impaired mental status.[42]

The human body is much better designed for losing heat, by way of sweat glands, breathing, and peripheral vasodilation, than for conserving it. Thermoregulation of the body is controlled by the hypothalamus, which during times of cold attempts to maintain the core temperature at the expense of the periphery. The body's response to cold is dependent on the heat produced as a result of metabolism and muscle function and the heat lost by convection, conduction, and evaporation, which together account for 90% of total heat loss.[1,13,42]

Environmental factors play an important role in frostbite injury. Wind promotes body-heat loss by increasing convection, which decreases skin-surface temperature (Figure 135-1). Wind may in fact have such a cooling effect on the skin that it may freeze even though the ambient temperature is above 0° C. Frostbite injury usually occurs over hours, but this time can be greatly reduced when the wind velocity is increased. Extremities can sustain freezing injury in 1 hour under conditions of 0° F with a 10-mph wind exposure, whereas only 10 minutes of exposure is required to cause injury when the wind velocity increases to 40 mph.[16] Robson and Smith[42] give another example of the major effect wind velocity has on injury. "The chilling effect of a +20° F temperature combined with a 45 mile/hour wind is identical to that of a −40° F temperature coupled with a 2 mile/hour breeze." Wind exposure also affects a moving body, such as a downhill skier or snowmobiler, subjecting the individual to the same heat loss as a high-velocity wind.[39]

Humidity and wetness increase the risk of frostbite injury. Wet clothing in contact with skin conducts heat away from the body.[19] Wet skin freezes at an environmental

Estimated wind speed (mph)	Actual Thermometer Reading (°F)											
	50	40	30	20	10	0	−10	−20	−30	−40	−50	−60
	Equivalent temperature (°F)											
Calm	50	40	30	20	10	0	−10	−20	−30	−40	−50	−60
5	48	37	27	16	6	−5	−15	−26	−36	−47	−57	−68
10	40	28	16	4	−9	−24	−33	−46	−58	−70	−83	−95
15	36	22	9	−5	−18	−32	−45	−58	−72	−85	−99	−112
20	32	18	4	−10	−25	−39	−53	−67	−82	−96	−110	−124
25	30	16	0	−15	−29	−44	−59	−74	−88	−104	−118	−133
30	28	13	−2	−18	−33	−48	−63	−79	−94	−109	−125	−140
35	27	11	−4	−21	−35	−51	−67	−82	−98	−113	−129	−145
40	26	10	−6	−21	−37	−53	−69	−85	−100	−116	−132	−148
(Wind speeds greater than 40 mph have little additional effect)	**Little danger** (for properly clothed person) Maximum danger of false sense of security			**Increasing danger** Danger from freezing of exposed flesh			**Great danger**					
	Trenchfoot and immersion foot may occur at any point on this chart											

Figure 135-1. Wind chill factor index. (From Gamble WB: Perspectives in frostbite and cold weather injures. In Habal MB [editor]: *Advances in plastic and reconstructive surgery*, vol 10, St. Louis, 1994, Mosby.)

temperature of 2° C compared with dry skin, which freezes at temperatures of −5° to −10° C. A body immersed in water loses approximately 25 times more heat than a body in air.[11]

Cold objects in contact with bare skin, such as metal, glass or cold packs, can rapidly conduct heat away from tissue, leading to frostbite injury. This conduction of heat away from tissue is even more pronounced when the cold object is wet. Liquefied gas, including propane, butane, and freon, may produce extensive subcutaneous fat and muscle injury in as little as 60 seconds.[39]

Mobility generates heat, which protects the body against cooling. Immobilization, especially in the hands and extremities, leads to loss of this protective mechanism and greater injury.[42] This is often seen in the elderly and patients with neurologic disorders. However, overexertion can also increase heat loss through exhalation of warm air from the lungs and evaporation of heat from the skin surface in the form of perspiration.

Inadequate protective clothing often increases the risk of frostbite. Clothing protects the body from environmental factors and conserves heat by minimizing the radiation of body heat into the environment. Mittens, for example, decrease the total body surface area exposed to circulating air and therefore decrease heat loss as compared with gloves, which increase the amount of circulating air between the fingers. Constrictive clothing however, such as tight gloves, leads to decreased peripheral blood flow, loss of air insulation, and rapid cooling.[42]

One of the most important factors determining an individual's susceptibility to frostbite injury is an altered mental state.[20] Impaired cerebral function is the major predisposing factor in civilian frostbite injury because it impedes our primary defense, the decision to seek shelter. It is an all too common story that loss of one's senses leads to frostbite injury, secondary to a decrease in the individual's awareness of a cold weather environment. Mental incapacitation is most often the result of alcohol or drug use, but it may also be caused by psychoses, senility, confusion, and fatigue.

In addition to the effect on mental capacity, alcohol causes peripheral vasodilation, which increases blood flow to the body surface and gives a false sense of warmth when, in reality, the body is undergoing accelerated cooling.[42] Alcohol hastens the development of hypothermia and acts as a diuretic, effectively dehydrating the individual, which increases blood viscosity while decreasing tissue perfusion.[13]

High altitudes also increase the extent of injury by reducing plasma volume and decreasing the partial pressure of oxygen, leading to hypoxemia. The type of frostbite experienced by World War II pilots and by mountain climbers can occur quickly in environmental temperatures below 0° F with very-high-velocity winds. These conditions result in an instantaneous, deep freeze injury.

Smoking increases a person's susceptibility to cold injury because of the vasoconstricting effects of nicotine and a decrease in oxygen binding caused by carbon monoxide. Risk of frostbite injury also increases with previous frostbite injury and the presence of other disease states, such as peripheral vascular disease, scleroderma, or malnutrition.[19]

Susceptibility to injury is believed to decrease as a person becomes acclimated to cold environments. Risk appears to be lower in individuals born in the north compared with those from the south. Eskimos, for instance, appear to maintain warmer extremity temperatures than Caucasians and Orientals.[39] It is hypothesized that acclimated individuals are able to closely monitor their peripheral temperature and more economically distribute heat.[21]

Race may also be a factor determining susceptibility to cold injury. Studies done on military personnel have shown blacks appear to have a 2.8 to 6 times greater risk of cold injury than Caucasians.[13] It is hypothesized that blacks fail to increase heat production as markedly as Caucasians as a result of a difference in the cutaneous vascular shunting mechanism.[47]

Tissue injury in frostbite can be attributed to two mechanisms, direct cellular damage secondary to ice-crystal formation and indirect cell damage secondary to vascular compromise, ischemia, and necrosis.[42,52] The causative mechanism most important in cold injuries remains controversial. Is it the direct cellular injury when the tissue freezes or the indirect microcirculatory injury during reperfusion that plays a larger role in frostbite injury? Simply stated, does tissue freezing or thawing play a greater role in the ultimate tissue damage? The answer to this question is necessary to determine the degree to which frostbite injury is reversible and therefore the degree to which treatment modalities may potentially alter the course of tissue damage. Weatherly-White et al[50] supported the theory of reversible injury with transplantation of a full-thickness skin graft from a frostbitten ear to an uninjured site.[42,50] The graft survived on the new site in contrast to a graft from an uninjured ear transplanted to a frostbitten recipient bed that did not survive. The authors concluded that vascular compromise plays a significant role in frostbite injury. A progressive tissue-damage theory was supported by Gage,[12] who stated that even with extensive ice-crystal formation, tissue can recover from borderline injury if given an adequate blood supply. Both studies support the existence of a reversible component of frostbite injury and therefore the potential to halt the progression of tissue damage if blood flow can be restored. Correction of the vascular compromise component of frostbite injury has become the cornerstone for proposed treatment.

The development of frostbite injury is a complicated and detailed process. Cold exposure leads to peripheral cooling, which activates the hypothalamic thermoregulatory response, causing release of catecholamines and subsequent vasoconstriction of the periphery to conserve core body temperature. Oxidative processes are increased, converting more glycogen to glucose and providing energy for muscular shivering, which in turn produces more heat. When glycogen is depleted from the liver, shivering becomes the rate-limiting step in the thermoregulatory process.

Regulation of body temperature is dependent on the extremities, which encompass 50% of the total body surface area. The skin of the extremities contains numerous arteriovenous anastomoses, which by shunting blood flow (100 ml/min) can dissipate heat during exertion or warm the extremity during cold exposure. If an individual remains in positive heat balance during cold exposure, the "hunting response" described by Sir Thomas Lewis, also known as *cold-induced vasodilation,* acts to warm the periphery.[13] This physiologic survival mechanism allows for transient extremity vasodilation alternating with periods of vasoconstriction in 5- to 10-minute cycles in which arteriovenous channels found in fingertips, toes, ears, and the nose open and close, attempting to rewarm the cooled part while decreasing the core temperature. Once the body reaches a negative heat balance and the core temperature becomes compromised, the hunting response ceases and extremity arteriovenous anastomoses close to minimize peripheral heat loss until the body is rewarmed.[13] Peripheral vasoconstriction causes local tissue temperatures to drop to the tissue-freezing point of −2° C.[7] As the tissue freezes, circulation slows and eventually ceases. This cooling of tissue by the closing of arteriovenous shunts as the body reaches a negative heat balance represents the first phase of frostbite injury.

The second phase of cold injury is direct cellular trauma by freezing. The degree of cellular damage depends on the final freezing temperature reached, the rate of cooling and rewarming, and the duration of exposure to freezing temperatures. During tissue freezing, ice crystals that form may be intracellular or extracellular, depending on the rate of cooling. Rapid cooling produces intracellular ice crystals, which for the most part are lethal to cell membranes. The one exception is the formation of very small intracellular ice crystals as seen with supercooling for cell preservation systems, which does not damage the cells. Slow cooling, as seen in clinical frostbite, results in extracellular ice crystal formation. This leads to the development of an osmotic gradient. Water is pulled from the intracellular space, increasing extracellular volume. Extracellular crystals slowly enlarge, with the incorporation of available free water producing a hyperosmolar environment with hypertonic cells.[13,28] Cell dehydration leads to disruption of electrolyte balance, denaturation of lipid-protein complexes, intracellular enzyme instability, cell membrane damage, and eventual cell death (Figure 135-2).[6,28,31,52] Direct freezing is responsible for the initial separation of vascular endothelium from the internal elastic lamina. Marzella et al[27] demonstrated this separation immediately after freezing. Therefore direct endothelial injury appears to be the initial event in the cascade of vascular destruction seen with frostbite injury.[6]

The third phase of cold injury occurs during the rewarming process itself by indirect microvascular damage (Figure 135-3). Water crystals melt as the temperature rises, leading to movement of water intracellularly. There is an initial return of blood flow immediately after thawing through the previously frozen tissue. The main site of injury in frostbite appears to be the endothelial cells of the microcirculation, which are damaged by the direct effects of freezing, as mentioned in phase two, and indirectly during the rewarming process.[23,26,27,34,52] Endothelial cell damage leads to increased capillary permeability, with subsequent extravasation of fluid into the interstitial space

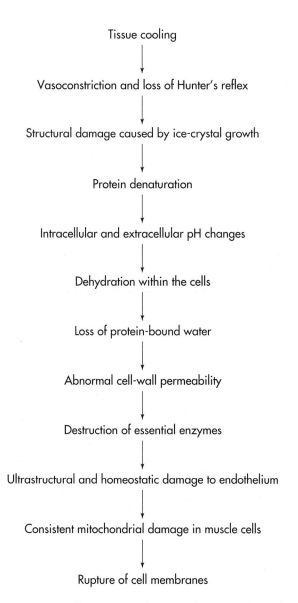

Figure 135-2. Progression of tissue changes with cooling. (From Gamble WB: Perspectives in frostbite and cold weather injures. In Habal MB [editor]: *Advances in plastic and reconstructive surgery,* vol 10, St. Louis, 1994, Mosby.)

resulting in tissue edema (Figure 135-4). Swelling within the interstitial space creates cell hypoxia secondary to the increased diffusion distance between cells.[52] Extravasation of fluid out of the vascular space increases blood viscosity. This sludging of blood flow, along with end arterial vasoconstriction and arteriovenous shunting, produces local tissue ischemia, cell damage, and death.

This reperfusion injury is thought to be similar to the no-reflow phenomenon seen after ischemia-reperfusion injury, which involves the activation of neutrophils and subsequent production of oxygen-free radicals that cause tissue injury

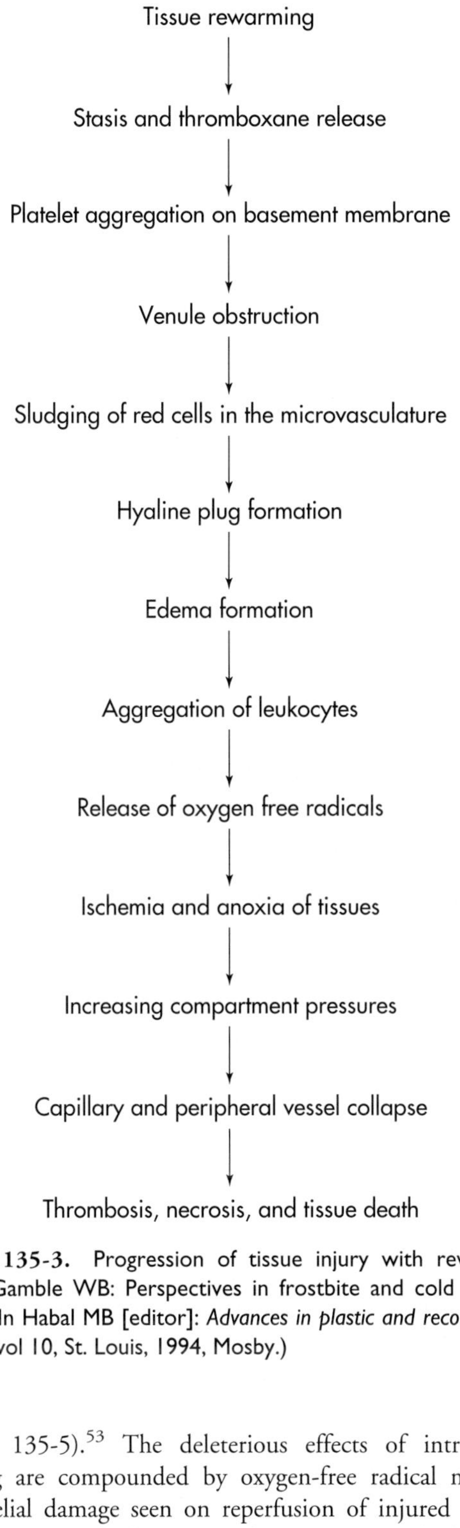

Tissue rewarming

↓

Stasis and thromboxane release

↓

Platelet aggregation on basement membrane

↓

Venule obstruction

↓

Sludging of red cells in the microvasculature

↓

Hyaline plug formation

↓

Edema formation

↓

Aggregation of leukocytes

↓

Release of oxygen free radicals

↓

Ischemia and anoxia of tissues

↓

Increasing compartment pressures

↓

Capillary and peripheral vessel collapse

↓

Thrombosis, necrosis, and tissue death

Figure 135-3. Progression of tissue injury with rewarming. (From Gamble WB: Perspectives in frostbite and cold weather injures. In Habal MB [editor]: *Advances in plastic and reconstructive surgery,* vol 10, St. Louis, 1994, Mosby.)

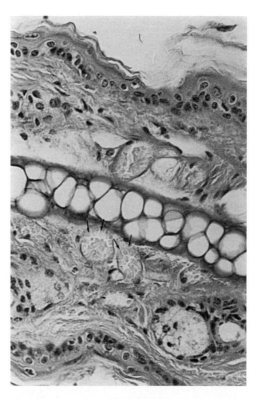

Figure 135-4. A PAS stain of hairless mouse ear 3 hours after thawing demonstrating extravasation of erythrocytes through discontinuities in the basement membrane. (From Bourne MH, Prepkorn MW, Clayton F, Leonard LG: *J Surg Res* 40:26-35, 1986.)

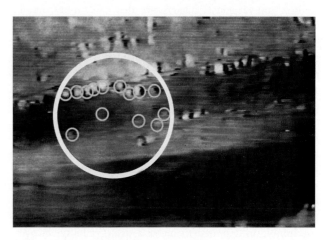

Figure 135-5. Magnification of 100-μm venular segments demonstrating neutrophil adherence to endothelial cells. (From Zamboni WA, Roth AC, Russell RC: *Plast Reconstr Surg* 91[6]:1110-1123, 1993.)

(Figure 135-5).[53] The deleterious effects of intracellular swelling are compounded by oxygen-free radical mediated endothelial damage seen on reperfusion of injured tissue.[49] Endothelial damage from direct freezing exposes the basement membrane, activating leukocyte aggregation and the production of oxygen-free radicals from endothelial cells and neutrophils. The role of neutrophils in frostbite was investigated by Manson,[26] whose animal model of frostbite demonstrated increased tissue survival with the use of oxygen-free radical scavengers. Superoxide dismutase and deferoxamine appeared to protect tissues from free-radical injury if given before reperfu-

sion. In Manson's study, overall tissue survival improved, but there was no evidence of actual endothelial cell protection.[26] This supports the belief that initial endothelial cell injury is the result of direct freezing and not indirect damage sustained on vascular reperfusion.[6,27]

Mileski et al[32] also demonstrated the role of neutrophils in endothelial cell injury. Neutrophils are thought to adhere to one another and to endothelial cells by specific neutrophil-binding molecules known as CD11/CD18 and ICAM, respectively. This binding results in the release of proteases and free-radical products that are believed to cause the endothelial damage seen after reperfusion. Mileski demonstrated decreased tissue loss and edema with the use of anti-CD11 and CD18 molecule antibodies that block the neutrophil-binding molecules. These molecules, known as *monoclonal antibody 60.3 (Mab60.3),* decrease tissue loss and edema. Histologically, control animals not given MAb60.3 revealed microvascular occlusion and thrombosis not seen in MAb60.3-treated animals. By blocking neutrophil adhesion, fewer proteases and oxygen metabolism byproducts are produced to cause cellular injury. The greatest benefit was seen when the antibody was given at the time of rewarming rather that after the tissue had rewarmed, supporting the role of neutrophil-mediated injury early in the reperfusion phase. This brings up the question of whether neutrophils play a role in injury early or late in reperfusion. Mileski's study supports early involvement of neutrophils, with a greater positive effect of Mab60.3 when given early compared with later in the rewarming process. Other studies support the role of neutrophils later in the inflammatory stages of rewarming.[27,54]

Prostaglandin E2 (PGE2), a vasodilator found in the endothelium, and thromboxane (TX), a vasoconstrictor and platelet aggregator found in platelets, have also been implicated in the reperfusion phase of frostbite injury. There appears to be a temperature-dependent balance between PGE2/TX. A decrease in temperature appears to increase TXA2/B2 levels. Robson and Heggers[41] hypothesize that cold injury may be similar to the inflammatory-mediated response, which occurs by progressive dermal ischemia in burn wounds. They found the blisters formed after frostbite injury, as with those associated with burn wounds, contained prostanoids PGE2, PGF2, and TXA2/B2. These prostanoids are released after injury as a protective mechanism to produce clot formation and platelet and neutrophil aggregation. Levels of PGF2 and TXA2/B2 vasoconstricting and platelet aggregating substances were markedly elevated, whereas the levels of vasodilating and platelet antiaggregating substance, PGE2, were low. This theory is supported by the Raine et al[40] study on the treatment of rabbit-ear frostbite by blocking the arachidonic acid cascade and hence the production of TXA2/B2 and PGF2. Thromboxane inhibition appeared to increase tissue viability. Heggers et al[15] have also demonstrated improved survival in clinical trials with aloe vera, a topical inhibitor of thromboxane, and ibuprofen, a systemic inhibitor of prostaglandins.

The presence of a thrombogenic process involved in frostbite injury is supported by various ultrastructural and microscopic examinations of frozen tissue after rewarming that demonstrate thrombi within the microcirculation. Intravascular cellular aggregation appears soon after blood flow is restored, forming thrombi within capillaries, venules, and arterioles (Figure 135-6).[26,33,35,51] The composition of these thrombi includes platelet aggregates,[12] neutrophil-neutrophil aggregates,[32] clumped erythrocytes,[21] and fibrin.[21,42,52,54] A signifi-

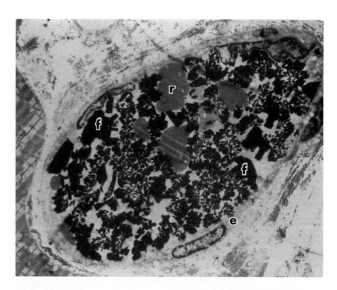

Figure 135-6. A blood vessel filled with fibrin clot (f) after a frostbite injury, as seen on electron microscopy. *e,* Endothelium; *r,* erythrocytes. (From Zook N, Hussman J, Brown R: *Ann Plast Surg* 40[3]:249, 1998.)

cant number of thrombi were observed in vivo almost immediately after thawing and continued to be seen within venules up to 1 hour after injury. It is hypothesized that freezing causes direct endothelial damage, exposing the basement membrane and allowing platelets to adhere to microfibrils, the basement membrane, and collagen. This induces thromboxane A2 synthesis and activates the coagulation cascade, resulting in fibrin thrombi that block the microcirculation and lead to further ischemic injury. According to Lange and Boyd,[23] in less than 2 hours, irreversible stasis leads to extravasation, edema, and irreversible microvascular damage.

NATURAL HISTORY

Frostbite injury can be classified into first, second, third, and fourth degree based on the physical findings observed during the initial presentation and after rewarming rather than on the full extent of actual tissue injury (Table 135-1). First- and second-degree injuries are considered superficial, whereas third- and fourth-degree injuries are considered deep.[16,42] Frostbite classification is attempted clinically, but the grading of damage is arbitrary and usually retrospective.[13] It is often difficult on initial evaluation to make the distinction between superficial and deep injury. The grading becomes an ongoing process throughout the nonoperative treatment course.

A careful history must be obtained from the patient at the initial consultation, including the weather conditions, the temperature of the environment where injury occurred, the presence or lack of protection, the duration of exposure, and any prior cold injuries.[13] The length of time that passes between injury and rewarming should be noted because it appears to be

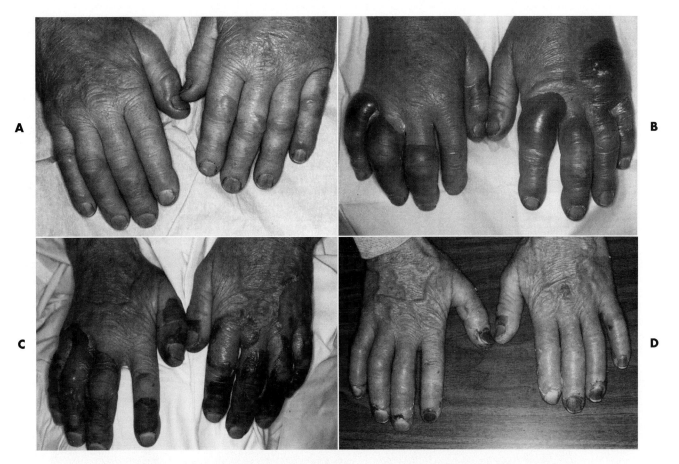

Figure 135-7. A, A patient with indeterminate depth of injury 5 hours after rewarming. **B,** Blister formation 75 hours after rewarming, indicating a second- or third-degree frostbite injury. **C,** The results 7 days after injury, after blister debridement, with second-degree injury. **D,** Frostbitten areas are reepithelialized at 15 days.

directly proportional to the severity of the injury and the need for eventual surgical intervention.[5]

Patients initially experience swelling, redness, and tingling or a painful cold sensation in the areas of injured tissue. This progresses to numbness and then loss of sensation believed to be caused by vasoconstriction-induced ischemia.[1] The skin feels stiff and has a white, waxy appearance with a grey/blue or purple, mottled tint secondary to vasoconstriction.

Circulation temporarily returns as the tissue thaws and becomes erythematous and swollen. Blood flow caused by vasodilation progresses distally, giving a purple or burgundy appearance. Throbbing pain begins hours to days after injury and may last 2 to 3 weeks, or as long as wounds remain open. Causalgia with a sensory deficit is common after injury secondary to ischemic neuritis and can last indefinitely, with diminished touch, pain, and temperature sensation. Superficial frostbite involving only the skin produces clear or bloody blisters that slough after 7 to 15 days and are followed by complete reepithelialization from the basal cell layer within 4

weeks. Substantial edema, which is usually seen beyond the area of injury, occurs within the first few hours of injury and lasts days to months. Edema can be a good prognostic sign because it indicates a minor injury of a superficial degree, especially when the edema persists more than 48 hours (Figure 135-7). Persistent edema is a sign that the microcirculation is patent, allowing for continued release of fluid into the surrounding tissue. Deeper frostbite injury involves subcutaneous tissue and is characterized by very little edema formation because of widespread circulatory thrombosis.[12] Edema, however, may be seen in the surrounding unfrozen tissue in which the circulation remains open. Blister formation does not occur in deep injuries, especially in fourth-degree frostbite (Figure 135-8).

Tissue with partial-thickness injury and a normal blood supply may reepithelialize or be grafted, whereas full-thickness avascular areas mummify to a dry gangrenous state. Deep frostbite injury usually results in extensive tissue loss, with demarcation between viable and nonviable tissue evident

Table 135-1.
Classification of Frostbite Injury

INJURY	SYMPTOMS	SIGNS	OUTCOME
First degree	Redness, pain tingling	White, yellow, firm plaque; minimal edema/erythema	No tissue necrosis; spontaneous healing
Second degree	Blistering, pain	Superficial clear or milky blisters; edema/erythema	Minimal tissue loss; spontaneous healing
Third degree	Purple/red skin	Deep, hemorrhagic blisters of partial or full thickness	Tissue necrosis common
Fourth degree	Mummification; insensate	Deep cyanosis; no blisters or edema	Gangrene

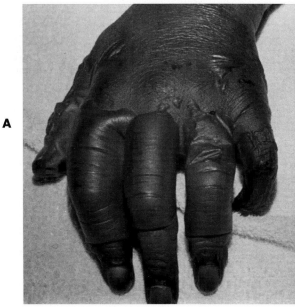

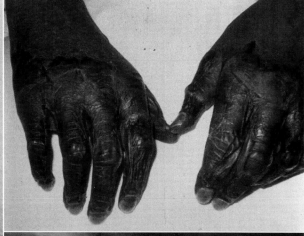

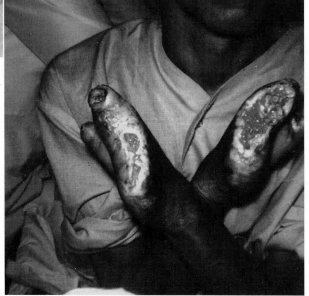

Figure 135-8. **A,** A patient with minimal edema and hemorrhagic blisters 24 hours after injury. **B,** Mummification of digits by 6 weeks. **C,** The patient after amputation of necrotic fingers 8 weeks after injury.

between 22 and 45 days after injury. The necrotic area sloughs, or autoamputates, revealing viable tissue beneath.

The prognostic clinical signs of a less-severe frostbite injury include warm tissue with relatively normal color, preservation of sensation, the presence of clear blisters that extend to the ends of digits, and edema lasting longer than 24 hours. Signs of more severe damage are the absence of edema, with cyanotic tissue that does not blanche under pressure, and continued loss of sensation.

INVESTIGATIONS

Diagnostic studies have been used to aid physicians in differentiating viable from nonviable tissue. Reliable studies would be useful in monitoring the efficacy of various adjunctive treatments and allowing for early amputation and rehabilitation, resulting in the economic benefits of a shortened hospital stay and earlier return to work. Unfortunately, many diagnostic modalities have been tried with varying success. Plain film radiography is not sensitive in assessing tissue damage. Abnormalities are not seen on plain films for weeks to months after injury. Transcutaneous O_2 levels have been used to estimate the chance for wound healing at various levels of amputation. In one study, a partial O_2 pressure of greater then 20 mmHg at the amputation site resulted in a 92% chance of wound healing. Ultrasonic and laser Doppler studies have been used for evaluation of tissue viability and the need for escharotomy,[13,33,49] however ischemia at the cellular level cannot be assessed. Arteriography has been used to assess blood flow in large vessels but fails to assess the microvascular network of the tissue.[9]

Nuclear scans measure the uptake or redistribution of isotope by frostbitten tissue and provide an indication of blood flow in the microvasculature. Xenon 133 nuclear scans have shown variable efficacy but are limited because of the uptake of isotope by adipose tissue, which complicates the evaluation and causes a great variation in the time necessary for isotope uptake.[13,43] Scintigraphy with technetium methylene diphosphonate (99mTc MDP) has been relatively successful at assessing bone perfusion and distinguishing between viable and nonviable bone. However, soft tissue perfusion, which is usually of greatest importance, is not well demonstrated. Salimi et al[43] used 99 technetium pertechnetate (99mTcO$_2$) imaging to demonstrate a persistent perfusion defect in nonviable tissue and increased soft tissue uptake in viable tissue. From this positive clinical experience with scintigraphy, Salimi recommends an initial scan within 24 to 48 hours of injury and a repeat scan 7 to 10 days later to assess the efficacy of treatment and as an early determinant of the amputation level. Ikawa[17] recommends the use of Tc-99m-phosphate in determining tissue viability as early as 3 days after injury. He postulates that radiophosphate images the intermediate zone of stasis and external zone of hyperemia. It is within the intermediate zone that the line of demarcation is determined.

Infrared thermography has shown some potential for diagnostic significance. This test has been able to indicate loss of peripheral blood flow and predict tissue viability within 2 to 3 mm of the demarcation line when used within 24 hours of injury. Thermography is noninterventional and relatively portable, making it a safe and easy test. It has also been used for the evaluation of late sympathetic vasospasm.[13]

Magnetic resonance imaging (MRI) and magnetic resonance angiography (MRA) have more recently been used for early determination of tissue viability. Barker et al[3] compared the results seen with MRI/MRA and those with Tc99 bone scan and found that both studies reliably predicted the extent of injury that correlated with the eventual line of tissue demarcation. The MRI/MRA, however, appeared to provide direct visualization of occluded vessels and better demarcation between ischemic and viable tissue compared with the bone scan. The ability to determine the amount of surrounding soft tissue loss was also believed to be superior with MRI/MRA studies. This paper also addressed the increased cost of MRI/MRA compared with bone-scan studies. A shortened hospital stay and thus lowered hospital costs, however, would be possible with earlier identification of nonviable tissue using MRI/MRA and therefore outweigh the higher testing costs.

OPERATIONS

MANAGEMENT

The goals of treating frostbite injury include the preservation of reversibly damaged tissue and the return of function to the injured part. The difficulty in treating frostbite lies in determining what injured tissue is reversibly damaged and will survive versus what tissue is irreversibly damaged and must be amputated. This determination can be extremely difficult. The initial treatment is directed toward preserving reversibly damaged tissue. Late treatment is usually focused on surgically removing necrotic tissue and correcting the resulting defects. The physician must be able to distinguish between viable and nonviable tissue to determine the required level of amputation. This demarcation may take weeks to months to be defined, as exemplified by the layman's adage "frostbite in January, amputation in July."

The treatment of frostbite injury dates back several centuries to the time of Alexander the Great when injured tissue was covered with oil. Other treatments through time have included heating the injured tissue by the fire, and dressing the tissue with alcohol, mercuric chloride, chloral hydrate with camphor, tincture of lead, and opium. Massage, electrical stimulation, and wool/gauze wraps have also been used. Snow and ice were once advocated to slowly rewarm the injured tissue. This method was later found to be more harmful to the tissue than simple rewarming.[31,39] Soon after World War II, Entin and Baxter[9] studied the rewarming of tissue at a series of different temperatures and found maximum tissue salvage at temperatures between 38° and 42° C. This discovery has become the foundation for present-day emergency treatment, resulting in improved survival of frostbitten tissue.

Adjunctive treatment for frostbite injury has been studied in great lengths, both experimentally and clinically. The Korean War was the turning point in frostbite research. Heparin, systemic vasodilators, cortisone, and sympathectomy were used in clinical studies of human frostbite and found to have little benefit. Some of these treatment modalities appeared beneficial in animal studies; however, human frostbite injury is too dissimilar for comparison. The slow freezing seen with human frostbite injury has not been duplicated in animal models.[6,12] Also, the timing of treatment in animal models is more easily controlled than with human frostbite cases. Animals in experimental frostbite studies were treated before, during, or immediately after rewarming. Most patients, however, are seen after the rewarming process is complete or near completion.

Adjunct treatments have been used to prevent the progressive microvascular thrombosis that occurs after the initial direct injury. A number of anticoagulant therapies have been proposed. The vasodilation of vessels and presence of red blood cell thrombi seen after tissue thawing led to the use of intravenous low-molecular-weight dextran (LMWD). Theoretically, LMWD decreases blood viscosity, reduces red blood cell clumping, and halts the zone of injury progression.[12,13,35] Experimental models showed that LMWD reversed or prevented circulatory stasis if given within 2 hours after thawing and decreased tissue loss if given within 1 hour.[34] Dextran also appeared to increase capillary blood flow and inhibit intravascular red blood cell aggregation if given before freezing.[34,51] Unfortunately, treatment before injury is of no benefit in the clinical treatment of patients. Weatherly-White et al[50] demonstrated protection of tissue in a rabbit-ear model with 1 gm/kg/day of LMWD. A report by Barat et al[2] on 847 cases of cold injury sustained during the Indo-Pakistan conflict demonstrated decreased tissue loss with the use of LMWD along with the vasodilator isoxsuprine hydrochloride and the antiinflammatory agent oxyphenbutazone. Other animal studies using LMWD demonstrated an increase in edema in the injured extremities and no significant decrease in tissue loss.[35]

The return of blood flow after tissue rewarming is accompanied by diffuse thrombosis within the microcirculation. Heparin was examined as a possible treatment to prevent this thrombi formation and restore adequate circulation but the results were contradictory. Early studies of heparin showed no clinical benefits,[50] whereas some later experimental models demonstrated tissue protection with the administration of heparin.[23,24,34] Heparin given within 1 hour after freezing, with maintenance of heparinization for the next 5 days, was shown to be effective in experimental animal models.[34] Lange and Lowe[24] performed a clinical experiment using human volunteers who were subjected to localized dry ice burns to the forearms. There was no tissue loss in patients heparinized immediately after the injury compared with the tissue necrosis seen in control patients. In contrast, angiogram studies of the vascular damage to rabbit ears after frostbite injury displayed no benefit to the vasculature after heparin treatment.[25]

Angiographic observation of frostbite-injured tissue during reperfusion has demonstrated vasospasm and arteriovenous fistula formation, which are believed to increase the capillary thrombosis after frostbite injury. This led to the examination of vasodilating techniques, such as surgical or medical sympathectomy, to decrease vasospasm and prevent ischemia.[7] Surgical sympathectomy was advocated as a beneficial treatment in the mid-1900s. Proponents demonstrated benefit in animal models, including increased resolution of edema, decreased tissue loss, faster demarcation between viable and nonviable tissue, and faster healing.[15,18,22,48] However, other studies showed increased edema and no decrease in tissue loss after surgical sympathectomy.[25] Medical sympathectomy with intraarterial reserpine was shown by Porter et al[38] to decrease vasospasm and by Golding[14] to increase resorption of edema and improve healing. However, Bouwman et al[7] and Snider and Porter[46] demonstrated no beneficial effects to patients with the use of medical sympathectomy. Sympathectomy, although practiced to a large extent 30 years ago, is no longer considered a widely appropriate treatment for acute frostbite injury. A general consensus of the literature on sympathectomy, however, is that it offers some protection against a second frostbite injury. An injured part initially treated by sympathectomy is more resistant to frostbite during a second exposure.[7,14]

Newer fibrinolytic agents that act on free plasminogen have been tested, including streptokinase and urokinase. A study by Salimi et al[44] showed a significant increase in tissue survival if intravenous streptokinase was given from 12 to 48 hours after injury, with the greatest benefit by treatment within the first 12 to 24 hours. Rapid rewarming and streptokinase appeared to have an additive effect.[13,44] Streptokinase, however, may be severely allergenic and probably should not be used clinically. Recombinant tissue plasminogen activator (r-tPA) therapy has been suggested for the treatment of frostbite for its fibrinolytic effect to restore blood flow. Sirr infused intraarterial r-tPA into the dominant extremity of 14 patients suffering from bilateral frostbite.[45] Patients who received r-tPA showed signs of reperfusion distally on bone scan. All 10 patients treated with only supportive care required amputation compared with one of the four patients treated with r-tPA. The single r-tPA patient who required amputation had more significant soft tissue injury compared with the other three patients. Unfortunately, the numbers in this study are too small to hold much statistical significance.

Prostaglandin derivatives appear to play a role in the microcirculatory damage of frostbite injury. Prostaglandins $F_{2\alpha}$ and thromboxane A2 accelerate the progression of Jackson's zones of tissue damage from a state of hyperemia, in which tissue recovers, to a state of coagulation, in which tissue becomes necrotic. Blocking the production of prostaglandins and thromboxanes may halt this progression and result in increased tissue survival. These prostaglandins have been identified in the blister fluid in frostbite injury, similar to the blisters of second-degree thermal injury.[29,42] Tissue survival was significantly improved in an experimental frostbite model by Raine[40] after treatment with prostaglandins and thromboxane-blocking agents. McCauley et al[29] performed a clinical trial in 38 frostbite-injured patients placed on a protocol that included treatment with a topical thromboxane inhibitor and systemic antiprostaglandins and demonstrated no significant tissue loss.

The initial treatment of frostbite injury is focused on conservative medical management. The most important initial treatment is to leave the tissue frozen if there is any chance the patient may be exposed to freezing conditions a second time.[39] Although the length of time that tissue remains frozen has been shown to increase the extent of injury, it appears to be less harmful than a refreeze injury.[31] If tissue is initially rewarmed but refreezes while in transport to a treatment facility, the cumulative injury sustained from a freeze-thaw-freeze scenario leads to even greater tissue damage.[39]

Wet and/or constricting clothing should first be removed. The exposed area should be elevated during transport and on arrival at the hospital. Evaluation and treatment of systemic hypothermia must be performed concomitant with the treatment of local tissue injury.[42] Intravenous rehydration with lactated Ringer's is initiated to replenish intravascular volume and to decrease stasis caused by hemoconcentration. Frequently, cold-injured patients will be acidotic and require administration of $NaHCO_3$. Total body rapid rewarming should be initiated in a moving water bath of 40° to 42° C (104° to 108° F).[19,20] The rate of tissue rewarming affects the severity of cell damage. Rapid rewarming decreases the duration of tissue exposure, decreasing extracellular crystal formation, which leads to less cell damage. A thermometer should be placed in the bath to ensure water temperature remains within the suggested range. Approximately 15 to 30 minutes of rewarming are usually required to restore core temperature. The end point of rewarming can be judged clinically by the development of reactive hyperemia of the injured soft tissue. Once normal temperatures are achieved, rewarming is promptly ceased to avoid thermal injury in susceptible tissue. The involved area may be extremely painful and edematous after thawing, with throbbing and tingling sensations that usually require parenteral analgesics such as meperidine or morphine. Tetanus prophylaxis should be initiated as has commonly been done since World War I.[22]

Frostbite management after rewarming consists mostly of local tissue care and the prevention of infection. Some advocate leaving tissue exposed,[16] whereas others cover the injured part with nonconstricting bulky or light dressings. Common wound protocol includes the separation of digits, protection of injured extremities from damage with cradles or sterile sheets, and constant elevation.[16] Some authors use topical silver nitrate (0.5%) or silver sulfadiazine (1%) to penetrate eschar and protect tissue from infection.[16,33] The majority of patients, especially those not ensured of a warm environment on discharge, are admitted for treatment and observation.

The protocol developed by McCauley et al[29] for the prevention of dermal ischemia after frostbite appears promising in clinical trials (Box 135-1). The protocol includes rapid rewarm-

Box 135-1.
University of Chicago Frostbite Protocol

1. All patients with frostbite injuries are admitted to the UCBC.
2. Upon admission, the affected areas will be rapidly rewarmed in warm water (104° to 108° F) for 15 to 30 minutes. Patients presenting 24 hours postinjury will not be rewarmed.
3. Upon completion of rewarming, the affected parts will be treated as follows:
   A. White blisters will be debrided and topical treatment with aloe vera (Dermaide Aloe) every 6 hours will be instituted
   B. Hemorrhagic blisters will be left intact and topical aloe vera (Dermaide Aloe) every 6 hours will be instituted
   C. Elevation of the affected parts with splinting as indicated
   D. Tetanus prophylaxis
   E. Analgesia intravenously or intramuscularly, morphine or Demerol as indicated
   F. Unless contraindicated by medical history:
      Aspirin: 1. Adults: 325 mg orally every 6 hours for 72 hours
      2. Children: 125 mg orally every 6 hours for 72 hours
   G. Penicillin: 1. Adults: 500,000 units every 6 hours intravenously until edema resolves
      2. Children: 50,000 units/kg/day in four divided doses until edema resolves
   H. Daily hydrotherapy

From: McCauley RL, Hing DN, Robson MC, Heggers JP: *J Trauma* 23:143-147, 1983.

ing, intravenous or intramuscular narcotics, tetanus prophylaxis, and elevation of the affected areas; these are all widely accepted practice in the treatment of frostbite. Several other steps, including the use of topical antithromboxane agents, systemic antiprostaglandin agents, and prophylactic antibiotics, are more controversial.[29]

Prostaglandin $F_{2\alpha}$ (PGF2) and thromboxane A2 (TXA2) as mentioned earlier have been found in increased concentrations within frostbite blisters. McCauley et al[29] suggest that clear or white blisters should be debrided to decrease the amount of PGF2 and TXA2 in contact with the tissue. Hemorrhagic blisters that are deeper and involve the dermal plexus are left intact because debridement could convert the injury to a full-thickness loss. Instead, fluid is aspirated from these deeper blisters. The use of topical antithromboxane agents such as aloe vera after superficial blister debridement is recommended to decrease the effects of thromboxane, theoretically decreasing platelet aggregation and smooth muscle vasoconstriction.[39]

Aloe vera inhibits thromboxane A2 and has been shown with topical application to decrease tissue loss.[42] Other authors argue that blister debridement should not be done unless the blisters interfere with motion of the extremity. Arguments against debridement focus on increasing the chance for bacterial contamination.[16] McCauley also uses systemic aspirin or ibuprofen to improve dermal microcirculation by blocking prostaglandins. Common dosages of ibuprofen are 400 to 600 mg orally three times per day (12 to 16 mg/kg/day).[13] Antiprostaglandin agents are also thought to decrease systemic thromboxane levels. Reduction of these systemic mediators may help stop progressive vasoconstriction that leads to stasis, coagulation, and eventual necrosis.

McCauley et al[29] recommend the use of parental penicillin, although prophylactic antibiotic use remains controversial.[12,16] They propose that normal skin possesses an antistreptococcal precipitate that is inactivated during the edema phase of frostbite injury, and therefore prophylactic penicillin may guard against infection during this time.[29] Others recommend treatment with culture-specific antibiotics if the patient develops a secondary infection.

Continuing care of cold-injured patients includes daily whirlpool baths, which will cleanse the wounds and assist in debridement of eschar. Tissue should be minimally manipulated to avoid further trauma. Necrotic tissue should be surgically debrided every 2 to 3 days[5] to prevent infection or facilitate epithelial regeneration. Daily cleansing should be continued until partial-thickness areas are healed and full-thickness areas have demarcated. Hydrotherapy theoretically increases blood flow and encourages active and passive joint motion in a safe environment. Physical and occupational therapy are instituted early to promote active motion[5,42] with extremity splinting in a functional position when at rest.[16] A wrist extension splint may be adequate for mild hand injuries but a safe-position splint is commonly used in most cases to avoid flexion deformities of the interphalangeal (IP) joints. Concomitant skeletal injuries are managed accordingly after rewarming, but traction should not be used on the tissue of insensate extremities to prevent further damage.[33] The goal of conservative treatment is to prevent functional loss or anatomic deformities until spontaneous healing or surgical intervention is complete.

The second phase of treatment includes debridement of nonviable tissue days to months after the injury. Debridement is delayed until the extent of tissue damage is more definitive, allowing preservation of the maximum amount of tissue. However, injured areas are watched closely because delaying debridement also increases the infection rate. Early surgical intervention is warranted with the development of infection or a compartment syndrome. The injured part must be followed initially for any signs of excess swelling, which may compromise arterial inflow or venous return in distal areas. The presence of vascular compromise, either venous or arterial, should be determined clinically by evaluating color, capillary refill, pulses with the use of Doppler flow probe, and compartment pressure measurements.[34] Increased compartment pressures

will be seen early with venous obstruction and late with arterial compromise. Escharotomy is recommended for distal vascular compromise. For common digital frostbite injuries, Robson et al[42] recommend mid-axial line incisions with careful preservation of underlying structures.

Minor injury involving only superficial skin layers often does not require surgical debridement. Full-thickness loss often requires debridement and definitive closure. Surgical reconstruction is initiated after all nonviable tissue has been excised. Options for wound closure include primary closure; split- and full-thickness skin grafts; and local, distant, pedicled, and free flaps. The first option, primary closure, is often used after digit amputation. Skeletal shortening must be sufficient to allow a loose approximation of distal skin flaps. If primary closure is not possible because of lack of sufficient skin, the wound is given time to granulate and it is then covered with a split-thickness skin graft. Full-thickness skin grafts are used to cover areas in which minimal graft contracture and maximum durability are desired. Donor-site morbidity must be considered when choosing full-thickness versus split-thickness skin grafts. Composite grafts of skin and underlying subcutaneous fat or cartilage may be used in patients with frostbite injury to the tip of the nose or helical rim of the ear.

Severe frostbite injury that results in loss of soft tissue or autoamputation may leave exposed bone, tendon, nerve, or vessels, which requires flap coverage. Local or regional flaps are preferred to preserve digital length, cover underlying structures, and provide a thicker, sensate padding. Local flaps can be rotated or advanced to close small defects but may be difficult to move because of decreased elasticity in the previously injured soft tissue. Distant, pedicled groin or abdominal wall flaps can be used to close larger hand defects. The groin flap based on the superficial circumflex vascular pedicle can be thinned distally, providing good hand coverage with minimal donor-site morbidity. Abdominal wall flaps are truly random, do not have an axial feeding vessel and leave a more noticeable donor-site deformity. The radial forearm fasciocutaneous flap can be based distally on the radial artery and vena comitans as an island pedicle flap and rotated distally to cover hand soft tissue defects. Various free tissue transfers can be used to close large soft tissue defects, such as the deltoid, lateral arm, scapular, temporalis, and toe-to-hand transfer.

The goal of reconstruction is to regain partial or full function of the injured or lost part. All major reconstructive procedures require a motivated, dependable, and compliant patient who is willing to face the challenges and work toward a functional rehabilitation. The surgeon must consider the patient's age, career goals, and future requirements in choosing the type of secondary reconstruction. The most important function for rehabilitation is usually opposition, which is lost in cases of thumb amputation caused by frostbite injury. The thumb provides one third to one half of total hand function; therefore reconstruction of a functioning thumb is the first priority. The pinching mechanism has been reestablished by lengthening the first metacarpal, deepening the first web space,

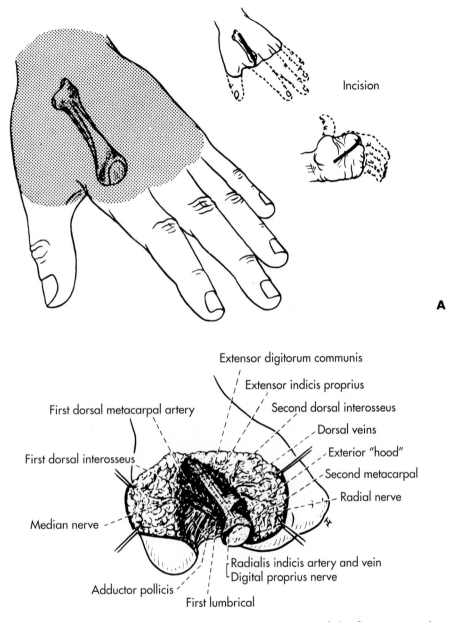

First dorsal metacarpal artery

Extensor digitorum communis

Extensor indicis proprius

Second dorsal interosseus

Dorsal veins

Exterior "hood"

Second metacarpal

Radial nerve

First dorsal interosseus

Median nerve

Radialis indicis artery and vein
Digital proprius nerve

Adductor pollicis

First lumbrical

Incision

A

Figure 135-9. A, The anatomy and incisions for phalangization of the first metacarpal, as described by Brown et al.

Continued

and digital pollicization to the first metacarpal position (Figure 135-9).

Toe-to-hand transfers have been used for reconstruction of the thumb with excellent functional results. Pisarek,[37] in a patient with bilateral complete digit amputations, transplanted the right second toe to the right thumb position and the second and third toes from the contralateral foot in an opposing position. The left hand was reconstructed with a complex of the right third through fifth toes serving as opposing digits (Figure 135-10). The functional results were reported as excellent, with no donor-site problems 1 year later. Minimal donor-site functional defects have been recorded after

toe-to-hand transfers, but the possible effect on long-term ambulation and lifestyle should be considered before surgery. The patient must be willing to sacrifice a toe or toes to gain hand function.

The intrinsic muscles of the hand must also be considered when restoring hand function. The intrinsics are sensitive to frostbite injury and often develop atrophy and fibrosis.[16] Flatt[10] reported intrinsic muscle-belly fibrosis in patients with third- and fourth-degree frostbite. Early, aggressive, active physiotherapy and functional splinting is required treatment for function preservation. Unfortunately, the benefits of intrinsic release measures are limited.

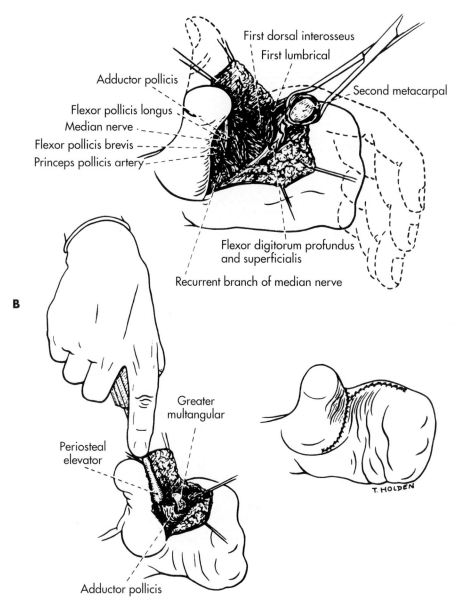

Figure 135-9, cont'd. B, The second metacarpal is removed and the web space deepened. (From Brown H, Welling R, Sigman R, et al: *Plast Reconstr Surg* 45[3]:294-297, 1970.)

OUTCOMES

Individuals often experience late sequelae of cold injury for months to years after the injury. Blair et al[4] followed 100 veterans of the Korean Conflict for 4 years after injury. Chronic symptoms in descending order of frequency were hyperhidrosis, pain, cold sensitivity, numbness, abnormal skin color, and joint stiffness. Late sequelae, including peripheral neuropathies, paraesthesias, and skin changes, have frequently been reported and are believed to be secondary to sympathetic overactivity.[12,39] Skin changes include hypopig-

mentation and erythrocyanosis and are more common in blacks than Caucasians.[42] Nails can become ridged and curved secondary to ischemia. Surgical sympathectomy has not shown benefit for acute frostbite, but has been shown to decrease the sympathetic overactivity leading to these late sequelae of frostbite, including pain, vasoconstriction on exposure to cold, hyperhidrosis, and trophic skin changes. The benefit of sympathectomy has been attributed to the down-regulation of sympathetic activity.[1,18] However, reports that sympathetic overactivity spontaneously resolves support the recommendation of a 2-year waiting period before intervention.[16]

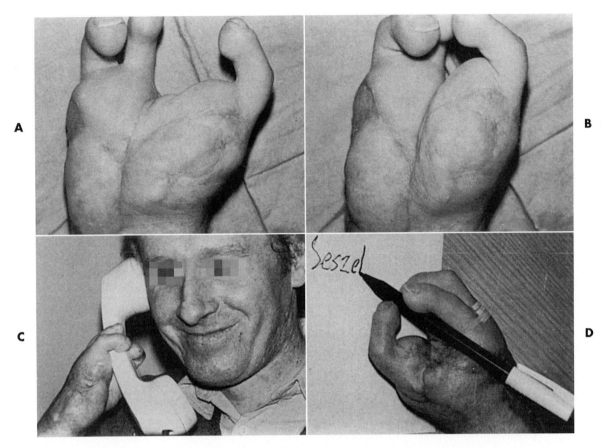

Figure 135-10. A-D, The appearance and function of a reconstructed right hand after toe-to-hand transfer. (From: Pisarek W: *Br J Plast Surg* 43:244-246, 1990.)

The late musculoskeletal sequelae of frostbite include demineralization of bone, which occurs in 50% of moderate to severe frostbite injury cases from weeks to years after injury.[30] There are two theories to explain the progressive bone and joint damage, including direct injury to vulnerable chondrocytes within the cartilage growth plate,[16] and vascular damage and subsequent tissue ischemia.[30] It is likely that these changes are secondary to a combination of the above theories. Increased density and lytic lesions are also seen, followed by later development of marginal spurs and flexion contractures of the distal interphalangeal (DIP) joint.[30,42] Patients may suffer from dull, achy, stiff joints or episodic attacks of severe pain for months after the injury. Degenerative joint changes are seen most often in DIP joints, followed by the proximal interphalangeal (PIP) and metacarpophalangeal (MCP) joints. Severe frostbite injury in children causes premature closure of phalangeal epiphyses approximately 6 to 12 months after injury. Premature closure leads to shortening of digits, joint laxity, skin redundancy, and angular deformities, usually in a radial direction (Figure 135-11). The sequelae may persist, but function is usually normal and surgery is rarely required.[16]

Because of the complex and unexplainable aspects of frostbite pathophysiology, the lack of successful diagnostic modalities or treatment protocols, and the associated morbidity of frostbite injury, we must place emphasis on the prevention of injury. The key to prevention involves eliminating risk factors. Probably the most important risk factor to avoid, as mentioned previously, is the use of any substances that alter one's level of consciousness. Avoiding exposure to high winds, damp conditions, cold objects, and volatile liquids and gases is also important in the elimination of cold injury. The next step is public education about cold injuries. Public and medical awareness of the causes of cold injury has improved over the years, leading to a decrease in incidence and delay of treatment. Applying appropriate treatment regimens early increases the chance of tissue survival, with decreased morbidity. However, many patients are still seen long after injury or rewarming has occurred, at which time the efficacy of early treatment has already diminished greatly. Patients and community physicians should be educated about the benefits of seeking immediate care of frostbitten tissue after a cold-exposure injury.

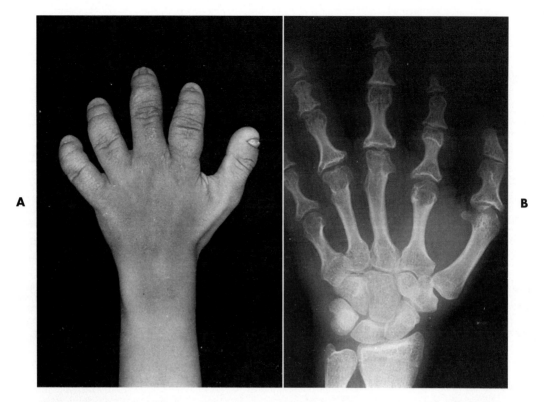

Figure 135-11. A, A 16-year-old female who suffered frostbite injury at 22 months of age. Note abnormal nail growth, shortening of metacarpals and phalanges, and skin redundancy. **B,** Radiographic illustration of metacarpal and phalangeal shortening, especially of the distal phalanges.

REFERENCES

1. Bangs C: Hypothermia and frostbite, *Emerg Med Clin* 2:475-487, 1984.
2. Barat AK, Puri HC, Ray N: Cold injuries in Kashmir, December 1971, *Ann R Coll Surg Engl* 60:332-335, 1978.
3. Barker JR, Haws MJ, Brown RE, et al: Magnetic resonance imaging of severe frostbite injures, *Ann Plast Surg* 38(3):275-279, 1997.
4. Blair JR, Schatzki R, Orin KD: Sequelae to cold injury in one hundred patients: follow-up study four years after occurrence of cold injury, *JAMA* 163:1203, 1957.
5. Boswick TA, Thompson JD, Jonas RA: The epidemiology of cold injury, *Surg Gynecol Obstet* 149:326-332, 1979.
6. Bourne MH, Piepkorn MW, Clayton F, Leonard LG: Analysis of microvascular changes in frostbite injury, *J Surg Res* 40:26-35, 1986.
7. Bouwman DL, Morrison S, Lucas CE, Ledgerwood AM: Early sympathetic blockade for frostbite: is it of value? *J Trauma* 20:744-749, 1979.
8. Brown H, Welling R, Sigman R, et al: Phalangizing the first metacarpal: case report, *Plast Reconstr Surg* 45(3):294-297, 1970.
9. Entin MA, Baxter H: The influence of rapid rewarming on frostbite in experimental animals, *Plast Reconstr Surg* 9:511, 1952.
10. Flatt AE: Frostbite of the extremity: a review of current therapy, *J Iowa Med Soc* 52:53-55, 1962.
11. Fritz RL, Perrin DH: Cold exposure injuries: prevention and treatment, *Clin Sports Med* 8:111-128, 1989.
12. Gage AM, Gage AA: Frostbite, *Trauma Emerg Med* 7(9):25-30, 1981.
13. Gamble WB: Perspectives in frostbite and cold weather injuries. In Habal MB (editor): *Advances in plastic and reconstructive surgery,* vol 10, St. Louis, 1994, Mosby.
14. Golding MR, Mendoza MF, Hennigar GR, et al: On settling the controversy on the benefit of sympathectomy for frostbite, *Surgery* 56:221-231, 1964.
15. Heggers JP, Robson MC, Manavalen K, et al: Experimental and clinical observations on frostbite, *Ann Emer Med* 16:191-197, 1987.
16. House JH, Fidler MO: Frostbite of the hand. In Green DP (editor): *Operative hand surgery,* ed 3, New York, 1993, Churchill Livingstone.
17. Ikawa G, dos Santos PA, Yanagerski KT: Frostbite and bone scanning: the case of 99m labeled phosphate in demarcating the line of viability in frostbite victims, *Orthopedics* 9:1257-1261, 1986.
18. Kapur BM, Gulati SM, Talwar JR: Low molecular dextran in the management of frostbite in monkeys, *Indian J Med Res* 56:1675-1681, 1968.
19. Knize DM: Cold injuries. In Converse JM (editor): *Plastic Reconstructive Surgery,* vol 1, Philadelphia, 1977, WB Saunders.
20. Knize DM, Weatherly-White RC, Paton BC, Owens JC: Prognostic factors in the management of frostbite, *J Trauma* 9:749, 1969.

21. Kulka JP: Vasomotor microcirculatory insufficiency: observations on nonfreezing cold injury of the mouse ear, *Angiology* 12:491-506, 1961.

22. Kyosola K: Clinical experiences in the management of cold injuries: a case study of 110 cases, *J Trauma* 14:32-36. 1974.

23. Lange K, Boyd LJ: The functional pathology of frostbite and the prevention of gangrene in experimental animals and humans, *Science* 1945;102:151-152, 1945.

24. Lange K, Lowe L: Subcutaneous heparin in the Pitkin menstruum for the treatment of experimental human frostbite, *Surg Gynecol Obstet* 82:256-260, 1946.

25. Lazarus HM, Hutto W: Electrical burns and frostbite patterns of vascular injury, *J Trauma* 22:581-585, 1982.

26. Manson PN, Jesudass RR, Marzella L, et al: Evidence for an early free radical–mediated reperfusion injury in frostbite, *Free Radic Biol Med* 10:7-11, 1991.

27. Marzella L, Jesudass RR, Manson PN, et al: Morphologic characterization of acute injury to vascular endothelium of skin after frostbite, *Plast Reconstr Surg* 83:67-75, 1989.

28. Mazur P: Theoretical and experimental effects of cooling and warming velocity on the survival of frozen and thawed cells, *Cryobiology* 2:181-192, 1966.

29. McCauley RL, Hing DN, Robson MC, Heggers JP: Frostbite injuries: a rational approach based on the pathophysiology, *J Trauma* 23:143-147, 1983.

30. McKendry RJ: Frostbite arthritis, *Can Med Assoc* 125(10):1128-1130, 1981.

31. Merryman HT: Mechanics of freezing in living cells and tissues, *Science* 124(3221):515-521, 1956.

32. Mileski WJ, Raymond JF, Winn RK, et al: Inhibition of leukocyte adherence and aggregation for the treatment of severe cold injury in rabbits, *J Appl Physiol* 79(3):1432-1436, 1993.

33. Mills WJ: Summary of treatment of cold injured patients, *Alaska Med* 25:33-38, 1983.

34. Mundth ED, Long DM, Brown RB: Treatment of experimental frostbite with low molecular weight dextran, *J Trauma* 4:246-257, 1964.

35. Penn I, Schwartz S: Evaluation of low molecular weight dextran in the treatment of frostbite, *J Trauma* 4:784-790, 1964.

36. Pirozynski WJ, Webster DR: Muscle tissue changes in experimental frostbite, *Ann Surg* 136:993-998, 1952.

37. Pisarek W: Transfer of the third, fourth and fifth toes for one-stage reconstruction of the thumb and two fingers: case report, *Br J Plast Surg* 43:244-246, 1990.

38. Porter JM, Wesche DH, Rosch J, et al: Intra-arterial sympathetic blockade in treatment of clinical frostbite, *Am J Surg* 132:625-630, 1976.

39. Purdue GF, Hunt JL: Cold injury: a collective review, *J Burn Care Rehabil* 7:331-342, 1986.

40. Raine TJ, London MD, Goluch L, et al: Anti-prostaglandins and anti-thromboxanes for treatment of frostbite, *Surg Forum Plast Surg* 557-779,

41. Robson MC, Heggers JP: Evaluation of hand frostbite as a clue to pathogenesis, *J Hand Surg [Am]* 6:43-47, 1981.

42. Robson MC, Smith DJ: Cold injuries. In McCarthy JG: *Plastic surgery: general principles*, vol 1, Philadelphia, 1990, WB Saunders.

43. Salimi Z, Vas W, Tang-Baiton P, et al: Assessment of tissue viability in frostbite by 99mTC pertechnetate scintigraphy, *AJR* 142:415-419, 1984.

44. Salimi Z, Wolverson MK, Herbold DR, et al: Treatment of frostbite with IV streptokinase: an experimental study in rabbits, *Am J Roentgenol* 149:773-776, 1987.

45. Skolnick AA: Early data suggest clot-dissolving drug may help save frostbitten limbs from amputation, *JAMA* 267(15):2008-2010, 1992.

46. Snider RL, Porter JM: Treatment of experimental frostbite with intra-arterial sympathetic blocking drugs, *Surgery* 77:557-561, 1975.

47. Sumner DS, Cibley TL, Doolittle WH: Host factors in human frostbite, *Mil Med* 193:454-461, 1974.

48. Ulate SM, Kapur BM, Talwar JR: Sympathetectomy in the management of frostbite: an experimental study, *Indian J Med Res* 58:343-351, 1970.

49. Vogel JE, Dellon AL: Frostbite injuries of the hand, *Clin Plast Surg* 16:565-576, 1989.

50. Weatherly-White RCA, Sjostrm B, Paton BC: Experimental studies in cold injury. II. The pathogenesis of frostbite, *J Surg Res* 4:17-22, 1964.

51. Webster DR, Bonn G: Low molecular weight dextran in the treatment of experimental frostbite, *Can J Surg* 8:423-427, 1965.

52. Zacarian SA, Stone D, Clater M: Effects of cryogenic temperature on microcirculation in the golden hamster cheek pouch, *Cryobiology* (1):27-39, 1970.

53. Zamboni WA, Roth AC, Russell RC: Morphologic analysis of the microcirculation during reperfusion of ischemic skeletal muscle and the effect of hyperbaric oxygen, *Plast Reconstr Surg* 91(6):1110-1123, 1993.

54. Zook N, Hussman J, Brown R: Microcirculatory studies of frostbite injury, *Ann Plast Surg* 40(3):246-255, 1998.

Index

14 Index

Child—cont'd
auricular reconstruction for microtia—cont'd
low hairline and, 1046-1049
proportional and dimensional evaluation of auricle, 1053-1055
second-stage operation, 1027-1040
secondary reconstruction and, 1040, 1044-1046, 1047
subtotal or partial, 1051-1053
congenital nevus, 997-1021
blue nevus, 999-1000
epidermal nevus, 1001
large and giant nevi, 1006-1018
Mongolian spot, 999
neural nevus, 1000-1001
nevus of Ota and nevus of Ito, 1000
nevus spilus, 1001
operations for, 1003-1006
sebaceous nevus, 1001-1003
Spitz nevus, 1003
surgical outcomes in, 1018-1020
craniomaxillofacial surgery in, 609-611
cyst and cystlike lesions of skin and subcutaneous tissue, 1133-1143
branchial cleft anomalies, 1140-1142
dermoid, 1133-1138
epidermal cyst, 1143-1144
frontonasal encephalocele, 1140
lymphatic malformations of lateral neck, 1142
nasal glioma, 1138-1140
parotid gland lesion, 1142
pilomatrixoma, 1144-1146
thyroglossal duct cyst, 1142-1143
facial trauma, 941-969
condylar head injuries, 950-953
cranial reconstruction with bone loss, 961-966
dental and alveolar bone injuries, 943-944
fracture exposure in, 966
frontal bone and frontal sinus fractures, 960-961
Le Fort fractures, 953-955
mandibular body, symphysis, and ramus injuries, 944-950, 951
nasal fracture, 959
nasoorbital ethmoidal fracture, 959-960
orbital fractures, 955-956
outcomes in, 966-968
subcondylar fractures, 953
zygoma fractures, 956-959
free tissue transfer in, 177
hamartoma, 1129-1133
hemangiomas and vascular malformations of head and neck, 973-995
aesthetic results, 993
arteriovenous malformations, 977-978
capillary hemangioma, 974-976, 977
chemotherapy in, 980-982
complications of surgery, 991-993
costs of care, 994
embolization and sclerotherapy in, 986-991, 992, 993
laser therapy in, 983-986
patient satisfaction after treatment, 994
physical functioning after treatment, 993
port-wine stain, 977, 978, 979
pressure therapy in, 982-983
quality of life and, 994
radiation therapy in, 983, 984
steroid therapy in, 980, 981-982
thermal therapy/cryotherapy in, 983, 984
juvenile xanthogranuloma, 1145
prominent ears, 1057-1065
anesthesia in, 1059
anterior approaches to cartilage, 1059
for conchal hypertrophy, 1063-1064
indications for, 1057
nonsurgical treatment in, 1058
open otoplasty, 1059-1063
posterior approaches to cartilage, 1059, 1060
rhabdomyosarcoma in, 1156
salivary gland tumor in, 1367-1368, 1379
selection for plastic surgery, 144
Child abuse, thermal burn and, 365, 366
Chimerism, 231
Chin
assessment before aesthetic surgery, 2432, 2433
genioplasty, 2683-2703
aesthetic results of, 2698-2701
after mandibular retrusion correction, 888, 892
complications of, 2697-2698
cost of care in, 2701
indications for, 2683-2690

Chin—cont'd
genioplasty—cont'd
informed consent in, 2688-2689
in mandibular prognathism, 894
in maxillary vertical excess, 875, 883-884
operations in, 2690-2697
patient satisfaction in, 2701-2702
physical function after, 2701
ptosis after mandibular reconstruction, 1234-1235
Chloramine, 390
Chlorate burn, 390
Chlorinated hydrocarbons, 392, 397
Chlorine gas, 390
Chloroprocaine, 217
Chlorpromazine
after blepharoplasty, 2543
after replantation of hand or finger, 2141
Choke vessel, 267, 270
Cholesteatoma, 1542-1543
Chondritis in burned ear, 1497, 1511
Chondroblastoma, 2304
Chondrocutaneous advancement flap of Antia and Buch, 1500-1502
Chondrocyte, 90, 91, 232
Chondroitin sulfate, 39
Chondromalacia, 1947
Chondromyxoid fibroma, 2304
Chondron, 90
Chondronecrosis, 1113
Chondroplasty, abrasion, 1947
Chondrosarcoma, 2304-2305
extracranial, 1548-1549
mandibular, 1247, 1251
of upper extremity, 2294
Chopart's amputation, 510-512
Chopart's joint, 478
Chorda tympani nerve, 1357
Chordee, 533
epispadias and, 538-539
in Peyronie's disease, 542
Chordoma, extracranial, 1546-1547
Chromatolysis, 81
Chromic acid burn, 390-391
Chromic collagen suture, 152
Chromic gut suture, 152
Chromium, 240
Chromium picolinate, 2787
Chromophore, 32, 189, 2459, 2460
Chronic fracture dislocation of proximal interphalangeal joint, 1871-1872
Chronic rejection, 229-230
Cigarette smoking
after hand or finger replantation, 2132
Buerger's disease and, 2327-2328
delayed wound healing and, 69-70
effects on flap, 271
free tissue transfer and, 177-178
frostbite and, 2411
lip cancer and, 1214
oral cavity cancer and, 1067
risk for thrombosis in microsurgical hand surgery, 2149
Ciprofloxacin, 2033
Circular graft in hair transplantation, 2495-2496
Circumferential bone wire technique
in Le Fort fracture, 954
in mandibular fracture, 947-949
Circumflex scapular artery, 1264-1265
Cisplatin, 1073
Citanest; see Prilocaine
Claforan; see Cefotaxime
Clamp
microsurgical, 164, 165
in thumb reconstruction, 2194
Clarkson repair of bilateral cleft lip and palate, 785-786
Class I major histocompatibility complex molecule, 227-228
Class I occlusion
after mandibular prognathism correction, 893
after maxillary retrusion correction, 887
after maxillary vertical excess repair, 877
after skeletal open bite repair, 880
Angle's classification of, 871, 873
in hemifacial microsomia, 913, 916
Class II major histocompatibility complex molecule, 228
Class II malocclusion
Angle's classification of, 871, 873
in mandibular retrusion, 888, 889
in maxillary vertical excess, 875, 876
skeletal open bite and, 878-879
in vertical maxillary deficiency, 884

Class III malocclusion
Angle's classification of, 871-872, 873
mandibular prognathism and, 892, 894
maxillary retrusion and, 886
tight lip deformity and, 844
Clavicular fracture, 2076, 2086-2088
Claviopectoral fascia of breast, 2769
Claw hand deformity
after thermal injury, 438
biomechanics of, 1638
low ulnar nerve palsy and, 2009-2010
Clear cell chondrosarcoma, 2305
Cleft
craniofacial, 741-754
cranial, 750-752
general surgical principles in, 741
lateral facial, 748-750
morphogenesis of, 742
oral-nasal, 744-746
oral ocular, 746-748
outcomes in, 752-753
laryngeal, 1325
Cleft lip and palate, 799-807
alveolar cleft management in, 809-817
bone grafting in, 810-814
indications for, 809-810
outcomes in, 814-816
bilateral, 769-797
analysis of defect, 769-770, 771
author's preferred technique in, 786-788, 789-792
bilateral synchronous *versus* unilateral asynchronous repair, 775
combined upper and lower lip z-plasty in, 785-786
epidemiology and etiology of, 770-772
management issues and principles, 774
management of nasal defect in, 788-795
management of premaxillary segment, 775-778
management of prolabial lip segment, 775
one-stage *versus* two-stage repair, 775
outcomes in, 795-796
postoperative management of, 788
straight line closure in, 779-781, 782
timing of repair, 770-774
upper lip z-plasty in, 782-785
z-plasty in, 781-782
classification of, 770, 771
cleft-orthognathic surgery for, 851-867
indications for, 851
orthodontic objectives in, 852-858
outcomes in, 858-865
fetal surgery for, 112-115
genetics of, 613-614
indications for surgery, 799-800
operations for, 800-804
orthodontics for, 649
outcomes in, 804-806
pharyngeal dysfunction in, 1289
secondary cleft lip and nasal deformities, 835-849
assessment of, 835-836
constricted upper lip, 844-845
long upper lip, 845-847
muscular diastasis, 847
secondary bilateral cleft nose repair, 847-848
secondary unilateral cleft lip repair, 836-840
secondary unilateral cleft nose repair, 840, 841, 842
short upper lip, 844
surgical outcomes in, 848
whistle deformity of lip, 840-843
unilateral repair of, 755-767
alveolar cleft and, 762-763
cleft lip nose and, 762
design of skin incisions in, 759-760, 761
economic issues in, 764-765
evolution of surgical principles of, 755-758
indications for, 755
muscle repair and, 760-761
primary evaluation in, 759
revisional surgery and, 763-764
velopharyngeal insufficiency after repair of, 819-833
evolution of surgical solutions, 819-824
future directions in outcomes research, 830-831
historical controls in primary cleft palate surgery, 829-830
long-term outcomes in, 828-829
methodology and shortcomings of previous cleft lip and palate outcome research, 827-828
nosology of, 819
patient satisfaction and, 830
prosthetic management of, 824
secondary procedures and, 827, 829
sphincter pharyngoplasty for, 824-827

Elbow—cont'd
  median neuropathy at, 2123-2125
  peripheral nerve blocks and, 1701
  secondary brachial plexus reconstruction and, 2084
  tuberculosis of, 2038
  upper extremity compression syndromes and, 2119
Elderly
  auricular reconstruction in, 1049-1050
  delayed wound healing in, 68-69
  free tissue transfer in, 177
Electrical injuries, 375-385
  assessment and initial therapy, 376-377
  extremity trauma, 380-382, 383-384
  indications for reconstructive surgery, 375-376
  lip and oral commissure trauma, 378-380, 382-383
  neck trauma, 382
  scalp and skull trauma, 377-378, 382, 1525
  to thumb, 439
Electrical stimulation after brachial plexus reconstruction,
    2085
Electrocautery
  in blepharoplasty, 2535
  in excision of burn wound, 2393
  in hair transplantation, 2495
  in surgical escharotomy, 2389
  in transpalpebral corrugator resection, 2569
Electrochemical series of metals, 252
Electrodiagnostic tests
  in brachial plexus injury, 2077
  in upper extremity compression syndromes, 2119
Electrolarynx, 1345
Electromagnetic radiation, 409, 1107
Electromagnetic spectrum, 186, 2458
Electromyography
  in brachial plexus injury, 2077
  before free muscle transplantation, 2166
  in reflex sympathetic dystrophy, 2356-2357
  before temporomandibular joint ankylosis release, 905
Electron, 184, 185
Electron beam energy, 410
Electroporation, 376
Electrosurgery
  for benign and premalignant skin conditions, 295
  for skin cancer, 321
Electrothermal burn, 376
Elliot flap, 2511
Elliptic incisional/excisional biopsy, 296-298
Elongation, 651
Embolism of hand, 2325-2326
Embolization
  of arteriovenous malformation, 978-980
  of vascular lesions, 986-991, 992, 993
Embryology
  of bone, 658
  cranial vault development and suture formation,
      622-624
  in craniofacial cleft, 742
  of ear, 1057
  of salivary gland, 1355
  of skin, 29
  of temporomandibular joint, 898
  of upper limb, 1655-1665
    genetic encoding and molecular responses,
        1661-1663
    hand and phalangeal formation, 1657-1659
    muscle development, 1661, 1662
    peripheral nerve development, 1659
    peripheral vascular development, 1659-1661
    skeletal development, 1659, 1660
EMG; see Electromyography
Emotional stress, reflex sympathetic dystrophy and, 2343
Employees, 124-125
Enamel, 1093
Encephalocele, frontonasal, 1140, 1149
Enchondroma, 2303
End-end anastomosis, 166-167, 178
End-side anastomosis, 167-168, 169, 178
Endochondral bone, 92, 93, 658-659
Endochondral ossification, 651
Endoforehead fixation technique, 2616
Endomorph, 2859
Endomysium, 85, 86
Endonasal approach in secondary rhinoplasty, 2676
Endoneurium, 79, 80, 172, 2104
Endoprosthetic replacement, 2314-2315
Endorphins, reflex sympathetic dystrophy and, 2353-2354
Endoscope, 195
Endoscopic access device, 2570-2571
Endoscopic breast augmentation, 2757-2767
  evolution of, 2758
  indications for, 2757-2758

Endoscopic breast augmentation—cont'd
  outcomes in, 2765-2766
  transaxillary, 2759-2761
  transumbilical, 2761-2765
Endoscopic retractor, 199-201
Endoscopically assisted abdominoplasty, 2806
Endoscopy, 195-210
  aesthetic results and, 209
  applications and indications for, 196-199
  in breast reduction, 2732
  in carpal tunnel release, 2121-2122
  contraindications for, 199
  economic issues in, 209
  fetal, 109-111
  fiberoptic endoscopic examination of swallowing, 1125
  in forehead rejuvenation, 2569-2574, 2580
  history of, 195, 196
  informed consent in, 199
  potential benefits of, 195-196
  safety and complications in, 208-209
  subpectoral transaxillary augmentation mammoplasty,
      204-209
    access incision and tunnel in, 205
    anatomy and, 204, 205
    muscle division and release in, 206
    patient evaluation for, 204
    patient preparation for, 204
    pocket dissection in, 205-206
    postoperative care in, 207, 208
    secondary procedures and, 207, 208
    sizers and implants in, 206-207
  in subperiosteal facelift, 2609-2630
    aesthetic results of, 2629
    anatomic and clinical analysis of face, 2609-2610
    BEAL rhytidectomy, 2622-2628
    complications of, 2628-2629
    endoscope-assisted biplanar facelift, 2621-2622
    forehead rejuvenation, 2612-2613
    full endoscopic total forehead lift, 2613-2617
    indications for, 2610-2611
    informed consent in, 2612
    patient evaluation in, 2611
    physical functioning after, 2629
    SMILE facelift, 2619-2621
  technique in, 199-203
    basic approach, 201-203
    optical cavity, 199-201
Endosteum, 93
Endotenon, 88
Endotenon sheath, 1714
Endothelins, 270
Endothelium
  in blood vessel, 83, 84
  damage in rewarming process, 2412, 2413
  in regulation of blood flow to flap, 268-270
Endotracheal tube
  for general anesthesia, 220
  for inhalation injury, 362
Endpoints in laser skin resurfacing, 2468
Endurance in hand therapy, 1713-1714
Energy density, 186
Energy for laser system, 183
Enflurane, 220
Enophthalmos
  after facial trauma, 938
  following skull base surgery, 1575
  orbital hypertelorism correction and, 722
  orbital surgery for, 1456
Entamoeba histolytica, 402-403
Enterobacteriaceae, 2033
Enterococci, 2033
Enteromesenteric bridge, 467, 468
Environmental factors
  in frostbite, 2410
  in vasospastic disorders of hand, 2328
Enzymatic debridement, 148, 1822
Enzymatic escharotomy, 2388
Eosinophilic granuloma, 2307-2308
EPB; see Extensor pollicis brevis tendon
Ephedrine after flap transfer, 223
Epibulbar dermoid, 912
Epicranium, 2508
Epidermal cyst, 1143-1144
Epidermal growth factor
  blood vessel repair and, 84
  bone healing and, 95
  cellular and matrix effects of, 43
  epithelialization and, 45
  fetal healing and, 102

Epidermal growth factor—cont'd
  tendon healing and, 89
  wound healing and, 41
Epidermal nevus syndrome, 1001, 1002
Epidermal tumors, 298-303
  actinic keratosis, 301
  Bowen's disease, 301
  cutaneous horn, 300
  epidermodysplasia verruciformis, 302
  epithelial cysts, 302-303
  erythroplasia of Queyrat, 301
  giant condyloma acuminatum, 301-302
  keratoacanthoma, 299-300
  Paget's disease, 301
  porokeratosis, 302
  seborrheic keratosis, 299
  verruca vulgaris, 298-299
Epidermis, 37, 357, 1167
  aging and, 31-32
  effects of radiation therapy on, 68
  phenol peel and, 2437, 2438
  plantar, 506
  of scalp, 2508
  structure and function of, 23-25
  sun exposure and, 32
Epidermodysplasia verruciformis, 302
Epidermoid inclusion cyst, 2280
Epiglottis, 1328
  adenoid cystic carcinoma of, 1325
Epiglottoplasty, 1331
Epilepsy, Dupuytren's contracture and, 2058
Epimysium, 85, 86
Epinephrine
  absorption of local anesthetic and, 1700
  in liposuction, 2842
  in tumescent anesthetic solution, 218
Epineural repair, 172, 2107
Epineurium, 79, 80, 172, 2104
Epiphora
  after blepharoplasty, 2544
  following skull base surgery, 1575
  pediatric facial trauma and, 966
Epiphyseal growth plate of toe, 2175
Epispadias, 537-540
Epitendinous suture in flexor tendon repair, 1969, 1970
Epitenon, 88
Epitenon fibroblast, 1965-1966
Epitenon sheath, 1714
Epithelial cyst, 302-303
Epithelial nonodontogenic cyst, 1239-1240
Epithelial odontogenic cyst, 1237-1239
Epithelial odontogenic malignant tumor, 1244
Epithelialization, 39, 44-46, 98
  after laser resurfacing, 2470
  diabetes mellitus and, 67
  effects of radiation therapy on, 68
Epithelioid angiosarcoma, 2332
Epithelioid cell nevus, 306
Epithelioid sarcoma, 2291, 2292
Epithelioma, sebaceous, 1145
Epithelium of fingernail, 1751
Epitope, 228
EPL; see Extensor pollicis longus tendon
Eponychium, 1751, 1752
  reconstruction of, 1765-1766
Epoxy resin exposure, 398
Epsom salts for hydrofluoric acid exposure, 393
Equipment
  for abdominoplasty, 2809
  in microsurgery, 164, 165
  in thumb reconstruction, 2194
Erbium:yttrium aluminum garnet laser, 190, 191
  in hair transplantation, 2499
  for skin resurfacing, 2460, 2463-2464, 2466-2468,
      2476-2478
  wound management and, 2470
Erectile dysfunction, 540
Erich arch bars, 1101, 1102
Erythema
  after chemical peel, 2453
  after laser resurfacing, 2475
  in brown recluse spider bite, 405
  in frostbite, 2415
  radiation-therapy related, 411-412
Erythrocyte, diabetes mellitus and, 499
Erythromycin for brown recluse spider bite, 405
Erythroplakia, 1214
Erythroplasia, 1067
Erythroplasia of Queyrat, 301, 318
Eschar, 2387